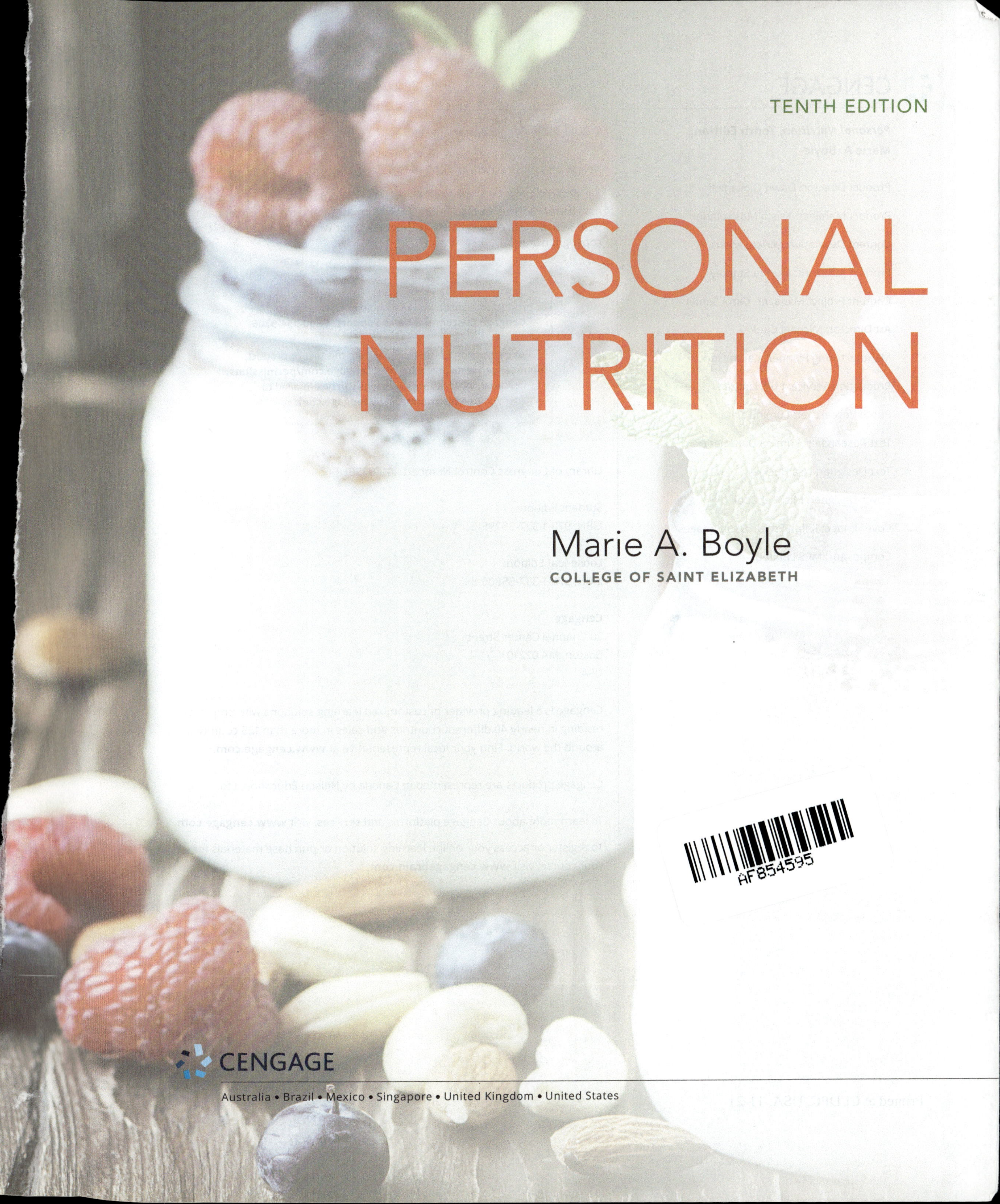

TENTH EDITION

PERSONAL NUTRITION

Marie A. Boyle

COLLEGE OF SAINT ELIZABETH

CENGAGE

Australia • Brazil • Mexico • Singapore • United Kingdom • United States

CENGAGE

***Personal Nutrition*, Tenth Edition**
Marie A. Boyle

Product Director: Dawn Giovaniello

Product Manager: Krista Mastroianni

Content Developer: Miriam Myers

Product Assistant: Marina Starkey

Content Project Manager: Carol Samet

Art Director: Michael Cook

Manufacturing Planner: Karen Hunt

Production Service: MPS Limited

Photo Researcher: Lumina Datamatics

Text Researcher: Lumina Datamatics

Text Designer: Lisa Buckley

Cover Designer: Michael Cook

Cover Image: Ralph Smith/Getty Images

Compositor: MPS Limited

Library of Congress Control Number: 2017935638

Student Edition:
ISBN: 978-1-337-55795-5

Loose-leaf Edition:
ISBN: 978-1-337-55806-8

Cengage
20 Channel Center Street
Boston, MA 02210
USA

Printed at CLDPC, USA, 11-21

In memory of Jesse, Dylan, Kate, McCauley, and Elvis—my twinkling stars in the night sky—and to all those who surround themselves with lives even more fleeting than their own. And to Maggie, Rex, and Tess—may there always be time for footprints in the sand.

—MARIE A. BOYLE

About the Author

MARIE A. BOYLE, PhD, RD, received her BA in psychology from the University of Southern Maine and her MS and PhD in nutrition from Florida State University in Tallahassee, Florida. She is author of the community nutrition textbook *Community Nutrition in Action: An Entrepreneurial Approach*. She is Professor of Nutrition at the College of Saint Elizabeth in Morristown, New Jersey. Her other professional activities include serving as an author and reviewer for the Academy of Nutrition and Dietetics. She coauthored the current Position Paper of the Academy of Nutrition and Dietetics on *Nutrition Security in Developing Nations: Sustainable Food, Water, and Health,* and serves as editor-in-chief of the *Journal of Hunger and Environmental Nutrition* by Taylor & Francis Publishers. She is a member of the Academy of Nutrition and Dietetics, the American Public Health Association, and the Society for Nutrition Education and Behavior.

Contents in Brief

Contents

12 The Life Cycle: Conception through the Later Years 361

13 Food Safety and the Global Food Supply 399

Preface

This 10th edition of *Personal Nutrition* reflects the same vision we had in writing the first edition of this book some 30 years ago—that is, to apply basic nutrition concepts to personal, everyday life. The text is designed to support the many one- to four-credit introductory nutrition courses available to students today from a variety of majors, and offers all readers the opportunity to develop practical skills in making decisions regarding their personal nutrition and health. Our challenge has been to teach facts about nutrition, to nurture critical thinking skills, and to motivate readers to apply what they learn in daily life.

Chapter Content

Chapter 1 introduces the basic nutrients the body needs and provides a personal invitation to eat well for optimum health. It assists readers in becoming sophisticated consumers of new information about nutrition, and explores the factors that affect food choices, including the media, advertising, and cultural factors. Chapter 2 describes in detail the MyPlate food guide and related nutrition tools, and the *2015–2020 Dietary Guidelines for Americans* needed to create healthy eating patterns. It provides the newly revised food label for understanding the nutrition information, terminology, and health claims found on labels. Chapter 2 also includes a section on various international and ethnic cuisines that highlights the multicultural heritage of our country. Chapter 3 provides a colorfully illustrated introduction to the workings of the human body, with an emphasis on the body's digestion and absorption of nutrients from foods. Chapters 4 through 8 present the nutrients and show how they all work together to nourish the body. Chapters 7 and 8 take a functional approach in presenting the roles of vitamins and minerals and spotlights the emerging importance of the antioxidant nutrients and phytochemicals; both chapters include colorful food photos depicting excellent food sources for individual vitamins and minerals. Chapter 9 discusses the impact of the beverages we drink on our nutritional health. In-depth coverage of alcohol in Chapter 9 provides students with important information on alcohol's relationship to nutrition and health, helping them make informed and responsible decisions. Chapter 10 discusses weight management issues and compares major weight-loss programs. Chapter 11 addresses the relationships between nutrition and personal fitness. Chapter 12 describes the special nutrition needs and concerns that arise during the various stages of the life cycle from conception through the older adult years. Chapter 13 addresses consumer concerns about the safety of our food supply, provides a glimpse at some of the problems and advantages of current food technologies, illustrates the global benefits derived when consumers choose locally grown, seasonal foods as much as possible, and presents a brief overview of hunger and food insecurity—both at home and abroad.

Features

The *Savvy Diner* features throughout the text motivate readers to make good health a priority and provide suggestions for making the best food and lifestyle choices for healthy living and disease prevention. This feature includes practical tips for today's students that offer health benefits for a lifetime. Topics include "Whole Grains for Health," "Nourish the Heart," "Never Say 'Diet,'" "An Eating Pattern for Longevity," and "Color Your Plate for Health." The *Savvy Diner* features provide practical suggestions for healthy eating and reinforce the recommendations made in the *Dietary Guidelines for Americans.* These features include tips for consuming heart-healthy diets, eating more beans, preserving vitamins in foods, seasoning foods without excess sodium, dining out defensively, sports nutrition basics for athletes, and practicing home food safety.

The *Nutrition Action* features are magazine-style essays that keep you abreast of current topics important to nutrition-conscious consumers. The *Nutrition Action* features address topics such as fast food, smart snacking, food allergies, dietary supplements and medicinal herbs, diet and blood pressure, and aging well with physical activity. The *Nutrition Action* sections reflect the latest issues in the field. For example, "Carbohydrates—Friend or Foe?" helps consumers choose healthful carbohydrates while making sense of the carbohydrate debate; "Diet Confusion: Weighing the Evidence" helps readers make sense of the current weight-loss scene; and "Eat Fresh Eat Local" includes the earth-friendly benefits of eating fresh and locally grown organic foods.

The *Ask Yourself* sections at the beginning of each chapter contain a set of true or false questions designed to provide readers with a preview of the chapter's contents. Answers to the questions are also provided.

Scorecards are hands-on features that allow readers to evaluate their own nutrition behaviors and knowledge in many areas. Some of the *Scorecards* assist readers in assessing their longevity, overall diet, fruit and vegetable consumption, weight status, physical activity habits, and food safety know-how.

The final special feature of each chapter is the *Spotlight.* Each addresses a common concern people have about nutrition. *Spotlight* topics include nutrition and the media, ethnic cuisines, alternative sweeteners, diet and heart disease, the benefits derived from vegetarian diets, nutrition and cancer prevention, osteoporosis, fetal alcohol syndrome, eating disorders, athletes and nutritional supplements, and child obesity. The Chapter 13 *Spotlight* covers the many factors that influence nutrition and food insecurity among the people of the world, and underscores that the practical suggestions offered throughout this book for attaining the ideals of personal nutrition are the very suggestions that best support the health of the whole earth as well. The *Spotlights* continue in their question-and-answer format to encourage readers to ask further questions about nutrition issues. We encourage you to ask us questions, too, in care of the publisher.

The appendixes have also been updated. Appendix A presents aids to calculations, including how to calculate the percentage of calories from fat in one's diet. Appendix A also provides a series of photos depicting the *Choose Your Foods: Food Lists for Diabetes and Weight Management*, and sample USDA Healthy Eating Patterns at various calorie levels that complement the *Dietary Guidelines for Americans.* Appendix B includes *Eating Well with Canada's Food Guide*, which interprets Canada's *Guidelines for Healthy Living*, including recommendations for physical activity.

A *Diet and Wellness Plus* assignment follows the appendixes. The glossary of terms that follows the appendixes provides a quick reference to the nutrition terminology defined in the margins of the text and can be used as a review tool.

Notable Changes in the 10th Edition

Nutrition is a subject that is forever changing. This edition incorporates the many recent changes that have taken place in the field of nutrition. Since the last edition was published, we have more robust research findings examining healthy eating patterns and the prevention of chronic diseases such as heart disease and certain types of cancer, as well as increasing consumer interest in environmentally friendly food choices. Additionally, we have been challenged by the increasing cultural, ethnic, and generational diversity of our society, recent advances in biotechnology, and the parallel trends toward supersized food portions and obesity. The *2015–2020 Dietary Guidelines for Americans* report describes healthy eating patterns, while emphasizing that all segments of our society—from home to school to work to communities—have a role to play in supporting healthy choices for all. Nevertheless, nutrition claims bombard us frequently in advertising and articles about nutrition and fitness on television, radio, and the Internet, and in newspapers and magazines. It is important that consumers have the knowledge to evaluate the nutrition issues and controversies. This 10th edition of *Personal Nutrition* provides a sieve through which to separate the valid nutrition information from the rest.

For all chapters and special chapter features:

- We have reviewed and updated content.
- Several new photos enhance student interest and reinforce the real-life applications of the material.
- The learning objectives have been augmented and refined to specify key student outcomes for each major section of each chapter.
- Some web links to sources of nutrition information on a variety of nutrition topics are included in the chapters; others are available to instructors through the companion website.
- *Diet & Wellness Plus* activities for each chapter have been revised and made available in MindTap. Visit www.cengagebrain.com to access MindTap, a complete digital course that includes access to *Diet & Wellness Plus* exercises and more.
- We've created several new figures and tables and updated others.
- **Chapter 1**
  - Included the latest trend information on consumer sources of nutrition information.
  - Updated the discussion regarding healthy lifestyle choices and disease prevention.
  - Revised the Nutrition Action feature to reflect the MyPlate and *Dietary Guidelines for Americans* messages.
  - Enhanced the discussion regarding nutrition misinformation and credible nutrition resources.
- **Chapter 2**
  - Created a new photo-illustrated graphic depicting nutrient density and the small shifts in food choices that can yield healthy eating patterns over time.
  - Created new graphic illustrating both a healthy eating pattern and the food and beverage components to be limited according to the *Dietary Guidelines for Americans.*

    - Reorganized information on MyPlate; included table to provide summary information of dietary intake goals, key nutrients, and strategies for choosing nutrient-dense items from each food group.
    - Revised the section on *Dietary Guidelines for Americans*, including new tables, figures, photos, and discussion to reflect the 2015–2020 edition; added new graphic demonstrating how the U.S. diet measures up to the recommended dietary guidelines.
    - Included discussion and illustration of approved food label changes, including newly approved Daily Values; included labels showing nutrient claims, health claims, and structure/function claims.
    - Added new tips for enjoying foods from many cultures.
- **Chapter 3**
    - Expanded discussion on prebiotics, probiotics, and intestinal microflora.
    - Added discussion regarding choking with a new graphic illustrating the prevention of choking.
- **Chapter 4**
    - Added a new figure that identifies common sources of added sugars and demonstrates how Americans exceed recommended limits for added sugars.
    - Enhanced the discussion of health benefits of various types of fiber; introduced a discussion of fermentable fiber.
    - Revised content on glycemic index of foods.
    - Strengthened the chapter discussion regarding diabetes.
    - Reorganized material in chapter *Spotlight* to include sweeteners approved for consumer use.
- **Chapter 5**
    - Reorganized major "Fat in the Diet" section; added new figure that identifies sources of saturated fat in the diet and demonstrates how Americans exceed recommended limits for saturated fats.
    - Strengthened discussion of omega-3 fats in the diet; updated recommendations for pregnant women regarding consumption of fish.
    - Revised recommendations and discussion for cholesterol according to the 2015–2020 *Dietary Guidelines for Americans.*
    - Added a new figure for a healthy Mediterranean eating pattern.
    - Added new information regarding lipoproteins and heart disease risk.
- **Chapter 6**
    - Updated food allergy feature and discussion of gluten intolerance and celiac disease.
    - Updated *Spotlight* including new tips for creating healthy vegetarian eating patterns reflecting the goals of the *Dietary Guidelines for Americans.*
    - Included new USDA Healthy Eating Patterns for Vegetarians, located in Appendix A.
- **Chapter 7**
    - Created summary tables for vitamin groups based on the functional roles they play in the body.
    - Included information on the vitamins of public health concern from the *Dietary Guidelines for Americans.*
    - Added a new text section regarding phytochemicals and functional foods with tips for optimizing intakes in the daily diet.

- Expanded *Nutrition Action* feature "Choosing a Vitamin-Mineral Supplement or Herbal Remedy"; developed new figures and discussion regarding dietary supplement use among U.S. adults; created new figure demonstrating structure/function labels used on supplements.
- Updated recommendations for reducing risk for cancer from major professional organizations; added discussion of prebiotics and probiotics.

- **Chapter 8**
  - Created summary tables for mineral groups based on the functional roles they play in the body.
  - Included information on the minerals of public health concern from the *Dietary Guidelines for Americans*.
  - Added a new figure that identifies major sources of sodium in the diet and demonstrates how Americans exceed recommended limits for sodium.
  - Updated *Nutrition Action* feature "Diet and Blood Pressure—Beyond Just the Salt Shaker"; enhanced DASH eating plan guidance with a new chart.
  - Revised *Spotlight* feature "Osteoporosis"; updated recommendations for prevention, and included tips for adding more calcium to the diet.
- **Chapter 9**
  - Enhanced discussion of fructose-versus glucose-based sports drinks and sports performance; updated discussion regarding energy drinks.
  - Modified content regarding fetal alcohol spectrum disorder.
- **Chapter 10**
  - Added new figure and maps regarding current prevalence of obesity.
  - Revised opening discussion and section on "What Is a Healthy Weight?"
  - Created new tables describing characteristics of successful dieters and the elements of behavior change.
  - Included new pharmaceutical options for weight loss.
  - Updated discussion and summary table comparing popular weight-loss diets.
  - Revised discussion of eating disorders, including summary table comparing the incidence and characteristics of various eating disorders.
- **Chapter 11**
  - Updated photos of people exercising; added new feature discussing the nutritional needs of active individuals versus competitive athletes.
  - Enhanced discussion of anaerobic versus aerobic metabolism, and expanded content regarding fuel use and duration/intensity of physical activity.
  - Included information about cardiorespiratory fitness and added new discussion and illustration regarding neuromotor exercise.
  - Updated recommendations regarding hydration and protein needs; added a new figure illustrating the color of urine in relation to hydration.
  - Added new table for carbohydrate recommendations for various levels of physical activity.
  - Added new Savvy Diner feature regarding sports nutrition for athletes, including MyPlates for athletes at various levels of training.
  - Added new graphic and discussion to introduce creation of SMART goals.
  - Revised Spotlight on supplements and athletes and added new table of ergogenic aids.

- **Chapter 12**
  - Revised risk factor criteria and discussion of gestational diabetes.
  - Added new American Academy of Pediatrics recommendations regarding use of juice during infancy and childhood.
  - Included new information and graphic regarding sugar-sweetened beverage consumption by children and teens.
  - Updated *Spotlight* feature—"Addressing Weight Problems in Children and Adolescents."
  - Updated discussion regarding the aging of the population.
  - Revised recommendations for reducing the risk of chronic diseases; added new graphics showing prevalence of chronic health conditions as well as functional limitations among older adults.
  - Created new Savvy Diner feature illustrating the concepts included in the new MyPlate for Older Adults graphic.
  - Created new photo-illustrated figure highlighting the many elements of successful aging.
- **Chapter 13**
  - Updated discussions of problem foods needing special handling for food safety.
  - Expanded *The Savvy Diner* feature on local foods and sustainable food system approaches; added tips for reducing one's ecological footprint.
  - Updated statistics, diagrams, and discussions in chapter *Spotlight* on global food insecurity issues.

We welcome you to the fascinating subject of nutrition. We hope that the book speaks to you personally and that you find it practical for your everyday use. We hope, too, that by reading it, you may enhance your own personal nutrition and health.

Student and Instructor Resources

In addition to the text, an array of teaching and learning resources are available for both instructors and students.

Instructor Companion Site Everything instructors need in one place! This collection of book-specific lecture and class tools is available online via www.cengage.com/login. Access and download PowerPoint presentations, images, an instructor's manual, chapter references, videos, and more.

Cengage Learning Testing Powered by Cognero This flexible online system allows instructors to author, edit, and manage test bank content from multiple Cengage Learning solutions; create multiple test versions in an instant; and deliver tests from an LMS, a classroom, or wherever the instructor wants.

MindTap Nutrition MindTap is well beyond an eBook, a homework solution or digital supplement, a resource center website, a course delivery platform or a Learning Management System. MindTap is a personal learning experience that combines all your digital assets—readings, multimedia, activities, and assessments—into a singular learning path to improve student outcomes. The learning plan for each chapter features activities that incorporate *Diet and Wellness Plus,* the market-leading diet analysis software, to help students directly relate nutritional concepts to their own lives.

Diet & Wellness Plus *Diet & Wellness Plus* helps you understand how nutrition relates to your personal health goals. Track your diet and activity, generate reports, and analyze the nutritional value of the food you eat. *Diet & Wellness Plus* includes over 75,000 foods as well as custom food and recipe features. The Behavior Change Planner helps you identify risks in your life and guides you through the key steps to make positive changes.

Global Nutrition Watch Global Nutrition Watch is a student-friendly website that provides one-stop access to the most current information about nutrition for classroom discussion and research projects. Global Nutrition Watch provides thousands of trusted nutrition sources, is updated daily, and is searchable by topic or key word, making it easy to find the most current news related to nutrition.

Acknowledgments

We are grateful to the many individuals who have made contributions to the development of this 10th edition of *Personal Nutrition*. We thank our family and friends for their continued support and encouragement throughout this endeavor and countless others. We appreciate the insights provided by our colleagues—especially to all those individuals who have contributed their expertise to previous editions of this text—including Eleanor Whitney, Sara Long Roth, Diane Morris, Gail Zyla, and Kathleen Morgan. Their insights are reflected in this new edition, still. We thank Kathy Roberts for her thorough revision of Chapter 12. We are grateful to Dr. Anne Buison Pellizzon for her scholarly edits to Chapter 10, and to Jennifer Doane for her expertise and thorough revision of Chapter 11. We thank Amber Bowitz, too, for assistance with updates to the Spotlight features in Chapters 7, 8, and 11. We appreciate the hard work and expertise of the team of authors who prepared ancillary material for this edition. Special thanks go to the editorial team and their staff: Krista Mastroianni, Product Manager; Miriam Myers, Senior Content Developer; Lori Hazzard, MPS Limited; and Carol Samet, Senior Content Project Manager. Their guidance ensured the highest quality of work throughout all facets of this production. We appreciate the work of Lumina Datametrics for their work on the student and instructor resources. Our gratitude goes to Tom Ziolkowski, Executive Marketing Manager, and his team for their fine efforts in marketing this book. Our thanks to the many sales representatives who will introduce this new book to its readers. Our appreciation goes to other members of the production team: MPS Limited, artist, Geeta Kamath of Lumina Datamatics for photo research, and everyone at MPS Limited for their hard work and diligence in producing a text to be proud of. Last, but not least, we owe much to our colleagues who provided expert reviews of this text—not only for their ideas and suggestions, many of which made their way into the text, but also for their continued enthusiasm, support, and interest in *Personal Nutrition*. Thanks to all of you:

Debra Boardley, *University of Toledo*
Dori Cinque, *SUNY Suffolk County Community College*
Jeanne Freeland-Graves, *University of Texas*
Art Gilbert, *University of California, Santa Barbara*
Beth Goehring, MS MA, *Contra Costa College*
Joanne Gould, *Kean University*
Laura M. Horn, MEd, RD, LD, *Cincinnati State Technical and Community College*
Gustavo Ibarra, *Salt Lake Community College*
Judy Kaufman, *Monroe Community College*
Zaheer Ali Kirmani, *Sam Houston State University*
Colleen McCrief, MS, RDN, *The Sage Colleges*
Elizabeth Koester Morton, *University of South Carolina*
Pam Massey, *University of Wisconsin–Fox Valley*
Lorrie Miller Kohler, *Minneapolis Community and Technical College*
Rosa A. Mo, *University of New Haven*
Kristen S. Montgomery, PHD RN, *University of North Carolina at Charlotte*
Esther Okeiyi, *North Carolina Central University*
Caren L. Rojas, MA RD, *Western Michigan University*
Kathleen C. Sailsbery, *Morgan Community College*
Brandy Sarrette, RD, LDN, *Springfield Technical Community College*
Robin S. Schenk, *Buffalo State, SUNY*
Karen Schuster, *Florida State College at Jacksonville*
Denise L. Signorelli, *College of Southern Nevada*
Tricia Steffen, *Nova Southeastern University*
Melissa Wdowik, *University of North Carolina at Charlotte*
Sharman Willmore, *Cincinnati State Technical and Community College*
Kathryn A. Witt, *Messiah College*
Lisa Wright, MT (ASCP) CMA, *Bristol Community College*
Linda O. Young, *University of Nebraska–Lincoln*
Maureen Zimmerman, *Mesa Community College*

—Marie Boyle
January 2018

PERSONAL NUTRITION

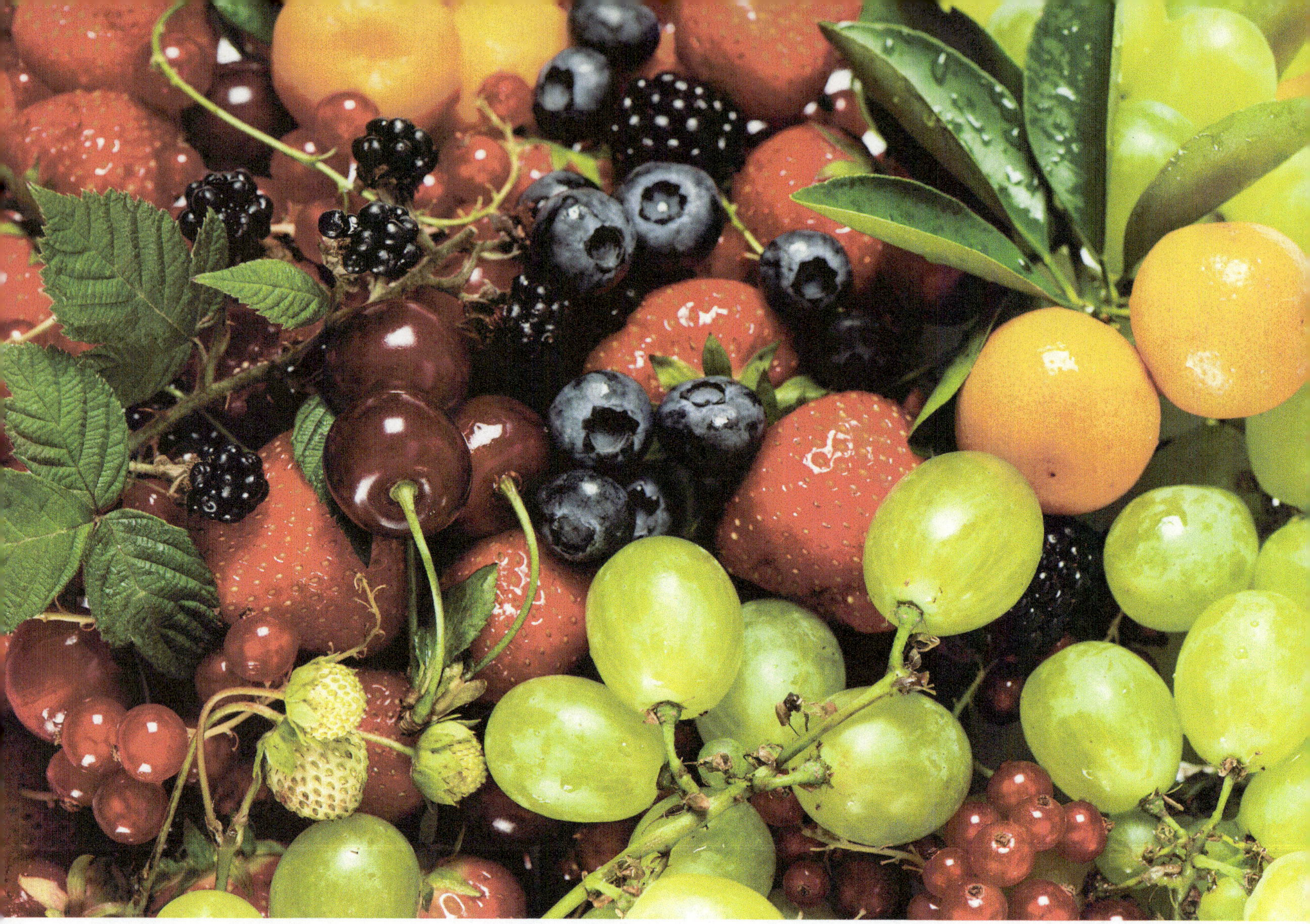

LiliGraphie/Shutterstock.com

AskYourself . . .

Which of the following statements about nutrition are true, and which are false? For each false statement, what is true?

1. The way people choose to live and eat can affect their health and quality of life as they age.
2. Healthy diets cost more than relatively unhealthy diets.
3. Most people obtain information about nutrition from health professionals.
4. The more current a dietary claim, the more you can trust its accuracy and reliability.

Answers found on page 4.

ChapterObjectives

1.1 List the six classes of nutrients.

1.2 Identify lifestyle factors that impact risk for chronic disease.

1.3 List several national nutrition-related objectives aimed at improving the nation's health.

1.4 Describe lifestyle practices associated with longevity and health.

1.5 Identify different factors that influence personal food choices.

1.6 Identify tips for stocking a healthy food pantry.

1.7 List strategies for choosing healthy meals when dining away from home.

1.8 Distinguish between reliable science-based nutrition information and nutrition/health fraud.

The Basics of Understanding Nutrition

CHAPTER 1

Stroll down the aisle of any supermarket, and you'll see all manner of foods touted with such claims as "low-fat," "low-carb," "low-calorie," and "fat-free." Flip through the pages of just about any magazine, and you're likely to find advice on how to lose weight. Walk into any gym, and you'll probably hear members discussing the merits of one performance-enhancing food or another. All this boils down to the fact that nutrition has become part and parcel of the American lifestyle.

> Tell me what you eat, and I will tell you what you are.
>
> — Jean Anthelme Brillat-Savarin (1755–1826, French Politician and Gourmet; Author of *Physiology of Taste*)

It wasn't always that way, however. The field of nutrition is a relative newcomer on the scientific block. Although Hippocrates recognized diet as a component of health back in 400 B.C., only in the past hundred years or so have researchers begun to understand that carbohydrates, fats, and proteins are needed for normal growth. The discovery of the first vitamin occurred in the early 1900s. It wasn't until 1928, when an organization called the American Institute of Nutrition was formed, that nutrition was officially recognized as a distinct field of study.[1]* It took several more decades before nutrition achieved its current status as one of the most talked-about scientific disciplines.

Today we spend billions of dollars each year investigating the many aspects of **nutrition**, a science that encompasses the study not only of vitamins, minerals, and other nutrients, but also of such diverse subjects as the effects of alcohol, caffeine, and pesticides. In addition, nutrition scientists continually expand our understanding of the impact food has on our bodies by examining research in chemistry, physics, biology, biochemistry, genetics, immunology, and other nutrition-related fields. A number of other disciplines also make valuable contributions to the study of nutrition. These related fields include psychology, anthropology, epidemiology, geography, agriculture, ethics, economics, sociology, and philosophy.

nutrition the study of foods, their nutrients and other chemical components, their actions and interactions in the body, and their influence on health and disease.

*Reference notes for each chapter are in MindTap and in the Instructor Companion Site.

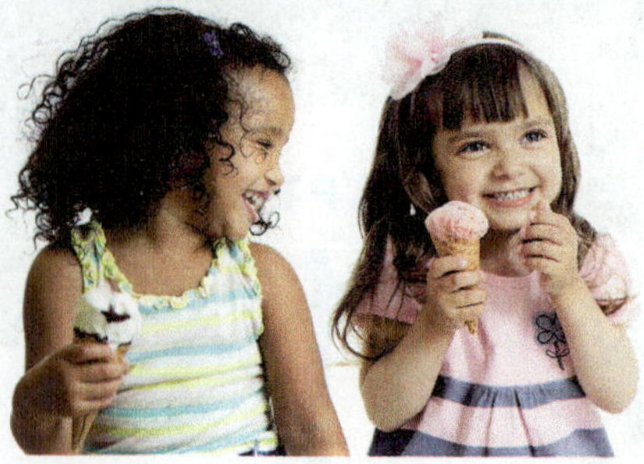

Andrey_Kuzmin/Shutterstock.com

The scientific discipline of nutrition investigates how the foods you eat and your lifestyle habits affect your health over a lifetime.

Even though science has shown us that, to some extent, we really are what we eat, many consumers have become more confused than ever about how to translate the steady stream of new findings about nutrition into a lifestyle of healthy eating. Reportedly, people of all ages make food-purchasing decisions based on claims regarding nutrition and health.[2] Each additional nugget of nutrition news that comes along raises new concerns: Is caffeine bad for me? Should I take vitamin supplements? Do diet pills work? Can a sports drink improve my performance? Do pesticides really pose a hazard?

Some manufacturers and media outlets feed the confusion by offering health-conscious consumers unreliable products and misleading dietary advice, often making unsubstantiated claims for a number of nutritional products, including supplements touted as fat melters, muscle builders, and energy boosters. Unfortunately, misinformation runs rampant in the marketplace. Americans spend billions of dollars annually on medical and nutritional **health fraud** and **quackery**.[3] Consider, for example, that college athletes alone may spend hundreds of dollars a month on nutritional supplements, even though most of the products pitched to serious exercisers are useless and, in some cases, potentially harmful. At the same time, the sale of weight-loss foods, products, and services—not all of them sound—has become a $60 billion industry.[4]

To be sure, the widespread interest in nutrition has generated some positive changes in the marketplace. Whereas the sale of fresh fruit, low-fat yogurt, and salads in fast-food chains was virtually unheard of at one time, those eateries couldn't survive in the current nutrition-conscious environment without offering such healthy fare. (See the Nutrition Action feature later in this chapter for tips on eating healthfully at fast-food outlets.) By the same token, food manufacturers and grocers have responded to consumer concerns about health, wellness, and sustainability by providing shoppers with an unprecedented number of organic and locally sourced products and precooked fresh, retail meals at the supermarket.[5]

With the amount of nutrition information and the number of food alternatives always on the rise, choosing a healthy diet can seem like a daunting task. Fortunately, you don't need a degree in nutrition to put the principles of the science to use in your own life. A basic understanding of nutrition can go a long way in helping you protect your health (and your wallet). This book lays the foundation you need to take nutrition science out of the laboratory and move it into your kitchen, both today and tomorrow. The first steps are understanding the nature of the nutrients themselves and exploring the current thrust of the field of nutrition.

health fraud conscious deceit practiced for profit, such as the promotion of a false or an unproven product or therapy.

quackery health fraud; a quack is a person who practices health fraud (quack = to boast loudly).

ASK YOURSELF ANSWERS: **1.** True. **2.** False. People can save money when they switch from a typical high-fat diet to the whole-grain, produce-rich diet recommended by health experts. **3.** False. Most Americans look first to television for nutrition information, then to magazines, and then to the Internet. **4.** False. If a nutrition claim is too new, it may not have been adequately tested. Findings must be confirmed many times over by experiments and evaluated in light of other knowledge before they can be translated into recommendations for the public.

1.1 The Nutrients in Foods

Almost any food you eat is mostly water, and some foods are as high as 99 percent water. The bulk of the solid materials consists of carbohydrates, fats, and proteins. If you could remove these materials, you would be left with a tiny residue of minerals, vitamins, and other compounds. Water, carbohydrates, fats, proteins, vitamins, and some of the minerals found in foods represent the six classes of **nutrients** (see Table 1-1). The other compounds may include food additives, pigments, phytochemicals, and other substances.

A complete chemical analysis of your body would show that it is made of materials similar to those in most foods, in roughly the same proportions. For example, if you weigh 150 pounds (and if that is a desirable weight for you), your body contains about 90 pounds of water and about 30 pounds of fat. The other 30 pounds consist mostly of proteins, carbohydrates, and the major minerals of your bones—calcium and phosphorus. Vitamins, other minerals, and incidental extras constitute only a fraction of a pound.

Scientists use the term **essential nutrient** to describe the nutrients that the body must obtain from food. About 40 nutrients are known to be *essential*; that is, they are compounds that the body cannot make for itself but are indispensable to life processes. How can you be sure you're getting all of the nutrients you need? The rest of this chapter, along with the diet-planning tools presented in Chapter 2, will help you design a diet that supports good health.

TABLE 1-1 The Six Classes of Nutrients

- carbohydrates
- fats
- proteins
- vitamins
- minerals
- water

The energy-yielding nutrients:

- carbohydrates
- fats
- proteins

The Energy-Yielding Nutrients

Upon being broken down in the body, or digested, three of the nutrients—carbohydrates, proteins, and fats—yield the **energy** that the body uses to fuel its various activities. In contrast, vitamins, minerals, and water, once broken down in the body, do not yield energy but perform other tasks, such as maintenance and repair. Each gram of carbohydrate and protein consumed supplies your body with 4 calories, and each gram of fat provides 9 calories (see Figure 1-1). Only one other substance that people consume supplies calories, and that is alcohol, which provides 7 calories per gram. Alcohol is not considered a nutrient, however, because it does not help maintain or repair body tissues the way nutrients do.

The body uses energy from carbohydrates, fats, and proteins to do work or generate heat. This energy is measured in **calories**—familiar to almost everyone as markers of how "fattening" foods are. If your body doesn't use (release) the energy you obtained from a food soon after you've eaten it, it stores that energy, usually as body fat, for later use. If a person eats excess amounts of proteins, fats, or carbohydrates fairly regularly, the stored fat builds up over time and leads to obesity. Too much of any food, whether lean meat (a protein-rich food), potatoes (a high-carbohydrate food), or butter (a fatty food), can contribute excess calories that result in making someone overweight.

FIGURE 1-1 Caloric Values of Carbohydrates, Proteins, Fats, and Alcohol

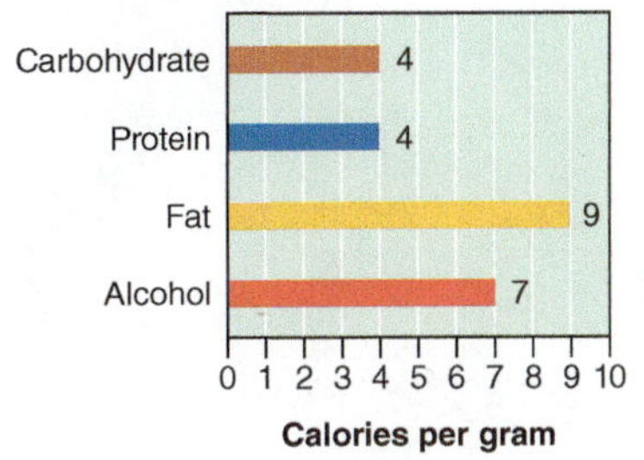

Vitamins, Minerals, and Water

Unlike carbohydrates, fats, and proteins, **vitamins** and **minerals** do not supply energy or calories. Instead, they regulate the release of energy and other aspects of **metabolism**. As Table 1-2 shows, there are 13 vitamins, each with its special role to play. Vitamins are divided into two classes: water-soluble (the B vitamins and vitamin C) and fat-soluble (vitamins A, D, E, and K). This distinction has many implications for the kinds of foods that provide the different vitamins and how the body uses them, as you will see in Chapter 7.

The minerals also perform important functions. Some, such as calcium, make up the structure of bones and teeth. Others, including sodium, float about in the body's fluids, where they help regulate crucial bodily functions, such as heartbeat and muscle contractions.

nutrients Substances obtained from food and used in the body to promote growth, maintenance, and repair. The nutrients include carbohydrates, fats, proteins, vitamins, minerals, and water.

essential nutrient A nutrient that must be obtained from food because the body cannot make it for itself.

energy The capacity to do work, such as moving or heating something.

calorie The unit used to measure energy.

vitamins Organic, or carbon-containing, essential nutrients that are vital to life but needed only in relatively minute amounts (*vita* = life; *amine* = containing nitrogen).

minerals Inorganic compounds, some of which are essential nutrients.

metabolism Collective term for all of the chemical and physical reactions occurring in living cells, including the reactions by which the body obtains and uses energy from foods.

TABLE 1-2 The Vitamins and Minerals

The Vitamins		The Minerals	
The Water-Soluble Vitamins:	**The Fat-Soluble Vitamins:**	**The Major Minerals:**	**The Trace Minerals:**
B vitamins	Vitamin A	Calcium	Chromium
Thiamin	Vitamin D	Potassium	Manganese
Riboflavin	Vitamin E	Chloride	Copper
Niacin	Vitamin K	Sodium	Molybdenum
Vitamin B_6		Magnesium	Fluoride
Folate		Sulfur	Selenium
Vitamin B_{12}		Phosphorus	Iodine
Biotin			Zinc
Pantothenic acid			Iron
Vitamin C			

NOTE: A number of trace minerals are currently under study to determine possible dietary requirements for humans. These include arsenic, boron, cadmium, cobalt, lead, lithium, nickel, silicon, tin, and vanadium.

Often neglected but equally vital, **water** is the medium in which all of the body's processes take place. Some 60 percent of your body's weight consists of water, which carries materials to and from cells and provides the warm, nutrient-rich bath in which cells thrive. Water also transports hormonal messages from place to place. When energy-yielding nutrients release energy, they break down into water and other simple compounds. Without water, you could live only a few days.

Each day your body loses water in the form of sweat and urine. Therefore, you must replace large amounts of it—on the order of 2 to 3 quarts a day. To be sure, you don't

water Fluid that provides the medium for life processes.

Calorie Value of Carbohydrates, Fats, and Proteins

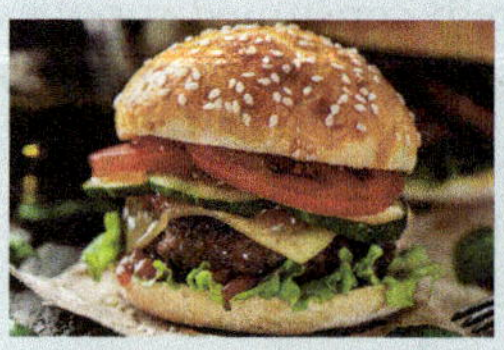

Vankad/Shutterstock.com

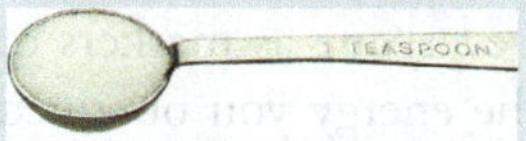

James R. T. Bossert/Shutterstock.com

Remember that 1 gram is a very small amount. For instance, 1 teaspoon of sugar weighs roughly 4 grams.

If you know the number of grams of carbohydrates, fats, and proteins in a food, you can calculate the number of calories in it. Simply multiply the carbohydrate grams by 4, the fat grams by 9, and the protein grams by 4. Add the totals together to obtain the number of calories. For example, a deluxe fast-food hamburger contains about 45 grams of carbohydrate, 27 grams of protein, and 39 grams of fat:

45 grams of carbohydrate × 4 calories	= 180 calories
39 grams of fat × 9 calories	= 351 calories
27 grams of protein × 4 calories	= 108 calories
Total:	639 calories

The percentage of your total energy intake from carbohydrates, fats, and proteins can then be determined by dividing the number of calories from each energy nutrient by the total calories and then multiplying your answer by 100 to get the percentage:

$$\text{calories from carbohydrates} = \frac{45 \times 4 \text{ cal/g}}{639} = 0.281 \times 100 = 28\%$$

$$\text{calories from fats} = \frac{39 \times 9 \text{ cal/g}}{639} = 0.548 \times 100 = 55\%$$

$$\text{calories from proteins} = \frac{27 \times 4 \text{ cal/g}}{639} = 0.168 \times 100 = 17\%$$

See Appendix A for help with figuring percentages and other calculations.

need to *drink* that much water daily, because the foods and other beverages you consume do supply some of the water you need.

1.2 Nutrition and Health Promotion

In the past, scientists investigating the role that diet plays in health focused on the consequences of getting too little of one nutrient or another. Until the end of World War II, in fact, nutrition researchers concentrated on eliminating diseases caused by deficiency (lack or absence) of a particular vitamin or mineral.

These days, the focus is just the opposite. Deficiency diseases have been virtually eliminated in America because of our abundant food supply and the practice of fortifying food with essential nutrients (adding iodine to salt, for example). Nevertheless, diseases related to **malnutrition**, in the form of dietary excess and imbalance, run rampant. Many of the major killers, such as heart disease, some types of cancer, stroke, and diabetes, are influenced by a number of factors, including a person's genetic makeup, eating and physical activity habits, exposure to tobacco, and other lifestyle practices (see Table 1-3). Five of the leading causes of death—heart disease, cancer, stroke, diabetes, and hypertension—have been linked to diet (see Figure 1-2). Another three are associated with excessive alcohol consumption: accidents, suicide, and liver disease.[6] **Overnutrition** contributes to other ills as well, including obesity and dental disease. Because obesity and a sedentary lifestyle are linked with chronic diseases, such as diabetes, heart disease, and certain cancers, it can be projected that increased rates of obesity will lead to increased deaths each year, not to mention hospitalizations, disabilities, time lost from jobs, and poor quality of life for many Americans.[7]

This is not to say that diet is the sole culprit causing these diseases. Figure 1-3 puts nutrition (a factor you can control) in perspective with respect to heredity (a factor you cannot control). It illustrates the point that some diseases are much more related

TABLE 1-3 **Factors Contributing to Deaths in the United States**

Factors	Percentage of Deaths
Tobacco	18
Poor diet/inactivity	15
Alcohol	4
Microbial agents	3
Toxic agents	2
Motor vehicles	2
Firearms	1
Sexual behavior	1
Illicit drugs	1

SOURCE: A. H. Mokdad and coauthors, Actual causes of death in the United States, 2000, *Journal of American Medical Association* 291 (2004): 1238–45, with corrections from *Journal of the American Medical Association* 293 (2005): 298.

malnutrition Any condition caused by an excess, deficiency, or imbalance of calories or nutrients.

overnutrition Calorie or nutrient overconsumption severe enough to cause disease or increased risk of disease; a form of malnutrition.

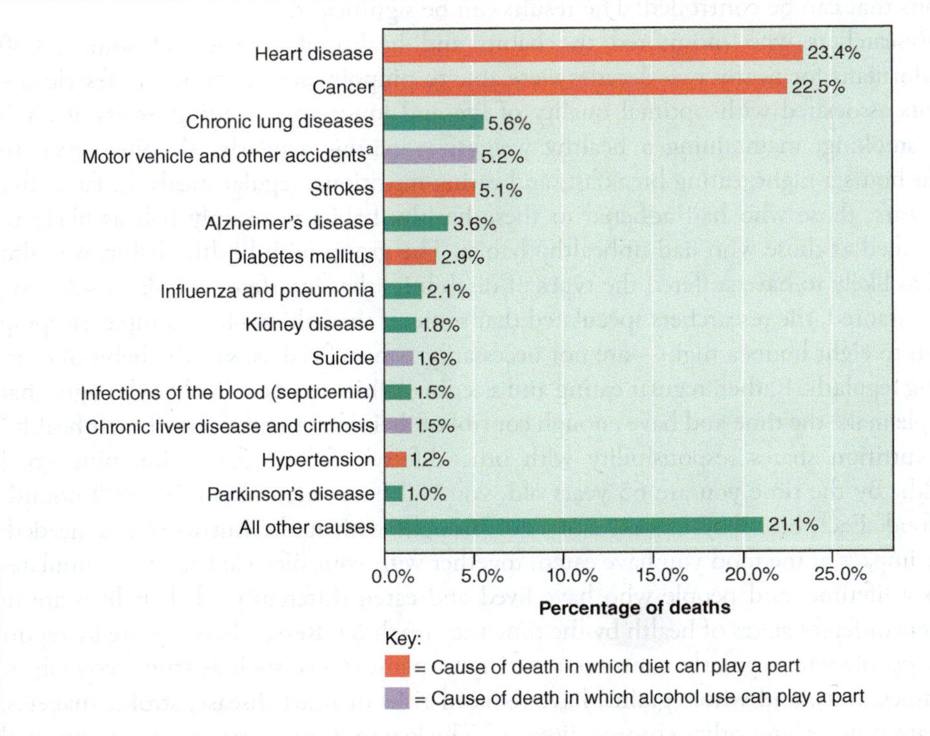

FIGURE 1-2

The Leading Causes of Death in the United States

[a] The leading cause of death for people aged 15 to 24 is motor vehicle and other accidents, followed by suicide, homicide, cancer, and heart disease. About half of all accident fatalities are alcohol related.

SOURCE: Table C from p. 9 of Centers for Disease Control & Prevention, *National Vital Statistics Reports*, Vol 65, No. 5. June 30, 2016.

FIGURE 1-3

Nutrition and Disease

Not all diseases are equally influenced by diet. Some are purely hereditary, such as sickle-cell anemia. Some may be inherited (or the tendency to develop them may be inherited) but may be influenced by diet, such as some forms of diabetes. Some are purely dietary, such as the vitamin and mineral deficiency diseases. Good nutrition alone is certainly not enough to prevent many diseases, but it helps.

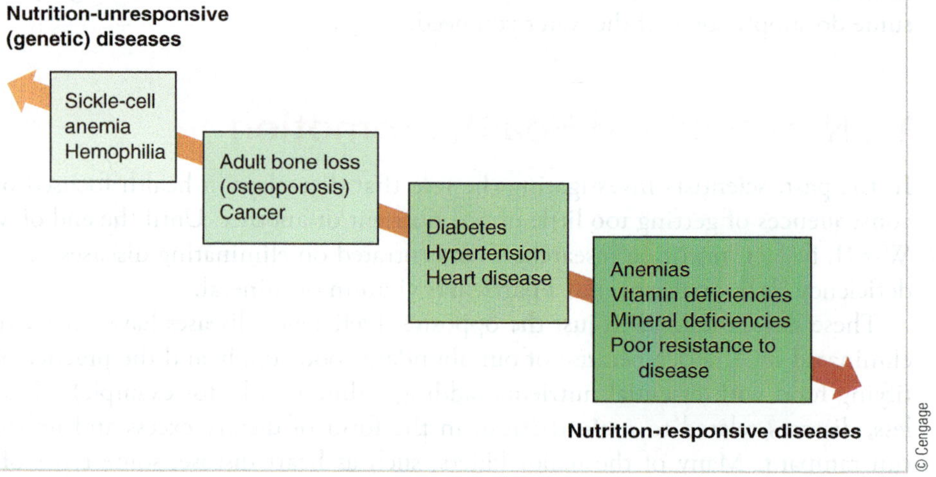

to nutrition than others and that some are not responsive to nutrition at all. At one extreme are diseases that can be completely cured by supplying missing nutrients, and at the other extreme are certain genetic (inherited) diseases that are unaltered by nutrition. Most diseases fall in between, being influenced by inherited susceptibility but responsive to dietary manipulations that help counteract the disease process. Thus, diabetes may be managed by means of a special diet; cardiovascular disease may respond favorably to a heart-healthy diet.

A number of environmental, behavioral, social, and genetic factors work together to determine a person's likelihood of suffering from a **degenerative disease**. For example, diet notwithstanding, someone who smokes, doesn't exercise regularly, and has a parent who suffered a heart attack is more likely to end up with heart disease than a nonsmoker who works out regularly and does not have a close relative with heart disease. The way to alter disease risk is to concentrate on changing the daily habits that can be controlled. The results can be significant.

Researchers who monitored the habits and health of a group of some 7,000 Californians for nearly two decades were able to pinpoint seven common lifestyle elements associated with optimal quality of life and longevity: avoiding excess alcohol; not smoking; maintaining a healthy weight; exercising regularly; sleeping seven to eight hours a night; eating breakfast; and eating nutritious, regular meals. In fact, after 20 years, those who had adhered to these healthy habits were only half as likely to have died as those who had unhealthy habits. The group with healthy habits was also half as likely to have suffered the types of disabilities that interfere with day-to-day living. Granted, the researchers speculated that some of the habits—for example, sleeping seven to eight hours a night—are not necessarily as beneficial as, say, the habit of exercising regularly. Rather, regular eating and sleeping habits are most likely to be signs that people make the time and have enough control of their lives to take care of their health.[8]

Nutrition shares responsibility with other lifestyle factors for maintaining good health. By the time you are 65 years old, you will have eaten about 100,000 pounds of food. Each bite may or may not have brought with it the nutrients you needed. The impact of the food you have eaten, together with your lifestyle habits, accumulates over a lifetime, and people who have lived and eaten differently all their lives are in widely different states of health by the time they reach 65. Researchers repeatedly report that people who regularly consume a variety of plant foods, such as fruits, vegetables, legumes, nuts, and whole grains, have reduced risks of heart disease, stroke, diabetes, certain cancers, and other chronic diseases.[9] The key to disease prevention and optimal

degenerative disease Chronic disease characterized by deterioration of body organs as a result of misuse and neglect. Poor eating habits, smoking, lack of exercise, and other lifestyle habits often contribute to degenerative diseases including heart disease, cancer, osteoporosis, and diabetes.

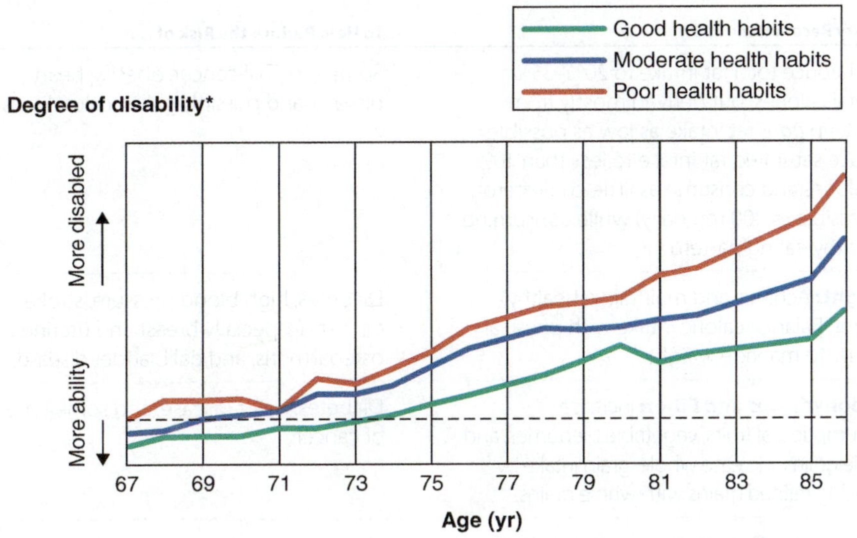

FIGURE 1-4

Healthy Aging

In a study of more than 1,700 people, those who smoked the least, maintained a healthy weight, and exercised regularly not only lived longer but also postponed disability. As shown here, people with the best health habits delayed the onset of even minimal disability to about age 73, compared with age 66 for those with the poorest health habits.

*The dashed line represents minimal disability, defined as having some difficulty performing the everyday tasks of daily living (such as bathing, dressing, eating, walking, toileting, and getting outside).

SOURCE: Based on Figure 2 from p. 4 of the following article: J. F. Fries, The theory and practice of active aging. *Current Gerontology and Geriatrics Research* 2012, no 3 (2012): 420637. doi:10.1155/2012/420637.

health is not in eating or avoiding a certain food, but rather in creating a lifestyle that includes time for preparing nutritious meals and enjoying regular physical activity.

A person who practices good health habits can expect to delay the onset of even minimal disability by several years, compared with a person who practices few or none of them (see Figure 1-4).[10] If you believe in accepting the things you cannot control and controlling the things you can, you are in luck. Your nutritional health can be controlled, and because nutrition is involved in at least half of the preceding lifestyle recommendations, it clearly plays a key role in maintaining good health. This chapter's Scorecard feature, "The Longevity Game," further demonstrates this point.

Table 1-4 summarizes ways to improve health with sound nutrition practices. As you read Table 1-4, keep in mind that although everyone can benefit from eating a nutritious diet that complies with the guidelines, some people stand to gain more than others. Those who have high blood cholesterol levels, for instance, are already at risk for heart disease, thereby making it especially important for them to eat a health-promoting diet and maintain a healthy weight. By the same token, those who have close relatives with, say, diabetes, would do well to keep their weight down and pay particular attention to the other nutrition guidelines that help stave off that condition. (The chapters that follow explain the link between diet and chronic diseases in more detail and offer advice on how to follow each dietary recommendation.)

1.3 A National Agenda for Improving Nutrition and Health

Some people do things that are not good for their health. They overeat, smoke, refuse to wear a helmet when riding a bicycle, never wear seat belts when driving, fail to take their blood pressure medication—the list is endless. These behaviors reflect personal choices, habits, and customs that are influenced and modified by social forces. We call these *lifestyle behaviors*, and they can be changed if the individual is so motivated. **Health promotion** focuses on changing human behavior: getting people to eat healthy diets, be physically active, get regular rest, develop leisure-time hobbies for relaxation, strengthen social networks with family and friends, and achieve a balance among family, work, and play.[11]

health promotion Helping people achieve their maximum potential for good health.

TABLE 1-4 **Eating to Beat the Odds**

Dietary Recommendation	To Help Reduce the Risk of . . .
Fat: Reduce total fat intake to 20%–35% of total calories, but derived mostly from oils. Keep *trans* fat intake as low as possible. Reduce saturated fat intake to less than 10% of calories and consume as little cholesterol as possible (<300 mg daily) while consuming a healthy eating pattern.[a]	Some types of cancer, obesity, heart disease, and possibly gallbladder disease.
Weight: Achieve and maintain a healthy weight. Balance caloric intake with physical activity to manage weight.	Diabetes, high blood pressure, stroke, cancers (especially breast and uterine), osteoarthritis, and gallbladder disease.
Carbohydrates and Fiber: Increase consumption of fruits, vegetables, legumes, and whole grains. Increase whole-grain intake by replacing refined grains with whole grains.[b]	Diabetes, heart disease, and some types of cancer.
Sodium and Potassium: Limit daily intake of salt.[c] Increase food sources of potassium such as fresh fruits and vegetables.[d]	High blood pressure and stroke.
Alcohol: Avoid completely or drink only in moderation.[e]	Heart disease, high blood pressure, liver disease, stroke, some forms of cancer, and malformations in babies born to mothers who drink alcohol during pregnancy.
Sugar: Choose and prepare foods and beverages with little added sugars or caloric sweeteners. Aim for less than 10% of total calories from sugars.[b]	Tooth decay and gum disease.
Calcium and Vitamin D: Maintain adequate calcium and vitamin D intakes.[d]	Osteoporosis (adult bone loss) and bone fractures.

[a] The intake of saturated fat, *trans* fat and cholesterol can be reduced by substituting fish, poultry without skin, lean meats, and low-fat or fat-free dairy products for fatty meats and whole-milk products; by choosing more vegetables, fruits, whole-grain cereals, and legumes; by using oils to replace solid fats where possible; and by limiting egg yolks and fried or other fatty foods. Solid fats are fats with a high content of saturated and/or *trans* fatty acids (discussed in Chapter 5), which are usually solid at room temperature.
[b] Refined grains (discussed in Chapter 4) are processed grains and grain products that are not whole grain. Added sugars are those incorporated into foods and beverages during processing or preparation, or consumed separately.
[c] Limit the use of salt in cooking, and avoid adding it to foods at the table. Highly processed, salty, salt-preserved, and salt-pickled foods should be consumed sparingly.
[d] Choose foods that provide more potassium, dietary fiber, calcium, and vitamin D, which are nutrients of concern in American diets. These foods include vegetables, fruits, whole grains, and milk and milk products. Specific nutrient recommendations are provided at the back of this book.
[e] *Moderate drinking* is defined as no more than one drink a day for the average-sized woman and no more than two drinks a day for the average-sized man. A *drink* is any alcoholic beverage that delivers ½ ounce of pure ethanol: 5 ounces of wine, 12 ounces of beer, or 1½ ounces of hard liquor (whiskey, scotch, etc.). There are many circumstances in which people should avoid alcohol.

SOURCES: Adapted from U.S. Department of Health and Human Services and U.S. Department of Agriculture, *2015–2020 Dietary Guidelines for Americans*, 8th ed. (Washington, DC: U.S. Government Printing Office, 2015); and Institute of Medicine, *Dietary Reference Intakes for Energy, Carbohydrate, Fiber, Fat, Fatty Acids, Cholesterol, Protein, and Amino Acids* (Washington, DC: National Academy Press, 2002).

The relative importance of certain dietary recommendations is underscored by their appearance in the U.S. Department of Health and Human Services' official health promotion strategy for improving the nation's health, laid out in the year 2010. Called *Healthy People 2020*, the plan of action presents a national health promotion and disease prevention agenda for the next 10 years.[12] The report sets health objectives for the year 2020 with four broad goals designed to help all Americans achieve their full potential by attaining high-quality, longer lives free of preventable

1.4 Eating Pattern for Longevity

Need proof that good dietary choices can have a profound effect on your health and longevity? Look no farther than the Okinawans! These people dwell on a group of islands—known collectively as Okinawa—that lie southwest of mainland Japan. Okinawans enjoy one of the longest life spans of anyone on Earth, and they do so while maintaining a very high quality of life. This fact has sparked much interest in the Okinawan culture and resulted in the 25-year Okinawa Centenarian Study that began in 1976 to investigate what makes these people so healthy.[13] Researchers studied more than 600 Okinawan centenarians and numerous others in their 70s, 80s, and 90s.

When the study began, researchers were surprised to find that many centenarians were still very active, devoid of health problems, and looked years younger than their chronological age. Upon further investigation, they also discovered that these people have low levels of cancer-causing free radicals, low cardiovascular risks, extremely healthy bone densities, and a lower prevalence of dementia than those of the same age in other countries. Indeed, Okinawan elders have among the lowest mortality rates in the world from many chronic diseases, including cancer, stroke, osteoporosis, and heart disease. Although there is no magic bullet that results in the Okinawans' longevity and health, Okinawan centenarians have a number of variables in common.[14]

1 Enough Is Enough.

Okinawan elders have an average body mass index (BMI) that ranges from 18 to 22. The Okinawans stay lean by eating a low-calorie diet and practicing calorie control in a cultural habit known as *hara hachi bu* (eating until they are only 80 percent full) and keeping physically active every day. In contrast, middle-aged Okinawans, who have a less traditional lifestyle, have an average BMI of 26, the highest in Japan and similar to that of Americans. As discussed in Chapter 10, a BMI of 25 or greater is considered overweight and places you at greater risk for chronic diseases, especially heart disease and stroke.

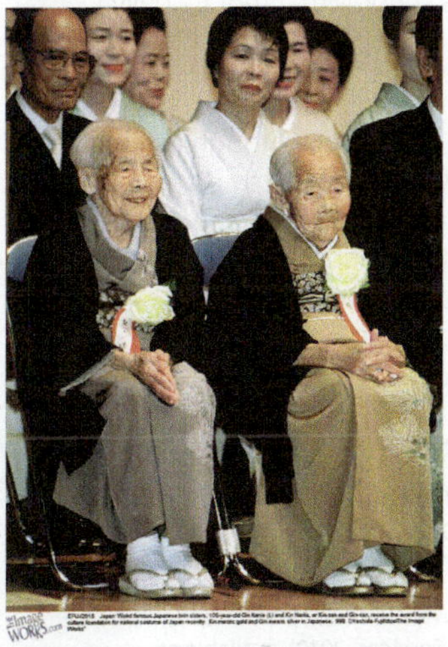

Yoshida-Fujifotos/The Image Works

Okinawan twin sisters—Gin Kanie and Kin Narita at age 106—celebrate with family and friends. Okinawan centenarians maintain optimistic attitudes and strong social bonds throughout their lives.

2 Moderation and a Healthy Lifestyle Are Key Cultural Values.

Okinawan elders never smoke. They consume a diet that is 80 percent plant-based and naturally high in unrefined whole grains, soy, vegetables, and fruits—all of which are rich in antioxidants and phytochemicals. They consume higher intakes of good fats from fish, nuts, and vegetable oils, and they have rather low amounts of less healthy fats in their diet. They keep active every day throughout their lives with a variety of activities, such as gardening, traditional dance, and martial arts. In fact, many of those studied still participated in competitive games and karate past the age of 100!

Even though these concepts may seem rather simple, the average American is not following suit. With high stress, sedentary lifestyles, and diets high in saturated fats and low in protective nutrients such as antioxidants, it seems that the American way of life is the opposite of the Okinawan path. It might be hard to drastically change your entire lifestyle to follow that of the Okinawans; however, making some dietary changes would be a good place to start. Who knows, maybe you, too, can live to be a centenarian! Here is a general overview of the Okinawan elders' way of eating:

- They eat about 500 calories less per day than Americans.
- They eat plenty of whole grains, seven servings (3.5 cups) of vegetables, and about four servings (2 cups) of fruits a day.
- They eat seaweed, coldwater fish, and other seafood choices at least three times a week.
- They include soy foods in their daily diet, and consume poultry, eggs, pork, beef, and other meats in moderation.
- They drink plenty of water and tea, and drink alcohol in moderation.
- They consume very few sweets.

3 Psychological and Spiritual Health Matters.

Okinawans put family first. They keep socially engaged, maintaining strong bonds with friends and family. They have an easygoing approach to life. Centenarians score high on optimistic attitudes and adaptability. They possess a strong sense of purpose, which translates roughly to "that which makes one's life worth living."

United States Department of Health & Human Services

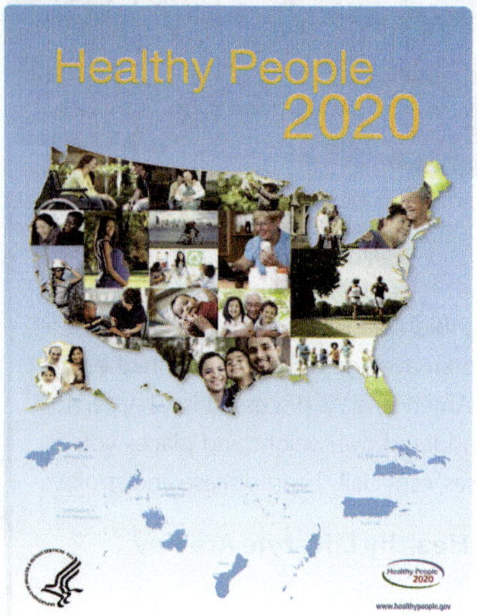

United States Department of Health & Human Services

disease, by eliminating health disparities, by creating social and physical environments that promote good health, and by promoting healthy behaviors across the life span. Table 1-5 lists the nutrition-related objectives considered to be top health priorities for the present decade.

TABLE 1-5 ***Healthy People 2020*** **Nutrition-Related Objectives for the Nation**[a]

Nutrition and Weight Status Objectives

- Increase the proportion of adults who are at a healthy weight.
- Reduce the proportion of adults who are obese.
- Reduce the proportion of children and adolescents who are overweight or obese.
- Increase the contribution of fruits to the diets of the population aged 2 years and older.[b]
- Increase the contribution of total vegetables to the diets of the population aged 2 years and older.[b]
- Increase the contribution of dark green vegetables, orange vegetables, and legumes to the diets of the population aged 2 years and older.[b]
- Increase the contribution of whole grains to the diets of the population aged 2 years and older.[b]
- Reduce consumption of calories from solid fats and added sugars in the population aged 2 years and older.[b]
- Reduce consumption of saturated fat in the population aged 2 years and older.[c]
- Reduce consumption of sodium in the population aged 2 years and older.[c]
- Increase consumption of calcium in the population aged 2 years and older.[c]
- Reduce iron deficiency among young children, females of childbearing age, and pregnant women.
- Reduce household food insecurity and in so doing reduce hunger.
- Increase the number of states that have state-level policies that incentivize food retail outlets to provide foods that are encouraged by the *Dietary Guidelines for Americans*.
- Increase the number of states with nutrition standards for foods and beverages provided to preschool-aged children in child care.
- Increase the proportion of schools that offer nutritious foods and beverages outside of school meals.
- Increase the proportion of physicians who regularly measure the body mass index of their patients.
- Increase the proportion of physician office visits that include counseling or education related to weight reduction, nutrition, or physical activity.
- Increase the proportion of worksites that offer nutrition or weight management classes or counseling.

Physical Activity Objectives

- Reduce the proportion of adults who engage in no leisure-time physical activity.
- Increase the proportion of adults who meet the objectives for aerobic physical activity and for muscle-strengthening activity.
- Increase the proportion of the nation's public and private schools that require daily physical education for all students.

Food Safety Objectives[d]

- Reduce infections caused by key pathogens transmitted commonly through food.
- Reduce severe allergic reactions to food among adults with a food allergy diagnosis.
- Increase the proportion of consumers who practice four essential food safety behaviors when handling food: washing hands, avoiding cross-contamination, cooking foods thoroughly, and chilling foods promptly.
- Improve food safety practices associated with foodborne illness in food service and retail establishments.

[a] The complete list of *Healthy People 2020* objectives may be viewed online at www.healthypeople.gov.
[b] See Table 2-4 and Figure 2-12 for specific recommendations.
[c] Recommendations: < 10% of calories from saturated fat; 2,300 mg or less of sodium and 1,300 mg of calcium for children (ages 9 to 18); 1,000 mg of calcium for adults (ages 19 to 50); and 1,200 mg of calcium for adults over 50.
[d] See Chapter 13 for more on the topic of food safety.

SOURCE: U.S. Department of Health and Human Services, Office of Disease Prevention and Health Promotion, *Healthy People 2020* (Washington, DC: U.S. Department of Health and Human Services, 2010), available at www.healthypeople.gov.

SCORE Card The Longevity Game (Obj. 1.4)

You cannot look into a crystal ball to find out how long you will live—but you can get a rough idea of the number of years you're likely to live based largely on your lifestyle today as well as certain givens, such as your family history. To do so, play the Longevity Game.

Start at the top line: age 78.8, the average life expectancy for adults in the United States today. For each of the 11 lifestyle areas, add or subtract years as instructed. If an area doesn't apply to you, go on to the next one. If you are not sure of the exact number to add or subtract, make a guess. Don't take the score too seriously, but do pay attention to those areas in which you lose years; they could point to habits you might want to change.

START WITH	**78.8**
1. Exercise	______
2. Relaxation	______
3. Driving	______
4. Blood pressure	______
5. 65 and working	______
6. Family history	______
7. Smoking	______
8. Drinking	______
9. Gender	______
10. Weight	______
11. Age	______
12. Seat belts	______
YOUR FINAL SCORE:	

1. Exercise. If you work out on a daily basis, add 3 years. If you don't get much exercise at home, on the job, or at play, subtract 3 years.
2. Relaxation. If you have a laid-back approach to life (you roll with the punches), add 1 year. If you're aggressive, hard-driving, or anxious (suffer from sleepless nights, bite your nails, etc.), subtract 1 year. If you consider yourself unhappy, subtract another year.
3. Driving. Drivers involved in an accident or violation in the past 3 years should subtract 2 years. If you have been convicted of driving while intoxicated (DWI), subtract 5 years. If your record is free of accidents and violations over the last 2 years, add 1 year.
4. Blood pressure. Although high blood pressure is a major risk factor for common conditions (heart attacks and strokes), it can be lowered effectively through changes in lifestyle and/or medication. The problem is that rises in blood pressure cannot be felt, so many people don't know they have high blood pressure and therefore never receive treatment. If your blood pressure is checked regularly with a normal reading, add 3 years. If you have high blood pressure, subtract 3.
5. 65 and working. If you are at the traditional retirement age or older and still working, add 2 years.
6. Family history. If any grandparent has reached age 85, add 2 years; if all grandparents have reached age 80, add 4. If a parent or sibling suffered from or died of a stroke or heart attack before age 50, subtract 3.
7. Smoking. Cigarette smokers who finish more than two packs a day, subtract 8; one or two packs a day, subtract 6; one-half to one pack, subtract 3.
8. Drinking. If you drink three cocktails (or beers or glasses of wine) a day, subtract 1 year.
9. Gender. Women live longer than men. Females add 3 years; males subtract 3 years.
10. Weight. If you generally follow a healthy diet, you will probably remain healthy longer, entitling you to add 2 years.
11. Age. How long you have already lived can help predict how much longer you'll survive. If you're under 30, the jury is still out. But if your age is 30 to 39, add 2 years; 40 to 49, add 3 years; 50 to 69, add 4 years; 70 or over, add 5 years.
12. Seat belts. Do you always buckle up, even if it's a short trip? If you use a seat belt, add 1 year. If you don't, subtract 1 year.

SOURCE: Based on "The Longevity Game," by Northwestern Mutual Life Insurance Company.

NOTE: The Longevity Game uses statistics from the U.S. Decennial Life Tables 1999 to 2001, U.S. Centers for Disease Control and Prevention (CDC). The outcome may not provide accurate results for individuals with chronic illnesses and conditions.

The goals of the *Healthy People 2020* nutrition topic area promote health and reduce chronic disease risk through the consumption of healthy diets and achievement and maintenance of healthy body weights. Several *Healthy People 2020* objectives focus on risk reduction and specify targets for the intake of nutrients such as

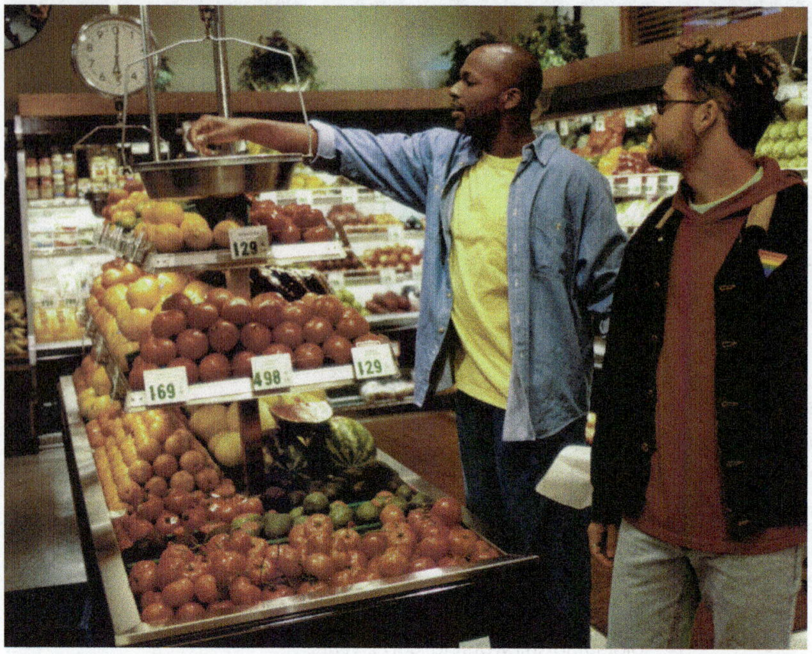

Doug Menuez/Forrester Images/Getty Images

Numerous factors influence your food choices. Examining your health beliefs, priorities, food preferences and attitudes can help you understand why you select the foods you do.

sodium and calcium and of foods such as fruits, vegetables, and whole-grain products. Other risk-reduction objectives set targets to reduce the prevalence of obesity, to reduce consumption of calories from solid fats and added sugars, to increase the proportion of schools that do not sell or offer calorically sweetened beverages to students, and to reduce the proportion of people who engage in no leisure-time physical activity. Each *Healthy People* objective has a target for specific improvements to be achieved by the year 2020.

How are Americans doing in terms of meeting the Healthy People objectives? About half of all American adults—117 million people—suffer from one or more preventable diseases related to poor-quality **eating patterns** and physical inactivity, and more than two-thirds of adults and nearly one-third of children and adolescents are overweight or obese.[15] On average, the U.S. diet is low in vegetables, fruit, and whole grains, and is high in sodium, calories, unhealthy types of fat, and added sugars.[16] About one-third of adults engage in no leisure-time physical activity.

The *Healthy People 2020* objectives represent some of the priorities for maintaining good health. Much of the practical information presented later in this chapter and in those that follow is aimed at guiding you toward developing eating and lifestyle habits that will help you achieve these goals.

1.5 Understanding Our Food Choices

The choices you make about what to eat can have a profound impact on your health, both now and in your later years. Healthy eaters resist disease and other stresses better than people with poor dietary habits and are more likely to enjoy an active, vigorous lifestyle for a greater number of years. Even so, the nutritional profile of various foods ranks as only one of many factors that influence your eating habits (see Table 1-6). Whether or not you realize it, each time you sit down to a meal, you bring to the table such factors as your own personal preferences, cultural traditions, and economic considerations. These influences exert as great an impact on your eating habits as do **hunger**—the physiological need for food—and **appetite**—the psychological desire for food, which may be stimulated in response to the sight, smell, or thought of

eating pattern The combination of foods and beverages that constitute an individual's complete dietary intake over time; may describe a usual way of eating or a combination of foods recommended for consumption.

hunger The physiological need for food.

appetite The psychological desire to eat, which is often but not always accompanied by hunger.

TABLE 1-6 Many Factors Influence Personal Food Choices

- Hunger, appetite, and food habits
- Nutritional knowledge, health beliefs/concerns, and practices
- Availability, convenience, and economy
- Advertising and the media
- Early experiences, social interactions, and cultural traditions
- Personal preference, taste, and psychological needs
- Values, such as political views, environmental concerns, and religious beliefs

food even when you're not hungry. The following sections examine some of the most influential factors in making food choices.

Availability Our diets are limited by the types and amounts of food available through the food supply, which in turn are influenced by many forces. Because we have the geographic area, climate, soil conditions, labor, and capital necessary to maintain a large agricultural industry, Americans enjoy what is arguably the most abundant food supply in the world. In addition, unlike many other less wealthy countries, the United States and Canada have the resources needed to import and distribute a wide variety of foods from other countries—everything from kiwi from New Zealand to mangoes from the tropics.

History has shown, however, that when it comes to health, an abundant food supply can be a double-edged sword. Access to many types of foods allows people to choose high-calorie diets, which can contribute to obesity and increased risk for heart disease and other problems. That's one of the reasons why degenerative diseases are sometimes referred to as *diseases of affluence*.

Income, Food Prices, and Convenience As most college students know firsthand, the amount of money available to spend on food can mean the difference between ordering pizza every night and resigning yourself to a steady diet of peanut butter and jelly sandwiches. Extremely low incomes can make it difficult for people to buy enough food to meet their minimum nutritional needs, thereby putting them at risk of **undernutrition**.

We know that a balanced diet of nutritious foods is associated with reduced risk of chronic diseases and death, particularly from heart disease and cancer. One reason people may not choose nutritious foods over foods that are low in nutrients is cost. If you are like most Americans, you think it's "more expensive" to eat healthy foods like fruits and vegetables. But is the cost of a healthy diet really significantly higher than the standard American diet of "convenience" foods, snacks, bakery items, soft drinks, and other less nutritious foods? Compare the cost of convenience foods with the same foods made from scratch (most convenience foods cost more).

A consumer's *perception* of the cost of various foods can also play a role in his or her choices. For example, two barriers that prevent people from adopting healthy eating habits are the beliefs that it would be too expensive and inconvenient. Table 1-7 lists the most frequently cited roadblocks to healthy eating.[17] In fact, 40 percent of consumers who answered one survey said that fruits, vegetables, seafood, and other elements of a nutrient-rich diet would strain their budgets. In reality, some research has shown that switching from a high-fat diet to one that is lower in fat can *reduce* food costs.[18] When measured on the basis of weight or average portion size, grains, vegetables, fruit, and dairy foods are less expensive than most protein foods and foods high in saturated fat, added sugars, and/or sodium. In other words, with healthy foods, you get fewer calories but more nutrients per dollar.[19] Just cutting back on the amount of meat and poultry—the source of much of the fat in the American diet and the category in which many of our food dollars are spent—goes a long way in trimming food budgets. See the accompanying Box, "You *Can* Afford to Eat Nutritious Foods—Tips for Supermarketing," for more smart food shopping tips.

Research has found that not only is a diet of nutritious foods less costly, but it also promotes weight loss.[20] In one study, overweight children and their parents were encouraged to consume more "nutrient-dense" foods like fruits and vegetables (high in nutrients and low in fat and calories) and less "empty-calorie" foods (low in nutrients and high in fat and/or calories). After one year, food costs decreased, and the children and parents were 5 to 8 percent less overweight than they were at the beginning of the study![21]

TABLE 1-7 Perceived Barriers to Healthy Eating

- Healthy foods are not always available from fast-food and take-out restaurants.
- It costs more to eat healthy foods.
- I'm too busy to take the time to eat healthfully.
- I hear too much conflicting information about which foods are good for me and which foods are not.
- I don't want to give up the foods I like.
- Healthy foods don't taste as good.
- The people I usually eat with do not eat healthy foods.

undernutrition Severe underconsumption of calories or nutrients, leading to disease or increased susceptibility to disease; a form of malnutrition.

THE SAVVY Diner

1.6 You *Can* Afford to Eat Nutritious Foods—Tips for Supermarketing

Want to save money and consume a more nutritious diet? Nutritious eating starts with healthy food shopping. With preparation and some label-reading skills, you can leave the grocery store with a supply of healthy basics like these:

- Fat-free or low-fat milk, yogurt, cheeses, and cottage cheese
- Light or reduced-fat margarines; olive oil
- Eggs/egg substitutes
- Whole-grain breads, bagels, and English muffins
- Low-fat flour tortillas, soft corn tortillas
- Plain cereals (dry or cooked)
- Whole-grain rice and pasta (remember, it's what you put on these grain products that increases the fat/calorie content)
- Fresh, frozen, or canned fruits packed in juice
- Fresh, frozen, or canned vegetables
- Dried or canned beans and peas
- Skinless, white-meat chicken or turkey; frozen veggie burgers
- Fish and shellfish (not battered and fried)
- Beef: round, sirloin, chuck, loin, and extra lean ground beef
- Pork: leg, shoulder, tenderloin
- Low-fat or nonfat salad dressings, salsa, herbs, and spices
- Nuts and seeds (unsalted, raw, or dry-roasted varieties)
- Whole-grain crackers, unsalted popcorn[22]

The next time you shop for groceries, keep in mind these smart shopping tips:

1. Buy local foods and fresh foods in season. Use the local newspaper to find the best seasonal buys and special sale items.
2. Shop from a list to help avoid buying unnecessary items. Keep a running list in your kitchen, and note items that you need to replace.
3. Read the ingredients list and Nutrition Facts label on packaged foods; compare amounts of fat, sodium, calories, and nutrients in similar products. Ingredients are listed in order of quantity.
4. Use "sell by" and "best if used by" dates to ensure quality and freshness. Buy only the amount you or your family will eat before the food spoils.
5. Shop the perimeter of the grocery store to find many fresh whole foods: fresh produce; low-fat dairy products; lean meats, poultry, and fish; and whole-grain breads. Maneuver down the aisles only for specific items on your list, such as canned tomato products, spices, and canned or dry beans.[23]

Advertising and the Media Television and radio commercials, as well as magazine and newspaper ads and the Internet, play an extremely powerful role in influencing our food choices and our knowledge of nutrition. Additionally, in a recent consumer survey, some 78 percent of shoppers report interest in reading nutrition labels.[24] Given today's health-conscious environment, food manufacturers promote the nutritional merits of their products more than ever before.

Unfortunately, advertising is not always created with the consumers' best interests in mind. Much of the food advertising that we're exposed to, from the earliest ages, is aimed at selling products that aren't the optimal choices for regular inclusion in a healthy diet.[25] For example, the great majority of television commercials geared toward children and aired on Saturday mornings promote high-fat, sugary foods, such as candy and sugar-coated cereals.[26] In fact, the food industry spends more than $11 billion overall for food, beverage, and fast-food advertising. This amount dwarfs the almost $5 million spent by the government in its campaign to encourage people of all ages to increase their consumption of fruits and vegetables.[27] As a result, commercials promoting good nutrition are relatively few and far between.

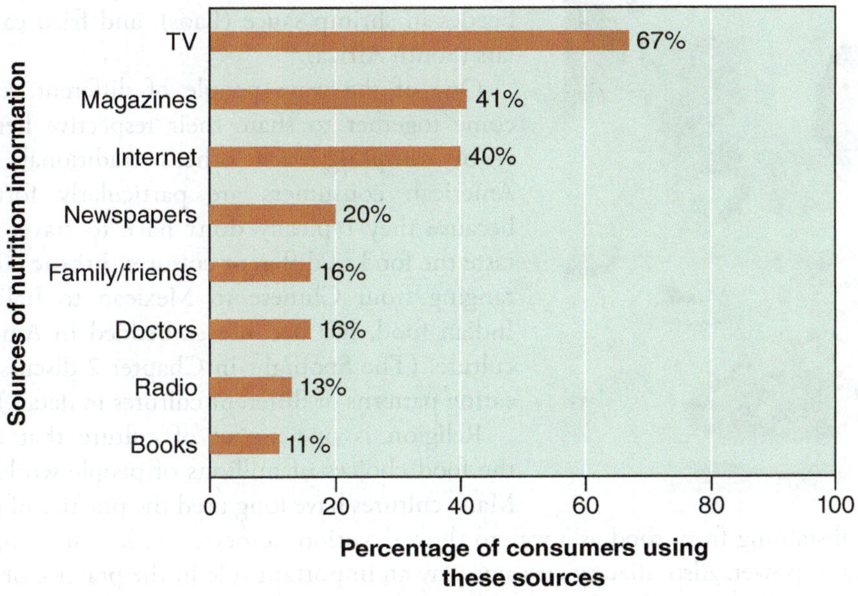

FIGURE 1-5

Consumer Sources of Nutrition Information*

*NOTE: Consumers could cite more than one source.

SOURCE: Based on the Academy of Nutrition and Dietetics, *Nutrition and You: Trends 2011*, Academy of Nutrition and Dietetics, 2011.

Along with advertising, the media rank among the most influential sources of diet and nutrition information, which in turn affects our food choices. Consider that most Americans look first to television as a source of nutrition information; then to magazines, the Internet, newspapers, doctors, family or friends, radio; and finally to books (see Figure 1-5).[28] Unfortunately, the reliability of the information delivered by the media varies considerably. The Spotlight at the end of this chapter will help you learn how to evaluate the nutrition information you receive via the media.

Social and Cultural Factors

People's social and cultural groups have a significant impact on their food choices. **Social groups** such as families, friends, and coworkers tend to exert the most influence. The family, particularly the wife/mother, plays one of the most powerful roles in determining our food choices. That makes sense, because the family is the first social group people encounter, as well as the one to which they typically belong for the longest period of time. The values, attitudes, and traditions of our family can have a lasting effect on our food choices. Think of the holiday food traditions in your own family. Treasured recipes or rituals surrounding holiday meals are often passed from one generation to the next.

Friends, coworkers, and members of other social networks also influence our food choices and eating behavior. For instance, many weight-loss programs feature group sessions made up of people who are in the same boat. Thus, they can support one another in their efforts to lose weight. Social pressure can also push us to eat meals we might not choose on our own. For example, if you are a guest in another country or in a friend's home, choosing not to partake of the food and drink that's offered might be considered rude. By the same token, it's natural to join your friends on a spontaneous trip for ice cream or pizza even when you're not hungry.

Culture also determines our food choices, to a large extent. Many of our eating habits arise from the traditions, belief systems, technologies, values, and norms of the culture in which we live. For example, in the United States and Canada, the idea of eating insects is generally considered repulsive. However, many people throughout the rest of the world relish dishes prepared with various bugs, including locust dumplings

social group A group of people, such as a family, who depend on one another and share a set of norms, beliefs, values, and behaviors.

culture Knowledge, beliefs, customs, laws, morals, art, and literature acquired by members of a society and passed along to succeeding generations.

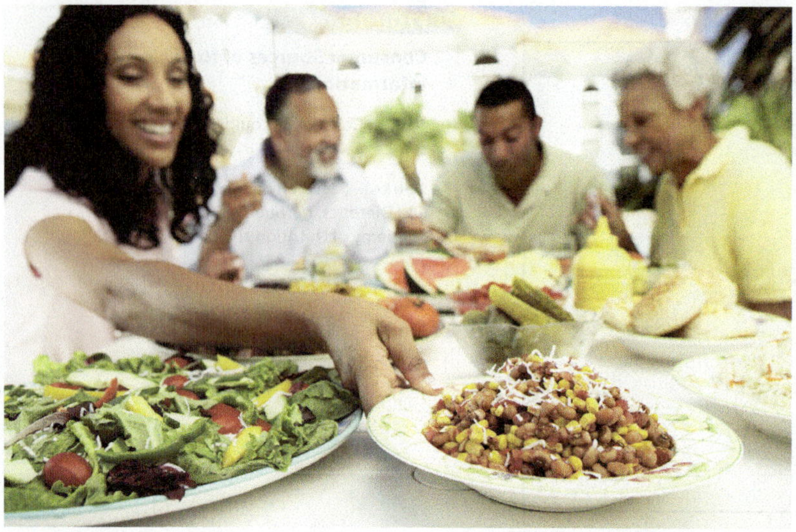

Monkey Business Images/Shutterstock.com

The act of eating is complex. We derive many benefits—both physical and emotional—when we eat foods.

(northern Africa), red-ant chutney (India), water beetles in shrimp sauce (Laos), and fried caterpillars (South Africa).[29]

One of the ways people of different cultures come together to share their respective heritages is by sampling each other's traditional foods. American consumers are particularly fortunate because they typically don't have to travel far to taste the food of different cultures. **Ethnic cuisine**, ranging from Chinese to Mexican to Italian to Indian food, has become embedded in American culture. (The Spotlight in Chapter 2 discusses the eating patterns of different cultures in detail.)

Religion is one aspect of culture that affects the food choices of millions of people worldwide. Many cultures have long used the practice of giving and abstaining from food as a way to show devotion, respect, and love to a supreme being or power. Also, dietary customs play an important role in the practice of many of the world's major religions. As Table 1-8 shows, many religions specify which foods their followers may eat and how those foods must be prepared.

Personal Values or Beliefs

Some people adopt a certain way of eating or making food choices based on a larger worldview. For instance, many environmentally conscious people, believing that raising animals for human consumption strains the world's supply of land and water, choose to abstain from meat as

ethnic cuisine The traditional foods eaten by the people of a particular culture.

TABLE 1-8 Dietary Practices of Selected Religious Groups

Religious Group	Dietary Practices
Buddhist	Dietary customs vary depending on sect. Many are lacto-ovovegetarians, because of restrictions on taking a life. Some eat fish, and most eat no beef or poultry. Monks fast at certain times of the month and avoid eating solid food after the noon hour.
Hindu	All foods thought to interfere with physical and spiritual development are avoided. Many are lacto-vegetarians and/or avoid alcohol. The cow is considered sacred—an animal dear to the Lord Krishna. Beef is never consumed, and often pork is avoided.
Jewish	*Kashrut* is the body of Jewish law dealing with foods. The purpose of following the complex dietary laws is to conform to the Divine Will as expressed in the Torah. The term *kosher* denotes all foods that are permitted for consumption. To "keep kosher" means to follow dietary laws in the home. A lengthy list of prohibited foods, called *treyf*, includes pork and shellfish. The laws define how birds and mammals must be slaughtered, how foods must be prepared, and when they may be consumed. For example, dairy foods and meat products cannot be eaten at the same meal. During Passover, special laws are observed, such as the elimination of any foods that can be leavened.
Mormon	Alcoholic beverages and hot drinks (coffee, tea) are avoided. Many also avoid beverages containing caffeine. Mormons are encouraged to limit meat intake and emphasize grains in the diet. Mormons fast on the first Sunday of every month.
Muslim	Overeating is discouraged, and consuming only two-thirds of capacity is suggested. Dietary laws are called *halal*. Prohibited foods are called *haram*, and they include pork and birds of prey. Laws define how animals must be slaughtered. Alcoholic drinks are not allowed. Fasting is required from sunup to sundown during the month of Ramadan.
Roman Catholic	Meat is not consumed on Fridays during Lent (40 days before Easter). No food or beverages (except water) are to be consumed 1 hour before taking communion.
Seventh-Day Adventist	Most are lacto-ovovegetarians. If meat is consumed, pork is avoided. Tea, coffee, and alcoholic beverages are not allowed. Water is not consumed with meals, but is drunk before and after meals. Followers refrain from using seasonings and condiments. Overeating and snacking are discouraged.

SOURCE: From M. Boyle, *Community Nutrition in Action: An Entrepreneurial Approach*, 7th ed. (Boston, MA: Cengage Learning, 2017), 613. © 2017.

much as possible in an effort to preserve Earth's resources. Others may choose to boycott certain manufacturers' items for political reasons, perhaps because they disagree with a company's advertising practices.

Today, many people make food choices based on sustainability issues, animal welfare concerns, and the benefits of purchasing locally produced, seasonally available, and organically grown food.[30] *Sustainability* in the food system is defined as a society's ability to shape its economic and social systems to maintain both natural resources and human life, and it involves building locally based, self-reliant food systems.[31] When consumers purchase foods that have been produced locally, a greater proportion of the profits remains with local farmers, providing them with a livable income while supporting local economies.[32] Additionally, the purchase of locally produced foods protects the environment by reducing the use of fossil fuel (for transporting food) and packaging materials.[33]

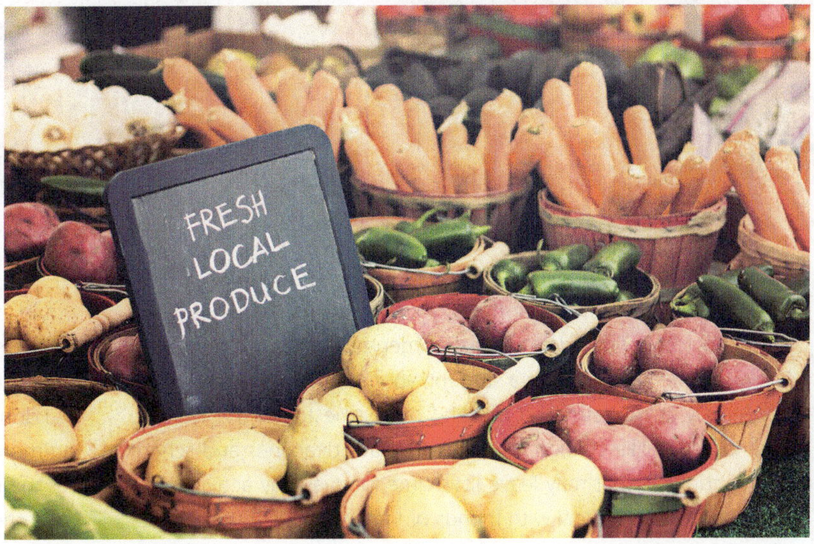

Arina P. Habich/Shutterstock.com

Visit your local farmers' market for foods that have been produced locally. See the Nutrition Action feature in Chapter 13 for more about the benefits of purchasing locally produced, seasonally available, and organically grown foods.

Other Factors That Affect Our Food Choices

One of the main reasons you choose to eat certain foods is your preference for certain tastes.[34] Just about everyone enjoys sweet foods, for example, because humans are born with an affinity for sugar.[35] In addition, we usually prefer foods that have happy associations for us: foods prepared for special occasions, those given to us by a loved one when we were children, or those eaten by an admired role model. By the same token, intense aversions to certain foods—perhaps foods you were given when you were sick or foods you were forced to eat as a child—can be strong enough to last a lifetime. Your parents may have taught you to prefer certain foods and pass up others for reasons of their own, without even being aware they were doing so.

Food habits are also intimately tied to deep psychological needs, such as an infant's association of food with a parent's love. Yearnings, cravings, and addictions with profound meaning and significance sometimes surface as food behavior. Some people respond to stress—positive or negative—by eating; others use food to fill a void, such as lack of satisfying personal relationships or fulfilling work.

The influences on people's eating habits are as many and varied as the individuals themselves. Our food choices reflect our own unique cultural legacies, philosophies, and beliefs. To think of food as nothing more than a source of nutrients would deny food's rich symbolism and meaning and take away much of the pleasure of breaking bread with friends and family. As you read this book and consider ways to improve your own eating habits, take time to reflect on your unique background and think about how you can integrate your knowledge of nutrition into your cultural heritage and philosophies.

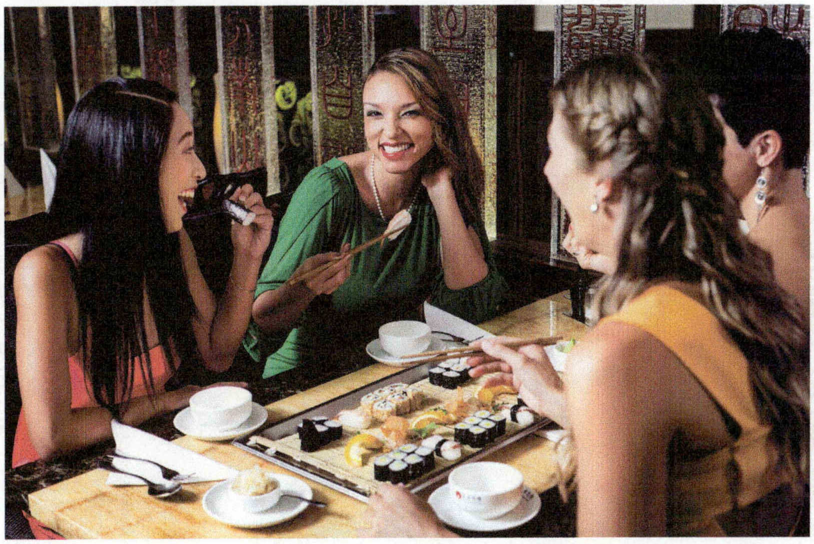

Kzenon/Shutterstock.com

Even at many American-style restaurants, you can experience other cultures by sampling from the various ethnic cuisines found on the menu. Many of the nation's public markets maintain a public space that builds upon the economic, social, and cultural assets within the surrounding communities. The markets provide an opportunity to sample the foods, crafts, and other aspects of diverse cultural groups.

Nutrition ACTION

1.7 Good and Fast—A Guide to Eating on the Run, or Has Your Waistline Been Supersized?

Contrary to popular belief, your professors do not conspire to plan due dates for assignments, quizzes, and exams on the same day. As a student, your schedule can get hectic, especially at midterm and the end of a semester. In the working world, much like college, you will also have deadlines and scheduling conflicts that may leave little time for everyday activities like sitting down to a meal with friends or family. Even if your life is not hectic, chances are you've stood in line for a burger and fries, a slice of pizza, a taco, or a muffin and coffee at least once this week. Consumers spend almost 50 percent of their food budget on restaurant meals, compared with only 25 percent in 1955.[36]

Seven out of 10 consumers say they are trying to eat healthier when dining out and to pay more attention to the nutritional content of their food choices.[37] Even though a meal eaten on the run fits easily into a busy schedule, it's not necessarily as simple to work it into the dietary guidelines recommended by major health organizations. Eating away from home is not an invitation to forget about good nutrition, eat more ("supersize"), or eat differently than you would at home.[38] Can you eat away from home and still eat healthfully? It is possible, but it takes some planning.

Fast food does not have to be an unhealthy option, as long as you don't supersize. Fast foods commonly contain more fat (including more saturated fat), less fiber, more cholesterol, and more calories than meals made at home.

Portion sizes of foods have been on the increase since the early 1970s.[39] In the 1950s, a single-serve bottle of a soft drink was 6 ounces. Today, a single-serve bottle is 20 ounces. A typical bagel purchased today is, at 4 to 7 ounces, almost twice the size bagels used to be, at 2 to 3 ounces.[40]

Along with the larger portions come more calories. Could these larger portions be contributing to the obesity epidemic in the United States? Yes! When people are served more food, they eat more.[41] Is it any coincidence, then, that as portion sizes have increased over the past two decades, the incidence of overweight and obesity among adults and children also has increased?[42] We don't think so.

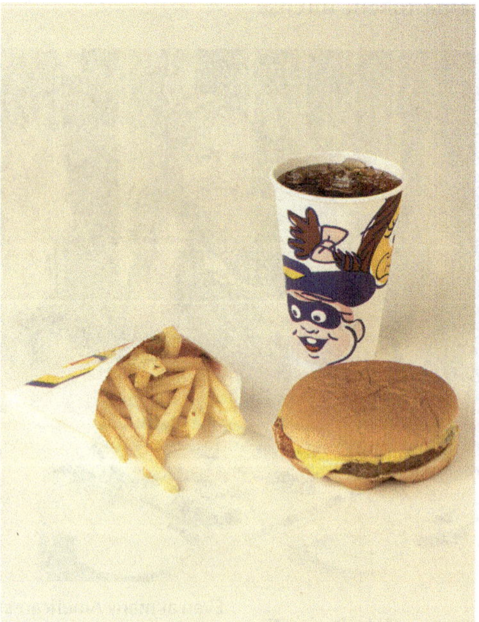

Felicia Martinez Photography/PhotoEdit

Cheeseburger
Small fries
Small soft drink
670 calories
23 g fat
7.5 g saturated fat

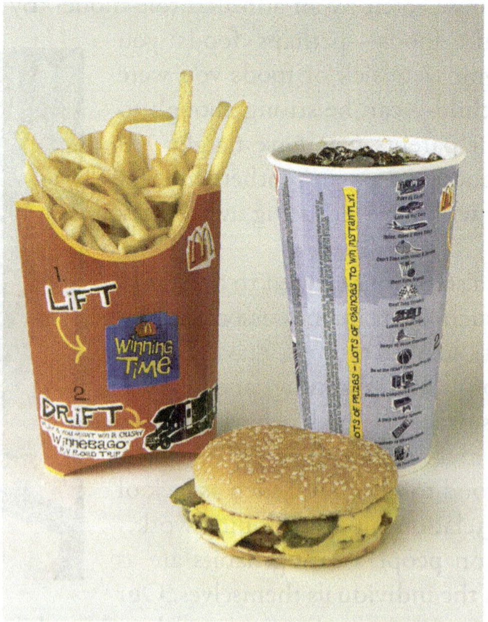

Felicia Martinez Photography/PhotoEdit

Double cheeseburger
Supersize fries
Supersize soft drink
1,220 calories
48 g fat
14.5 g saturated fat

The enlarging size of American food portions is linked to a practice used by the food industry called "value" marketing. Consumers are prompted by point-of-purchase displays and verbally by employees to spend a little extra money to "upgrade" to larger portions, leaving the customer with the feeling of "What a deal I got!"[43] For the food sellers, costs to increase portion sizes are small, but the profit margin is huge.

So, how do you, the typical harried college student, get fast meals without increasing the calories and fat in your daily diet? Remember these strategies the next time you find yourself in a time crunch and in line at the closest fast-food restaurant.

Strategy 1: Don't supersize. It's a great marketing ploy to get you to buy more, but you will also be eating more fat, cholesterol, and salt—and weighing more as a result. Think small. Stick with smaller burgers, sliced meat, or grilled chicken sandwiches with mustard, catsup, lettuce, onion, and tomatoes.

Strategy 2: Think grilled, not fried. Frying foods adds about 50 percent more fat and/or calories compared with items that have not been fried. (At Wendy's, a grilled chicken sandwich has 7 grams of fat versus 20 for a deep-fried, crispy chicken sandwich.[44]) If you cannot live without French fries, get them on occasion; but most of the time, try to substitute a salad (ask for dressing on the side) or a baked potato with low-fat toppings.

Strategy 3: Hold the mayo. Each spoonful of mayonnaise adds about 100 calories, nearly all of which are from fat. Most fast-food sandwiches contain more than just one spoonful of mayo in their toppings and special sauces. The same goes for tartar sauce. Order a fish sandwich without it, and you'll trim at least 70 fat-laden calories (the amount in just 1 tablespoon) from your meal. Ask for lots of lettuce and tomatoes and less sour cream and guacamole on your nachos and tacos. A tablespoon of either sour cream or guacamole adds about 25 calories to Mexican fare. A few extra chunks of tomato, in contrast, supply a negligible number of calories, no fat, and a good deal of vitamin C.

Strategy 4: Avoid all-you-can-eat restaurants. No explanation necessary. Remember moderation and variety.

Strategy 5: "Just say no." Did you know that a 16-ounce soft drink adds 200 calories to a meal and nothing else? A medium chocolate shake can add 350 calories to a meal, and a large shake can add 770 calories. Wash your meal down with low-fat milk instead of a milk shake, and you'll cut the fat and calorie count at least in half. Better yet, in the continuing effort to get enough fluids, drink water instead.

Strategy 6: Balance fast-food meals with other food choices during the day.[45] If you cannot avoid fast food, then adjust your portion sizes and food choices at other meals. Increasing physical activity will help counterbalance extra calories.

Strategy 7: Split your order—share with a friend. A half portion is often adequate. Or split dessert. Frequently a few bites can satisfy a sweet tooth.

Strategy 8: Bring your lunch. You'll save money and spend less time planning a healthy lunch than you would likely spend in the drive-through line. Try taking leftovers in a microwavable container. Make double batches when you cook, and put some in the freezer in single-serving containers for lunch.

Strategy 9: Choose grab-and-go foods. Keep these foods handy for a fast and nutritious snack: baby carrots, fresh fruit, dried fruit, fruit juices (not fruit drinks), low-fat yogurt, string cheese, and low-fat, unsalted popcorn.

Strategy 10: If all else fails, go for the obvious low-calorie choices. For example, Subway sells subs with 6 grams of fat or less. Don't let the word *chicken* or *fish* fool you. Many health-conscious consumers have heard the advice to choose skinless poultry and fish instead of relatively high-fat red meat—but when it comes to chicken nuggets and fish patties coated with batter and deep fried, it is a different story. Six chicken nuggets, for example, typically contain as many calories (about 300) as an entire burger. What's more, many chicken and fish sandwiches chalk up as much fat as a pint and a half of ice cream. Even rotisserie-style chicken contains a large amount of fat and calories if you don't remove the skin before eating it. When ordering a pizza, hold the sausage and pepperoni, and ask for mushrooms, green peppers, and onions instead. Pizza is an excellent source of calcium—the bone-building mineral that many Americans don't get enough of—as well as protein, carbohydrates, and a number of vitamins and minerals. Still, two slices of pepperoni pizza can easily contain 100 more calories and twice as much fat as the same amount topped with onions, green peppers, and mushrooms.

SPOTLight

1.8 How Do You Tell If It's Nutrition Fact or Nutrition Fiction?

Most people want to eat a healthy diet and lower their chances of cancer and other chronic diseases. Frequently, however, information they read or hear about healthy eating from one source is contradicted by another. It's not always easy to distinguish accurate information from misinformation. Do you know which of the following statements are true or false? Check your answers with the correct answers at the end of this section.*

1. It is difficult for busy people to eat a balanced diet.
2. People who graduate from college are smart enough not to be victimized by nutrition misinformation.
3. Sugar is a major cause of hyperactivity in children.
4. No special training is legally required for a person to offer nutrition information to the public.
5. Most health food retailers have been educated about the research done regarding the products they sell.
6. Protein and/or amino acid supplements help bodybuilders, recreational weight lifters, and other athletes improve their performance by increasing muscle size.
7. Most nutrition-related books and magazine articles undergo prepublication review by experts.
8. Cigarette smoking is the leading cause of preventable death in the United States.
9. Herbal products are as safe and effective as many drugs prescribed by physicians.
10. It is illegal for manufacturers of dietary supplements to print false information on their product labels.

You've just watched a television commercial for a vitamin supplement that is guaranteed to produce a laundry list of benefits, including fewer colds, a better complexion, and a decreased risk of cancer. Should you buy it? You've just read a magazine article with a plan for quick weight loss. Should you believe it? Someone who plays the same sport as you says that improving your diet will help your game. Where do you go for help?

We all find ourselves faced with such decisions at one time or another. It's crucial to know how to protect ourselves from nutrition misinformation. Health fraud costs consumers almost $30 billion each year, and money down the drain is just one problem stemming from misleading nutritional information. Although some fraudulent claims about nutrition are harmless and may make for a good laugh, others can be harmful. False claims about nutritional products have been known to bring about malnutrition, birth defects, mental retardation, and, in extreme cases, even death.

Negative effects due to following false nutritional claims can happen in two ways. First, the product in question may cause direct harm. Even a seemingly innocuous substance such as vitamin A can cause severe liver damage over time if taken in large enough amounts. Second, using bogus nutritional remedies can cause problems because such remedies can build false hope and might keep a consumer from obtaining sound, scientifically tested medical treatment. A person who relies on a so-called anticancer diet as a cure for the disease, for example, might forgo possible lifesaving interventions such as surgery or chemotherapy.

The following questions and answers will help you learn to evaluate the nutrition information that you see in the media. They will help you develop the skills necessary to view nutrition claims with a skeptic's eye or, at the very least, to help you decide when to find a qualified professional to help you evaluate the information. Table 1-9 lists sources of credible nutrition information.

Judging by what I've read on the Internet, it seems as though nutritionists are always changing their minds. One week the headlines say to take vitamin E to help prevent heart disease, and the next week they say that vitamin E may not, in fact, prevent the disease. Why is there so much controversy?

Part of the confusion stems from the way the media interpret findings of scientific research. A good case in point is the controversy over whether a high-fiber diet protects against colon and rectal cancers—diseases that affect some 135,000 Americans each year.

The fiber and colon cancer connection dates back to the early 1970s, when scientists observed that colon cancer was extremely uncommon in areas of the world where the diet consisted largely of unrefined foods and little meat. Researchers theorized that dietary fiber may protect against colon cancer by binding bile (a chemical substance needed in fat digestion) and speeding the passage of wastes and potentially harmful compounds through the colon. Since then, other studies have also suggested that those who eat a high-fiber diet have a lower risk of colon and rectal cancers.[46]

*Adapted from Quackwatch. Consumer Health I.Q. Test. Available at www.quackwatch.org/04ConsumerEducation/iq.html.

TABLE 1-9 Credible Nutrition Resources on the Web
www.healthfinder.gov Scroll down to myhealthfinder for online screening checkups; go to Health Topics A to Z and scroll to Everyday Healthy Living for more information on healthy lifestyles; this site offers many links to other reliable health-related sites.
www.cdc.gov/healthyliving The Centers for Disease Control and Prevention (CDC) website provides links for healthy living topics.
www.cdc.gov/nutrition/index.html The Centers for Disease Control and Prevention (CDC) maintains a nutrition home page that includes many links.
www.eatright.org/Public The Academy of Nutrition and Dietetics home page includes many nutrition resources and links. Search the Food menu for tips on eating out, food shopping, and other topics.
www.fruitsandveggiesmorematters.org This site provides healthy resources and encourages fruit and vegetable consumption.
www.hc-sc.gc.ca A Canadian health and nutrition information home page.
www.healthypeople.gov Provides updates on the *Healthy People 2020* initiative.
www.nutrition.gov This resource provided by the United States Department of Agriculture (USDA) provides easy access to all online government information on nutrition and dietary guidance.
http://fnic.nal.usda.gov The Food and Nutrition Information Center (FNIC) provides credible, accurate, and practical information about nutrition and health. Click on Dietary Guidance and then scroll down to Fraud and Nutrition Misinformation.
http://publications.usa.gov This resource developed by the Federal Citizen Information Center (FCIC) provides access to consumer issues including food and health information.
www.health.nih.gov A search engine from the National Institutes of Health (NIH) with access to health information; many database links are available, such as PubMed and clinical trials.
www.nlm.nih.gov/medlineplus/healthfraud.html This government site provides health fraud resources including how to report fraud cases.
http://ndb.nal.usda.gov Click on "Start your search here" for free food analyses. Just type in the food you want to analyze, and get a breakdown of its calories, fat, fiber, protein, vitamins, and minerals.
www.health.gov This website sponsored by the U.S. Department of Health and Human Services (HHS) is a portal to websites of a number of multi-agency government health initiatives pertaining to health and nutrition.

However, a flurry of headlines later threatened to pull the pedestal out from under the popular fiber theory, asking, "Fiber: Is It Still the Right Choice?" A Harvard-based study published in the *New England Journal of Medicine*, one of the most prestigious medical journals, suggested that fiber did nothing to prevent cancer.[47] The 16-year trial of almost 90,000 nurses—called the Nurses' Health Study—found that nurses who ate low-fiber diets (less than 10 grams daily) were no more likely to develop colon cancer than those eating higher levels of fiber (about 25 grams daily). As a result, the researchers concluded that the study provided no support for the theory that fiber could reduce risk of colon cancer.

The news was surprising and reinforces the need for research studies to be duplicated. All studies have some limitations, and a number of questions can be raised regarding conclusions of the Nurses' Health Study. For example, the study relied on participants to recall their eating habits accurately.

Is this type of self-reported dietary information reliable? Back in 1980, the nurses were asked for information about their intakes of "dark" breads. However, food labels at that time did not list the fiber content of breads, and some wheat breads on the shelf had amounts of fiber similar to those found in white bread. Did the nurses mistakenly consider "dark" bread to be the same as 100 percent whole-wheat bread?

Another question is, "What are the optimal levels of fiber intake for colon cancer protection?" Some experts believe it may take more than 25 grams of fiber a day to show cancer-protective effects, which might explain the lack of effect noted in the Nurses' Health Study.

This fiber story illustrates how news reports based on only one study can leave the public with the impression that scientists cannot make up their minds. It seems as if one week scientists are saying fiber is good, and the next week the word is that fiber doesn't do any good at all. The truth is that health experts and major health organizations continue to urge adults to get about 28 grams of fiber a day. (The average fiber intake today is about 16 grams.)

Contrary to what some headlines imply, reputable scientists do not base their dietary recommendations for the public on findings of one or two studies. Scientists are still conducting research to determine whether fiber does in fact help prevent colon cancer, and, if so, what types of fiber and in what amount. Scientists design their research to test theories, such as the notion that eating a high-fiber diet is associated with lower risk of cancer. Other factors, however, often complicate the matter at hand. The study of fiber and colon cancer is complicated by many other factors linked with colon cancer development, including inactivity, obesity, saturated fat intake, low calcium or folate intakes, and others.

So, should you hang on to your high-fiber cereals and vegetables? Yes, according to the American Institute for Cancer Research. Its analysis of more than 7,000 research studies provides evidence that increased intake of fiber may be associated with decreased incidence of colon cancer.[48] Most important, however, the health benefits of fruits, vegetables, legumes, and whole grains go beyond possible protection from colon cancer.[49] Diets rich in fiber from these foods are also strongly associated with reduced risks of heart disease, high blood pressure, type 2 diabetes, and diverticular disease, a condition that can lead to painful inflammation of the large intestine. Fiber also promotes a feeling of fullness after you eat, which can help with weight control.

How can I tell if a nutrition news story is noteworthy and a source of credible nutrition information?

You can critique nutrition news you read by asking a series of questions. Consider the following points as a checklist for separating the bogus news stories from those worth your attention:

- Where is the study published? The study described in the news story should have been published in a journal that uses experts in the field to review research results (called *peer review*). These reviewers can point out flaws in research design and may challenge researchers' conclusions before the study is published.
- How recent is the study? Be sure that the report is about recent research. The science of nutrition continues to develop from the results of new studies that employ state-of-the-art methods and technology, and benefits from the scrutiny of experts current in the particular field of study.
- What research methods were used to obtain the data? Are the reported results from an **epidemiological study** or an **intervention study**? Epidemiological studies examine populations to determine food patterns and health status over time. These population studies are useful in uncovering **correlations** between two factors (for example, whether a high calcium intake early in life reduces the incidence of bone fractures later in life). However, they are not considered as conclusive as intervention studies. A correlation between two factors may *suggest* a cause-and-effect relationship between the factors, but it *does not prove* a causal relationship.

  Intervention studies examine the effects of a specific treatment or intervention on a particular group of subjects and compare the results to those of a similar group of people not receiving the treatment. An example is a cholesterol-monitoring study in which half of the subjects follow dietary advice to lower their blood cholesterol and half do not. Ideally, intervention studies should be randomized and controlled—that is, subjects are assigned to either an experimental group or a control group using a random selection process. Each subject has an equal chance of being assigned to either group. The **experimental group** receives the "treatment" being tested; the **control group** receives a **placebo** or neutral substance. If possible, neither the researcher nor the participants should know which subjects have been assigned to which group until the end of the experiment. A randomized, controlled study helps ensure that the results were actually due to the treatment, and it minimizes chances that the results are due to a placebo effect or bias on the part of the researcher.
- What was the size of the study? To achieve *validity*—accuracy in results—studies generally must include a sufficiently large number of people (for example, intervention studies of 50 or more people). This reduces the chances that the results are simply a coincidence and helps researchers generalize the conclusions of the study to a wider population.
- Who were the subjects? Was the study done with animals or humans? Look for similarities between the subjects in the study and yourself. The more you have in common with the participants (age, diet pattern, gender, and so forth), the more pertinent the study results may be for you.
- Does a consensus of published studies support the results reported in the news? Even if an experiment is carefully designed and carried out perfectly, its findings cannot be considered definitive until they have been confirmed by other research. Testing and retesting reduce the possibility that the outcome was simply the result of chance, error, or oversight on the part of the experimenter.

When making dietary recommendations for the public, experts pool the results of different types of studies, such as analyses of food patterns of groups of people and carefully controlled studies on people in hospitals or clinics. Before drawing any conclusions, they then consider the evidence from all the research. The bottom line is that if you read a report on the Internet or watch one on television that advises making a dramatic change in your diet based on the results of one study, don't take it to heart. The findings may make for a good story, but they're not worth taking too seriously.

Why doesn't the government do something to prevent the media from delivering misleading nutrition information?

The **First Amendment** guarantees freedom of the press. Accordingly, people may express whatever views they like in the media, whether sound, unsound, or even dangerous. This freedom is a cornerstone of the U.S. Constitution and to deny it would be to deny democracy. By law, writers cannot be punished for publishing misinformation unless it can be proven in court that the information has caused a reader bodily harm.

Fortunately, most professional health groups maintain committees to combat the spread of health and nutrition misinformation. For more information on separating nutrition fact from nutrition fiction, visit these websites:

- **www.fda.gov/ForConsumers/ProtectYourself/HealthFraud/default.htm**
- **www.nlm.nih.gov/medlineplus/healthfraud.html**

Is the Internet a reliable source of nutrition and health information?

Information is rampant on the Internet.[50] In a sense, the Internet is information, and the information is continually being revised and *created.* Internet information exists in many forms (facts, statistics, stories, opinions), is created for many purposes (to entertain, to inform, to persuade, to sell, to influence), and varies in quality from good to bad.

The information you find on the Internet is only as good as its source. One method for determining whether information is reliable and of good quality is the CARS checklist. The acronym *CARS* stands for *credibility, accuracy, reasonableness,* and *support.*[51]

- ***Credibility.*** Check credentials of the author (if it lists one!) or sponsoring organization. Is the author or organization respected and well known as a source of sound, *scientific* information? Evidence of a lack of credibility includes no posted author and even the presence of misspelled words or bad grammar. Websites should be from credible web addresses ending in .edu (an educational institution), .gov (government agency), or .org (nonprofit). Use caution on websites that end in .com (commercial) or .net (networks).

- ***Accuracy.*** Check to ensure the information is current, factual, and comprehensive. If important facts, consequences, or other information is missing, the website may not be presenting a complete story. Evidence of a lack of accuracy includes no date on the document, the use of sweeping generalizations, and the presence of outdated information. How often is the site updated? Reliable sites are updated regularly and post those dates on the site. Watch out for testimonials masquerading as scientific evidence—a common method for promoting questionable products on the Internet.
- ***Reasonableness.*** Evaluate the information for fairness, balance, and consistency. Does the author present a fair, balanced argument supporting his or her ideas? Are the author's arguments rational? Has he or she maintained objectivity in discussing the topic? Does the author have an obvious—or somewhat hidden—conflict of interest? Evidence of a lack of reasonableness includes gross generalizations ("Foods not grown organically are all toxic and shouldn't be eaten") and outlandish claims ("Kombucha tea will cure cancer and diabetes").
- ***Support.*** Check to see whether supporting documentation is cited for scientific statements. Does the website refer to legitimate scientific publications? Is the source of information clearly presented? An Internet document that fails to show its sources is suspect.

How can I tell whether a product is bogus?

It's not always easy. Given that many misleading claims are supposedly backed by scientific-sounding statements, it is difficult for even informed consumers to separate fact from fiction (see Figure 1-6). The general rule of thumb is: If it sounds too good to be true, it probably is. The following red flags can help you spot a quack:

- *The promoter claims that the medical establishment is against him or her and that the government won't accept this new "alternative" treatment.* If the government or medical community doesn't accept a treatment, it's because the treatment hasn't been proven to work. Reputable professionals don't suppress knowledge about fighting disease. On the contrary, they welcome new remedies for illness, provided the treatments have been carefully tested.
- *The promoter uses testimonials and anecdotes from satisfied customers to support claims.* Valid nutrition information comes from careful experimental research, not from random tales. A few people's reports that the product in question "works every time" are never acceptable as sound scientific evidence.
- *The promoter uses a computer-scored questionnaire for diagnosing "nutrient deficiencies."* Those computers are programmed to suggest that just about everyone has a deficiency that can be reversed with supplements the promoter just happens to be selling, regardless of the consumer's symptoms or health.
- *The promoter claims that the product will make weight loss easy with guaranteed results.* Unfortunately, there is no simple way to lose weight. Again, if a claim sounds too good to be true, it probably is.

FIGURE 1-6

Red Flags of Nutrition Quackery

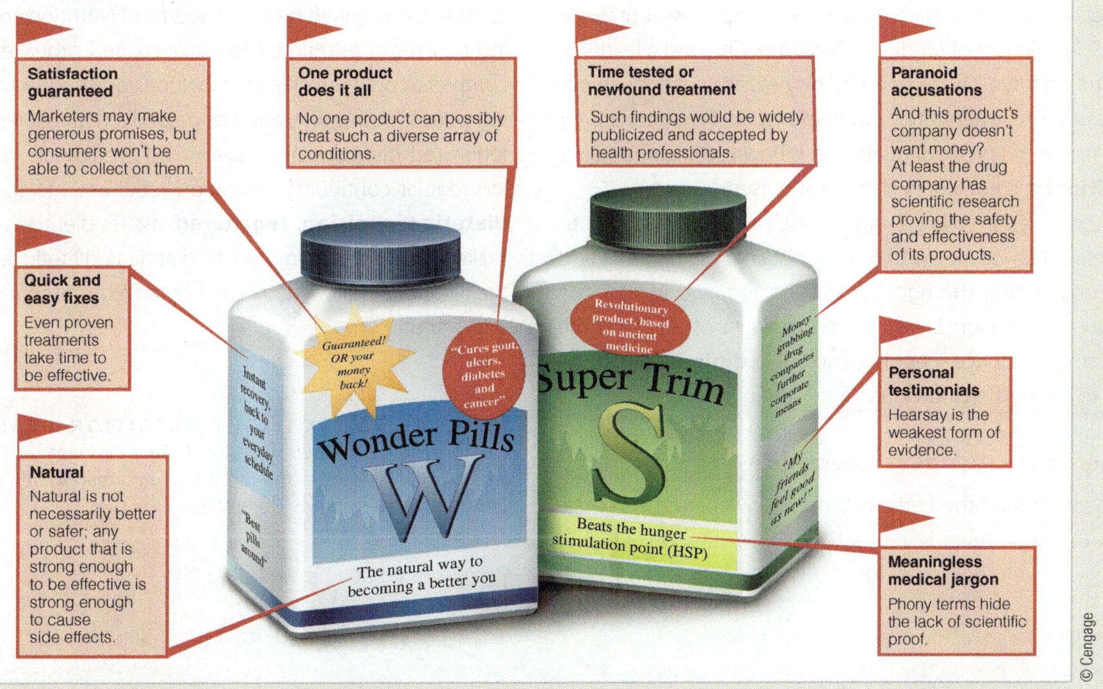

SOURCE: From Whitney/Rolfes, *Understanding Nutrition*, 14th ed. (Boston, MA: Cengage Learning, 2017), p. 34.

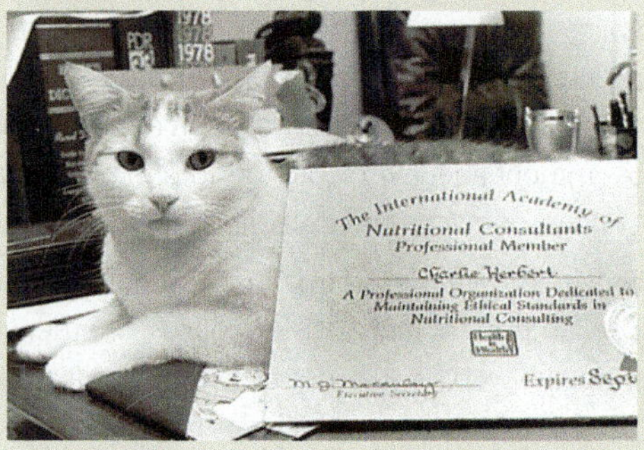

Marilynne Herbert

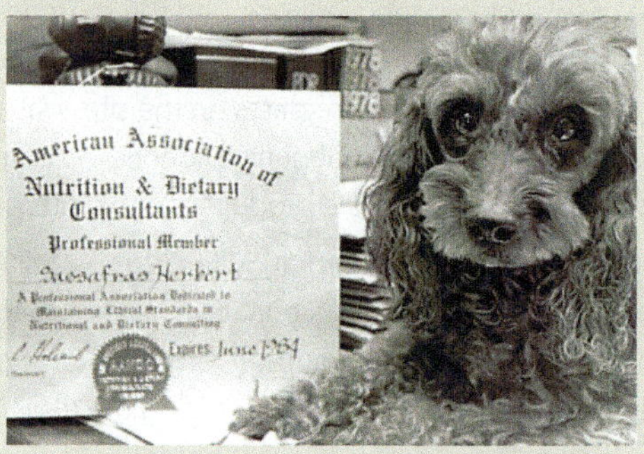

Marilynne Herbert

Charlie and Sassafras display their professional credentials.

- *The promoter claims that the product is a "cure-all" for all kinds of ailments—even for conditions that have no cure (e.g., arthritis).* The broader the claims, the less likely they are to be true.
- *The recommendations are based on a single study.* Every study should be viewed as preliminary until it becomes just one addition to a significant body of evidence pointing in the same direction.
- *The promoter promises that the product is made with a "secret formula" available only from this one company.* Legitimate health professionals share their knowledge of proven treatments so that others can benefit from it.
- *The treatment is available only through the back pages of magazines, over the phone, or by mail-order ads in the form of news stories or 30-minute commercials (known as infomercials) in talk-show format.* Results of studies on credible treatments are reported first in medical journals and then administered by a health professional. If information about a treatment appears only elsewhere, it probably cannot withstand scientific scrutiny.

If I do buy a product, say, to help me lose weight, but I still need some advice about dieting, should I check with a nutritionist?

To answer that question, first consider the following story. Charlie Herbert was able to become a professional of the International Academy of Nutrition Consultants. Another member of the household, Sassafras Herbert, met all the requirements for membership in the American Association of Nutritional and Dietary Consultants, a "professional association dedicated to maintaining ethical standards in nutritional and dietary consulting." The only qualification for membership is a $50 fee, regardless of your background (or even your species). Charlie Herbert is a cat, and Sassafras is a poodle. The two obtained their "credentials" with the help of the late Victor Herbert, M.D., former professor of medicine, at Mount Sinai School of Medicine, New York City, and a leader in combating nutrition fraud. Dr. Herbert had his pets added to the membership rosters of those organizations to demonstrate how easy it is for anyone to get fake nutrition credentials. This is because in some states, the term **nutritionist** is not legally defined at present.

Before you pay a fee or follow a nutritionist's advice, inquire about the person's credentials. Some "nutritionists" obtain their diplomas and titles without undergoing the rigorous training required to obtain a legitimate degree in nutrition. Lax state laws make it possible for some irresponsible correspondence schools—also called **diploma mills**—to grant degrees to unqualified individuals for nothing more than a fee.

How can I check a nutritionist's credentials?

You can call the institution the person claims has awarded the degree. To find out about the existence or reputation of an institution of higher learning, you can check the directory of colleges and universities called *Accredited Institutions of Postsecondary Education*, published by the American Council on Education **(www.acenet.edu)**. Be suspicious of diplomas or degrees issued by institutions that cannot prove that they have **accreditation** from the Council on Education.

Another option is to find out whether the person is a **registered dietitian/nutritionist (RD/RDN)**. The RD, an especially meaningful credential, has a standard definition: a professional who has fulfilled coursework required by the Academy of Nutrition and Dietetics, including courses in nutrition, food science, and other related subjects; has completed an internship that includes on-the-job training for counseling people about diet; and has passed a national registration exam. All registered dietitians must keep their credentials current by completing regular continuing education requirements. In some instances, a **dietetic technician, registered**, assists dietitians in helping people make healthy food choices. Like dietitians, dietetic technicians maintain their national registration credential through continuing professional education.

ANSWERS TO SPOTLIGHT NUTRITION HEALTH IQ TEST: All are false except numbers 4, 8, and 10. Seven correct answers suggest that you are fairly well informed about nutrition information. Ten correct answers suggest that you are very well informed.

Miniglossary

accreditation Approval; in the case of hospitals or university departments, approval by a professional organization of the educational program offered. There are phony accrediting agencies; the genuine ones are listed in a directory called *Accredited Institutions of Postsecondary Education.*

control group A group of individuals with characteristics that match those of the group being treated in an intervention study but who receive a placebo or no treatment at all.

correlation A simultaneous change in two factors, such as a decrease in blood pressure with regular aerobic activity (a direct or positive correlation) or the decrease in incidence of bone fractures with increasing calcium intakes (an inverse or negative correlation).

dietetic technician, registered (DTR) Nutrition professionals who work as part of health care and food service management teams. DTRs have completed at least a two-year associate's degree at a U.S. regionally accredited college or university and an accredited dietetic technician program, and passed a national examination.

diploma mill A correspondence school that grinds out degrees (sometimes worth no more than the paper they are printed on) the way a grain mill grinds out flour.

epidemiological study A study of a population that searches for possible correlations between nutrition factors and health patterns over time.

experimental group The participants in a study who receive the real treatment or intervention under investigation.

First Amendment The amendment to the U.S. Constitution that guarantees freedom of the press.

intervention study A population study examining the effects of a treatment on experimental subjects compared to a control group.

nutritionist A person who claims to be capable of advising people about their diets. Some nutritionists are registered dietitians, whereas others are self-described experts whose training is questionable.

placebo An inert, harmless "treatment" given to the control group in a study that the group's members cannot recognize as different from the actual treatment or intervention given to the experimental group.

registered dietitian/nutritionist (RD/RDN) A professional who has graduated from a nutrition and dietetics program accredited by the Accreditation Council for Education in Nutrition and Dietetics (ACEND) of the Academy of Nutrition and Dietetics, has completed an internship program or the equivalent to gain practical skills, has passed a registration examination, and maintains competencies through continuing education. Most states require licensing for dietitians, thereby requiring anyone who wants to use the title "dietitian" to receive permission to do so by passing a state examination.

WHAT'S ONLINE

MINDTAP From Cengage

Visit www.cengagebrain.com to access MindTap, a complete digital course that includes Diet & Wellness Plus, interactive quizzes, videos, and more.

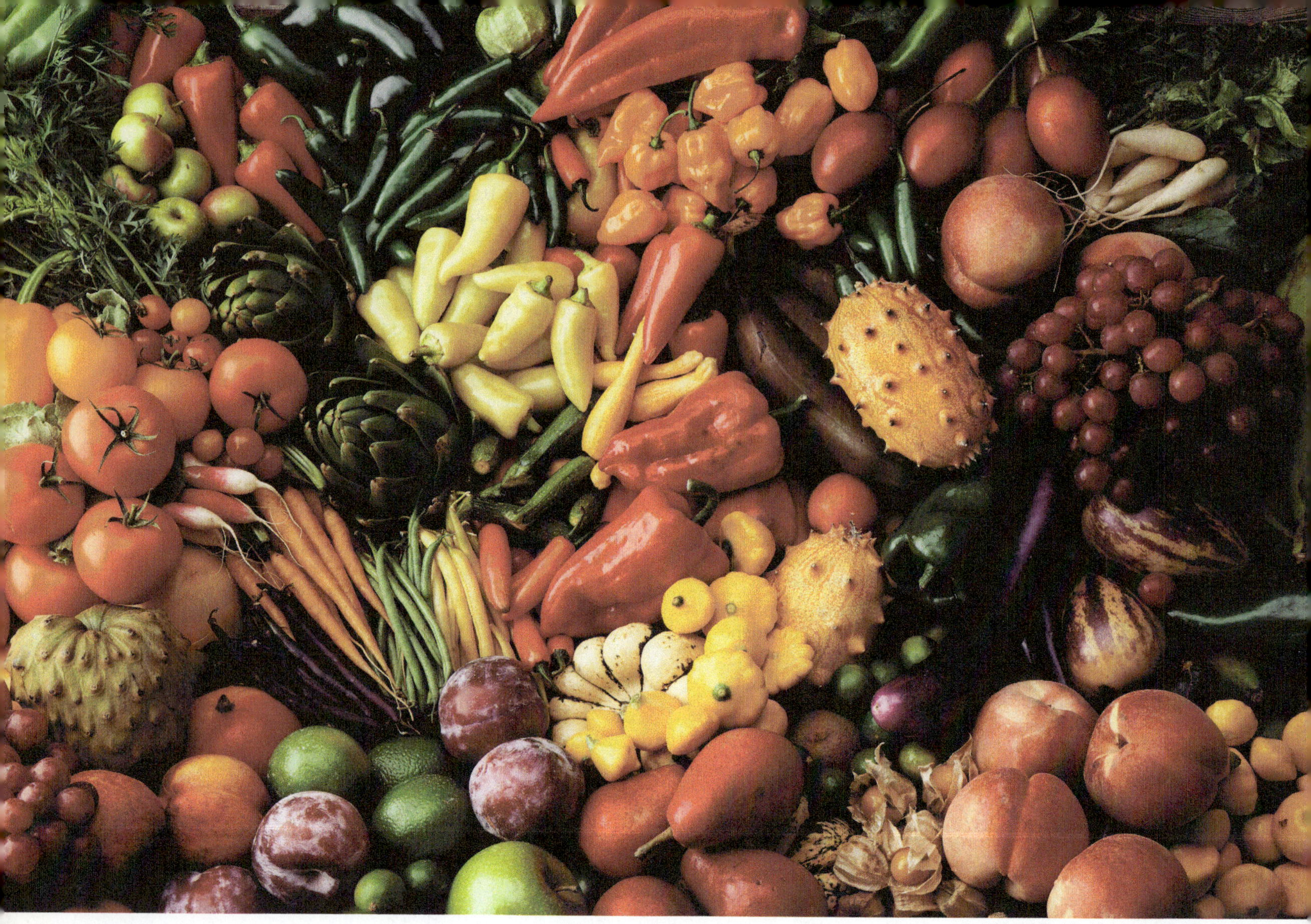

David Solzberg/Stock Food Creative/Getty Images

AskYourself . . .

Which of the following statements about nutrition are true, and which are false? For each false statement, what is true?

1. It is wise to eat the same foods every day.
2. When it comes to nutrients, more is always better.
3. A person's energy needs are based on his or her age, gender, weight, and physical activity levels.
4. If a food label claims that a product is low in fat, you can believe it.

Answers found on page 30.

ChapterObjectives

2.1 List and describe six characteristics of planning a healthy diet.

2.2 Describe the purpose of each of the four categories of nutrient intake values that make up the Dietary Reference Intakes (DRI) for nutrients.

2.3 Describe three major goals for building healthy eating patterns as emphasized by the *Dietary Guidelines for Americans*.

2.4 Explain how the MyPlate Food Guide incorporates the principles of diet planning to help consumers make healthy meal choices.

2.5 List four nutrients whose intakes are low enough to be of public health concern in the United States.

2.6 List the information found on food labels that is useful when making comparisons between similar products based on health goals.

2.7 Discuss tips for incorporating ethnic food choices into a healthy eating pattern.

The Pursuit of a Healthy Diet

CHAPTER 2

For most people, eating is so habitual they give hardly any thought to the foods they choose to eat. Yet, as Chapter 1 emphasized, the foods you select can have a profound effect on the quality, and possibly even the length, of your life. Given all the statistics and government mandates presented so far, however, designing a healthy diet may seem like a complicated matter involving a rigid regimen that excludes certain foods from the diet. Fortunately, that's not the case. The government, as well as many major health organizations, has devised dietary guidelines and tools (such as food labels) to help you build healthy eating patterns. This chapter provides an overview of some of the best guides and tools and shows you how to use them.

> If the doctors of today will not become the nutritionists of tomorrow, the nutritionists of today will become the doctors of tomorrow.
>
> —Thomas Edison (1847–1931, American inventor)

As you read the following pages, keep in mind that one of the biggest misconceptions about planning a healthy diet is believing that some foods (say, carrots and celery sticks) are "good," whereas others, like cookies and candy, are "bad." People who categorize foods this way often feel guilty every time they "splurge" on a so-called bad food.

All of your food and beverage choices matter, but the overall **eating pattern** is what really counts. A healthy eating pattern is not a rigid diet prescription, but rather a flexible framework that can accommodate personal and cultural food preferences and seasonal availability while fitting within your budget. The trick is choosing a healthy balance of foods. The ideal pattern contains primarily foods that supply adequate nutrients, fiber, and calories without an excess of added sugars, solid fats, sodium, or alcohol.

eating pattern An individual's complete dietary intake of foods and beverages over time.

2.1 The ABCs of Eating for Health

We all make choices every day about what foods and beverages we will consume and how physically active we will be. You can create a healthy eating pattern that meets nutrient needs and stays within your calorie budget—at home, in the grocery store, or while dining out—by keeping in mind the following six dietary principles:

- **Adequacy** (to provide enough of the essential nutrients, fiber, and energy—in the form of calories)
- **Balance** (to avoid overemphasis on any food type or nutrient at the expense of another)
- **Calorie control** (to supply the amount of energy you need to maintain a healthy weight—not more, not less)
- **Nutrient density** (to create a healthy eating pattern that meets nutrient needs and stays within calorie limits)
- **Moderation** (to avoid excess amounts of unwanted constituents, such as solid fats and added sugars)
- **Variety** (to incorporate a wide selection of different foods from within and among the different food groups rather than eating the same foods day after day)

Equally important, be sure that your diet suits you—that it consists of foods that fit your personality, family and cultural traditions, lifestyle, and budget. At best, your diet can be a source of both pleasure and good health.

Adequacy

Adequacy characterizes a diet that provides all of the nutrients and energy (calories) in amounts sufficient to maintain health. Any nutrient can be used to demonstrate the importance of dietary adequacy. For example, iron is an essential nutrient that your body loses daily; it must be replaced continually by iron-rich foods. If your diet does not provide adequate iron—that is, if it lacks food sources of the mineral—you can develop a condition known as *iron-deficiency anemia*. If you add iron-rich foods such as meat, fish, poultry, and legumes to your diet, the condition is likely to disappear soon. (More information about iron appears in Chapter 8.)

Balance

Balance promotes adequacy in the diet. Balancing the whole diet is a juggling act that, if successful, provides enough, but not too much, of each of the 40-odd nutrients the body needs for good health. As you will see later in the chapter, you can design an eating pattern that is both adequate and balanced by using food group plans that help you choose from various groups the specific amounts of foods that should be eaten each day.

To appreciate the importance of balance, consider a second essential nutrient. Calcium plays a vital role in building a strong frame that can withstand the gradual bone loss that occurs with age. Thus, adults are advised to consume three cups of milk or milk products (the best sources of this bone-building mineral) daily to meet their calcium needs. Foods that are rich in calcium typically lack iron, however, and vice versa; so you have to balance the two in your diet.

adequacy The characteristic of a diet that provides all of the essential nutrients, fiber, and energy (calories) in amounts sufficient to maintain health.

balance A feature of a diet that provides a number of types of foods in harmony with one another, such that foods rich in one nutrient do not crowd out of the diet foods that are rich in another nutrient.

calorie control A feature of a diet that achieves balance between calories consumed in foods and beverages and calories expended through physical activity.

nutrient density A measure of the nutrients a food supplies relative to the number of calories it provides. The higher the level of nutrients and the fewer the number of calories, the higher the nutrient density.

moderation The attribute of a diet that provides no unwanted constituent in excess.

variety A feature of a diet in which a wide selection of foods from within and among the different food groups are consumed; the opposite of *monotony.*

ASK YOURSELF ANSWERS: **1.** False. It is unwise to eat the same foods day in and day out; your diet will lack variety and probably will not supply all the nutrients your body needs. **2.** False. Too much or too little of a nutrient is often equally harmful. **3.** True. **4.** True.

Calorie Control To maintain a healthy weight, energy intakes should not exceed energy needs. Calorie control helps ensure a balance between energy we take in from food and energy we expend in activity. A cup and a half of ice cream, for example, has about the same amount of calcium as a cup of milk, but the ice cream may provide more than 500 calories, whereas the milk may supply only 90. When it comes to iron, a 3-ounce serving of beef pot roast provides about twice the amount of the mineral as a 3-ounce serving of canned tuna. But whereas the beef supplies 280 calories, the tuna adds only about 100 calories to the diet. The choice of which one to eat depends on personal preferences as well as the nutrient and calorie content of the other foods in the total diet.

Nutrient Density Nutrient density helps those who are trying to ensure optimal intakes of nutrients without excess calories by emphasizing foods that are rich in nutrients (protein, vitamins, and minerals) but relatively low in calories and added fats and sugars. Such foods are referred to as nutrient dense. A healthy eating pattern focuses on nutrient-dense foods—vegetables, fruits, whole grains, fat-free or low-fat milk and milk products, lean meats and poultry, seafood, eggs, beans and peas, and nuts and seeds that are prepared without added solid fats, sugars, and sodium. A baked potato, for example, contains more iron and vitamin C for its calories than French fries. Hence, it is more nutrient dense. Figure 2-1 shows how every food choice is an opportunity to move toward a healthy eating pattern. Remember, too, that many beverages add calories to the diet without providing essential nutrients. Figure 2-2 compares the nutrient density of selected beverages.

Moderation Another characteristic of a healthy diet is moderation. In other words, try to eat meals that do not contain excessive amounts of any one nutrient, such as solid fats, which are major sources of saturated fatty acids (discussed in Chapter 5), the culprits linked to a number of chronic diseases. That's not to say that you

FIGURE 2-1

Make Food Choices Nutrient Dense

Every food and beverage choice is an opportunity to move toward a healthy eating pattern. Small shifts in food choices—over the course of a week, a day, or even a meal—can make a big difference. Here are some ideas for small shifts that can help you adopt a healthy eating pattern. What are healthy shifts? When you can, swap out a food or ingredient for a healthier option. For example, you could:

SOURCE: Adapted from U.S. Department of Agriculture and U.S. Department of Health and Human Services, *Dietary Guidelines for Americans*, 2015. 8th ed. (Washington, DC: U.S. Government Printing Office, 2015); Office of Disease Prevention and Health Promotion, *2015–2020 Dietary Guidelines for Americans, Shift to Healthier Food & Beverage Choices*, March 2016.

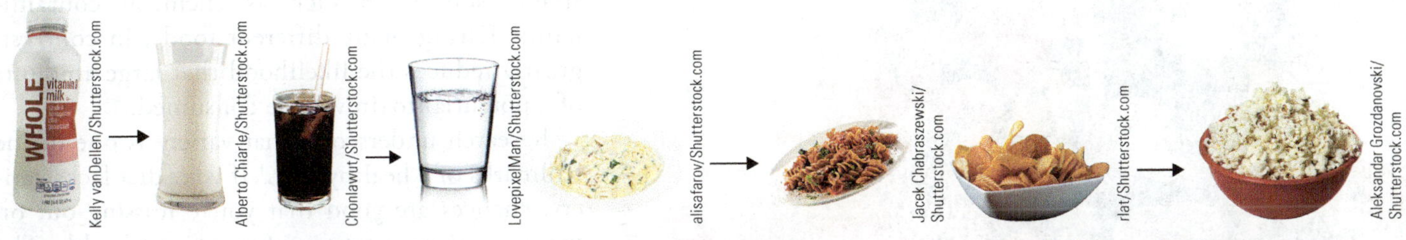

Shift from whole milk to low-fat milk in your breakfast cereal

Shift from soda with added sugars to water during lunch

Shift from a cream-based pasta dish to one with a lighter sauce and more vegetables for dinner.

Shift from refined grains to whole grains. Have plain popcorn for a snack instead of potato chips.

FIGURE 2-2

Nutrient Density of Selected Beverages

Compare the nutrient contributions made by the three beverages shown here. The figures show that 1% low-fat milk and whole milk are good sources of several essential nutrients, whereas the cola beverage simply provides calories (from sugar). Note that the low-fat milk is more nutrient dense per 100 calories than the whole milk.

[a]The Daily Values, used on food labels, are based on 2,000 calories a day for adults and children over 4 years old, and are useful for making comparisons among foods in terms of their nutrient composition.

[b]A good source of this nutrient (more than 10 percent of the recommended intake).

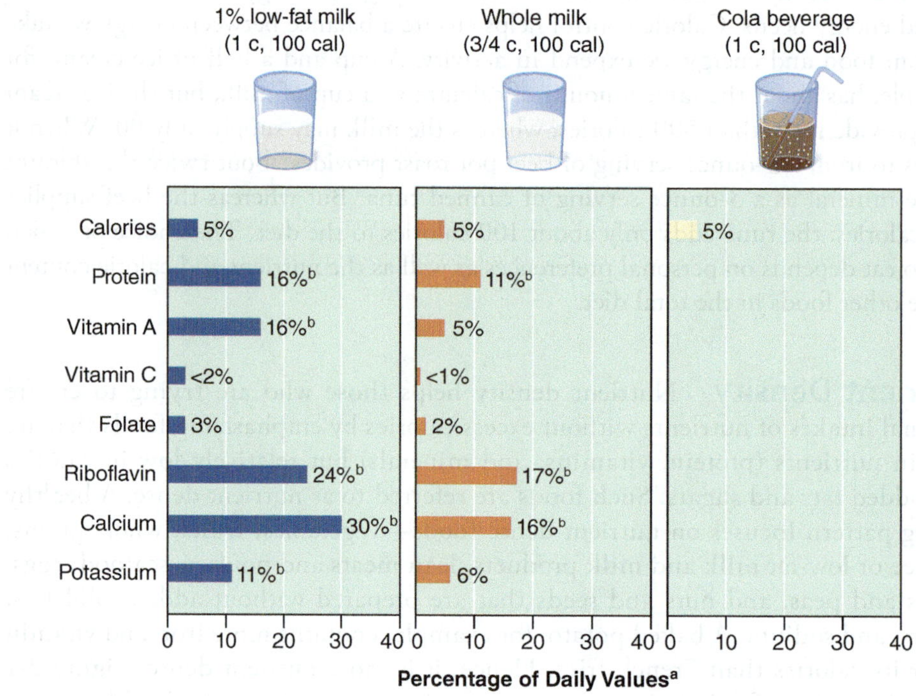

© Cengage

should choose only foods that supply little or no fat. Such an approach is unrealistic and will only lead to frustration. Practice moderation by choosing such foods only on occasion (milkshake versus low-fat milk) and regularly choosing the most nutrient-dense foods from all food groups without exceeding overall calorie needs.

Variety Aside from avoiding the monotony of eating the same foods day after day, we need variety in our diet for several reasons. First, some foods are better sources of nutrients needed in such small amounts that we don't consciously plan diets around them. Second, variety improves nutrient adequacy, as foods within a specific food group may contain different amounts of nutrients. For example, when selecting fruits, oranges are an excellent source of vitamin C, but a slice of cantaloupe would be a better choice for vitamin A. Finally, a limited diet can supply excess amounts of undesirable substances such as chemical contaminants. Eating many different foods, in contrast, greatly reduces the likelihood that large amounts of a potential toxin will be consumed.

Research underscores that variety is one of the hallmarks of a healthy diet.[1] If your diet lacks variety, chances are good that you're missing out on many nutrients necessary for optimal health. The Japanese, incidentally, recognize variety as such an important part of healthy eating that their dietary guidelines recommend consuming a good combination of various foods *every* day to achieve a balance of essential nutrients.[2]

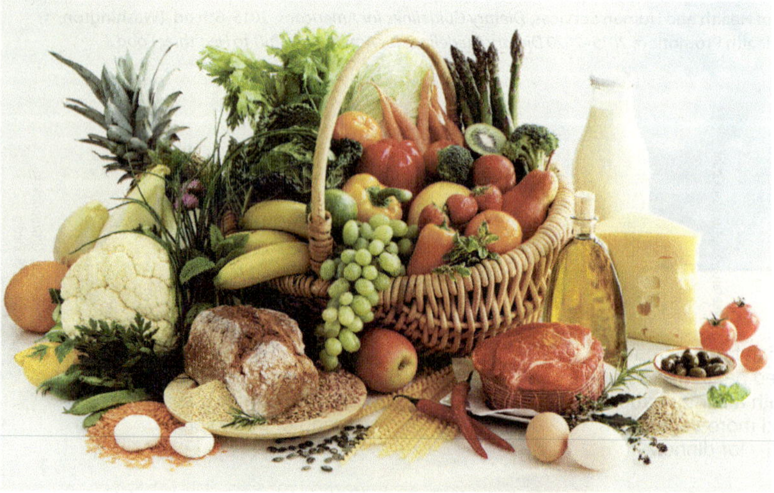

Maximilian Stock Ltd./Getty Images

Variety fosters good nutrition.

2.2 Nutrient Recommendations

At this point, knowing that foods are made of so many different combinations of nutrients, you may be wondering how to determine whether you are eating the right balance of nutrients. Obviously, if your diet lacks any of the essential nutrients, you may develop deficiencies. Even if you don't develop a full-blown deficiency disease, when you are less than optimally nourished, you may get sick more easily and suffer other health problems. To help prevent such problems and provide a benchmark for people's nutrient needs, experts in Canada and the United States devised the **Dietary Reference Intakes (DRI)** for planning and assessing diets of healthy people in both countries.[3]

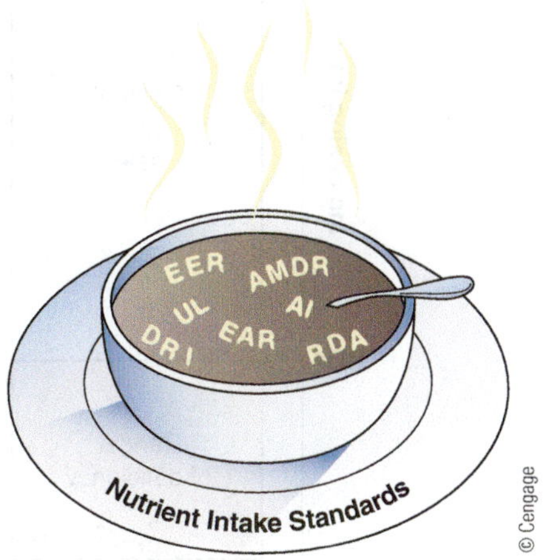

The Dietary Reference Intakes (DRI)

A committee of nutrition experts selected by the National Academy of Sciences (NAS) sets forth the DRI—a set of daily nutrient standards based on the latest scientific evidence regarding diet and health. The DRI for all age groups are listed at the back of this book. The DRI are defined in the Miniglossary and include:

- Estimated Average Requirements (EAR)
- Recommended Dietary Allowances (RDA)
- Adequate Intakes (AI)
- Tolerable Upper Intake Levels (UL)
- Estimated Energy Requirements (EER)
- Acceptable Macronutrient Distribution Ranges (AMDR)

Although the DRI are widely used, many people have misconceptions about their meaning and intent. To get a proper perspective about the DRI, consider the following facts:

- The DRI estimate the energy and nutrient needs of *healthy* people. People with certain medical problems often have different nutritional needs.
- Separate recommendations are made for different groups of people. For instance, the DRI committee issues one set of recommendations for children ages 4 through 8, another set for adult men, another for pregnant women, and so on.
- The DRI may evolve over time because of new scientific evidence indicating a need for reevaluation of current concepts and recommended intakes.[4]
- The DRI take into account differences among individuals and establish a range within which the nutritional needs of virtually all healthy people in a particular age and gender group will be covered (see Figure 2-3).

The DRI for Nutrients

The DRI aim to prevent nutrient deficiencies in a population as well as reduce risk for chronic diseases such as heart disease, cancer, and osteoporosis. To understand the process of developing the DRI, consider the following discussion. Suppose we were the committee members, and we were called upon to set the DRI for nutrient X. First, we would determine the **requirement**—how much of that nutrient the average healthy person needs to prevent a deficiency. To do so, we would review scientific research and explore how the body stores the nutrient, what the consequence of a deficiency might be, what causes depletion of the nutrient, and what other factors affect a person's need for nutrient X. We would also consider current concepts regarding the amount of the nutrient needed for reducing risk of chronic disease (for example, optimal calcium intake and reduced risk of bone

Dietary Reference Intakes (DRI) A set of reference values for energy and nutrients that can be used for planning and assessing diets for healthy people.

requirement The minimum amount of a nutrient that will prevent the development of deficiency symptoms. Requirements differ from the RDA and AI, which include a substantial margin of safety to cover the requirements of different individuals.

FIGURE 2-3

The Correct View of the DRI

This figure shows that people with intakes below the EAR are likely to have dietary adequacy of 50 percent or less. People with intakes between the EAR and RDA are likely to have adequacy between 50 and 97 to 98 percent. Intakes between the RDA or AI and the UL are likely to be adequate. At intakes above the UL, the risk of harm increases.

People often think that more is better when it comes to nutrients. Too much of a good thing can be dangerous, however, so the RDA and AI fall within an optimal margin of safety, and the UL helps people avoid harmful excesses of nutrients.

SOURCE: Adapted from Institute of Medicine, *Dietary Intakes for Energy, Carbohydrate, Fiber, Fat, Fatty Acids, Cholesterol, Protein, and Amino Acids* (Washington, DC: National Academy Press, 2002).

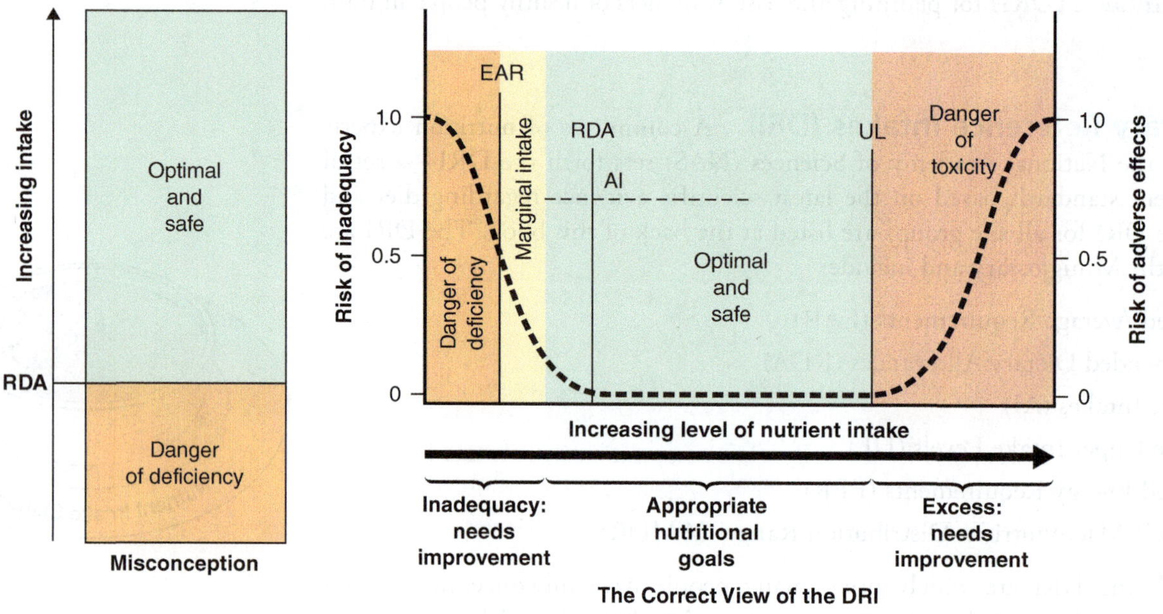

fractures later in life). However, we know that people vary in the amount of a given nutrient they need. Mr. A might need an average of 40 units of nutrient X daily for optimal health; Ms. B might need 35; Mr. C, 60; and so on.

Our next task would be to determine what amount of nutrient X to recommend for the general public. In other words, what amount of nutrient X would we consider optimal for covering most people's needs without posing a hazard? One option would be to set it at the average requirement for nutrient X (shown in Figure 2-4 at 45 units). This is the **Estimated Average Requirement (EAR)**: the amount of a

FIGURE 2-4

Nutrient Requirements Vary from Person to Person

Each square represents a person with different nutrient needs. For example, the squares labeled A, B, and C represent Mr. A, Ms. B, and Mr. C. The EAR is the amount of a nutrient estimated to meet the needs of half of the people in a particular age and gender group. The RDA for the nutrient is the amount that covers about 98 percent of the population.

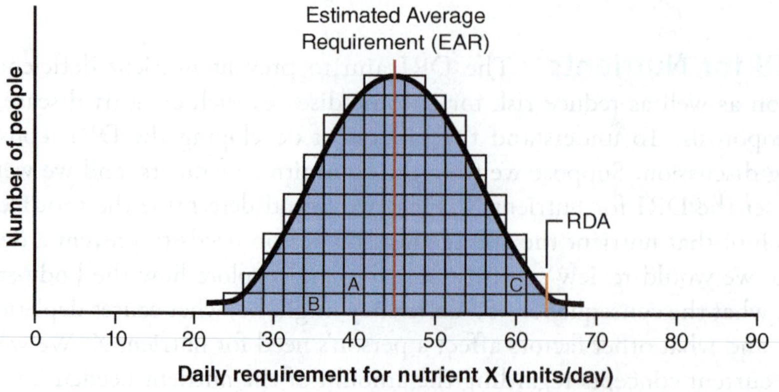

nutrient that is estimated to meet the requirement for the nutrient in half of the people of a specific age and gender. But if we did so and people took us literally, half the population—Mr. C and everyone else whose requirement is greater than 45—would eventually develop deficiencies.

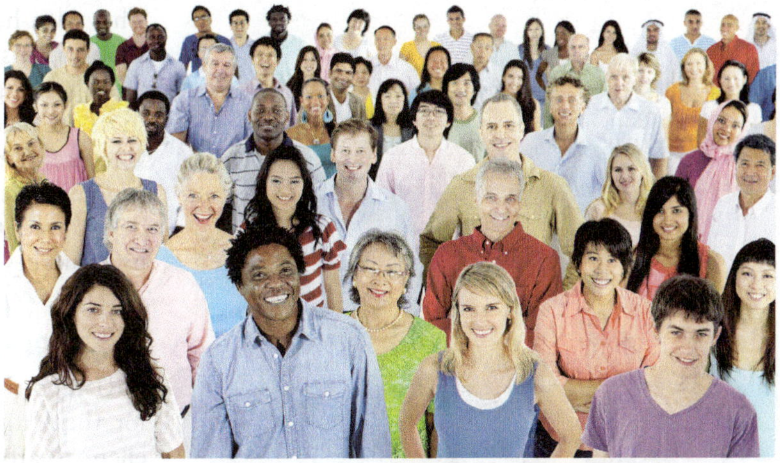

People vary in the amount of a given nutrient they need. The challenge of the DRI is to determine the best amount to recommend for everybody.

Instead, we use the EAR to set the **Recommended Dietary Allowance (RDA)**. To benefit the most people, the RDA is set at a point high enough to cover most healthy people without creating an excess in people who do not require as much nutrient X. In this case, a reasonable choice might be 63 units, which would add a generous safety margin to ensure that just about all healthy people are covered (see Figure 2-4).

If sufficient scientific evidence is not available for us to set an EAR—the requirement for nutrient X—that is needed to establish an RDA, an **Adequate Intake (AI)** is provided instead of an RDA.* Because sufficient scientific evidence is lacking, the AI is based on our best estimate of the need for nutrient X in practically all apparently healthy individuals of a specific age and gender. Individuals may use both the RDA and the AI as goals for nutrient intake.

For healthy individuals, no established benefits result from consuming amounts of a nutrient that exceed the recommended intake (the RDA or AI). However, the DRI include a **Tolerable Upper Intake Level (UL)**, which is the maximum daily intake of a nutrient that is unlikely to pose risk of *adverse* effects in healthy people. The UL exceeds the RDA and is not intended to be a recommended level of intake (refer to Figure 2-3). The need to set ULs is the result of more and more people using large doses of nutrient supplements and the increasing availability of **fortified foods**. Individuals can use the UL to determine whether their levels of nutrient intakes may pose risks of adverse effects over time.

The DRI represent a major shift in thinking about nutrient requirements for humans, from prevention of nutrient deficiencies to prevention of chronic disease.

fortified foods Foods to which nutrients have been added, either because they were not already present or because they were present in insignificant amounts; foods to which manufacturers have added 10 percent or more of the daily value for a particular nutrient. Examples: margarine with added vitamin A, milk with added vitamin D, certain brands of orange juice with added calcium, and breakfast cereals with added nutrients and nonnutrients.

Miniglossary of DRI Terms

EAR, Estimated Average Requirement The amount of a nutrient that is estimated to meet the requirement for the nutrient in half of the people of a specific age and gender. The EAR is used in setting the RDA.

RDA, Recommended Dietary Allowance The average daily amount of a nutrient that is sufficient to meet the nutrient needs of nearly all (97 to 98 percent) healthy individuals of a specific age and gender.

AI, Adequate Intake The average amount of a nutrient that appears to be adequate for individuals when there is not sufficient scientific research to calculate an RDA. The AI exceeds the EAR and possibly the RDA.

UL, Tolerable Upper Intake Level The maximum amount of a nutrient that is unlikely to pose any risk of adverse health effects to most healthy people. The UL is not intended to be a recommended level of intake.

EER, Estimated Energy Requirement The average calorie intake that is predicted to maintain energy balance in a healthy adult of a defined age, gender, weight, height, and level of physical activity, consistent with good health.

AMDR, Acceptable Macronutrient Distribution Range A range of intakes for a particular energy source (carbohydrates, fat, protein) that is associated with a reduced risk of chronic disease while providing adequate intakes of essential nutrients.

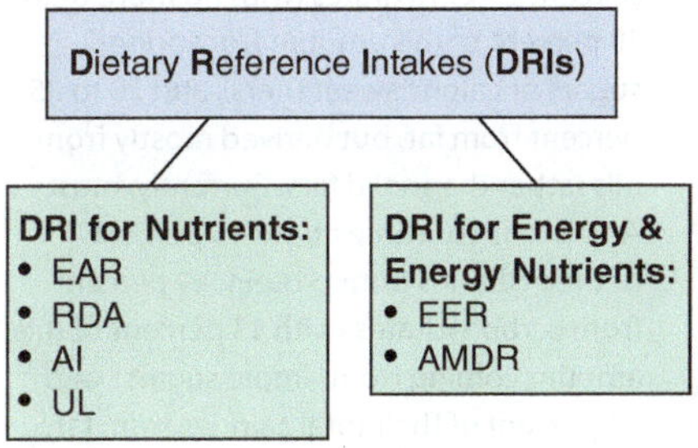

*This text refers to the nutrient recommendations (for example, RDA and AI) as DRI recommended intakes.

They also herald a new way of thinking about the role of dietary supplements in achieving good health—such that, for some individuals at higher risk, use of nutrient supplements may be desirable so as to meet recommended intakes. For example, older women who are at risk of osteoporosis may benefit from dietary calcium supplements to help maintain bone mineral mass. In addition, the development of the UL signals the widespread recognition that high intakes of nutrients can create a degree of risk.

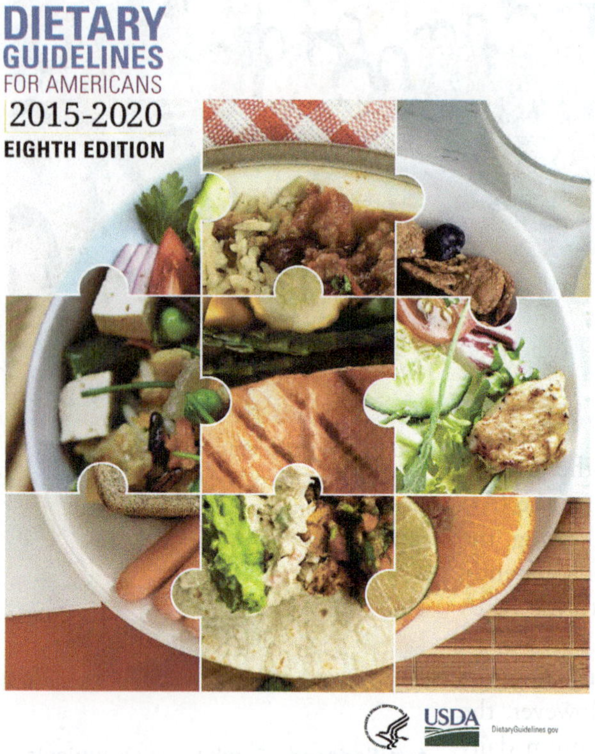

USDA

The *Dietary Guidelines* translate the DRI for energy and nutrients into food-based guidance that builds a healthy eating pattern to meet nutrient needs at appropriate calorie levels.

The DRI for Energy and the Energy Nutrients The DRI report on energy and the energy nutrients provides guidelines for the United States and Canada regarding the consumption of energy, carbohydrates, fiber, fat, fatty acids, cholesterol, and protein; it includes guidelines for physical activity as well. To meet the body's daily energy and nutritional needs while minimizing risk for chronic disease, consumption of the energy nutrients should resemble the pattern shown in Figure 2-5, and include mostly nutrient-dense foods such as a variety of fruits and vegetables every day.

To reduce the risk of chronic disease, the DRI report stresses the need to balance caloric intake with physical activity, recommending total calories to be consumed by individuals of given heights, weights, and genders for each of four different levels of physical activity (from sedentary to very active). For more about weight management and specific physical activity guidelines, see Chapters 10 and 11.

FIGURE 2-5

Recommended Dietary Intake Ranges for Energy Nutrients

A balanced diet is composed of approximately 10 to 35 percent protein, 45 to 65 percent carbohydrates (with no more than 10 percent of this amount from added sugars or caloric sweeteners), and 20 to 35 percent from fat, but derived mostly from oils rather than solid fats. Currently, most Americans consume about 15 percent of their calories from protein, 49 percent from carbohydrates (with 13 percent of this amount coming from simple sugars), and 34 percent of their total calories from fat.

Dietary Reference Intakes (DRI) for Carbohydrates, Fats, and Protein	
Carbohydrates	45 to 65 percent of total calories
Fats	20 to 35 percent of total calories
Protein	10 to 35 percent of total calories

© Cengage

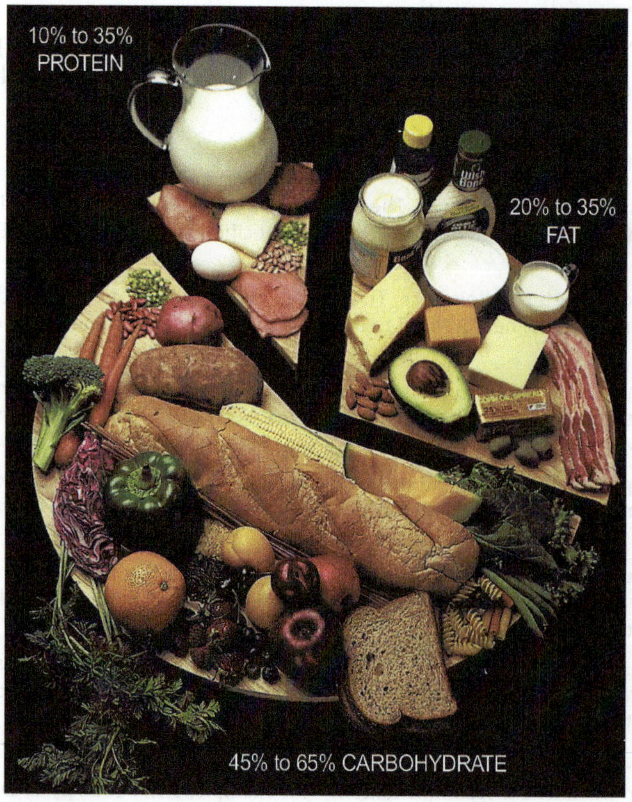

Felicia Martinez Photography/PhotoEdit

2.3 The Challenge of Dietary Guidelines

As Chapter 1 pointed out, health authorities are as concerned today about widespread nutrient excesses among Americans as they used to be about nutrient deficiencies. This is where dietary guidelines come into play. Among the most widely used of the guidelines are the *Dietary Guidelines for Americans*. The Eating Well with Canada's Food Guide recommendations presented in Appendix B are also commonly used.[5]

The *Dietary Guidelines for Americans* provide science-based advice to promote health and to reduce risk for chronic diseases through healthy eating patterns and physical activity. They emphasize variety, calorie control, moderation, and nutrient density. The guidelines also acknowledge that all segments of our society (homes, schools, workplaces, communities) have a role to play in supporting healthy food choices and opportunities for regular physical activity to help people achieve and maintain good health.

Table 2-1 presents the current *Dietary Guidelines for Americans*. These guidelines incorporate two general themes: maintaining calorie balance over time to achieve and maintain a healthy weight, and consuming more nutrient-dense foods and beverages. Americans currently consume too much sodium and too many calories from solid fats, added sugars, and refined grains. These replace nutrient-dense foods and beverages and make it difficult for people to achieve recommended nutrient intakes without exceeding their energy needs. For this reason, the *Dietary Guidelines* emphasize three major goals for building the healthy eating pattern shown in Figure 2-6:

- Balance calories with physical activity to manage weight.
- Consume a variety of nutrient-dense foods such as fruits, vegetables, whole grains, fat-free and low-fat (1%) milk products, seafood, lean

TABLE 2-1 The *2015–2020 Dietary Guidelines for Americans*

The *2015–2020 Dietary Guidelines for Americans* are built around five guidelines. Key recommendations for healthy eating patterns provide further guidance on how individuals can follow the five guidelines.[a]

The Guidelines:

1. *Follow a healthy eating pattern across the life span.* All food and beverage choices matter. Choose a healthy eating pattern at an appropriate calorie level to help achieve and maintain a healthy body weight, support nutrient adequacy, and reduce the risk of chronic disease.
2. *Focus on variety, nutrient density, and amount.* To meet nutrient needs within calorie limits, choose a variety of nutrient-dense foods across and within all food groups in recommended amounts.
3. *Limit calories from added sugars and saturated fats and reduce sodium intake.* Consume an eating pattern low in added sugars, saturated fats, and sodium. Cut back on foods and beverages higher in these components to amounts that fit within healthy eating patterns.
4. *Shift to healthier food and beverage choices.* Choose nutrient-dense foods and beverages across and within all food groups in place of less healthy choices. Consider cultural and personal preferences to make these shifts easier to accomplish and maintain.
5. *Support healthy eating patterns for all.* Everyone has a role in helping to create and support healthy eating patterns in multiple settings nationwide, from home to school to work to communities.

Key Recommendations:

- Consume a healthy eating pattern that accounts for all foods and beverages within an appropriate calorie level (see Figure 2-6).
- A healthy eating pattern limits saturated fats and *trans* fats, added sugars, and sodium:
  - Consume less than 10% of calories per day from added sugars.[b]
  - Consume less than 10% of calories per day from saturated fats.[c]
  - Consume less than 2,300 milligrams (mg) per day of sodium.[d]
- If alcohol is consumed, it should be consumed in moderation—up to one drink per day for women and up to two drinks per day for men—and only by adults of legal drinking age.[e]
- Meet the Physical Activity Guidelines for Americans (see Chapter 11).

[a] The *2015–2020 Dietary Guidelines for Americans* are intended for adults and children age 2 years and older, including those who are at increased risk of chronic disease.
[b] The recommendation to limit intake of calories from added sugars to <10% per day is a target based on the need to meet food group and nutrient needs within calorie limits. For most calorie levels, there are not enough calories available after meeting food group needs to consume 10% of calories from added sugars within calorie limits.
[c] The recommendation is a target based on evidence that replacing saturated fats with unsaturated fats is associated with reduced risk of cardiovascular disease.
[d] The recommendation to limit intake of sodium to less than 2,300 mg per day is based on the UL for individuals ages 14 years and older.
[e] It is not recommended that individuals begin drinking for any reason. There are many circumstances in which individuals should not drink, such as during pregnancy.

SOURCE: U.S. Department of Health and Human Services and U.S. Department of Agriculture, *2015–2020 Dietary Guidelines for Americans*, 8th edition, December 2015.

meats and poultry, eggs, beans and peas, soy products, and unsalted nuts and seeds.

- Consume fewer foods with sodium, saturated fats, *trans* fats, and added sugars.

Healthy eating and regular physical activity enable people of all ages to work productively, enjoy life, and feel their best. They also help children grow, develop, and do well in school. The focus of the *Dietary Guidelines* is disease prevention. The recommendations help people decrease their risk of some forms of cancer, heart disease, obesity, diabetes, high blood pressure, stroke, osteoporosis, and liver disease—the so-called **lifestyle diseases**. Following such recommendations certainly makes sense, given the potential health benefits they confer.

lifestyle diseases Conditions that may be aggravated by modern lifestyles that include too little exercise, poor diets, excessive drinking, and smoking. Lifestyle diseases are also referred to as *diseases of affluence*.

FIGURE 2-6

What's in a Healthy Eating Pattern?

SOURCE: Office of Disease Prevention and Health Promotion, *2015-2020 Dietary Guidelines for Americans, For Professionals: Talk to Your Patients & Clients about Healthy Eating Patterns*, March 2016 and *2015–2020 Dietary Guidelines for Americans, For Professionals: Recommendations At-A-Glance*, March 2016.

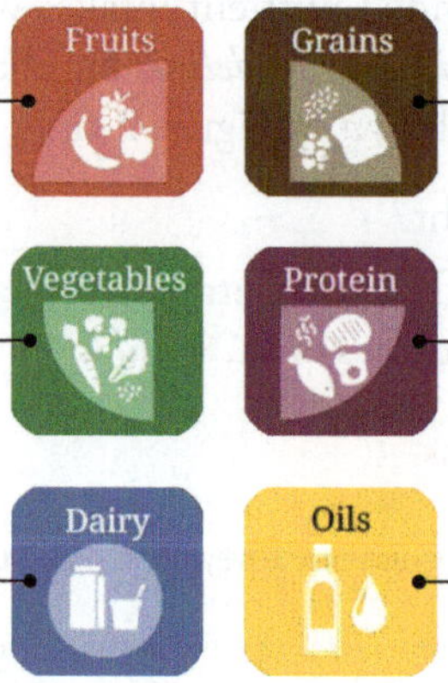

Fruits, especially whole fruits

Grains, at least half of which are whole grains

A variety of vegetables— dark green, red and orange, legumes (beans and peas), starchy, and other vegetables

A variety of protein foods, including seafood, lean meats and poultry, eggs, legumes (beans and peas), soy products, and nuts and seeds

Fat-free or low-fat dairy, including milk, yogurt, cheese, and/or fortified soy beverages

Oils, including those from plants (such as canola, corn, olive, peanut, safflower, soybean, and sunflower) and in foods (such as nuts, seeds, seafood, olives, and avocados)

The *Dietary Guidelines* also recommends limits on a few specific dietary components.

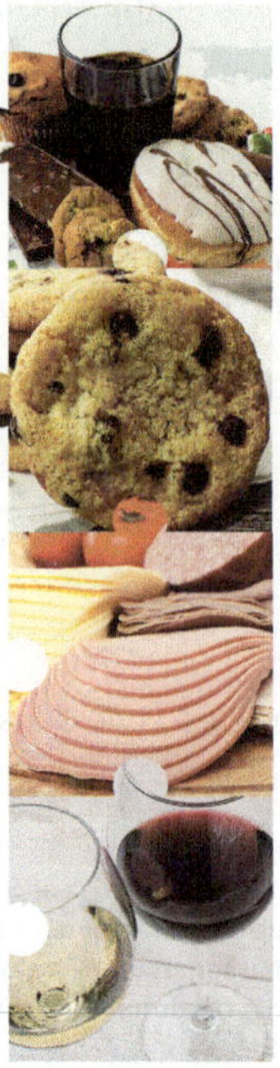

Ekaterina Markelova/Shutterstock.com

vm2002/Shutterstock.com

Olga Nayashkova/Shutterstock.com

Dima Sobko/Shutterstock.com

Added Sugars: Limit to less than 10% of total calories daily.
When sugars or syrups are added to foods as they're processed or prepared, they're called added sugars. (Natural sugars—in fruits, vegetables, and milk—are not added sugars.) Added sugars add calories without other nutritional value. When a person's diet is high in added sugars, it may be hard for them to achieve a healthy eating pattern.

Saturated & *Trans* Fats: Limit saturated fats to less than 10% of total calories daily by replacing them with unsaturated fats and limit *trans* fats to as low as possible.
Diets high in saturated and *trans* fats are associated with heart disease. Foods high in saturated fats include butter, whole milk, and meats that aren't labeled lean. *Trans* fats are in processed foods, like desserts, frozen pizza, and coffee creamer.

Sodium: Limit to less than 2,300 mg daily (for adults and children 14 years and older).
Most Americans get 50% more sodium than recommended. Diets high in sodium are associated with high blood pressure and heart disease.

Alcohol: Limit to no more than 1 drink daily for women and no more than 2 for men.
The *Dietary Guidelines* doesn't recommend that people start drinking alcohol for any reason and many people shouldn't drink, such as women during pregnancy. But for adults of legal drinking age who already do, moderation is essential.

Nutrition ACTION Grazer's Guide to Smart Snacking (Obj. 2.3)

It's 3:30 in the afternoon, and that sound you just heard is coming from your stomach. Physiologically speaking, the human digestive system is customized for us to eat about every four hours to maintain our energy level. So, it's not unreasonable to get a little hungry between meals or before we go to bed. In fact, it is now clear that healthy snacking can fit into any eating plan and is important to everyone's health.[6]

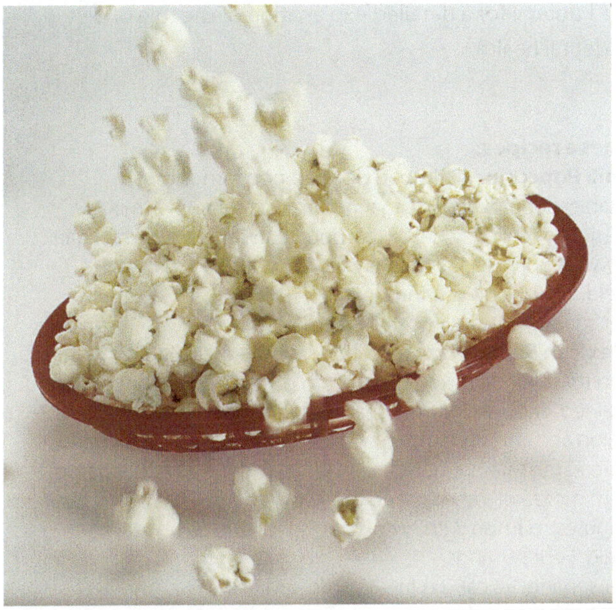

PhotoDisc/Getty Images

Still, although **grazing** is "in," many people feel a twinge of guilt now and then about between-meal munching. Perhaps parental warnings from childhood that snacks can spoil a meal linger in the back of many minds. Nevertheless, nutritious nibbling can make it easier for many people to eat healthfully.

Snacks can supply essential vitamins, minerals, and calories to diets of young children, who often cannot eat large portions at mealtime because of their small stomachs and appetites. Teenagers typically don't seem to have the time (or inclination) to eat regularly, due to busy school schedules, sports practices, music lessons, or other activities. Snacks account for approximately 25 percent of the calories they eat and are often more energy dense than their meals.[7]

Snacks also contribute to nutritional needs of adults, who may find that fitting meals into a busy schedule is difficult. Even older adults, whose lifestyles tend to be less hectic, can benefit from grazing. That's because lack of activity, certain medications, and isolation can blunt a formerly hearty appetite, making frequent, small meals more desirable than large breakfasts, lunches, and dinners. And, of course, a college student's busy life makes it difficult, if not impossible, to plan meals and snacks in advance, so snacking is a factor at any age.

The key to healthy snacking for everyone is to choose healthy, high-fiber, nutrient-dense foods instead of snacks that add unhealthful fats and calories to the diet and little else in the way of nutrients. A snack with a balance of carbohydrate, some fat, and some protein will satisfy hunger for a longer period of time than food with only carbohydrates or sugars (such as candy or soft drinks). How do you achieve this balance? Choosing snacks that contain at least two food groups can provide yummy and healthy snack possibilities.

Some snacks that appear nutritious may be deceiving. For example, fruit drinks, mixes, and punches are loaded with sugar (usually in the form of high-fructose corn syrup) and are more similar to soft drinks than to fruit juice. Fruit rolls and bars are nutritionally similar to jams and jelly, not fresh fruit. For these snacks, sugar is added and most of the nutrients are lost when the fruit is processed with heat. Energy and protein bars can also be deceiving because, like candy bars, many are loaded with sugar and fat. Even some varieties of microwave popcorn don't rate well as snacks, because they contain so much oil and salt. (You can easily make your own popcorn in the microwave oven without adding excessive extras.) Use Table 2-2 as a guide for choosing healthy snacks instead of calorie-dense snacks with little nutritional value. When you feel like snacking, try some of

TABLE 2-2 Snack Ideas from Each Food Group

Grains	Whole-grain cereal, whole-grain crackers, mini rice cakes, sliced whole-grain bread, mini bagels, graham crackers, whole-wheat tortillas
Vegetables	Veggie "matchsticks" (thin sticks) made from fresh carrots or zucchini, bell pepper rings, cherry tomatoes, steamed broccoli, green beans, sugar snap peas, avocados
Fruits	Apple slices, clementine sections, strawberry halves, bananas, pineapple, kiwi, peach, mango, nectarine, melon, grapes, berries, dried apricots
Dairy	Low-fat cheese slices or string cheese, fat-free or low-fat milk, low-fat cottage cheese, low-fat regular or Greek yogurt
Protein Foods	Hard-boiled eggs, peanut butter, bean dip, hummus, slices of lean turkey or chicken, shelled pumpkin seeds

SOURCE: www.ChooseMyPlate.gov

grazing Eating small amounts of food at intervals throughout the day rather than or in addition to eating regular meals.

(Continued)

the alternatives offered in Figure 2-7. These snacks provide at least two food groups and 100 to 250 calories per serving.[8] In addition, consider the following tips next time you're in the mood to grab a snack:

- Stock your refrigerator and kitchen cupboards with healthy foods like fruit juices, low-fat yogurt, fresh fruits and vegetables, plain popcorn, whole-grain crackers, and low-fat cheeses so that they are close at hand. Nibblers often reach for a snack just to have something to munch on rather than because of a desire for the food itself. If nutritious choices are easy to get to, chances are that's what you'll eat.
- Carry fresh fruit and crackers and cheese in your backpack or book bag so you won't have to resort to buying candy from a vending machine when you get the urge to munch.
- Create your own snacks. Mix together one cup each of whole-grain cereal, almonds, raisins, and sunflower seeds to take with you on your next bicycle trip or hike.
- Make new versions of old favorites, such as *Chili Popcorn* and *Mexican Snack Pizzas*.[9]
- Snack with a friend. If you're craving a candy bar or chips and nothing else will do, try splitting a bar or a bag with a friend. That way, you'll satisfy your craving without going too far overboard on calories, fat, or salt.
- Try to brush your teeth—or at least rinse your mouth thoroughly—after snacking to prevent tooth decay. (See Chapter 4 for a detailed explanation of the role of diet in dental health.)

FIGURE 2-7

Smart Snacking

As a general guideline, make snacks that include at least two food groups. Choose nutrient-rich snacks like the following:

- 1 to 2 tablespoons peanut butter on an apple, celery, or carrots
- A *small* handful of tortilla chips with salsa or low-fat bean dip
- ½ cup hummus with whole-grain pita bread wedges, or cut-up vegetables
- 1 cup cereal with low-fat milk or soy milk
- 1-ounce serving trail mix (nuts, seeds, dried fruits)
- Fruit and cheese: apples or grapes with 1 ounce low-fat mozzarella string cheese
- 3 tablespoons grated Parmesan cheese sprinkled on 3 cups hot popcorn
- Granola or snack bar (choose bars with 200 or fewer calories per bar, 5 or fewer grams of sugar per 100 calories, and at least 3 grams dietary fiber per bar)

Try these recipes:

- **Chili Popcorn:** Mix 1 quart popped popcorn with 1 tablespoon melted margarine. In a separate bowl, mix 1¼ teaspoons chili powder, ¼ teaspoon cumin, and a dash of garlic powder. Sprinkle seasonings over popcorn and mix well.
  Yield: Four 1-cup servings
  Per serving: 50 cal, 3 g fat, 42 mg sodium
- **Mexican Snack Pizzas:** Split two whole-grain English muffins and toast lightly. Mix ¼ cup tomato paste; ¼ cup canned, drained, chopped kidney beans; 1 tablespoon each chopped onion and chopped green pepper; and ½ teaspoon oregano. Spread mixture on muffin halves. Top with ¼ cup shredded part-skim mozzarella cheese and broil until cheese is bubbly (about 2 minutes). Garnish with ¼ cup shredded lettuce.
  Yield: Four servings
  Per serving: 95 cal, 2 g fat, 300 mg sodium

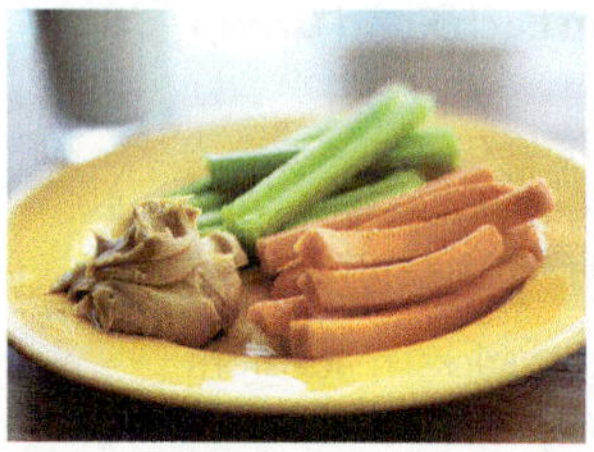
Joshua Resnick/Shutterstock.com

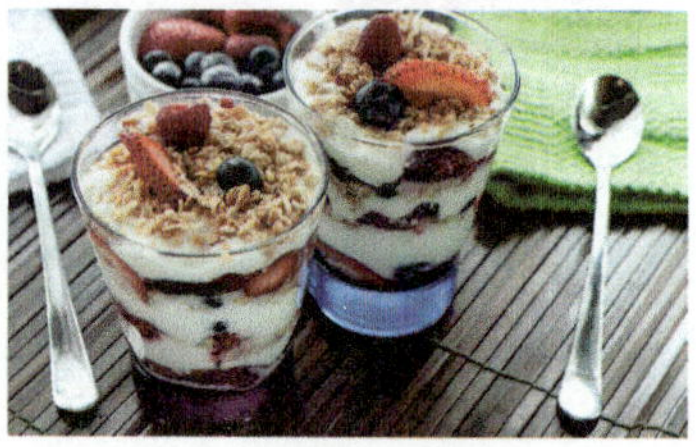
John S. Quinn/Shutterstock.com

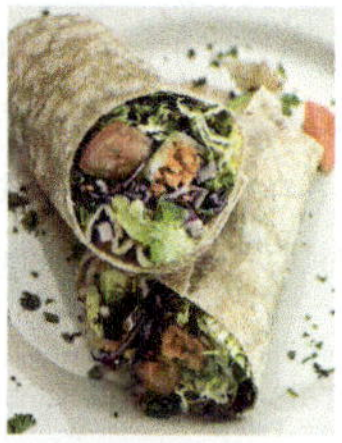
© iStockphoto.com/Juanmonino

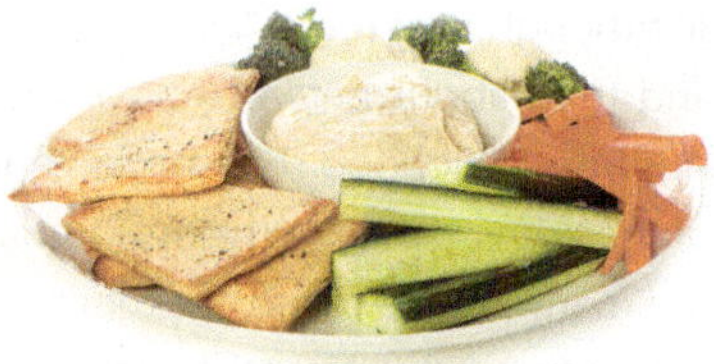
msheldrake/Shutterstock.com

Be creative:

- **Individual pizzas:** Spread heated tomato or pizza sauce on a toasted whole-grain English muffin half. Top with shredded low-fat mozzarella.
- **Fruit and yogurt smoothies:** Blend 1 container plain or flavored low-fat yogurt or low-fat Greek yogurt, 1 bag frozen berries or fruit of choice (partially thawed), and a banana for 30 seconds for a delicious smoothie.
- **Salad rolls:** Chop up a few different vegetables and roll them in a whole-wheat or spinach tortilla spread with ¼ cup hummus; top with salsa or reduced-fat salad dressing.
- **Fruit parfait:** Layer low-fat vanilla yogurt or ricotta cheese and berries in a tall glass. Top with a sprinkle of sliced almonds.
- **Snack kabobs:** Put cubes of low-fat cheese and cubes of fresh veggies or fruit on mini skewers.
- **Easy soup:** Microwave a cup of reduced-sodium tomato or vegetable soup and enjoy with 5 whole-grain crackers.
- **Anytime oatmeal:** Prepare one packet of instant oatmeal with low-fat milk; top with fresh fruit or unsweetened applesauce and sprinkle with cinnamon.
- **Frozen banana treat:** Peel a banana and dip it in yogurt. Roll in crushed cereal and freeze.
- **Homemade trail mix:** Mix 1 cup toasted oat cereal, ½ ounce chopped, unsalted nuts and/or seeds, and ¼ cup dried fruit.
- **Mini-sandwich:** Enjoy tuna or egg salad on a whole-grain dinner roll; or a pouch of tuna or salmon with whole-grain crackers or rice cakes.

SOURCE: Adapted from: ChooseMyPlate.gov, and Food, nutrition and health tips from the Academy of Nutrition and Dietetics: 25 healthy snacks for kids, Tearpad, 2012.

2.4 Introducing the MyPlate Food Planning Tool

Although the DRI and the *Dietary Guidelines* provide good frameworks for healthy eating, planning daily menus requires use of other, more specific tools. Dietitians and other nutrition experts often rely on a number of tools that you, too, can use to assess and plan your own diet.

One of the most helpful, easy-to-use diet-planning tools is the **food group plan**, which separates foods into specific groups and then specifies the amount of food from each group to eat each day either in household measures like cups or as **servings**. The MyPlate food guide is presented in detail in Figure 2-8 and Figure 2-9. This tool includes five food groups and presents tips for choosing foods from within each group.

The MyPlate food guidance system helps you implement the recommendations of the *Dietary Guidelines for Americans*, and provides a visual aid to assist in improving diet and lifestyle. MyPlate provides a visual reminder of a key nutrition principle: Fruits and vegetables form the foundation of a healthy diet and should fill at least half of a plate at every meal. MyPlate is designed to help you:

- Make smart choices from every food group;
- Find your balance between food and physical activity; and
- Get the most nutrition out of your calories by focusing on nutrient-dense foods in sensible portion sizes.

FIGURE 2-8

The MyPlate Food Guide

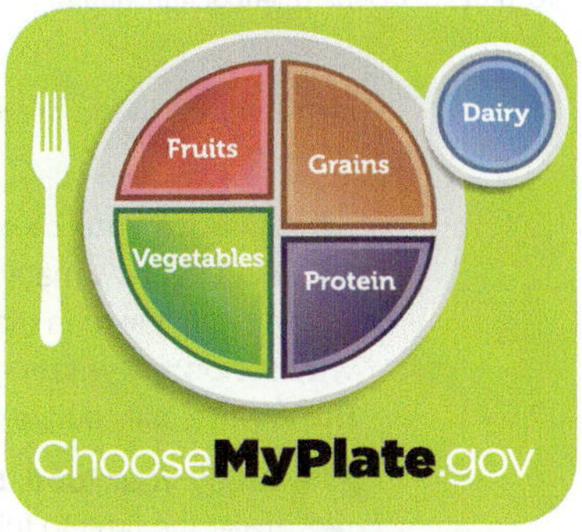

© Cengage

A healthy meal starts with more vegetables and fruits and smaller portions of protein and grains. Adjust the portions on your plate to get more of what you need without too many calories. Choose milk with your meal or add low-fat dairy products to your plate.

Some popular foods don't fit neatly into one MyPlate food group. For example, a slice of cheese pizza includes servings from several groups: the crust from the grains group, the tomato sauce from the vegetable group, and the cheese from the dairy group. For more information on menu planning with the MyPlate tool, go to www.ChooseMyPlate.gov.

Using MyPlate to Achieve a Healthy Lifestyle

MyPlate is designed to help consumers choose foods that supply a good balance of nutrients, and it aims to moderate or limit dietary components often consumed in excess, such as saturated fat, *trans* fat, added sugar, and sodium, in keeping with the U.S. government's *Dietary Guidelines for Americans*. MyPlate includes six key components that can help you achieve a healthy lifestyle, including:

1. **Activity.** The MyPlate website promotes regular physical activity and reduced sedentary activities. As part of an overall healthy eating pattern, balancing caloric intake with energy needs can help reduce the risk of chronic disease, help prevent weight gain, and help sustain weight loss. Adults should do at least 2 hours and 30 minutes each week of aerobic physical activity at a moderate level or 1 hour and 15 minutes each week of aerobic physical activity at a vigorous level. Some examples of moderate physical activity are walking briskly, swimming, and bicycling on level terrain. Some examples of vigorous physical activity are jogging, swimming continuous laps, and bicycling uphill.
2. **Variety.** MyPlate creates a foundation for good nutrition and health by guiding us to make food selections from all food groups and subgroups. Different foods contain different nutrients and other substances known to be protective against chronic diseases. No one food or single food group provides all essential nutrients in amounts necessary for good health.
3. **Proportionality.** MyPlate shows the proportions of foods that should make up a healthy diet. MyPlate illustrates the five food groups using a familiar mealtime visual, a place setting. The plate is split into four sections: red for fruits, green for vegetables, purple for protein, and orange for grains (refer to Figure 2-8). A separate blue section, shaped like a drinking glass, represents dairy foods. The MyPlate food guide advises you to eat more of some foods

food group plan A diet-planning tool, such as MyPlate, that groups foods according to similar origin and nutrient content and then specifies the amount of food a person should eat from each group.

serving The standard amount of food used as a reference to give advice regarding how much to eat (such as a 1-cup serving of milk); serving sizes also allow comparisons to be made when reading food labels.

FIGURE 2-9

Choose MyPlate: Ten Tips to a Great Plate

SOURCE: U.S. Department of Agriculture

Use the ideas in this list to *balance your calories*, to choose foods to *eat more often*, and to cut back on foods to *eat less often*.

1 Balance your calories
Find out how many calories you need for a day as a first step in managing your weight. Go to **www.ChooseMyPlate.gov** to find your calorie level. Being physically active also helps you balance calories.

2 Enjoy your food, but eat less
Take the time to fully enjoy your food as you eat it. Pay attention to hunger and fullness cues before, during, and after meals. Use them to recognize when to eat and when you've had enough.

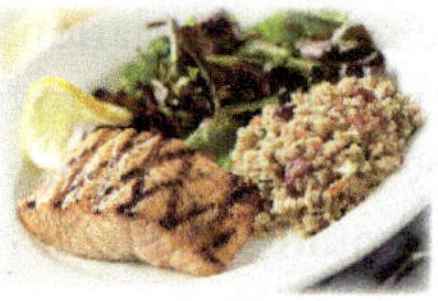

3 Avoid oversized portions
Use a smaller plate, bowl, and glass. Portion out foods before you eat. When eating out, choose a smaller size option, share a dish, or take home part of your meal.

4 Eat some foods more often
Eat more vegetables, fruits, whole grains, and fat-free or 1% dairy products. Make them the basis for meals and snacks.

5 Make half your plate fruits and vegetables
Choose red, orange, and dark-green vegetables like tomatoes, sweet potatoes, and broccoli, along with other vegetables for your meals. Add fruit to meals as part of main or side dishes or as dessert.

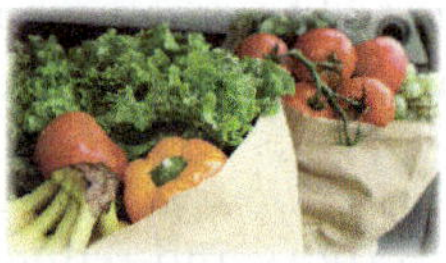

6 Switch to fat-free or low-fat (1%) milk
They have the same amount of calcium and other essential nutrients as whole milk, but fewer calories and less saturated fat.

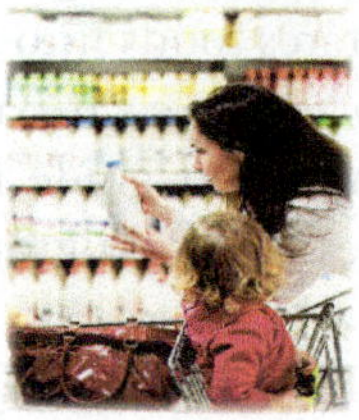

7 Make half your grains whole grains
To eat more whole grains, substitute a whole-grain product for a refined product—such as eating whole-wheat bread instead of white bread or brown rice instead of white rice.

8 Eat certain foods less often
Cut back on foods high in solid fats, added sugars, and salt. They include cakes, cookies, ice cream, candies, sweetened drinks, pizza, and fatty meats like ribs, sausages, bacon, and hot dogs. Use these foods as occasional treats, not everyday foods.

9 Compare sodium in foods
Use the Nutrition Facts label to choose lower sodium versions of foods like soup, bread, and frozen meals. Select canned foods labeled "low sodium," reduced sodium," or "no salt added."

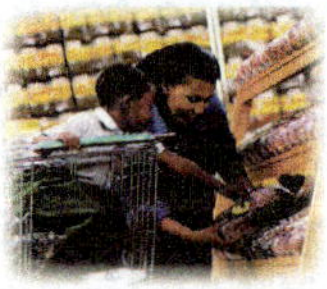

10 Drink water instead of sugary drinks
Cut calories by drinking water or unsweetened beverages. Soda, energy drinks, and sports drinks are major sources of added sugar and calories in many diets.

Source: Adapted from Center for Nutrition Policy and Promotion, Tip Sheet No. 1. June 2011. Go to www.ChooseMyPlate.gov

GRAINS Make half your grains whole	VEGETABLES Vary your veggies	FRUITS Focus on fruits	DAIRY Get your calcium-rich foods	PROTEIN FOODS Go lean with protein
Eat at least 3 oz of whole grain cereals, breads, crackers, rice, or pasta every day. 1 oz is about 1 slice of bread, about 1 cup of breakfast cereal, or 1/2 cup of cooked rice, cereal, or pasta.	Eat more dark-green veggies like broccoli, spinach, and other dark leafy greens. Eat more orange vegetables like carrots and sweet potatoes. Eat more dry beans and peas like pinto beans, kidney beans, and lentils.	Eat a variety of fruit. Choose fresh, frozen, canned, or dried fruit. Go easy on fruit juices.	Go low-fat or fat-free when you choose milk, yogurt, and other milk products. If you don't or can't consume milk, choose lactose-free products or other calcium sources such as fortified foods and beverages. 1 cup = 1 1/2 oz natural cheese, or 2 oz processed cheese.	Choose low-fat or lean meats and poultry. Bake it, broil it, or grill it. Vary your protein routine—choose more fish, beans, peas, nuts, and seeds. 1 oz = 1 oz meat, poultry, or fish; 1/4 cup cooked dry beans; 1 egg; 1 tbsp peanut butter; 1/2 oz nuts/seeds.
For a 2,000-calorie diet, you need the amounts below from each food group. To find the amounts that are right for you, go to www.ChooseMyPlate.gov.				
Eat 6 oz every day.	Eat 2 1/2 cups every day.	Eat 2 cups every day.	Get 3 cups every day; for kids aged 2 to 8, it's 2.	Eat 5 1/2 oz every day.

*Make the most of your fat choices from fish, nuts, and vegetable oils. Find your allowance for oils at www.ChooseMyPlate.gov.

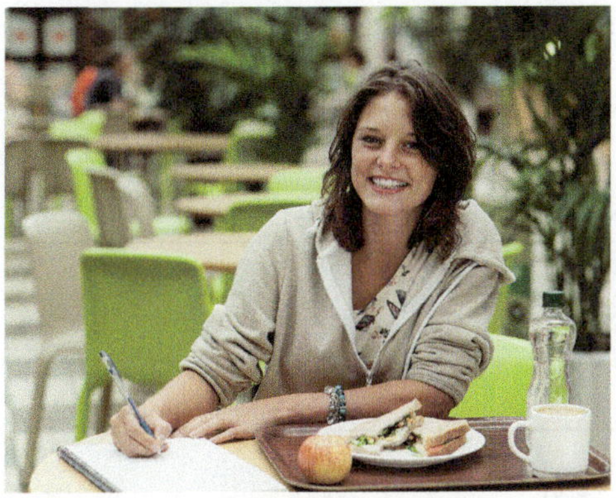

wavebreakmedia/Shutterstock.com

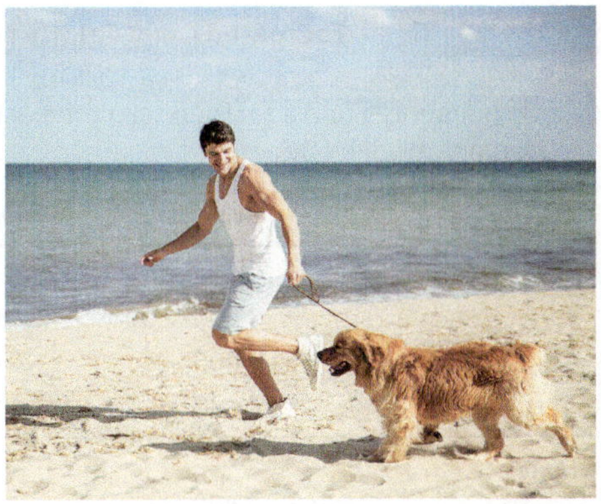

Dean Drobot/Shutterstock.com

The MyPlate Food Guidance System calls for eating a variety of foods to get the nutrients you need and at the same time the right amount of calories to maintain a healthy weight. Remember to balance the energy consumed with the energy expended in play.

(fruits, vegetables, whole grains, and fat-free or low-fat milk products), and eat less of others (such as foods high in refined grains and added sugars).

4. **Moderation.** Currently, many of the foods and beverages Americans eat and drink supply *empty calories*—calories from **solid fats** and/or **added sugars**. Solid fats and added sugars add calories to the food but few or no nutrients and are thus called *empty calories*. A small amount of empty calories is fine, but most people eat far more than is healthy. It is important to emphasize nutrient-rich foods in the diet and limit empty calories to the amount that fits your calorie and nutrient needs. Making better choices, like unsweetened applesauce or extra-lean ground beef, can help keep your intake of added sugars and solid fats low.
5. **Personalization.** One size doesn't fit all. MyPlate can help you choose the foods and amounts of food that are right for you. For a quick estimate of what and how much you need to eat, enter your age, gender, and physical activity level in the "Daily Checklist" online tool at www.ChooseMyPlate.gov. You can also print out a worksheet based on your personal food plan to help you track your progress. Use the SuperTracker "Food Tracker" at www.supertracker.usda.gov to get a personalized nutrition and activity plan. The Spotlight feature at the end of this chapter shows you how to sort ethnic foods into the MyPlate food groups.
6. **Gradual improvement.** Individuals can benefit from taking small steps to improve their diet and lifestyle every day (for example, taking the stairs instead of the elevator or escalator, or ordering a green salad instead of fries).

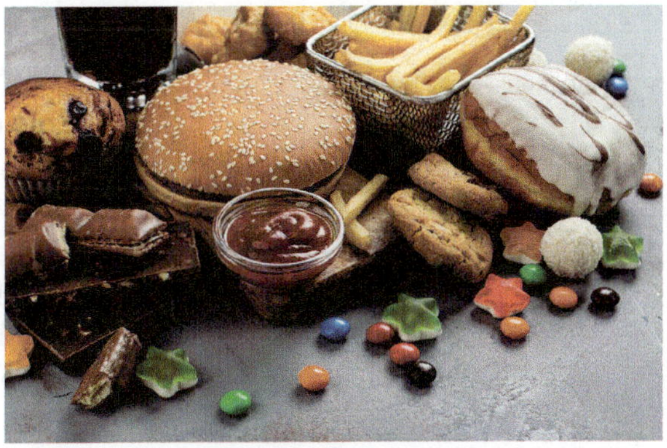

Ekaterina Markelova/Shutterstock.com

Choose nutrient-dense foods most often, and limit intakes of foods and beverages with solid fats or added sugars.

solid fats Fats that are solid at room temperature. These fats may be visible or may be a constituent of foods such as milk, cheese, meats, or baked products, and most have a high percentage of saturated fatty acids (see Chapter 5). Common solid fats include butter, beef fat, chicken fat, pork fat (lard), stick margarine, and shortening. The fat in whole milk is also considered to be solid fat because it is solid at room temperature but suspended in milk by the process of homogenization.

added sugars Sugars and other caloric sweeteners that are added to foods during processing or preparation. Added sugars do not include naturally occurring sugars such as those found in milk and fruits.

Use the Simplicity of MyPlate to Build a Healthy Eating Plan

You can determine the right amount of foods to eat to meet your personal energy needs and promote a healthy weight in three easy steps (see Figure 2-10).

Step 1: **Estimate Your Daily Energy Needs.** Use Table 2-3 to find your estimated daily energy needs, or go to www.ChooseMyPlate.gov and enter your age, gender, and usual activity level. If you are moderately physically active, you need fewer calories than those who are more active.

FIGURE 2-10

Making Use of MyPlate

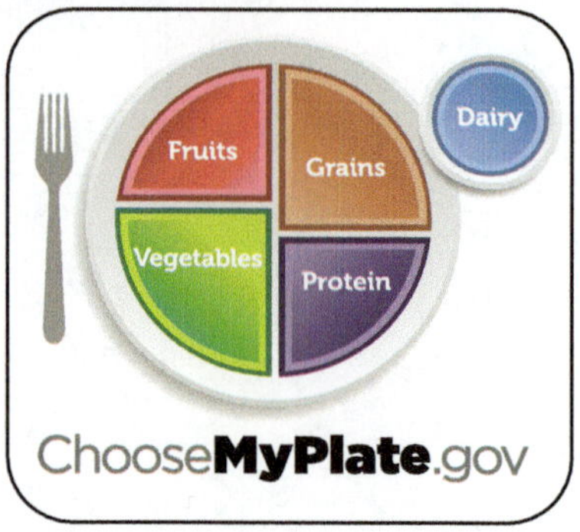

Making Use of MyPlate

- Estimate daily energy needs and balance food intake with physical activity.
- Note amount of food to eat from each food group.
- Plan meals and snacks.

TABLE 2-3 Estimated Daily Calorie Needs for Adults[a]

Find your gender and age. Then select the activity level that best describes your lifestyle (sedentary, moderately active, or active).

Activity Level:	Sedentary[b]	Moderate[c]	Active[d]
Females			
19–30	1,800–2,000	2,000–2,200	2,400
31–50	1,800	2,000	2,200
51+	1,600	1,800	2,000–2,200
Males			
19–30	2,400–2,600	2,600–2,800	3,000
31–50	2,200–2,400	2,400–2,600	2,800–3,000
51+	2,000–2,200	2,200–2,400	2,400–2,800

[a] The calorie levels in each gender and age group are based on people of average height and at a healthy weight. A range of calories is given to meet needs of different ages within the group. For adults, fewer calories are needed at older ages.

[b] **Sedentary:** less than 30 minutes a day of moderate physical activity in addition to daily activities.

[c] **Moderately active:** at least 30 minutes and up to 60 minutes a day of moderate physical activity in addition to daily activities.

[d] **Active:** 60 or more minutes a day of moderate physical activity in addition to daily activities.

NOTE: For more information, visit www.ChooseMyPlate.gov.

Step 2: **Build Your Daily Eating Plan.** Use your estimated number of calories to build a daily eating plan that incorporates all five food groups. How much food do you need to eat each day? MyPlate provides guidance by indicating an appropriate amount of food to eat from each food group that will supply not only necessary nutrients but also adequate amounts of calories. Table 2-4 specifies the amounts of foods from each group that are needed daily to create a healthy eating plan at several calorie levels.

TABLE 2-4 Build Your Eating Plan with Recommended Daily Amounts from Each Food Group

Find your calorie level at the top of the chart. Follow the column below your estimated calorie level to see how much food to eat from each of the food groups. (Estimated daily energy needs are shown in Table 2-3.) Recommended amounts for fruits, vegetables, and dairy are measured in cups and those for grains and meats, in ounces.

Calorie Level:	1,600	1,800	2,000	2,200	2,400	2,600	2,800	3,000
Grains	5 oz	6 oz	6 oz	7 oz	8 oz	9 oz	10 oz	10 oz
Vegetables	2 cups	2½ cups	2½ cups	3 cups	3 cups	3½ cups	3½ cups	4 cups
Fruits	1½ cups	1½ cups	2 cups	2 cups	2 cups	2 cups	2½ cups	2½ cups
Dairy	3 cups	3 cups	3 cups	3 cups	3 cups	3 cups	3 cups	3 cups
Protein Foods	5 oz	5 oz	5½ oz	6 oz	6½ oz	6½ oz	7 oz	7 oz
Oils	5 tsp	5 tsp	6 tsp	6 tsp	7 tsp	8 tsp	8 tsp	10 tsp
Daily Limit for Discretionary Calories (calories for other uses)*	130 cal	170 cal	270 cal	280 cal	350 cal	380 cal	400 cal	470 cal

**The Daily Limit for Discretionary Calories* (extra fats and added sugars) includes the balance of calories remaining in a person's estimated energy allowance after accounting for the number of calories needed to meet recommended nutrient intakes through consumption of foods in low-fat or no-added-sugar forms. The calories assigned to discretionary calories may be used to increase intake from the basic food groups; to select foods from these groups that are higher in fat or with added sugars; to add oils, solid fats, or sugars to foods or beverages; or to consume alcohol.

Step 3: **Let MyPlate Guide Your Food Choices.** Eating is one of life's great pleasures. Different people like different foods and like to prepare the same foods in different ways. Because you can build a healthy menu using many foods in many ways, you have lots of room for choice. MyPlate can provide a starting point to develop healthy eating patterns while still allowing for personal preferences in food choices. Make choices from each major food group and combine them however you like. Read food labels to identify foods that are higher in saturated fats, *trans* fats, added sugars, and sodium. Some items in each food group may be difficult to fit into a healthy eating plan on a regular basis.

If you consistently build your diet by choosing mostly nutrient-dense foods that are low in solid fat and added sugars, you may be able to meet your nutrient needs without using your full calorie allowance. If so, you may have what is called a **daily limit of calories for other uses**—or **discretionary calories**—for use in meeting the rest of your calorie needs (see Figure 2-11). Most discretionary calorie allowances are very small, between 100 and 300 calories, especially for those who are not physically active. Keep in mind that, for many people, the discretionary calorie limit is totally used up by the foods they choose with solid fats and added sugars, such as higher-fat meats, higher-fat cheeses, whole milk, and sweetened bakery products.

Using MyPlate to Meet Nutrient Needs

Using MyPlate to assess and plan your own diet requires an understanding of how much food to consume from the various food groups. For instance, one slice of bread, half a bagel, and ½ cup of pasta each count as 1 ounce from the Grains group. When it comes to vegetables, 1 cup of raw or cooked vegetables is equivalent to 2 cups of leafy raw vegetables. Figure 2-12 shows the recommended amounts of food to eat from each of the various food groups. Besides showing what foods are the equivalent of one serving from each food group, Figure 2-12 also lists the nutrients supplied by each of the five food groups.

daily limit of calories for other uses or **discretionary calories** The balance of calories remaining in a person's energy allowance, after accounting for the number of calories needed to meet recommended nutrient intakes through consumption of nutrient-dense foods.

FIGURE 2-11

Discretionary Calories in a 2,000-Calorie Diet

Your discretionary calorie limit can be used to:

- Eat additional nutrient-dense foods from each of the food groups, such as an extra container of fat-free yogurt or an extra piece of fruit;
- Select limited amounts of foods that are not in their most nutrient-dense form and/or contain solid fats or added sugars, such as whole milk, full-fat cheese, and sweetened cereal;
- Add fats or sweeteners to foods, such as sauces, gravies, sugar, syrup, butter, and jelly; or
- Eat or drink items that contain only fats, caloric sweeteners, and/or alcohol, such as candy, soda, wine, and beer.

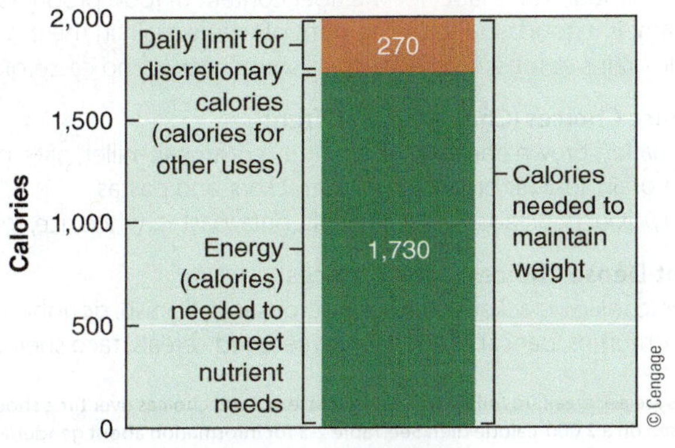

FIGURE 2-12

Making the Most of Your Personal Food Plan[a]

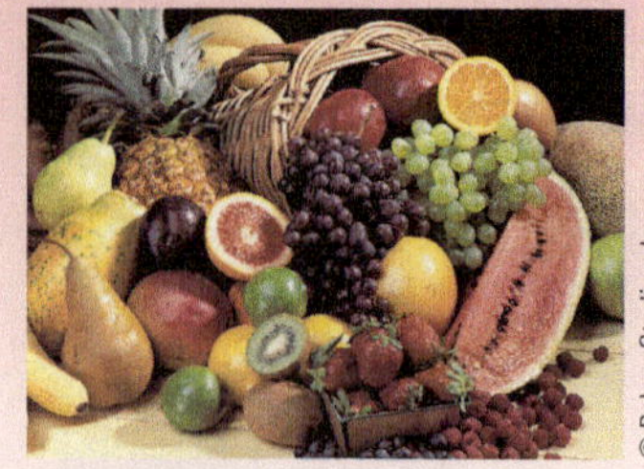

© Polara Studios, Inc.

Goal: 2 cups

½ cup is equivalent to:

- ½ cup fresh, frozen, or canned fruit
- 1 medium fruit
- ¼ cup dried fruit
- ½ cup fruit juice

Fruit Group Supplies vitamin C, beta-carotene, potassium, folate, magnesium, and fiber.

Tip: Choose a variety of whole or cut-up fruits more often as snacks or with meals, instead of juice.

- Use fruit in salads, toppings, desserts, and/or snacks regularly.
- Use fruit as a topping on cereal, pancakes, and other foods rather than sugars and syrups.
- Buy fruits that are dried, frozen, and canned (in water or juice) as well as fresh, so that you always have a supply on hand.

Nutrient-Dense Choices (Choose Most Often)

Apples, apricots, avocados, bananas, blueberries, cantaloupe, cherries, grapefruit, grapes, guava, honeydew, kiwi, mango, oranges, papaya, peaches, pears, pineapples, plums, raspberries, strawberries, watermelon, dried fruit, 100% fruit juices

Less Nutrient-Dense Choices (Limit Choices)

Canned or frozen fruit in syrup; juices, punches, and fruit drinks with added sugars

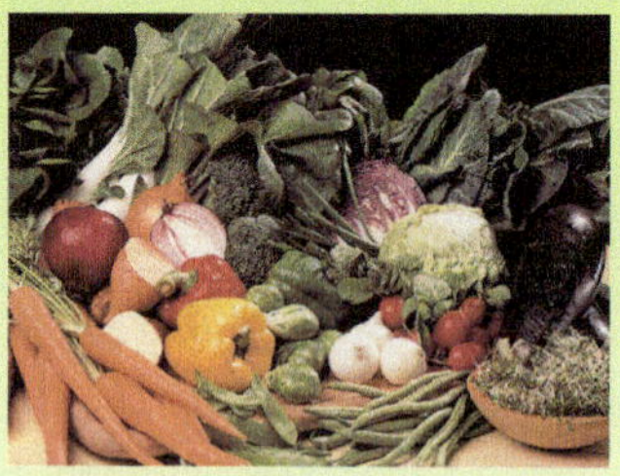

© Polara Studios, Inc.

Goal: 2½ cups

½ cup is equivalent to:

- ½ cup cut-up raw or cooked vegetables
- 1 cup raw leafy vegetable
- ½ cup vegetable juice

Vegetable Subgroups:

Dark-green vegetables	1½ cups/week
Red and orange vegetables	5½ cups/week
Legumes (dry beans)	1½ cups/week
Starchy vegetables	5 cups/week
Other vegetables	4 cups/week

Vegetable Group Supplies vitamin C, vitamin K, beta-carotene, potassium, folate, calcium, magnesium, and fiber.

Tip: Enjoy a colorful variety of vegetables every day. Choose from all five vegetable subgroups several times a week.

- Stock up on frozen vegetables for quick and easy cooking.
- Add dark green or red and orange vegetables to soups, stews, casseroles, and stir-fries.
- Use romaine, spinach, or other dark leafy greens as salad greens, and eat green salads often.
- Choose main dishes, side dishes, and salads that include cooked dry beans or peas.

Nutrient-Dense Choices (Choose Most Often)

Dark-green vegetables: Broccoli and leafy greens such as arugula, kale, bok choy, romaine lettuce; spinach, beet, collard, mustard, and turnip greens

Red and orange vegetables: Carrots, pumpkin, sweet potatoes, winter squash, red bell peppers, tomatoes, tomato juice, vegetable juice

Legumes: Black beans, black-eyed peas, chickpeas (garbanzo beans), kidney beans, pinto beans, soybeans and soy products, split peas, and lentils

Starchy vegetables: Cassava, corn, green peas, hominy, lima beans, and white potatoes

Other vegetables: Artichokes, asparagus, bamboo shoots, beets, Brussels sprouts, cabbage, cauliflower, celery, cucumbers, eggplant, green beans, iceberg lettuce, mushrooms, okra, onions, green bell peppers, snow peas, zucchini

Less Nutrient-Dense Choices (Limit Choices)

Baked beans, candied sweet potatoes, coleslaw, French fries, potato salad, refried beans, scalloped potatoes, tempura vegetables

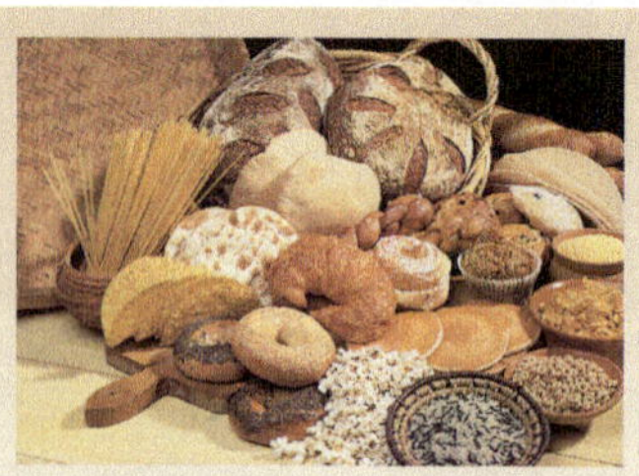

© Polara Studios, Inc.

Goal: 6 oz

1 ounce is equivalent to:

- 1 slice bread, 1 mini bagel, 6-inch tortilla, ½ English muffin
- 1 cup dry cereal
- ½ cup cooked rice, pasta, cereal
- 1 packet instant oatmeal
- 3 cups popcorn

Grain Group Supplies folate, niacin, riboflavin, thiamin, magnesium, selenium, iron, and fiber.

Tip: Make most (at least half) of your grain selections whole grains.

- Buy products that list a whole grain or a whole-wheat or other whole-grain flour first on the label's ingredient list.
- Check the Nutrition Facts label for the fiber content of food products.
- Fiber content is a good clue to the amount of whole grain in the product.
- Add whole grains to mixed dishes such as soups, stews, and casseroles.

Nutrient-Dense Choices (Choose Most Often)

Whole grains: Barley, brown and wild rice, bulgur, cornmeal, millet, oats, popcorn, quinoa, rye, wheat; whole-grain, low-fat breads, cereals, crackers, and pastas

Enriched grain products: Breads, bagels, cereals, grits, pastas, white rice, rolls, and tortillas

Less Nutrient-Dense Choices (Limit Choices)

Biscuits, cakes, cookies, crackers, cornbread, croissants, Danish, doughnuts, fried rice, French toast, granola, muffins, pancakes, pies, presweetened cereals, taco shells, waffles

[a] All goals are per day unless otherwise noted. Vegetable subgroup amounts are per week. To follow this eating pattern, food choices over time should provide these amounts of food from each group on average. Recommended amounts to eat are based on a 2,000-calorie diet. See Table 2-3 for information about gender/age/activity levels and appropriate calorie intakes. See Table 2-4 for more information on the food groups, amounts, and food intake patterns at other calorie levels, or go to www.ChooseMyPlate.gov.

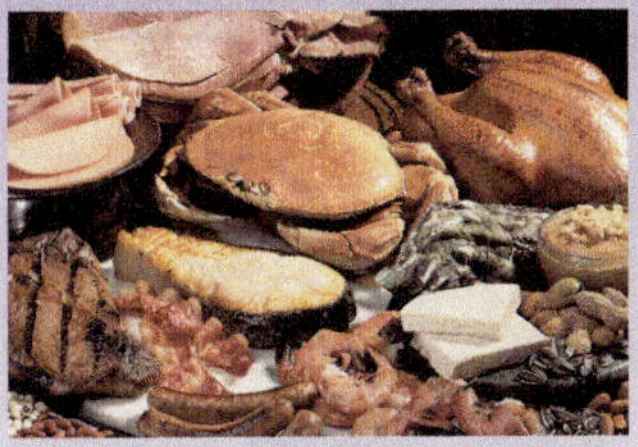

© Polara Studios, Inc.

Goal: 5½ oz

1 ounce is equivalent to:

- 1 oz cooked lean meats, poultry, or seafood
- 1 egg
- ¼ cup cooked legumes or tofu
- 1 tbsp peanut butter
- ½ oz nuts or seeds
- ½ cup split-pea soup

Protein Foods Subgroups:

Seafood	8 oz/week
Meats, poultry, eggs	26 oz/week
Nuts, seeds, soy products	5 oz/week

Protein Foods Group Supplies protein, essential fatty acids, zinc, iron, niacin, thiamin, phosphorus, magnesium, potassium, vitamin B_6, vitamin B_{12}, and fiber (legumes).

Tip: Make most choices lean or low-fat and choose from all three subgroups.

- Select meat cuts that are low in fat and ground beef that is extra lean (at least 90% lean).
- Trim fat from meat and remove poultry skin before cooking or eating.
- Drain fat from ground meats after cooking.
- Use preparation methods that do not add fat, such as grilling, broiling, poaching, or roasting.
- Select fish twice a week, especially fish rich in omega-3 fatty acids, such as salmon, trout, and herring.
- Choose legumes as a main dish often.
- Choose unsalted nuts as a snack, on salads, or in main dishes, to replace meat or poultry.

Nutrient-Dense Choices (Choose Most Often)

Lean meat, fish, shellfish, poultry (no skin), eggs, legumes, soy products (tofu, tempeh, textured vegetable protein), peanuts, peanut butter, unsalted nuts, and seeds (flaxseeds, pumpkin seeds, sesame seeds, sunflower seeds)

Less Nutrient-Dense Choices (Limit Choices)

Luncheon meats, ground beef, hot dogs, fried meats, fried fish, fried poultry, or fried eggs, poultry with skin, refried beans, sausages

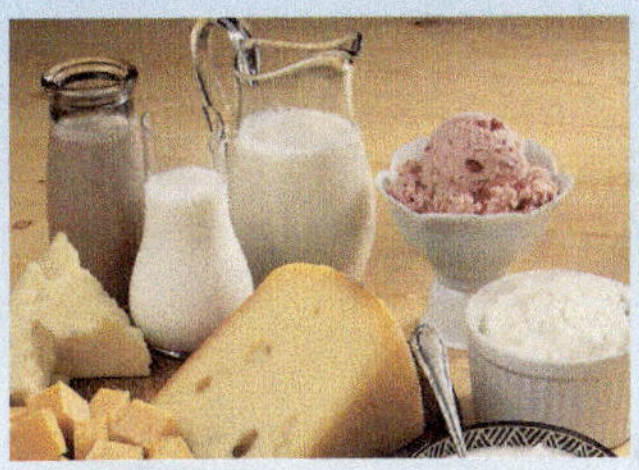

© Polara Studios, Inc.

Goal: 3 cups

1 cup is equivalent to:

- 1 cup low-fat/fat-free milk, yogurt
- 1½ oz low-fat or fat-free natural cheese
- 2 oz low-fat or fat-free processed cheese
- ⅓ cup shredded cheese

Dairy Group Supplies protein, calcium, potassium, riboflavin, vitamin B_{12}, vitamin A, and vitamin D.

Tip: Make fat-free or low-fat choices. Choose other calcium-rich foods or fortified cereals or beverages if milk products are not consumed.

- Drink fat-free or low-fat (1%) milk as a beverage.
- Use fat-free or low-fat milk or yogurt on cereal or as a snack.
- If you drink cappuccinos or lattes, ask for them with fat-free milk.
- Add fat-free or low-fat milk instead of water to oatmeal and hot cereals.
- Choose low-fat cheeses.

Nutrient-Dense Choices (Choose Most Often)

Fat-free or 1% low-fat milk and milk products such as buttermilk, cheeses, cottage cheese, yogurt; fat-free fortified soy milk

Less Nutrient-Dense Choices (Limit Choices)

Reduced-fat 2% milk, whole milk, reduced-fat and whole-milk products such as cheeses, cottage cheese, yogurt, chocolate milk, custards and puddings, ice cream, milkshakes, frozen yogurt, and fortified soy milk

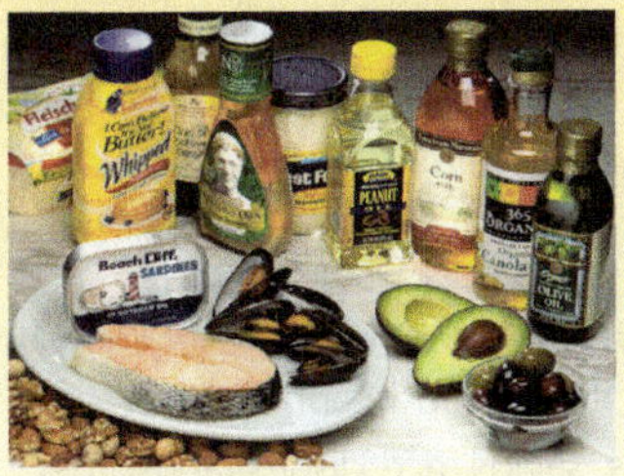

© Polara Studios, Inc.

1 tsp equivalent is:

- 1 tsp vegetable oil
- 1 tsp soft margarine
- 1 tbsp low-fat mayonnaise
- 2 tbsp light salad dressing

Oils Supplies vitamin E and essential fatty acids.

Tip: Choose most fats from sources of monounsaturated and polyunsaturated fatty acids, such as fish, nuts, seeds, and vegetable oils.

- Substitute vegetable oils for solid fats like butter, stick margarine, shortening, or lard.

Nutrient-Dense Choices (Choose Most Often)

Liquid vegetable oils such as canola, corn, flaxseed, olive, peanut, safflower, sesame, soybean, and sunflower oils; mayonnaise, oil-based salad dressing, and soft *trans*-free margarine; foods naturally high in oils, such as avocados, nuts, seeds, olives, fatty fish, and shellfish

Limit Solid Fats

Butter, animal fats, processed meats, fried foods, stick margarine, shortening, lard

THE SAVVY Diner

Color Your Plate for Health with a Variety of Fruits and Vegetables (Obj. 2.5)

The message is simple: *Eat plenty of fruits and vegetables every day for better health.* Most Americans, however, find this simple bit of nutritional advice challenging to put into practice. Overwhelming evidence points to the health benefits available from diets rich in fruits and vegetables because of the vitamins, minerals, and **phytochemicals** (*phyto* is the Greek word for "plant") found in plant foods.

In the classic sense, the naturally occurring phytochemicals—for example, lycopene, a pigment that makes tomatoes red and watermelon pink—are not vitamins, minerals, or nutrients because they do not provide energy or building materials. However, scientists who study them say that phytochemicals may have the potential to slow the aging process; boost immune function; decrease blood pressure and cholesterol; prevent cataracts; prevent, slow, or even reverse certain cancers; and strengthen our hearts and circulatory systems. (More about the food sources and beneficial effects of phytochemicals appears in Chapter 7.)

How can you incorporate fruits and vegetables into your diet to achieve the maximum health benefits? Aim for the amounts of fruits and vegetables recommended in MyPlate (about 2 cups of fruits and 2½ cups of vegetables on a 2,000-calorie diet).* Go to www.ChooseMyPlate.gov to determine your own recommended intake of fruits and vegetables. Also consider the following three steps in your daily food planning.

1 Color Your Plate with Health-Protective Foods.

Consume many differently colored fruits and vegetables. Select at least three differently colored fruits and vegetables a day. The red pigment in tomatoes has different bioactive properties than the orange pigments in carrots, sweet potatoes, melon, or winter squash. Add dark-green leafy vegetables such as kale, mustard greens, collards, and spinach, along with broccoli and Brussels sprouts. Fruits are a vital powerhouse of the **antioxidant nutrients** that act to squelch cell-damaging molecules in the body. Blueberries top the list for being one of the highest in antioxidants. Be sure to include citrus fruits such as oranges and grapefruit regularly, as they contain many compounds that have antioxidant and other vital health benefits.

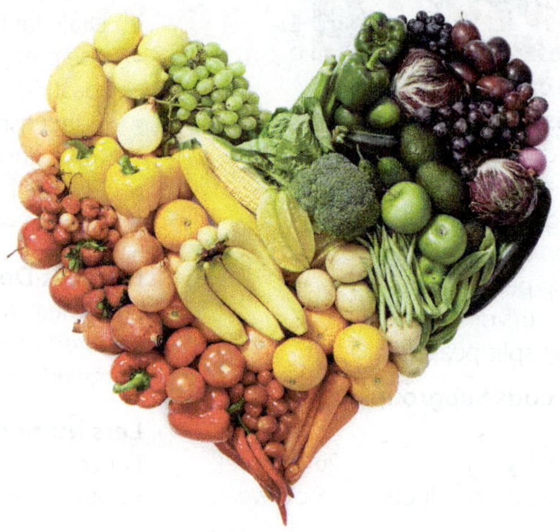

© iStockphoto.com/ansonsaw

Eating patterns rich in fruits and vegetables and low in saturated fat may reduce the risk of heart disease and some types of cancer—diseases associated with many factors.

2 Be Adventurous: Select from as Wide a Variety of Fruits and Vegetables as Possible.

Foods within each group of the MyPlate Food Guidance System have similar nutrient content. Choosing foods from each group offers a variety of the nutrients necessary for health, but variety within food groups is valuable, too. Even fruits that may seem like comparable foods often provide a number of different nutrients; no food has them all. For example, strawberries are higher in vitamin C than raspberries; but neither supply beta-carotene (a precursor of vitamin A); a pink grapefruit is high in beta-carotene, but a white grapefruit is not.

3 Make It Easy on Yourself!

Keep fruit and sliced vegetables in easy-to-reach places, such as sliced vegetables in the refrigerator and fresh fruit on the table. For convenience, keep a variety of fresh, frozen, and canned fruits and vegetables on hand to add to soups, salads, rice dishes, and other menu items. Frozen fruits and vegetables are processed right after harvesting and contain nutrient profiles similar to fresh produce. If using canned items, choose fruits packed in fruit juice (not in syrup) and remove excess salt from vegetables by rinsing before using them.

*In general, 1 cup fruit or 100% fruit juice, or ½ cup dried fruit is considered 1 cup from the fruit group; 1 cup raw or cooked vegetables or vegetable juice, or 2 cups raw leafy vegetables are considered as 1 cup from the vegetable group.

phytochemicals Nonnutritive compounds in plants that confer color and other characteristics. Some phytochemicals provide health-protecting benefits in the body.

antioxidant nutrients Vitamins and minerals that protect other compounds from damaging reactions involving oxygen by themselves reacting with oxygen. The antioxidant nutrients are vitamin C, vitamin E, and beta-carotene. The mineral selenium also has a role in antioxidant reactions in the body.

2.5 How Well Do We Eat?

How are consumers doing in following the nutrition recommendations presented in this chapter? The answer to this question is, "Needs improvement." Undoubtedly, trends such as eating away from home and increased portion sizes in restaurant and carryout items negatively affect American eating habits.

Figure 2-13 and Figure 2-14 provide insights into how the typical American diet compares to recommended intakes or limits.[10] In general, we eat too many calories and too much solid fat, added sugars, refined grains, and sodium. Solid fats and added sugars should make up only a small proportion of total calories in the diet. However, as illustrated in Figure 2-13, Americans consume about 35 percent of total calories from foods high in solid fats and added sugars—soft drinks, desserts, fatty meats, French fries, pizza, and whole-milk products, in contrast to a recommended limit of no more than 5 to 15 percent of total calories for most individuals.

In general, we do not meet recommendations for vegetables, fruit, dairy, oils, or whole grains, and exceed recommendations, leading to overconsumption of sodium, saturated fat, refined grains, solid fats, and added sugars. As shown in Figure 2-14, three-fourths of the population has an eating pattern that is low in vegetables, fruits, dairy, and oils, and half the population is not meeting the recommendation for whole grains. By eating fewer nutrient-dense foods from these food groups, consumers are at risk for lower than recommended levels of specific nutrients, including vitamin D, calcium, potassium, and dietary fiber. Some 70 percent of consumers exceed the recommended limits—less than 10 percent of calories per day—for both added sugars and saturated fat. Added sugars account for almost 270 calories, or more than 13 percent of calories per day in the average U.S. diet; average intake of saturated fat is 11 percent of calories. Most consumers also have sodium intakes above the Tolerable Upper Intake Level (2,300 mg). The average daily intake of sodium is 4,240 mg for men and 2,980 mg for women.

FIGURE 2-13

What We Eat vs. Recommended Limits

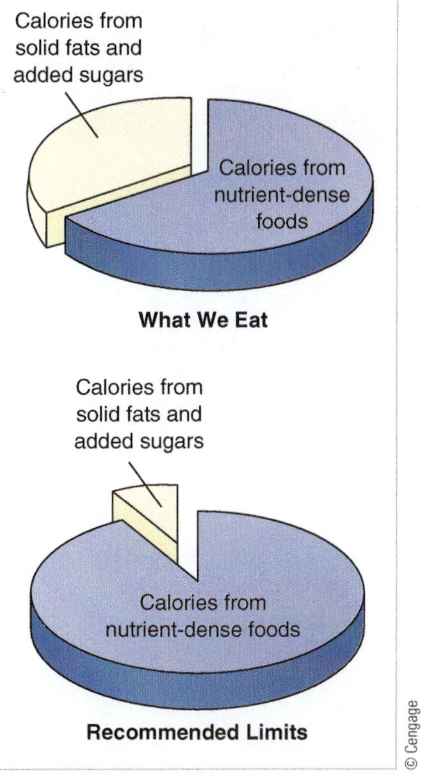

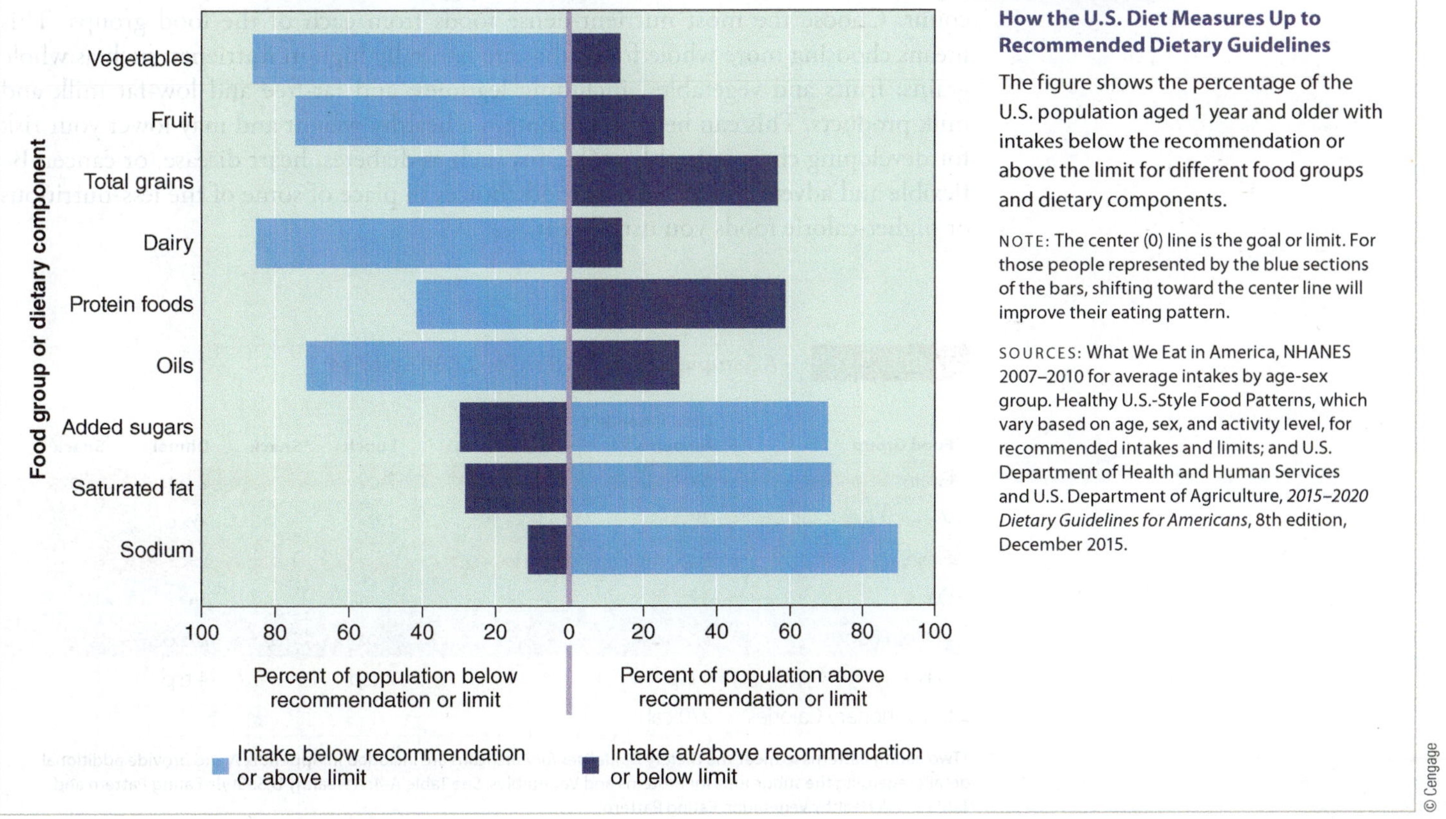

FIGURE 2-14

How the U.S. Diet Measures Up to Recommended Dietary Guidelines

The figure shows the percentage of the U.S. population aged 1 year and older with intakes below the recommendation or above the limit for different food groups and dietary components.

NOTE: The center (0) line is the goal or limit. For those people represented by the blue sections of the bars, shifting toward the center line will improve their eating pattern.

SOURCES: What We Eat in America, NHANES 2007–2010 for average intakes by age-sex group. Healthy U.S.-Style Food Patterns, which vary based on age, sex, and activity level, for recommended intakes and limits; and U.S. Department of Health and Human Services and U.S. Department of Agriculture, *2015–2020 Dietary Guidelines for Americans*, 8th edition, December 2015.

Using MyPlate to Improve Nutrient and Energy Intakes MyPlate can help you get the nutrients your body needs each day. The grains, fruits, and vegetables groups serve as the foundation of a healthy eating pattern because they supply the vitamins, minerals, and fiber lacking in many people's diets. When it comes to the dairy group, low-fat (1%) and fat-free dairy products make the best nutrient-dense choices. Although foods from the protein foods group provide protein, iron, zinc, and other nutrients, some items can contain large amounts of saturated fat and *trans* fat. Thus, choosing wisely from this group goes a long way in limiting the solid fat content of your diet. Because lean cuts of meat, skinless poultry, and fish rank lower in saturated fat than ground beef and chicken with skin, the leaner items should be chosen most often. Dry beans, which contain only a trace of fat, are good choices to add to the diet even more often.

In addition to the five food groups, we need a small amount of oil in our diet because oils provide vitamin E and essential fats. The Oils category includes vegetable oils and soft margarines containing no *trans* fat. Heart-healthy oils like olive, canola, and peanut oil are also good choices. (For more about fats, see Chapter 5.)

According to the Dietary Guidelines Advisory Committee, Americans can benefit from the practice of mindful eating, that is, "consciously" and carefully choosing all foods and beverages consumed.[11] You can improve your health with an eating pattern that is:

- Energy balanced and portion controlled
- Nutrient-dense
- Very low in solid fats and added sugars and low in sodium

A sample eating pattern is given in Table 2-5, and Table 2-6 translates that eating pattern into a nutritious menu.

You can follow the MyPlate guidelines to get enough nutrients without overdoing calories. The way to balance your energy needs is to make your food choices count. Choose the most nutrient-dense foods from each of the food groups. This means choosing more whole foods that are naturally high in nutrients, such as whole grains; fruits and vegetables, including legumes; and fat-free and low-fat milk and milk products. This can help you maintain a healthy weight and may lower your risk for developing chronic health problems, such as diabetes, heart disease, or cancer. Be flexible and adventurous! Try new food choices in place of some of the less-nutritious or higher-calorie foods you usually eat.

TABLE 2-5 A Sample Eating Pattern for 2,000 Calories[a]

Food Group	Recommended Amounts	Breakfast	Lunch	Snack	Dinner	Snack
Grains	6 oz	1½ oz	2 oz		2 oz	½ oz
Vegetables	2½ c		1 c		1½ c	
Fruits	2 c	½ c		1 c	½ c	
Dairy	3 c	1 c			1 c	1 c
Protein Foods	5½ oz		2 oz	1 oz	2½ oz	
Oils	6 tsp		2 tsp		4 tsp	
Discretionary Calories	270 cal					

[a] Two eating patterns to meet the *Dietary Guidelines for Americans* are included in Appendix A and provide additional details regarding the subgroups for Proteins and Vegetables. See Table A-4: A Healthy U.S.-Style Eating Pattern and Table A-5: A Healthy Vegetarian Eating Pattern.

TABLE 2-6 A Sample Menu for 2,000 Calories

The following menu provides about 1,830 calories, leaving about 170 extra calories to spend on additional nutrient-dense foods, or on foods with added sugars or fats.

Amounts	Menu Item	Calories
	Breakfast	
1½ oz whole grains	1½ c whole-grain cereal	162
1 c dairy	1 c fat-free milk	90
1 c fruit	1 c sliced banana	105
	Lunch	
2 oz whole grains	2 slices rye bread	160
2 oz protein foods	2 oz tuna, packed in water, drained	55
1 c vegetables	2 tbsp kidney beans	25
	6 baby carrots, shredded	25
	¼ c shredded Romaine lettuce	2
	2 slices tomato	10
1 tsp oils	1 tbsp low-fat mayonnaise	35
	1 tsp Dijon mustard	5
8 oz unsweetened beverage	1 c iced tea, unsweetened	0
	Snack	
½ c fruit	¼ c dried apricots	80
1 oz protein foods	½ oz almonds (12 almonds)	80
	Dinner	
	Spinach salad:	
½ c vegetables	1 c raw baby spinach leaves	8
½ oz protein foods	2 tbsp chickpeas	34
½ c fruit	½ c tangerine slices	30
2 tsp oils	2 tsp oil and vinegar dressing	60
	Pasta with meat sauce:	
2 oz enriched grains	1 c rigatoni pasta	197
1 c vegetables	½ c tomato sauce with	25
	½ c mixed frozen vegetables	25
2 oz protein foods	2 oz cooked ground turkey breast,	130
2 tsp oils	sautéed in 2 tsp oil	90
1 c dairy	1½ oz Parmesan cheese	190
	Snack	
1 c dairy	1 c fat-free yogurt parfait with ¼ c berries and ⅛ c low-fat granola	210
¼ c fruit		
½ oz grains		

The Savvy Diner feature on page 48 provides additional tips for including a variety of fruits and vegetables in your diet for maximum health benefits. By incorporating the tips and strategies for healthy eating found in Figure 2-12 into your eating plan, you will get the nutrients you need for good health. To get an idea of how your current diet compares with the recommendations of the interactive MyPlate website, try the Rate Your Plate Scorecard on page 53.

THE **SAVVY** Diner

Rules of Thumb for Portion Sizes—It's All in Your Hands (Obj. 2.4)

In the "more must be better" viewpoint of eating in the United States today, it can be difficult to balance the energy we take in through the food we eat with the energy we expend on a daily basis. This is evidenced by the larger and larger portion sizes we find in restaurants, on the grocery shelves, and in almost every aspect of eating in the United States today.

What's the difference between a *serving* and a portion? A *serving* is a standard amount of food used as a reference to give advice regarding how much food to eat (such as 1 cup milk or its equivalent). The amount of a food that is considered a serving usually stays the same. A *portion*, in contrast, is the amount of food *you* choose to eat, and it may vary from one meal or snack to the next based on your appetite or hunger. How do you determine how much food is in your portion? You can use the following images as a visual reference to "right-size" your portions and avoid consuming extra calories.

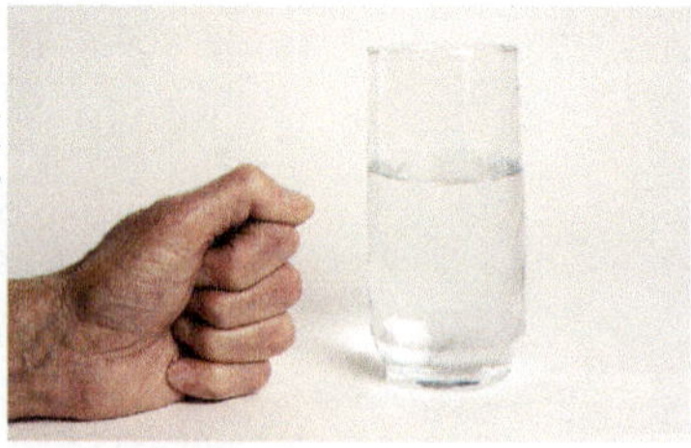

Felicia Martinez/Photography/PhotoEdit

One fist, clenched = 8 fl oz

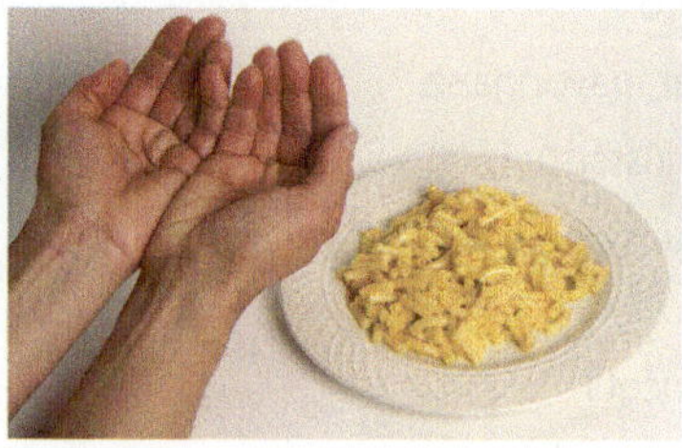

Felicia Martinez/Photography/PhotoEdit

Two hands, cupped = 1 cup

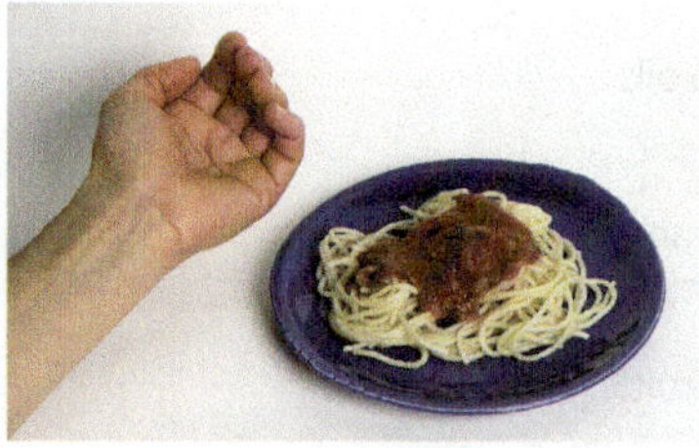

Felicia Martinez/Photography/PhotoEdit

One hand, cupped = 1/2 cup

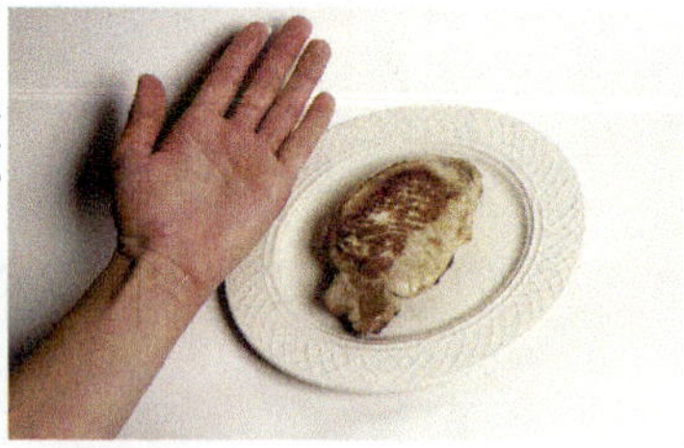

Felicia Martinez/Photography/PhotoEdit

Palm of hand = 3 oz

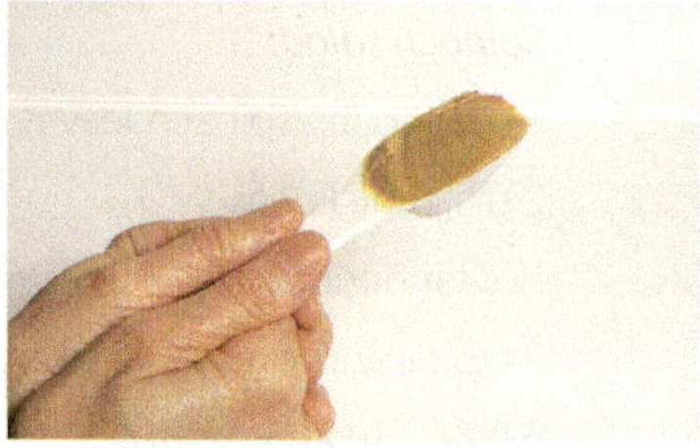

Felicia Martinez/Photography/PhotoEdit

Two thumbs together = 1 tbsp

SOURCE: Adapted from USDA, *Dietary Guidelines for Americans*, 5th ed., 2000.

Food Lists Although food group plans provide sufficient detail to help most healthy people plan a good diet, food lists take meal planning and portion control a step further. As their name implies, **food lists** are simply lists of categories of foods, such as fruit, with portions specified in a way that allows the foods to be mixed and matched or exchanged with one another in the diet (see Appendix A). For instance, you might strive to eat four servings of fruit each day, and the food list shows you that ½ cup of orange juice, a small banana, or a small apple each counts as a fruit.

food lists Lists of foods with serving sizes specified (formerly exchange lists). The foods on a single list are similar with respect to nutrient and calorie content and thus can be mixed and matched in the diet. Appendix A provides more details regarding Choose Your Foods: Food Lists for Diabetes and Weight Management.

Serving sizes within groups are determined by considering the calorie, protein, carbohydrate, and fat content of the food. For example, one fruit contains about 60 calories and 15 grams of carbohydrate. One starch, in contrast, provides about

SCORE Card

Rate Your Plate Using the MyPlate Food Guide (Obj. 2.4)

To see how your diet measures up to the recommendations in the MyPlate food plan, follow these steps:

Step 1: Write down everything you ate yesterday, including meals *and* snacks. Make note of portion sizes as well. (Refer to Figure 2-12 for help with conversions.)

Step 2: Identify the food group for each item you ate. (Refer to Figure 2-12 for help.)

Step 3: Using the five food groups, determine the amounts that are right for you. Go to "SuperTracker" at www.ChooseMyPlate.gov and type in your age, sex, weight, and activity level under the "Daily Checklist" and click on "Calculate Food Plan." This will give you a plan with a good estimate of the amount of food you need from each food group. In addition, it will give you the approximate number of calories you require.

Step 4: Circle the estimated amounts you should eat from the middle column. In the right column, write down the amounts you ate yesterday. (Refer to Figure 2-12 and the "Rules of Thumb for Portion Sizes" Box on page 52 for help with conversions.) Compare the two columns to see how your diet rates.

	Amount You Should Eat	Amount You Ate
Grain group servings (ounces)	5 6 7 8 9 10	________
Vegetable group servings (cups)	2 2½ 3 4	________
Fruit group servings (cups)	1½ 2 2½	________
Dairy group servings (cups)	3	________
Protein Foods group (ounces)	5 5½ 6 7	________
Solid Fats and Added Sugars	Use Discretionary Calorie Limit	________

Step 5: Decide what changes in your eating habits will make your overall eating pattern more healthy. If your diet is "unproportional," with too many foods coming from one food group, make gradual changes to develop a diet with more variety. The chapters that follow offer tips on how to do so.

80 calories, 15 grams of carbohydrate, 3 grams of protein, and a trace of fat. This breakdown makes food lists especially useful tools for people who follow carefully planned diets as a result of a health condition such as diabetes.

2.6 More Tools for Diet Planning

In 1990, Congress passed one of the most important pieces of legislation of the 20th century. Known as the Nutrition Labeling and Education Act, the law called for sweeping changes in the way foods are labeled in the United States.[12] For consumers, the law ensures that food companies provide the kind of nutrition information that best allows people to select foods that fit into a healthy eating plan (see Figure 2-15).

The Affordable Care Act, signed into law on March 23, 2010, mandated that the Food and Drug Administration (FDA) establish labeling requirements for restaurants, similar retail food establishments, and vending machines. Examples of these venues include fast-food outlets, bakeries, coffee shops, and certain grocery

FIGURE 2-15

How to Read a Food Label[a]

You can use food labels to help you make informed food choices for healthy eating practices. The food label allows you to compare similar products, determine the nutritional value of the foods you choose, and increase your awareness of the links between good nutrition and reduced risk of chronic, diet-related diseases.

[a]Manufacturers will need to use the new label by July 26, 2018, and small businesses will have an additional year to comply. During this transition time, you will see either the older Nutrition Facts label or the new label on products.

SOURCE: Food and Drug Administration

The package must always state the product name and the name and address of the manufacturer, packer, or distributor.

Claims such as "Good Source" or "High" can appear on labels but must follow legal definitions.

Approved health claims may be made but only in terms of total diet.

The net contents are shown in weight, measure, or count.

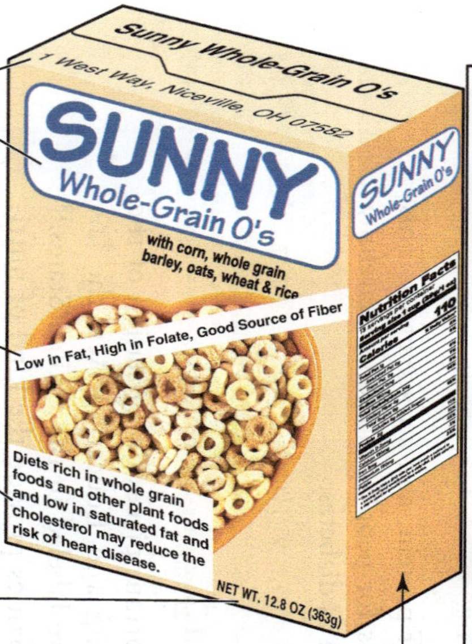

Ingredients in descending order of predominance by weight

Ingredients: Corn flour, whole-grain barley flour, sugar, whole-grain oat flour, whole wheat flour, brown sugar, whole-grain brown rice flour, oat hull fiber, modified corn starch, wheat starch, sunflower and/or canola oil, salt, caramel color, tri-sodium phosphate, beta-carotene & annatto (for color), mixed tocopherols (Vitamin E for freshness). Vitamins & Minerals: Calcium carbonate, ascorbic acid, reduced iron, zinc oxide, niacinamide, vitamin A palmitate, folic acid, vitamin D3, thiamin, riboflavin, vitamin B12.

Allergy information: Declaration that the product contains major food allergens

Contains Wheat

Old Food Label (1993–2016)

Nutrition Facts
Serving Size 1 cup (29g/1 oz)
Servings Per Container About 13

Amount per serving	
Calories 110	Calories from Fat 10
	% Daily Value*
Total Fat 1g	**2%**
Saturated Fat 0g	**0%**
Trans Fat 0g	
Cholesterol 0mg	**0%**
Sodium 160mg	**7%**
Total Carbohydrate 24g	**8%**
Dietary Fiber 4g	**16%**
Sugars 6g	
Protein 2g	
Vitamin A	10%
Vitamin C	8%
Calcium	13%
Iron	45%
Folate	25%

* Percent Daily Values are based on a 2,000 calorie diet. Your daily value may be higher or lower depending on your calorie needs.

		Calories: 2,000	2,500
Total Fat	Less than	65g	80g
Sat Fat	Less than	20g	25g
Cholesterol	Less than	300mg	300 mg
Sodium	Less than	2,400mg	2,400mg
Total Carbohydrate		300g	375g
Dietary Fiber		25g	30g

New Food Label (2016)

Nutrition Facts
13 servings per container
Serving size 1 cup (29g/1 oz)

Amount per serving	
Calories	**110**
	% Daily Value*
Total Fat 1g	**2%**
Saturated Fat 0g	**0%**
Trans Fat 0g	
Cholesterol 0mg	**0%**
Sodium 160mg	**7%**
Total Carbohydrate 24g	**9%**
Dietary Fiber 4g	**14%**
Total Sugars 6g	
Includes 6g Added Sugars	**12%**
Protein 2g	
Vitamin D 2mcg	10%
Calcium 130mg	10%
Iron 8mg	45%
Potassium 130mg	3%
Folate	25%

* The % Daily Value (DV) tells you how much a nutrient in a serving of food contributes to a daily diet. 2,000 calories a day is used for general nutrition advice.

Start here.

Note the number of servings in the package and the serving size. Find out how many **calories** are in a single serving.

Limit these nutrients.

The new design requires information about **added sugars**.

Get enough of these nutrients. The "get enough" section includes vitamin D, potassium, calcium, iron and fiber, based on evidence that Americans do not get enough of these nutrients.

Guide to the % Daily Value:
Quantities of nutrients as "% Daily Values" based on a 2,000-calorie energy intake.

- 5% or less is low—try to aim low in saturated fat, *trans* fat, cholesterol, sodium, and added sugars.
- 10% or more is good; 20% or more is high—look for foods that are good or high sources of vitamin D, calcium, iron, potassium, and dietary fiber.

The only vitamin now required to appear on the Nutrition Facts panel is vitamin D; vitamins A and C are no longer required. Four minerals are required as well: iron, calcium, potassium, and sodium. The actual amount (in milligrams or micrograms) in addition to the %DV must be listed for vitamin D, calcium, iron, and potassium. If a manufacturer makes a nutrition claim about another vitamin or mineral, however, the amount of that nutrient in a serving of the product must be stated on the panel. For instance, the cereal shown is touted as "High in Folate," so the percentage of the recommended intake for folate in a serving of the cereal (25%) is stated on the label. The manufacturer has the option of listing any other nutrients as well.

and convenience stores. Restaurants with 20 or more locations must now provide the calories, milligrams of sodium, and grams of saturated fat contained in their menu items.[13]

Food Labels Considering the great variety of packaged foods available, using the food label to understand the nutrients a food supplies or lacks is essential. The label is one of the most important tools you can use to eat healthfully.

By law, all labels must contain the following five components:

- The name of the food, also known as the statement of identity.
- The name of the manufacturer, packer, or distributor, as well as the firm's contact information.
- The net contents of the package, which tells you the quantity of the food product that is in the container and helps you compare prices.
- The **ingredients list**, with items listed in descending order of predominance by weight. The first ingredient listed makes up the largest proportion of all the ingredients in the food; the second, the second largest amount; and so on. If the first ingredient in the list is sugar, for example, you know the food contains more sugar than anything else. The list is especially useful in helping people identify ingredients they want to avoid for health, religious, or other reasons (see Figure 2-16).

Since 2006, federal law requires that the labels of most packaged foods marketed in the United States disclose—in simple-to-understand terms—when they are made with a major food allergen.* The law allows manufacturers a choice in how they identify the specific food source names of the major food allergens on the label (see Figure 2-15). They must be declared either in:

- The ingredients list, such as "casein (milk)" or "nonfat dry milk," or
- A separate "Contains" statement, such as "Contains milk," placed immediately after or next to the ingredients list.
- The **Nutrition Facts panel**, unless the package is small—no larger than 12 square inches of surface area (about the size of a small candy bar or a roll of breath mints). Small packages must carry contact information that consumers can use to obtain nutrition details. Other small containers (e.g., a can of tuna) are allowed to present fewer facts.

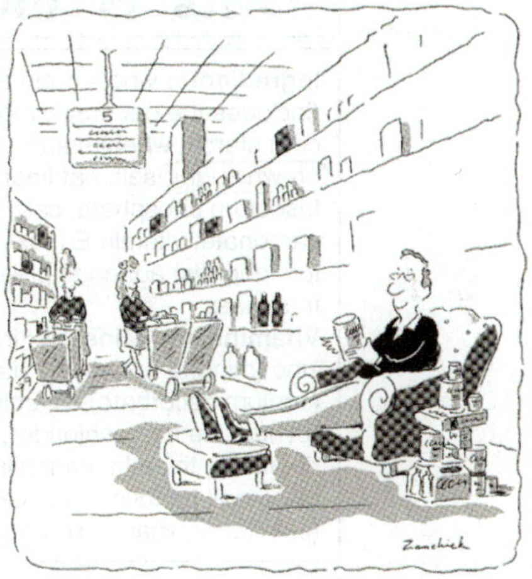

Courtesy: Modern Maturity Magazine

"Henry likes nothing more than to curl up with a good label."

The Food Label Makeover In July 2016, the FDA updated the Nutrition Facts panel—introduced more than 20 years ago—for packaged foods to reflect new dietary recommendations and public health concerns, including the link between diet and chronic diseases such as obesity and heart disease.[14] Key changes to the label (see Figure 2-15) include:

- Updating out-of-date serving size requirements, so they reflect the amounts people actually eat and drink. For example, a serving of ice cream for food labels

*According to the Food Allergen Labeling and Consumer Protection Act of 2004, any of the six foods that account for the majority of all food allergy reactions, namely milk, eggs, peanuts, tree nuts (almond, cashew, Brazil nut, pistachio, macadamia, walnut, pecan, hazelnut, pine nut), fish (e.g., bass, flounder, cod), and crustacean shellfish (e.g., crab, lobster, shrimp), plus two others (soybeans and wheat) are required to be declared on food labels if the product contains or was produced in a facility that may contain any of these basic eight foods.

ingredients list A listing of the ingredients in a food, with items listed in descending order of predominance by weight. All food labels are required to bear an ingredients list.

Nutrition Facts panel A detailed breakdown of the nutritional content of a serving of a food that must appear on virtually all packaged foods sold in the United States.

FIGURE 2-16

Using the Ingredients List on Food Labels

COURTESY: *Modern Maturity* magazine.

Oats 'N' More	Morning Krisps	
Ingredients: whole grain oats, (includes the oat bran), modified corn starch, wheat starch, brown sugar, salt, oat fiber, trisodium phosphate, calcium carbonate, vitamin E (mixed tocopherols) added to preserve freshness. **Vitamins and Minerals:** iron and zinc (mineral nutrients), vitamin C (sodium ascorbate), vitamin B_6 (pyridoxine hydrochloride), riboflavin, thiamin mononitrate, niacinamide, folic acid, vitamin A (palmitate), vitamin B_{12}, vitamin D.	**Ingredients:** Brown sugar, wheat, corn syrup, honey, hydrogenated soybean oil, salt, caramel color, soy lecithin. **Vitamins and Iron:** sodium ascorbate (vitamin C), ferric phosphate (iron), niacinamide, pyridoxine hydrochloride (vitamin B_6), riboflavin, vitamin A palmitate, thiamin hydrochloride, BHT (preservative), folic acid, vitamin B_{12}, and vitamin D.	The cereals shown contain sugars. Learn to read the ingredients list. Labels list ingredients in order of amount by weight with the greatest amount of an ingredient present in the food listed first. Check labels for sugar terms, in addition to sugar, such as: brown sugar, corn syrup, dextrose, fructose, glucose, high-fructose corn syrup, honey, invert sugar, levulose, mannitol, molasses, sorbitol, and sucrose.

used to be a half cup; the new serving is 1 cup and will better reflect what a consumer is likely to consume. For soft drinks, a serving used to be 8 ounces; now it will be 12 to 20 ounces.

- Emphasizing certain elements, such as calories, serving sizes, and percent Daily Value, that are important in addressing current public health concerns. The "Calories from Fat" line was removed, as the *type* of fat present is deemed more useful than the total fat information.
- Presenting calorie and nutrition information for the whole package, in addition to per serving, on certain products that contain more than one serving size but that could be consumed in one sitting (such as a pint of ice cream or a 24-ounce sweetened beverage).
- Requiring information about added sugars—sugars added by food manufacturers. The *Dietary Guidelines for Americans* recommend that people reduce their intake of calories from added sugars.
- Listing potassium and vitamin D on the label, if present in the food, because many people are not consuming adequate amounts. Calcium and iron continue to be required on the label, but listing vitamins A and C is now voluntary.
- Revising the daily values for a variety of nutrients such as sodium, potassium, calcium, dietary fiber, and vitamin D.

Using the Nutrition Facts Panel The Nutrition Facts panel must indicate the amount of certain mandatory nutrients that one serving of the food contains. You can use the Nutrition Facts panel to help you follow a healthy eating pattern by considering the following nutrition information that it provides:

1. Keep serving sizes in mind. Based on the amount of food most people eat at one time, the FDA has set forth a list of serving sizes for more than 100 food categories. Manufacturers must use these recommended serving sizes on food labels. For instance, the FDA might say that the serving size for product X must

always be 8 ounces. This procedure ensures that consumers can easily compare one brand of a product to another without having to make difficult calculations to compare nutrient quantities for different serving sizes.

2. Notice the total calories per serving.
3. Check out the nutrient information that must appear on the Nutrition Facts panel, including total fat, saturated fat, *trans* fat, cholesterol, sodium, total carbohydrates, dietary fiber, added sugars, protein, vitamin D, calcium, iron, and potassium (in that order). These nutrients were chosen to appear on the Nutrition Facts panel because they address health concerns.

   The FDA spelled out the ranking of the required nutrients to ensure that the label reflects the government's dietary priorities for the public. For example, fat falls near the top of the list because most consumers need to pay closer attention to the type of fat in their diet. Most Americans eat too much saturated fat and *trans* fat, which raises the risk of developing heart disease. Protein, in contrast, appears near the bottom of the label because the amount of protein most Americans eat does not rate as a major health concern. Note that only vitamin D, calcium, iron, potassium, and sodium must appear on the nutrition panel. Those are the only vitamins and minerals required to be on food labels, unless a manufacturer chooses to make a nutrition claim about another one. For instance, if a manufacturer says that a cereal is *high* in folate or fortified with niacin, the amount of folate or niacin in the product must appear on the label (see Figure 2-15).
4. Look for the percent Daily Values. The **Daily Values** for fats, protein, carbohydrates, and fiber are calculated according to what experts deem a healthy diet for adults (see Figure 2-17 on page 59). For instance, because the Daily Value for fat recommends that no more than 35 percent of total calories should come from fat, the % Daily Value tells you the percentage of fat that a serving of the food contributes to a 2,000-calorie eater's fat "allowance." A 2,000-calorie diet was chosen as a good point of reference because that's about the amount recommended for most moderately active women, teenage girls, and sedentary men. Of course, more calories may be appropriate for many men, teenage boys, and active women.

Using the Percent Daily Values (% DV)

To understand how the Daily Values for fats, sodium, carbohydrates, and fiber are calculated, let's go through an example. First, look for the grams of fiber and the % Daily Value for the cereal shown in Figure 2-15. The label shows that a serving supplies 4 grams of fiber, with a Daily Value of 14 percent. This means that a serving of the cereal contributes 14 percent of the total fiber that a person eating 2,000 calories a day should consume.

Now look at Figure 2-17, which indicates that someone eating 2,000 calories a day should take in 28 grams of fiber a day. Divide 4 (the number of fiber grams in a serving of the cereal) by 28. Multiply that number by 100 to obtain a percentage. The answer is 14—that is, 14 percent of the total fiber.

You can use the % Daily Values to get a good idea of how various foods fit into a healthy diet, regardless of the number of calories you eat. Consider a student who eats only 1,800 calories a day. If she snacks on two servings of potato chips with a Daily Value of 15 percent fat per serving, she has already taken in 30 percent of the fat that someone eating 2,000 calories should have in an entire day. Because she eats less than 2,000 calories, the potato chips contribute slightly more than 30 percent. Thus, the 30 percent Daily Value shows that potato chips add up to a lot of fat for one snack.

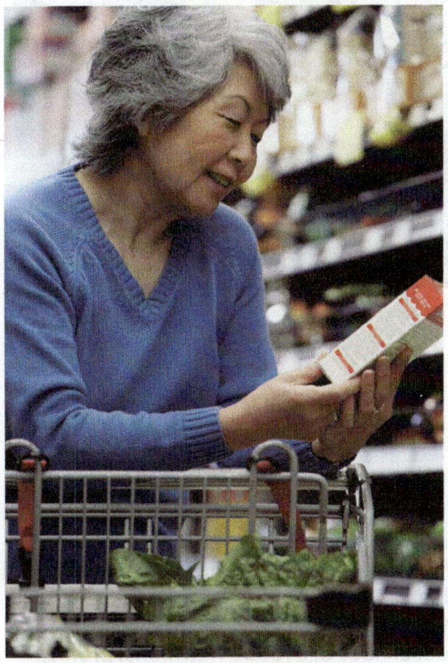

Noel Hendrickson/Blend Images

Learn to read food labels to help you achieve an overall healthy eating pattern.

daily value The amount of fat, sodium, fiber, and other nutrients health experts say should make up a healthy diet. The "% Daily Values" that appear on food labels tell you the percentage of a nutrient that a serving of the food contributes to a healthy diet.

In short, the % Daily Value column can give you a good idea of how different foods fit into your overall diet.

Some people find it easiest to bypass the % Daily Values and simply check the grams of total fat a serving of food supplies to see how much it adds to a daily fat tally. Let's say a man eats 2,000 calories a day and therefore should consume no more than 78 grams of fat a day. If he eats a muffin (15 grams of fat) and coffee with cream (10 grams) in the morning, he's already up to 25 grams of fat. That means he can have about 50 more grams during the rest of the day to stay within his fat "budget." Once you determine the maximum number of fat grams you should have in a day, you can use the food label to get a good idea of how many grams of total fat the items you buy add to your daily tally. To figure out your fat allowance, check Table 5-4 in Chapter 5.

You can also use the Daily Values to comparison-shop. For example, if you're looking for a high-fiber cereal to increase the amount of fiber in your diet, you can check the % Daily Value for fiber on the labels of several brands of cereal. If a serving of Brand X's cereal has a Daily Value of 20 percent for fiber and Brand Y supplies only 5 percent, you know that Brand X is a better source of fiber, whereas Brand Y is low in fiber.

The % Daily Values for vitamins and minerals are calculated using standard values designed specifically for use on food labels. These values are listed in Figure 2-17, and additional values can be found in Appendix A of this book. These standard values for nutrients were created to help manufacturers avoid a stumbling block they face as they label foods. Because manufacturers don't know whether you're an 18-year-old woman or a 30-year-old man, they don't know exactly what your nutritional needs are. You may recall that the DRI include a different set of vitamin and mineral recommendations for each gender and age group.

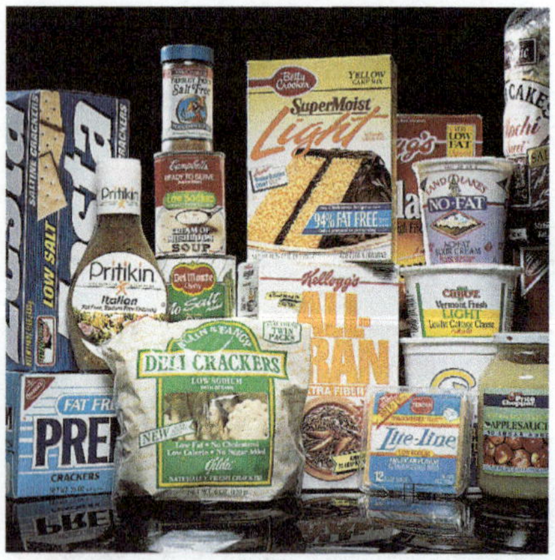

Charles Winters/Science Source

To help get around this problem, the nutrient recommendations used for vitamins and minerals on labels represent the highest of all the values to ensure that virtually everyone in the population is covered. For most nutrients, the highest recommendation is for an adult man. When it comes to iron, however, the DRI for women is the highest (women require more iron than men), so the women's DRI is used as the standard value on labels.

Nutrient Content Claims

By law, foods carrying terms called **nutrient content claims**—low-fat, low-calorie, light, and so forth—must adhere to specific definitions spelled out by the Food and Drug Administration. For instance, a serving of a food dubbed low-fat must contain no more than 3 grams of fat. An item touted as low-calorie may provide no more than 40 calories per serving. Table 2-7 lists the claims commonly used on food labels and their legal definitions.

nutrient content claims Claims such as "low-fat" and "low-calorie" used on food labels to help consumers who don't want to scrutinize the Nutrition Facts panel get an idea of a food's nutritional profile. These claims must adhere to specific definitions set forth by the Food and Drug Administration.

health claim A statement on the food label linking the nutritional profile of a food to a reduced risk of a particular disease, such as osteoporosis or cancer. Manufacturers must adhere to strict government guidelines when making such claims.

Health Claims

A statement linking the nutritional profile of a food to a reduced risk of a particular disease is known as a **health claim**. The FDA has set forth very strict rules governing the use of such health claims (see Table 2-8).[15] For example, if a food label bears health claims regarding calcium, a serving of the product must contain at least 20 percent of the Daily Value for calcium, among other restrictions. What's more, the manufacturers are allowed to imply only that the food "may" or "might" reduce risk of disease. They must also note the other factors, such as exercise, that play a role in prevention of the disease. Finally, they must phrase

FIGURE 2-17

Calculation Practice: Determining Personal Daily Values (DVs)

The Daily Values (DVs) and % Daily Values (% DVs) can help you choose foods and comparison-shop. As noted earlier, the DVs are designed for people requiring 2,000 calories to meet their energy needs. The Daily Values for carbohydrates, protein, and fat are calculated using "calculation factors" set forth by the FDA for food labeling purposes as listed in the following table:

Daily Values for Food Labels

Food labels must present the "% Daily Value" for these nutrients.

Food Component	Daily Value	Calculation Factors
Fat	78 g	35% of calories
Saturated fat	20 g	10% of calories
Cholesterol	300 mg	—
Carbohydrate (total)	275 g	55% of calories
Fiber	28 g	—
Added sugars	50 g	—
Protein	50 g	10% of calories
Sodium	2,300 mg	—
Potassium	4,700 mg	—
Vitamin D	20 μg	—
Calcium	1,300 mg	—
Iron	18 mg	—

NOTE: Daily Values were established for adults and children more than 4 years old. The values for energy-yielding nutrients are based on 2,000 calories a day.

To understand how the Daily Values for the energy nutrients are calculated if your energy needs differ from 2,000 calories, let's go through an example using the calculation factors. If a person's Estimated Energy Requirement (EER) is 1,800 calories, determine this person's DVs for carbohydrate, protein, and fat.

Carbohydrate:
55% of 1,800 calories = 0.55 × 1,800 = 990 calories
990 calories of carbohydrate = 248 grams of carbohydrate (990 calories ÷ 4 calories/gram)
DV for carbohydrate = 248 grams

Protein:
10% of 1,800 calories = 0.10 × 1,800 = 180 calories
180 calories of protein = 45 grams of protein (180 calories ÷ 4 calories/gram)
DV for protein = 45 grams

Fat:
35% of 1,800 calories = 0.35 × 1,800 = 630 calories
630 calories of fat = 70 grams of fat (630 calories ÷ 9 calories/gram)
DV for fat = 70 grams

the claim so that consumers can understand the relationship between the nutrient and the disease. For example, a health claim on a food low in fat, saturated fat, and cholesterol might read, "Whereas many factors affect heart disease, diets low in saturated fat and cholesterol may reduce the risk of this disease." The nutrient–disease relationships about which health claims can be made are listed in Table 2-8.[16]

Table 2-7 Definitions of Nutrient Content Claims

General Terms

- **Fresh, Raw:** Unprocessed, or minimally processed with no added preservatives.
- **Good Source of:** A serving of the food supplies 10% to 19% of the Daily Value for a particular nutrient.
- **Healthy:** A food is low in fat, saturated fat, *trans* fat, cholesterol, and sodium, and provides at least 10% of the Daily Value for vitamin D, potassium, protein, calcium, iron, or fiber.
- **High, Rich in, Excellent Source of:** Contains 20% or more of the Daily Value for a particular nutrient.
- **Less, Fewer, Reduced:** A serving provides at least 25% less of a nutrient or calories than the comparison food.
- **Light or Lite:** A serving provides one-third fewer calories than the comparison food; or 50% or less of the fat or sodium in the comparison food.
- **More, Extra:** A serving of the food contains at least 10% more of the Daily Value of a particular nutrient than the regular food.
- **Organic:** At least 95% of the product's ingredients have been grown and processed according to USDA regulations regarding the use of fertilizers, herbicides, fungicides, insecticides, preservatives, and other substances (see Chapter 13).

Energy Terms

- **Calorie-Free:** Less than 5 calories per serving.
- **Low-Calorie:** No more than 40 calories per serving.
- **Reduced Calorie:** Contains at least 25% fewer calories than the regular, unaltered product.

Carbohydrates: Sugar, Fiber, and Gluten

- **Sugar-Free:** Less than 0.5 g of sugar per serving.
- **High-Fiber:** 5 g or more fiber per serving.
- **Good Source of Fiber:** 2.5 g to 4.9 g per serving.
- **Gluten-Free, No Gluten, Free of Gluten:** A grain can be labeled gluten-free once it is processed to remove gluten* and the presence of any unavoidable gluten due to cross-contact is less than 20 parts per million (ppm).

Fat and Cholesterol Terms

- **Fat-Free:** Less than 0.5 g of fat per serving.
- **Low-Fat:** 3 grams of fat or less per serving.
- **Saturated Fat-Free:** Less than 0.5 g of saturated fat and less than 0.5 g *trans* fat per serving.
- **Low-Saturated Fat:** 1 gram or less saturated fat per serving and less than 0.5 g *trans* fat per serving.
- **Less Saturated Fat:** At least 25% less saturated fat and *trans* fat combined than the comparison food.
- ***Trans* Fat-Free:** Less than 0.5 g of *trans* fat and less than 0.5 g of saturated fat per serving.
- **Cholesterol-Free:** Less than 2 mg cholesterol and 2 g or less saturated fat and *trans* fat combined per serving.
- **Low in Cholesterol:** 20 mg or less of cholesterol and 2 g or less of saturated fat and *trans* fat combined per serving.
- **Reduced or Less Cholesterol:** At least 25% less cholesterol than the comparison food and 2 g or less saturated fat and *trans* fat combined per serving.
- **Percent Fat-Free:** An indication of the amount of a food's weight that is fat-free; can be used only on foods that are low-fat or fat-free to begin with, and must reflect the amount of fat in 100 g. For instance, a food that weighs 100 g with 3 g from fat can be labeled "97% fat-free." Note that this term refers to the amount of the food that is fat-free by weight, not calories. If that same food supplies 100 calories, the 3 g of fat contribute 27 of them (1 g of fat provides 9 calories). This means that 27 of the 100 calories, or 27% of the total calories, come from fat.
- "Lean" and "Extra Lean" describe the fat content of meat and poultry products:
  Lean: Less than 10 g of fat, 4.5 g of saturated fat and *trans* fat combined, and less than 95 mg of cholesterol per serving.
  Extra Lean: Less than 5 g of fat, 2 g of saturated fat and *trans* fat combined, and less than 95 mg of cholesterol per serving.

TABLE 2-7	Definitions of Nutrient Content Claims *(continued)*

Sodium Terms
- **Sodium-Free and Salt-Free:** Less than 5 mg of sodium per serving.
- **Very Low Sodium:** 35 mg or less sodium per serving.
- **Low in Sodium:** 140 mg sodium or less per serving.
- **Reduced Sodium:** At least 25% lower in sodium than the regular product.

*Gluten is the protein that occurs naturally in wheat, rye, barley, and crossbreeds of these grains, and is the ingredient that gives breads and other grain products their shape, strength, and texture. People with celiac disease cannot tolerate gluten and need to avoid products containing gluten.

SOURCE: Food and Drug Administration.

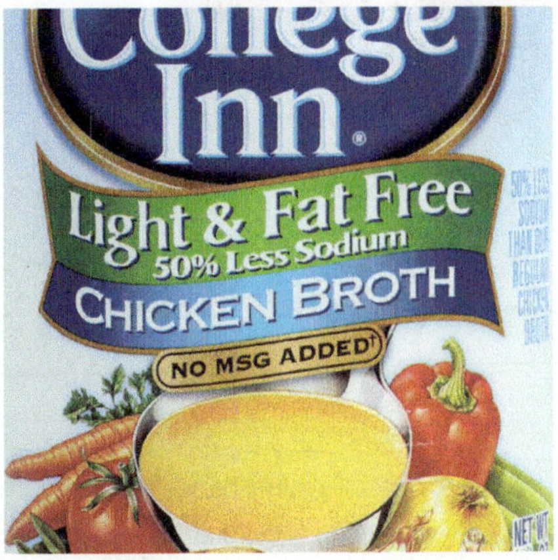

© Sam Kolich/Bill Smith Group/Cengage Learning

Nutrient claims characterize the level of a nutrient in the food—for example, "fat-free" or "less sodium." Nutrient content claims are strictly defined by the FDA.

TABLE 2-8	Health Claims on Food Labels

Approved health claims with significant scientific agreement:[a]
- Diets adequate in calcium and vitamin D, as part of a well-balanced diet, may reduce the risk of osteoporosis.
- Eating a healthy diet low in total fat may help reduce the risk of some types of cancers.
- Low-fat diets rich in fiber-containing grain products, fruits, and vegetables may reduce the risk of some types of cancer.
- Low-fat diets rich in fruits and vegetables may reduce the risk of some types of cancer.
- Diets low in sodium may reduce the risk of high blood pressure.
- Diets low in saturated fat and cholesterol, and as low as possible in *trans* fat, may reduce the risk of heart disease.
- Diets low in saturated fat and cholesterol and high in fruits, vegetables, and grain products that contain fiber may lower blood cholesterol levels and reduce your risk of heart disease.
- Diets low in saturated fat and cholesterol and rich in fruits, vegetables, and grain products that contain dietary fiber, particularly soluble fiber, may reduce the risk of heart disease.
- Diets that are low in saturated fat and cholesterol and that include soluble fiber in foods such as whole oats may reduce the risk of heart disease.
- Adequate folate in healthy diets may reduce a woman's risk of having a child with a brain or spinal cord birth defect.
- Sugar alcohols may reduce the risk of tooth decay.
- Drinking fluoridated water may reduce the risk of tooth decay.
- Diets low in saturated fat and cholesterol that include 25 grams of soy protein a day may reduce the risk of heart disease.
- Diets rich in whole-grain foods and other plant foods and low in total fat, saturated fat, and cholesterol may reduce the risk of heart disease and certain cancers.
- Diets low in saturated fat and cholesterol that include a daily total of at least 3.4 grams of phytosterols (plant sterols, plant stanols), eaten with meals or snacks may reduce the risk of heart disease.
- Diets containing foods that are good sources of potassium and low in sodium may reduce the risk of high blood pressure and stroke.

A sampling of qualified health claims:[b]
- Omega-3 fatty acids and reduced risk of heart disease
- Nuts such as walnuts and reduced risk of heart disease
- Calcium and reduced risk of high blood pressure
- Calcium and reduced risk of colorectal cancer
- Monounsaturated fat from olive oil and reduced risk of heart disease

[a]The FDA does not require these claims to carry disclaimers.
[b]FDA requires label disclaimers when these claims are used; for example, "Health claim: Although there is scientific evidence supporting the claim, the evidence is not conclusive."

SOURCE: Food and Drug Administration.

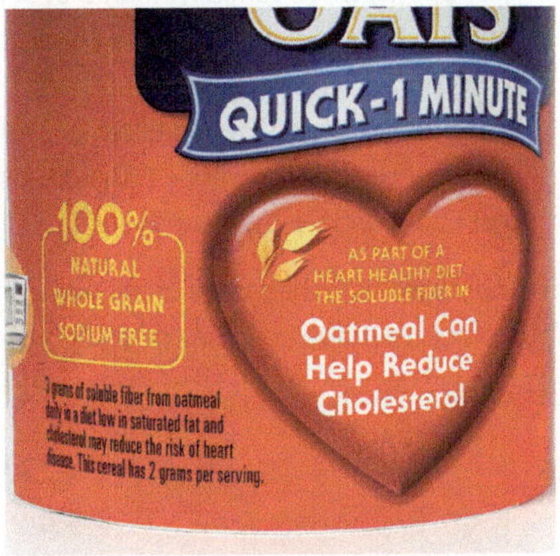

© Sam Kolich/Bill Smith Group/Cengage Learning

Health claims characterize the relationship of a food or food component to a disease—for example, "soluble fiber from oatmeal daily in a diet low in saturated fat and cholesterol may reduce the risk of heart disease." Such claims must follow FDA guidelines.

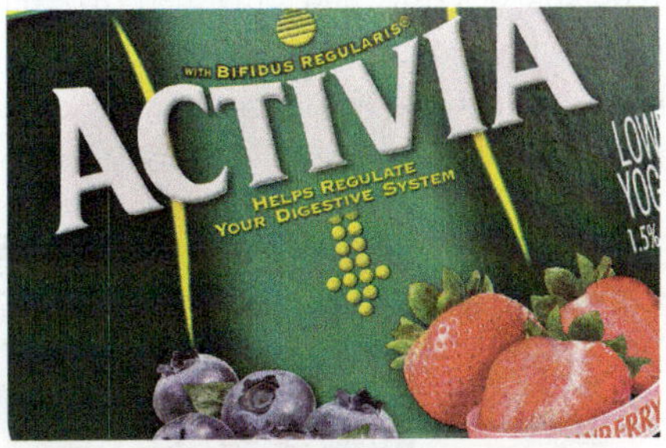

Q-Images/Alamy Stock Photo

Structure/function claims describe the effect that a nutrient or dietary ingredient has on the structure or function of the body, but cannot mention a disease or symptom. Examples include "calcium builds strong bones," or "probiotics help regulate your digestive system." These claims are not preapproved by FDA.

SPOTLight

2.7 A Tapestry of Cultures and Cuisines

American eating habits have become as diverse as the various ethnic and cultural groups that make up America's people. Throughout American history, immigrant groups—from Poles to Jews to Italians to Irish to Germans to Hispanics to African Americans to Asians—have had and continue to have profound effects on the collective American palate. As food writer and critic John Mariani has pointed out:

> [T]he United States—a stewpot of cultures—has developed a gastronomy more varied . . . than that of any other country in the world. . . . In any major American city one will find restaurants representing a dozen national cuisines, including northern Italian trattorias, bourgeois French bistros, Portuguese seafood houses, Vietnamese and Thai eateries, Chinese dim sum parlors, Japanese sushi bars, and German rathskellers.[17]

This Spotlight examines some of the more prevalent ethnic and regional food practices to see how they originated and how they fit into a healthy eating plan.

I love to eat Mexican food. Is it true that it is loaded with fat? Do the Mexican people eat a lot of high-fat food?

Although it's true that many menu selections in Mexican restaurants are loaded with high-fat ingredients such as cheese, ground beef, sour cream, guacamole, and fried tortillas, most dishes eaten regularly in Mexican American homes are much simpler. Breakfast, for example, might be tortillas (flat, thin corn, or wheat pancakes) served with refried beans, eggs, or cereal, and a beverage. Lunches and dinners often consist of beans and rice, bread or tortillas, meat/sausage (often as part of a stew), a vegetable or lettuce and tomato, and a beverage.

The traditional Mexican diet drawing largely from Spanish and Indian influences was even simpler, containing mostly vegetables, including beans, squash, and maize (corn). In addition, it often included cactus parts, agave (a plant with spiny-margined leaves and flowers), chili peppers, amaranth (a grain), avocado, and guava (a sweet, juicy fruit with green or yellow skin and red or yellow flesh).

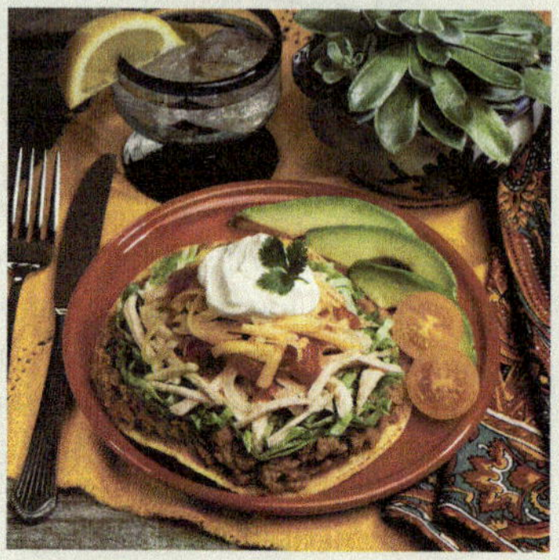

ClassicStock/Alamy Stock Photo

This type of diet is high in complex carbohydrates such as rice and vitamin A- and C-rich fruits and vegetables, making it a particularly healthy aspect of the traditional Mexican way of eating. Consider that no Mexican meal is complete without salsa, a low-fat condiment consisting of vitamin-rich tomatoes, chilies, and onions. Another plus of the Mexican diet is frequent use of beans, mostly the pinto variety, which rank as a particularly good source of fiber.

There are downsides to the Mexican diet, however. Most foods, even beans and rice, are typically fried rather than baked or broiled. For example, *frijoles refritos* (refried beans) are usually fried in lard and contain about 270 calories and 3 grams of fat per cup. Most flour tortillas are also made with lard, sometimes 1 or 2 teaspoons per tortilla. (Corn tortillas, in contrast, typically contain very little fat.) Another drawback of the Mexican diet is the frequent consumption of high-fat meats, such as *chorizo* (spicy pork or beef sausage) and eggs, which are used in dishes such as *chiles rellenos* (roasted mild green chili pepper stuffed with cheese, dipped in egg batter, and fried), *burritos* (warm flour tortillas stuffed with a mixture of egg, meat, beans, and/or avocado), and *chilaquiles* (tortilla casserole often made with eggs or meat).

Fortunately, health-conscious Mexican food lovers can take advantage of the popular cuisine with a little know-how. Instead of the usual American versions of Mexican fare, such as fried tortillas packed with ground beef smothered in cheese and sour cream, opt for corn tortillas filled with, say, regular, unfried pinto beans mixed with chopped onion and topped with a sprinkle of shredded cheese and a generous portion of lettuce, salsa, a dollop of fat-free plain yogurt or fat-free sour cream, and a garnish of sliced avocado. Or, instead of serving high-fat commercial tortilla chips with salsa, try making "no-fry" chips: Immerse several tortillas in warm water, drain quickly, cut into six to eight wedges, and place on a nonstick pan; bake in a 500-degree Fahrenheit oven for 3 to 4 minutes, flip, and continue to bake for another minute or two until golden brown.

Adventurous eaters who have access to a wide variety of exotic produce might want to try some of the different fruits and vegetables the Mexican people have enjoyed for decades, such as *jicama* (HE-cah-mah), a yam bean root vegetable that is tan outside and white inside, has a mild chestnut flavor, and is always eaten raw.[18] Figure 2-18 shows produce and other foods commonly eaten by Mexican Americans.

FIGURE 2-18

Mexican American Foods and MyPlate[a]

[a] Discretionary calorie limit can be used for bacon, butter, candy, cream cheese, fried pork rinds, lard, hard margarine, soft drinks, and sour cream.
[b] These foods are described in the Miniglossary.

SOURCE: Adapted from www.ChooseMyPlate.gov and the Pyramid Packet © 1993, Penn State Nutrition Center, 417 East Calder Way, University Park, PA 16801.

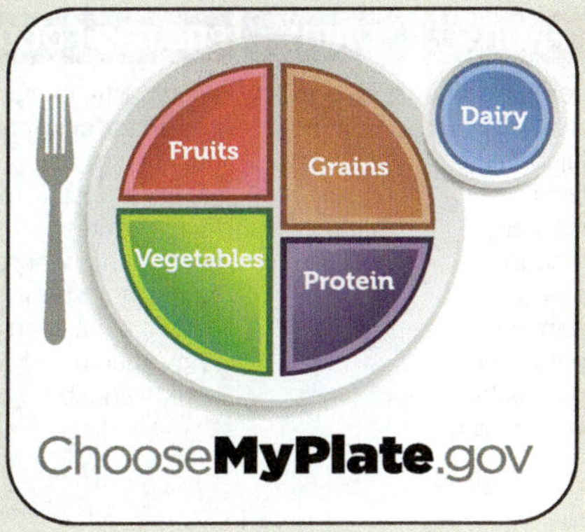

GRAINS	VEGETABLES	FRUITS	DAIRY	PROTEIN FOODS
bolillo[b], bread, cake, cereal, corn tortilla, crackers, flour tortilla, fried flour tortilla, graham crackers, macaroni, oatmeal, pastry, rice, sopa[b], spaghetti, sweet bread, taco shell	agave[b], beets, cabbage, carrots, cassava[b], chilis, corn, green tomatoes, iceberg lettuce, jicama[b], onion, peas, potato, prickly pear cactus leaves, purslane[b], squash, sweet potatoes, tomato, turnips	apple, avocado, banana, cherimoya[b], guava[b], mango, orange, papaya, pineapple, plantain[b], zapote[b]	cheddar cheese, custard, evaporated milk, ice cream, jack cheese, powdered milk, queso blanco, fresco, or mexicano[b]	beef, black beans, chicken, chorizo[b], eggs, fish, garbanzo beans, kidney beans, lamb, nuts, peanut butter, pinto beans, pork, refried beans

© Cengage

Are foods served in Chinese restaurants in the United States, such as chop suey, egg rolls, and fortune cookies, traditional Chinese foods? A Chinese American friend of mine says they aren't. Is she right?

Yes, it's true that chop suey and the like are American inventions. The traditional Chinese diet consists of much simpler, lower-fat dishes.

Overall, about 80 percent of the calories in traditional Chinese fare comes from grains, legumes, and vegetables while the other 20 percent comes from animal meats, fruits, and fat. In southern China, rice can be easily produced and provides the bulk of the complex carbohydrate in the diet. In northern areas, where wheat grows readily, noodles, dumplings, and steamed buns are staples. In all regions of the country, fruits and vegetables are eaten in abundance. Typically, they are not eaten raw, but rather are steamed, added to soups, or stir-fried in peanut or corn oil or (less frequently) lard. In addition, vegetables are often salted, pickled, and dried, a practice resulting from lack of the facilities needed to refrigerate and transport fresh produce across the country. As for meat and other protein foods, pork is considered the staple meat, though poultry, eggs, lamb, and fish are eaten when available. Tofu, or soybean curd, is another staple often added to stir-fries or fermented into sauces. Dairy foods, such as milk and cheese, have never been part of the Chinese diet.

Traditional Chinese meals follow basically the same pattern. Breakfast might be rice congee (rice gruel containing bits of meat), a salty side dish such as pickles, and tea. Lunch typically consists of soup, rice, and mixed dishes made with vegetables and fish, meat, or poultry; dinner is usually a larger version of lunch, occasionally followed by fresh fruit.

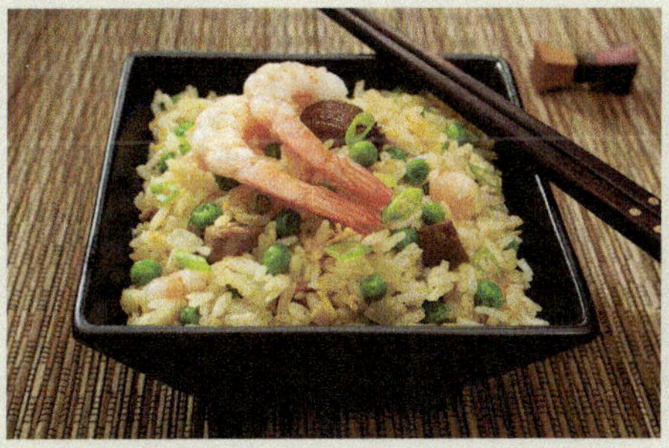

travellight/Shutterstock.com

Four schools of cooking have developed within China as a result of differences in climate, food production, religion, and custom: Peking, Shanghai, Szechwan or Hunan, and Cantonese. *Peking cooking* comes from the north and northeast part of China and is distinguished by use of garlic, leeks, and scallions. It has given rise to familiar dishes such as Peking duck and spring rolls. *Shanghai cuisine*, from the east and coastal areas, is characterized by "red cooking"—braising foods with large amounts of soy sauce and sugar. Pickled and salted vegetables are also frequently served with meat. In the west and central part of China, people favor the *Szechwan or Hunan cooking* style, in which chili peppers and hot pepper sauces are added liberally to dishes, and the food tends to be spicy and oily. The cuisine of southern China, known as *Cantonese cooking*, is the style Americans know best. Because foods are usually steamed or stir-fried and chicken broth is often used as a cooking medium, Cantonese food tends to be the least fatty. One popular example of Cantonese food is *dim sum*, dumplings stuffed with pork, shrimp, beef, sweet paste, or preserves and steamed or fried.[19]

The regional differences in cooking styles and eating habits among people living in rural China make the country fertile ground for scientific research into the effects of diet on disease. Another reason rural China is such an ideal place to conduct research is that most people residing in rural China today spend their entire lives within the vicinity of the community where they were born. In addition, eating habits are dictated by climate and environment because the country has little or no means of transporting foods from one region to another. Thus, scientists have been able to carefully study eating patterns and disease rates in an attempt to see how the two are related. One of the largest such studies was led by T. Colin Campbell, PhD, of Cornell University. Begun in 1983, the research was carried out in 130 villages located in 65 counties of rural China and included 6,500 adults. Findings suggest

FIGURE 2-19

A Chinese American MyPlate Food Guide[a]

[a] Discretionary calorie limit can be used for bacon fat, butter, coconut milk, duck sauce, honey, lard, maltose syrup, sesame paste, suet, and sugar.
[b] These foods are described in the Miniglossary.

SOURCE: Adapted from www.ChooseMyPlate.gov and the Pyramid Packet (1993) Penn State Nutrition Center, 417 East Calder Way, University Park, PA 16801.

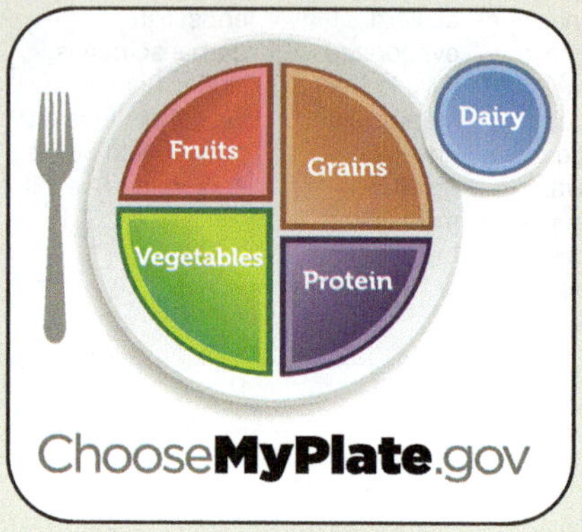

GRAINS	VEGETABLES	FRUITS	DAIRY	PROTEIN FOODS
amaranth[b], barley, bing[b], dumplings, fried rice, glutinous rice[b], mantou[b], noodles (including cellophane noodles[b], rice sticks[b], rice vermicelli[b]), rice congee, rice flour, steamed rice, sorghum, wonton wrappers	bamboo shoots, black mushroom, bok choy[b], cabbage, celery, chiles, Chinese broccoli[b], choy sum[b], eggplant, garlic, ginger, green beans, leek, mustard greens, okra, onions, Oriental radish[b], peas, pickled cucumber, potatoes, scallions, spinach, sprouts, taro[b], tomatoes, turnip, water chestnut, watercress, yard-long beans[b]	carambola, guava, jujube[b], litchi[b], longan[b], mango, orange, papaya, persimmon, pummelo, watermelon	buffalo milk, cow's milk, fish bones, soybean milk, yogurt	bean paste, beef, chestnuts, chicken, duck, eggs, fish (e.g., carp, catfish), lamb, legumes (e.g., mung beans, soybeans), shellfish and other seafood (e.g., shrimp, squid), squab

© Cengage

that the traditional, plant-based Chinese diet is associated with low rates of many of the chronic diseases that plague Americans, such as heart disease and some types of cancer.[20]

To be sure, Chinese food served in American Chinese restaurants is a far cry from the type rural Chinese people eat daily. Many Chinese restaurant meals are swimming in oil and contain much more meat and poultry and fewer vegetables than "real" Chinese food. Consider that a typical American Chinese meal might include wonton soup, barbecued spareribs, chicken lo mein, and fried rice—chalking up some 1,400 calories and more than 80 grams of fat. A typical meal eaten in rural China, in contrast, would likely contain a heaping portion of rice, along with fiber- and nutrient-rich vegetables and less than an ounce of meat or fish, and would thereby contain only a fraction of the fat.[21] Americans who want to enjoy both the flavor and health benefits of traditional Chinese cuisine can "stretch" one of the many delicious vegetable-based dishes with relatively large portions of rice and go easy on deep-fried appetizers such as egg rolls. People who enjoy cooking can also follow the Chinese people's lead and make low-fat, high-carbohydrate stir-fries with lots of vegetables, little oil, and small amounts of meat, poultry, or seafood. People who are sodium conscious may also want to go easy on soy sauce, which contains large amounts of the mineral, or try some of the reduced-sodium soy sauces on the market. Figure 2-19 shows Chinese foods placed into the five food groups of MyPlate.

How does Italian food rate? I've heard that olive oil in Italian pasta dishes is good for health.

Much of the Italian food served in the United States runs very high in fat and calories. Rich cream sauces in dishes such as fettuccine Alfredo; an abundance of cheese and sausage in entrees, including meat-topped pizza and lasagna; and liberal use of olive oil to prepare all manner of pasta and other Italian fare can chalk up extraordinary amounts of fat and calories.

With a little modification, however, the Italian food so many Americans love can easily fit into a healthy diet. For example, substituting vegetables for sausage and pepperoni on pizza and in pasta sauces and lasagna reduces saturated fat content considerably. Using reduced-fat cheeses, such as part-skim mozzarella and ricotta and low-fat cottage cheese, as substitutes for the high-fat versions called for in many Italian recipes also helps skim some of the fat. When it comes to olive oil, a staple in traditional Italian cuisine, it's true that using it instead of butter is preferable from a health standpoint. Figure 2-20 shows a food guide for common Italian American foods.

For reasons that are explained in detail in Chapter 5, olive oil and other vegetable oils are less likely than certain other types of fat, such as butter and lard, to boost blood cholesterol levels. Some scientists even believe that people can eat large amounts of fat— in the neighborhood of 35 to 40 percent of total calories—without raising their risk of heart disease, as long as the predominant fat is olive oil. This line of thinking stems from research conducted in southern Italy and the Greek island of Crete, as well as southern regions of other European nations, including France, North African areas such as Morocco and Tunisia, and Middle Eastern

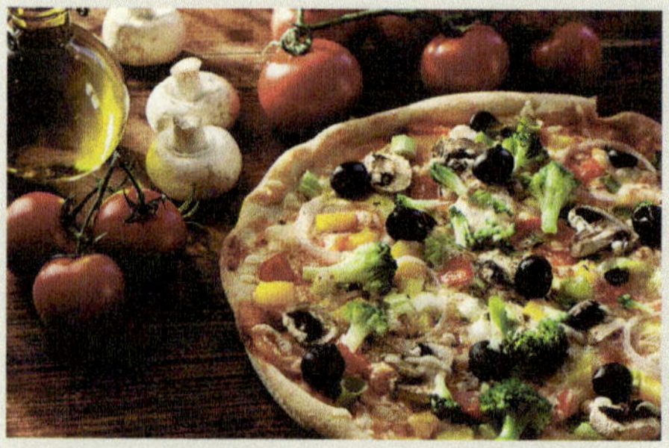

Vima/Shutterstock.com

FIGURE 2-20

An Italian American MyPlate Food Guide[a]

[a] Discretionary calorie limit can be used for butter, olives, olive oil, and heavy cream.

SOURCE: Adapted from www.ChooseMyPlate.gov and the Pyramid Packet (1993) Penn State Nutrition Center, 417 East Calder Way, University Park, PA 16801.

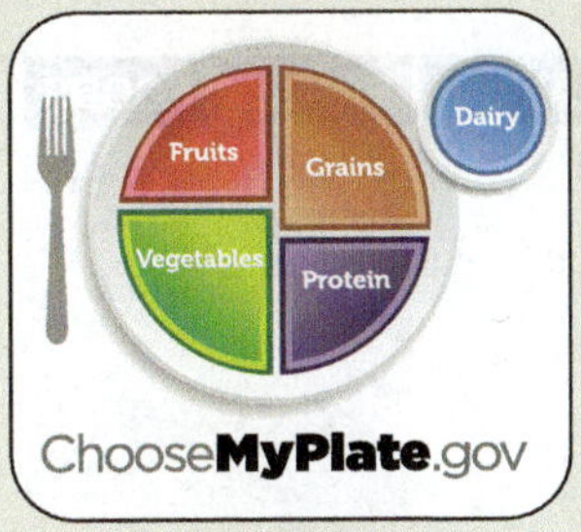

GRAINS	VEGETABLES	FRUITS	DAIRY	PROTEIN FOODS
Rice, linguini, macaroni, spaghetti, focaccia, polenta, Italian bread	Asparagus, artichokes, broccoli, cabbage, capers, carrots, cauliflower, celery, eggplant, mushrooms, onions, peppers, tomatoes, zucchini	Apples, figs, grapes, oranges, peaches, pears, strawberries	Cheeses: mozzarella, parmesan, provolone, ricotta	Beef, calamari, chicken, fava beans, lobster, mussels, lentils, shrimp, perch, sausage

countries such as Israel and Syria. Collectively known as the *Mediterranean region*, these countries share an overall dietary pattern that includes an abundance of fruits and vegetables; breads and other grains; beans, nuts, and seeds; low to moderate amounts of cheese, yogurt, fish, and poultry; small amounts of red meat; moderate consumption of wine; and liberal use of olive oil. Scientists are fascinated with this region because people living there historically have enjoyed long lives and low rates of chronic diseases. That was particularly true in Crete during the 1950s and 1960s. At that time, researchers found that residents of the island shared one of the lowest rates of heart disease and cancer ever recorded and one of the longest life expectancies. That held true despite the fact that their diets derived nearly 40 percent of calories from fat—well above the amount recommended by major U.S. health organizations.[22]

With this historical perspective in mind, some scientists recommend that Americans adopt a "Mediterranean diet" that includes lots of fruits, vegetables, and grains; little meat and other flesh food; moderate amounts of wine; and generous amounts of olive oil (see Figure 5-14 on page 142). This advice has sparked a good deal of controversy within the scientific community, however. Many nutrition experts question the wisdom of recommending such a diet in America, where excess fat from olive oil and other sources might contribute to the epidemic of obesity in this country. In addition, many experts point out that diet is not the only lifestyle factor that may have promoted the long, healthy lives of the people of Crete and Italy several decades ago. For example, the residents of this region farmed the land and thereby engaged in far more physical activity than the average American, a factor that probably played a role in their health and longevity. In addition, unlike many modern-day Americans, they enjoyed social support of extended networks of family and friends, another part of their lifestyle that probably contributed to their well-being. Given these caveats, major U.S. health organizations, including the Academy of Nutrition and Dietetics, the American Heart Association, and the U.S. Department of Health and Human Services, maintain that Americans should keep the amount of total fat—whether in the form of olive oil or anything else—to no more than 20 to 35 percent of total calories.

Our advice is that you consider adopting the aspects of the Mediterranean diet that virtually all nutrition experts advocate: Eat an abundance of produce, grains, and legumes combined with moderate amounts of dairy products and relatively smaller amounts of meats, poultry, and fish.

I have heard that the traditional Indian diet is vegetarian; is that true?

"Traditional Indian diet" can mean many different things. Other than the heavy use of vegetables and spices throughout India, Indian cuisines share few other characteristics. Geographic location, religious beliefs, and availability all contribute to the varied nature of the Indian diet. Furthering the diversity, Indian cooking rarely follows recipes, relying more on the skill of the cook and the availability of ingredients. These phenomena have resulted in a mix of cuisines that are both tasty and various.

The history of vegetarianism in India dates back thousands of years. Many believe it started with the introduction of Buddhism and Jainism in the sixth century B.C. These religions, which are closely related, are strong advocates of the sanctity of all forms of life and are therefore opposed to the slaughter of animals for consumption. However, it is not uncommon for those who live along the coast to incorporate fish into their diet. Likewise, the more northern territories are known to eat much more meat than their southern counterparts. These food choices are most likely due to availability and climate differences.

Nonetheless, the idea that the Indian diet is vegetarian is not far from the truth. Anthropology sources clearly show the predominance of vegetarianism, and even those who do partake in meat consumption do so in moderation, usually no more than one day a week. More often, meat consumption is reserved for special occasions like weddings and celebrations, averaging about four times a year. Another interesting fact is that women are less likely to eat meat than men. This practice stems from the belief that meat causes masculine traits such as aggressiveness.

This feature cannot possibly encompass the vast culture and history that influences Indian cuisine. With the second largest population in the world, India is a multifaceted land with traditions and beliefs that would take books upon books to explain. Even so, its cuisines are a good illustration of the history of India, as there are so many distinctive characteristics. Overall, the diet is based on complex carbohydrates and rich in fiber-full vegetables and fruits. In any Indian restaurant, you are

FIGURE 2-21

Fitting Indian Foods into the MyPlate Food Guide[a]

[a] Discretionary calorie limit can be used for ghee,[b] coconut oil, and similar items.
[b] These foods are described in the Miniglossary.

SOURCE: Adapted from www.ChooseMyPlate.gov and the Pyramid Packet (1993) Penn State Nutrition Center, 417 East Calder Way, University Park, PA 16801.

ChooseMyPlate.gov

GRAINS	VEGETABLES	FRUITS	DAIRY	PROTEIN FOODS
basmati rice, bulgur wheat, chapati[b], millet, rice, roti[b]	broccoli, cabbage, carrots, cauliflower, cucumber, eggplant, onions, plantains, potato, squash, tomatoes, turnips	bananas, chutney, dates, figs, grapes, mango, melon, papaya	lassi[b], milk, yogurt	almonds, beef, cashews, chicken, chickpeas, lamb, lentils, shrimp

bound to find a flavorful and healthy dish that will satisfy you! Some traditional Indian foods are shown in Figure 2-21.

As with most ethnic cuisines, the Americanization of Indian ingredients has not been very positive from a health perspective. With the addition of more animal-based protein sources and fat, and a decrease in fiber content, many of the advantages of the traditional Indian diet have been lost. However, those who prepare Indian cuisine in a traditional manner will receive the benefits of a high-carbohydrate, low-fat, low-cost diet that is as tasty as it is healthy.

What about "soul food" or "southern" cooking? Do most African Americans eat lots of it?

The term *soul food* was coined in the mid-1960s to promote ethnic pride and solidarity among African Americans, but the origins of soul food date back to a much earlier time in history. Black-eyed peas, grits (coarsely ground cornmeal), collard greens, okra, and other soul foods evolved from the traditional diet of West African slaves living in the South. When West Africans were brought to the United States to work the fields, their dietary habits revolved around foods provided by slave owners. Corn was commonly given as a staple, and it was prepared in many forms, such as grits, cornmeal pudding, and hominy (hulled, dried corn kernels with certain parts removed). Also, because salt pork was frequently a staple supplied to slaves, pork fat was used to fry and flavor greens, breads, stews, and other foods. In addition, some owners allowed their slaves to grow vegetables in small plots. Slaves who farmed such plots grew American vegetables, including cabbage, collard and mustard greens, sweet potatoes, and turnips, and the slaves introduced okra and black-eyed peas, two West African favorites, to the United States. The slaves who worked as cooks in the homes of slave owners made popular other southern favorites, such as fried chicken and fried catfish. Figure 2-22 shows traditional African American foods in the five food groups.

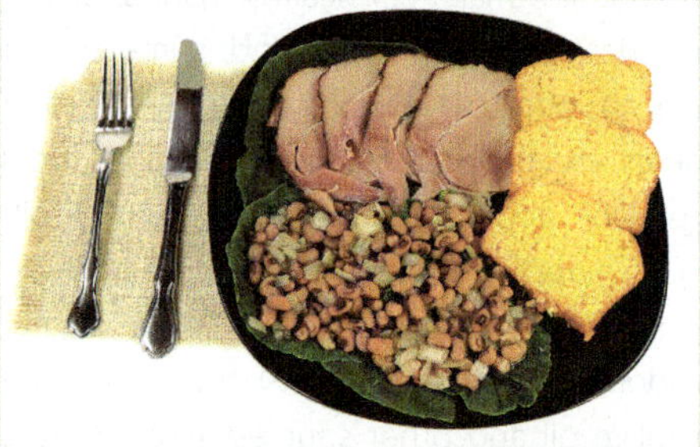

FIGURE 2-22

Traditional African American Foods and the MyPlate Food Guide[a]

[a] Discretionary calorie limit can be used for butter, candy, fruit drinks, lard, meat drippings, chitterlings,[b] soft drinks, and vegetable shortening.
[b] These foods are described in the Miniglossary.

SOURCE: Adapted from www.ChooseMyPlate.gov and the Pyramid Packet (1993) Penn State Nutrition Center, 417 East Calder Way, University Park, PA 16801.

ChooseMyPlate.gov

GRAINS	VEGETABLES	FRUITS	DAIRY	PROTEIN FOODS
biscuits, cookies, cornbread, grits[b], pasta, rice	beets, broccoli, cabbage, corn, green peas, greens, hominy[b], okra, potatoes, spinach, squash, sweet potatoes, tomatoes, yams	apples, bananas, berries, fruit juice, peaches, watermelon	buttermilk, cheese, milk	blackeyed peas, beef, catfish, chicken, crab, crayfish, eggs, kidney beans, peanuts, perch, pinto beans, pork, red beans, red snapper, salmon, sardines, shrimp, tuna, turkey

After emancipation, eating patterns of African Americans did not change significantly, and they represent much of what we think of as southern cuisine today. The underpinnings of this eating style, which is very high in fat, remain corn-based dishes, greens, pork, and pork products such as chitterlings (chitlins—pig intestines) and ham hocks. Food habits of African Americans around the country tend to be influenced more by economic status and geographic location than by heritage, although soul food remains a symbol of identity and heritage for many African Americans.[23]

I see many foods marked "kosher" in the supermarket, especially during Jewish holidays such as Passover. Are kosher foods better for health than regular food items? Do other religious groups eat special foods?

As pointed out in Chapter 1 (refer to Table 1-8), food is part of the symbolism and traditions of many major religions. In the predominantly Christian United States, however, most people's eating habits are not dictated by religion to a large extent.

Nevertheless, during the past few decades, "Jewish" foods have been growing in popularity among Americans of various religious backgrounds. For instance, bagels are now staple breakfast menu items in the United States.

Most traditional Jewish foods eaten in America come from a particular group known as *Ashkenazic Jews*—Jews from central and eastern European countries such as Russia, Germany, Poland, and Romania. (The other major group is Sephardic Jews, who come mainly from Spain and Portugal.) Although few Jewish people in the United States strictly abide by all dietary laws Judaism prescribes, many adhere to at least some rules of *kashrut*, biblical ordinances specifying which foods are *kosher*, or fit to eat.

Most people assume that the laws of kashrut were set forth to protect the health of the Jewish people. For example, a popular misconception is that kashrut forbids consumption of pork products because eating undercooked pork can cause serious illness. In truth, however,

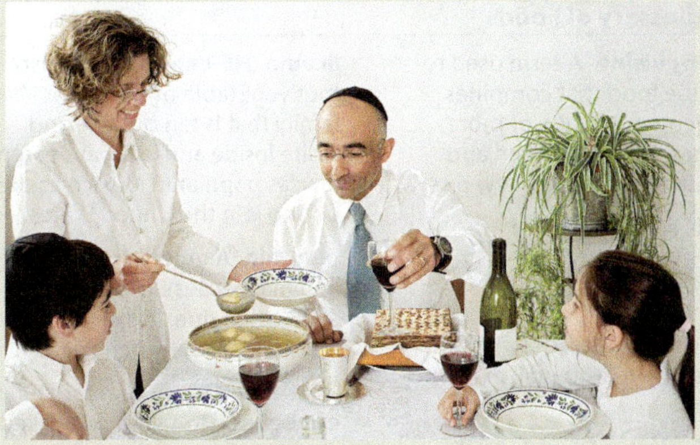

Noam Armonn/Shutterstock.com

Jewish dietary laws are considered divine commandments set forth to maintain spiritual, not physical, health. Foods labeled as kosher are not necessarily more healthy than their unmarked counterparts. Instead, the designation "kosher" indicates that a food has been prepared in accordance with the basic tenets of kashrut. For instance, one principle of kashrut is separation of milk and meat products, meaning that an item containing, say, both ground beef and cheese would not be kosher.

Another tenet is selection of appropriate meat, poultry, and seafood items. Only animals with cloven hooves that chew their cud are allowed to become food: cattle, sheep, goats, and deer. Chicken, turkey, goose, pheasant, and duck can be kosher, but birds of prey cannot. Seafood with both fins and scales can be kosher, whereas shellfish is forbidden.

Finally, as a result of the salting process used to prepare kosher animal foods, many traditional Jewish foods are high in sodium. Herring, smoked fish, canned beef, tongue, corned beef, and other deli-style meats are examples. Other traditional Jewish foods, many of which are high in fat, include schmaltz (chicken fat), knishes (potato pastry filled with ground meat or potato), cream cheese, and chopped liver.[24] Figure 2-23 shows how some traditional Jewish foods fit into the MyPlate food guide.

FIGURE 2-23

Fitting Jewish American Foods into the MyPlate Food Guide[a]

[a] Discretionary calorie limit can be used for cream cheese, honey, jelly, margarine, marmalade, preserves, schmaltz,[b] sherbet, sour cream, and sugar.
[b] These foods are described in the Miniglossary.

SOURCE: Adapted from www.ChooseMyPlate.gov and the Pyramid Packet (1993) Penn State Nutrition Center, 417 East Calder Way, University Park, PA 16801.

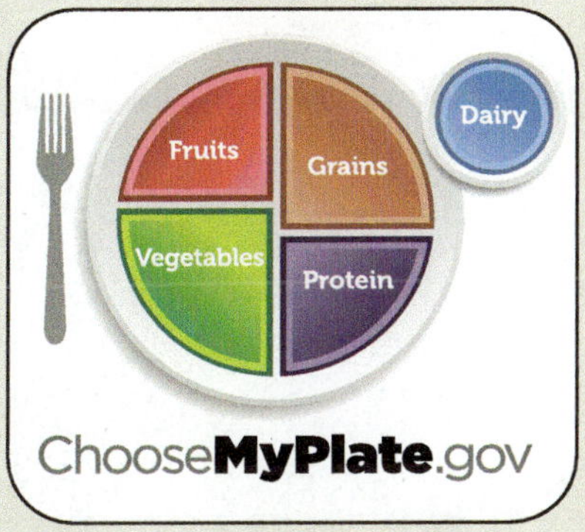

GRAINS	VEGETABLES	FRUITS	DAIRY	PROTEIN FOODS
bagel, barley, bialy[b], blintz, bulgur, challah[b], crepe, dumplings, hard rolls, honey cake, kasha[b], matzoh[b], noodle pudding, pastry, pita bread, pumpernickel bread, rye bread	artichokes, asparagus, beets/borscht, broccoli, Brussels sprouts, cabbage, carrot, cauliflower, corn, garlic, green beans, greens, leeks, olives, onion, peas, peppers, pickles, potatoes, sorrel, spinach, squash, sweet potatoes, tomatoes, turnips, yams	bananas, citrus fruits, dates, dried apples, dried apricots, dried pears, figs, grapes, melons, prunes, raisins	cottage cheese, edam cheese, farmer's cheese, gouda cheese, milk, Swiss cheese, yogurt	almonds, beef, beef tongue, brisket, chickpeas, chopped liver, corned beef, dry beans, eggs, gefilte fish[b], herring, lentils, lox[b], pastrami, poultry, salmon, sardines, smelt, smoked fish, split peas, tripe, veal

Miniglossary of Foods

fusion cuisine A term used to describe food that combines the elements of two or more cuisines—say, European and Oriental—to create a new one.

MEXICAN AMERICAN

amaranth A golden-colored grain.

agave (uh-GAH-vee) A plant with spiny-margined leaves and flower.

bolillo (buh-LEE-oh) A roll-like bread often used instead of tortillas or to make sandwiches.

burritos Warm flour tortillas stuffed with a mixture of egg, meat, beans, and/or avocado.

cassava A starchy root that is never eaten raw because it must be cooked to eliminate its bitter smell.

cherimoya A fruit with a rough green outer skin and sherbet-like flesh.

chilaquiles (chee-lah-KEE-lehs) Tortilla casserole often made with eggs or meat.

chiles rellenos (CHEE-lehs Ray-EN-yose) Roasted mild green chili peppers stuffed with cheese, dipped in egg batter, and fried.

chorizo (chuh-REE-zoh) Spicy beef or pork sausage.

guava A sweet, juicy fruit with green or yellow skin and red or yellow flesh.

jicama (HE-cah-mah) A crisp root vegetable of the bean family that is tan outside and white inside and is always eaten raw; as popular in Mexico as the potato is in the United States.

plantain A greenish, starchy banana; because it is starchy even when ripe, it is never eaten raw and is usually pan-fried.

purslane A leafy vegetable that can be used in salads or cooked like spinach.

queso blanco, fresco, or Mexicano Soft white cheese made of part-skim milk.

sopa Rice or pasta that is fried and cooked in consommé.

zapote (sah-POH-tay) An apple-sized fruit with green skin and black flesh.

CHINESE AMERICAN

bing Thin pancakes.

bok choy A vegetable with broad, white or greenish-white stalks and dark-green leaves; also called *Chinese chard.*

cellophane noodles Thin, translucent noodles made from mung beans.

Chinese broccoli A green leafy vegetable often stir-fried; also called *Chinese kale.*

choy sum A bright green vegetable commonly stir fried; also called *field mustard* or *Chinese flowering cabbage.*

dim sum Dumplings stuffed with pork, shrimp, beef, sweet paste, or preserves and steamed or fried.

glutinous rice Short-grained, opaque white rice that turns sticky when cooked.

jujube (JOO-joob) Chinese date.

litchi (LEE-chee) Small, round fruits with orange-red skin and opaque white flesh; also called *litchee* or *lychee.*

longan A small round fruit with smooth brown skin and clear pulp.

mantou Steamed bread.

Oriental radish A large, cylindrically shaped vegetable with smooth skin; also called *daikon.*

rice sticks Flat, opaque, wide noodles made from rice flour.

rice vermicelli (vur-mi-SEL-ee) Thin white noodles made from rice flour.

taro A starchy vegetable with brown, hairy skin and a pink-purple interior.

yard-long beans Thin, tender string beans that grow to as long as 18 inches.

INDIAN

chapatti A flat, unleavened bread made with finely milled whole-meal flour.

ghee A clarified butter without any milk solids or water.

lassi A milkshake-like drink made from yogurt.

roti An unleavened flatbread, resembling a tortilla, usually made from whole-wheat flour.

AFRICAN AMERICAN

chitterlings (chitlins) Pig intestine.

grits Coarsely ground cornmeal.

hominy Hulled, dried corn kernels.

JEWISH AMERICAN

bialy A flat breakfast roll that is softer than a bagel.

challah (KAH-luh) An egg-containing yeast bread, often braided, typically served on the Sabbath and holidays.

gefilte fish (guh-FIL-tuh) A chopped fish mixture often made with pike and whitefish as well as matzoh crumbs, eggs, and seasonings.

kasha Cracked buckwheat, barley, millet, or wheat that is served as a cooked cereal or potato substitute.

knish A potato pastry filled with ground meat, potato, or kasha.

kosher Fit, proper, or in accordance with religious law.

lox Smoked salmon.

matzoh A cracker-like bread eaten most often at Passover.

schmaltz Chicken fat.

WHAT'S ONLINE

MINDTAP From Cengage

Visit www.cengagebrain.com to access MindTap, a complete digital course that includes Diet & Wellness Plus, interactive quizzes, videos, and more.

10 tips
Nutrition Education Series

enjoy foods from many cultures

10 tips to wisely celebrate healthier foods and customs

As a diverse Nation, we can embrace our cultural traditions for the foods we love and still prepare them in healthier ways. This involves being creative with favorite recipes by substituting foods and ingredients that are less healthy with flavorful and appealing choices that still help remind us of our treasured food ways.

1 cook with others

Learn about cooking different traditional or regional foods from others who use authentic recipes and ingredients and explore ways to improve the nutrition of some of your own family favorites. Cooking dishes at home allows you to add variety to meals. If needed, adapt recipes by cutting back on gravies, creams, and sauces; adding more vegetables; or baking instead of frying.

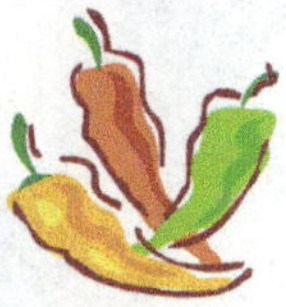

2 blend cultures

Many popular foods and beverages in America blend the cuisines of many cultures. Celebrate our Nation's diversity and be inspired by dishes that include more fruits, vegetables, whole grains, beans, seafood, lean meats, and low-fat dairy.

3 add a touch of spice

Combinations of herbs and spices often remind us of dishes from our own heritage or our favorite ethnic food. Add flavor to meals with herbs and spices, such as chili, garlic, ginger, basil, oregano, curry, or cilantro, which can replace salt and saturated fat.

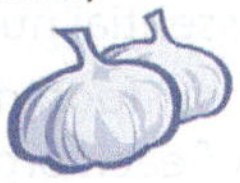

4 use familiar foods to create exotic dishes

Use foods you know and prepare new recipes, such as adding curry to chick peas, cilantro to brown rice, or mango to your salad or smoothie. Make half your plate fruits and vegetables.

5 find the salt and sodium and go with lower numbers

All packaged foods are labeled to show amounts of sodium. Use "low-sodium" soy sauce, or broth or canned beans labeled "no salt added." Check nutrition labels and use products that are lower in sodium or are salt-free.

6 think about beverages

Many cultures offer tasty beverages, such as fruit drinks, alcoholic drinks, rich coffees, and sweet teas. Consider using frozen fruits to create a great tasting smoothie, or adding spices, low-fat dairy, and small amounts of sugar to make beverages. When buying prepared beverages, choose items with less sugar and fat. To manage calories, drink water or other unsweetened beverages instead of sugary drinks.

7 delight in cultural gatherings

Celebrate traditions, especially those that help you stay physically active. Have fun with traditional dances, sports, and games that make you move. Balance what you eat with regular physical activity.

8 show children what's important

Children learn to cook from their elders. Show kids how meals and dishes from various traditions are prepared. Let them taste foods they made, as you share related stories and customs from your own heritage or expose them to other cultures, but consider ways to cut back on high-calorie foods and ingredients.

9 make smart choices when dining out

Eating out offers tempting new dishes that make it easy to overeat. Choose lower calorie dishes, such as stir fries, kabobs, or whole-wheat pastas with tomato sauce. Split a dish or ask for a take-home container at the start of a meal to save part of what's served on your plate.

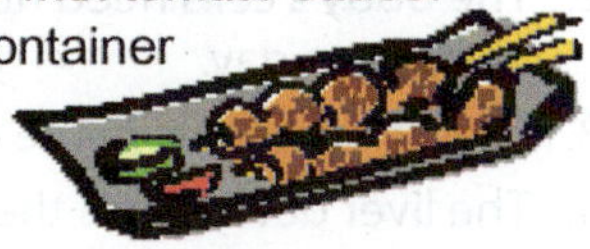

10 remember, all types of foods fit on MyPlate

MyPlate is designed to remind Americans to eat healthfully, using foods from the food groups. The MyPlate website provides practical information, tips, tools, and recipes that will help you build a healthier diet. Go to www.ChooseMyPlate.gov.

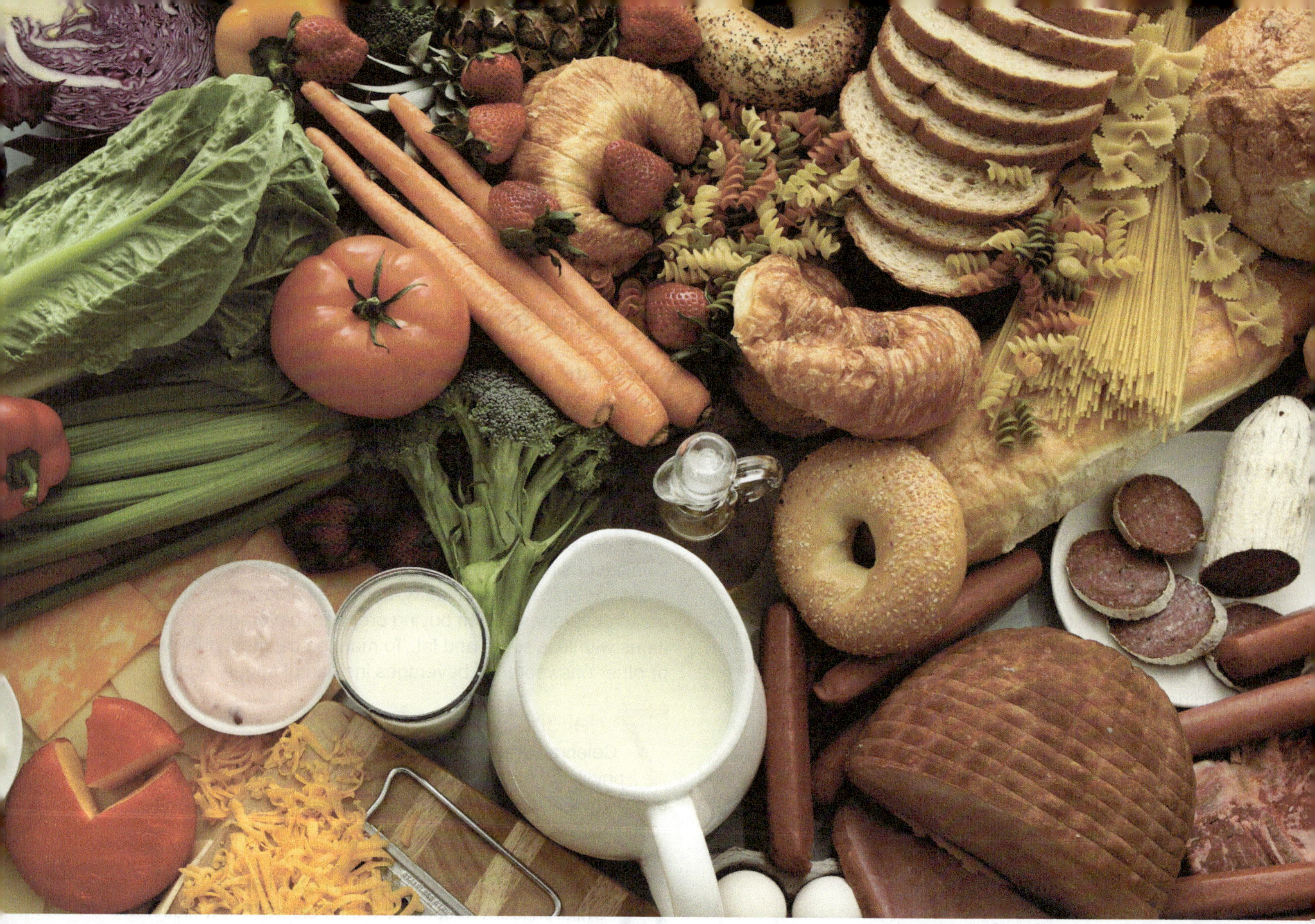

©iStockphoto.com/viafilms

AskYourself . . .

Which of the following statements about nutrition are true, and which are false? For each false statement, what is true?

1. Essential nutrients are those nutrients that can be made by the body.
2. The body's cells need nutrients 24 hours a day.
3. Digestion begins in the mouth.
4. The liver determines the metabolic fate of every nutrient absorbed.

Answers found on page 72.

ChapterObjectives

3.0 Define essential nutrients.

3.1 Explain how food moves through the digestive system, and identify the role of each organ involved in digestion, including accessory organs.

3.2 Outline how the metabolic processes of catabolism and anabolism allow the body to store and release energy as needed.

3.3 Recognize that most of the body's work is done automatically and is finely regulated to achieve a state of well-being.

3.4 Identify common digestive problems and strategies to prevent them.

Anatomy for Nutrition's Sake

CHAPTER 3

The body is composed of millions of **cells**, and not one of them knows anything about food.* Although you get hungry for meat, milk, or bread, each cell of your body sits in its place waiting until the nutrients it needs pass by. Each cell is a self-contained, living entity (see Figure 3-1); however, each depends on the rest of the body to supply its needs. The body cells' most basic needs, always, are for energy (or fuel), oxygen, and water.

Every cell in our body was once in the food we ate.

— Helen Guthrie

After energy, cells need a constant supply of nutrients to synthesize new cells and new cell parts. These necessary nutrients cannot be made by the cells and are, therefore, **essential nutrients**. Essential nutrients must be supplied by the foods we eat. Need for these nutrients is a limitation of our heredity that we cannot change, and this need underlies the first principle of nutrition: Whatever foods we choose, they must provide energy, water, and essential nutrients. In a sense, the body is merely a system organized to provide for these cellular needs.

Cells are organized into *tissues* designed to perform specialized tasks. For example, some cells are organized to form muscle tissue that helps move our bodies from place to place. Tissues can be organized to form *organs*. One organ, the heart, relies on muscle tissues, nerve tissues, and connective tissues to pump blood throughout the body. When several organs work together cooperatively, these organs are considered parts of a body *system*. One such system, the digestive system, consists of organs and tissues working together to supply necessary energy, water, and essential nutrients to every cell in our bodies.

cells The smallest units in which independent life can exist. All living things are single cells or organisms made of cells.

essential nutrients Compounds that must be obtained from food because they cannot be synthesized by the body in amounts sufficient to meet physiological needs.

*Material in this chapter was drawn generally from J. E. Hall, *Guyton and Hall Textbook of Medical Physiology*, 13th ed. (Philadelphia: Elsevier/Saunders, 2016); and L. Sherwood, *Human Physiology: From Cells to Symptoms*, 9th ed. (Belmont, CA: Cengage Learning, 2016).

FIGURE 3-1

A Typical Cell

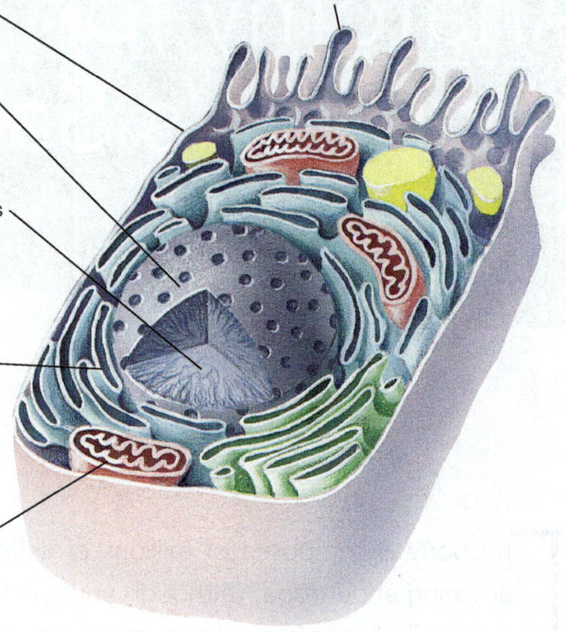

3.1 The Digestive System

You may eat meals only two or three times a day, but your body's cells need nutrients 24 hours a day. Providing the needed nutrients requires cooperation of millions of specialized cells. When the body's cells are deprived of fuel, specific nerve cells in the **hypothalamus** (part of the brain) detect this condition and generate nerve impulses that signal hunger to the conscious part of the brain. Hunger and appetite are experienced in the **cortex** of the brain—the thinking, outer layer (see Figure 3-2). Hunger (involuntary action) has primary control over how much we eat, while the type of food we look for and eat is determined by appetite (voluntary action).

The digestive system is made up of the gastrointestinal (GI) tract—also called the digestive tract—and the liver, pancreas, and gallbladder. The gastrointestinal tract provides the body with a constant supply of water and nutrients. Accomplishing this seemingly simple task entails:

- Passage of food through the GI tract
- Secretion of digestive juices and enzymes
- Digestion of the food
- Absorption of water and nutrients
- Circulation of blood through the body to distribute absorbed substances
- Control of these functions

hypothalamus (high-poh-THALL-uh-mus) A part of the brain that senses a variety of conditions in the blood, such as temperature, salt content, glucose content, and others, and signals other parts of the brain or body to change those conditions when necessary.

cortex An outer covering; in the brain, that part in which conscious thought takes place.

ASK YOURSELF ANSWERS: **1.** False: Essential nutrients cannot be made by the body and must be obtained from food. **2.** True. **3.** True. **4.** True.

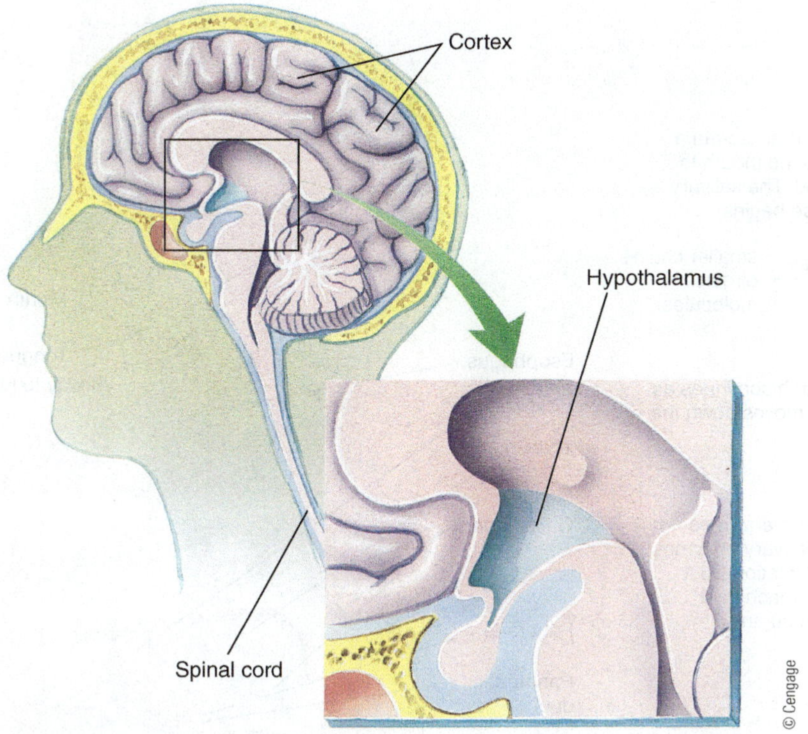

FIGURE 3-2
The Hypothalamus
The hypothalamus monitors the body's conditions and sends signals to the brain's thinking portion, the cortex, which decides on actions.

The Gastrointestinal Tract

Each part of the digestive tract has specific functions, as detailed in Figure 3-3. Some parts and functions involve basic passage of food; other parts serve as temporary storage units, and still other parts digest food and absorb the resulting nutrients.

The outer layer of the GI tract wall (called the *mesentery*) protects blood vessels, nerves, and lymphatic vessels. It also attaches the lower parts of the small intestine (jejunum and ileum) and part of the large intestine (transverse colon) to the abdominal wall to prevent the intestines from twisting.

Figure 3-4 shows a typical cross section of the intestinal wall. Movement of food through the GI tract is enabled by the different layers of smooth muscle. These muscles in the GI tract are longitudinal (up and down the length of the GI tract) and circular (around the GI tract). These two sets of muscles work together to spontaneously move food along the GI tract (see Figure 3-5). As food works its way along the GI tract, it is mixed with digestive juices and enzymes in preparation for the digestive process. Optimal food processing depends on the amount of time the food remains in each part of the GI tract. These functions are controlled by nervous and hormonal feedback systems, which are discussed later in this chapter.

The innermost layer of the GI tract wall, called the *mucosa*, is made up of cells that serve vital functions in the digestive process. Some cells secrete gastric juices, digestive enzymes, and **mucus** to protect the lining of the GI tract. These cells and their functions are also discussed later.

The Mouth Digestive processes begin in the mouth. The mouth is designed for physical breakdown of foods (mechanical digestion). Teeth cut off a bite-size portion and then, aided by the tongue, grind it finely enough to be mixed with

(*Text continues on page* 76.)

mucus (MYOO-kuss) A thick, slippery coating of the intestinal tract lining (and other body linings) that protects the cells from exposure to digestive juices. The adjective form is *mucous*, and the coating is often called the *mucous membrane*.

FIGURE 3-3

The Gastrointestinal Tract

Fiber	Carbohydrate
Mouth The mechanical action of the mouth and teeth crushes and tears fiber in food and mixes it with saliva to moisten it for swallowing.	The salivary glands secrete a watery fluid into the mouth to moisten the food. The salivary enzyme amylase begins digestion: $\text{Starch} \xrightarrow{\text{amylase}} \text{smaller chains of glucose molecules.}$
Esophagus Fiber is unchanged.	Digestion of starch continues as swallowed food moves down the esophagus.
Stomach Fiber is unchanged.	Stomach acid and enzymes start to digest salivary enzymes, halting starch digestion. To a small extent, stomach acid hydrolyzes maltose and sucrose.
Small intestine Fiber is unchanged.	The pancreas produces enzymes and releases them through the pancreatic duct into the small intestine: $\text{Polysaccharides} \xrightarrow[\text{amylase}]{\text{pancreatic}} \text{disaccharides.}$ Then enzymes on the surfaces of the small intestinal cells break disaccharides into monosaccharides, and the cells absorb them: $\text{Maltose} \xrightarrow{\text{maltase}} \text{glucose + glucose.}$ $\text{Sucrose} \xrightarrow{\text{sucrase}} \text{fructose + glucose.}$ $\text{Lactose} \xrightarrow{\text{lactase}} \text{galactose + glucose.}$
Large intestine (colon) Most fiber passes intact through the digestive tract to the colon. Here, bacterial enzymes digest some fiber: $\text{Some fiber} \xrightarrow[\text{enzymes}]{\text{bacterial}} \text{fatty acids, gas.}$ Fiber holds water; regulates bowel activity; and binds cholesterol and some minerals, carrying them out of the body as it is excreted with feces.	

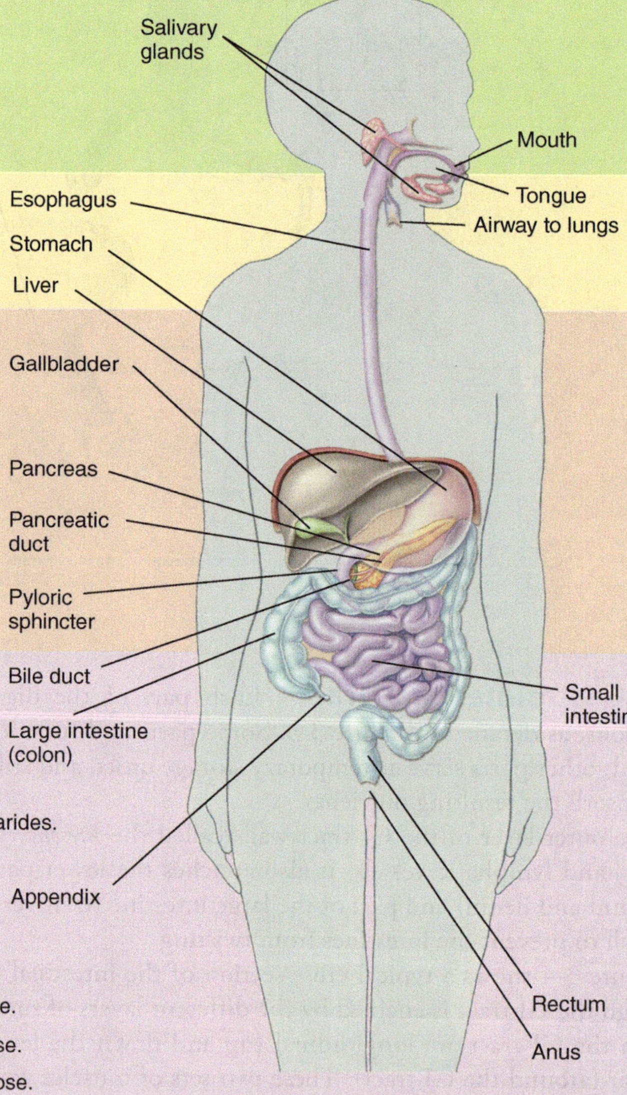

Fat	Protein	Vitamins	Minerals and Water
Mouth Glands in the base of the tongue secrete a fat-digesting enzyme known as lingual lipase. Some hard fats begin to melt as they reach body temperature.	In the mouth, chewing crushes and softens protein-rich foods and mixes them with saliva to be swallowed.	No action.	The salivary glands add water to disperse and carry food.
Esophagus Fat is unchanged.	No action.	No action.	No action.
Stomach The degree of hydrolysis is slight for most fats but may be appreciable for milk fats. The stomach's churning action mixes fat with water and acid. A gastric enzyme accesses and hydrolyzes a small percentage of fat.	Stomach acid works to uncoil protein strands and activate stomach enzymes. Then the enzymes break the strands into smaller fragments: $\text{Protein} \xrightarrow[\text{HCl}]{\text{pepsin}} \text{smaller polypeptides}$	Water-soluble vitamins need little action by the digestive organs except absorption in the small intestine. However, vitamin B12 requires "intrinsic factor" produced by the stomach in order to be absorbed.	The stomach secretes enough watery fluid to turn a moist, chewed mass of swallowed food into a liquid. Stomach acid acts on iron to make it more absorbable. Vitamin C and a factor in meat also increase iron absorption.
Small intestine The liver secretes bile; the gallbladder stores it and releases it through the common bile duct into the small intestine when fat arrives there. The bile emulsifies the fat, making it ready for enzyme action. The pancreas produces fat-digesting enzymes and releases them through the common bile duct into the small intestine. These enzymes split triglycerides into monoglycerides, free fatty acids, and glycerol, which are absorbed.	In the small intestine, the fragments of protein are split into free amino acids, dipeptides, and tripeptides with the help of enzymes from the pancreas and small intestine. Enzymes on the surface of the small intestinal cells break these peptides into amino acids, and they are absorbed through the cells into the blood. The large intestine carries any undigested protein residue out of the body. Normally, practically all the protein is digested and absorbed.	Bile emulsifies fat-soluble vitamins and aids in their absorption with other fats. Water-soluble vitamins are absorbed.	The small intestine, pancreas, and liver add enough fluid so that approximately 2 gallons are secreted into the intestine in a day. Many minerals are absorbed. Vitamin D aids in the absorption of calcium.
Large intestine (colon) Some fat and cholesterol, trapped in fiber, exit in feces.		Bacteria can produce vitamin K and biotin, which are absorbed.	More minerals and most of the water are absorbed.

FIGURE 3-4

Layers of the GI Tract

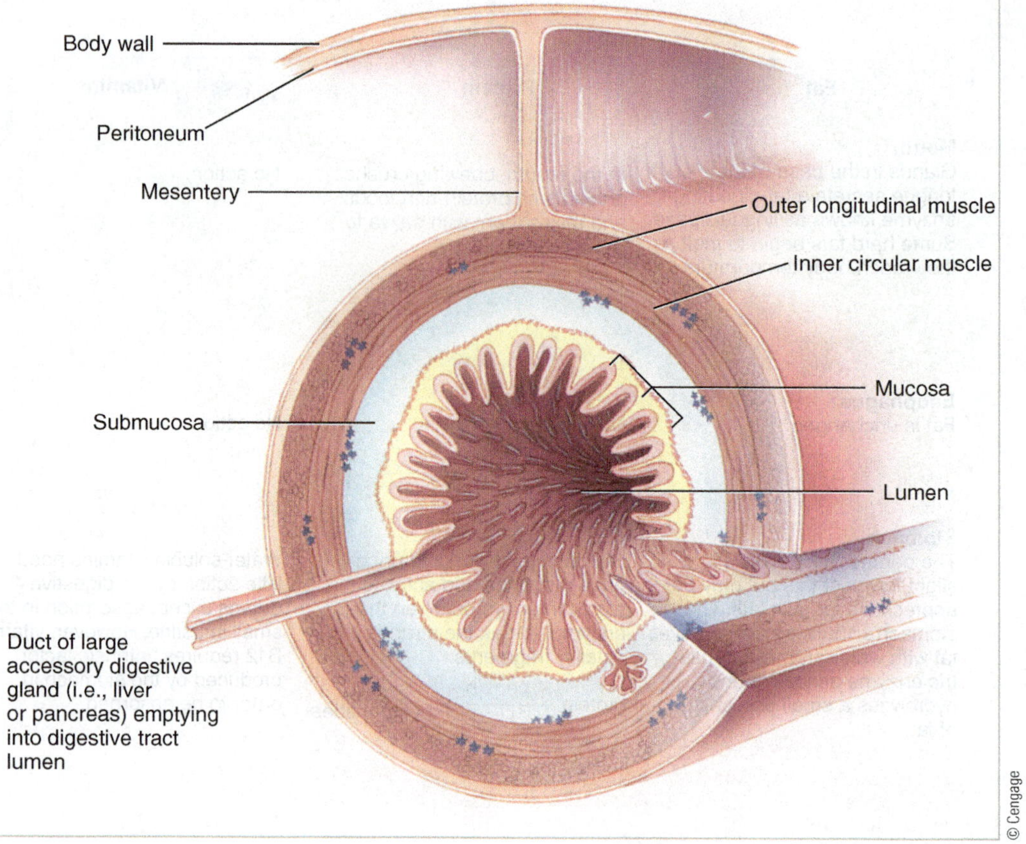

saliva and swallowed. The significance of chewing becomes apparent when eating raw fruits and vegetables. These foods have indigestible membranes covering the nutrient-containing portions, and these membranes must be broken down before the food can be digested. Chewing also exposes the surface area of food to digestive secretions. This is important because digestive enzymes act only on the surface of food particles. The mouth also contains three salivary glands that secrete salivary amylase (called *ptyalin*), which moistens food during chewing and makes it easier to swallow. This salivary amylase also begins the breakdown (chemical digestion) of complex carbohydrates (starch). This action is stopped when the carbohydrate units reach the stomach (as discussed later).

FIGURE 3-5

Peristalsis

As the wave of peristaltic contraction sweeps down the esophagus, it pushes the food bolus (a mixture of food particles and saliva) into the relaxed area ahead of it, propelling the bolus toward the stomach.

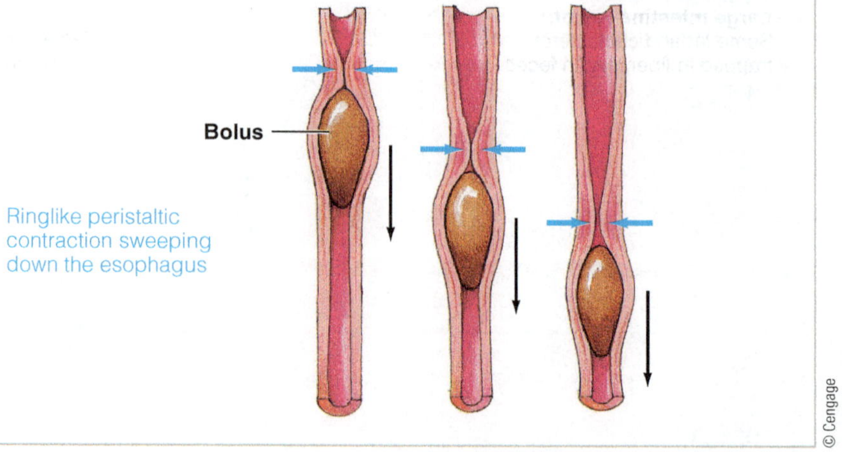

When food is chewed, the result is a mixture of food particles and saliva called a *bolus*. The food bolus must move from the mouth to the esophagus. This occurs through the process of swallowing, a seemingly simple act that is in actuality a very intricate process (see Figure 3-6) because the back of the throat (*pharynx*) is also a part of the respiratory system. The first part of the swallowing process is voluntary because we choose to chew and then, with the help of the tongue, move the bolus toward the pharynx. From there on, the process is pretty much automatic (involuntary) and as a rule cannot be stopped. The trachea (windpipe) closes and the pharynx propels the bolus toward the esophagus. This complete process occurs in less than two seconds!

The Esophagus No digestion takes place in the esophagus. Its purpose is strictly to serve as a vehicle for the food bolus as the bolus travels from the mouth to the stomach. During the swallowing process, a *sphincter* (circular band of muscle fibers that constricts a passage or closes a natural opening in the body) at the top of the esophagus relaxes to permit the bolus to enter. Longitudinal and circular muscle layers of the esophagus rhythmically push the bolus down the length of the esophagus to the stomach. This movement is called **peristalsis** (see Figure 3-5). A bolus passing through the esophagus is coated with mucus to make it slippery and easy to swallow. The mucus also protects the lining of the esophagus from being damaged by inadequately chewed foods.

At the lower end of the esophagus (between the esophagus and stomach), circular muscles form another sphincter called the *lower esophageal sphincter* (LES) or *gastroesophageal sphincter*. This sphincter, which is normally constricted or closed, plays an important role in protecting the esophagus from stomach acid that might otherwise splash back into the esophagus.

The Stomach The stomach carries out three jobs during digestion. It stores a sizeable amount of food until the food can be processed; forms a mixture of food and gastric secretions, which becomes a semiliquid blend called *chyme* (KIME); and controls movement of the chyme into the **small intestine** at a rate suitable for proper digestion and absorption by the small intestine.

An empty stomach has a volume of about 1½ ounces or 3 tablespoons. Eat some food, drink some fluids, and the stomach capacity can increase to about 1 liter (a little over 1 quart). How, you ask? The stomach is lined with deep folds (see Figure 3-7) that relax and flatten as we eat. Eating more than 1 liter (overeating) causes the stomach to stretch just a little too much and triggers discomfort.

peristalsis (pair-ih-STALL-sis) The wavelike squeezing motions of the stomach and intestines that push their contents along the digestive tract.

small intestine A long, tubular organ of digestion that is the site of nutrient absorption.

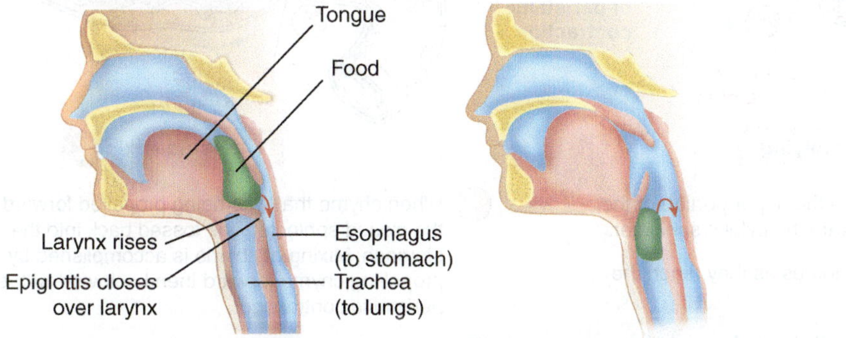

Swallowing. The epiglottis closes over the larynx, blocking entrance to the lungs via the trachea. The red arrow shows that food is heading down the esophagus normally.

Choking. A choking person cannot speak or gasp because food lodged in the trachea blocks the passage of air. The red arrow points to where the food should have gone to prevent choking.

FIGURE 3-6

Normal Swallowing and Choking

See this chapter's Spotlight feature for more information on choking and how to prevent it.

FIGURE 3-7

Simplified Anatomy of the Stomach

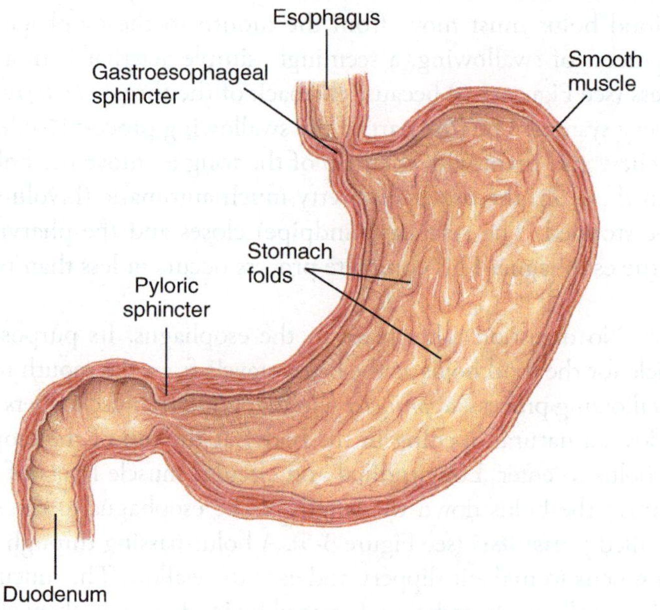

Food entering the stomach from the esophagus triggers peristalsis in the stomach, which causes the stomach to "churn," thereby mixing the food with hydrochloric acid (HCl) and other gastric secretions to form chyme. Each peristaltic wave pushes chyme toward the pyloric sphincter (see Figure 3-8) at the lower end of the stomach. The *pyloric*

FIGURE 3-8

Mixing of Stomach Contents and Emptying of the Stomach

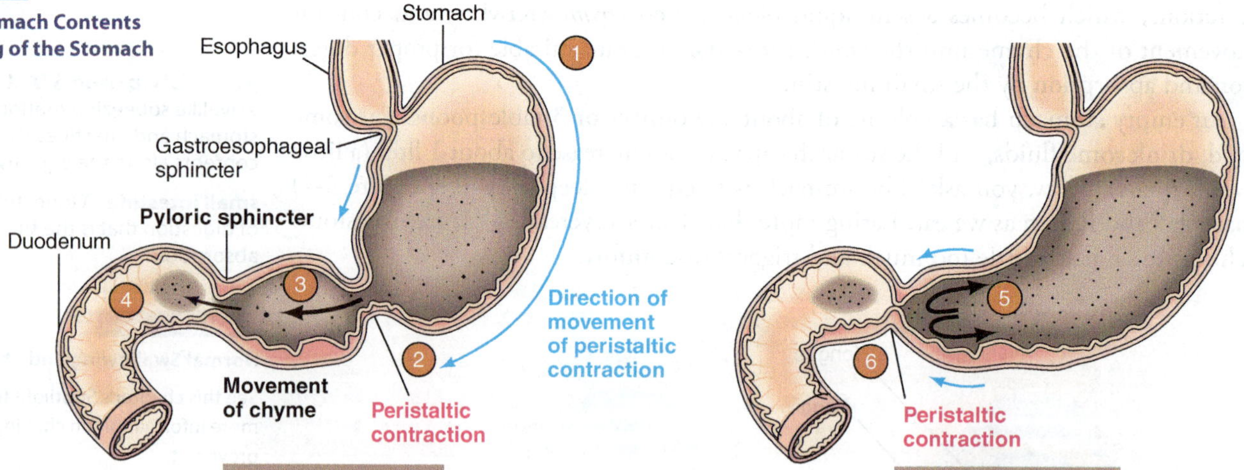

1. Peristaltic contractions begin in the upper portion of the stomach and sweep down toward the pyloric sphincter.
2. Contractions become more vigorous as they reach the lower part of the stomach.
3. These strong contractions propel chyme forward.
4. A small portion of chyme is pushed through the partially open sphincter into the small intestine. The stronger the contractions, the more chyme is emptied with each contraction.
5. When chyme that was being propelled forward hits the closed sphincter, it is tossed back into the stomach. Mixing of chyme is accomplished by propelling chyme forward then backward with each peristaltic contraction.
6. When the peristaltic contractions reach the pyloric sphincter, the sphincter is tightly closed and prevents emptying.

TABLE 3-1 Primary Functions of Selected Digestive Enzymes

Enzyme	Enzyme Function	Enzyme Source
A. Carbohydrate Digestion		
Amylase	Breaks down starch into smaller chains of glucose molecules	Produced in the salivary glands (salivary amylase) and the pancreas (pancreatic amylase)
Sucrase	Splits the disaccharide sucrose into glucose and fructose	Produced in the small intestine
Lactase	Splits the disaccharide lactose into glucose and galactose	Produced in the small intestine
Maltase	Splits the disaccharide maltose into two molecules of glucose	Produced in the small intestine
B. Fat Digestion		
Lipase	Breaks down fats into fragments of fatty acids and glycerol	Produced in salivary glands (lingual lipase) and the pancreas (pancreatic lipase) The action of lipase is enhanced by bile
C. Protein Digestion		
Pepsin	Separates protein into shorter chains of amino acids	Produced by the stomach
Trypsin	Splits short chains of amino acids into molecules containing one, two, or three amino acids	Produced by the pancreas

sphincter or **pylorus** is a circular muscle surrounding the lower end of the stomach and is normally almost completely closed. It controls the exodus of stomach contents, allowing only a little at a time to be squirted forcefully into the small intestine. Gradually, the stomach empties itself by this method. The complicated chemical breakdown that takes place beyond the stomach requires that only small amounts be processed at a time.

Several digestive secretions are produced in the stomach (see Tables 3-1 and 3-2). One such secretion is mucus. The stomach produces two types: One is thick and forms a protective barrier for the stomach lining, and the other is thin and watery to mix with food particles forming part of the chyme. Intrinsic factor is also produced by specialized

pylorus (pie-LORE-us) Muscle that regulates the opening of the bottom of the stomach.

TABLE 3-2 Digestive Tract Secretions and Their Actions

Salivary glands	Saliva (salivary fluid eases swallowing) Salivary amylase (enzyme that breaks down starch)
Esophagus	Mucus (protects lining of esophagus; mucus coats bolus and eases swallowing)
Stomach gastric glands	Gastric juice (mixes with bolus) Hydrochloric acid (uncoils protein) Pepsin (enzyme that breaks down protein) Intrinsic factor (essential for absorption of vitamin B_{12}) Mucus (thick coating that protects the stomach wall from these secretions)
Intestinal cells	Enzymes (break down carbohydrate, fat, and protein) Mucus (thin coating that protects the intestinal wall)
Liver and gallbladder	Bile (emulsifier that separates fat into particles small enough for enzymes to break down)
Pancreas	Bicarbonate (neutralizes acidic fluid from stomach so intestinal and pancreatic enzymes can work on its contents) Enzymes (break down carbohydrate, fat, and protein)

cells in the stomach. It is necessary for absorption of vitamin B_{12} in the small intestine. Even though HCl does not really digest anything, it facilitates digestion in several ways. HCl activates pepsinogen, which is the inactive form of the enzyme pepsin. Pepsin can function only in this acidic environment, where it begins the chemical breakdown of proteins. Large food particles are digested into smaller particles by breaking down muscle fiber and connective tissues. HCl also kills bacteria. Carbohydrate digestion that began in the mouth stops because the action of salivary amylase is halted by the stomach's acidic environment. Carbohydrates are chemically digested in the small intestine.

It takes approximately four hours for a meal to empty from the stomach. Liquids pass through the stomach quickly, while solids stay in the stomach until they are mixed thoroughly with stomach secretions. Carbohydrates tend to move through the stomach more quickly than proteins, and fatty foods may stay in the stomach for as long as six hours. The rate of stomach emptying (also controlled by the central nervous system and hormonal mechanisms) plays an important role in digestion and absorption of nutrients from foods. If the stomach is too slow to empty, digestion and absorption are reduced. Likewise, if the stomach empties too quickly, before food particles are thoroughly mixed with stomach secretions, very few nutrients are digested and the acidic chyme may damage the lining of the small intestine.

The Small Intestine The small intestine is the organ of digestion and absorption; it finishes the job that the mouth and stomach started. It is actually about 20 feet long, but it is called *small* because its diameter is small compared with that of the large intestine.

Chyme must touch the walls of the small intestine to make contact with the secretions and to be absorbed at the proper places. At the end of the small intestine, a circular muscle (similar in function to the pylorus at the end of the stomach) controls the flow of the contents going into the large intestine (colon). It is called the *ileocecal valve.*

The small intestine works with the precision of a laboratory chemist. As the thoroughly liquefied and partially digested nutrient mixture (chyme) arrives there, hormonal messages tell the gallbladder to send its **emulsifier**, called **bile**, in amounts matched to the amount of fat present. Other **hormones** notify the pancreas to release **bicarbonate** in amounts precisely adjusted to neutralize stomach acid as well as **enzymes** of the appropriate kinds and quantities to continue dismantling whatever large molecules remain. Such messages also maintain peristalsis so the contents will be passed along to the next region. Peristalsis is stimulated by the presence of roughage or fiber and is quieted by the presence of fat, which requires a longer time for digestion.

Meanwhile, as the pancreatic and intestinal enzymes act on bonds that hold the large nutrients together, smaller and smaller units make their appearance in the intestinal fluids. Finally, units that cells can use—glucose, glycerol, fatty acids, and amino acids, among others—are released.

Once the digestive system has broken down food to its nutrient components, it must deliver those nutrients to the rest of the body. The cells lining the small intestine absorb nutrients from the mixture and deposit them in the blood and **lymph**. Every molecule of nutrient must traverse one of these cells if it is to enter body fluids. The cells are selective: They can recognize nutrients needed by the body. The cells are also extraordinarily efficient: They absorb enough nutrients to nourish all the body's other cells.

The intestinal tract lining is composed of a single sheet of cells, and the sheet pokes out into millions of finger-shaped projections called **villi**. Each villus has its own capillary network and a lymph vessel so that as nutrients move across the cells, they can immediately mingle into the body fluids. Every villus cell has a brush-like covering of tiny hairs, called **microvilli**, that can trap nutrient particles. Figure 3-9 provides a close look at these details.

The lining of the small intestine, villi and all, is wrinkled into thousands of folds, making its absorbent surface area enormous. If the folds and the villi that cover them

emulsifier (ee-MULL-sih-fire) A compound with both water-soluble and fat-soluble portions that can attract lipids into water to form an emulsion.

bile A compound made from cholesterol by the liver, stored in the gallbladder, and secreted into the small intestine. It emulsifies lipids to ready them for enzymatic digestion.

hormone A chemical messenger, secreted by one organ (a gland) in response to a condition in the body, that acts on another organ or organs to change that condition.

bicarbonate A chemical that neutralizes acid; a secretion of the pancreas.

enzyme A protein catalyst. A catalyst is a compound that facilitates (speeds up the rate of) a chemical reaction without itself being altered in the process.

lymph (LIMF) The fluid outside the circulatory system that bathes the cells; derived from the blood by being pressed through the capillary walls; similar to the blood in composition but without red blood cells.

villi (VILL-ee, VILL-eye) Fingerlike projections of the sheet of cells that line the GI tract; the villi make the surface area much greater than it would otherwise be (singular: *villus*).

microvilli (MY-croh-VILL-ee, MY-croh-VILL-eye) Tiny hairlike projections on each cell of the intestinal tract lining that can trap nutrient particles and translocate them into the cells (singular: *microvillus*).

FIGURE 3-9

Details of the Lining of the Small Intestine

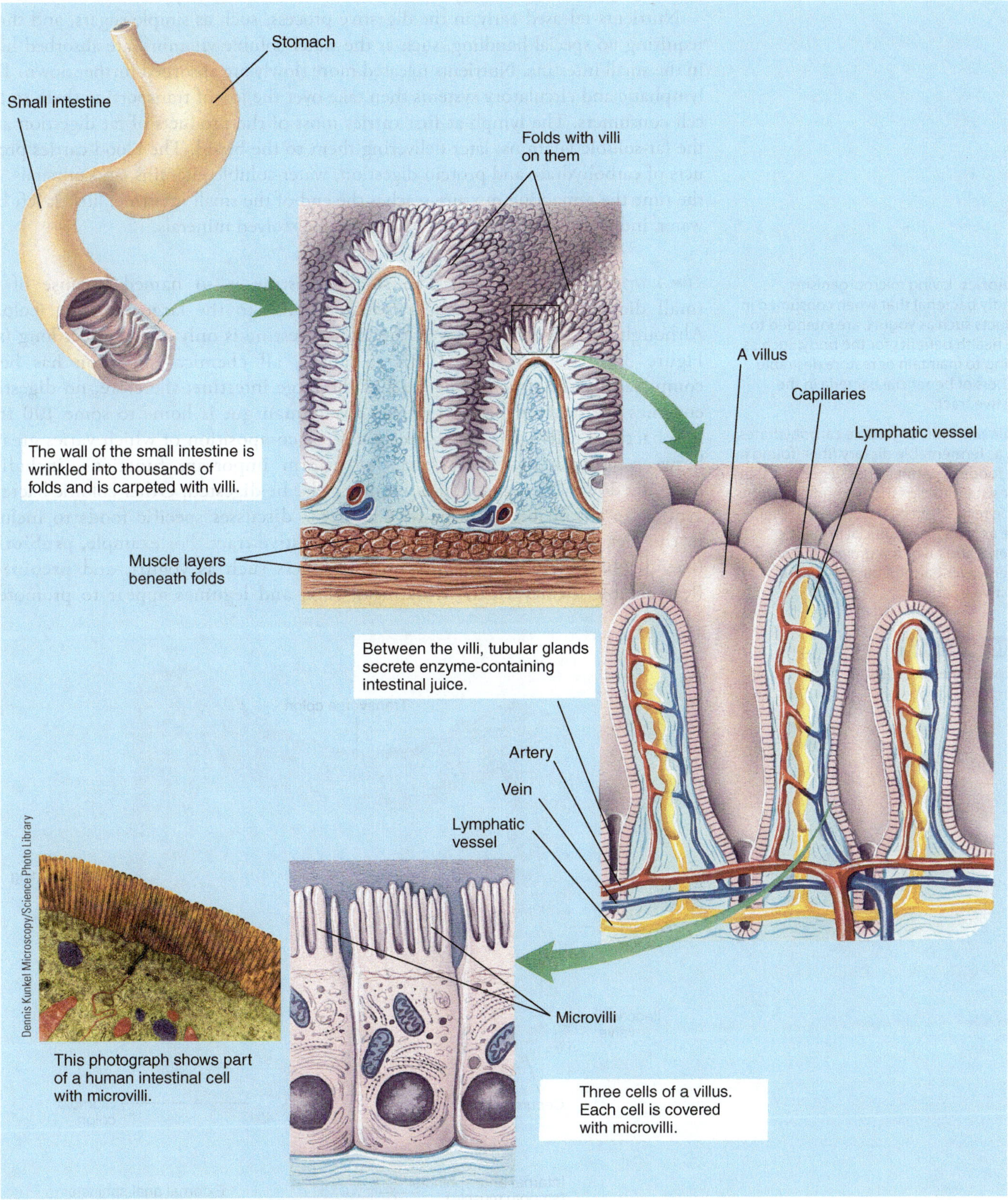

were spread out flat, the total area would equal the size of a tennis court. The billions of cells of that surface, although they weigh only 4 to 5 pounds total, absorb enough nutrients in a few hours a day to nourish the other 150 or so pounds of body tissues.

Nutrients released early in the digestive process, such as simple sugars, and those requiring no special handling, such as the water-soluble vitamins, are absorbed high in the small intestine. Nutrients released more slowly are absorbed further down. The lymphatic and circulatory systems then take over the job of transporting them to the cell consumers. The lymph at first carries most of the products of fat digestion and the fat-soluble vitamins, later delivering them to the blood. The blood carries products of carbohydrate and protein digestion, water-soluble vitamins, and minerals. By the time the remaining mixture reaches the end of the small intestine, little is left but water, indigestible residue (mostly fiber), and dissolved minerals.

probiotics Living microorganisms (friendly bacteria) that when consumed in products such as yogurt, are intended to have health benefits for the body, such as helping to maintain or restore desirable numbers of beneficial bacteria in the digestive tract.

prebiotics Non-digestible carbohydrates, such as fermentable dietary fiber (found in such foods as oatmeal, flax, legumes), that are resistant to digestion in humans, but can be fermented by intestinal bacteria, serve as food for beneficial probiotic bacteria, and favor the growth of beneficial bacteria over harmful bacteria in the digestive tract.

The Large Intestine (Colon) The small intestine is so named because of its small diameter, and the same rationale applies to the large intestine (colon). Although the diameter is larger, the large intestine is only about 5 feet long (see Figure 3-10). Under normal circumstances, all chemical digestion has been completed by the time chyme reaches the large intestine; therefore, no digestive enzymes are secreted here. However, the human gut is home to some 100 trillion bacterial cells—the gut *microbiota*—the composition of which varies greatly between individuals. These bacteria perform important functions, including breaking down fibers that could not otherwise be digested. Other colonic bacteria synthesize absorbable vitamin K. Chapter 7 discusses specific foods to include in the diet to enhance the health of the digestive tract. For example, **probiotics** (friendly bacteria) in fermented milk products such as yogurt, and **prebiotics** (fermentable dietary fiber) in oatmeal, flax, and legumes appear to promote a

FIGURE 3-10

Large Intestine (Colon)

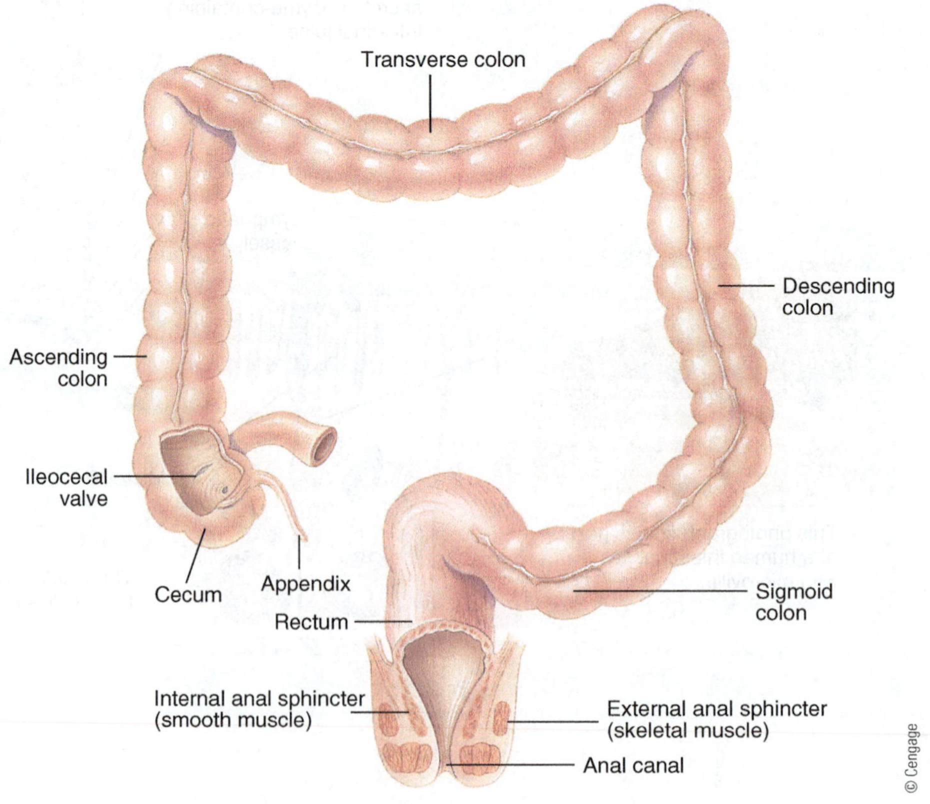

healthy digestive tract. Probiotics are also associated with outcompeting potentially disease-causing bacteria in the digestive tract.

Because the primary functions of the large intestine are to absorb dissolved minerals and water and eliminate waste products, cells lining the colon are specialized for absorbing these minerals and retrieving water for recycling. The final waste product is mixed with mucus produced in the large intestine to protect the innermost lining against abrasion and irritation from the chyme. Fecal material, a smooth paste of a consistency suitable for excretion, is stored in the colon until excretion. This system can adjust to whatever mixture of foods is presented. Fecal material normally consists of water, undigested fiber, bile pigments, bacteria, and a small amount of salt.

The colon has the same type of mixing and peristaltic movements as in other sections of the digestive tract, but they are more sluggish and occur less frequently. Commonly occurring after a meal, as the rectum fills with feces, the defecation reflex is set in motion and waste products are eliminated.

In addition to feces being eliminated via the colon, sometimes intestinal gas (*flatus*) passes out. Most intestinal gas is produced by bacterial fermentation. The quantity and quality of the gas depends on the types of foods eaten and characteristics of intestinal bacteria.

Accessory Organs of Digestion Organs outside the digestive tract—the liver, gallbladder, and pancreas—also contribute digestive juices through a common duct into the small intestine (see Figure 3-11). Presence of these digestive juices and

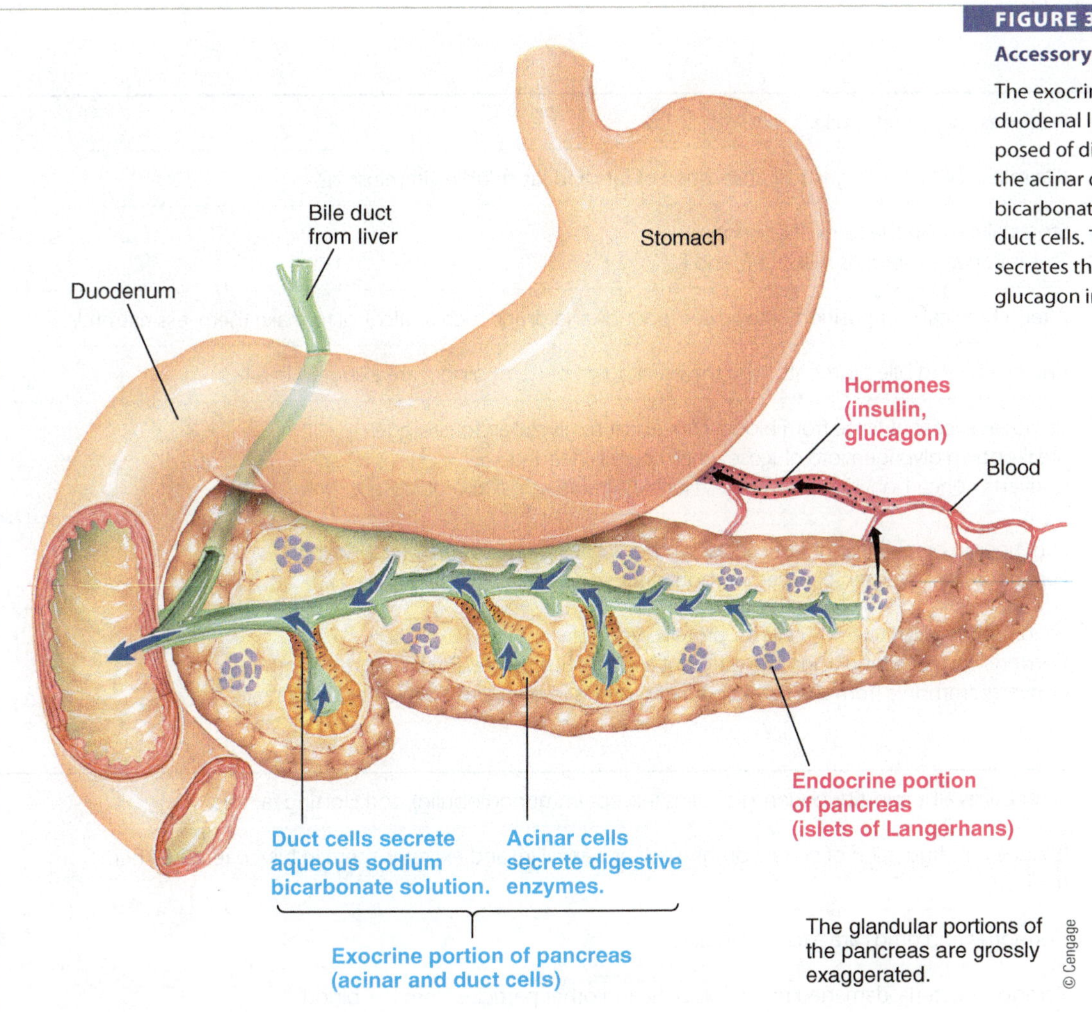

FIGURE 3-11

Accessory Organs of Digestion

The exocrine pancreas secretes into the duodenal lumen a digestive juice composed of digestive enzymes secreted by the acinar cells and an aqueous sodium bicarbonate solution secreted by the duct cells. The endocrine pancreas secretes the hormones insulin and glucagon into the blood.

enzymes requires ancillary cells that specialize in protecting the digestive system. They do so by secreting a layer of thick, viscous mucus.

Liver The **liver** determines the metabolic fate of every nutrient we digest and absorb, in addition to performing a wide variety of other functions, most of them essential for life (see Table 3-3). The liver produces about one liter of bile each day. *Bile*, made up of water, bile salts, bile pigments, and cholesterol, is slightly alkaline, which helps neutralize acidic chyme in the intestinal tract. Bile salts are not digestive enzymes, but do play a role in the digestion of fats. Bile salts are emulsifying agents, which break down large globules of fat into tiny globules of fat. This improves the efficiency of fat digestion by increasing the surface area of fat. Bile salts also play a role in absorption of fat-soluble vitamins. The bile pigments and cholesterol are waste products and are eventually eliminated from the body.

Gallbladder The gallbladder is a sac, attached to the liver (see Figure 3-3), where bile is stored and concentrated. Bile empties from the gallbladder into the uppermost part of the small intestine (*duodenum*) via the common bile duct. Entry of bile into the small intestine is controlled by the sphincter of Oddi. When the small intestine is empty, the sphincter is closed and bile is backed up into the gallbladder for

liver The large, lobed organ that lies under the ribs and filters the blood, in the process removing, processing, and readying for redistribution many of its materials.

TABLE 3-3 **Functions of the Liver**

Digestive Functions	
Secretion	Produces and secretes bile.
Synthesis of bile salts	Bile salts facilitate fat digestion, absorption of fats and fat-soluble vitamins.
Storage	Stores glucose in the form of glycogen. Stores iron and vitamins A, B_{12}, D, E, and K.
Detoxification	Alters chemical composition of toxic compounds and drugs such as alcohol to make them less harmful.
Excretion	Cholesterol and bile pigments from the breakdown of hemoglobin are excreted in bile.
Carbohydrate metabolism	Removes excess glucose from blood, converts it to glycogen for storage. Breaks down glycogen into glucose when more is needed. Converts noncarbohydrate molecules (such as amino acids) into glucose.
Fat metabolism	Functions in breakdown of fatty acids, synthesis of cholesterol and phospholipids. Functions in conversion of excess carbohydrates and proteins into fats.
Protein metabolism	Sends amino acids to body cells for protein synthesis. Converts certain amino acids into different amino acids as needed for protein synthesis. Converts ammonia from the breakdown of proteins into urea to be excreted in urine.
Nondigestive Functions	
Synthesis of plasma proteins	Synthesizes albumin, fibrinogen, globulins (except immunoglobulin), and clotting factors.
Detoxification	Changes configuration of certain drugs (such as penicillin) and excretes them in bile to remove them from the body.
Excretion	Hormones and drugs are excreted in bile.
Filtration	Removes bacteria, damaged red blood cells, and other particles from the blood.

concentration and storage until it is needed. When chyme with fatty content enters the small intestine, a hormone (cholecystokinin [koh-lee-sis-toh-KYE-nin]) stimulates the gallbladder to contract and the sphincter to open, thus allowing bile to flow into the small intestine.

Pancreas A gland having both endocrine and exocrine functions, the **pancreas** lies behind the stomach and upper portion of the small intestine (see Figure 3-11). The islets of Langerhans (which are scattered on the surface of the pancreas) perform the **endocrine** functions of the pancreas. These cells help regulate blood glucose levels through secretion of the hormones **insulin** and glucagon into the blood. The principal functions of the pancreas, however, are **exocrine**.Bicarbonate and digestive enzymes that act on carbohydrates, proteins, and fats are secreted into the duodenum. Pancreatic amylase breaks down starch and other complex carbohydrates into simpler sugars called *disaccharides* (see Chapter 4).

3.2 Metabolism: Breaking Down Nutrients for Energy

All nutrients leaving the digestive system by way of blood are collected in thousands of **capillaries** in the membrane that supports the intestine. These converge into **veins** and then into a single large vein. This vein conveys its contents to the liver and there breaks up once again into a vast network of capillaries that weave among liver cells, allowing them access to newly arriving nutrients.

Liver cells process these nutrients. They convert sugars from carbohydrate mostly into the body's primary sugar, *glucose*. If there is a surplus, they store some as glycogen (discussed in Chapter 4) and convert the remainder to fat. They reassemble fatty acids and glycerol from dietary fat into larger fats and package them with protein for transport to other parts of the body. As for amino acids from protein, liver cells alter these as needed, making glucose from some if necessary and fat from others if there is an excess, or converting one amino acid into another for use in making proteins.

Nutrients that leave the digestive tract by way of lymph are packaged as **chylomicrons** that circulate throughout the body, allowing cells to withdraw fats from them. Some also find their way into blood and circulate through the liver, which removes them, alters their components, and releases new products, including other **lipoproteins**.

The new products of liver **metabolism**—glucose, fat packaged with protein (lipoproteins—see Chapter 5), and amino acids—are released into the bloodstream again and circulated to all other cells of the body. Surplus fat is then removed by cells specialized for its storage; these fat cells are located in deposits all over the body.

The glycogen stored in the liver provides a reserve supply of the body's sugar, glucose, and thus can sustain cell activities if intervals between meals become so long that glucose absorbed from ingested foods is used up. When the body is depending solely on liver glycogen, however, the supply is used up within 3 to 6 hours. Similarly, fat cells store reserves of fat, the body's other principal energy nutrient.

Unlike the liver, however, fat cells have virtually infinite storage capacity and can continue to supply fat for days, weeks, or even months when no food is eaten. (Chapter 10 contains more about fasting, and Chapter 11 contains more about energy production.)

pancreas A gland that secretes the endocrine hormone insulin and also produces the exocrine secretions that aid digestion in the small intestine. (See also *endocrine; exocrine.*)

endocrine (EN-doh-krin) A term to describe a gland secreting or a hormone being secreted into the blood.

insulin A hormone from the pancreas that helps glucose get into cells.

exocrine (EX-oh-krin) Describes glands that secrete chemical messengers through a duct into a body cavity or onto the surface of the skin; *exo* means "out."

capillaries Minute, weblike blood vessels that connect arteries to veins and permit transfer of materials between blood and tissues.

veins Blood vessels that carry used blood from the tissues back to the heart.

chylomicron (KIGH-loh-MY-cron) A type of lipoprotein that transports newly digested fat—mostly triglyceride—from the intestine through lymph and blood.

lipoproteins (LIP-oh-PRO-teens) Clusters of lipids associated with protein that serve as transport vehicles for lipids in blood and lymph (see Chapter 5).

metabolism (meh-TAB-o-lism) Total of all chemical reactions that go on in living cells.

These storage systems for glucose and fat ensure cells will not go without energy nutrients even if the body is hungry for food, except under extreme conditions. Body stores also exist for many other nutrients, each with a characteristic capacity. For example, the third energy nutrient, protein, is held in an available pool (amino acids in the liver and blood) that is rather rapidly depleted during protein deficiency conditions (see Chapter 6). Liver and fat cells store many vitamins, and bones provide reserves of calcium, sodium, and other minerals that can be drawn on to keep blood levels constant and to meet cellular demands.

The breakdown of body compounds is known as *catabolism*. These reactions usually release energy. Glycogen can be broken down to glucose, triglycerides to fatty acids and glycerol, and protein to amino acids. When the body needs energy, it breaks any or all of the four basic units—glucose, fatty acids, glycerol, and amino acids—into even smaller units. When the body does not require energy, the end products of digestion (glucose, amino acids, glycerol, and fatty acids) are used to build body compounds in a process called *anabolism*. Anabolic reactions involve conversion of glucose to glycogen or fat, conversion of amino acids to body proteins or fat, and synthesis of body fat from glycerol and fatty acids. Catabolism and anabolism are examples of **energy metabolism**.

3.3 Other Systems

In addition to the digestive system, the body has many more systems: bones, muscles, nerves, lungs, reproductive organs, and others. All of these systems cooperate so each cell can carry on its own life. Each assures, through hormonal or nerve-mediated messages, that its needs will be met by the others, and each contributes to the welfare of the whole by doing its specialized work. Most of the body's work is done automatically and is finely regulated to achieve a state of well-being. We would do well to "listen" to our bodies and to cultivate an understanding and appreciation of the body's needs. Then we can make decisions to promote health.

energy metabolism All reactions by which the body obtains and expends the energy from food or body stores.

Nutrition ACTION Do Your Genes Affect What's in Your Jeans? (Obj. 3.3)

As you study the material in this text, you will learn that our bodies need protein to build and repair cells, that fats supply more than twice as much energy as carbohydrates, and that the "typical American" diet (Western diet) can be wholly or partially linked to chronic diseases such as heart disease (the leading cause of death in the United States), some cancers (second leading cause of death in the United States), osteoporosis, overweight, obesity, and type 2 diabetes. But you may not know why.

As humans, 99 percent of our genetic physiology and metabolic heritage dates back roughly 40,000 years! What does this mean to present-day humans? Why is this important? And most importantly, why should you care? Think about this: If our bodies are "programmed" the way our distant hunter-gatherer ancestors' were, nearly all of our metabolism and physiology are fine-tuned to conditions that existed more than 10,000 years ago, before the development of agriculture and the domestication of animals we currently use for food. Our physiology most certainly predates fast foods, convenience foods, and sedentary workplaces and lifestyles. Our **gene** pool has been programmed to perform in ancient surroundings significantly unlike those in which we now live.

If you're still thinking, "So what?" take a look at this comparison between the eating patterns of our ancient ancestors and those of today.

Food/Nutrient	Ancient Ancestors' Eating Habits	The Way We Eat Today
Grains (wheat, rice, corn, oats, barley)	Rarely used	40–90% of total caloric intake
Meat	30% total calories (undomesticated wild game, fish)	12% total calories (domesticated animals)
Fruits	50% total calories	6% total calories
Vegetables	(>100 different species of uncultivated plant foods, roots, tubers)	5% total calories
Fiber	>100 g/d	<20 g/day
Milk & milk products	Nonexistent after weaning	1.8 c/day (or 14% total calories)
Fats	~35% total calories (varied with latitude)	20–35% total calories
Saturated fats	5–7.5% total calorie intake	11–15% total calorie intake
Sugar	Honey when available	20 to 30 tsp/day
Sodium	600 mg/day	~4,000 mg/day
Potassium	7,000 mg/day	~3,000 mg/day
Energy intake	Feast–famine	Food abundance (food available 24 hr/day)
Energy expenditure	Obligatory for survival (probably ≥3,000 cal/day)	Sedentary (<30 min/d of moderate-intensity physical activity, ~2,000 cal/day)

What does all of this information mean? You will learn what it means as you read this text for your class, but to give you a sneak peek of information to come, consider the impact that our ancestors' lifestyles and eating habits might have on the chronic degenerative diseases that are the most common ailments of today.

gene A unit of a cell's inheritance; made of a chemical, DNA, that is copied faithfully so that every time the cell divides, both its offspring get identical copies. Genes direct the cells' machinery to make the proteins that form each cell's structures and enable the cell to do its work.

Some of you may be thinking, "Yeah, but Stone Age humans didn't live as long as we do!" Though this is true, the major contributors to our increased life expectancy are better sanitation (purer water, adequate sewage disposal), safer food, and an effective system of quarantine and immunization. Chronic degenerative diseases do cause death later in life, but they begin much earlier in life, usually in our late teens and early 20s. We do not have to expend energy (as compared to our ancestors) to obtain our food, making calories accessible at the lowest cost in human history without reciprocal energy expenditure.

(Continued)

Disease	Protective Attributes of Ancient Habits and Eating Patterns
Heart disease	High intake of very lean animal protein. Habitual physical activity reduces incidence of atherosclerosis. Fiber from fruits and vegetables is predominantly soluble fiber, which protects against heart disease. Saturated fat intake was negligible and *trans* fats nonexistent.
Hypertension	High dietary potassium intake along with low dietary sodium intake. Habitual physical activity decreases blood pressure. Decreased blood pressure reduces risk of heart disease..
Cancer	Humans are the only free-living primates that consume cereal grains. Fruits and vegetables provide more potential cancer prevention (phytochemical protection from free radicals), but consumption of fruits and vegetables has largely been replaced by consumption of cereal grains. Habitual physical activity reduces risk of some cancers (especially breast cancer).
Osteoporosis	Wild plant foods (fruits and vegetables) contain considerable calcium and do not contain chemicals that bind calcium and keep it from being absorbed in the small intestine. Habitual physical activity increases bone density and muscular strength, and reduces incidence of age-related fractures. High intake of dietary potassium (fruits and vegetables) and low intake of dietary sodium counteract the effects of high animal protein intake that increases urinary calcium loss.
Diabetes/insulin resistance	Habitual physical activity can decrease serum glucose levels. Higher-fiber diets can help control blood glucose levels.
Obesity	Our ancestral genes were not selected for a sedentary lifestyle. Inactivity has a greater impact on weight gain than consuming large amounts of calories alone.

Certainly, the foods we consume today are very different from the foods of the ancient past. As Dr. Michael Eades, founder of the Arkansas Center for Health and Weight Control in Little Rock, observed, "The same thing that caused our ancestors to survive is killing us now."

SOURCES:

M. V. Chakravarthy and F. W. Booth, Eating, exercise, and "thrifty" genotypes: Connecting the dots toward an evolutionary understanding of modern chronic diseases, *Journal of Applied Physiology, 96* (2004): 3–10.

L. Cordain et al., Origins and evolution of the Western diet: Health implications for the 21st century, *American Journal of Clinical Nutrition, 81* (2005): 341–54.

S. B. Eaton, The ancestral human diet: What was it and should it be a paradigm for contemporary nutrition? *Proceedings of the Nutrition Society, 65* (2006): 1–6.

S. B. Eaton and S. B. Eaton III, Paleolithic vs. modern diets: Selected pathophysiological implications, *European Journal of Nutrition, 39* (2000): 67–70.

S. B. Eaton et al., Review: Evolutionary health promotion, *Preventive Medicine*, 34 (2002): 109–18.

Foods Found in Modern Diets Generally Unavailable to Our Prehistoric Ancestors

Food Group	Foods
Dairy	Whole milk Low-fat milk Cheese Butter
Cereal grains	Whole grains Refined grains Refined sugars High-fructose corn syrup (used in soft drinks, etc.) Syrups
Refined vegetable oils	Salad and cooking oils Shortening Margarine
Alcohol	Alcoholic beverages

SOURCE: Adapted from L. Cordain et al., Origins and evolution of the Western diet: Health implications for the 21st century, *American Journal of Clinical Nutrition, 81* (2005): 41–54.

SPOTLight

3.4 Gut Feelings—Common Digestive Problems

Americans have come a long way since Hippocrates proclaimed, "Passing gas is necessary to well-being," or the Emperor Claudius decreed, "All Roman citizens shall be allowed to pass gas whenever necessary." Digestive problems such as choking, hiccupping, burping/belching, flatulence, heartburn, constipation, diarrhea, and hemorrhoids are common, yet most people don't know what causes them or how to avoid them. It is important to understand how your GI tract works and what you can do to keep it healthy.

What causes a person to choke?

Pieces of food or small objects can cause choking if they get caught in your throat and block your airway (see Figure 3-6). Oxygen cannot get to your lungs and brain if your airway is blocked. And, if your brain goes without oxygen for more than 4 minutes, you could experience brain damage or die. When you or someone else is choking, quick action can be lifesaving. How can you prevent yourself or someone else from choking?

- Be extra careful when eating foods that are easy to choke on. This includes foods like hot dogs, nuts, grapes, raw carrots, popcorn, and hard or sticky candy.
- Sit down while eating, take small bites, and don't talk or laugh with your mouth full. Does this sound like something your mom would say? Well, mom was right! In addition to describing good manners, this advice will help prevent choking.
- If babies or toddlers can pick something up, they will probably put it in their mouth, so help keep them safe by picking up anything off the floor that might be dangerous to swallow. This includes items like pen caps, coins, beads, batteries, and toys with small parts. Keep hazards out of their reach, and supervise them when they eat.
- Learn the Heimlich maneuver—a technique that uses abdominal thrusts for dislodging an object from the trachea (see Figure 3-12). Check for first aid classes on your campus.

What are hiccups?

Hiccups occur when the muscle at the base of the lungs (diaphragm) spasms. This causes a person to take a short, quick breath that is interrupted by the closing of the epiglottis. The sound we hear when hiccupping is the vocal cords slamming closed after the spasm.

What causes hiccups?

Hiccups can be associated with a variety of ailments, but there is often no obvious cause. Usually hiccups disappear after several minutes, but

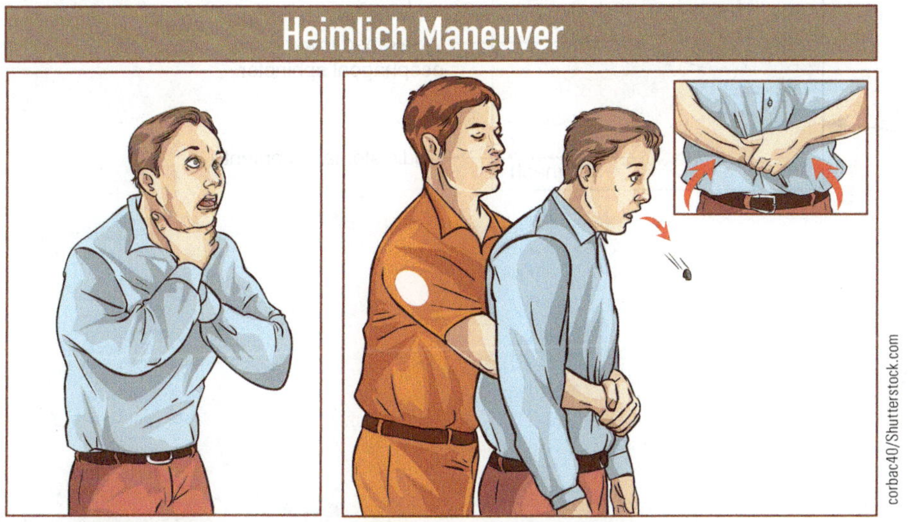

FIGURE 3-12

The Heimlich Maneuver: A First Aid Procedure for Choking

Named after Dr. Henry Heimlich, who first described the procedure in 1974, the Heimlich maneuver is an emergency procedure for removing food or other foreign object that is lodged in the upper airway (trachea) and preventing a person from breathing.

A. Use the universal signal for choking to signal for help, by holding both hands on the throat.

B. The Heimlich maneuver uses abdominal thrusts to expel the trapped object. Consider taking a first aid class to learn more about this and other life-saving procedures.

a health care provider should be consulted if hiccups continue for more than a few days. Some common causes of hiccups include:

- Hot and spicy foods and liquids
- Noxious fumes
- Pneumonia
- Swallowing air
- Excess smoking and drinking alcohol
- Emotions such as shock, excitement, and stress
- Nerve irritation
- Surgery, especially abdominal surgery
- Mental health issues

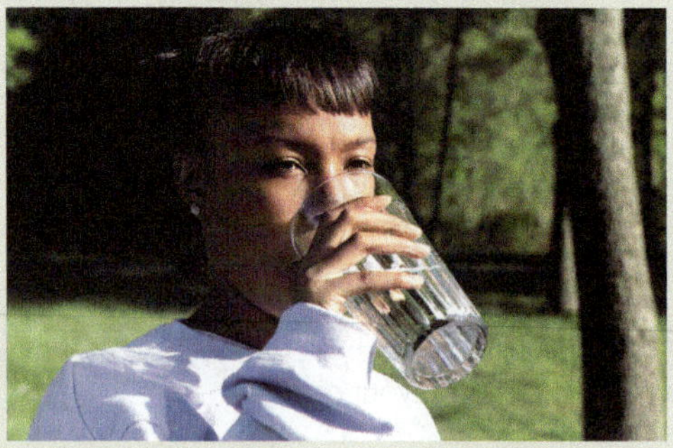
Frank Siteman/PhotoEdit

Is there a "cure"? How do I get rid of them?

There is no one sure way to get rid of hiccups, but there are several common suggestions (home remedies) that may or may not be effective:

- Hold your breath and count slowly to 10.
- Breathe repeatedly into a paper bag for a short time.
- Drink a glass of cold water quickly.
- Eat a teaspoon of sugar or honey.

Does heartburn mean that your heart is on fire?

Heartburn by any other name is called pyrosis or acid indigestion. It is not a heart problem, but a gastrointestinal condition that gets its name from the painful burning sensation that occurs in the esophagus just below or behind the sternum or breastbone. Almost everyone has occasional heartburn. But if heartburn becomes frequent and ongoing, a more serious problem may be at hand . . . *gastroesophageal reflux disease* (GERD). GERD occurs when the muscles (sphincter) between the esophagus and stomach do not close tightly enough, allowing acidic contents of the stomach to back up (or reflux) into the esophagus and irritate it (see Figure 3-13). Other symptoms of heartburn or GERD are:

- Burning in the throat—or hot, sour, acidic, or salty-tasting fluid at the back of the throat
- Difficulty swallowing
- Feeling of food "sticking" in the middle of the chest or throat
- Chronic cough, sore throat, or chronic hoarseness

Some foods we eat or drink can initiate heartburn and so can some over-the-counter and prescription medications. Examples include:

- Certain foods such as fatty foods, spicy foods, chocolate, caffeine, onions, tomato sauce, carbonated beverages, and mints
- Alcohol
- Large meals

FIGURE 3-13

Gastroesophageal Reflux

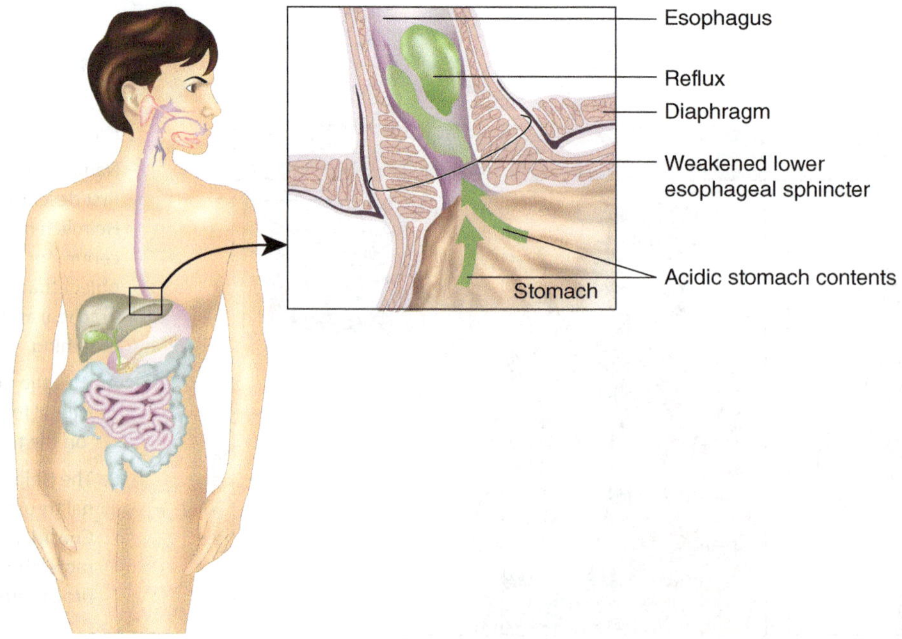

© Cengage

- Lying down too soon after eating
- Certain medications, including sedatives, antidepressants, and calcium channel blockers for high blood pressure
- Cigarette smoking
- Aspirin
- Other anti-inflammatory medications like ibuprofen (Motrin®, Advil®, Nuprin, etc.)

Smoking and consumption of high-fat-content foods tend to cause the lower esophageal sphincter (LES) to relax and allow acid to reflux into the esophagus. Pregnancy, obesity, and wearing clothing too tight around the waist can also cause increased pressure in the abdomen, leading to reflux. The best thing to do if you experience any of these symptoms is to see your health care provider, who may recommend over-the-counter remedies or prescribe medication.

How does gas get into my digestive tract?

Everyone has gas. Belching or burping is nature's way of getting rid of air we've swallowed when eating or drinking. If we eat or drink too rapidly, chew gum, smoke, or wear loose-fitting dentures, even more air may get into the stomach.

Any gas remaining in the stomach moves into the small intestine, where two things take place: It is absorbed in the small intestine; and a small amount finds its way into the large intestine, where it joins up with undigested foods and/or the gas produced by the friendly bacteria that live in our large intestine. All of this gas is released through the rectum. Gas from swallowed air is odorless, but the friendly, helpful bacteria that live in our large intestine to make vitamin K and biotin, and break down fibers in the carbohydrates we eat, sometimes produce small amounts of sulfur that does have an unpleasant odor.

Foods That May Cause Gas Include:

- Beans
- Broccoli
- Cabbage
- Brussels sprouts
- Onions
- Artichokes
- Asparagus
- Pears
- Apples
- Peaches
- Whole grains
- Bran
- Soft drinks
- Fruit drinks
- Milk and milk products
- Sorbitol (in sugar-free candies and gum)

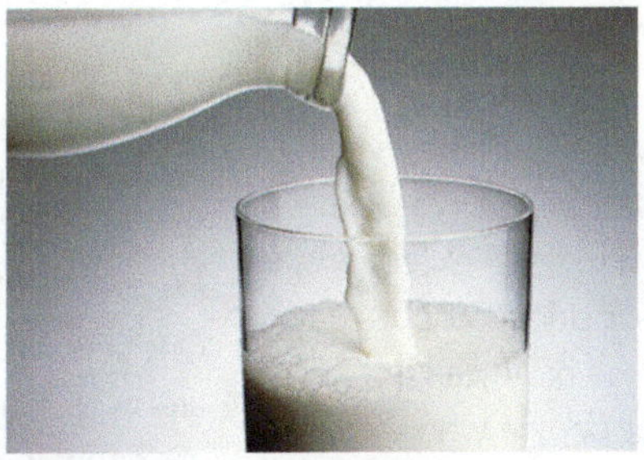
© Linux Patrol/Shutterstock.com

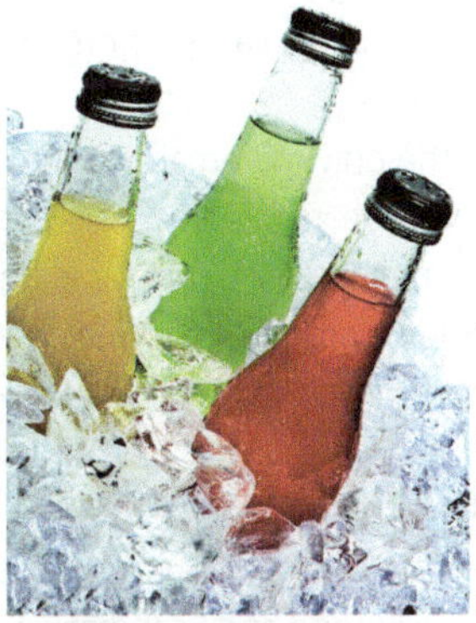
Tischenko Irina/Shutterstock.com

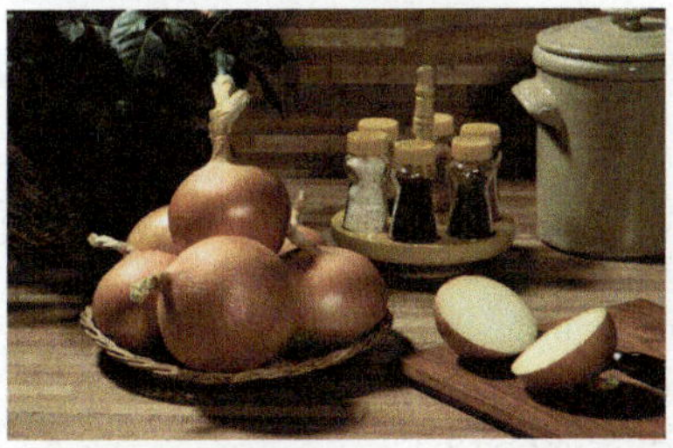
Photolink/Getty Images

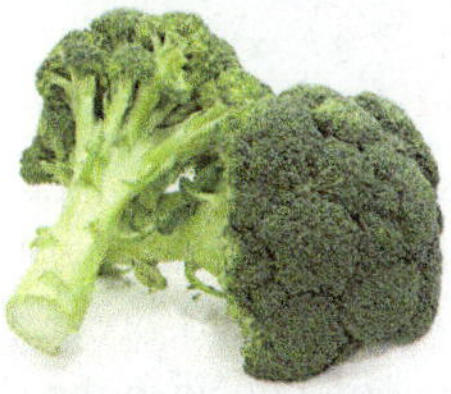
©iStockphoto.com/egal

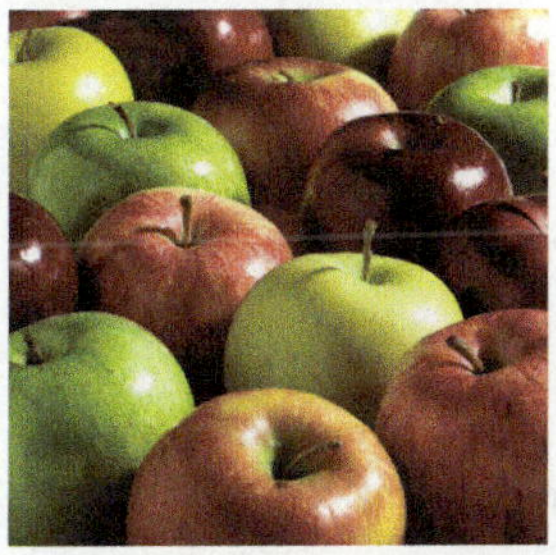
Purestock/Getty Images

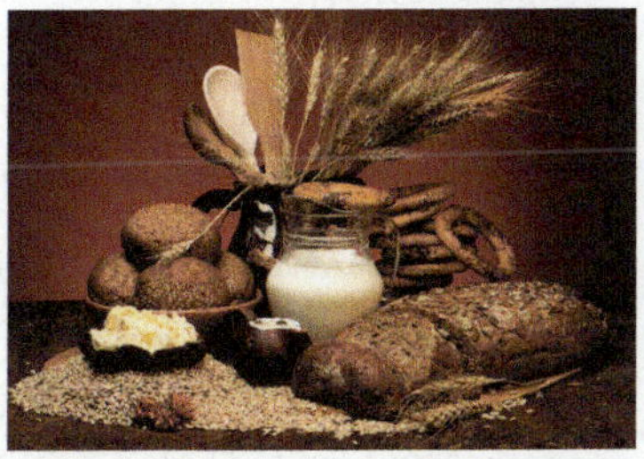
©iStockphoto.com/MargarytaVakhterova

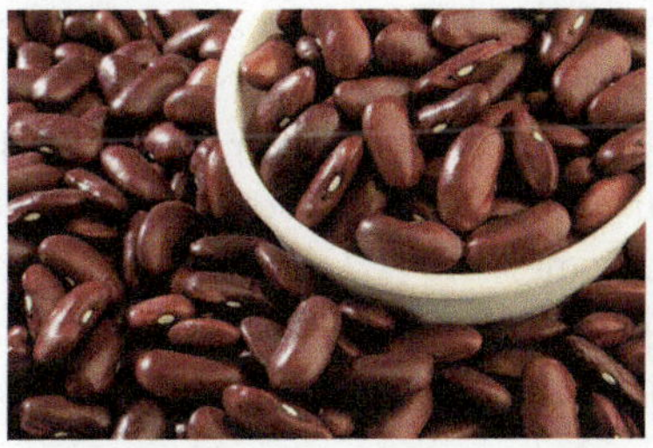
Cedric Carter/Dreamstime.com

I've heard that intestinal gas is caused by the types of food I eat. Is this true?

It's true and false. As you've learned from reading this chapter (and will learn in Chapter 4), humans do not digest and absorb some types of carbohydrates. We simply do not make the necessary digestive enzymes to break down fiber. Another interesting note is foods that produce gas in one person may not cause gas in another, and the amount of gas caused by certain foods varies from person to person. Trial and error is the only way to learn how specific foods affect you and your gas production.

My roommate says she has gas and diarrhea when she drinks milk. How can that happen? Isn't milk supposed to be good for us?

What is most likely happening is your roommate cannot digest the disaccharide lactose, the natural sugar in milk and some milk products such as cheese and ice cream. This occurs because a person has low to no levels of lactase, the enzyme necessary to break down lactose into its two absorbable components, the monosaccharides galactose and glucose. Nutrients are commonly broken down and absorbed in the small intestine. When a nutrient has been broken down only partially (maldigestion) and has not been absorbed, it causes all kinds of havoc when it reaches the large intestine. Fluid is pulled from surrounding tissues to "water down" or dilute the intact or partially intact lactose in the colon, thus causing a bloated feeling and diarrhea, along with gas and abdominal cramping caused from intestinal bacteria that digest lactose.

Humans are the only mammals that regularly drink milk past weaning. And, for many years, scientists believed that people who experienced lactose maldigestion or intolerance were the "exceptions," while in truth they were the "rule" because this included about 70 to 90 percent of the world's population (mostly those of African or Asian descent). The more recent genetic theory is that people who tolerate lactose do so because their prehistoric ancestors migrated to parts of the world where dairy cattle could be raised safely and economically, primarily northern Europe and Scandinavia.

What causes constipation?

Constipation is the most common GI complaint in the United States. Constipation is defined as experiencing bowel movements three times a week or less. Stools are usually hard, dry, small in size, and difficult to eliminate. More than 4 million people in the United States report having frequent constipation, and over half believe it serious enough to visit their physician. To understand what causes constipation, it will help to review the section of this chapter on the large intestine (see Figure 3-10). As what's left over after digestion and absorption passes through the colon, water is absorbed, forming stool. As muscle contractions push the stool toward the rectum, it becomes more and more solid in consistency. When the colon absorbs too much water or if the muscle contractions are slow-moving, stools can become hard and dry. Frequent causes of constipation include:

- Lack of fiber in the diet
- Lack of physical activity (particularly in older adults)
- Not enough liquids
- Medications (e.g., pain medications, antacids, blood pressure medications, antidepressants, iron supplements, diuretics, antispasmodics, anticonvulsants)
- Milk
- Changes in life or routine (e.g., pregnancy, aging, travel)
- Over-the-counter laxative abuse
- Ignoring the urge to have a bowel movement

How is constipation treated?

Constipation is a symptom, not a disease. Most constipation is temporary and not serious. Treatment depends on the cause, severity, and duration of the constipation, but in most cases dietary and lifestyle changes will help relieve symptoms and assist in preventing them from recurring:

- Diet: 20 to 35 grams of fiber each day helps the body form soft, bulky stools. See Chapter 4 to find out what foods are high in fiber.
- Lifestyle changes: Increasing water consumption and other liquids, daily exercise, and not ignoring the urge to have a bowel movement will help prevent constipation.
- Laxatives: Most cases of mild constipation do not require use of laxatives. But if the constipation is of long duration, a physician should be consulted for the best treatment to retrain a persistently lethargic bowel.

What if constipation becomes serious?

One serious complication of constipation is hemorrhoids. Hemorrhoids are swollen and inflamed veins around the anus or lower rectum. They are either internal (inside the anus) or external (under the skin around the anus). Hemorrhoids may result from straining to have bowel movements, pregnancy, aging, chronic constipation or diarrhea, and anal intercourse. They are usually not dangerous or life-threatening, but the itching and irritation can be annoying. About half the U.S. population develops hemorrhoids by the time they are 50, but not everyone experiences symptoms. The most common symptom of internal hemorrhoids is bright red blood covering the stool, on toilet paper, or in the toilet bowl. Hemorrhoids are common in pregnant women. Hormonal changes and pressure of the fetus on the abdomen cause hemorrhoidal vessels to enlarge.

How are hemorrhoids treated?

Initial treatment is to relieve symptoms:

- Tub baths several times a day in plain, warm water for about 10 minutes
- Application of hemorrhoidal cream or a suppository to the affected area for a limited time

Preventing hemorrhoids from occurring or recurring requires relieving the pressure and straining of constipation. Increasing fiber and fluids (not alcohol) in the diet will result in softer, bulkier, easier-to-pass stools.

SOURCES:

G. Bloom and P. W. Sherman, Dairying barriers affect the distribution of lactose malabsorption, *Evolution and Human Behavior* 26 (2005): 301.e1–301.e33.

Constipation. National Digestive Diseases Information Clearinghouse, http://digestive.niddk.nih.gov/ddiseases/pubs/constipation/index.htm.

Dehydration. National Digestive Diseases Information Clearinghouse, http://digestive.niddk.nih.gov/ddiseases/pubs/diarrhea/index.htm.

Gas in the digestive tract. National Digestive Diseases Information Clearinghouse, http://digestive.niddk.nih.gov/ddiseases/pubs/gas/index.htm.

Hemorrhoids. National Digestive Diseases Information Clearinghouse, http://digestive.niddk.nih.gov/ddiseases/pubs/hemorrhoids/index.htm.

Hiccups. eMedicineHealth, www.emedicinehealth.com/hiccups/article_em.htm.

Jeffries M. How hiccups work, Howstuffworks. http://health.howstuffworks.com/hiccup.htm.

Medical encyclopedia: hiccups, MedlinePlus, www.nlm.nih.gov/medlineplus/ency/article/003068.htm.

Lactose intolerances. National Digestive Diseases Information Clearinghouse, digestive.niddk.nih.gov/ddiseases/pubs/lactoseintolerance/index.htm.

WHAT'S ONLINE

MINDTAP From Cengage

Visit www.cengagebrain.com to access MindTap, a complete digital course that includes Diet & Wellness Plus, interactive quizzes, videos, and more.

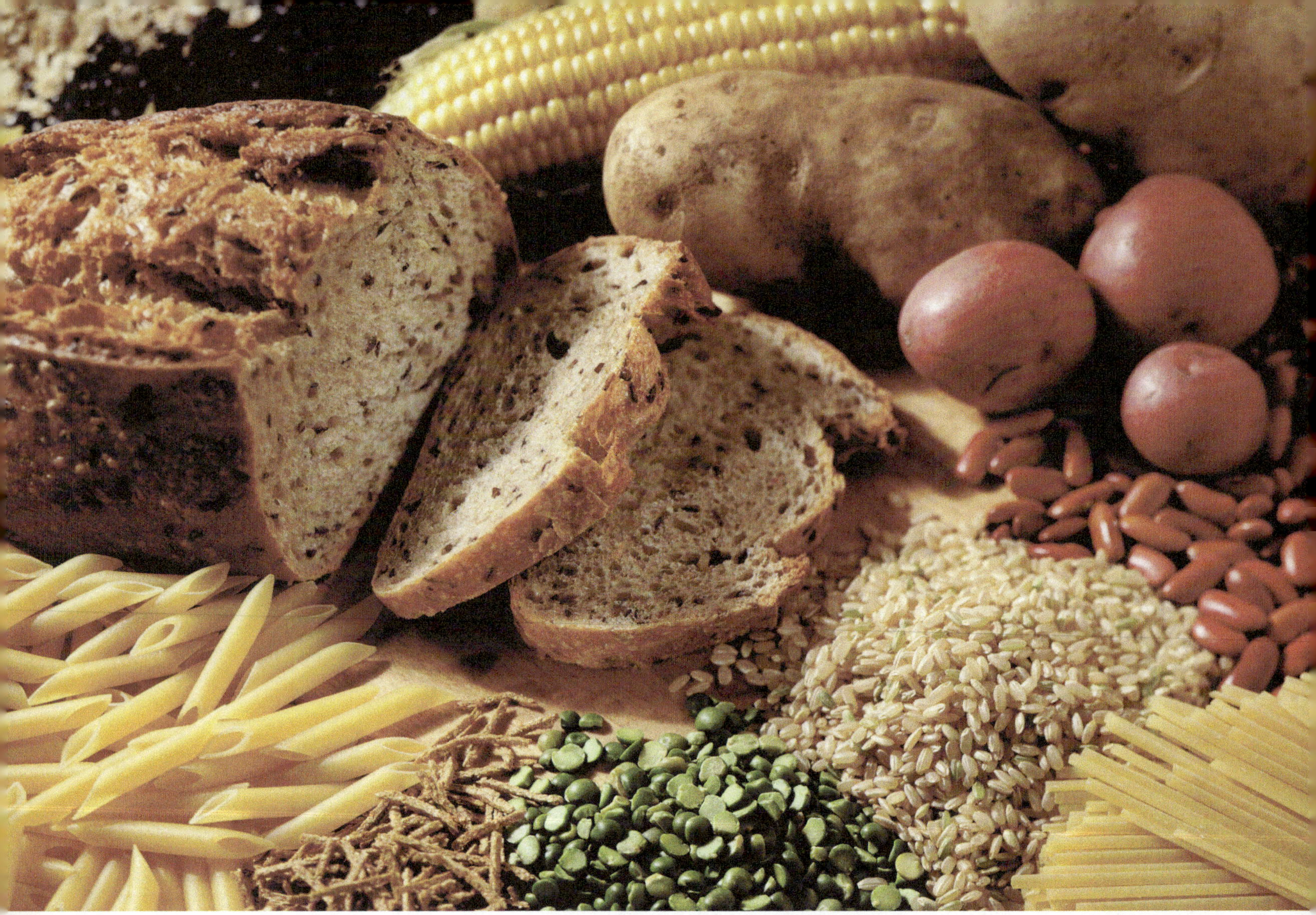

John E. Kelly/Getty Images

AskYourself . . .

Which of the following statements about nutrition are true, and which are false? For each false statement, what is true?

1. Foods high in complex carbohydrate (starch and fiber) are good choices when you are trying to lose weight.
2. People with diabetes should never eat sugar.
3. The brain demands the sugar glucose to fuel its activities.
4. Breads that are brown in color have more fiber than white bread.

Answers found on page 96.

ChapterObjectives

4.1 Describe how carbohydrates are used in the body.

4.2 Identify major food sources of the monosaccharides, disaccharides, and polysaccharides common in nutrition.

4.3 Describe the health benefits associated with complex carbohydrates, including the two major types of dietary fibers.

4.4 List the dietary recommendations for total carbohydrates, dietary fiber, and added sugars in the diet.

4.5 Summarize carbohydrate digestion and explain how the body maintains a normal blood glucose level.

4.6 Differentiate between type 1 and type 2 diabetes, including risk factors for each.

4.7 Identify strategies for reducing added sugars in the diet.

4.8 List examples of alternative sweeteners approved for use in the diet.

The Carbohydrates: Sugar, Starch, and Fiber

CHAPTER 4

Once upon a time, bread, potatoes, pasta, and other starchy foods were placed on the dieter's list of most-fattening or "illegal" foods. Today, carbohydrate bashing is still a popular pastime. This unattractive image undoubtedly comes from the practice of serving many carbohydrate-rich foods laden with fat: potatoes with sour cream and butter, vegetables or pasta with rich cream sauces, toast with butter, and salads with fat-rich dressings. People who need to lose weight must limit high-calorie foods, but they are ill advised to try to avoid all **carbohydrates**. Excess calories *are* fattening, and the fat, not the carbohydrate, raises the calorie count the most.

This chapter invites you to learn to distinguish between certain carbohydrates, such as the refined carbohydrates found in many snack crackers and baked goods, versus the complex carbohydrates found in whole grains, fruits, vegetables, and legumes, and others, such as the concentrated sugars of sweetened beverages, candies, and cookies. Because some foods are healthier carbohydrate choices than others, you will learn that the key to building a healthy plate is to make smart carbohydrate choices.

Rabbit said, "Honey or condensed milk with your bread?" [Pooh] was so excited that he said, "Both," and then, so as not to seem greedy, he added, "But don't bother about the bread, please."

—From *Winnie the Pooh*, by A. A. Milne (1882–1956)

4.1 Carbohydrate Basics

The primary role of carbohydrates is to provide the body with energy (calories). For certain body systems (for example, the brain and the nervous system), carbohydrates are the preferred energy source. Carbohydrates are the ideal fuel for the body. There are only two alternative calorie sources: protein and fat. Protein-rich foods are usually

carbohydrates Compounds made of single sugars or multiple sugars and composed of carbon, hydrogen, and oxygen atoms [*carbo* = carbon (C); *hydrate* = water (H_2O)].

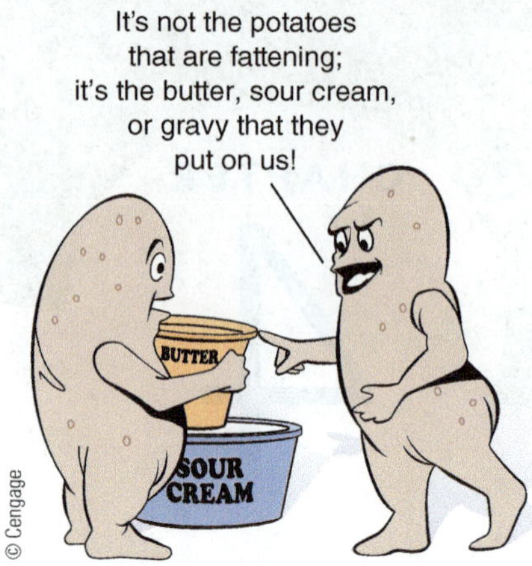

TABLE 4-1 Roles of Carbohydrates

- Provide energy (4 calories per gram); glucose provides a quick source of energy; glucose is the preferred fuel for the brain and nerves.
- Provide an energy reserve: Glycogen in muscle and liver can be broken down to glucose.
- Serve as raw materials: Sugars can be converted into other body compounds such as amino acids—the building blocks of protein.
- Fibers:
  - Contribute to digestive tract health.
  - Maintain normal bowel function.
  - Lower blood cholesterol by binding bile.
  - Slow the absorption of glucose.
  - Provide bulk and satiety (feeling of fullness).
  - Enhance weight loss and maintenance of a healthy body weight.
- Contribute flavor and texture to foods: Sugars provide sweetness.

more expensive and provide no advantage over carbohydrates when used to provide fuel for the body. Fat-rich foods might be less expensive, but fat cannot be used efficiently as fuel by the brain and nerves, and diets high in solid fats are associated with many chronic diseases. Thus, of all the possible food-energy sources, carbohydrates are preferred; they provide about half of the fuel used by muscles and other tissues; the remaining fuel comes from fat.

The brain and nervous system are sensitive to the concentration of glucose in the blood. Normal blood glucose levels are important for a feeling of well-being. When your blood glucose level becomes too high, you get sleepy; when the concentration falls too low, you get weak and shaky. Only when blood glucose is within the normal range can you feel energetic and alert. The person who wants to feel energetic and alert all day should make the effort to eat so as to maintain blood glucose levels in the normal range to fuel the critical work of the brain and nervous system. Table 4-1 lists a few of the vital functions of carbohydrate in the body and in foods you eat.

Carbohydrate-rich foods are obtained almost exclusively from plants. Milk is the only animal-derived food that contains significant amounts of carbohydrate. Carbohydrates are divided into two categories: **complex carbohydrates** and **simple carbohydrates**. Complex carbohydrates include starch and fiber. Starches make up a large part of the world's food supply, mostly as grains. For example, such staples as wheat, rice, and corn are rich sources of starch. Fiber is found abundantly in plants, especially in the outer portions of cereal grains, and in fruits, legumes, and most vegetables. Simple carbohydrates include naturally occurring sugars in fresh fruits, in some vegetables, in milk and milk products, and as added sugars in concentrated form, such as in honey, corn syrup, or sugar in the sugar bowl. All of these carbohydrates have characteristics in common, but they are of different merit nutritionally. Table 4-2 introduces the different types of carbohydrates.

complex carbohydrates Long chains of sugars (glucose) arranged as starch or fiber; also called *polysaccharides* (*poly* = many; *saccharide* = sugar unit).

simple carbohydrates (sugars) The single sugars (*monosaccharides*) and the pairs of sugars (*disaccharides*) linked together.

monosaccharides The single sugars (glucose, fructose, and galactose); *mono* = one.

glucose (GLOO-koce) The building block of carbohydrate; a monosaccharide used in both plant and animal tissues as quick energy.

fructose (FROOK-toce) Fruit sugar; the sweetest of the monosaccharides.

galactose (guh-LACK-toce) A monosaccharide that occurs bonded to glucose in the sugar of milk.

disaccharide A double sugar (sucrose, maltose, and lactose); *di* = two.

sucrose (SOO-krose) A disaccharide composed of glucose and fructose.

maltose A disaccharide composed of two glucose units.

lactose A disaccharide composed of glucose and galactose; commonly known as *milk sugar.*

ASK YOURSELF ANSWERS: 1. True. **2.** False. People with diabetes need to watch the total carbohydrate in their diets, but they can choose foods with sugar as a small portion of that total. **3.** True. **4.** Not always. A brown color does not always mean the bread is high in fiber. The color can come from molasses or caramel. To be high in fiber, the label must say *whole-grain* or *whole-wheat,* not simply *wheat* bread. *Whole-grain* flour should be listed first in the ingredients list.

TABLE 4-2 Categories and Sources of Carbohydrate

Carbohydrate Type	Common Names	Examples of Food Sources
Monosaccharides		
Glucose ●	Dextrose, blood sugar	Fruits, sweeteners
Fructose ■	Fruit sugar, levulose	Fruits, honey, high-fructose corn syrup
Galactose ▲	—	Part of lactose, found in milk
Disaccharides		
Sucrose (glucose + fructose) ●—■ = ● + ■	Table sugar	Beet and cane sugar, fruit, most sweets
Lactose (glucose + galactose) ●—▲ = ● + ▲	Milk sugar	Milk and milk products
Maltose (glucose + glucose) ●—● = ● + ●	Malt sugar	Sprouted seeds
Polysaccharides		
Starches ●–●–●–●–●–●–●	Dextrins*	Potatoes, legumes, corn, wheat, rye, and other grains
Dietary fiber ●⁄●⁀●⁄●⁀●⁄●	Roughage, bulk:	Whole grains, legumes, fruits, vegetables
Insoluble fibers	cellulose, hemicellulose	Wheat products, brown rice, vegetables, legumes, seeds
Soluble fibers	pectins, gums, mucilages, some hemicelluloses	Oat products, barley, legumes, fruits, vegetables, seeds

*Starch can be broken down during food processing to shorter chains of glucose units known as *dextrins*. The word *dextrins* sometimes appears on food labels, because dextrins can be used as thickening agents in foods.

4.2 The Simple Carbohydrates: Monosaccharides and Disaccharides

All carbohydrates are composed of single sugars—known as **monosaccharides**—alone or in various combinations, and all carbohydrates but fiber can be converted to **glucose** in the body. Green plants make glucose from carbon dioxide and water through a process known as *photosynthesis* in the presence of chlorophyll and sunlight, as illustrated in Figure 4-1.

Glucose is not a very sweet sugar, but plants can rearrange its atoms to form another sugar, **fructose**, which is sweet to the taste. Fructose is found mostly in fruits, in honey, and as part of another sugar—table sugar. Glucose and fructose are the most common monosaccharides in nature.

Some sugars are double sugars—known as **disaccharides**—made by bonding two monosaccharides together. When glucose and fructose are bonded together, they form **sucrose**, or table sugar, the product most people refer to when they use the term *sugar*. The sweet taste of sucrose comes primarily from the fructose in its structure. It occurs naturally in many fruits and vegetables. Sugar cane and sugar beets are two sources from which sucrose is purified and granulated to various extents to provide the brown, white, and powdered sugars available in the supermarket. Sucrose is one of the two most caloric ingredients of candy, cakes, pastries, frostings, cookies, presweetened ready-to-eat cereals, and other concentrated sweets. (The other major calorie contributor is fat, discussed in Chapter 5.)

Another disaccharide, **maltose**, consists of two glucose units. It occurs in barley and sprouting seeds and is produced during the digestion of starch in the human body. Finally, **lactose**, the major sugar in milk, is a disaccharide made by mammals from galactose and glucose units. A human baby is born with the digestive enzymes necessary to split lactose into its two simple sugars—glucose and **galactose**—so that the body can absorb them. Lactose also facilitates the absorption of calcium and promotes the growth of beneficial bacteria in the intestines. Breast milk, which contains

FIGURE 4-1

Photosynthesis

Plants use chlorophyll and the sun's energy to make glucose through a process called photosynthesis. Water, absorbed by the plant's roots, and carbon dioxide, absorbed through the plant's leaves, combine to form a glucose molecule.

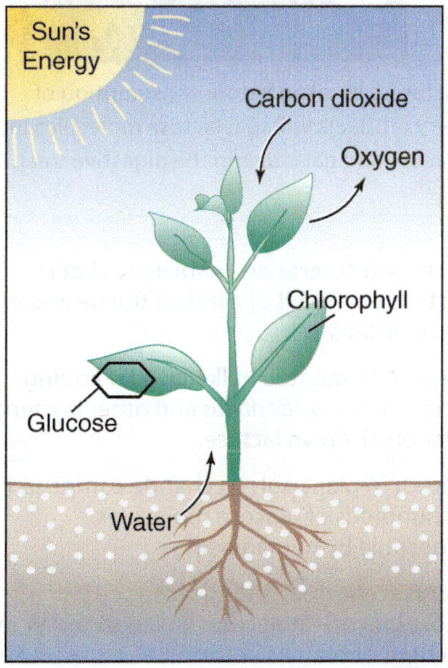

TABLE 4-3 Lactose in Selected Dairy Products	
Dairy Product	**Lactose (grams)**
Cheese (1 oz)	
Parmesan or cream	0.8
Cheddar or American	0.5
Milk (1 c)	12.0
Lactose-reduced, low-fat milk (1 c)	3.0
Buttermilk (1 c)	9.0–11.0
Yogurt, low-fat (1 c)*	11.0–15.0
Cottage cheese, low-fat (1 c)	7.0–8.0
Ice cream (1 c)	9.0
Sherbet (1 c)	4.0

*Choose yogurt with "active cultures"—the bacteria in these products digest the lactose found in yogurt for their own use.

© Cengage

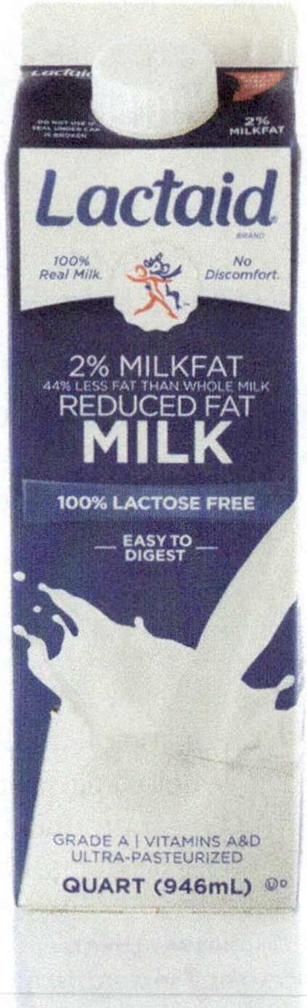

LunaseeStudios/Shutterstock.com

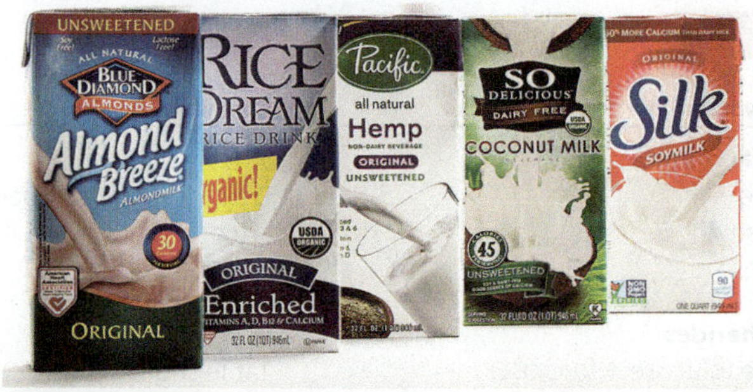

Bob Chamberlin/Los Angeles Times/Getty Images

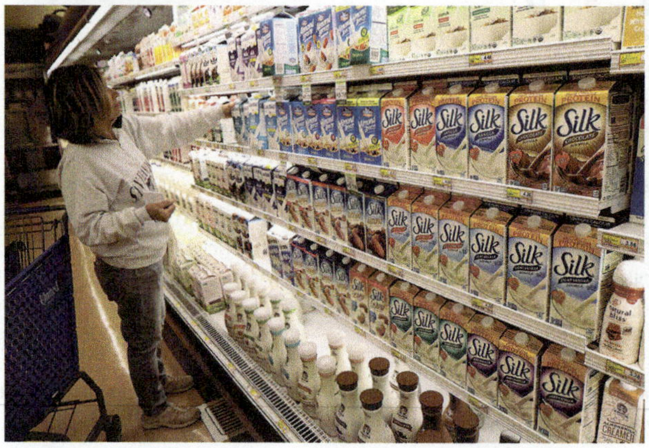

Justin Sullivan/Getty Images News/Getty Images

Lactose-reduced milk, enzyme solutions containing lactase for treating dairy products, and lactase tablets can help reduce the symptoms of lactose intolerance. Milk substitutes (soy, almond, or rice-based beverages) can be good choices, too. Check the Nutrition Facts panel to find brands that are fortified with the calcium and vitamin D found in milk.

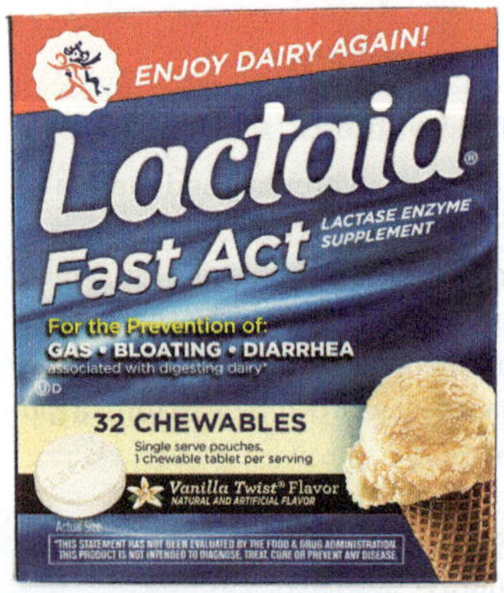

Keith Homan/Shutterstock.com

Lactase pills taken before consumption of dairy products will split lactose molecules into glucose and galactose in the digestive tract.

lactose intolerance Inability to digest lactose as a result of a lack of the necessary enzyme lactase.

kefir A fermented milk made by adding *Lactobacillus acidophilus* and other bacteria that break down lactose.

starch A plant polysaccharide composed of hundreds of glucose molecules, digestible by human beings.

polysaccharide A long chain of 10 or more glucose molecules linked together in straight or branched chains; another term for *complex carbohydrates*.

lactose, is an ideal food for babies because it provides a simple, easily digested carbohydrate to meet an infant's energy needs.

When you eat a food containing lactose, the enzyme *lactase* in your small intestine first splits the double sugar into single sugars so that they can enter your bloodstream. Many people lose the ability to digest lactose during or after childhood. Thereafter, these people may experience nausea, bloating, abdominal pain or cramping, diarrhea, or excessive gas after drinking milk or eating lactose-containing products. These symptoms result because when the intestinal bacteria use the lactose for energy, they produce acids and gas that irritate the intestine. This condition, called **lactose intolerance**, is inherited by about 70 percent of the world's people. It is most common in African Americans, Mediterranean peoples, Native Americans, and Asians, and less common in people of northern European origin.[1] It also can develop temporarily in people who are malnourished or sick, making it necessary for them to choose lactose-reduced milk products until they return to a healthy state.

Many people with lactose intolerance are able to consume small amounts of lactose without symptoms.[2] For them, fermented milk products, such as yogurt and **kefir**, aged cheeses, cottage cheese, or specially prepared milk products that have been treated with an enzyme to reduce lactose may be tolerated. Table 4-3 shows the lactose contents of fermented dairy products compared with the lactose content of milk.

4.3 The Complex Carbohydrates: Starch and Fiber

Complex carbohydrates include starch and fiber. All starchy foods are plant foods. **Starch** is a **polysaccharide** made up of many glucose units bonded together—3,000 or so in each molecule of starch. Shorter carbohydrate chains composed of 3 to 10 glucose molecules are called *oligosaccharides*.

TABLE 4-4 Types of Carbohydrates Found in Selected Foods in the MyPlate Food Guide

	Sugar	Starch	Fiber
Grains Group			
Bread, cooked grains	✓		✓
Vegetable Group			
Corn, peas	✓	✓	✓
Green beans	✓		✓
Potato	✓	✓	✓
Tomato	✓		✓
Fruit Group			
Apple, banana	✓ (mostly fructose)		✓
Orange juice	✓ (mostly fructose)		
Dairy Group			
Milk	✓ (lactose)		
Protein Group			
Meat, poultry, fish, eggs			
Legumes	✓		✓

© Cengage

FIGURE 4-2

A Wheat Kernel

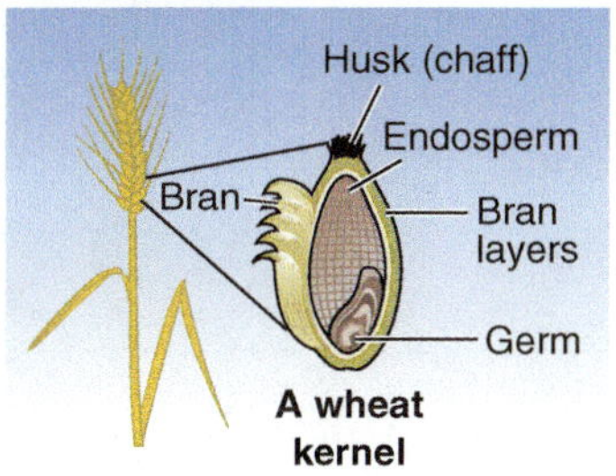

© Cengage

Seeds such as grains, peas, and beans are the richest starch sources. Most societies have a primary or **staple grain** that provides most of the people's food energy. In many Asian nations, the staple grain is rice. In Canada, the United States, and Europe, the staple grain is wheat. If you consider all the food products made from wheat—bread (and other baked goods made from wheat flour), cereals, and pasta—you will realize how pervasive this grain is in the food supply. The staple grains of other peoples include corn, millet, rye, barley, and oats.

A second important source of starch is the legume family, including dried beans and peas such as butter beans, kidney beans, pinto beans, navy beans, black-eyed peas, chickpeas, lentils, and soybeans. These vegetables are about 40 percent starch by weight and contain abundant protein. Root vegetables (such as yams) and tubers (such as potatoes) are other sources of starch that are important in many societies. Table 4-4 shows the types of carbohydrates found in foods from the USDA MyPlate food guidance system.

staple grain A grain used frequently in the diet; for example, corn (in Mexico), or rice (in Asia), or wheat (in the United States).

refined grains Grains that have been milled to remove the husk, bran, and germ from the grain—leaving only the endosperm—to yield a finer texture and improved shelf life. The process also removes dietary fiber, iron and other minerals, and many B vitamins. Many refined grain products can be high in solid fats and added sugars (e.g., cookies and cakes). The recommended amount of refined grains is no more than 3 ounce-equivalents per day.

enriched Refers to the process by which the B vitamins thiamin, riboflavin, niacin, folic acid, and the mineral iron are added to refined grains and grain products at levels specified by law.

fortified Term for foods to which nutrients have been added. Typically, commonly eaten foods are chosen for fortification with added nutrients to help prevent a deficiency (iodized salt, milk with vitamin D) or to reduce the risk of chronic disease (juices with added calcium).

whole grain A grain that is milled in its entirety (all but the husk), not refined. Whole grains include whole wheat, bulgur, corn (and popcorn), brown or red rice, whole rye, oats, barley, sorghum, triticale and millet. Amaranth, buckwheat, and quinoa are similar in nutrient content to whole grains.

The Bread Box: Refined, Enriched, and Whole-Grain Breads

For many people, grains supply much of the carbohydrate, or at least most of the starch, in a day's meals. Because grains have such a primary place in the diet, be sure that the grains you choose—wheat, rice, oats, or corn—contribute the nutrients you need. Also, be sure to learn the meanings of the words associated with the flours that make up the grain products you use: **refined**, **enriched**, **fortified**, and **whole grain**. This discussion of the nutritional differences between different breads provides an example of an important principle of nutrition: Foods that are far removed from their original state of wholeness may lack significant nutrients.

The part of the wheat plant that is made into flour and then into bread and other baked goods is the *kernel.* The wheat kernel (a whole grain) has four main parts (see Figure 4-2). The *germ* is the part that grows into a wheat plant, and it contains concentrated food to support the new life. It is especially rich in protein, vitamins, and minerals. The *endosperm* is the soft, white inside portion of the kernel containing starch and protein. The *bran,* a protective coating around the kernel (which is similar in function to the shell of a nut), is also rich in nutrients and fiber. The *husk,* commonly called *chaff,* is unusable for most purposes except for animal feed.

In earlier times, people milled wheat by grinding it between two stones, sifting out the inedible chaff, but retaining the nutrient-rich bran and germ as well as the endosperm. Improved milling machinery made it possible to remove the dark, heavy germ and bran as well, leaving a whiter, smoother-textured flour. People came to look on this flour as more desirable than the crunchy, dark-brown, "old-fashioned" flour, but initially were unaware of the nutrition implications. Bread eaters suffered a tragic loss of needed nutrients when they turned to white bread. A 1936 U.S. survey revealed that many people were suffering from deficiencies of the nutrients iron, thiamin, riboflavin, and niacin, which they had formerly received from bread. The Enrichment Act of 1942 standardized the return of these four lost nutrients to commercial flour. This legislation was amended in 1996 to include folic acid, a form of the B vitamin folate, which is considered important in the prevention of certain birth defects. Today, you can assume that almost all breads, grains such as rice, wheat products such as macaroni and spaghetti, and cereals (both cooked and ready to eat) have been enriched. Figure 4-3 shows that although enrichment makes refined bread comparable to whole-grain bread with respect to the enrichment nutrients, it does not do so with respect to other important nutrients. Therefore, although the enrichment of flour and other cereal products does improve them, it doesn't improve them enough: Whole-grain products are still preferable to enriched

FIGURE 4-3

Nutrients in Whole-Grain, Enriched White, and Unenriched White Breads

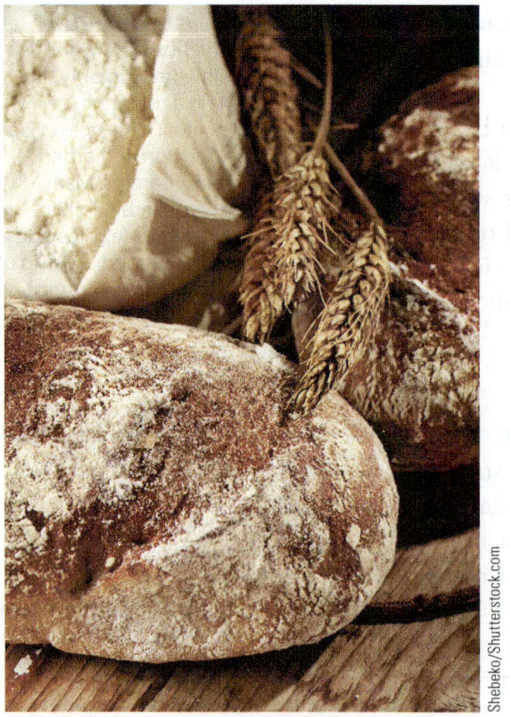

The nutrients present in the wheat plant at harvest are not always present in the wheat products you eat.

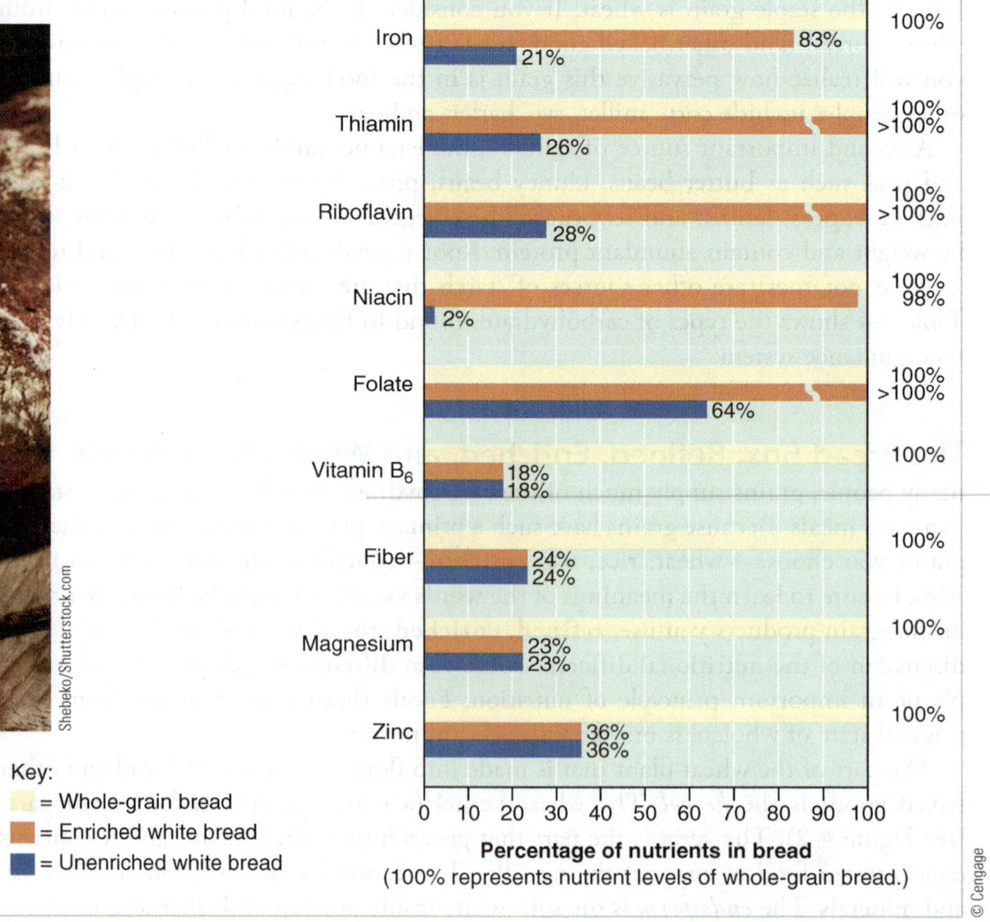

products. If bread is a staple food in your diet—that is, if you eat it every day—you are well advised to learn to like the hearty flavor of whole-grain breads.

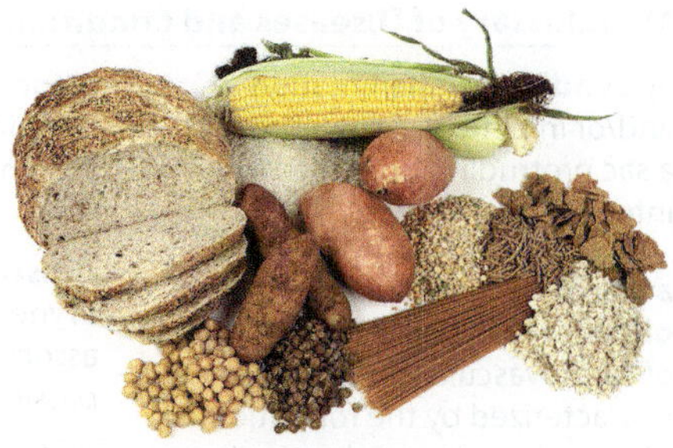

Robyn Mackenzie/Shutterstock.com

Foods such as potatoes, dried beans and peas, rice and whole-grain breads, cereals, and pastas are especially nutritious because of their starch, fiber, vitamin, and mineral content—and because they are virtually fat- and cholesterol-free.

Dietary Fiber

The **fibers** of a plant form the supporting structures of its leaves, stems, and seeds. Most fibers are polysaccharides, just as starch is, but with different bonds between the glucose units—bonds that cannot be broken by human digestive enzymes. The term fiber is used by almost everyone as though it represents a single entity. However, many compounds, mostly carbohydrates, make up fiber.* Such compounds are familiar to us as the strings of celery, the skins of corn kernels, and the membranes separating the segments in citrus fruits. When isolated from plants, fiber may be used to thicken jelly (citrus pectin), to keep salad dressing from separating (guar gum), to provide bulk (wheat and other brans), and to create other effects on food texture and consistency.

Unlike starch, fiber cannot be digested by human enzymes. However, some soluble fibers can be easily fermented by the bacteria that reside in the human digestive tract, but contribute little or no energy to the body. Fiber has two forms, **insoluble fiber** and **soluble fiber,** each of which exerts important effects on people's health.

fibers The indigestible residues of food, composed mostly of polysaccharides (sometimes called "roughage"). The best known of the fibers are cellulose, hemicellulose, pectin, and gums.

insoluble fiber Fiber category that includes the fiber types called cellulose, hemicellulose, and lignin. Insoluble fibers do not dissolve in water.

soluble fiber Fiber category that includes the fiber types called pectin, gums, mucilages, some hemicelluloses, and algal substances (for example, carrageenan). Soluble fibers either dissolve or swell when placed in water.

The Health Effects of Fiber

Many health experts encourage consumers to eat more fiber. According to recent evidence, inadequate levels of fiber in the diet are associated with several diseases (see the Miniglossary), whereas the consumption of recommended levels of fiber offers many health benefits.[3] Recall that dietary fiber is found only in plant foods, such as fruits, vegetables, legumes, and whole grains.

Table 4-5 shows the health benefits from consuming the two types of fiber. As you can see from the table, not all fibers are created equal. Because fibers have different effects in the body, it is best to eat a variety of high-fiber foods to get both types.

TABLE 4-5 Health Benefits and Sources of Dietary Fibers

Type of Fiber	Action in the Body	Possible Health Benefits	Food Sources
Soluble (more fermentable):[a] Gums, pectins, beta-glucans, mucilages, psyllium[b], inulin[b], some hemicelluloses, algal substances (e.g., carrageenan)	• Increase satiety • Lower blood cholesterol by binding bile • Slow glucose absorption • Fermentable fibers yield small fatty aids as energy source for cells of colon • Promote healthy colonic bacteria	• Help with weight management • Lower risk of heart disease • Improve blood glucose tolerance and lower risk of diabetes • Lower risk of colon and rectal cancer	Barley, rye, oats, oat bran, apples, citrus, legumes, seaweeds, many vegetables (broccoli, carrots, corn, potatoes), seeds, fibers used as food additives
Insoluble (less fermentable): Cellulose, hemicellulose, lignins, resistant starch[c]	• Increased bulk enlarges and softens stools and aids intestinal motility • Speed transit time through intestines • Increased bulk increases feeling of fullness	• Reduce risk of constipation, hemorrhoids, appendicitis, diverticulitis • Lower risk of colon and rectal cancer • Help with weight management	Wheat bran, whole-grain products, brown rice, fruits, legumes, many vegetables (cabbage, brussels sprouts, carrots), nuts, seeds, fibers used as food additives

[a]Fermentable fibers are more easily digested by bacteria in the colon and may yield health-protective fatty acids that may serve as an energy source for colonic cells.
[b]Psyllium is derived from seed husks and used as a food additive (e.g., in cereals) and in bulk-forming laxatives and contains both soluble and insoluble fibers. Inulin is derived from chicory root and used as a food additive.
[c]Resistant starch—such as that found in seeds, legumes, unprocessed whole grains, or under-ripe bananas—escapes digestion and absorption in the small intestine and functions as insoluble fiber that is fermented by intestinal bacteria to promote a healthy colon.

*The woody material of heavy stems and bark is the noncarbohydrate lignin, which is classed by some as a fiber.

Miniglossary of Diseases and Conditions Associated with Lack of Fiber in the Diet

appendicitis Inflammation and/or infection of the appendix, a sac protruding from the large intestine.

atherosclerosis (ATH-er-oh-skler-OH-sis) A type of cardiovascular disease characterized by the formation of fatty deposits, or plaques, in the inner walls of the arteries.

colon cancer Cancer of the large intestine (colon), the terminal portion of the digestive tract.

constipation Hardness and dryness of bowel movements associated with discomfort in passing them.

diabetes A disease characterized by insufficiency or relative ineffectiveness of insulin that renders a person unable to regulate the blood glucose level normally.

diverticulosis (dye-ver-tik-you-LOH-siss) Outpocketings of weakened areas of the intestinal wall that can rupture, like blowouts in a tire, causing dangerous infections.

hemorrhoids (HEM-or-oyds) Swollen, hardened (varicose) veins in the rectum, usually caused by the pressure resulting from constipation.

obesity Body weight that is high enough above normal weight to constitute a health hazard (see Chapter 10).

FIGURE 4-4

Diverticulosis

The outpocketings or pouches of intestinal linings that balloon through the weakened intestinal wall muscles are known as diverticula. *Diverticulitis* refers to the painful inflammation of the diverticula.

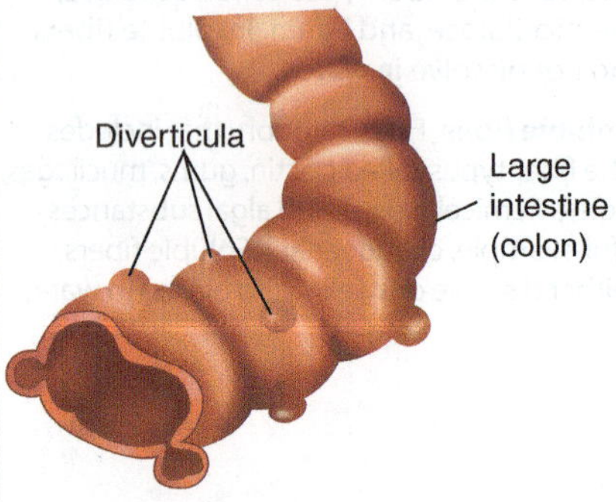

Both types of fiber, soluble and insoluble, can help with weight control. In the stomach, they convey a feeling of fullness because they absorb water, and some of them delay the emptying of the stomach so that you feel full longer. Also, if you eat many high-fiber foods, you are likely to eat fewer empty-calorie foods such as sweets. In fact, producers of some diet aids base the success of their products on the ability of certain fibers in the products to provide bulk and make you feel full.

Insoluble fiber (the type in wheat bran, for example) holds water in the colon, thereby increasing bulk and stimulating the muscles of the digestive tract so that they retain their health and tone. The toned muscles can more easily move waste products through the colon for excretion. This reduces risk for constipation and hemorrhoids (in which veins in the rectum swell, bulge out, become weak, and bleed). Insoluble fibers may improve symptoms associated with diverticulosis (in which the intestinal walls become weak and bulge out in places in response to the pressure needed to excrete waste when bulk is inadequate) and decrease the risk of diverticulitis (see Figure 4-4).[4] These types of fiber may also speed up the passage of food through the digestive tract, thus shortening the time of exposure of the tissue to agents in food that might cause certain cancers, such as colon cancer.[5]

Soluble fiber (the type in legumes, barley, and oats, for example) is credited with reducing the risks of heart and artery disease—atherosclerosis—by lowering the level of cholesterol in the blood. Certain soluble fibers can bind bile (a compound made from cholesterol) in the digestive tract and cause it to be excreted, thus lowering the body's total cholesterol level. As a result, the liver uses its own cholesterol to make new bile for digestion. It also appears that the products of bacterial fermentation of soluble fiber in the colon are absorbed into the body and may inhibit the liver's production of cholesterol.[6] Cholesterol levels may also decrease if food sources of soluble fiber (for example, barley, legumes, and oatmeal) are used as part of a healthy diet.[7]

Soluble fibers also improve the body's handling of glucose, even for people with diabetes, perhaps by slowing the digestion or absorption rate of carbohydrates.[8] Blood glucose levels therefore stay moderate, helping to prevent symptoms of diabetes or hypoglycemia. The list of fiber's contributions to human health is impressive!

When people choose high-fiber foods in hope of receiving some of these benefits, they must choose with care. Wheat bran, which is composed mostly of cellulose, has no cholesterol-lowering effect, whereas oat bran and the fibers found in legumes, carrots, apples, and grapefruits do lower blood cholesterol. In contrast, the fiber of wheat bran in whole-wheat bread is one of the most effective stool-softening fibers, and thus can help to prevent constipation and hemorrhoids. If one practical conclusion were to be drawn from what we know about fiber, it would have to be that all whole-plant foods seem to contain many kinds of fibers. To obtain the greatest benefits from fiber, therefore, eat a variety of fiber-rich foods rather than taking doses of purified fiber, such as bran, from a single source.

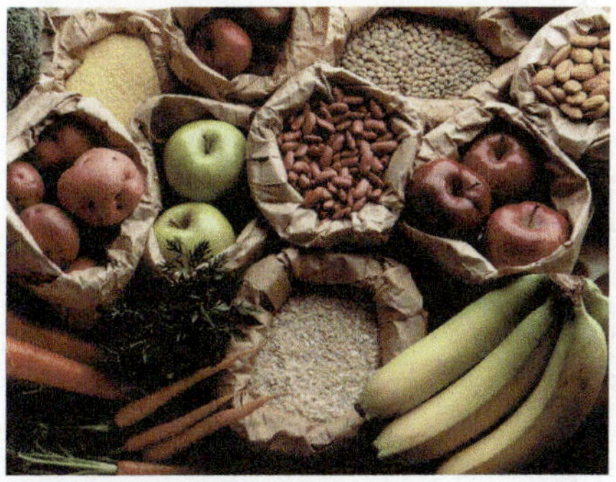

© PhotoDisc/Getty Images

We are advised to increase our intakes of complex carbohydrates. Choose plenty of whole foods like these . . .

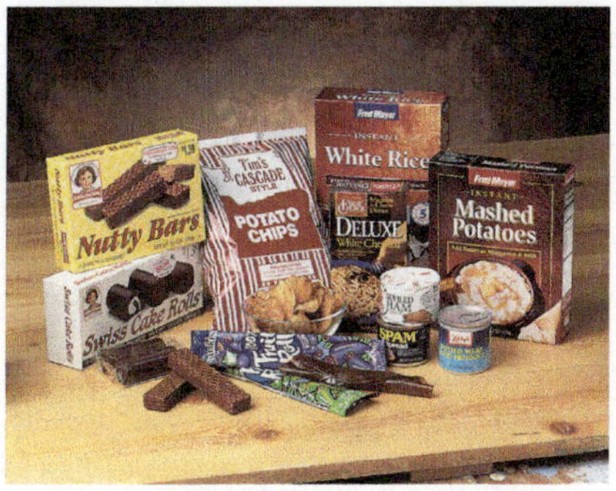

© Polara Studios, Inc.

. . . and fewer foods like these—foods that no longer resemble the original farm-grown products.

4.4 Guidelines for Choosing Carbohydrates

As it happens, most of the recent nutrition guidelines have had one point in common: They tend to favor a return to a diet of more plant-based **whole foods**. Generally speaking, the more a food resembles the original, farm-grown product, the more nutritious it is likely to be. During processing, some nutrients may be lost, and food producers often add nutrient-poor ingredients such as sugar, salt, and fat. For example, a potato contains 20 milligrams of vitamin C, but the same number of calories in French fries contains only about 7 milligrams, and the same number of calories in potato chips contains only 2 milligrams of vitamin C. People who change their diet and begin to eat fewer processed foods and more whole-food, plant-based products can expect many health benefits.

Complex Carbohydrates in the Diet

Complex carbohydrates are thought to be our most valuable energy nutrient. The *Dietary Guidelines for Americans* include the following recommendations concerning intakes of complex carbohydrates in the diet:

- Consume more fruits, especially whole fruits.
- Eat a variety of vegetables, especially dark-green and red and orange vegetables and legumes (beans and peas).
- Consume at least half of all grains as whole grains. Increase whole-grain intake by replacing refined grains with whole grains.[9]

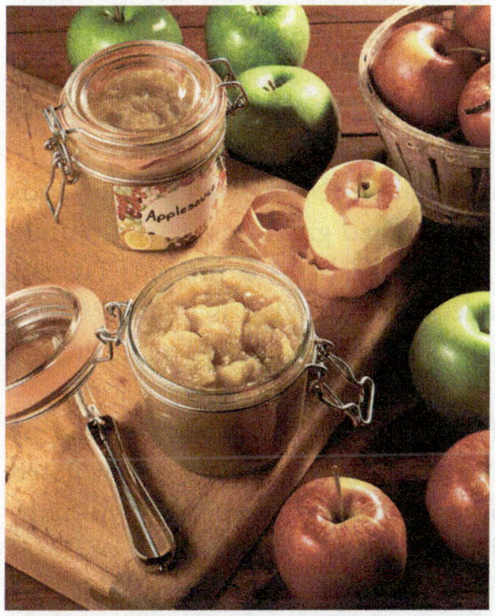

Spencer Jones/Getty Images

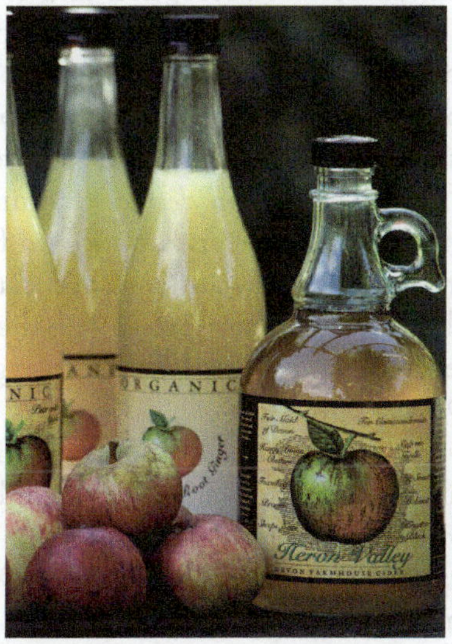

Mark Bolton/Corbis Documentary/Getty Images

A whole food has the nutritional advantage over its processed forms: large whole apple with peel—4 g fiber; ½ c applesauce—1.5 g fiber; ¾ c apple juice—0.2 g fiber.

whole food A food that is altered as little as possible from the plant or animal tissue from which it was taken; examples are milk, oats, potatoes, and apples.

TABLE 4-6 **Recommendations for Carbohydrates in the Diet**

	Total Carbohydrate	Added Sugars	Fiber	Men	Women
Dietary Guidelines	45%–65% of total calories	< 10% of total calories	Choose foods that provide more dietary fiber.		
DRI Committee	45%–65% of total calories	Minimize intake of added sugars	Adequate Intake (AI)		
			Adults under 50 years	38 g	25 g
			Adults over 50 years	30 g	21 g
Current Intake	49%	13%	16 g		

Likewise, the MyPlate food guide illustrates the goal of healthy eating as a shift away from a diet based on high-protein, higher-fat foods to one that uses more of the beneficial complex carbohydrates. Thus, the MyPlate graphic reflects this shift visually and encourages you to eat proportionally more servings of whole grain products, vegetables, and fruit (see Figure 2-8 and Figure 2-9 in Chapter 2). Table 4-6 lists the current recommendations for choosing carbohydrates for a healthy eating pattern.

Grain products are low in fat, unless fat is added in processing, in food preparation, or at the table. According to the *Dietary Guidelines*, at least half of the recommended grain servings consumed should be whole grains, particularly because of their fiber content. Today, less than 5 percent of Americans consume the minimum recommended amount of whole grains.[10] See the Savvy Diner feature that follows for more benefits and tips for making half your grains whole.

Fiber in the Diet Undoubtedly, including fiber in a daily meal plan has benefits—but how much is enough? How much is too much? Even fiber has potential to cause harm if taken in excess.

Because fiber carries water out of the body, too much fiber can cause dehydration and intestinal discomfort. Also, iron is mainly absorbed early in the digestive process; thus, because fiber speeds the movement of foods through the digestive system, it may limit the opportunity for absorption of iron and other nutrients. Binders in some fibers link chemically with minerals such as calcium and zinc, making them unavailable for absorption and carrying them out of the body (more about this in Chapter 8). Too much bulk from the diet could reduce the total amount of food consumed and cause deficiencies of both nutrients and energy. The malnourished, some older adults, and children, because they eat small amounts of food anyway, are especially vulnerable to these concerns.

The *Dietary Guidelines* recommend increasing intakes of fiber-rich whole foods and limiting the consumption of foods that contain refined grains, especially refined grain foods that contain solid fats and added sugars.[11] Table 4-6 presents current fiber recommendations.[12] The diet can supply adequate fiber if it is high in fruits, vegetables, legumes, and whole grains—the same recommendations made in the *Dietary Guidelines*.

The wholesale addition of purified fiber to foods is ill advised because it can be taken so easily to extremes. People whose fiber intake consists of only one isolated type of fiber are deprived of the benefits the other types of fiber provide. In contrast, if you include a variety of whole grains, legumes, nuts, fruits, and vegetables in your diet, you get the various types of fiber you need, together with a package of other benefits as well: water, minerals, vitamins, the energy nutrients, and other beneficial substances.

THE SAVVY Diner

Whole Grains for Health (Obj. 4.4)

Fruits, vegetables, and foods made from whole grains should form the foundation of a nutritious diet. Why the emphasis on whole-grain foods? Vitamins, minerals, fiber, and other protective substances, including hundreds of phytochemicals, contribute to the health benefits of whole-grain foods. Refined grains are low in fiber and in the protective substances that accompany the fiber in whole grains. A diet rich in whole grains may help protect you against many chronic diseases, including diabetes, heart disease, and certain cancers, and it can also be an effective tool for managing your weight.

Evidence suggests that people consuming diets rich in whole-grain foods, including fiber-rich cereals, have improved insulin sensitivity and are less likely to develop **metabolic syndrome,** a clustering of risk factors associated with the development of type 2 diabetes and heart disease.[13] These risk factors include excess body weight (especially around the abdomen), insulin resistance (reduced ability of the hormone insulin to regulate blood glucose), high levels of fat particles in the blood (known as *triglycerides*), low levels of the body's good form of cholesterol (known as *HDL cholesterol*), and increased blood glucose levels. Recent data show that an estimated 33 percent of adults in the United States have metabolic syndrome.[14] Metabolic syndrome can also be found among children, especially in those who are overweight.

How can you incorporate whole grains into your diet to achieve the maximum health benefits and protection from chronic diseases? Very easily! Consider the following three tips:

1 Count to Three.

Consume three or more servings of whole-grain products per day, with the rest of the recommended grains coming from enriched or whole-grain products.* Go to www.ChooseMyPlate.gov to determine your own recommended intake of whole grains. In general, at least half the grains you eat should come from whole grains.

2 Keep It Varied.

Whole grains differ from refined grains in the amount of fiber and nutrients they provide, and different whole-grain foods differ in the amount and type of fiber and nutrients they contain. Therefore, choose a variety of whole grains. Experiment with new or unfamiliar grains like quinoa, bulgur (cracked wheat), barley, buckwheat, and amaranth. The following tips can get you started on building a healthy foundation for your diet by selecting a variety of whole grains daily.

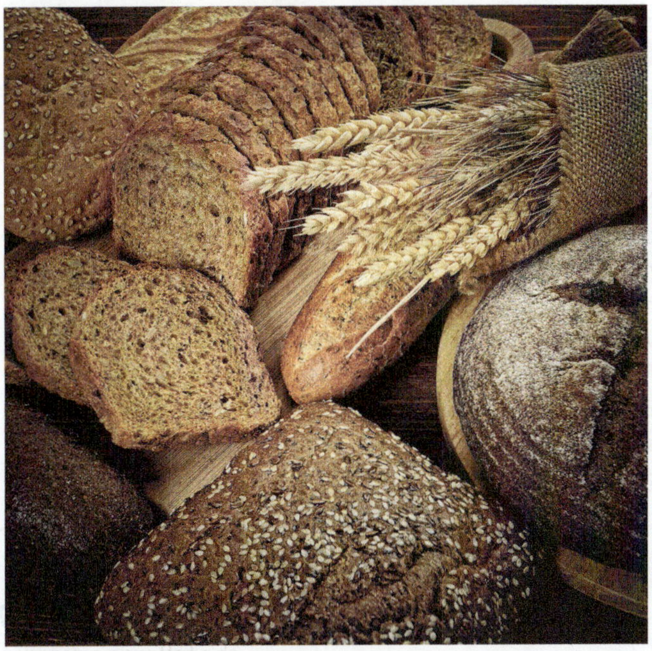

Scorpp/Shutterstock.com

Enjoy the hearty flavor of whole grains. Make at least half of your daily grain choices whole grains.

- Start your day with a high-fiber selection—a warm bowl of oatmeal with fresh fruit, bran cereals or shredded wheat with sliced fruit, low-fat apple bran muffin, buckwheat pancakes, or whole-grain English muffin.
- Whole grains are naturally low in fat and added sugars. Keep them that way by going easy on the fats and sugars you add as spreads, seasonings, or toppings, such as butter, margarine, oil, gravy, sauces, sugar, jams, and jellies.
- Whenever possible, substitute whole-grain flour for at least one-fourth of the all-purpose flour called for in baking.
- Make a fiber-rich snack mix from ready-to-eat whole-grain cereals, fat-free popcorn, and unsalted nuts, or enjoy air-popped or light microwaved popcorn.

metabolic syndrome A cluster of interrelated symptoms, including obesity, high blood pressure, abnormal blood lipids, and insulin resistance; highly associated with development of type 2 diabetes and heart disease.

*One serving of whole grains from the Grains group equals the following: 1 slice whole-grain bread; ½ whole-grain English muffin, bun, or bagel; 1 ounce whole-grain dinner roll; 1 cup (1 ounce) ready-to-eat whole-grain cereal; ½ cup cooked cereal (oatmeal); ½ cup cooked brown rice or whole-wheat pasta; 5 to 6 whole-grain crackers; 3 cups popped popcorn.

(Continued)

- Try whole-wheat pasta or brown rice, and order sandwiches on whole-grain breads or whole-wheat tortillas for a change.
- Combine whole grains with other tasty, nutritious foods in mixed dishes. Try brown rice stuffing (cooked brown rice, onion, celery, and seasonings) in baked green peppers or tomatoes; whole-grain barley in vegetable soup; bulgur in vegetarian chili.

3 Check the Label.

Choose whole grains and whole-grain foods over highly processed grains and cereals by doing some investigative shopping in the grocery store. Compare products by examining the ingredients list and Nutrition Facts panel (also refer to Figure 2-15 in Chapter 2). Buy products that list a whole-grain or whole-wheat or other whole-grain flour *first* on the label's ingredient list. Look for brown rice, oatmeal, whole oats, bulgur, popcorn, whole rye, graham flour, hulled barley, whole wheat, whole-grain corn. If the label states "wheat flour," "enriched flour," or "degerminated cornmeal," the product is not whole grain. Believe it or not, food products labeled with the words *multigrain, stone-ground, 100% wheat, seven-grain,* or *bran* are usually *not* whole-grain products! Read the ingredient list to see if it is a whole grain.

Sample Ingredients List for a Whole-grain Food

Ingredients: Whole-wheat flour, water, wheat gluten, soybean and/or canola oil, yeast, salt, honey

Check the Daily Value listed in the Nutrition Facts panel to find out if a food is high or low in fiber. The "% Daily Value" for fiber provides a good clue about the amount of whole grain in the product. A percent Daily Value (% DV) of 5 percent for fiber is low, whereas 20 percent or more is high. Use the Nutrition Facts panel to help you choose products with a higher % Daily Value.

The level of whole grains in ready-to-eat cereal also depends on the sugar content. The more sugar, the less grain and fiber. For example, an ounce of unsweetened oat cereal may contain 3 grams of fiber, but the same amount of its sweetened counterpart may contain 13 grams of sugar and only 1 gram of fiber. Read the food label's ingredient list, looking for terms that indicate added sugars (sucrose, high-fructose corn syrup, honey, and molasses) that add extra calories. Choose grain products with fewer solid fats and added sugars. For more information about whole-grain foods, go to: www.wheatfoods.org or www.wholegrainscouncil.org.

Added Sugars: Use Discretion

The *Dietary Guidelines for Americans* includes the following recommendation concerning intakes of **added sugars** in the diet:[15]

- Limit added sugars to less than 10 percent of calories per day.

The MyPlate food guide distinguishes between naturally occurring sugars, such as those found in fruits, and concentrated added sugars containing *empty calories,* as found in soft drinks or other calorically sweetened foods.

The World Health Organization recommends that we limit our intake of added sugars to 10 percent of calories.[16] The Dietary Reference Intakes (DRI) committee recommends that we choose most often the naturally occurring sugars present in nutrient-dense dairy products and fruits and minimize our intake of added sugars.[17] For people who otherwise meet their nutrient needs, maintain a healthy body weight, and still need additional calories to meet energy needs, the DRI committee sets the *maximum* intake for added sugars at 25 percent of total calories or less, because diets high in added sugars tend to displace intakes of vitamin A, calcium, iron, zinc, and other essential vitamins and minerals. For most people, 3 to 12 teaspoons of sugar per day represent the maximum allowance for one's intake of empty calories. Table 4-7 shows the amounts of sugar in some common products.

Currently, adults in the United States consume an average of 270 calories a day from added sugars, or more than 13 percent of total calories from sugar.[18] Added sugar intakes are highest in children, adolescents, and young adults, particularly men aged 19 to 30, with some individuals having added sugar intakes as high as 55 teaspoons of sugar a day. The major sources of added sugars in the American diet (see Figure 4-5) include: regular soft drinks; sugars and candy; cakes, cookies, pies; fruit drinks; dairy products (such as ice cream, sweetened yogurt, and sweetened milk); and sweetened grains (such as waffles and cinnamon toast).[19] A later section of this chapter offers pointers on using discretion in "Keeping Sweetness in the Diet."

added sugars Sugars and other caloric sweeteners that are added to foods during processing or preparation. Added sugars do not include naturally occurring sugars such as those found in milk and fruits.

TABLE 4-7 Sugar in Selected Foods

Food	Teaspoons of Sugar per Serving (1 tsp = 4 grams)	Food	Teaspoons of Sugar per Serving (1 tsp = 4 grams)
Fruit drink, lemonade (12 oz)	12	Cereal, Sugar Pops (¾ c)	4
Chocolate shake (10 oz)	9	Shredded wheat (¾ c)	0
Chocolate (2 oz)	8	Fruit, canned in heavy syrup (½ c)	4
Cola (12 oz)	8	Gelatin dessert (½ c)	4
Jelly beans (10)	7	Chocolate milk, 2% (1 c)	3
Yogurt, fruit flavored (1 c)	7	Corn, canned (½ c)	3
Apple pie (⅙ of pie)	6	Ice cream, ice milk, or frozen yogurt (½ c)	3
Cake, frosted (1⁄16 of cake)	6	Syrup or honey (1 tbsp)	3
Angel food cake (1⁄12 of cake)	5	Dairy creamer (1 tbsp)	2
Applesauce, sweetened (½ c)	5	Doughnuts, plain (1)	2
Fig bars (1)	5	Catsup (1 tbsp)	1
Fudge (1 oz)	5	Chewing gum (2 sticks)	1
Sherbet (½ c)	5	Cookie, Oreo type (1)	1
Doughnuts, glazed (1)	4	Sugar, jam, or jelly (1 tsp)	1

FIGURE 4-5

Sources of Added Sugars in the U.S. Diet

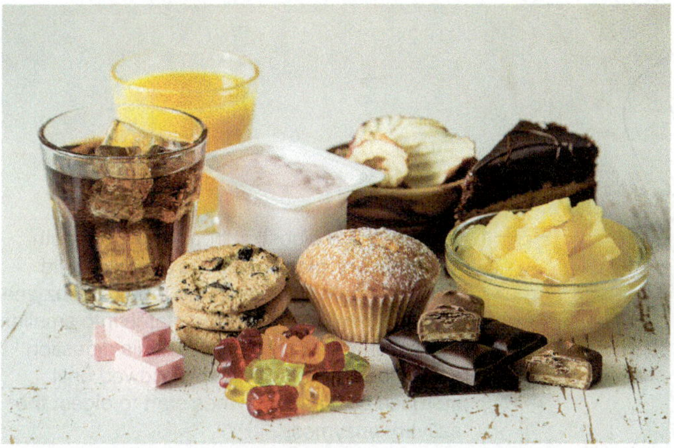

A sampling of foods providing added sugars to the diet. Small amounts of added sugars can be included as part of a nutrient-dense diet and be within your MyPlate calorie allowance:

- 3 tsp for 1,600 calories
- 5 tsp for 1,800 calories
- 8 tsp for 2,000 calories

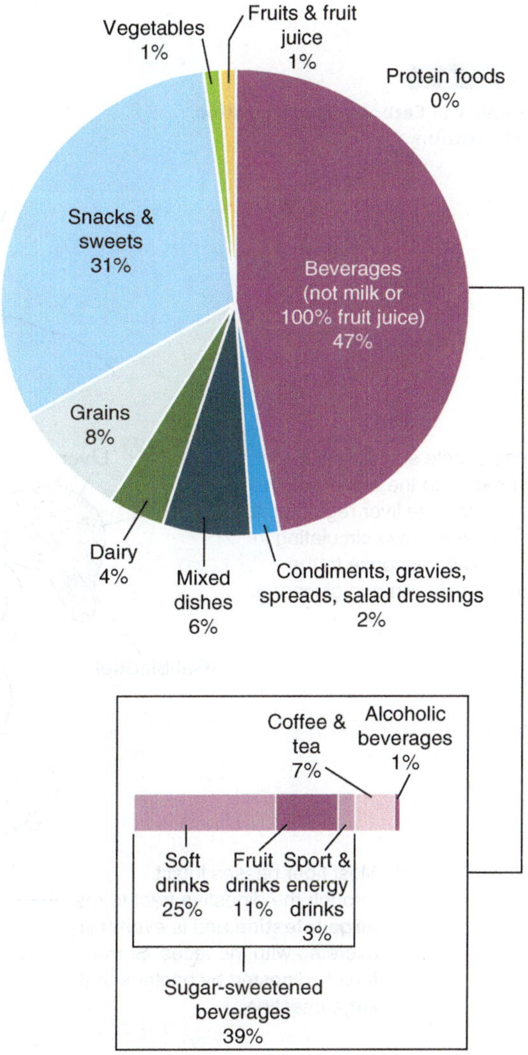

4.5 How the Body Handles Carbohydrates

digestive system The body system composed of organs and glands associated with the ingestion and processing of food for absorption of nutrients into the body. Refer to Chapter 3 for a review of the structure and function of the many body organs discussed in this section.

digestion The process by which foods are broken down into smaller, absorbable products.

absorption The passage of nutrients or substances into cells or tissues; nutrients pass into intestinal cells after digestion and then into the circulatory system (for example, into the bloodstream).

glycogen (GLEYE-ko-jen) A polysaccharide composed of chains of glucose, manufactured in the body and stored in liver and muscle. As a storage form of glucose, liver glycogen can be broken down by the liver to help maintain the blood glucose level when carbohydrate intake is inadequate.

Just as glucose is the original unit from which the many different carbohydrate foods are made, so is glucose the basic carbohydrate unit that each cell of the body uses for energy. Cells cannot use lactose, sucrose, or starch—they require glucose. The task of the **digestive system**, then, is to disassemble the disaccharides and starch into monosaccharides that can be absorbed into the blood. Following absorption, the liver converts to glucose any carbohydrates that were not absorbed in the form of glucose, so the cells can use them. The cells can then store the glucose, use it for current energy needs, or convert it to fat.

The first digestive enzymes to work on starch are those in the saliva; they begin taking the starch apart, and the enzymes in the stomach and intestines continue digestive action (see Figure 4-6). The enzymes release the individual glucose units, which are absorbed across the intestinal wall into the blood. Cooking facilitates the digestive process by spreading out the tightly packaged chains of glucose so that during **digestion** the digestive enzymes can break down the chains into glucose units for **absorption**. One to four hours after a meal, all the starch has been digested and absorbed and is circulating to the cells as glucose.

If the blood delivers more glucose than the cells need, the liver and muscles take up the surplus to build the polysaccharide **glycogen** (see Figure 4-7). The muscles hold two-thirds of the body's total store of this carbohydrate and use it during exercise.

FIGURE 4-6

A Summary of Carbohydrate Digestion and Absorption

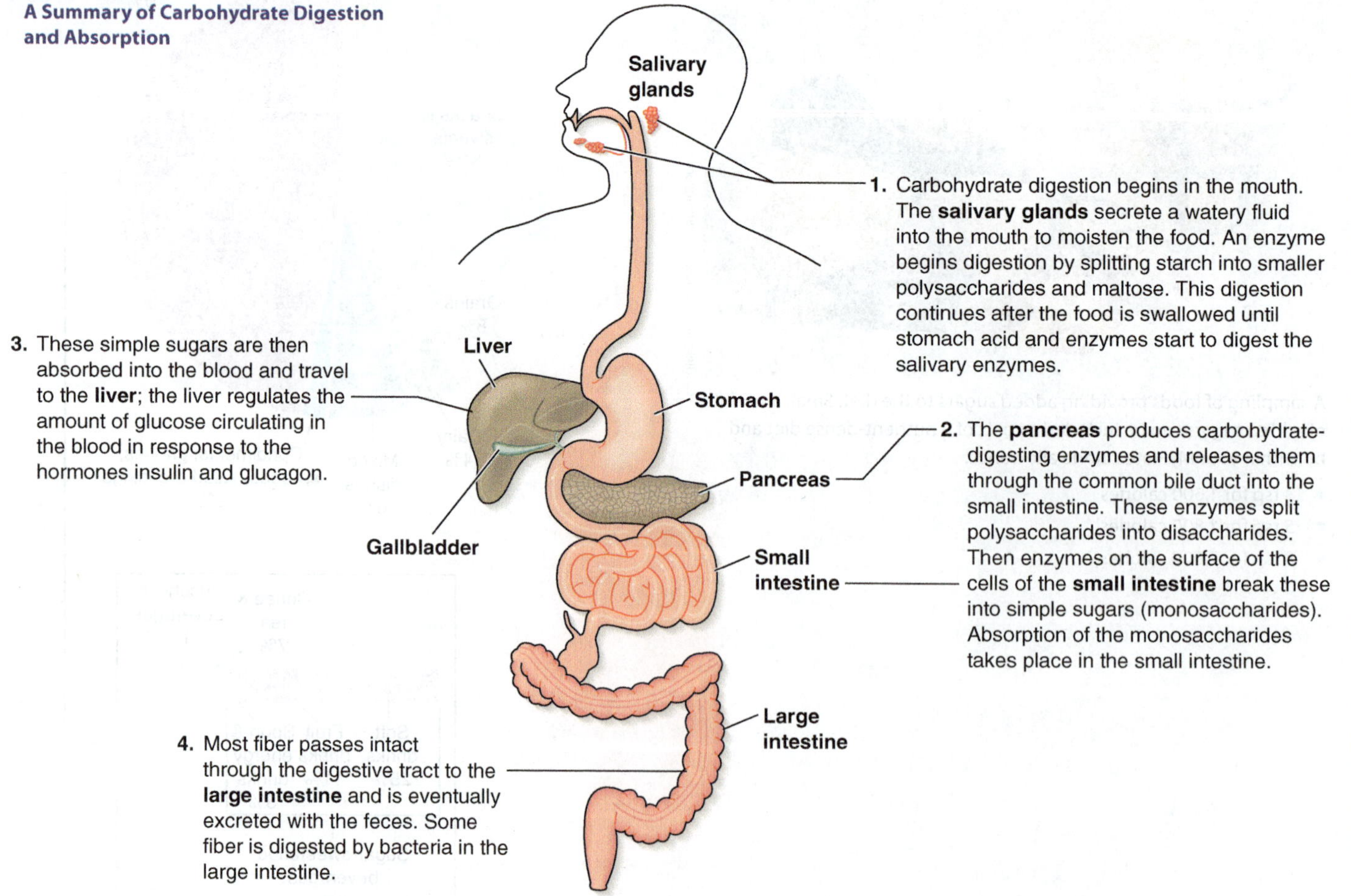

FIGURE 4-7

Feasting and Fasting

In A, the person is storing energy. In B, the person is drawing on stored energy.

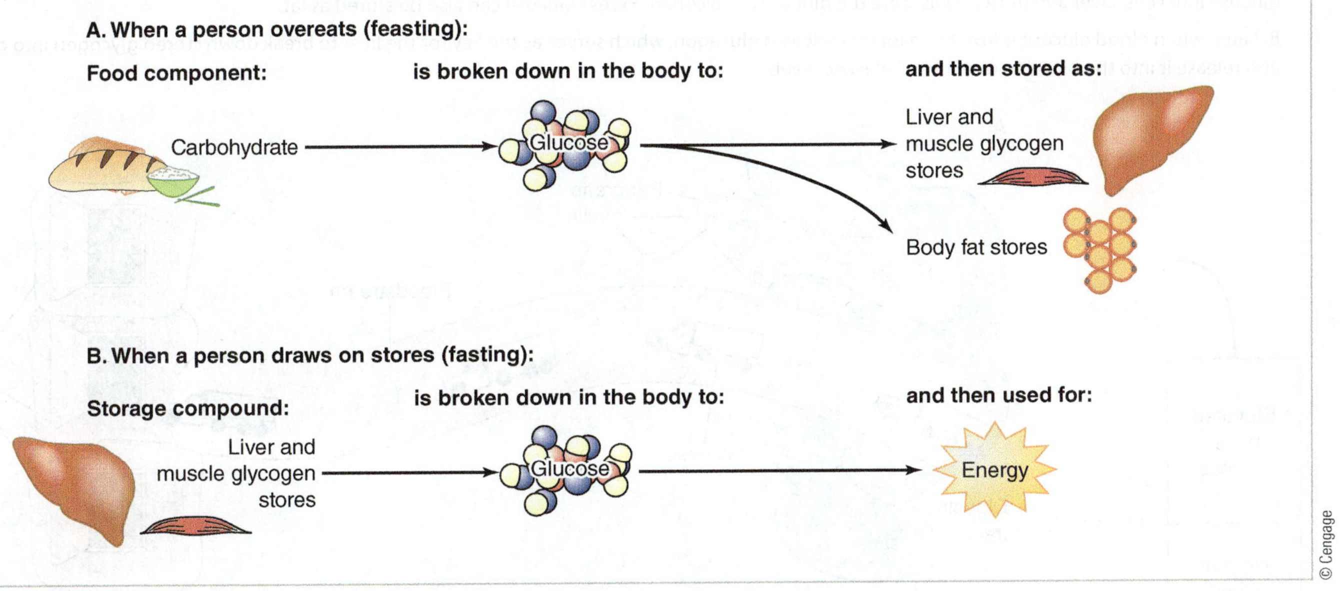

Chapter 11 explores the relationship between glycogen and physical activity and offers tips on how to make the most of glycogen stores. The liver stores the remaining one-third of the body's glycogen, making it available as needed to help maintain the blood glucose level.

Maintaining the Blood Glucose Level

After the glycogen stores are full and the cells' immediate energy needs are met, the body takes a third path for using carbohydrates. For example, perhaps you have eaten a dinner that includes enough carbohydrates to fill your glycogen stores. Now, you watch a movie, eat popcorn, and drink a cola. Your digestive tract delivers glucose from the popcorn and soda to your liver; your liver breaks these extra energy compounds into small fragments and puts them together into the more permanent energy-storage compound: fat (see Figure 4-7). The fat is then released from the liver, carried to the fatty tissues of the body, and deposited there. (Fat cells, too, can utilize excess glucose to make fat for storage.) Unlike the liver cells, however, which can store only about half a day's glucose needs as glycogen, the fat cells can store unlimited quantities of fat.

Maintaining a normal blood glucose level depends on two safeguards, as shown in Figure 4-8. When it gets too high (for example, immediately after a meal), the blood glucose level can be corrected by siphoning off the excess glucose and converting it into liver glycogen, muscle glycogen, or body fat. When it gets too low (for example, following an overnight fast), it can be replenished by drawing on liver glycogen stores.

When the blood glucose level rises, the body adjusts by storing the excess. The first organ to detect the excess glucose is the pancreas, which releases the hormone **insulin** in response. Most of the body's cells respond to insulin by taking up glucose from the blood to make glycogen or fat. Thus, the blood glucose level is quickly brought back down to normal as the body stores the excess. Insulin's opposing hormone, released by the pancreas when blood glucose is too low, is **glucagon,** which draws forth glucose from storage, making it available to supply energy. Insulin and glucagon both work to maintain the concentration of glucose in the blood within the normal range—neither too high nor too low.

insulin A hormone secreted by the pancreas in response to high blood glucose levels; it assists cells in drawing glucose from the blood.

glucagon (GLOO-kuh-gahn) A hormone released by the pancreas that signals the liver to release glucose into the bloodstream.

FIGURE 4-8

Blood Glucose Regulation

A. When a person eats, blood glucose rises. High blood glucose stimulates the pancreas to release insulin. Insulin serves as a key for entrance of blood glucose into cells. Liver and muscle cells store the glucose as glycogen. Excess glucose can also be stored as fat.

B. Later, when blood glucose is low, the pancreas releases glucagon, which serves as the key for the liver to break down stored glycogen into glucose and release it into the blood to raise blood glucose levels.

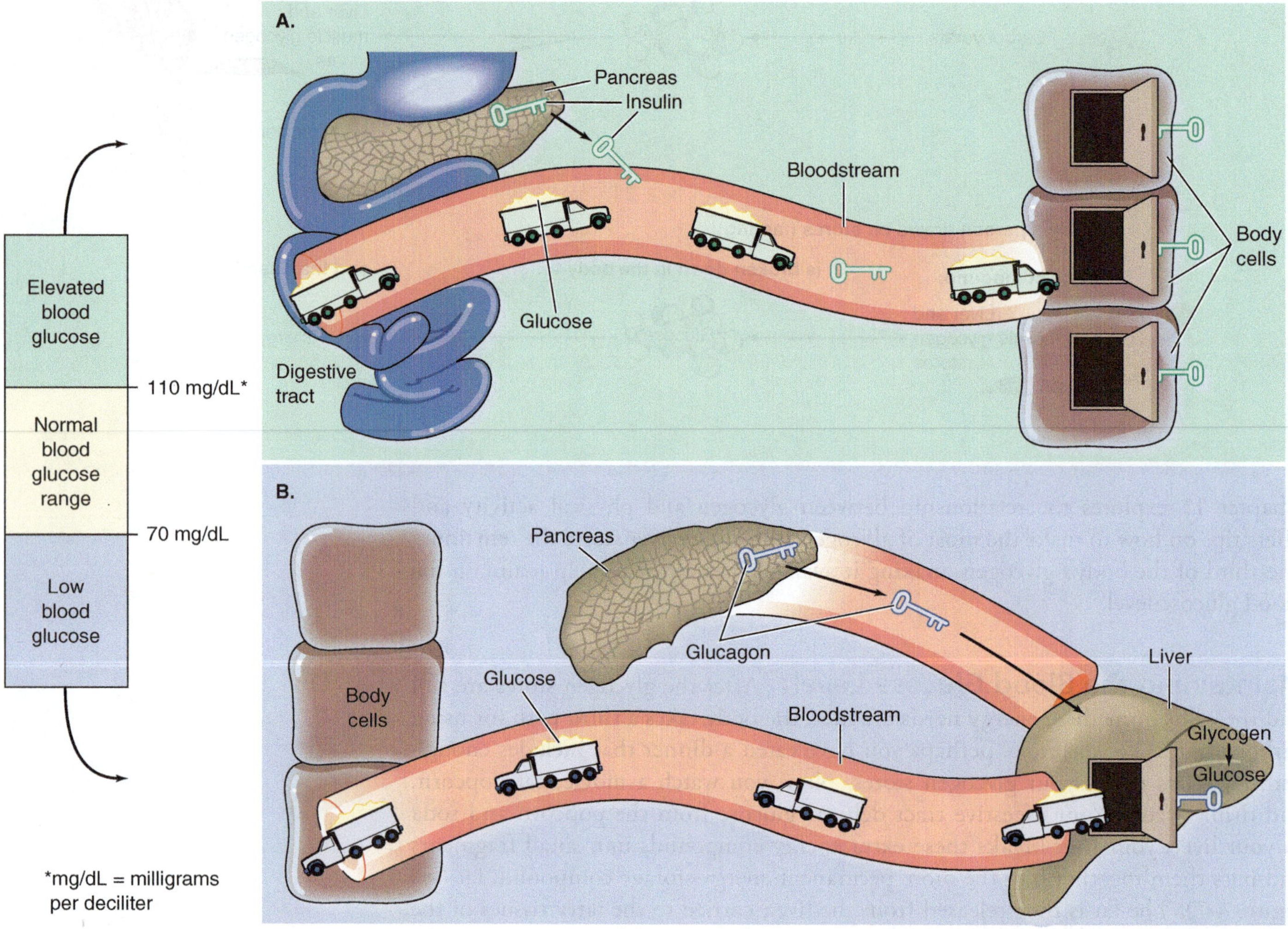

Obviously, when the blood glucose level falls and stores are depleted, a meal or a snack can replenish the supply. An appropriate choice is to eat a balanced meal containing foods that offer carbohydrates (including fiber), protein, and fat, for the following reasons:

- The carbohydrates in the meal provide a quick source of glucose.
- The protein in the meal stimulates glucagon secretion, which opposes insulin and prevents it from storing glucose too quickly.
- The soluble fibers and fat in the meal slow down digestion so that a steady stream of glucose is received rather than a sudden flood.[20]

By these standards, a bowl of whole-grain cereal and fresh fruit with low-fat yogurt for breakfast (offering complex carbohydrate, protein, and fat) is a good choice. Eating well-spaced, carefully chosen meals that provide the balance of protein, carbohydrates, and fat recommended in the *Dietary Guidelines* can prevent rapid rises and falls in the blood glucose level.

4.6 Hypoglycemia and Diabetes

In some people, conditions develop in which the body is unable to maintain normal blood glucose levels without careful medical and dietary interventions. The following discussions help you appreciate the difficulties of the person with **hypoglycemia,** whose insulin response is excessive, or the person with **diabetes,** whose insulin response is slow or ineffective.

Hypoglycemia Suppose that your blood glucose falls, your glycogen reserves are exhausted, but you do *not* eat. Gradually, your body will shift into a fasting state, breaking down its muscle to provide amino acids to the liver. In this state, the liver converts some of these amino acids into glucose to fuel the brain, and the fat released from the muscle cells is used to fuel other cells. (Chapter 10 describes this state, **ketosis**, in more detail.) Most times when this happens, the transition is smooth and not noticeable. At other times, though, when your blood glucose level falls rapidly or below what is normal for you, you may experience symptoms of glucose deprivation to the brain, such as irritability, weakness, and dizziness. Your muscles may become weak, shaky, and trembling, and your heart may race in an attempt to speed more fuel to your brain. Although *true* hypoglycemia is rare, the symptoms of low blood sugar may occur in people who do not eat often enough to keep their blood sugar levels from dropping. The treatment consists of eating balanced meals and learning to eat more frequently throughout the day (see the sample menu on page 115).

People who suspect they might have *true* hypoglycemia should consult a physician for diagnosis and treatment. It is a serious condition in which abnormal amounts of insulin are secreted. As a result, the person's blood glucose level is constantly too low. This type of hypoglycemia causes symptoms such as headache, confusion, fatigue, nervousness, sweating, or unconsciousness. People with hypoglycemia are told to avoid alcohol and snacks high in simple sugars. They usually benefit from eating six small, evenly spaced meals a day that include a variety of complex carbohydrates and lean protein foods. These foods will increase blood sugar levels slowly and more gradually than highly refined carbohydrates.

Diabetes Because you know how the blood glucose level is maintained, you can appreciate the problem of people with diabetes whose insulin response is slow or ineffective. Most adults with diabetes fall into this category (see Table 4-8).[21] Even if the blood glucose level rises too high (**hyperglycemia**), glucose still fails to get into cells and the blood glucose level stays too high for an abnormally long time. The kidneys may respond by shifting some glucose into the urine so that it can be excreted. Short-term effects of hyperglycemia may include thirst, frequent urination, weakness, lack of ability to concentrate, hunger, and blurred vision. People with diabetes must be careful to eat regularly scheduled, balanced meals—providing a constant, steady, moderate flow of glucose to the bloodstream—so the body's insulin response can keep up with the need to process the glucose.

The most common type of diabetes, type 2 diabetes, is usually diagnosed in people over the age of 40 and results from genetic factors, too little insulin, or cellular resistance to insulin.[22] As noted in Figure 4-9, the incidence of type 2 diabetes is rising, mostly because the U.S. population is aging, sedentary, and gaining excess weight.[23] Obesity is considered a major risk factor for this type of diabetes, especially when the excess fat is carried around the abdomen. Usually, eating a healthy diet, exercising, and losing weight can normalize blood glucose levels for people with type 2 diabetes. For others, oral medications and sometimes insulin shots are necessary.

hypoglycemia (HIGH-po-gligh-SEEM-ee-uh) An abnormally low blood glucose concentration, below 60 to 70 mg/100 mL.

diabetes (dye-uh-BEET-eez) A disorder (technically termed *diabetes mellitus*) characterized by insufficiency or relative ineffectiveness of insulin, which renders a person unable to regulate the blood glucose level normally.

ketosis Abnormal amounts of ketone bodies in the blood and urine; ketone bodies are produced from the incomplete breakdown of fat when glucose is unavailable for the brain and nerve cells.

hyperglycemia An abnormally high blood glucose concentration, often a symptom of diabetes.

TABLE 4-8 **Distinctions between the Two Major Types of Diabetes**

	Type 1 Diabetes	Type 2 Diabetes
Incidence	5%–10% of cases	90%–95% of cases
Age of Onset	< 30	> 40*
Insulin Deficiency	Yes; pancreas unable to make insulin to meet needs.	In some cases there may be insufficient insulin, or cells may be unresponsive to insulin.
Risk Factors	Genetic predisposition plus environmental factor (for example, viral infection).	Genetic predisposition plus obesity, family history, aging.
Treatment	Insulin injections, diet, and physical activity.	Weight loss, diet, and physical activity; oral drugs or insulin sometimes needed.

*The incidence of type 2 diabetes is increasing among children. In the majority of cases, the children are overweight or obese and have a family history of type 2 diabetes.

Type 2 diabetes, which in the past occurred only in adults, is now affecting an increasing number of children and adolescents. Obesity in children and teens seems to play a major role in the early development of type 2 diabetes.[24]

People with type 2 diabetes (those whose bodies make insulin but whose cells resist responding to it) tend to become obese, storing more fat than normal and being constantly hungry. This happens because the liver takes the glucose from the blood that the cells cannot take up, converts it to fat, and then ships it out to the fat cells for storage. Because their body cells are resistant to the insulin produced by the pancreas, insulin does not move glucose into cells effectively, and the message that energy fuels are coming in from food is delayed, causing the person with diabetes to be constantly hungry. Unfortunately, the larger the fat cells become, the more resistant they may be to insulin, thus making the diabetes worse. People with diabetes in their family are urged not to gain excess weight, for it is likely to precipitate the onset of the disease.

People with the less common type of diabetes, type 1, produce no (or very little) insulin and require insulin injections to control their blood sugar levels. Type 1 diabetes is more likely to be diagnosed during childhood and has been linked to a possible

FIGURE 4-9

Prevalence of Diagnosed Diabetes by State, United States, 1994 and 2014

This series of maps displays the increasing prevalence (existing cases) of diagnosed diabetes among the adult populations of states between 1994 and 2014. In 1994, 26 states had a prevalence of less than 4.5 percent and only 1 state had a prevalence of 6 percent or greater. However, by 2014, all states had a prevalence of 6 percent or greater, and 27 of the states had a prevalence of 9 percent or higher.

SOURCE: Centers for Disease Control and Prevention.

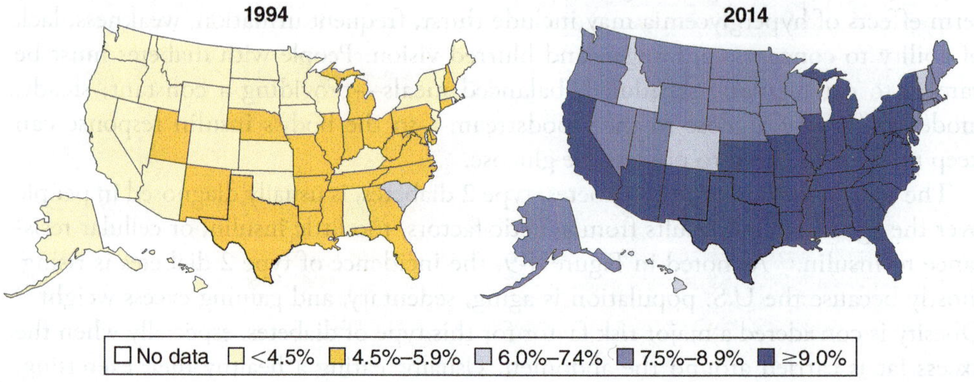

Nutrition ACTION Carbohydrates—Friend or Foe? (Obj. 4.5)

With the low-carbohydrate trend now on its way out, many people are wondering, "What are they going to tell us next about carbohydrates?" The answer to that question might lie in an older theory concerning the glycemic effect of carbohydrates, which is making its way back into the spotlight. The **glycemic effect** refers to the effect of food on a person's blood glucose and insulin response: how fast and how high the blood glucose rises and how quickly the body responds by bringing it back to normal. This phenomenon is the basis of many diets, including the "South Beach" and "Nutrisystem" plans, and it relates to the effect particular carbohydrates have on raising or lowering blood glucose and the time it takes to do so.

A Closer Look at the Glycemic Effect of Foods

Researchers rank carbohydrate foods according to how fast each is digested into glucose and how much the food causes blood glucose to rise (see Figure 4-10). In general, legumes produce the most even blood glucose response, dairy products next, and fruits and cereals next.

In rating this effect with a scale called the **glycemic index (GI)**, foods that quickly raise blood glucose are given a higher score, and lower scores are assigned to those that don't. Some believe this can help people pick "good carbohydrates" that are digested more slowly and therefore increase **satiety**. Nevertheless, many others are quick to point out that there are well-known flaws in this system. For example, foods of different glycemic index scores when eaten together behave much differently than when eaten alone, therefore voiding practical use of these scores.

A glycemic index ranks foods on the basis of the extent to which the foods raise the blood glucose level as compared with pure glucose. The blood glucose response to foods with a *high* glycemic index (such as white bread, cornflakes, waffles, and jelly beans) is fast and high. As shown in Table 4-9, foods with a *low* glycemic index *tend* to be wholesome, fiber-rich foods (such as fruits, legumes, whole oats, bran cereals) and dairy products. Because these foods are more slowly digested, they release glucose gradually into the blood.

The effect of a food on the blood glucose level is important to people with abnormalities of blood glucose regulation, notably diabetes and hypoglycemia. Rapid swings in blood glucose can also affect the performance of an athlete during an endurance event or an office employee following lunch.[25] However, a problem with using the glycemic index as a tool for food selection is that the actual glycemic index of a food can vary from person to person, as well as from meal to meal, depending on the overall composition of the meal. Due to the high variability of the index, it may take some experimenting on an individual's part to learn what combinations of foods yield the most satisfying effects.

FIGURE 4-10

Glycemic Effect of Carbohydrates

Researchers rank foods according to how fast each is digested into glucose and how much the food causes blood glucose to rise following ingestion. In general, legumes produce the most even blood glucose response, whereas pure sugar produces the greatest rise in the blood glucose level.

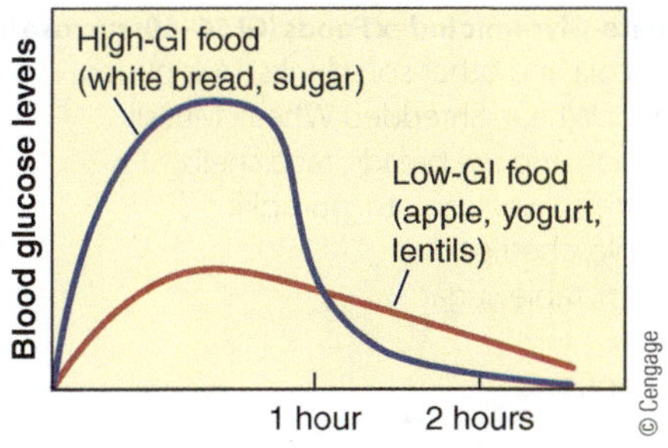

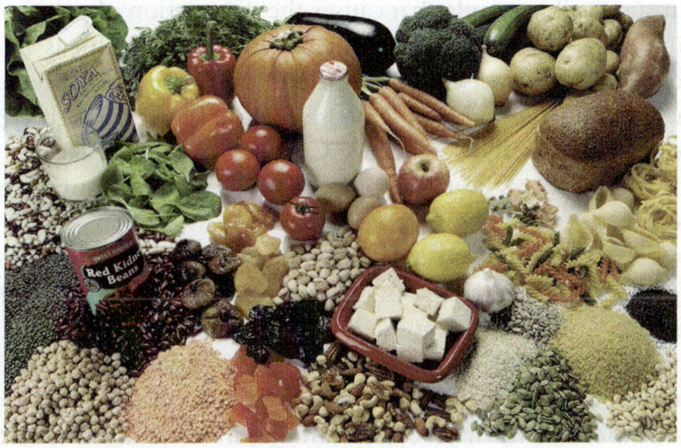

Buntrock, Gerrit/StockFood

glycemic effect (also called *glycemic response*) The effect of food on a person's blood glucose and insulin response; how fast and how high the blood glucose rises and how quickly the body responds by bringing it back to normal.

glycemic index (GI) A ranking of foods based on their potential to raise blood glucose levels.

satiety (sah-TIE-eh-tee) The feeling of fullness and satisfaction that occurs after a meal.

(Continued)

TABLE 4-9 Glycemic Index of Selected Foods
High Glycemic Index Foods (GI = 70–100; glucose has a GI of 100) • French, white, and other soft-textured breads or bagels • rice (medium-grain white or brown), rice milk, rice crackers • certain cereals (Cheerios, Corn Flakes, Rice Krispies), instant oatmeal • waffles, doughnuts • mashed potatoes, baked potato • regular soft drinks, sports drinks, jelly beans • pretzels, corn chips • watermelon
Intermediate-Glycemic Index Foods (GI 56–69; sucrose has GI of 65) • honey, cola and other soft drinks, fruit punch • Cream of Wheat, Shredded Wheat, Muesli • sourdough and rye breads, taco shells • french fries, sweet potato, pumpkin • pineapple, cherries • ice cream, table sugar • popcorn • raisins, apricots
Low-Glycemic Index Foods (GI 55 or lower; fructose has GI of 15) • whole-grain, heavy-textured breads, corn tortilla, chapatti • long-grain brown rice, barley, pasta • bran cereals, whole oats • apples, oranges, pears, banana, grapefruit, grapes, peaches, strawberries, mango, plantain, dates, apple juice, orange juice • carrots, green peas, yams, broccoli, vegetable soup • baked beans, lentils, other legumes, tomato juice • milk, yogurt, soy milk • cashews, peanuts, soybeans, hummus

However, many nutrition professionals agree about the theory of so-called good carbohydrates. These "good carbohydrates" are usually thought of as containing little added sugar and having adequate amounts of complex carbohydrates and fiber—which often create a better GI score. In fact, this belief is a major underpinning of the new dietary guidelines, which recommend increasing intakes of fruits, vegetables, and whole grains.

Here is a comparison of glycemic index, carbohydrate, fiber, fat, and calorie content of two similar meals:

Meal 1	***Meal 2***
White bread	Wheat bread
Carrots	Black-eyed peas
Baked white potato	Sweet potato
Soda	Skim milk
Chicken breast	Chicken breast
Watermelon	Peaches
Total: GI 492, 4g fat, 9g fiber, 77g carb., 620 calories	**Total: GI 341, 3g fat, 11g fiber, 84g carb., 663 calories**

As shown by the second meal, a lower glycemic index does not necessarily mean that the meal will be lower in calories and/or higher in fiber. This illustrates why use of the GI as a "dieting" tool might be up for debate.

Overall, people are wise to choose diets rich in fruits, vegetables, legumes, whole grains, low-fat dairy, unsalted nuts, fish, and lean meats. Quite often, such a diet will have a low glycemic index, plus an array of other healthful attributes. Here are some nutrition "do's" that ensure a healthy diet:

- Choose foods minimally processed and with fiber intact.
- Forgo items with sugar added.
- Look for "whole grain" as the main ingredient.

Whether it is the glycemic index or any other way of dealing with carbohydrates, these principles will not steer you and your diet wrong no matter what the current fad happens to be!

Diabetes Information on the Web

The American Diabetes Association

- **www.diabetes.org**

National Diabetes Education Program

- **www.ndep.nih.gov**

National Diabetes Information Clearinghouse

- **www.diabetes.niddk.nih.gov**

Government websites:

- **www.healthfinder.gov**
- **www.cdc.gov/diabetes/index.htm**

viral or allergic reaction in susceptible people that causes the destruction of pancreatic cells that produce insulin. The person who does not produce any insulin is likely to experience a sudden onset of the disease. Such a person may lose weight rapidly because, without insulin, the cells cannot store glucose or fat. Thus, the two types of diabetes have opposite effects on body weight. See Chapter 12 for a discussion of *gestational diabetes*—a form of diabetes seen only in pregnancy. To determine your own risk for diabetes, take the test in the box on page 115.

The American Diabetes Association eased its restriction on sugar use in the diets of people with diabetes because sucrose-containing foods do not seem to exert any higher glycemic response than do some starchy foods.[26] However, according to their guidelines, any foods containing sucrose must be used in place of other carbohydrate-containing foods and should not exceed 5 to 10 percent of the total carbohydrate calories. Many people with diabetes learn to count carbohydrates and estimate the caloric content of foods by using the food lists presented in Appendix A. Additional online resources are listed in the margin.

A Sample Meal Plan for Keeping Blood Sugar Levels on an Even Keel

Breakfast

Spread ¼ cup low-fat ricotta cheese on 2 halves of a small cinnamon-raisin bagel. Top with 2 tbsp raisins and sprinkle with cinnamon. Heat under broiler for 1 to 2 minutes.

Midmorning Snack

Mix 1 sliced fresh peach with 1 cup low-fat plain yogurt and top with ¼ cup low-fat granola.

Lunch

Stuff a whole-wheat pita with ¾ cup Zesty Vegetable Tuna (see recipe), and top with shredded lettuce. Enjoy 1 cup fresh melon cubes as a side dish.

Midafternoon Snack

Spread 2 tbsp hummus over 4 slices whole-grain melba toast.

Dinner

¾ cup Quick Kidney Bean Salad (see recipe)
3 oz grilled chicken breast
1 cup steamed broccoli florets
1 medium baked sweet potato
2 tsp butter

Evening Snack

Combine ¾ cup fat-free milk, 1 frozen peeled banana, and 1 tbsp peanut butter, and blend for 1 to 2 minutes until smooth.

Zesty Vegetable Tuna

one 6-oz can water-packed tuna
½ cup chopped green pepper
½ cup chopped red pepper
½ cup shredded carrots
3 tbsp light mayonnaise
2 tbsp Dijon mustard
3 tbsp balsamic vinegar

Combine last three ingredients, then add remaining ingredients.

Makes 3 servings.

Quick Kidney Bean Salad

one 16-oz can kidney beans, rinsed and drained
½ cup chopped celery
½ cup chopped onion
⅓ cup orange juice
2 tbsp cider vinegar

Mix all ingredients in a bowl and refrigerate until chilled.

Makes 4 servings.

SOURCE: Adapted from "Getting Even with Low Blood Sugar," *Health Wise* 5 (1999): 6.

What Is Your Risk for Diabetes?

1. I have given birth to a baby weighing more than nine pounds.
   Yes = 1 No = 0 ________
2. I have a sister or a brother with diabetes.
   Yes = 1 No = 0 ________
3. I have a parent with diabetes.
   Yes = 1 No = 0 ________
4. My weight is equal to or above that listed in the At-Risk Weight Chart shown at right.
   Yes = 1 No = 0 ________
5. I am under 65 years of age and I get little or no exercise during a typical day.
   Yes = 1 No = 0 ________
6. I am between 45 and 64 years of age.
   Yes = 1 No = 0 ________
7. I am 65 years or older.
   Yes = 9 No = 0 ________

Total: ________

At-Risk Weight Chart

If you weigh the same or more than the weight listed here for your height (BMI > 27), you may be at risk for diabetes.

Height, without shoes (feet/inches)	Weight, without clothing (pounds)	Height, without shoes (feet/inches)	Weight, without clothes (pounds)
4′10″	128	5′8″	177
4′11″	133	5′9″	183
5′0″	138	5′10″	188
5′1″	143	5′11″	193
5′2″	147	6′0″	198
5′3″	152	6′1″	204
5′4″	157	6′2″	210
5′5″	162	6′3″	218
5′6″	167	6′4″	221
5′7″	172		

SCORING

3–9 points: Chances are you are at low risk for diabetes now. Maintain a healthy weight, eat nutritious low-fat meals, and exercise regularly to keep risk low.

10 or more points: You are at high risk for diabetes. See your doctor to be tested.

SOURCE: American Diabetes Association. For more information about diabetes, call 1-800-DIABETES or go to www.diabetes.org.

4.7 Sugar and Health

Sugar is often in the headlines and has been accused of contributing to a host of human ills, such as tooth decay, obesity, diabetes, heart disease, hyperactive behavior in children, and even criminal behavior. Nevertheless, research studies have not shown a direct link between sugar and any of these conditions, except tooth decay.[27] However, eating too many high-sugar foods could also mean that you are eating

Agnes Kantaruk/Shutterstock.com

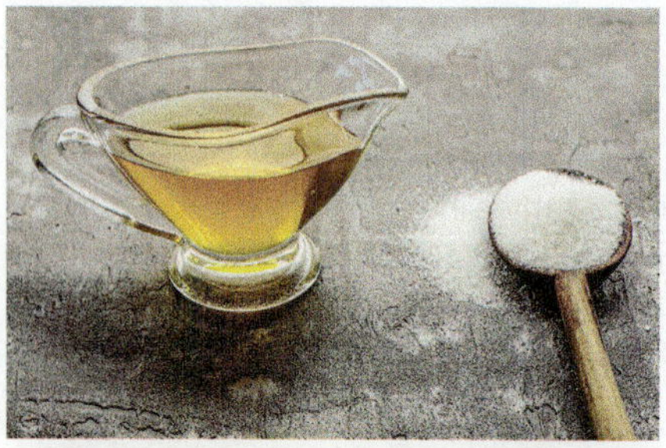

Deenida/Shutterstock.com

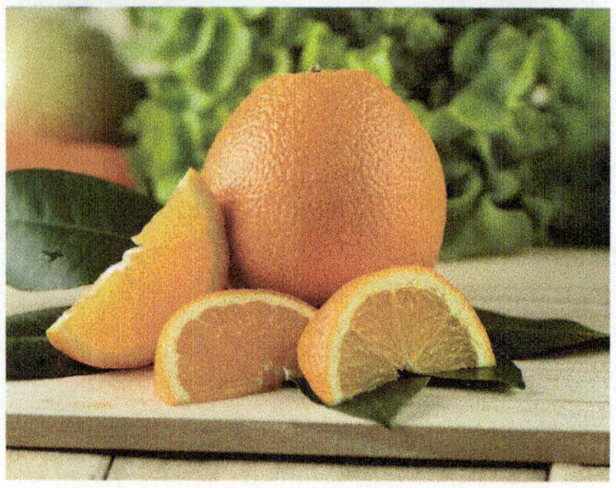

The honey and table sugar (sucrose) are concentrated sweeteners, each containing the simple sugars fructose and glucose. In the orange, these sugars are naturally occurring sugars. Compared with honey or sugar, the orange is more nutrient dense—providing vitamins, minerals, and fiber along with its sugars.

inadequate amounts of foods containing essential nutrients. Also, if you eat a lot of high-sugar foods without eating less of other foods, you might be getting too many calories. Excess calories from any energy nutrient, even protein, are stored as body fat. Evidence from population studies in many countries shows that obesity rates increase as sugar consumption increases. One reason may be that many sugary foods, such as candy bars, are also high in solid fat.

The dietary guideline to limit added sugar intake does not apply to *all* sugars in the diet. The diluted *naturally occurring* sugars found in milk and fruits should not be confused with concentrated refined sugars, such as table sugar, honey, and high-fructose corn syrup. These concentrated sweets should be used in moderation, so that they do not displace needed nutrients.

When people learn that fruit's energy comes from simple sugars, they may think that eating fruit is the same as consuming concentrated sweets such as candy or soft drinks. However, fruits differ from candy and soft drinks in important ways. Their sugars are diluted in large volumes of water, packaged in fiber, and mixed with many vitamins and minerals needed by the body (see Table 4-10). In contrast, concentrated sweets such as honey and table sugar are merely—as the popular phrase calls them—**empty-calorie foods**. How much sugar do *you* eat? Try the Carbohydrate Consumption Scorecard on page 119, which gives you the opportunity to check your diet for sugar and fiber.

empty-calorie foods Foods that supply calories but negligible nutrients.

Keeping Sweetness in the Diet

The taste of sweetness is a pleasure; the liking for it is innate. *The Dietary Guidelines* recommend that you "limit calories from added sugars and shift to healthier food and beverage choices."[28] To help with these tasks while still catering to the sweet tooth, consider the following tips:

- Use less of all sugars, including white sugar, brown sugar, honey, jelly, and syrups.
- Choose sensibly to limit your intake of beverages and foods that are high in added sugars, such as soft drinks, energy drinks, fruit drinks, candy, ice cream, cakes, cookies, and pies.

TABLE 4-10 Sample Nutrients in Fruits and Sugars

	Size of 100-Calorie Portion	Carbohydrate (g)	Fiber (g)	Vitamin A (μg)	Vitamin C (mg)	Folate (μg)	Potassium (mg)
Fruits							
Apricots	6	24	6	137	20	18	622
Apple	1 large	25	5	4	12	6	244
Cantaloupe	½ 5-in. melon	23	2	444	116	47	853
Orange	1¼ c sections	26	5	24	120	68	408
Pineapple	1¼ c chunks	24	2.5	2.5	30	20	219
Strawberries	2 c	20	6	4	164	50	478
Watermelon	1¼ c chunks	22	2	56	30	6	352
Sugars							
Cola beverage	8 oz	26	0	0	0	0	3
Honey	1½ tbsp	26	0	0	0	<1	22
Jelly	2 tbsp	26	0	0	<1	0	24
Sugar, white	2 tbsp	24	0	0	0	0	0
Sugar, brown	3 tbsp	24	0	0	0	0	90
Adult Dietary Reference Intake (DRI)		**> 130**	**21–38**	**700–900**	**75–90**	**400**	**4,700**

- Select fresh fruits to satisfy your urge for sweets.
- Learn to read the ingredients list. Check food labels for clues about added sugar content. If any of the following sugars appears first or second in the ingredients list, or if several names are listed, the food is likely to be high in sugar (see Figure 2-16 in Chapter 2). Examples of added sugars include agave syrup, brown sugar, coconut sugar, confectioner's sugar, corn syrup, dextrose, evaporated cane juice, fructose, high-fructose corn syrup, fruit juice concentrate, honey, malt syrup, maple syrup, molasses, nectars, powdered sugar, raw sugar, and white sugar.
- For dental health, remember that how frequently you eat sugar is as important as, and perhaps more important than, how much sugar you eat at one time (see the section that follows).
- Alternatives to sweet desserts might be whole-grain crackers, low-fat cheese, and fresh fruit with unsweetened yogurt. Snacks for children could include fruits, vegetables, string cheese, popcorn, homemade fruit juice pops, and other wholesome foods.
- Substitute fruit *juices* or water for fruit drinks, regular soft drinks, and punches that contain considerable amounts of added sugar.
- Buy *unsweetened* cereals so that you can control the amount of sugar added. Many cereals are presweetened. Check the Nutrition Facts panel for the grams of added sugar present. Many cereals list sugar first or second among their ingredients, indicating a high amount of added sugar.
- Experiment with reducing the sugar in your favorite recipes. Some recipes taste just the same even after a 50 percent reduction in sugar content.
- The sweet spices—allspice, anise, cardamom, cinnamon, ginger, and nutmeg—can replace substantial sugar in recipes. Use half as much sugar and increase one and a half times the amount of spice the recipe calls for. Increasing the amount of extracts like vanilla can enhance sweetness, too. Experiment with other extracts like maple, coconut, banana, and chocolate, or try adding dried fruit to baked goods for extra sweetness and nutrients as you decrease sugar.

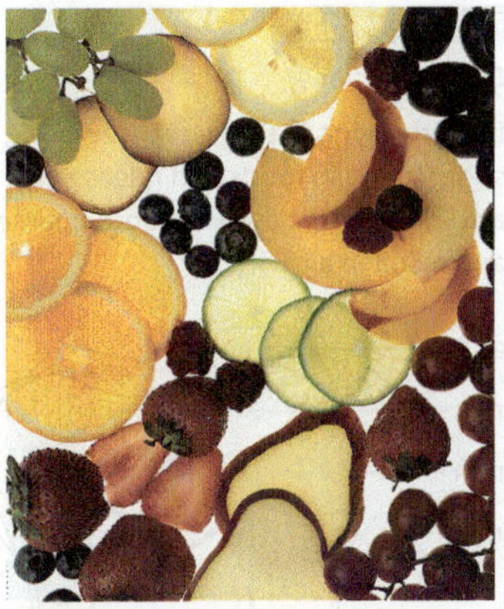
Tom McCarthy Photography

Naturally sweet foods such as fruit can satisfy your sweet tooth.

Still another alternative for reducing sugar intake is to use sugary foods that convey nutrients as well as calories. For example, rather than using table sugar as a topping, add raisins and banana slices, which are really very sweet. The person with nutrition sense and a taste for sweets can artfully combine the two by using sugar with creative imagination to enhance the flavors of nutritious foods.

You may wonder whether using artificial sweeteners to reduce some of the total sugar in your diet is a safe and recommended strategy. The Spotlight feature "Sweet Talk" at the end of this chapter will help you decide.

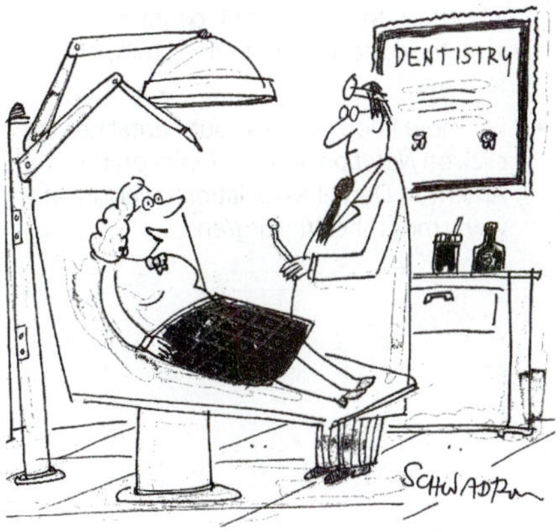

Harley Schwadron/Schwadron Cartoons

"Just pull my sweet tooth."

Keeping a Healthy Smile

For years, conventional wisdom has held that staying away from candy, cookies, sugary soda pop, and the like is the most important line of dietary defense against cavities. Even Aristotle asked, in about 350 B.C., "Why do figs when they are sweet, produce damage to the teeth?"[29]

These days, dentists advise that cutting down on the amount of sugar eaten is not the only way to prevent **dental caries.** Every bit as important (if not more) as when and how often a food is eaten is whether that food clings to the teeth and lingers in the mouth. It has to do with the mouth's level of acid. Each time you bite into a food, the bacteria that live in your mouth feed on the sugar in it and release an acid that eats away at tooth enamel. When a large number of bacteria living in a film referred to as **dental plaque** produce enough acid to dissolve a "hole" in the enamel over a period of time, the result is a cavity (see Figure 4-11).

dental caries Decay of the teeth; tooth cavities (*caries* = rottenness).

dental plaque A colorless film, consisting of bacteria and their by-products, that is constantly forming on the teeth.

FIGURE 4-11

Dental Caries

Bacteria living in the mouth feed on sugar found in foods and release an acid that can eat away at tooth enamel and result in a cavity.

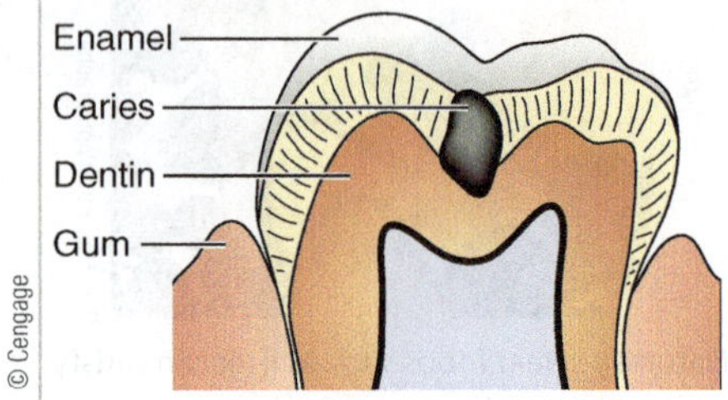

For optimal dental health, the American Dental Association (ADA) recommends the following:

- Eat a balanced diet.
- Keep snacking to a minimum, if possible. The ADA recognizes that some people, such as people with diabetes, may require snacks. For others, however, the ADA suggests limiting the number of snacks if brushing the teeth is not possible shortly after eating them.
- Eat sweets with meals rather than between them.
- Brush and floss thoroughly each day to remove dental plaque.
- Use an ADA-accepted fluoride toothpaste and mouth rinse, and talk to your dentist about the need for supplemental fluoride.
- Visit a dentist regularly.
- Do not allow an infant to sleep with a bottle in the mouth that contains sweetened liquids, fruit juices, milk, or formula.[32]
- For more information about dental health, click on *Nutrition* and *A-Z Topics* on the American Dental Association's website at www.mouthhealthy.org/en

Although consuming sugary items such as soft drinks boosts acid production in the mouth, so does munching on starchy foods such as crackers or pretzels. This happens because enzymes in the saliva can break the carbohydrate in the cracker or pretzel into the simple sugars that bacteria feast on. If a crumb or two from a starchy food gets caught between the teeth, it might provide enough carbohydrate for bacteria to feed on for hours, thereby prolonging the teeth's exposure to acid. In fact, some research indicates that even high-sugar foods such as chocolate bars and hot fudge sundaes are less likely to contribute to cavity formation than stickier, starchier items that are likely to linger in the mouth, such as potato chips and crackers.[30]

To be sure, the carbohydrate content and stickiness of a food are only two of the many factors that influence the food's effect on teeth. Another is how often you eat the food. Each time you eat a carbohydrate-containing food, your teeth are bathed in acids for about 20 minutes. Thus, the more often you eat, the longer your teeth are exposed to harmful acids.[31]

Yet another factor to consider is the combination of foods that you eat. Starchy, sugary foods tend to be less harmful to the teeth when eaten with a meal than when consumed alone. One reason may be that the mouth makes more saliva during a full meal. Saliva production is crucial, because even though it helps make the sugar that encourages bacteria to thrive, it also clears food particles from the mouth and neutralizes destructive acids before they can dissolve the teeth. One study at the University of Iowa's College of Dentistry studied people who nibbled on foods that have a strong tendency to produce acid, such as raisins and chocolate bars, and then chewed sugarless gum. They found that within 10 minutes, the gum helped stimulate the release of enough saliva to neutralize the acid flow that the sweets had caused.[33] In addition, some research suggests that, like sugarless chewing gum, foods such as cheese and peanuts help fight acid attacks that are stimulated by eating carbohydrate-rich foods.[34]

Of course, although saliva helps fight cavities, the best way to ensure good dental health is to brush your teeth as soon as possible after eating, or at least swish the mouth with water after a meal to help rinse the teeth and dislodge stuck particles. Flossing daily is also important because flossing rids the mouth not only of food but also of plaque—before it becomes so widespread that it produces tooth-threatening levels of acid. Regular visits to the dentist also play a role in maintaining dental health. In addition, drinking water containing fluoride, a mineral that helps strengthen tooth enamel, can prevent cavities. People whose drinking water does not supply fluoride should check with a dentist about the need for fluoride supplements.

Along with practicing good dental hygiene, eating a balanced diet helps keep the mouth healthy. One reason is that if the diet lacks essential nutrients, mouth tissues can become compromised, leaving them particularly vulnerable to infection. In fact, some experts believe that **periodontal disease** is especially severe among people who have poor diets.[35] Another reason to eat an adequate diet, particularly for children, is that it helps ensure proper tooth development.[36] Similarly, eating well should rank as a high priority for a pregnant woman, whose unborn baby's teeth, among other things, start forming after just six weeks and begin to harden between the first and second trimester of pregnancy.

Incidentally, parents should never allow an infant to sleep with a bottle filled with sweetened liquids, fruit juices, milk, or formula. Little ones allowed to do so often develop what is known as **nursing bottle syndrome.** As a baby sucks on a bottle, the tongue pushes outward slightly and covers the lower teeth. If the infant falls asleep with the bottle in the mouth, the liquid bathes the teeth, particularly the upper teeth not protected by the tongue, thereby literally soaking them in cavity-causing carbohydrates for hours at a time.

periodontal disease Inflammation or degeneration of the tissues that surround and support the teeth.

nursing bottle syndrome (also called *baby bottle tooth decay*) Decay of all the upper and sometimes the back lower teeth that occurs in infants given carbohydrate-containing liquids when they sleep. The syndrome can also develop in toddlers given bottles of liquid to carry around and sip all day.

SCORE Card

Carbohydrate Consumption—Rating Your Diet: How Sweet and Fiber-Rich Is It? (Obj. 4.7)

Now that you are aware of some of the sources of added sugars, as well as good sources of fiber, let's take a look at *your* diet.

Check Your Diet for Added Sugars

Check the box that most closely describes your eating habits to see how the foods you choose affect the amount of added sugars in your diet.

	Seldom or Never	1 or 2 Times a Week	3 to 5 Times a Week	Almost Daily
How often do you				
1. Drink soft drinks, sweetened fruit drinks, or other sweetened beverages?	☐	☐	☐	☐
2. Choose sweet desserts and snacks, such as cakes, pies, cookies, and ice cream?	☐	☐	☐	☐
3. Use canned or frozen fruits packed in heavy syrup or add sugar to fresh fruit?	☐	☐	☐	☐
4. Eat candy?	☐	☐	☐	☐
5. Add sugar to coffee or tea?	☐	☐	☐	☐
6. Use jam, jelly, or honey on bread or rolls?	☐	☐	☐	☐

How Did You Do?

The more often you choose the items listed, the higher your diet is likely to be in sugars. You may need to cut back on sugar-containing foods and beverages, especially those you checked as "3 to 5 times a week" or more. This does not mean eliminating these foods from your diet. You can moderate your intake of sugars by choosing foods that are high in sugar less often and by eating smaller portions.

Check Your Diet for Fiber

To reap the benefits of fiber, healthy adults need between 21 and 40 grams of fiber a day. The Daily Value (DV) used on food labels is 28 grams per day. Most Americans get about 16 grams a day. To figure how much fiber you consume in a day, write down the number of servings you eat in a typical day for each of the following food categories. Next, multiply by the factor shown. (This number represents the average amount of fiber from a serving in that food group.) Then add up the total and determine how you compare to the recommended goal.

Food Group	**Number of Servings**	**Amount (g)**
Vegetables (½ c cooked; 1 c raw)	_______ × 2 g	= _______
Fruits (1 medium; ½ c cut; ¼ c dried)	_______ × 2 g	= _______
Dried beans, lentils, split peas (½ c cooked)	_______ × 8 g	= _______
Nuts, seeds (¼ c; 2 tbsp peanut butter)	_______ × 2 g	= _______
Whole grains (1 slice bread; ½ c rice, pasta; ½ bun, bagel, muffin)	_______ × 2 g	= _______
Refined grains[a] (1 slice bread; ½ c rice, pasta; ½ bun, bagel, muffin)	_______ × 1 g	= _______
Breakfast cereals[b] (1 oz)	_______ × g	= _______
		Total = _______

[a] *Refined grains* refers to products made with white or wheat flour (not whole-wheat flour); white rice, or other processed grains.
[b] Check the Nutrition Facts panel on the cereal you eat to determine the number of grams of fiber in a 1-ounce serving.

Scoring

21–40: Good news! Your fiber intake meets the recommended goal.

17–20: You consume more fiber than the average American. Another serving from the fruit, vegetable, and whole-grain categories would help bring your fiber intake into the recommended goal area.

11–16: Your intake is similar to the average American intake. Consider adding a serving of legumes and additional servings of fruits, vegetables, and whole grains to your daily diet.

0–10: Your fiber intake is too low. Try getting at least five servings of fruits and vegetables, along with three servings of whole-grain foods each day. Add a high-fiber cereal to your morning routine, and consider adding legumes to some of your weekly meals.

SPOTLight

4.8 Sweet Talk—Alternatives to Sugar

It all started back in 1879—the year that a substance called saccharin was first discovered and found to be able to sweeten foods without adding calories. Since that time, the sale of **nonnutritive sweeteners** for use as tabletop sweeteners—such as Splenda and Equal—and in artificially sweetened soft drinks, yogurt, and numerous other products has soared.[37] The most common and popular nonnutritive sweeteners approved for use in the United States today are acesulfame-K, aspartame, neotame, saccharin, stevia, and sucralose. Despite the ever-growing popularity of such sweeteners, doubts about their safety have stirred a good deal of controversy over the years. In addition, confusion about the characteristics of the various alternatives to sugar (see Table 4-11) and their role in managing problems such as obesity, diabetes, and tooth decay prevails among the millions of Americans who use them. The following discussion about sugar substitutes will help put matters into perspective.

Is it true that small amounts of saccharin cause cancer?

This assertion has never been proven. It's true that some studies of saccharin (the sweetener in Sweet'N Low) have found that it can cause bladder cancer in laboratory rats. A human, however, would have to drink 850 cans of soft drinks a day to take in a dose equivalent to what the rats in those studies were given. Moreover, some research suggests that although very high doses of saccharin may promote bladder cancer in rats, the sweetener does not have the same effect on mice, hamsters, monkeys, or humans.[38] In addition, investigations of large groups of people have yet to establish any clear-cut link between saccharin consumption and the risk of cancer. One study, conducted by the National Cancer Institute and involving more than 9,000 men and women, showed no association between saccharin use and bladder cancer.[39] As the American Medical Association's Council on Scientific Affairs has stated, "In humans, available evidence indicates that the use of artificial sweeteners, including saccharin, is not associated with an increased risk of bladder cancer."[40] The government removed saccharin from a list of potential cancer-causing agents, and in December 2000, federal legislation was signed to remove the saccharin warning label that had been required on saccharin-sweetened foods and beverages in the United States since 1977.[41]

Does aspartame cause headaches?

Not in most people. Although the U.S. Food and Drug Administration (FDA) has received numerous complaints from consumers who claim to suffer from headaches, nausea, anxiety, and other symptoms after consuming aspartame-containing foods or beverages, scientific studies have never confirmed that the sweetener is truly the culprit. Scientists at Duke University, who conducted carefully controlled research into the matter, concluded that tablets containing the amount of aspartame in about 4 liters of diet soft drinks were no more likely to prompt headaches in people than **placebo** pills administered for the sake of comparison.[42] Furthermore, numerous scientific investigations carried out both before and after aspartame first appeared on the market have indicated that the product brings about adverse health effects in only a small group of people with a rare metabolic disorder known as **phenylketonuria,** or PKU.

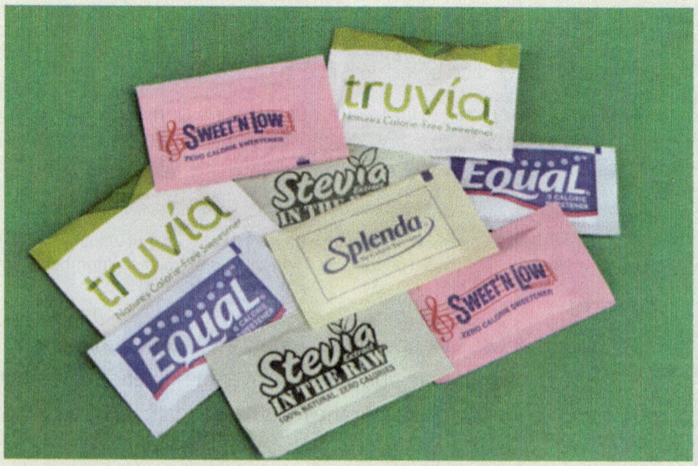

NoDerog/Getty Images

Aspartame, sucralose, stevia, and other sugar substitutes are used to sweeten a wide variety of products.

nonnutritive sweeteners Synthetic or natural ingredients added to foods and beverages to provide sweetness with negligible, if any, calories (sometimes referred to as artificial sweeteners or sugar substitutes), such as aspartame, saccharin, stevia, and sucralose.

placebo (plah-SEE-bo) A sham treatment given to a control group; an inert, harmless "treatment" that the group's members cannot recognize as different from the real thing. Using a placebo minimizes the chance that an effect of the treatment will appear to have occurred due to the healing effect of the *belief* in the treatment (known as the *placebo effect*), rather than the treatment itself.

phenylketonuria (FEN-il-KEY-toe-NYOO-ree-ah) or PKU An inborn error of metabolism, detectable at birth, in which the body lacks the enzyme needed to convert the amino acid phenylalanine to the amino acid tyrosine. If it is not detected and treated, derivatives of phenylalanine accumulate in the blood and tissues, where they can cause severe damage, including mental retardation.

People born with PKU must carefully control their consumption of phenylalanine (one of the two amino acids that make up aspartame) to prevent health problems as severe as mental retardation. The American Medical Association's Council on Scientific Affairs, the Centers for Disease Control and Prevention, the Food and Drug Administration, the Academy of Nutrition and Dietetics, and numerous other health organizations all consider the sweetener safe for use except by people with PKU.[43]

I have heard a lot about Splenda as a sweetener. Why is it so popular?

Splenda (sucralose) is billed as the sweetener that is "made from sugar so it tastes like sugar." Although taste is purely subjective, it is true that Splenda is a derivative of sugar (sucrose). Splenda is the result of a multistep process that selectively substitutes three atoms of chlorine for three hydroxyl groups (OH groups) on the sugar molecule, resulting in a sweetener 600 times sweeter than regular sugar. Splenda provides no calories. Because Splenda is stable, even when used at extremely high or low temperatures, it can be used in a variety of frozen and cooked foods that some of its competitor sweeteners cannot.

Splenda's marketing has gone well beyond simply claiming sugar-like qualities. Its manufacturer has produced "Splenda Granular" that mimics the characteristics and quality of regular sugar; it is intended for use in cooking and specifically baking. Because a molecule of sucralose is 600 times sweeter than a molecule of sucrose, the actual amount of Splenda you would need is much smaller. Therefore, bulking agents are added to allow use of Splenda cup for cup in place of sugar when cooking. A similar product that combines half regular sugar with half "Splenda Granular" is available for baking. Although this product contains calories, the baking results are claimed to be superior, and it also can be measured cup for cup like regular sugar.

Products that use Splenda claim that the taste is superior to other nonnutritive sweeteners, but that is for consumers to decide. The real advantage to using Splenda is its availability in a form that is highly interchangeable with regular sugar.

Can the use of nonnutritive sweeteners bring about weight loss?

If only it were that simple! Obviously, because artificially sweetened foods typically contain fewer calories than their sugar-sweetened counterparts, substituting a low-calorie alternative for a sugar-laden food can allow a person to enjoy sweet-tasting foods and still save calories. But simply *adding* foods sweetened with sugar substitutes to the diet will not do the trick. Moreover, eating artificially sweetened foods to create an excuse to splurge on a different high-calorie food defeats the purpose. A person who drinks diet soda to justify eating an ice cream sundae later is reaping little, if any, benefit. In other words, it's *how* you fit nonnutritive sweeteners into the rest of your diet that really counts. The Academy of Nutrition and Dietetics takes the position that individuals who desire to lose weight may choose to use nonnutritive sweeteners, but they should do so as part of a sensible weight management program that includes a nutritious diet and regular physical activity.[44] (See Chapter 10 for healthy weight-management guidelines.)

On the flip side, some consumers may be under the impression that nonnutritive sweeteners bolster the appetite. A report that aspartame sends mixed signals to the brain and thereby increases appetite as well as food consumption spawned the notion that nonnutritive sweeteners can interfere with weight loss.[45] However, that report was based on comparisons of the effects of drinking plain water and drinking aspartame- and sugar-sweetened water, rather than consuming actual foods or beverages that are typically sweetened with aspartame. Moreover, the researchers did not measure how much food people ate after drinking the liquids. Thus, the study did not show how consuming aspartame-sweetened foods influences appetite and eating behavior in the real world.

Since that time, many more investigations into the relationship between appetite and foods and beverages sweetened with the substance have indicated that aspartame either lessens or doesn't affect feelings of hunger or the amount of food ultimately eaten.[46] So for now, at least, it appears that aspartame's impact on appetite need not concern people who are trying to lose weight.

I have heard that foods sweetened with sugar substitutes do not contribute to tooth decay. Is this true?

Not necessarily. As pointed out earlier, any carbohydrate-containing food, be it sugar sweetened or otherwise, can promote tooth decay. When you eat a sugary food, the millions of bacteria lurking on the surfaces of your teeth and between them feast on the sugar and, in the process, release an acid that eats away at tooth enamel. Once inside the mouth, carbohydrates can be devoured by cavity-causing bacteria because enzymes in the saliva break the complex carbohydrates into simple sugars—on which bacteria thrive.

Should people with diabetes eat foods sweetened only with sugar substitutes?

That depends. It is often assumed that sugar from foods is the major culprit behind the high blood sugar (glucose) characteristic of diabetes and should, therefore, be off-limits for people with this disease. But it's not that simple. The total amount of carbohydrate, including both simple and complex, exerts the most influence on blood glucose levels. What's more, many other factors, including the amount of fat and fiber in a food, affect the body's blood glucose response to it. That's why people with diabetes do not have to limit themselves to only artificially sweetened foods. Sugar-containing items can be incorporated into a carefully designed eating plan.

Another reason blanket statements about the use of sugar substitutes are not made for people with diabetes is that the various types of sweeteners behave differently in the body. A group of sugar substitutes known as **alternative sweeteners** (fructose, sorbitol, mannitol, and

alternative sweeteners Nutritive (calorie-containing) sweeteners such as fructose and the sugar alcohols (e.g., sorbitol, mannitol, and xylitol) that are absorbed more slowly and metabolized differently than other sugars in the body.

TABLE 4-11 **How Sweet It Is: Sweeteners Approved for Use in the United States**

Name (Trade Name) and Chemical Composition	How Many Times Sweeter than Sucrose	ADI (mg/kg body weight) and (Estimated Equivalent)[a]	Approved Uses	Characteristics[b]
Acesulfame-potassium or ace-K (Sunett, Sweet One) Potassium salt	200	ADI: 15 (23 packets of sweetener)	General-purpose sweetener in beverages and foods (except meat and poultry); used as a tabletop sweetener.	Heat stable; noncaloric because it is not metabolized by the body.
Aspartame (NutraSweet, Equal, others) Amino acids (aspartic acid and phenylalanine)	200	ADI: 50 (75 packets of sweetener)	General-purpose sweetener in all foods and beverages; warning to people with PKU: Contains phenylalanine.	Degrades during heating; although it is digested as protein and supplies calories, it is so sweet that only small amounts, which contribute negligible calories, are needed to sweeten foods.
Monk fruit extract (luo han guo) *luo han* = monk, *guo* = fruit (Monk Fruit in the Raw, Nectresse, others) Cucurbitane glycosides from monk fruit extract	150–300	No ADI determined	GRAS[c]; general use as a food ingredient, tabletop sweetener, or component of other sweetener blends.	Heat stable; may have an aftertaste at high levels.
Neotame Derived from aspartic acid and phenylalanine with additional side group attached	10,000	ADI: 0.3 (23 packets of sweetener)	General-purpose sweetener, except in meat and poultry.	Noncaloric, heat stable; because of the intense sweetness of a small amount of neotame, the level of exposure to phenylalanine is considered insignificant, and thus no special labeling is required for people with PKU.
Saccharin (Sweet'N Low)	400	ADI: 15 (45 packets of sweetener)	Tabletop sweeteners; wide range of foods, beverages, cosmetics, and pharmaceutical products.	Noncaloric; heat stable; limited to <12 mg/fluid ounce in beverages, 20 mg/serving in individual packets, or 30 mg/serving in processed foods.
Stevia (SweetLeaf, PureVia, Truvia, Sun Crystals, Stevia in the Raw) Steviol glycosides (stevioside and rebaudioside A)	300	ADI: 4 (9 packets of sweetener)	GRAS[c]; for use as general-purpose sweetener; used in yogurt, ice cream, candies, cereals, energy bars, beverages, and as a tabletop sweetener.	GRAS status given to purified steviol glycoside extracts; noncaloric, heat stable; a small, shrubby perennial with small white flowers; native to Paraguay and Brazil.
Sucralose (Splenda) Derived from a chlorinated form of sugar	600	ADI: 5 (23 packets of sweetener)	General-purpose sweetener for all foods; tabletop sweetener.	Noncaloric, heat stable; although sucralose is made from sugar, the body does not recognize it as sugar, and the sucralose molecule is excreted in the urine essentially unchanged.

[a]The Acceptable Daily Intake (ADI) is the estimated amount of a sweetener that an individual can consume daily over their life span without adverse effects. The Estimated Equivalent is the number of tabletop sweetener packets that a 60 kg (132 pound) person would need to consume to reach the ADI.
[b]In addition to the characteristics listed, all of the nonnutritive sweeteners have a synergistic effect when combined with other sweeteners. In other words, together they enhance each other's sweetness, yielding a combined sweetness greater than the sum of each individual substance's sweetness.
[c]GRAS = Generally Recognized As Safe.

SOURCE: Adapted from: Position of the Academy of Nutrition and Dietetics: Use of nutritive and nonnutritive sweeteners, *Journal of the Academy of Nutrition and Dietetics* 112 (2012): 739–757.

xylitol), for instance, provide calories but were formerly recommended for people with diabetes because the body generally absorbs them more slowly than it does table sugar. Most of these alternative sweeteners, however, have side effects that detract from their desirability. Some research suggests, for example, that large amounts of fructose may contribute to increases in blood cholesterol levels, making fructose a poor choice for the many people whose diabetes goes hand in hand with heart disease. By the same token, some people experience diarrhea after consuming large amounts of sorbitol or mannitol, and, according to the American Diabetes Association, those sweeteners' overall effect on blood glucose control is insignificant. Products with sorbitol and mannitol may carry the following warning on the label because high intakes increase the risk of malabsorption: "Excess consumption may have a laxative effect." Thus, the role sugar substitutes play in the overall diet is a decision that should be made individually with the help of a dietitian and a physician.[47]

Isn't it true that sugar-free chewing gum is calorie free?

No. Some sugar-free chewing gum is sweetened with caloric alternative sweeteners, such as xylitol and sorbitol, also known as sugar alcohols. The sugar alcohols can be derived from fruits or commercially produced from dextrose and are absorbed more slowly and metabolized differently than other sugars in the human body. The sugar alcohols are not readily used by bacteria ordinarily found in the mouth and, therefore, are associated with less cavity formation. Although the sugar alcohols are used as sugar substitutes, they do add calories (about 1.5 to 3 calories per gram) to a food product. The common sugar alcohols found on food labels include erythritol, isomalt, lactitol, maltitol, mannitol, sorbitol, and xylitol. Xylitol may actually inhibit the production of tooth-damaging acid by the caries-producing bacteria in the mouth and prevent them from adhering to the teeth. For this reason, the FDA authorizes use of the health claim on food labels that sugar alcohols do not promote tooth decay. Sugar alcohols are found in a wide variety of chewing gums, candies, and dietetic foods.

Some manufacturers sweeten chewing gum with nonnutritive sweeteners or a combination of sweeteners (for example, both xylitol and aspartame). Chewing gum sweetened with nonnutritive sweeteners provides negligible calories and also does not promote tooth decay.

I've never heard of neotame. What is it?

Neotame is a derivative of two amino acids, aspartic acid and phenylalanine, and is approximately 7,000 to 13,000 times sweeter than table sugar. The FDA approved it for use in the United States in July 2002. And although neotame contains phenylalanine, it is considered safe for use by individuals with PKU. It was approved as a tabletop sweetener and for use in soft drinks, juices, dairy foods, yogurts, jellies, chewing gum, confections, baked goods, sauces, and cereals.[48]

My roommate's parents own a health food store and told me that stevia and monk fruit extract are better to use than artificial sweeteners or sugar because they are more natural products. I've never heard of them. What are they?

Stevia (STEE-vee-uh) is a plant that belongs to the daisy family and is native to Brazil and Paraguay. It has long been used in South America and Asia as a tabletop sweetener and in beverages, candy, gum, baked goods, dairy products, and frozen desserts. The main ingredient in stevia is stevioside, which is 200 to 300 times sweeter than sugar and virtually calorie free. The FDA approved stevia as a tabletop sweetener and food additive in foods and beverages in 2008.[49]

Monk fruit is a small, round, sweet green fruit native to China and Southeast Asia that has been used for centuries in Asian culture and by monks as a sweetener for tea, foods, or in herbal remedies. Monk fruit contains naturally occurring sweet compounds called mogrosides and is 150 to 300 times sweeter than sucrose. The sweetener is digested and absorbed with a yield of 1 calorie/gram. However, it is so sweet that only small amounts, which contribute negligible calories, are needed to sweeten foods. The FDA approved monk fruit extract as a tabletop sweetener and food additive in foods and beverages in 2009.[50]

WHAT'S ONLINE

MINDTAP From Cengage

Visit www.cengagebrain.com to access MindTap, a complete digital course that includes Diet & Wellness Plus, interactive quizzes, videos, and more.

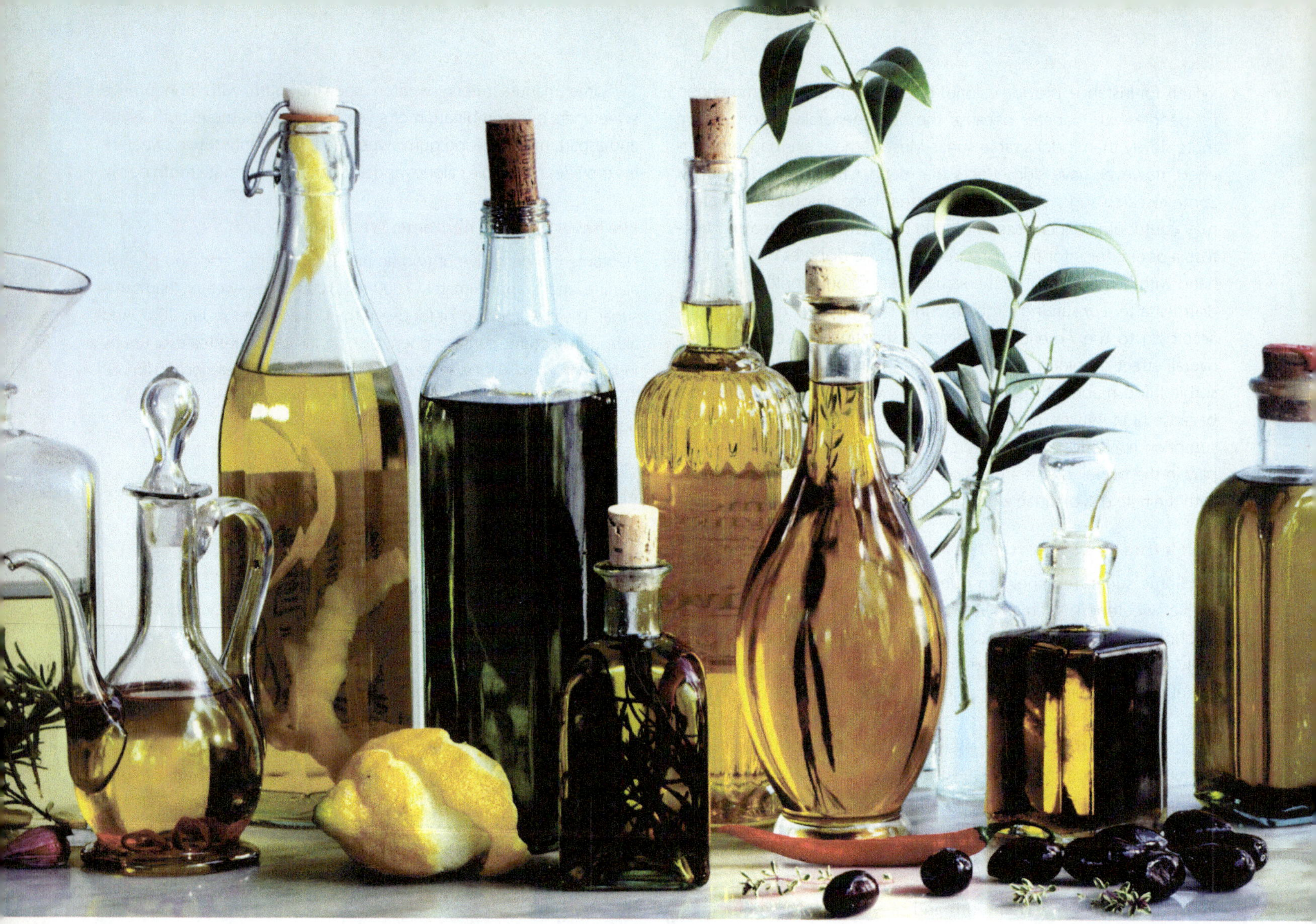

Maximilian Stock Ltd./Getty Images

AskYourself . . .

Which of the following statements about nutrition are true, and which are false? For each false statement, what is true?

1. The body can store fat in virtually unlimited amounts.
2. A person's blood level of cholesterol is a predictor of that person's risk of having a heart attack.
3. For the health of your heart, the fat you should most avoid eating is cholesterol.
4. All the foods you eat should contain less than 10 percent of calories from saturated fat.

Answers found on page 126.

ChapterObjectives

5.1 Describe the functions of fat in the body.
5.2 Describe the differences among saturated fat, polyunsaturated fat, and monounsaturated fat.
5.3 Describe food sources and roles of phospholipids and cholesterol.
5.4 Summarize fat digestion, absorption, and transport in the body.
5.5 Discuss dietary recommendations for fats in the diet.
5.6 List strategies for including heart-healthy fats in the diet.
5.7 Describe components of a heart-healthy lifestyle.

The Lipids: Fats and Oils

CHAPTER 5

While you and your friend are visiting a health fair at a local shopping mall, you learn that your blood cholesterol level is high. Your friend, a registered dietitian, urges you to see your health care provider to request a blood test to determine the level of triglycerides and the ratio of "good" to "bad" cholesterol in your blood. As you leave the mall, you notice a bookstore display with one diet book that urges you to cut your fat intake to virtually nothing to reduce cancer risk and another book touting the benefits of a high-fat diet for weight loss. Then you stop at the window of a health food store. Your friend points to the freshly ground peanut butter, mentioning to you that it is not hydrogenated; meanwhile, you stare at the bottles of antioxidant and fish oil supplements that line the wall. Later, during the evening news, you see a television commercial featuring a margarine that promises to reduce your blood cholesterol level. "What does all of this mean?" you ask.

> The ultimate reality of nutrition rests with the chemistry of the food we eat and its effects on the processes of life.
>
> — R. M. Deutsch (1928–1988, nutrition author and educator)

Actually, you may know more than you think you know about **lipids**, more commonly called **fats** and **oils**. The most obvious dietary sources of fat are oil, butter, margarine, and shortening. Other food sources that supply fat to the diet are meats, nuts, mayonnaise, salad dressings, eggs, bacon, gravy, cheese, ice cream, and whole milk. You may also know that egg yolk and liver are high in cholesterol, and you probably know that the cholesterol in the body is in some way related to heart disease. However, you may be confused by the many terms related to the fat in your diet. This chapter explores the terminology of fat and describes how fats can both contribute to health and detract from it.

lipids A family of compounds that includes triglycerides (fats and oils), phospholipids (lecithin), and sterols (cholesterol).

fats Lipids that are solid at normal room temperature.

oils Lipids that are liquid at normal room temperature.

5.1 A Primer on Fats

Because most people have the impression that fat is bad for them, it may come as a surprise to learn that fats are valuable. More than valuable, some are absolutely essential, and some fats *must* be present in the diet for you to maintain good health. Even if you wanted to, it would be impossible to remove all the fat from your diet, because at least a trace of fat is found in almost all foods.

FIGURE 5-1

A Fat Cell

Within the fat cell, lipid is stored in a droplet. This droplet can enlarge, and the cell membrane will grow to accommodate its swollen contents.

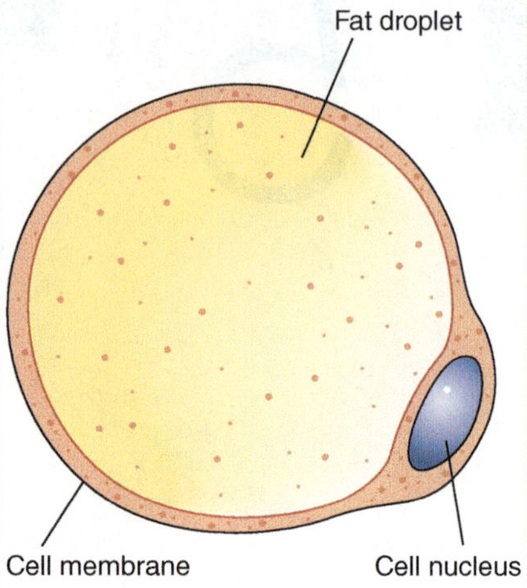

The Functions of Fats in the Body

Fat is the body's chief storage form for the energy (or calories) from food eaten in excess of immediate need. Fats provide the majority of the energy needed to perform much of the body's work during rest as well as during extended bouts of light to moderately intense exercise.

Fat serves as an energy reserve. Whenever you eat, you store some fat, and within a few hours after a meal, you take the fat out of storage and use it for energy until the next meal. Both glucose and fat are stored after meals, and both are released later when needed as energy to fuel the cells' work. However, whereas excess carbohydrate and protein can be converted to fat, the process does not work in reverse. Fat cannot be converted back into protein and carbohydrate. Fat can serve only as an energy fuel for cells equipped to use it.

The body has scanty reserves of carbohydrate and virtually no protein to spare, but it can store fat in practically unlimited amounts (see Figure 5-1). A pound of body fat is worth 3,500 calories, and a person's body can easily carry 30 to 50 pounds of fat without appearing fat at all.

Both fats and oils are found in your body, and both help to keep your body healthy. Table 5-1 summarizes the major functions of fats in the body. Fat is important to all your body's cells as a major component of cell membranes. Natural oils in the skin provide a radiant complexion; in the scalp they help to nourish the hair and make it glossy. Fat insulates the body and cushions the vital organs. It serves as a shock absorber. The fat under the skin also provides insulation from extremes of temperature, thus achieving internal climate control.

TABLE 5-1 The Functions of Fats

Fats in the Body
- Provide a concentrated source of energy to fuel the body's work
- Serve as the body's chief energy reserve
- Form the major components of cell membranes
- Nourish skin and hair
- Insulate the body from extremes of temperature
- Cushion the vital organs to protect them from shock
- Provide raw materials for body compounds such as bile and vitamin D

Fats in Foods
- Provide calories
- Provide satiety
- Carry fat-soluble vitamins and essential fatty acids
- Contribute aroma and flavor

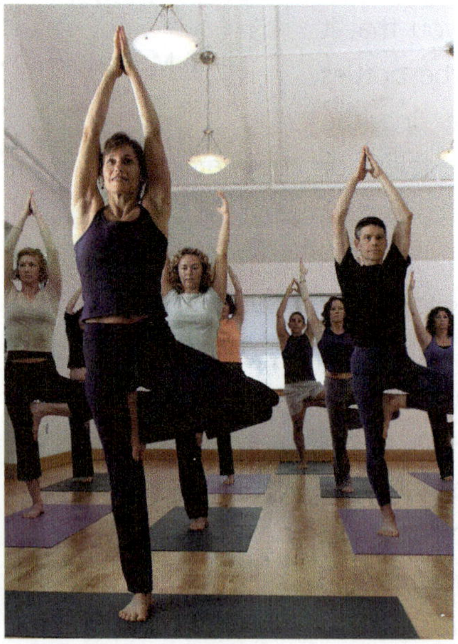

Muscles derive fuel from fat.

The Functions of Fats in Foods

Fat is a nutrient found in many foods. As the most concentrated source of calories, fat contains more than twice as many calories, ounce for ounce, as protein or carbohydrate. High-fat foods may therefore deliver many *unneeded* calories in only a few bites to the person who is not expending much physical energy. Fats in foods also provide **satiety** by slowing the rate at which the stomach empties. This is the reason you feel fuller longer after eating meals that include fat. Table 5-1 summarizes the functions of fats in foods.

satiety The feeling of fullness or satisfaction that people experience after meals.

ASK YOURSELF ANSWERS: **1.** True. **2.** True. **3.** False. For the health of your heart, the fats you should most avoid eating are saturated fat and *trans* fat. **4.** False. Your *total* diet, not individual foods, should contain less than 10 percent of calories from saturated fat.

Fat is important for another reason. Some essential nutrients are soluble in fat and therefore are found mainly in foods that contain it. These nutrients are the essential fatty acids (to be described shortly) and the fat-soluble vitamins—A, D, E, and K (described in Chapter 7). Fat also carries many dissolved compounds that give foods their aroma and flavor. This accounts for the aromatic smells associated with foods that are being fried, such as onions or French fries. It also helps explain why a plain doughnut is more flavorful than a plain roll—it is higher in fat.

FIGURE 5-2

A Triglyceride

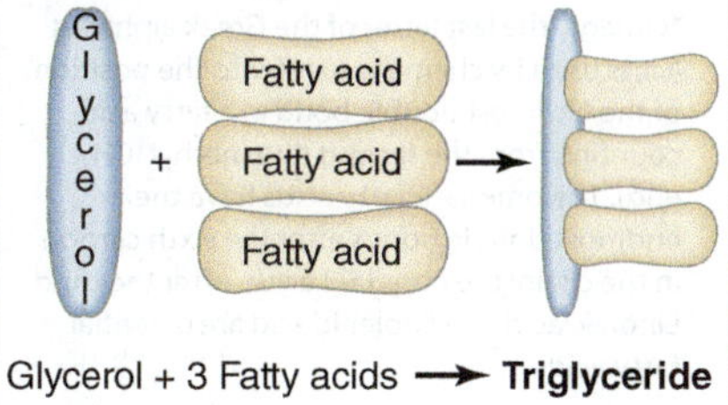

5.2 A Closer View of Fats

When the energy from any of the energy-yielding nutrients is to be stored as fat, it is first broken into fragments: small molecules made of carbon, hydrogen, and oxygen. These fragments are then linked together into chains known as **fatty acids,** the major building blocks of triglycerides, which are the chief form of fat found in the body. **Triglycerides** are composed of three fatty acids that are attached to the compound **glycerol,** which is why glycerol is known as the "backbone" of triglycerides (see Figure 5-2).

About 95 percent of the lipids in foods and in the human body are triglycerides. Other members of the lipid family are the **phospholipids** (of which **lecithin** is one) and the **sterols** (**cholesterol** is the best known of these).

Saturated versus Unsaturated Fats

Fatty acids differ from one another in two ways: in chain length and in degree of saturation. *Chain length* refers to the number of carbon atoms that are hooked together in the fatty acid.* Chain length is significant because it affects the solubility of fat in water; short-chain fatty acids are somewhat soluble in water. Milk, butter, and cheese are rich in short-chain fatty acids; in contrast, vegetable oils and red meat contain triglycerides with long-chain fatty acids, which are insoluble in water.

More significant than chain length, the other way fatty acids differ from one another is in their degree of saturation. *Saturation* refers to the chemical structure—specifically, to the number of hydrogen atoms the fatty acid chain is holding. If every available bond from the carbons is holding (or attached to) a hydrogen atom, we say the chain is a **saturated fatty acid**—filled to capacity, or *saturated,* with hydrogen (see Figure 5-3).

Sometimes, especially in the fatty acids in plants and fish, there is a place in the chain where hydrogens are missing and can easily be added. This is known as an "empty spot," or point of unsaturation (see Figure 5-3). A chain that possesses a point of unsaturation is an **unsaturated fatty acid.** If there is one point of unsaturation, it is a **monounsaturated fatty acid.** If there are two or more points of unsaturation, it is a **polyunsaturated fatty acid.**

The Essential Fatty Acids

The human body can synthesize all the fatty acids it needs from carbohydrate, fat, or protein, except two—**linoleic acid** and **linolenic acid** (see Figure 5-4). These two cannot be made from other substances in the body or from each other, and they must be supplied by the diet; they are, therefore,

*Short-chain fatty acids contain up to 6 carbons, medium-chain fatty acids contain 8 to 12 carbons, and long-chain fatty acids contain more than 12 carbons.

fatty acids Basic units of fat composed of chains of carbon atoms with an acid group at one end and hydrogen atoms attached all along their length.

triglycerides (try-GLISS-er-ides) The major class of dietary lipids, including fats and oils. A triglyceride is made up of three units known as *fatty acids* and one unit called *glycerol.*

glycerol (GLISS-er-all) An organic compound that serves as the backbone for triglycerides.

phospholipid (FOSS-foe-LIP-id) A lipid similar to a triglyceride but containing phosphorus; one of the three main classes of lipids.

lecithin (LESS-ih-thin) A phospholipid, a major constituent of cell membranes; manufactured by the liver and also found in many foods.

sterols (STEER-alls) Lipids with a structure similar to that of cholesterol; one of the three main classes of lipids.

cholesterol (koh-LESS-ter-all) One of the sterols, manufactured in the body for a variety of purposes.

saturated fatty acid A fatty acid carrying the maximum possible number of hydrogen atoms (having no points of unsaturation). Saturated fats are found in animal foods such as meat, poultry, and full-fat dairy products as well as in tropical oils such as palm and coconut.

unsaturated fatty acid A fatty acid with one or more points of unsaturation. Unsaturated fats are found in foods from both plant and animal sources. Unsaturated fatty acids are further divided into monounsaturated fatty acids and polyunsaturated fatty acids.

monounsaturated fatty acid A fatty acid containing one point of unsaturation; found mostly in vegetable oils such as olive, canola, and peanut.

polyunsaturated fatty acid (sometimes abbreviated PUFA) A fatty acid in which two or more points of unsaturation occur; found in nuts and vegetable oils such as safflower, sunflower, and soybean as well as in fatty fish.

linoleic (lin-oh-LAY-ik) acid, linolenic (lin-oh-LEN-ik) acid Polyunsaturated fatty acids, essential for human beings.

FIGURE 5-3

The Types of Fatty Acids

*Omega, the last letter of the Greek alphabet (ω), is used by chemists to refer to the position of the endmost double bond in a fatty acid counting from the far end (the methyl [CH_3] end). The omega-6 fatty acids have their endmost double bonds after the sixth carbon in the chain; the omega-3 acids, after the third. Linoleic acid and linolenic acid are essential fatty acids.

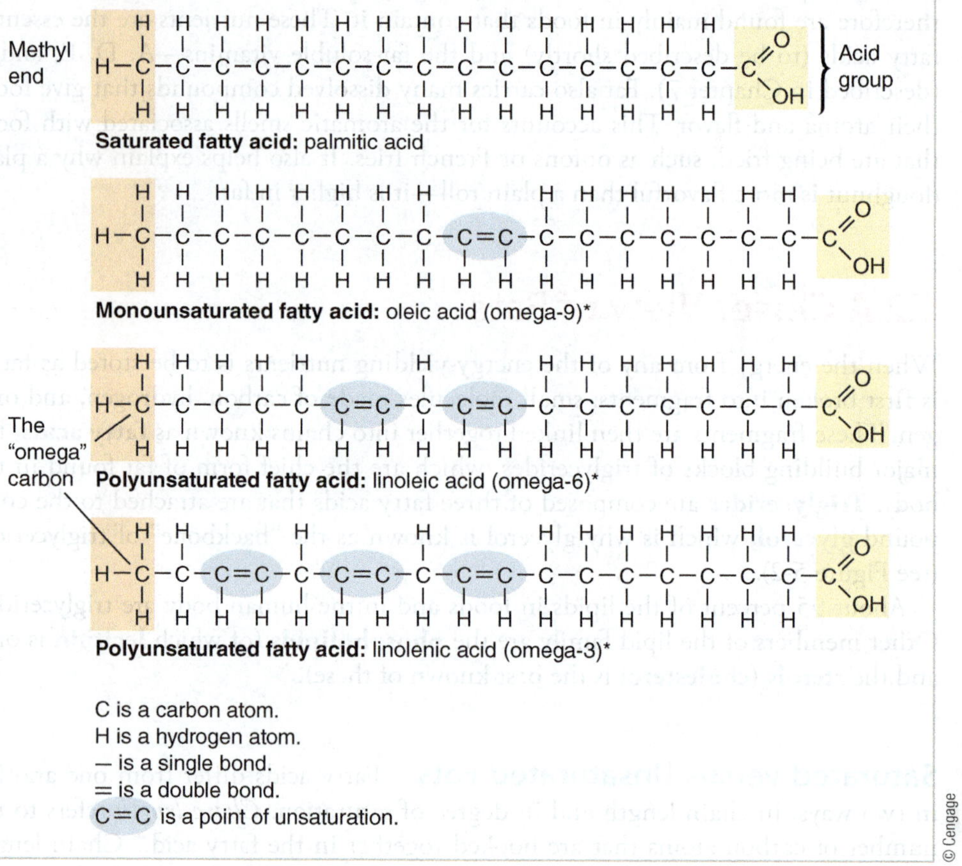

FIGURE 5-4

The Essential Fatty Acids

Linoleic acid and linolenic acid are essential fatty acids and must be supplied by the diet. The fatty acids in fish oils include eicosapentaenoic (EYE-kossa-PENTA-ee-NOH-ic) acid (EPA) and docosahexaenoic (DOE-cosa-HEXA- ee-NOH-ic) acid (DHA), both of which are omega-3 fatty acids with roles in disease prevention and human development.

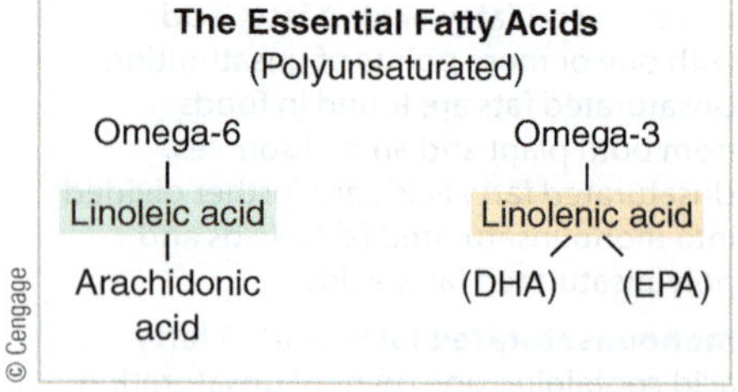

essential fatty acid A fatty acid that cannot be synthesized in the body in amounts sufficient to meet physiological need.

omega-6 fatty acids Polyunsaturated fatty acids that have their endmost double bonds after the sixth carbon in the chain.

omega-3 fatty acids Polyunsaturated fatty acids that have their endmost double bonds after the third carbon in the chain.

essential fatty acids. Linoleic acid and linolenic acid are polyunsaturated fatty acids, widely distributed in the food supply, especially in plant and fish oils. Fortunately, they are readily stored in the adult body, making deficiencies unlikely. Still, deficiency symptoms can appear in people deprived of these acids; these symptoms include a characteristic skin rash and, in children, poor growth.

Omega-6 versus Omega-3 Fatty Acids

One further classification system for unsaturated fatty acids identifies the fatty acids as either **omega-6 fatty acids** or **omega-3 fatty acids** (see Figure 5-3). Of the two essential fatty acids, linoleic acid is an omega-6 fatty acid, related to a whole series of others. Linolenic acid is an omega-3 fatty acid, with a similar family of its own.

Of interest in relation to dietary fat are findings about the omega-3 fatty acids found in fish oils, which offer a protective effect on health. Interest in fish oils was first kindled when someone thought to ask why the Eskimos of Greenland, who eat a diet very high in fat, have such a low rate of heart disease. The trail led to the abundance of fish they eat, then to the oils in those fish, and finally to the omega-3 fatty acids—EPA and DHA—in the oils. Now scientists are unraveling the mystery of what those fatty acids do.[1]

People who eat two to three meals of oily coldwater fish (such as salmon or bluefish) a week tend to have lower blood cholesterol and triglyceride levels, slower clot-forming rates, and less inflammation in body tissues.[2] Numerous studies have documented other connections as well. Diets rich in omega-3 fatty acids seem to bring about enhanced defenses against cancer (via the immune response) and reduced inflammation in arthritis and asthma sufferers.[3] See the

Spotlight feature later in this chapter for more about the benefits of omega-3 fats and fish in the diet.

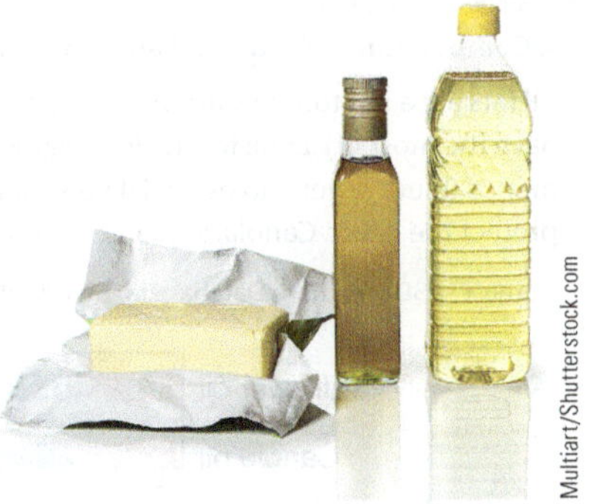

The more unsaturated a fat, the more liquid it is at room temperature. The more polyunsaturated the fat is, the sooner it melts.

Characteristics of Fats in Foods The amount of unsaturated fatty acids in a fat affects the temperature at which the fat melts. The more unsaturated a fat, the more liquid it is at room temperature. In contrast, the more saturated a fat (the more hydrogen it has), the firmer it is. Thus, of three fats—beef fat, chicken fat, and corn oil—beef fat is the most saturated and the hardest; chicken fat is less saturated and somewhat soft; and corn oil, which is the most unsaturated, is a liquid at room temperature. If your health care provider tells you to use monounsaturated fats or polyunsaturated fats, you can usually judge which ones to choose by their hardness at room temperature. Fats and oils contain mixtures of saturated, monounsaturated, and polyunsaturated fatty acids; the fatty acids that predominate determine whether the fat is solid or liquid at room temperature. Most fats with a high percentage of saturated or *trans* fatty acids are solid at room temperature and are referred to as **solid fats**, while those with more unsaturated fatty acids are usually liquid at room temperature and are referred to as oils.[4] Solid fats are found in most animal foods but also can be made from vegetable oils through the process of hydrogenation, as the following describes. Figure 5-5 compares the most common fats and oils with regard to their various types of fat. As shown in Figure 5-5, animal fats tend to have a higher proportion of saturated fatty acids (seafood being the major exception), and plant foods tend to have a higher proportion of monounsaturated and/or polyunsaturated fatty acids (coconut oil, palm kernel oil, and palm oil being the exceptions).

Because fats differ chemically, they behave differently in foods. To control their characteristics, food manufacturers sometimes alter them—and sometimes the alterations have health consequences, as described later in this chapter.

Points of unsaturation in fatty acids are like weak spots, in that they are vulnerable to attack by oxygen. When the unsaturated points react with oxygen, the oils become rancid. This is why unprocessed oils should be stored in tightly covered containers. If they are to be stored for long periods, they must be refrigerated to prevent spoilage.

One way to prevent spoilage of oils containing unsaturated fatty acids is to change them chemically by **hydrogenation,** but this causes them to lose their unsaturated character and the health benefits that go with it. When food producers want to use a polyunsaturated oil such as corn oil to make a spreadable margarine, they hydrogenate the oil. Hydrogen is forced into the oil, some of the unsaturated fatty acids accept the hydrogen, and the oil becomes harder. The spreadable margarine that results is more saturated than the original oil but not as saturated as butter.

A second way to prevent spoilage of oils is to add a chemical that will compete for the oxygen and thus protect the oil. Such an additive is called an **antioxidant**. Examples are the well-known additives BHA and BHT,* which are listed on the labels of many processed foods, such as breakfast cereals and snack foods, and the natural antioxidants vitamin C and vitamin E. A third alternative, as previously mentioned, is to keep the product refrigerated.

Another way in which the food industry alters natural fats and oils is by adding an **emulsifier** to a food product to allow fats and water to mix and remain mixed in that product. Mayonnaise, margarines, salad dressings, and cake mixes often list an emulsifier on their labels. Monoglycerides and diglycerides are good emulsifiers, as is lecithin, which is an emulsifier found in egg yolk.

solid fats Fats that are usually solid at room temperature. Most solid fats contain saturated fats, cholesterol, and/or *trans* fats. Examples include butter, beef fat, chicken fat, pork fat (lard), stick margarine, and shortening.

hydrogenation (high-drah-jen-AY-shun) The process of adding hydrogen to unsaturated fat to make it more solid and more resistant to chemical change.

antioxidant (an-tee-OKS-ih-dant) A compound that protects other compounds from oxygen by itself reacting with oxygen.

emulsifier A substance that mixes with both fat and water and can break fat globules into small droplets, thereby suspending fat in water.

*BHA and BHT are butylated hydroxyanisole and butylated hydroxytoluene.

FIGURE 5-5

A Comparison of Saturated and Unsaturated Fatty Acids in Dietary Fats and Oils

All fats are a mixture of saturated, monounsaturated, and polyunsaturated fatty acids (though we usually call them by the name of the fatty acid they have the most of). Look for the least saturated (red), and a good mixture of everything else (for example, canola oil). Polys (yellow and green) and monos (blue) lower cholesterol if you eat them in place of saturated fats. Alpha-linolenic acid (green) is an omega-3 polyunsaturated fat that may protect the heart. Canola, soy, and flaxseed oil are good sources.

SOURCE: USDA Nutrient Database for Standard Reference (Release 14), the National Sunflower Association, and the Flax Council of Canada.

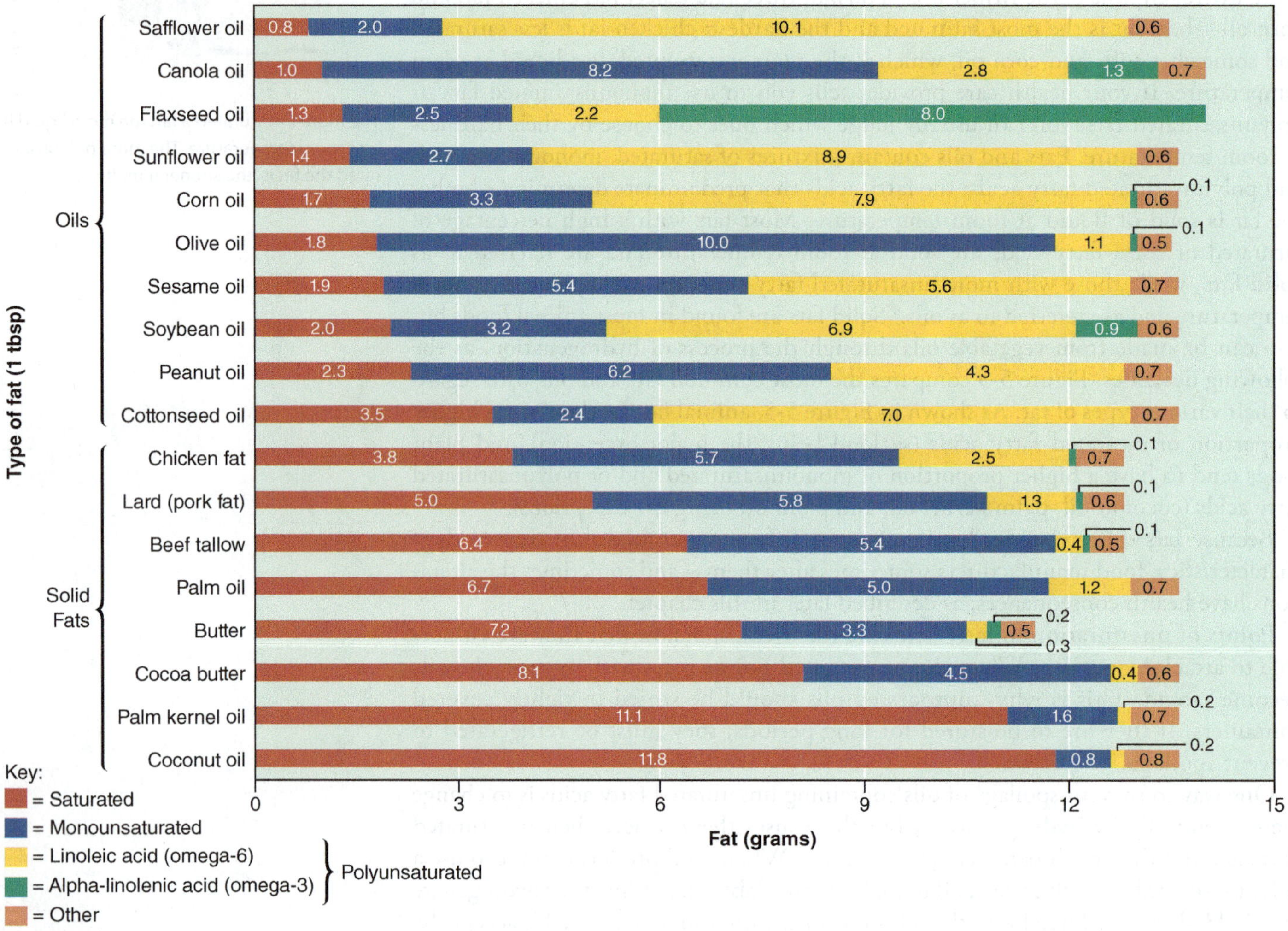

FIGURE 5-6

A Phospholipid: Lecithin

This phospholipid (lecithin) consists of a water-soluble head and a fat-soluble tail. Thus, lecithin can travel back and forth across lipid-containing cell membranes to the watery fluids on both sides. A phospholipid is a phosphorus-containing fat.

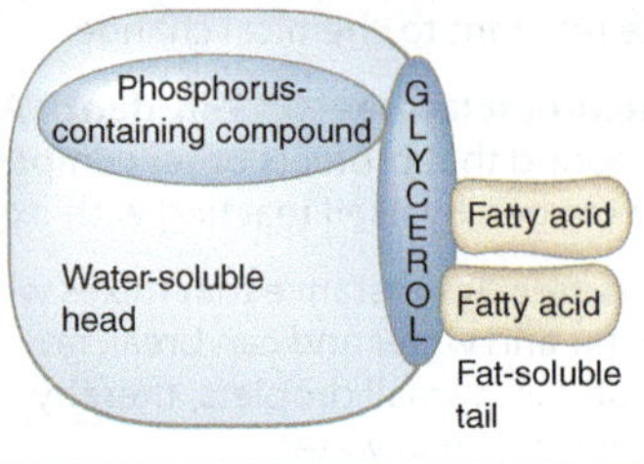

5.3 The Other Members of the Lipid Family: Phospholipids and Sterols

Lecithin and other phospholipids are important components of cell membranes. Because of the way the phospholipids are constructed, with a water-soluble head and a fat-soluble tail, they serve as emulsifiers in the body by joining with both water and fat (see Figure 5-6). Thus, they help fats travel back and forth across the lipid-containing membranes of cells into the watery fluids on both sides. Because it functions as an emulsifier, lecithin is often used as a food additive and thus appears in the ingredients list on food labels. Food manufacturers add lecithin to foods such as mayonnaise, margarine, chocolate, salad dressings, and frozen desserts to keep the fats evenly dispersed with the other ingredients. Lecithin is widespread in food and is also made by the liver in abundant quantities; therefore, most people's diets contain adequate amounts.

Sterols, such as cholesterol, are large molecules with a multiple-ring structure, as shown in Figure 5-7. Cholesterol is found only in animal foods and is also made in the body, where it is an important compound with many functions. It is a part of **bile**, which is necessary in the digestion of fats, and it is the starting material from which the sex hormones and many other hormones are made. In the skin, one of cholesterol's derivatives is made into vitamin D with the help of sunlight. It is also an important lipid in the structure of brain and nerve cells. In fact, cholesterol is a part of every cell. Still, although it is widespread in the body and necessary to the body's function, it also is the major component of the plaque that narrows the arteries in the killer disease atherosclerosis. (See the Spotlight at the end of this chapter for more on heart disease.) Five foods contribute up to 70 percent of the cholesterol in the U.S. diet: eggs (30 percent), beef (16 percent), poultry (12 percent), cheese (6 percent), and milk (5 percent).

FIGURE 5-7

Cholesterol

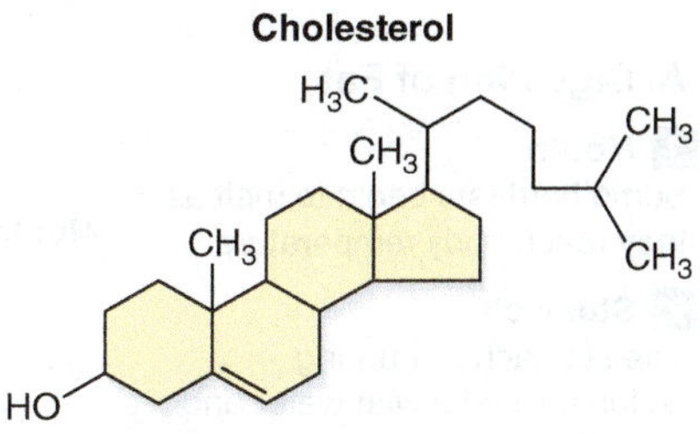

Sterols such as cholesterol have a multiple-ring structure. Cholesterol can be:

- Incorporated as an integral part of the structure of cell membranes
- Used to make bile for digestion
- Used to make sex hormones (estrogen and testosterone)
- Made into vitamin D
- Deposited in the artery walls, leading to plaque buildup and heart disease

5.4 How the Body Handles Fat

A summary of lipid digestion is shown in Figure 5-8. After digestion in the upper small intestine, the products of fat digestion—fatty acids, glycerol, and **monoglycerides**—must enter the bloodstream to be of use to the body's cells. The shortest free fatty acids pass into the cells that line the intestine by simple diffusion. Because these short-chain fatty acids are somewhat water-soluble, they can, without any further processing, enter the body's capillaries. Like the products of carbohydrate digestion, short-chain fatty acids are transported from these capillaries through collecting veins to the capillaries of the liver. The liver cells pick them up and convert them to other substances the body needs. The glycerol follows the same path as the short-chain fatty acids because it, too, is water-soluble.

The larger products of fat digestion (long-chain fatty acids, cholesterol, and phospholipids) are insoluble in water, a difficulty that must be overcome. The body's fluids—**lymph** and blood—are watery and will not accept these larger molecules as they are. The longer-chain fatty acids do pass into the intestinal cells, but there they reconnect with glycerol or with monoglycerides, forming new triglycerides. Then the cells package them for transport before releasing them into the lymph system.

The cells allow triglycerides and other lipids to form and combine with special proteins to make **chylomicrons**, one of the four types of **lipoproteins** found in the blood (see Figure 5-8, Part C). Within the body, the larger fats always travel in the form of lipoproteins. In this ingenious configuration, the water-soluble proteins enable the fats to travel in the watery body fluids. That way, when the tissues of the body need energy from fat, they can extract the energy they need from the lipoproteins in the blood and lymph. The lipoprotein remnants that remain are picked up by the liver, which dismantles them and reuses their parts. The characteristics of the four types of lipoproteins circulating in the blood are shown in Figure 5-9.

Lipoproteins are very much in the news these days. In fact, the health care provider who measures your blood lipid profile is interested not only in the types of fats in your blood (triglycerides and cholesterol) but also in the lipoproteins that carry them. One distinction among types of lipoproteins is very important because it has implications for the health of the heart and blood vessels: That distinction is between low-density lipoproteins (**LDL**) and high-density lipoproteins (**HDL**). The more protein in the lipoprotein molecule, the higher its density.

bile A mixture of compounds, including cholesterol, made by the liver, stored in the gallbladder, and secreted into the small intestine. Bile emulsifies lipids to ready them for enzymatic digestion and helps transport them into the intestinal wall cells.

monoglyceride (mahn-oh-GLISS-er-ide) A glycerol molecule with one fatty acid attached to it. A *diglyceride* is a glycerol molecule with two fatty acids attached to it.

lymph (LIMF) The body fluid that transports the products of fat digestion toward the heart and eventually drains back into the bloodstream; lymph consists of the same components as blood with the exception of red blood cells.

chylomicron (KIGH-low-MY-krahn) A type of lipoprotein that transports newly digested fat (mostly triglyceride) from the intestine through lymph and blood.

lipoproteins (LYE-poh-PRO-teenz) Clusters of lipids associated with protein that serve as transport vehicles for lipids in blood and lymph. The four main types of lipoproteins are chylomicrons, VLDL, LDL, and HDL.

VLDL (very-low-density lipoprotein) Lipoprotein that carries fats packaged or made by the liver to various tissues in the body.

LDL (low-density lipoprotein) Lipoprotein that carries cholesterol (much of it synthesized in the liver) to body cells. A high blood cholesterol level usually reflects high LDL.

HDL (high-density lipoprotein) Lipoprotein that carries cholesterol in the blood back to the liver for recycling or disposal.

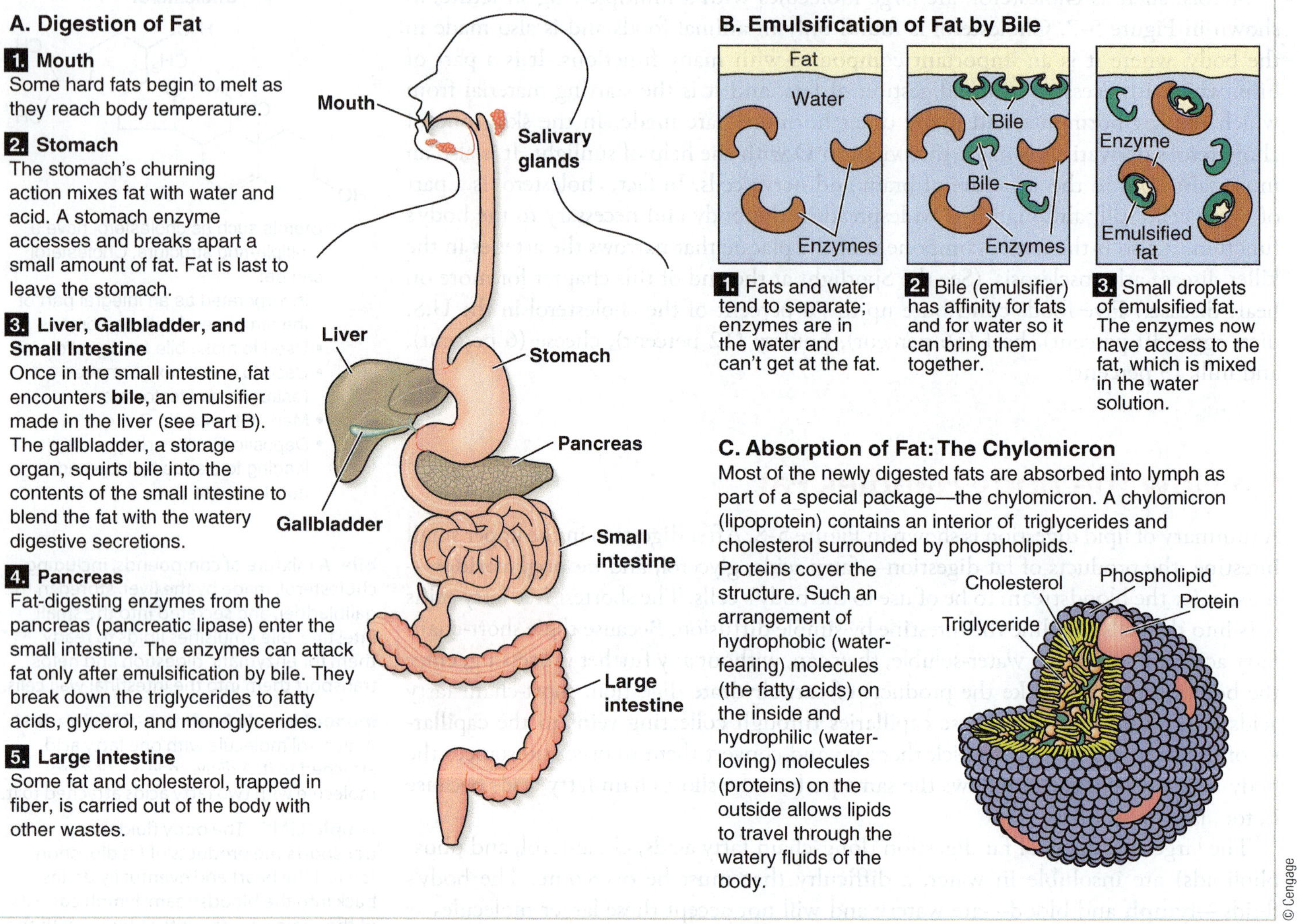

FIGURE 5-8

A Summary of Lipid Digestion and Absorption

Of course, the intestine also processes the few other dietary fats, such as phospholipids and cholesterol, that may have entered the body in food. These fats enter the circulation the same way the triglycerides do, and they also travel packaged in chylomicrons. After transport, they end up in the liver as part of the chylomicron remnants.

"Good" versus "Bad" Cholesterol A silent, symptomless risk factor for heart disease is much talked about but little understood: elevated blood cholesterol levels. Blood cholesterol levels may be high for any of a number of reasons. Some people inherit tendencies to make too much cholesterol or to fail to destroy it on schedule. Others have high blood cholesterol for any or all of the following lifestyle reasons: eating too much saturated fat and ***trans* fat**, exercising too little, or carrying too much weight.[5] The blood lipid profile mentioned earlier can give you an idea of your standing as to this risk factor. (Table 5-9 in the Spotlight at the end of this chapter shows how to interpret your blood lipid profile.)

The underlying cause of most heart disease is atherosclerosis: a narrowing of the arteries caused by a buildup of cholesterol-containing plaque in the arterial walls (this chapter's Spotlight further discusses atherosclerosis and heart disease). The initiating

***trans* fat** A type of fatty acid created when an unsaturated fat is hydrogenated. Found primarily in margarines, shortenings, commercial frying fats, and baked goods, *trans* fatty acids have been implicated by research as culprits in heart disease.

FIGURE 5-9

The Lipoproteins

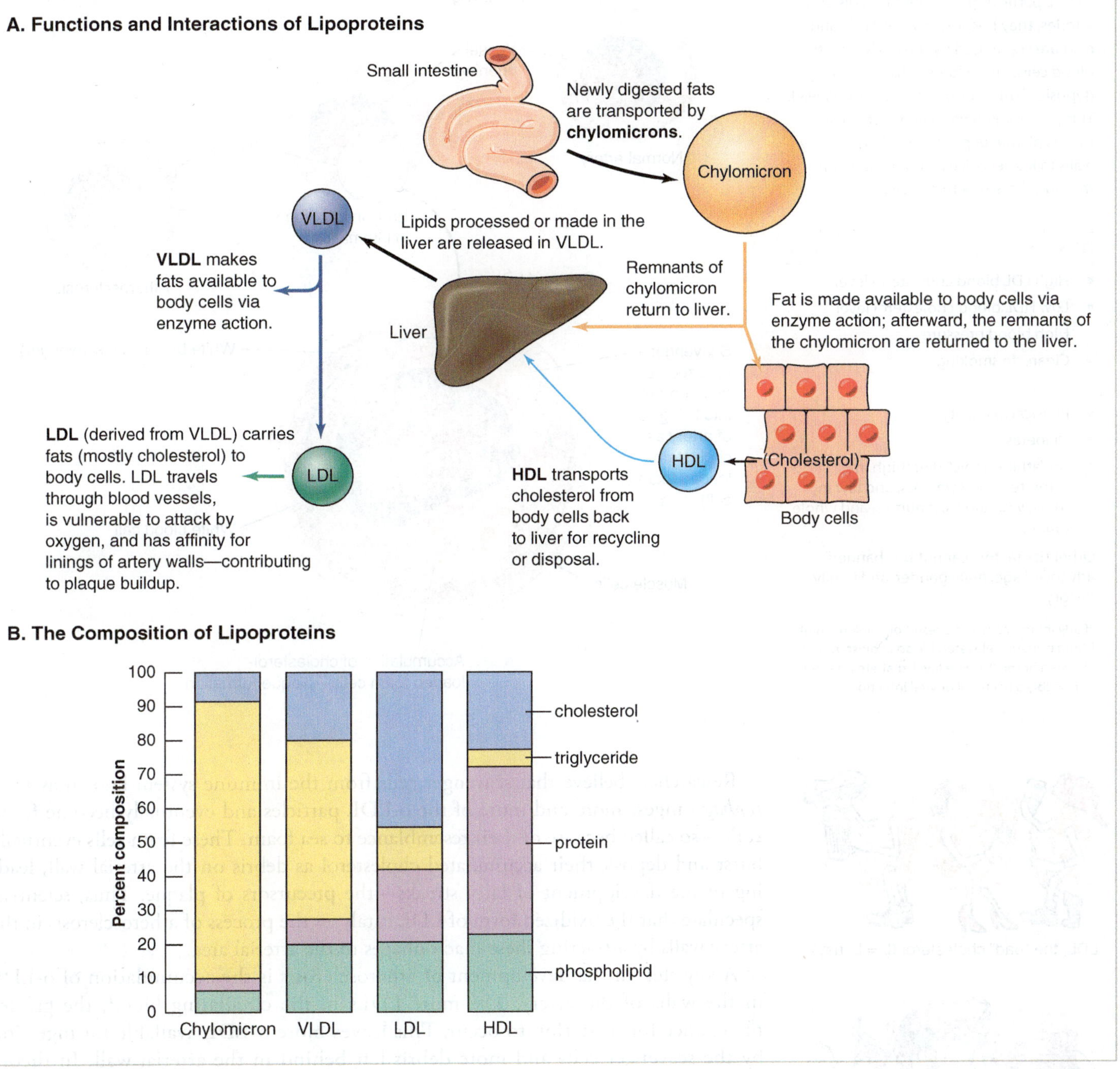

step in the process of atherosclerosis is some form of injury to or inflammation of the artery wall.[6] High blood pressure, high blood cholesterol levels, and cigarette smoke are potential sources of injury, as are the other causes listed in Figure 5-10 (see also Table 5-8 later in this chapter). Raised LDL concentrations in the blood are a sign of high heart attack risk because LDLs in the blood tend to deposit cholesterol in the arteries.

Researchers now theorize that LDL-cholesterol is damaging to the artery walls once it has been oxidized. Circulating LDL-cholesterol is more likely to settle along the linings of the artery walls after it first reacts with an unstable form of oxygen to become **oxidized LDL-cholesterol** (o-LDL; see Figure 5-10).

oxidized LDL-cholesterol (o-LDL) The cholesterol in LDLs that is attacked by reactive oxygen molecules inside the walls of the arteries; o-LDL is taken up by scavenger cells and deposited in plaque.

FIGURE 5-10

Atherosclerosis

As LDL particles penetrate the walls of the arteries, they become oxidized LDL and next are scavenged by the body's white blood cells. These foam cells are then deposited into the lining of the artery wall. This process, known as atherosclerosis, causes plaque deposits to enlarge, artery walls to lose elasticity, and the passage through the artery to narrow.

Leading Risk Factors for Heart Disease

- High LDL blood cholesterol level
- Low HDL blood cholesterol level
- High blood pressure
- Cigarette smoking
- Obesity
- Physical inactivity
- Diabetes
- An "atherogenic" diet (high in saturated and *trans* fats, and low in fruits, vegetables, legumes, and whole grains)

Other risk factors cannot be changed: advanced age, male gender, and family history.

*Early injury may be the result of smoking, high blood pressure, elevated blood cholesterol, elevated homocysteine level, diabetes, genetics, or possibly a bacterial or viral infection.

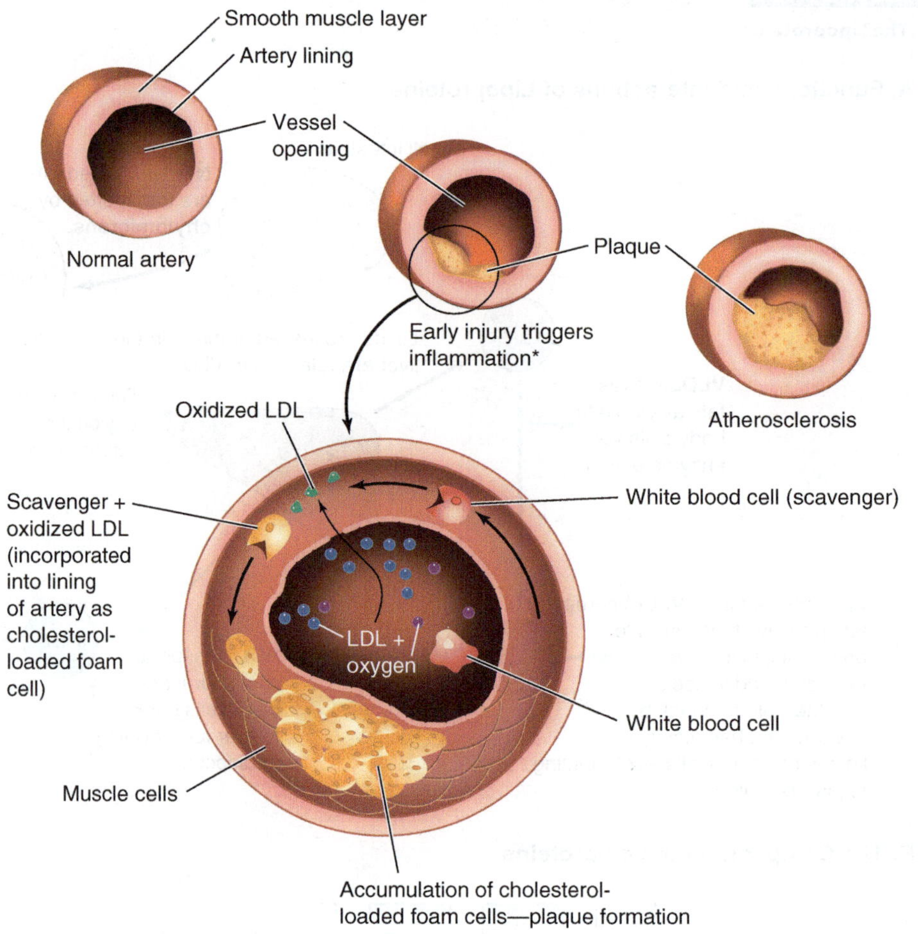

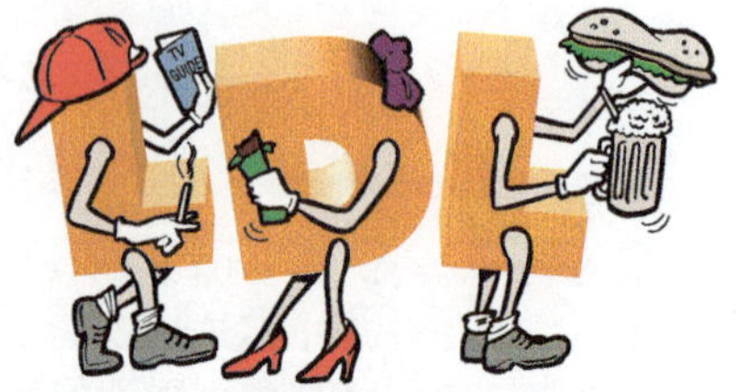

LDL, the "bad" cholesterol (L = Lousy)

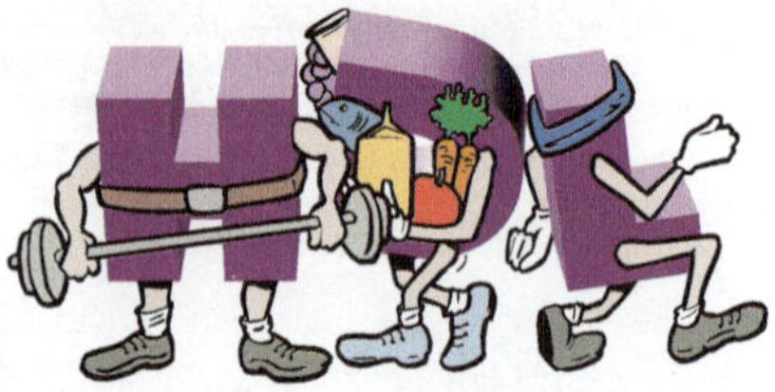

HDL, the "good" cholesterol (H = Healthy)

foam cells Cells from the immune system containing scavenged oxidized LDL-cholesterol; thought to initiate arterial plaque formation.

Researchers believe that scavenger cells from the immune system known as *macrophages* ingest more and more of the o-LDL particles and eventually become **foam cells**—so called because of their resemblance to sea foam. These foam cells eventually burst and deposit their accumulated cholesterol as debris on the arterial wall, leading to the development of fatty streaks—the precursors of plaque. Thus, scientists speculate that the oxidized form of LDL catalyzes the process of atherosclerosis in the artery walls by attracting these macrophages to the arterial area.

A key step in the development of atherosclerosis is the accumulation of o-LDL in the walls of the artery. The more LDLs in the circulating blood, the greater the chance for oxidation to occur. This leaves more o-LDL available for ingestion by the scavenger cells and more debris left behind in the arterial wall. In theory then, steps to reduce the total amount of LDL circulating in the blood (reducing saturated fat and *trans* fat in the diet) or steps to prevent the oxidation of LDL-cholesterol (ample antioxidants in the body) would reduce the formation of foam cells and cause less injury to arterial walls. Thus, the process of atherosclerosis could be slowed or possibly prevented. See Table 5-2 for the effects of various types of fat on blood lipids.

Most blood cholesterol is carried in LDL and correlates *directly* with heart disease risk, but some is carried in HDL and correlates *inversely* with risk. In fact, the most potent single predictor of heart attack risk may be the HDL level. Research indicates that an acceptable total blood cholesterol reading of 200 milligrams per deciliter (mg/dL) or below may not be protective against heart disease if the HDL level is low.

TABLE 5-2 The Effects of Various Kinds of Fat on Blood Lipids

Type of Fat[a]	Dietary Sources	Effects on Blood Lipids
Saturated Fat	All animal meats, beef tallow, butter, cheese, coconut, cocoa butter, coconut oil, cream, cream cheese, hydrogenated oils, lard, palm oil, stick margarine, shortening, sour cream, whole milk, and ice cream	Increases total cholesterol Increases LDL-cholesterol
Polyunsaturated Fat	Almonds, corn oil, cottonseed oil, fish, liquid/soft margarine, mayonnaise, pumpkin seeds, safflower oil, salad dressing, sesame oil, soybean oil, sunflower oil, sunflower seeds, walnuts	If used to *replace* saturated fat in the diet, polyunsaturated fat may: Decrease total cholesterol Decrease LDL-cholesterol Decrease HDL-cholesterol[b]
Monounsaturated Fat	Almonds, avocados, canola oil, cashews, filberts, hazelnuts, macadamia nuts, olive oil, olives, peanut butter, peanut oil, peanuts, pecans, pistachios, sesame seeds	If used to *replace* saturated fat in the diet, monounsaturated fat may: Decrease total cholesterol Decrease LDL-cholesterol without decreasing HDL-cholesterol
Omega-3 Fat	Canola and soybean oils, chia seeds, ground flaxseed, flaxseed oil, oily coldwater fish (salmon, mackerel, tuna, herring), soy foods, walnuts, wheat germ	If used to *replace* saturated fat in the diet, omega-3 fat may: Decrease total cholesterol Decrease LDL-cholesterol Increase HDL-cholesterol Decrease triglycerides
***Trans* Fat**	Margarine (hydrogenated), cake, cookies, doughnuts, crackers, chips, meat and dairy products, hydrogenated peanut butter, nondairy creamer, shortening, many fast foods, foods fried in partially hydrogenated oils or shortening	Increases total cholesterol Increases LDL-cholesterol

[a] All fats, whether classified as mainly saturated fat, monounsaturated fat, or polyunsaturated fat, contain mixtures of saturated and unsaturated fats and provide the same number of calories: 9 calories per gram.
[b] If consumed in large amounts (>10% of total calories).

Raised HDL concentrations relative to LDL represent cholesterol on its way out of the arteries back to the liver—and a reduced risk of heart attack.

Some cases of elevated blood cholesterol do not respond adequately to changes in lifestyle. In such cases, cholesterol-lowering drugs are prescribed. However, for many people, a few simple changes in diet can improve cholesterol readings, as discussed in the Savvy Diner feature later in this chapter.

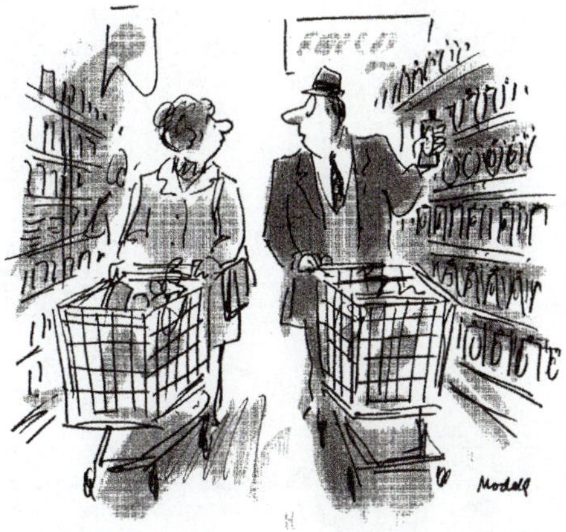

"Excuse me, but which is it that practically kills you—polysaturated or polyunsaturated!?"

5.5 Fat in the Diet

The type of fat consumed may be more important in influencing the risk of heart disease than is the total amount of fat in the diet.[7] Some researchers warn, however, that diets rich in any type of fat can be calorie-dense and could worsen the global problem of obesity. The question of what kind of fat to include in the diet can be puzzling. Research has potentially linked the fat in the diet to several diseases, including certain types of cancer, heart disease, arthritis, and gallbladder disease. The remainder of this chapter helps you apply what you have learned about fats—that is, how to choose foods that supply enough but not too much of the right kinds of fat to support a healthy weight and optimal health and provide pleasure in eating. The current recommendations for dietary fat intake are listed in Table 5-3.

TABLE 5-3 Dietary Recommendations for Fats in the Diet*

From the *Dietary Guidelines for Americans*:

- Keep total fat intake between 20 to 35 percent of calories, with most fats coming from sources of polyunsaturated and monounsaturated fatty acids, such as fish, nuts, and vegetable oils.
- When selecting and preparing meat, poultry, dry beans, and milk or milk products, make choices that are lean, low-fat, or fat-free.
- Consume less than 10 percent of calories as saturated fat, replacing these calories with those from monounsaturated or polyunsaturated fatty acids.
- Individuals should limit intake of *trans* fats to as low as possible by limiting foods that contain synthetic sources of *trans* fats, such as partially hydrogenated oils in margarines, and by limiting other solid fats.
- Reduce intake of solid fats (major sources of saturated and *trans* fatty acids).
- Eat as little dietary cholesterol as possible while consuming a healthy eating pattern, because foods that are higher in dietary cholesterol, such as fatty meats and high-fat dairy products, are also higher in saturated fats.
- Consume two 4-ounce servings of seafood per week as a source of omega-3 fatty acids.

From the American Heart Association:

- Saturated fat: less than 5% to 6% of total calories
- Avoid *trans* fat

From the DRI Committee:

An *Acceptable Macronutrient Distribution Range (AMDR)* for:

- Total fat: 20%–35% of total calorie intake
- Polyunsaturated fats:
  - Omega-6 fats: 5%–10% of total calorie intake
    Adequate intake of linoleic acid (essential omega-6 fatty acid):

Men	Women
17 g/day	12 g/day

  - Omega-3 fats: 0.6%–1.2% of total calorie intake
    Adequate intake of linolenic acid (essential omega-3 fatty acid):

Men	Women
1.6 g/day	1.1 g/day

On Food Labels: Daily Values (DV) for a 2,000-Calorie Diet:

Total Fat	Saturated Fat	Cholesterol
78 g	20 g	300 mg

* Refer to Table 5-2 for dietary sources of various types of fat.

Today, the average American diet includes about 34 percent of its calories from fat, about 11 percent of calories from saturated fat, and about 1 percent of calories from *trans* fat. The Institute of Medicine recommends that *total* fat not exceed 20 to 35 percent of the day's total calories and that it come mostly from polyunsaturated and monounsaturated fat sources such as fish, nuts, and vegetable oils.[8] Saturated fat should be kept low and contribute less than 10 percent of calories. *Trans* fat consumption should be avoided. Table 5-4 shows you how to determine your daily fat allowance.

To reduce the intake of both saturated fat and *trans* fat, the *Dietary Guidelines for Americans* recommends limiting consumption of foods high in solid fat and replacing them with foods that are rich in monounsaturated fat and polyunsaturated fat. For example, when preparing foods at home, solid fats such as butter and lard can be replaced with vegetable oils such as canola or olive oil (see Figure 5-5). Foods high in solid fats include many cheeses, creams, whole milk, ice creams, well-marbled cuts of meats, regular ground beef, bacon, sausages, poultry skin, and many baked goods such as cookies, crackers, doughnuts, pastries, and croissants.

"Fat on the plate" includes visible fats and oils, such as butter, the oil in salad dressing, and the fat you trim from a steak. It also refers to some you cannot see, such as the fat that marbles a steak or that is hidden in such foods as nuts, cheese, biscuits, crackers, doughnuts, cookies, muffins, avocados, olives, fried foods, and chocolate.

TABLE 5-4 **How to Determine Daily Fat Allowances**

We are advised to choose a diet that is low in saturated fat and cholesterol and moderate in total fat. The DRI committee has set an acceptable range of from 20 to 35 percent of total calories from fat. Recommended intake for saturated fat is less than 10 percent of total daily calories. Every single food you eat does not need to conform to these allowances if you balance higher-fat items with lower-fat foods throughout the day.

If you usually eat this many calories:	Your total fat intake should be no more than 20 to 35 percent of calories:		Your saturated fat intake should be no more than:
	20% of Total Calories from Fat[a] (g/day)	35% of Total Calories from Fat[a] (g/day)	10% of Total Calories (g/day)
1,500	33	58	17 or less
1,800	40	70	20 or less
2,000[b,c]	40	78	20 or less
2,400[d]	53	93	27 or less
2,500	55	95	28 or less
3,000[e]	67	117	33 or less

[a] The DRI committee set an Acceptable Macronutrient Distribution Range for fat intake at 20% to 35% of total calories. For more discussion about AMDR, see Chapter 2.
[b] Percent Daily Values on Nutrition Facts labels are based on a 2,000-calorie diet.
[c] Values for 2,000 calories are rounded to the nearest 5 grams to be consistent with the Nutrition Facts label.
[d] Estimated Energy Requirement (EER) for 19-year-old women; subtract 7 calories per day for females for each year of age above 19. EER values are determined at four physical activity levels; the values shown here are for "active" females.
[e] Estimated Energy Requirement (EER) for 19-year-old men; subtract 10 calories per day for males for each year of age above 19. EER values are determined at four physical activity levels; the values shown here are for "active" males.

Calculation Practice

Use Table 5-4 to find the total daily fat allowance, based on your daily calorie intake, that will keep your fat grams within the acceptable range. To find a reasonable calorie intake for yourself, see the DRI table at the back of this book. Or, use the following quick method to determine your calorie allowance: Multiply your body weight in pounds by 15 (if you're active) or 13 (if you're sedentary). If you are active and weigh 150 pounds, you expend about 2,250 calories (150 × 15) in a typical day.

Example: If you eat 1,800 calories per day, multiply 1,800 by 10 percent *to determine the maximum number of calories that should come from saturated fat* in one day (1,800 × 0.1 = 180 calories from saturated fat). Because 1 gram of fat provides 9 calories, divide the calories from saturated fat by 9 to see the maximum amount of saturated fat you can have per day (180 ÷ 9 = 20 grams of saturated fat per day):

Total daily calories × 0.10 = total saturated fat calories
Total saturated fat calories ÷ 9 = total saturated fat grams

Likewise, *to determine an acceptable range (20% to 35% of calories) for total fat intake:*

Total daily calories × 0.20 = total fat calories
Total fat calories ÷ 9 = total fat grams

To determine maximum amount of calories from fat:

Total daily calories × 0.35 = total fat calories
Total fat calories ÷ 9 = total fat grams

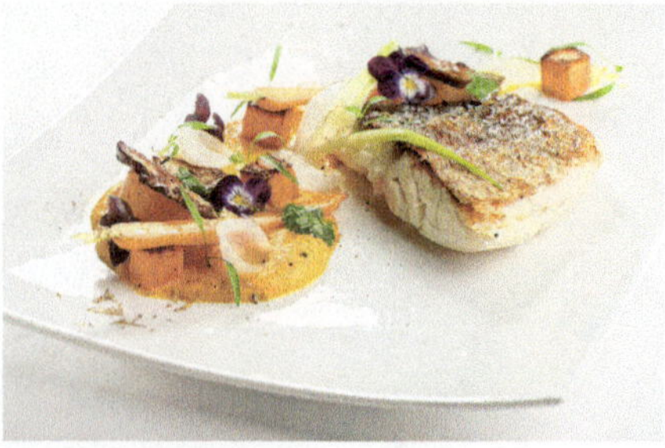

Visionsi/Shutterstock.com

A 3-ounce portion of lean beef, chicken, or fish is roughly the size of a deck of playing cards or the palm of the average woman's hand.

Most of the solid fat, especially saturated fat, in our diet comes from animal products (see Figure 5-11). Meats probably conceal most of the fat that people unwittingly consume. Many people, when choosing a serving of meat, don't realize that they are electing to eat a large amount of fat. When selecting beef or pork, look for the words *loin* or *round* on the label—these words represent lean cuts from which the fat can be trimmed. Table 5-5 shows a few examples of the differences in the saturated fat content of different forms of commonly eaten foods. Note that lower-saturated fat choices can be made within the same food group (for example, low-fat milk versus whole milk). The Scorecard feature later in this chapter will help you rate your own dietary selections for fat.

The *Trans* Fatty Acid Controversy—Is Butter Better?

The heart of the butter versus margarine controversy is a convincing body of research suggesting that a certain type of fat found in margarine may be as likely to boost blood levels of "bad" LDL-cholesterol as the saturated fat found in butter.[9] What's more, the research suggests that in large amounts, *trans* fatty acids lower "good" HDL-cholesterol in the blood.[10]

FIGURE 5-11

Sources of Saturated Fats in the U.S. Diet

The main sources of saturated fats in the U.S. diet include mixed dishes containing cheese, meat, or both, such as burgers, sandwiches, and tacos; pizza; rice, pasta, and grain dishes; and meat, poultry, and seafood dishes. Although some saturated fats are naturally present in foods, others are added during preparation or processing. Healthy eating patterns can accommodate nutrient-dense foods with small amounts of saturated fats, as long as calories from saturated fats do not exceed 10 percent of calories per day, intake of total fat calories remains within the recommended range, and total calorie intake remains within limits for a healthy weight. When possible, foods high in saturated fats should be replaced with foods high in unsaturated fats. See also the discussion of healthy eating patterns in Chapter 2.

SOURCE: U.S. Department of Agriculture and U.S. Department of Health and Human Services, *Dietary Guidelines for Americans, 2015*, 8th ed. (Washington, DC: U.S. Government Printing Office, 2015).

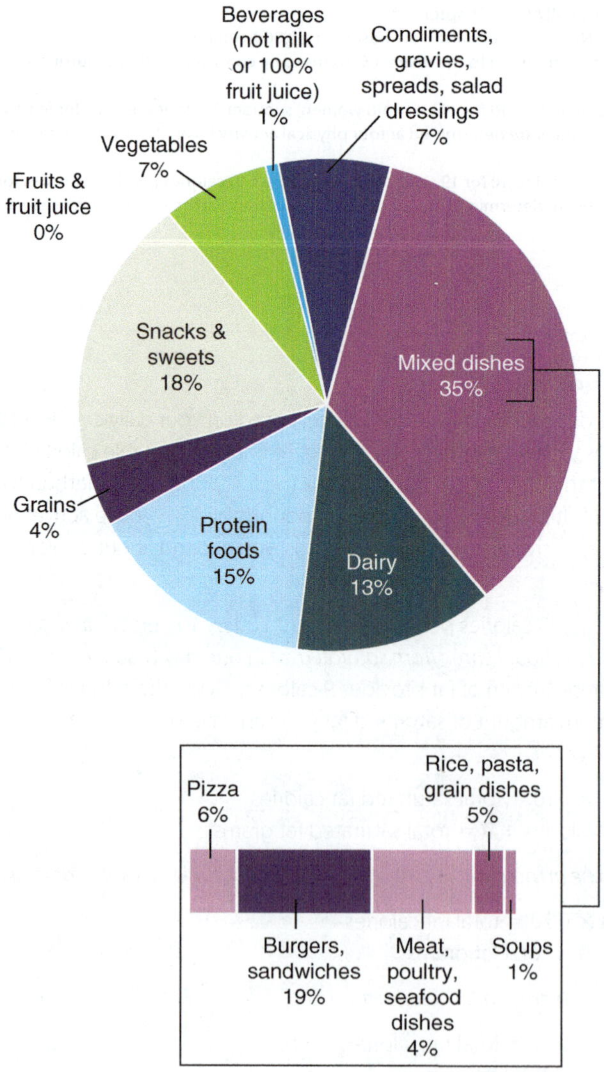

TABLE 5-5 **Compare the Saturated Fat and Calorie Content of Selected Foods**

Food Category	Portion	Saturated Fat (grams)	Calories
Added fat			
Butter	1 tbsp	7	100
Olive oil	1 tbsp	2	119
Cheese			
Regular cheddar cheese	1 oz	6.0	114
Low-fat cheddar cheese	1 oz	1.2	49
Milk			
Whole milk	1 cup	4.6	146
Low-fat (1%) milk	1 cup	1.5	102
Fat-free (skim) milk	1 cup	0	90
Frozen desserts			
Regular ice cream	½ cup	4.9	145
Low-fat frozen yogurt	½ cup	2.0	110
Meat, Poultry, Fish			
Regular ground beef (25% fat)	3 oz (cooked)	6.1	236
Extra lean ground beef (5% fat)	3 oz (cooked)	2.6	148
Spareribs	3 oz (cooked)	9.5	337
Ham, extra lean	3 oz (cooked)	1.5	123
Fried chicken (leg with skin)	3 oz (cooked)	3.3	212
Roasted chicken (breast, no skin)	3 oz (cooked)	0.9	140
Fish fillet, breaded, fried	3 oz (cooked)	2.4	197
Salmon	3 oz (cooked)	1.2	125
Snack Items			
Potato chips	10 chips	3.1	155
Mixed nuts	2 tbsp	1	100

SOURCE: U.S. Department of Agriculture, Agricultural Research Service, Nutrient Data Laboratory, 2016, USDA National Nutrient Database for Standard Reference, Release 28.

The alleged culprit, *trans* fatty acid, is formed when margarine is processed. To make margarine, manufacturers take a highly unsaturated vegetable oil and partially hydrogenate (add hydrogen to) it. Hydrogenation gives the spread its relatively solid consistency and helps protect against rancidity. During the hydrogenation process, however, a chemical "fluke" occurs. Hydrogenating the oil creates a new chemical configuration, known as a *trans* fatty acid, in which hydrogen atoms of the fat lie on opposite sides of the point of unsaturation in the carbon chain instead of side by side (see Figure 5-12). (Recall that the body of a fatty acid molecule consists of a chain of carbon atoms to which hydrogen is attached, as shown in Figure 5-3.)

Because *trans* fatty acids are formed whenever oils are hydrogenated, margarine is only one of the foods on the market that contain *trans* fatty acids. Shortenings and products made with partially hydrogenated fat such as many commercially prepared baked and fried foods are among the foods containing *trans* fatty acids. Fueling the controversy even further, an analysis by researchers at Harvard University suggested that more than 30,000 American deaths each year are attributable to *trans* fatty acids.[11]

In January 2006, the Food and Drug Administration (FDA) began requiring that manufacturers list the *trans* fat content on a separate line within the Nutrition Facts

FIGURE 5-12

Types of Unsaturated Fatty Acids: Cis versus Trans

Unsaturated fatty acids are either in *cis* form or in *trans* form, depending on the way in which the hydrogen atoms are attached to the points of unsaturation in the carbon chain. If the hydrogen atoms are attached to the same side of the points of unsaturation, the arrangement is called *cis*. If the hydrogen atoms are attached to different sides, the arrangement is called *trans*.

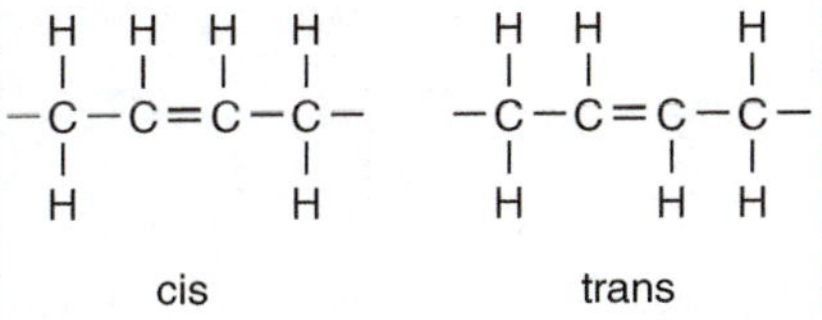

cis = same
trans = across

panel on all food products. Manufacturers can label a product "*trans* fat free" if the food contains less than 0.5 gram of *trans* fat and less than 0.5 gram of saturated fat per serving.[12]

In June 2015, in response to increasing pressure to eliminate the use of artificial *trans* fat, the U.S. FDA moved forward on banning the use of *trans* fats in foods. The FDA published a final determination in the *Federal Register* stating: "Partially hydrogenated oils, which are the primary dietary source of industrially produced *trans* fatty acids, are not *generally recognized as safe* (GRAS)* for any use in food based on current scientific evidence establishing the health risks associated with the consumption of *trans*-fat, and therefore . . . partially hydrogenated oils are food additives."[13] As a result, food manufacturers will no longer be permitted to use partially hydrogenated oils in food products without prior FDA approval.

Understanding Fat Replacers Fat-free ice cream, cookies, cakes, and salad dressings have long been the stuff that dieters' dreams are made of. The food industry makes such fatless fare a reality. With innovations in food chemistry, the food industry can now concoct new recipes or ingredients that yield low-fat or nonfat products that retain the characteristic flavor and mouth feel of fat. The types of fat-reduction ingredients currently in use are listed in Table 5-6.

Some manufacturers of fat-free cakes and cookies, for example, make those products by substituting egg whites for whole eggs and fat-free milk for whole milk, as well as by removing the butter from their recipes. The end products are sweets that contain fewer calories and fewer grams of fat per serving than traditional desserts.[14]

Another technique manufacturers use to replace fat is to add starches, gums, and gels to their products. For example, cellulose gel, a complex carbohydrate, is used as a filler to make fat-free salad dressings.[15] Food companies add starches and gums—also complex carbohydrates—to items such as sauces and yogurts to skim fat from those foods. That's because starches and gums hold water and impart a smooth, creamy texture similar to that of fat, and they add form and structure to foods.

TABLE 5-6 Types and Uses of Fat Replacers

Types and Uses of Fat Replacers
Carbohydrate based: Carrageenan (a seaweed derivative), fruit purees, gels derived from cellulose or starch, guar gum, xanthan gum, maltodextrins made from corn, polydextrose
Uses: Dairy products, frozen desserts, salad dressings, baked goods, cake and cookie mixes, frostings
Protein based: Whey protein concentrate, microparticulated protein products made from whey, or milk and egg-white protein
Uses: Cheese, butter, salad dressings, mayonnaise, sour cream, dairy products, ice cream, baked goods
Fat based: Mono- and diglycerides; Salatrim (found in reduced-fat baking chips) contains long-chain fatty acids, which are partially absorbed, and short-chain fatty acids (providing 5 calories per gram); olestra (noncaloric artificial fat made from fatty acids and sucrose)
Uses: Savory snacks, chocolate confections, bakery products

*A substance is GRAS if it is generally recognized "among qualified experts as having been adequately shown through scientific procedures to be safe under the conditions of its intended use." GRAS items are not food additives and can be lawfully used without FDA review and approval.

Yet another approach is the development of fat replacers made of mixtures of food proteins such as egg white, whey, and milk protein that are cooked and blended to form tiny round particles that trap water. Inside the mouth, the particles roll over one another, and the tongue perceives them as a creamy, smooth liquid similar to fat. Foods made with fat replacers contain considerably less fat and fewer calories than their traditional fat-containing counterparts.[16]

An artificial fat approved for use in salty snacks and crackers is **olestra** (sold under the brand name Olean). The olestra molecule resembles a triglyceride but is structured in a way that prevents it from being broken down by digestive enzymes in the body, thereby allowing it to pass through the digestive tract completely unabsorbed (see Figure 5-13). Olestra interferes with the absorption of the fat-soluble vitamins (A, D, E, and K), as well as beta-carotene. To compensate for this effect, olestra must be fortified with the fat-soluble vitamins. Consumption of large amounts of olestra can cause nutrient losses, abdominal cramping, and loose stools.[17]

Certainly, the variety of fat-free foods and fat replacers provides consumers with viable alternatives to fattier fare. Nevertheless, many experts view the fat-free boom with skepticism. Although reduced-fat foods can help lower the overall fat content of the diet, they *do* provide calories, and they are *not* a replacement for a healthy diet rich in whole grains, fresh fruits, and vegetables. When included in a heart-healthy diet, however, they can help consumers reach and adhere to the goal of taking in no more than 20 to 35 percent of total calories as fat.[18]

FIGURE 5-13

Olestra: A Fat-Free Fat

Compare the structure of olestra to that of a triglyceride. Whereas triglycerides have 3 fatty acids attached to a glycerol core, olestra has from 6 to 8 fatty acids on a sucrose core. The extra fatty acids make it too large to be digested or absorbed by the body, which is why it adds no fat or calories to the diet. Thus a 1-ounce bag of potato chips, which typically has 10 grams of fat and 150 calories, has 0 grams of fat and 60 calories when Olean is added in place of fat.

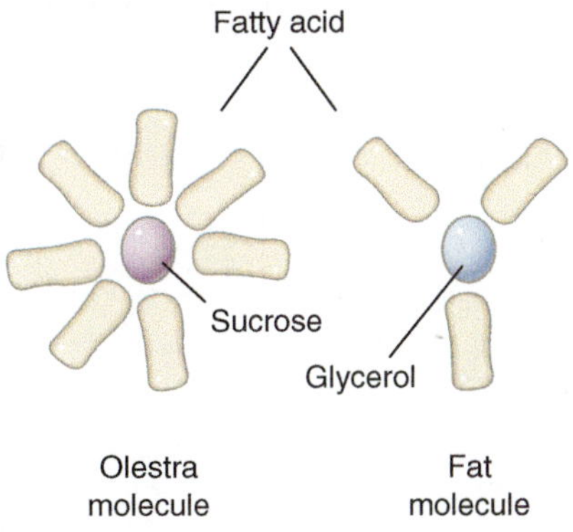

5.6 Fat Can Be Healthy

Think that all fat is evil? Think again. Researchers are finding that people living in Greece, France, Italy, and other countries around the Mediterranean Sea have only a fraction of the heart disease and related deaths experienced by people living in Western, industrial countries like the United States.

What causes this difference? Genetic differences aside, other factors suggest that nutritional differences may play a role because dietary patterns in countries around the Mediterranean Sea vary significantly from those in industrialized countries like the United States, Canada, and northern European countries. What do people who live around the Mediterranean Sea eat that protects them from coronary heart disease? The traditional "Mediterranean diet" is rich in fruits, vegetables, grains, fish, and beans, whereas most American diets include much more meat and other animal products known to be high in saturated fat. Thus, the Mediterranean diet is high in the vitamins, minerals, fiber, and **phytochemicals** that keep bodies healthy, and low in saturated fat, because Mediterranean people consume so little meat and butter (see Figure 5-14). Most Americans don't eat enough whole-grain products, fruits, and vegetables to get the necessary vitamins, minerals, fiber, and phytochemicals that will protect their bodies from coronary heart disease and other chronic diseases.

Study the pyramid in Figure 5-14, and you will see that the Mediterranean diet is not fat free. About 30 to 35 percent of total calories are provided by fat. The key is the *type* of fat eaten. Only about 7 to 8 percent of total calories come from saturated fat, whereas average Americans consume about 11 percent of their calories from saturated fat. As you already know, saturated fat and *trans* fat are the major dietary risk factors for heart disease.[19] What do these Mediterranean people use instead of animal fat (butter, meats, ice cream)? They use olive oil and other fats from plant sources that are higher in monounsaturated and polyunsaturated fats.[20]

olestra An artificial fat derived from sucrose and fatty acids combined in such a way that the body cannot break them down. Sold under the brand name Olean, olestra does not contribute calories to food.

phytochemicals (FIGHT-oh-KEM-ih-kulz) Physiologically active compounds found in plants that appear to help promote health and reduce risk for cancer, heart disease, and other conditions. Also called *phytonutrients* (*phyto* = plant).

FIGURE 5-14

The Mediterranean Food Pyramid

SOURCE: Adapted with permission. Copyright © 2010 Oldways Preservation & Exchange Trust, http://oldwayspt.org.

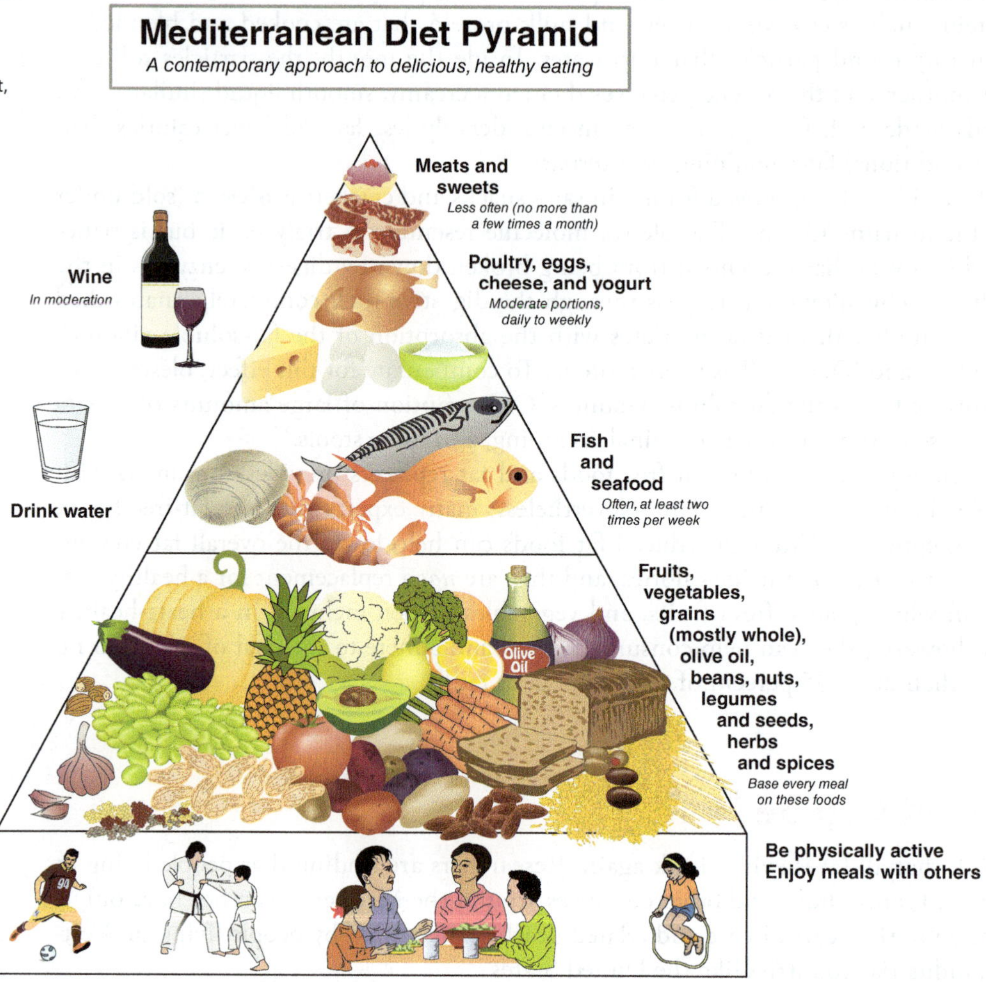

Olive oil is high in oleic acid, a monounsaturated fatty acid that seems to keep the heart healthy. Oleic acid helps keep "good" HDL-cholesterol (the artery cleaner) high while lowering levels of "bad" LDL-cholesterol (the artery clogger). It also contains a good ratio of omega-3 fatty acids to omega-6 fatty acids. This is a good thing. Keep in mind, though, that olive oil is still a fat. It provides as many calories as any other pure fat. Therefore, olive oil can promote overweight and obesity if too much is consumed. Other vegetable oils high in monounsaturated fats are peanut and canola oils.

Other Sources of Omega-3 Fatty Acids Another place to find omega-3 fats is fish, especially oily coldwater fish like salmon, cod, farmed catfish, lake trout, herring, bluefish, sardines, albacore tuna, mackerel, and shellfish (see Table 5-7). Eating these fish at least two times a week as part of a balanced diet can help reduce blood clot formation (which can lead to heart attack and stroke), decrease risk of arrhythmias (which can lead to sudden cardiac death), decrease triglyceride levels, decrease growth rate of atherosclerotic plaque, improve the health of the arteries, and slightly lower blood pressure (another risk factor for heart disease).[21]

TABLE 5-7 Sources of Omega-3 Fats for the Diet[a]

Common Seafood Varieties[a,b]	EPA + DHA[c] mg/4 oz
Salmon: Atlantic, Chinook, Coho	1,200–2,400
Anchovies, herring	2,300–2,400
Mackerel: Atlantic and Pacific (not king)	1,350–2,100
Tuna: bluefin and albacore	1,700
Sardines: Atlantic and Pacific	1,100–1,600
Oysters[d]: Pacific	1,550
Trout: freshwater	1,000–1,100
Tuna: white (albacore) canned	1,000
Mussels[d]: blue	900
Salmon: pink and sockeye	700–900
Squid	750
Pollock: Atlantic and walleye	600
Crab[d]: blue, king, snow	200–550
Tuna: skipjack and yellowfin	150–350
Flounder and sole	350
Clams[d]	200–300
Tuna: light canned	150–300

Common Seafood Varieties	EPA + DHA mg/4 oz
Catfish	100–250
Cod: Atlantic and Pacific	200
Scallops[d]: bay and sea	200
Haddock and hake	200
Lobster[d]: Northern	200
Crayfish[d]	200
Tilapia	150
Shrimp[d]	100

Other Sources of Omega-3 Fats	Omega-3 Content (linolenic acid)[e] grams/tbsp
Flaxseed oil	8.0
Walnuts, ¼ c	2.7
Flaxseeds, ground	1.9
Walnut oil	1.4
Canola oil	1.3
Canola oil mayonnaise	1.0
Soybeans, cooked, ½ c	1.0
Soybean oil	0.9
Tofu, ½ c	0.7
Olive oil	0.1

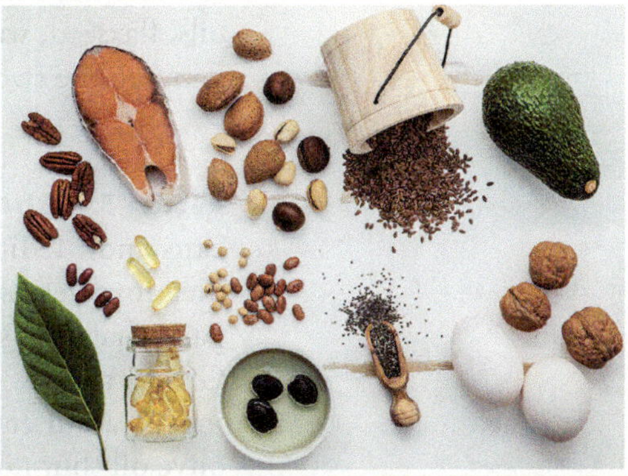

Omega-3 fats occur naturally in some foods and are added to certain fortified foods. Choose a variety of sources, including:

- Fish and other seafood (especially cold-water fatty fish, such as salmon, herring, mackerel, tuna, and sardines)
- Nuts (pecans, hazelnuts, and especially walnuts) and seeds (ground flaxseeds, chia seeds, pumpkin seeds)
- Oils (such as flaxseed oil, soybean oil, and canola oil)
- Fortified foods (such as certain brands of eggs (up to 200 milligrams per egg), yogurt, juices, milk, and soy products (beans, milk, tofu)
- Green leafy vegetables

Omega-3 supplements include cod liver oil, fish oil, krill oil, and algal oil (a vegetarian source from marine algae), but the *Dietary Guidelines* advises using food sources over supplements, unless under medical supervision.

[a] EPA and DHA values are for cooked, edible portion rounded to the nearest 50 mg. Ranges are provided when values are comparable. Values are estimates.
[b] Methylmercury is a heavy metal toxin found in varying levels in nearly all fish and shellfish. However, some fish and shellfish contain higher levels of mercury that may harm the developing nervous system of an unborn baby or young child. The Food and Drug Administration (FDA) and the Environmental Protection Agency (EPA) advise women who may become pregnant, pregnant women, lactating women, and young children to avoid some types of fish, including shark, swordfish, king mackerel, marlin, orange roughy, or tilefish, because they contain high levels of mercury. Women who are pregnant or breastfeeding should also limit white (albacore) tuna to 4 ounces per week. Instead, choose up to 12 ounces a week of a variety of fish and shellfish that are lower in mercury, such as shrimp, canned light tuna, salmon, flounder, pollock, or catfish. For updates on the mercury status of fish and shellfish, go to the Center for Food Safety at www.fda.gov/Food.
[c] A total of 1,750 mg of EPA and DHA per week (an average of 250 mg per day) is the goal amount for consumers to achieve at the recommended two 4-ounce seafood meals per week.
[d] Cooked by moist heat.
[e] Dietary Reference Intake (DRI) for omega-3 fats (linolenic acid): Men: 1.6 g/day; Women: 1.1 g/day

SOURCE: USDA, Nutrient Data Laboratory, USDA National Nutrient Database for Standard Reference, Release 28; P. M. Kris-Etherton, W. S. Harris, & L. J. Appel, Fish consumption, fish oil, omega-3 fatty acids, and cardiovascular disease, *Circulation* 106 (2002): 2747–57; and Institute of Medicine, *Seafood Choices* (Washington, DC: National Academies Press, 2006).

The FDA approved a claim for a reduced risk of heart disease for foods, such as fish, that contain the EPA and DHA omega-3 fatty acids: "Supportive, but not conclusive research shows that consumption of EPA and DHA omega-3 fatty acids may reduce the risk of coronary heart disease."[22]

Other places to find omega-3 fatty acids are ground flaxseed, flaxseed oil, chia seeds, canola oil, soy products, pecans, and walnuts. The type of omega-3 fatty acid in these plant foods is less potent than that found in fish oils, but they are good sources nonetheless.[23] Research has demonstrated that people who eat nuts tend to eat more dietary fat, but the fat is primarily monounsaturated. Also, nuts contain insoluble fiber, another dietary component that protects us from coronary heart disease.[24]

Current Western intakes of omega-3 fats are well below the levels that experts consider optimal.[25] Health experts now advise us to decrease consumption of foods rich in omega-6 fatty acids, such as vegetable oils (corn, safflower, sesame, sunflower), and increase the intake of omega-3 fatty acids (those found in fish, canola and soybean oils, flaxseed, walnuts, other nuts, and soy foods) to achieve a more healthful balance between the two types of fats.

What's Your Meal Mentality? Another difference between how Americans and Mediterranean people eat is the way meals are eaten. The Mediterranean diet involves a wide variety of foods served in several small courses at a slower pace that tends to prevent overeating. Note that one of the dietary guidelines in Greece advises everyone to "eat slowly, preferably at regular times of the day, and in a pleasant environment." Overall, the traditional Mediterranean diet emphasizes olive oil (but no other vegetable oils, hydrogenated oils, or tropical oils); less animal protein (particularly red meats); poultry, eggs, and sweets only a few times a week; and daily use of cheese, yogurt, fruits, vegetables, and whole-grain products. Still, other factors undoubtedly contribute to the lower incidence of heart disease in the Mediterranean region.

In understanding the paradox of how a moderate-fat diet (about 30 to 35 percent of calories from mostly monounsaturated fats) can coexist with a low incidence of heart disease, it is important to note that people from the Mediterranean region in general are more physically active, have the social and emotional support found in extended networks of family and friends, and consume more of each day's calories earlier in the day than people in the United States and Canada. Any one of these factors may also be significant in maintaining lower incidence of heart disease in the region. In addition to these possible lifestyle changes, a healthful change in eating patterns (with a Mediterranean twist) for most people in the United States and Canada would be to adopt a diet that is lower in saturated and *trans* fat and higher in complex carbohydrates and fiber (fruits, vegetables, whole grains, and legumes).

THE SAVVY Diner

Nourish the Heart (Obj. 5.6)

Heart disease rarely develops from a single risk factor. Clusters of risk factors usually occur, and a small increase in one risk factor, such as blood pressure, becomes more critical when combined with other risk factors, such as obesity. Luckily, a similar pattern happens in reverse: Even moderate changes in one risk factor can decrease several others at the same time. For example, a weight loss of just 5 to 10 pounds can reduce blood pressure in overweight people. Likewise, becoming physically active can lower blood pressure, increase HDL ("good" cholesterol), and help control weight.

In the past few years, attention has focused on reducing heart disease risk by both *reducing* contributory factors in the diet—notably, saturated fat and *trans* fat—and by *increasing* the intake of protective factors, such as fiber and the antioxidant vitamins. How does this translate into a heart-healthy lifestyle? What foods should you eat, for example, to achieve the goal of reducing your saturated fat intake to less than 10 percent of total calories, while also increasing your intake of the protective fibers and antioxidant nutrients? This feature offers some general tips that will help you make the heart-healthy food choices needed to achieve these goals. See this chapter's Spotlight for more tips on how to raise your HDL ("good" cholesterol) level and lower your LDL ("bad" cholesterol) level.

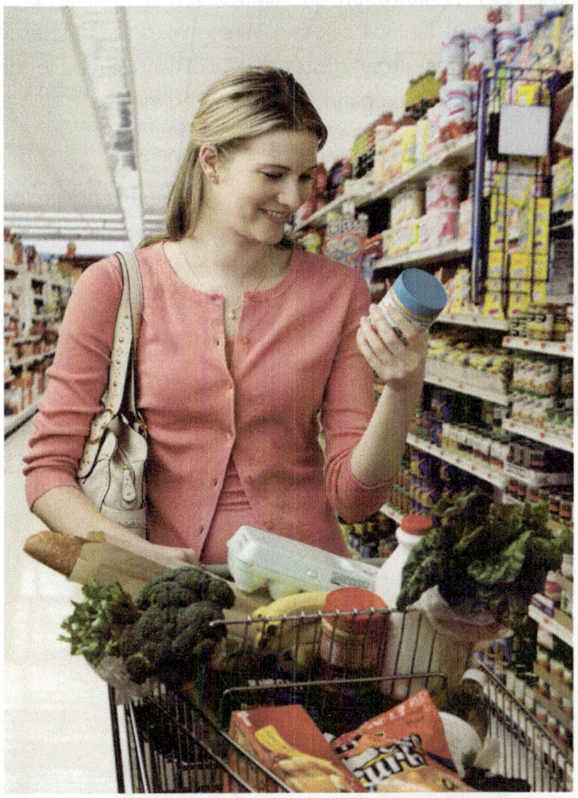

micro10x/Shutterstock.com

Be a savvy supermarket shopper. Read food labels to compare the total fat, saturated fat, and *trans* fat content of similar foods. Identify the amount of calories from added sugars and solid fats contained in the foods and beverages you consume at www.supertracker.usda.gov/foodapedia.aspx.

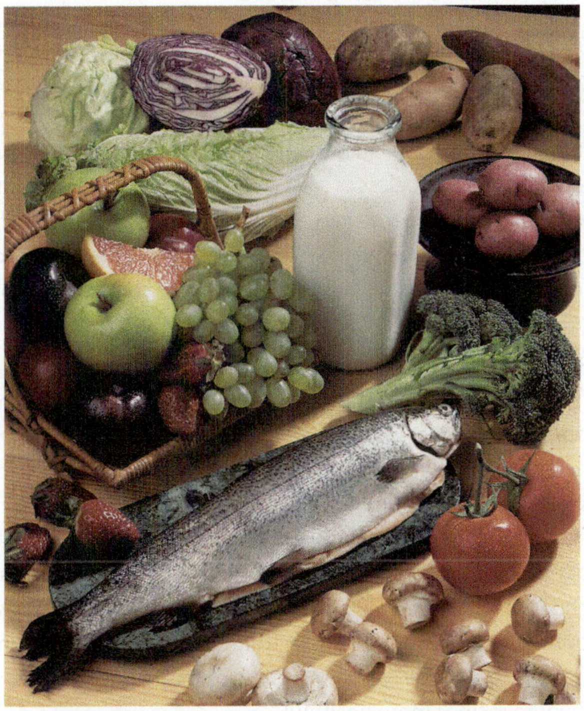

© Polara Studios, Inc.

Enjoy a variety of nutritious foods for the health of your heart.

1 Become a Savvy Supermarket Shopper.

Learn to read food labels to help you choose nutritious, heart-healthy food products. Read manufacturers' labels to determine both the amounts and the types of fat contained in foods. When comparing foods, look at the Nutrition Facts panel, and choose the food with the lower amounts of saturated fat, *trans* fat, and cholesterol (see Figure 2-15 on page 54). For saturated fat and cholesterol, keep in mind that 5 percent of the Daily Value (% DV) or less is low and 20 percent or more is high. There is no % DV for *trans* fat, but we are advised to avoid *trans* fat while consuming a nutritionally adequate diet.

(Continued)

2 Choose Fats Sensibly.

It is not the food but how you prepare it that often determines the total fat (and calories) in a food. Compare the fat in 3 ounces of broiled chicken (3 grams fat, 141 calories) versus 3 ounces of fried chicken (18 grams fat, 364 calories). What makes the difference in calories? Fat. This feature suggests a variety of ways to reduce added fats in your diet when preparing home-cooked meals:

- Use nonstick sprays rather than fat to coat pans.
- Try reducing the fat in recipes a little at a time, and notice that you can do so and still have a tasty meal. If you reduce fat by one tablespoon of butter or oil, you lower the total fat in the product by about 12 grams and at least 100 calories. Or, to reduce the fat even more, try substituting unsweetened applesauce or fruit purees for the oil called for in your favorite cake, quick bread, or cookie recipe.

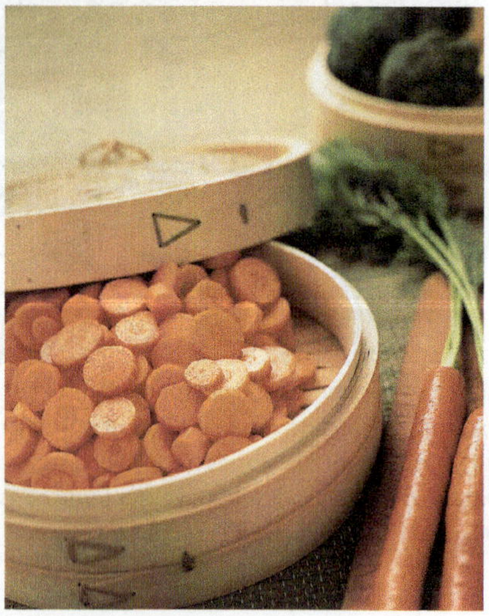
Thomas Del Brase/Getty Images

Bake, broil, poach, or steam.

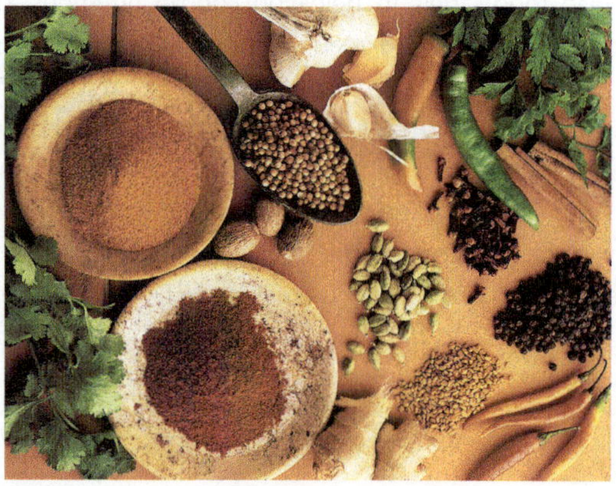
James Jackson/Getty Images

Season with herbs and spices.

- When you sauté a vegetable such as onion in butter, margarine, or oil, try reducing the amount used and substituting water, fat-free vegetable or chicken broth, or wine in its place.
- Prepare broths, soups, and stews ahead of time, refrigerate them, and then skim off hardened fat from the surface.
- Prepare lean cuts of meat, remove visible fat from meat, remove skin from poultry, and cook meats on a rack so that the invisible fat can drain off.
- For flavor in sauces and dressings, experiment with herbs and spices, onions or garlic, salsa, ginger, lemon juice, plain fat-free yogurt with lemon juice, mustard, or butter-flavored granules as replacements for butter, margarine, or oil.
- Try using fruit jam instead of butter on your bagel or toast. Most fruit jams contain half the calories per teaspoon of butter. Or, try the whipped varieties of butter, margarine, or cream cheese, which contain about half the calories of the regular types.

3 Keep Blood Cholesterol at or Below the Recommended Levels.

Among the most influential diet-related factors that raise blood cholesterol levels are saturated fat and *trans* fat intakes. For every 1 percent reduction in a high blood cholesterol level, there is a 2 to 3 percent reduction in the risk of heart attack. As it turns out, the changes in diet that reduce blood cholesterol concentrations mostly do so by reducing LDL-cholesterol. Dietary modifications that help lower LDL-cholesterol include:

- Substitute highly monounsaturated fats (canola or olive oils) and highly polyunsaturated fats (vegetable oils and fish oils) for saturated fats in the diet, because both lower LDL-cholesterol levels in the blood; refer to Table 5-2 on page 135. Choose fats and oils with 2 grams or less of saturated fat per tablespoon, such as liquid and tub margarines and olive or canola oils.[26] Shop for margarine with liquid vegetable oil as the first ingredient. Look for the canola- or olive-oil-based margarines containing zero *trans* fat.
- Replace saturated fats and *trans* fats with unsaturated fats from vegetables, legumes (beans), and nuts. Choose healthful portions of skinless poultry, lean meat, and fish, especially fish rich in omega-3 fatty acids (like salmon). Limit foods high in saturated fat and *trans* fat, such as full-fat milk products, fatty meats, tropical oils (coconut or palm), and partially hydrogenated vegetable oils. Eat fewer high-fat desserts (such as cheesecake, ice cream, brownies, pies, pastries, and cakes with butter cream frosting). Choose fruits as desserts most often. Use the tips in the Recipe Modification box to make your own favorite recipes more healthful.

Recipe Modification

Use this substitution information to modify your own favorite recipes. They'll be more healthful but will still look and taste as good as your originals!

Instead of:	Substitute:
1 whole egg	2 whipped egg whites or ¼ cup egg substitute
Whole milk	Fat-free or 1% milk
Evaporated milk	Evaporated nonfat or low-fat milk
Heavy cream	Evaporated nonfat or low-fat milk
Sour cream	Reduced-fat or fat-free sour cream or plain yogurt
Solid shortening (baking)	Vegetable oil, margarine
Solid shortening (stir-frying)	Peanut or olive oil
Mayonnaise	Reduced-fat or fat-free mayonnaise
Cream cheese	Reduced-fat or fat-free cream cheese
Regular cheese	Cheese made from part-skim milk (mozzarella, Swiss lace, farmer) or reduced-fat cheeses
Salad dressing	Fat-free salad dressings or reduced-calorie dressings
White sauce (made with cream and butter)	Use low-fat milk and cornstarch or flour by blending the starch into cold liquid to eliminate the need for fat

- Add bulk. People on high-fiber diets have been shown to excrete more cholesterol and fat than those on low-fiber diets. A 5 percent decrease in total cholesterol can be achieved with a 5- to 10-gram increase in soluble fiber intake.[27] One reason for this is that the high-fiber diet decreases food's transit time through the digestive tract, allowing less time for cholesterol to be absorbed. When cholesterol from the diet is thus reduced, the body must turn to its own supply for making necessary body compounds. Diets high in fiber are typically low in saturated fat—another advantage of emphasizing fiber. The various dietary fibers have varying effects on blood cholesterol. Soluble fiber, such as that found in rolled oats, oat bran, and psyllium-fortified cereals, has favorable effects on blood cholesterol, whereas wheat bran does not appear to be effective.[28] Apples, pears, peaches, oranges, and grapes are good sources of pectin, another type of cholesterol-lowering fiber.

- Eat generous amounts of fruits and vegetables—at least five to nine servings a day—as a source of antioxidants and other protective compounds in the diet. Antioxidants, such as beta-carotene, vitamins C and E, and the mineral selenium, strengthen the body's natural defenses against cell damage by blocking the potentially damaging free radicals that arise as a part of numerous normal cell activities. **Free radicals**, the chemical compounds that oxidize LDL-cholesterol, become a problem when they are too plentiful. Antioxidants in the body may reduce the amount of LDL-cholesterol that becomes oxidized because the antioxidants (particularly vitamin E) can neutralize the highly reactive oxygen before it gets a chance to oxidize the LDL particle, thereby lessening the buildup of plaque in the artery walls.[29] Scientists are now exploring the potential abilities of all the antioxidant substances found in foods to protect against heart disease.[30]

free radicals Highly toxic compounds created in the body as a result of chemical reactions that involve oxygen. Environmental pollutants such as cigarette smoke and ozone also prompt the formation of free radicals.

4 Balance Energy Intake with Energy Needs.

For heart health, maintain a healthy body weight and a level of physical activity that keeps you fit and matches the number of calories you eat.[31] Walk or do other activities on most days. Moderate exercise, such as brisk walking, may both lower LDL levels and raise HDL levels if the activity is consistently pursued for long enough periods.

It seems that the factors affecting the health of the heart are all tangled together, but all evidence points to the same general recommendations. For good health and to avoid heart disease, do not smoke; reduce blood pressure and weight, if necessary; exercise regularly; and eat a heart-healthy diet.

SCORE Card Rate Your Fats and Health IQ (Obj. 5.6)

How Often Do You?	Often	Sometimes	Rarely
Trim or drain the fat from meats, remove the skin from chicken, and serve fish-based meals?	10	5	1
Incorporate sources of healthy fats in your overall eating pattern (e.g., salmon and other fatty fish, unsalted nuts, avocados, olive oil)?	10	5	1
Eat high-fat foods such as bacon, sausage, regular franks, and luncheon meat several times a week?	1	5	10
Limit whole eggs or egg yolks to seven per week?	10	5	1
Read food labels when shopping?	10	5	1
Choose low-fat or fat-free milk, yogurt, cheese, and sour cream?	10	5	1
Bake, rather than fry, foods?	10	5	1
Maintain a healthy weight?	10	5	1
Think "eating right" and make trade-offs when eating out?	10	5	1
Choose doughnuts, croissants, or sweet rolls for breakfast?	1	5	10
Choose reduced-fat or fat-free products when available?	10	5	1
Routinely add margarine, butter, salad dressing, and sauces to foods?	1	5	10
Balance a high-fat dinner by choosing low-fat foods for breakfast and lunch?	10	5	1
Plan physical activity (walking, running, swimming, bike riding) into your schedule on most days of the week?	10	5	1
TOTAL	______	______	______

Scoring

113–150: You practice heart-healthy habits. Keep up the good work.
75–112: Not a bad score, but there's room for improvement.
5–74: Too low a score! Learn more about the relationships between fats and health.

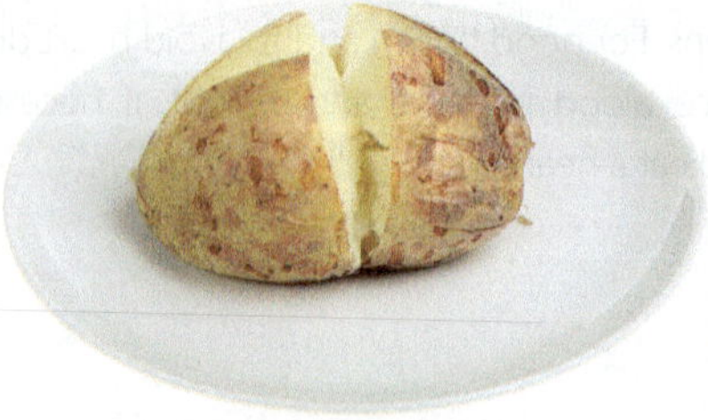

Joe Gough/Shutterstock.com

Large plain potato (200 calories); add 2 tablespoons fat-free sour cream or yogurt seasoned with chives (235 calories, <1 gram fat, 0 grams saturated fat).

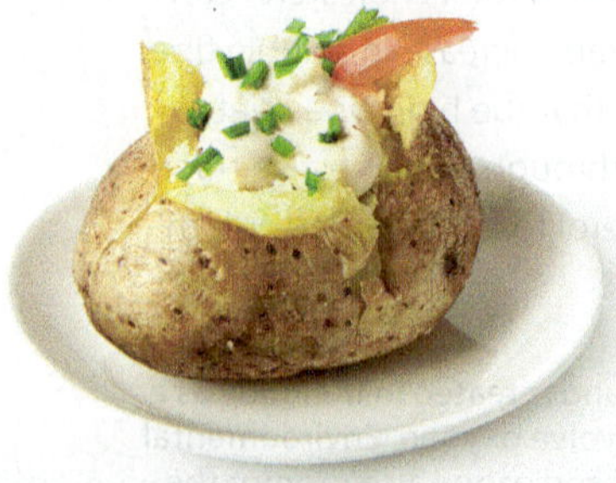

Timolina/Shutterstock.com

Large potato with 2 tablespoons sour cream and 1 tablespoon butter (350 calories, 16.5 grams fat, 10 grams saturated fat).

SOURCE: Adapted from American Dietetic Association and Mosby Great Performance, *Healthy Eating for the Whole Family* (St. Louis, MO: Mosby-Year Book, 1995), 5.

SPOT Light

5.7 Diet and Heart Disease

More than one of every three people who die in the United States each year die of heart and blood vessel disease. The underlying condition that contributes to most of these deaths is atherosclerosis, which leads to closure of the arteries that feed the heart and brain and thus to heart attacks and strokes. In terms of direct health care costs, lost wages, and lost productivity, heart disease costs the United States more than $315 billion a year. There is little wonder, then, that much effort has been focused on preventing it.

The twin demons that lead to most forms of heart disease are atherosclerosis and hypertension. Atherosclerosis, the subject of this Spotlight, is the narrowing of the arteries caused by a buildup of cholesterol-containing plaque in the arterial walls. Hypertension (which is discussed in the Nutrition Action feature of Chapter 8) is high blood pressure, and each of these conditions aggravates the other.

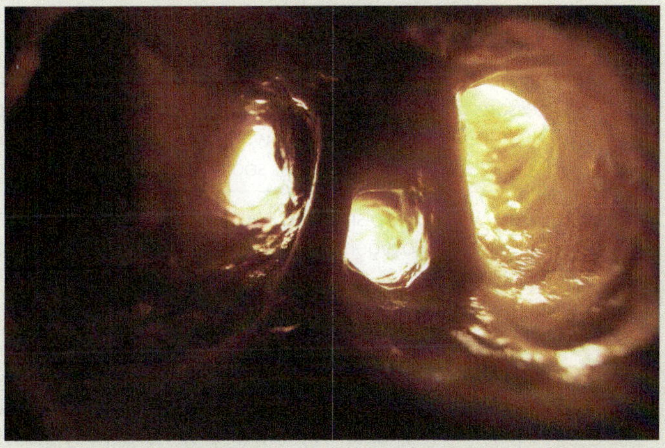
Jean-Claude Revy/ISM/Phototake

A normal artery provides open passage for blood to circulate.

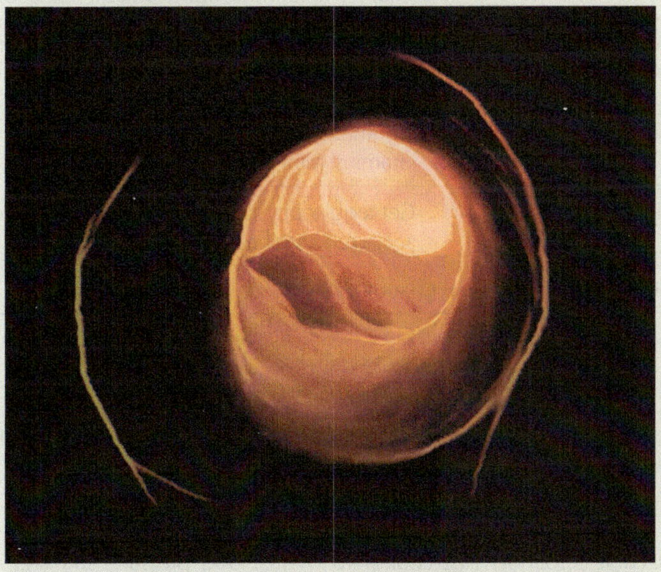
Zephyr/Science Source

Plaques along an artery narrow the passage and obstruct blood flow.

How can I know whether I have atherosclerosis?

No one is free of atherosclerosis. The question is not whether you have it, but how far advanced it is and what you can do to retard or reverse it. As already mentioned, atherosclerosis usually begins with the accumulation of soft mounds of lipids, known as *plaques,* along the inner walls of the arteries, especially at the branch points. These plaques gradually enlarge, making the artery walls lose their elasticity and narrowing the passage through them. Most people have well-developed plaques by the time they are 30.

Normally, the arteries expand with each heartbeat to accommodate the pulses of blood that flow through them. Because arteries that are hardened and narrowed by plaques cannot expand, the blood pressure rises. The increased pressure puts a strain on the heart and further damages the artery wall. At damaged points, plaques are especially likely to form; thus, the development of atherosclerosis is a self-accelerating process.

Hypertension makes atherosclerosis worse. A stiffened artery, already strained by each pulse of blood surging through it, is stressed even more if the internal pressure is high. Hypertension causes injured places within the blood vessels to develop more frequently, and plaques grow faster. Hardened arteries also fail to let blood flow freely through the body's blood pressure–sensing organs, the kidneys, which respond as if the blood pressure were too low and raise it further.

How can I slow the process down?

Learn your risk factors, and control the ones you can. Among the many factors linked to heart disease are smoking, gender (being male), age (men older than 45 and women older than 55), postmenopausal status in women, heredity, diabetes, high blood pressure, lack of exercise, obesity, high blood cholesterol level, and low HDL-cholesterol level (see Table 5-8). Some of the risk factors are also powerful *predictors* of heart disease. If you have none of the risk factors, the statistical likelihood of your developing heart disease may be only 1 in 100. If you have three major risk factors, your chance may rise to more than 1 in 20. Some of the factors that have emerged as powerful predictors of risk are high

TABLE 5-8 Leading Risk Factors for Heart Disease

Heart disease rarely develops from a single risk factor. Clusters of risk factors usually occur, and a small increase in one risk factor, such as blood pressure, becomes more critical when combined with other risk factors. Luckily, a similar pattern happens in reverse: Even moderate changes in one risk factor can decrease several others at the same time. For example, a weight loss of just 5 to 10 pounds can reduce blood pressure in overweight people. Or, becoming physically active can lower blood pressure, increase HDL ("good" cholesterol), and help control weight.

Risk Factors You Can Change

Risk Factor	How to Minimize the Risk
High LDL-cholesterol	Consume a diet emphasizing vegetables, fruits, and whole grains; include low-fat dairy products, poultry, fish, legumes, nontropical vegetable oils, and nuts; limit intake of sweets, sugar-sweetened beverages, and red meats; avoid *trans* fats.
Low HDL-cholesterol	Avoid *trans* fat; lose weight if necessary; do not smoke; and maintain a physically active lifestyle.
High blood pressure	Control high blood pressure with medication and a heart-healthy diet. Maintain a healthy weight. Losing just 5 to 10 pounds may lower your blood pressure. Compare sodium in soups, frozen meals, and other foods—and choose the foods with less sodium.
Cigarette smoking	Stop smoking. Nicotine constricts blood vessels and forces your heart to work harder. Carbon monoxide reduces oxygen in blood and damages the lining of blood vessels.
Diabetes	Maintain proper weight. Losing excess weight helps control blood sugar level. Eat high-fiber foods. Limit solid fats and added sugars. Get regular physical activity.
Physical inactivity	Increase physical activity by seeking ways to be more physically active every day. Aim for the equivalent of 150 minutes (2 hours and 30 minutes) of moderate-intensity aerobic activity (such as brisk walking) each week. See Chapter 11 for more physical activity guidelines.
Obesity	Maintain a healthy weight and be physically active. Being only 10% overweight increases heart disease risk. See Chapter 10 for more about weight management.
"Atherogenic" diet	To lower LDL-cholesterol, keep saturated fat to less than 5% to 6% of daily calories. For someone eating 2,000 calories a day, that's about 13 grams of saturated fat. Substitute olive and canola oils for saturated fat. Avoid *trans* fat. Limit consumption of foods with solid fats and added sugars. Increase soluble fiber intake by eating whole grains, legumes, fruits, and vegetables. Eat a variety of fruits and vegetables each day to receive the beneficial antioxidants, vitamins, minerals, and phytochemicals they contain.
Stress	Get regular physical activity. Avoid excessive caffeine and alcohol. Practice relaxation techniques. Maintain good social relationships.
Risk Factors You Cannot Change	
Age	Men over age 45 and women over age 55 are at increased risk.
Gender	Men are at higher risk. Estrogen may protect women before menopause.
Genetics	Risk is increased if you have a father or brother under age 55 or a mother or sister under 65 who had heart disease.

LDL-cholesterol, low HDL-cholesterol, high blood pressure, smoking, obesity, and physical inactivity.[32]

What can I do to reduce my risk?

Obviously, some risk factors cannot be altered. Being born male or inheriting a predisposition to develop high blood cholesterol or high blood pressure are factors beyond your control. Even so, you can make conscious choices that may reduce your risk of developing heart disease. Let's examine one of the two major risk factors related to diet—high blood cholesterol—with an eye toward learning which dietary and lifestyle changes will help reduce your heart disease risk.

To what extent does a high blood cholesterol level raise the risk of developing heart disease?

The likelihood of a person developing or dying from heart disease increases as total blood cholesterol level rises. Figure 5-15 presents this relationship graphically, showing that the number of deaths from heart disease increases steadily among those with elevated blood cholesterol levels, particularly when the level rises above 200 milligrams per deciliter. Individuals with a blood cholesterol level in the neighborhood of 300 milligrams per deciliter run four times the risk of dying from heart disease compared with those whose cholesterol level is lower than 200 mg/dL. Having a low HDL-cholesterol value is also recognized

FIGURE 5-15

Relationship between Blood Cholesterol Level and Death Rate from Heart Disease

People with blood cholesterol levels of 300 mg/dL are four times as likely to die from heart disease as those with blood cholesterol levels below 200 mg/dL.

SOURCE: Data from 361,662 men screened for the Multiple Risk Factor Intervention Trial (MRFIT). Adapted from National Cholesterol Education Program, *Report of the Expert Panel on Population Strategies for Blood Cholesterol Reduction* (Bethesda, MD: U.S. Department of Health and Human Services, Public Health Service, National Institutes of Health, National Heart, Lung, and Blood Institute, NIH Publication No. 90-3046, November 1990), 7.

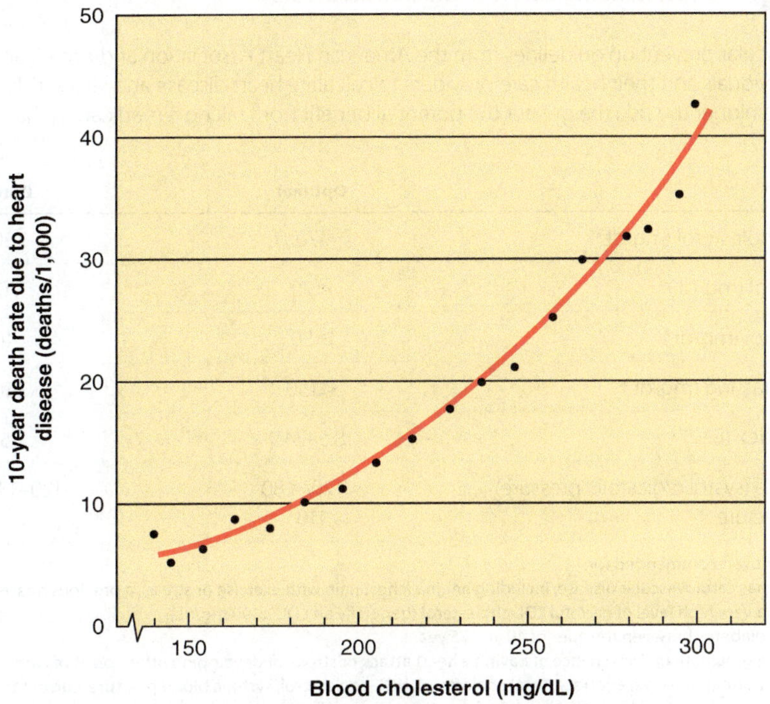

as being a risk factor for heart disease.[33] A low HDL value is defined as one below 40 mg/dL. A combined effort to lower LDL-cholesterol and raise HDL-cholesterol delivers a double punch in the fight against heart disease.

Reducing high blood cholesterol levels, particularly the "bad" LDL-cholesterol level, is thus an important strategy for lowering the risk of heart disease. This is especially true for people having one or more of the other major heart disease risk factors, such as smoking. Table 5-9 provides information for determining what to do if your blood cholesterol level is high and whether you might need to seek treatment.

Should children, like their parents, modify their fat intake for heart health?

The *Dietary Guidelines for Americans* supports the Institute of Medicine's recommendations for 30 to 40 percent of calories from fat for ages 1 to 3 years, 25 to 35 percent of calories from fat for ages 4 to 18 years, and 20 to 35 percent of calories from fat for adults.[34]

The current *Dietary Guidelines* and experts from major health and professional organizations also recommend that children aged 2 and older eat diets containing no more than 10 percent of total calories from saturated fat daily. The reason is that hardening of the arteries often begins in childhood.

The panel also advised that children or teens should get their blood cholesterol measured if they have one parent with a high blood cholesterol level. For children and adolescents, a total of 200 milligrams per deciliter or more is considered high, 170 to 199 is borderline high, and less than 170 is acceptable. In addition, children born to families with a history of premature heart disease should have both total blood cholesterol and HDL-cholesterol checked.[35]

What sorts of dietary changes should I make to reduce my total blood cholesterol and LDL-cholesterol levels?

Probably the most significant dietary changes you can make are to reduce the amounts of saturated fat and *trans* fat that you eat; high intakes of these fats are related to high blood levels of LDL-cholesterol.[36] The goals to work toward are to reduce your intake of saturated fat to less than 10 percent of total calories, and to avoid *trans* fatty acid consumption. People with elevated levels of LDL-cholesterol, existing heart disease, diabetes, or combinations of risk factors are advised to reduce their intake of saturated fat even further, to less than 5 to 6 percent of total calories.[37] See this chapter's Savvy Diner feature for more specifics on reducing your LDL-cholesterol level. Table 5-10 lists a variety of resources for understanding and improving heart health.

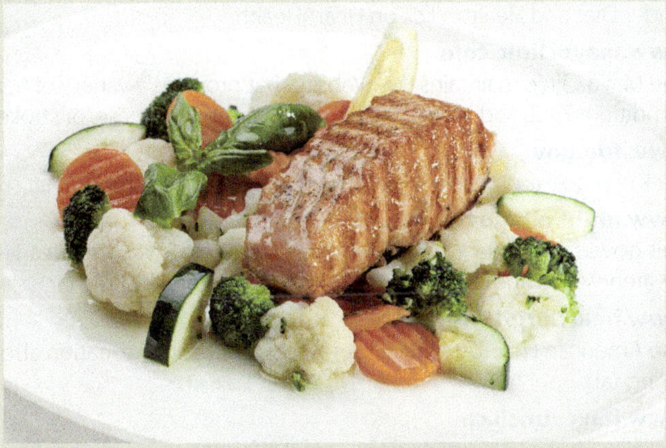

puhhha/Shutterstock.com

Choosing fish rich in omega-3 fatty acids may help reduce the risk of heart disease.

TABLE 5-9 Understanding Cardiovascular Risk Factors

The cardiovascular prevention guidelines from the American Heart Association and American College of Cardiology aim to initiate a discussion between individuals and their health care providers to calculate heart disease and stroke risk, rather than focusing on a specific cholesterol "number." The higher the risk, the greater the potential benefit from taking a medication that lowers cholesterol (a family of drugs called statins).[a, b]

Risk Factors	Optimal	Borderline	High Risk
Total blood cholesterol (mg/dL)[c]	170	200–239	≥240
LDL-cholesterol (mg/dL)[d]	<70	70–159	160–189
HDL-cholesterol (mg/dL)	≥50	40–49	<40
Triglycerides, fasting (mg/dL)[e]	<150	150–199	200–499
Body mass index (BMI)[f]	18.5–24.9	25–29.9	≥30
Blood pressure (systolic/diastolic pressure)	<120/<80	120–139/80–89[g]	≥140/≥90[h]
Systolic pressure	110		

[a] Taking a statin is now recommended for:

1. Individual who has cardiovascular disease, including angina (chest pain with exercise or stress), a previous heart attack or stroke, or other related condition.
2. Individual with a very high level of harmful LDL-cholesterol (generally an LDL ≥190 mg/dL).
3. Individual with diabetes between the ages of 40 and 75 years.
4. Individual with a greater than 7.5% chance of having a heart attack or stroke or developing other forms of cardiovascular disease in the next 10 years. A risk calculator uses nine pieces of information—sex, age, race, total cholesterol, HDL-cholesterol, systolic blood pressure, current treatment for high blood pressure, diagnosis of diabetes, and smoking habit—to gauge an individual's chances of developing heart disease over the next 10 years.

[b] A downloadable spreadsheet enabling estimation of 10-year and lifetime risk for cardiovascular disease and a web-based calculator are available at my.americanheart.org/cvriskcalculator.

[c] Total cholesterol is the level of all the lipids in your blood, including your LDL-cholesterol and HDL-cholesterol. Generally, a lower total cholesterol level is better.

[d] Ideally, the level of bad (LDL) cholesterol should be <70 milligrams per deciliter of blood (mg/dL); ≥190 mg/dL LDL indicates a very high risk.

[e] ≥500 mg/dL triglycerides indicates very high risk.

[f] See the BMI chart on the inside back cover of this book

[g] These values indicate prehypertension.

[h] These values indicate hypertension. Physicians use these values to determine treatment.

SOURCE: Adapted from: N. J. Stone, J. Robinson, A. H. Lichtenstein, et al., 2013 ACC/AHA Guideline on the Treatment of Blood Cholesterol to Reduce Atherosclerotic Cardiovascular Risk in Adults: A report of the American College of Cardiology/American Heart Association Task Force on Practice Guidelines. *Circulation.* 2013.

TABLE 5-10 Nutrition on the Web

www.healthfinder.gov
Search for information on atherosclerosis, heart disease, and stroke.

www.eatright.org
The Academy of Nutrition and Dietetics home page includes many nutrition resources and links.

http://fnic.nal.usda.gov/
Under Diet and Health, click on Heart Health.

www.mayoclinic.com
The Mayo Clinic maintains this website that provides a variety of health information. Go to Patient Care & Health Info. Click on Diseases & Conditions A–Z, and look up atherosclerosis, heart disease, or stroke.

www.fda.gov
Click on Food and search for information on olestra and other fat substitutes and labeling of *trans* fatty acids in foods.

www.nhlbi.nih.gov
This government website is a clearinghouse for the National Heart, Lung, and Blood Institute (NHLBI). Under Public, click on the Education and Awareness tab and the Resources tab for more information, including a 10-Year Heart Attack Risk Calculator.

www.heart.org/HEARTORG
The American Heart Association provides practical information about diet, physical activity, and cardiovascular risk reduction under the Healthy Living tab.

www.flaxcouncil.ca
The Flax Council of Canada gives useful information on the health benefits of flaxseed.

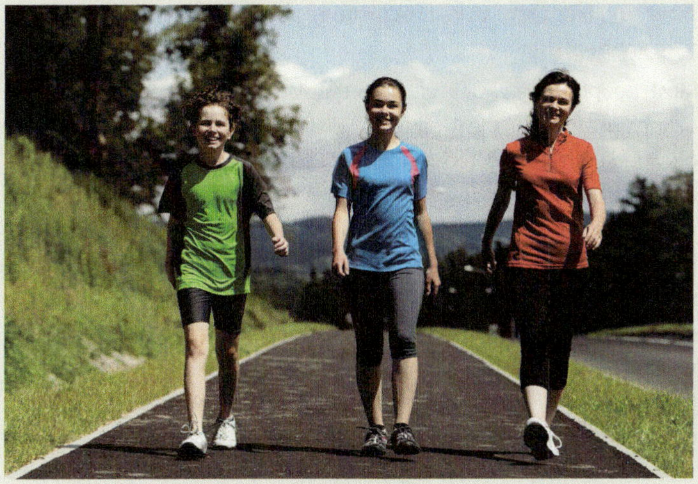

Jacek Chabraszewski/Shutterstock.com

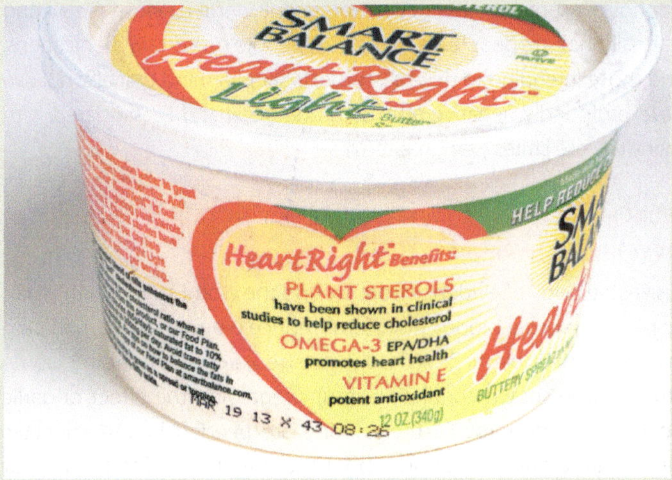

© Sam Kolich/Bill Smith Group/Cengage Learning

Another powerful influence on LDL levels is not a dietary factor at all—it is regular *physical activity.* Moderate exercise, such as walking, may lower LDL levels if the activity is consistently pursued for long enough periods. Increase physical activity by seeking ways to be more physically active every day. Aim for the equivalent of 150 minutes (2 hours and 30 minutes) of moderate-intensity aerobic activity (such as brisk walking) each week.[38]

Should I also reduce my dietary cholesterol intake?

Dietary cholesterol can raise LDL levels, depending on the amount consumed and on the body's ability to compensate by making less. The *Dietary Guidelines* recommend that individuals eat as little dietary cholesterol as possible while consuming a healthy eating pattern. In general, foods that are higher in dietary cholesterol, such as fatty meats and high-fat dairy products, are also higher in saturated fats. On average, men consume 333 milligrams of cholesterol and women consume about 224 milligrams daily.

What factors determine my HDL-cholesterol level?

One is gender. Women have higher HDL-cholesterol levels than men. However, heart disease is the major cause of death among women after menopause, when low levels of estrogen lead to a decrease in HDL levels along with an increase in LDL levels. Another factor, interestingly, seems to be smoking habits. Nonsmokers have uniformly higher HDL levels than do smokers. Still another factor is weight reduction for those who are overweight.[39]

If any dietary factors are significant, one important one may be to include some fish in the diet.[40] Eat fish such as salmon, trout, and herring in place of meat or poultry twice a week. Another may be including soy foods and foods containing soluble fibers that lower LDL levels.

Can the addition of plant sterols to the diet help reduce blood cholesterol levels?

Certain brands of margarine contain phytosterols (plant stanols or plant sterols), which are compounds derived from plant oils that may actually reduce blood cholesterol when consumed as part of a low-fat diet.[41] A *phytosterol* is a phytochemical that is structurally similar to the steroid hormones (for example, estrogen). Examples of margarines containing phytosterols include Benecol and Promise Activ. Benecol uses a stanol ester derived from pine trees, and Promise Activ uses one made from soy. These compounds block the absorption of dietary cholesterol from the intestine. The FDA has given the manufacturers approval to use labels stating that the products "promote healthy cholesterol levels." Margarines containing these compounds, however, typically cost more than regular margarine, and the safety of their long-term daily use is not known.

What about alcohol? I've heard that moderate alcohol intake can be beneficial, at least with respect to heart disease risk.

The evidence with regard to alcohol and blood lipids points to a possible protective mechanism between moderate alcohol consumption and heart disease risk factors.[42] Investigators have reported that the consumption of moderate amounts of alcohol appears to raise HDL levels.[43] *Moderate drinking* is defined as no more than one drink a day for most women, and no more than two drinks a day for most men. A strong association between moderate alcohol consumption and low rates of heart disease was first observed in France and then in other wine-drinking areas of the Mediterranean. Researchers have since identified antioxidants and other compounds in red wine that decrease blood clotting, and this may help explain part of the "French paradox," or how a region with high fat intakes could have such low rates of heart disease. Researchers are quick to point out, however, that other factors certainly may contribute to the paradox. For example, the French consume about 57 percent of their day's calories before 2 p.m., whereas most Americans have consumed only about 38 percent of their calories by that time.[44] Also, the French mostly consume their wine with meals, and they eat more fruits and vegetables and leaner cuts of meat.

Scientists warn that caution is needed in recommending moderate alcohol consumption to the public. Many people need to refrain from alcohol consumption altogether (pregnant women, those recovering from alcoholism, people under age 21, people on certain medications, and those intending to drive a vehicle).[45] Keep in mind that alcohol can have profoundly negative effects on the body and is associated with many disease states (see Chapter 9).

What about garlic? I've heard that garlic pills and whole cloves help lower blood cholesterol.

A sizeable body of evidence from around the world suggests that garlic may help lower blood cholesterol, reduce blood pressure, and help arteries remain elastic.[46] Although the research is promising, some studies have shown conflicting results regarding the effect of garlic on blood cholesterol. Further studies are needed before scientists can come to any conclusions about the usefulness of fresh garlic or garlic pills (which vary a great deal in composition) in lowering blood cholesterol levels. See Chapter 7 for more about the phytochemical benefits derived from garlic and its relatives (leeks, onions, chives, scallions, and shallots).

What about eating chocolate? Are there any health benefits derived from chocolate?

Some evidence suggests that modest consumption of dark chocolate or cocoa is associated with health benefits in the form of reduced risk for heart disease. However, chocolate is high in calories (a 3-ounce chocolate bar can contain more than 400 calories), so the benefits need to be balanced with caloric intake to prevent weight gain. The predominant fat in chocolate is stearic acid, a saturated fat that has been shown to not raise blood cholesterol. The beneficial effects from dark chocolate are attributed to its phytochemicals, in particular the flavonoids, which act as antioxidants. The benefits most frequently associated with consumption of dark chocolate include reducing inflammation; decreasing total cholesterol; decreasing LDL-cholesterol; protecting against blood clot formation; and decreasing blood pressure.[47] Many foods and beverages that are less calorie-dense (berries, citrus fruit, grapes, soy foods, and tea) contain flavonoids, and chocolate is considered a minor source. See Chapter 7 for more about phytochemicals, and see Chapter 9 for more about the flavonoids found in both tea and cocoa.

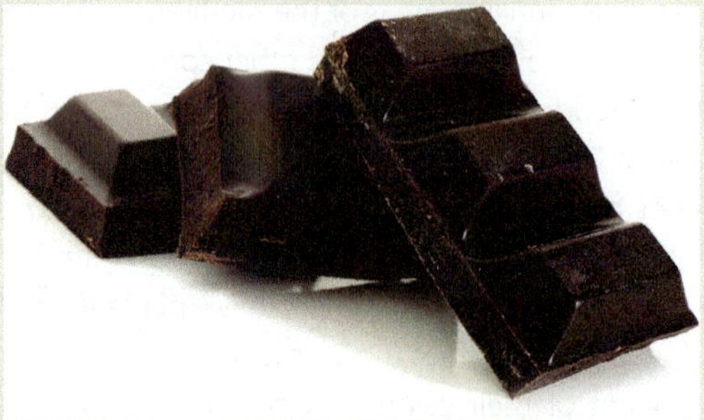

Nikola Bilic/Shutterstock.com

How do I translate these recommendations into a heart-healthy lifestyle?

Most people have a difficult time translating the dietary recommendations into actual meal patterns. This chapter's Savvy Diner feature provided many tips for reducing your LDL-cholesterol level. Consider the following suggestions as well.[48]

The American Heart Association guidelines recommend eating a heart-healthy diet that emphasizes fruits, vegetables, and whole grains, while including low-fat dairy products, poultry, fish, legumes, nontropical vegetable oils, and nuts and limiting red meat, sweets, and sugar-sweetened beverages. Following this pattern should help people limit their saturated fat, *trans* fat, and sodium to the recommended levels even if they do not count grams.[49]

Based on a 2,000 calories per day diet, a heart-healthy eating pattern should include:

- *Fruits: 4 to 5 servings a day.* One serving equals 1 medium fruit; ¼ cup dried fruit; ½ cup fresh, frozen, or canned fruit; or ½ cup fruit juice.
- *Vegetables: 4 to 5 servings a day.* One serving equals 1 cup raw leafy vegetable, ½ cup cut-up raw or cooked vegetable, or ½ cup vegetable juice.
- *Whole grains, preferably high fiber: 6 to 8 servings a day.* One serving equals 1 slice bread; 1 oz dry cereal; or ½ cup cooked rice, pasta, or cooked cereal.
- *Fat-free or low-fat milk and milk products: 2 to 3 servings a day.* One serving equals 1 cup milk or yogurt or 1½ ounces of cheese.
- *Lean meats, poultry, and fish: 6 or fewer ounces a day.*
- *Nuts, legumes, and seeds: 4 to 5 servings a week.* One serving equals ⅓ cup or 1½ ounces nuts, 2 tablespoons peanut butter, 2 tablespoons or ½ ounce seeds, or ½ cup cooked legumes.
- *Fats and oils: 2 to 3 servings of healthy oils per day; limit trans and saturated fat.* One serving of fats and oils equals 1 teaspoon soft margarine, 1 teaspoon vegetable oil, 1 tablespoon mayonnaise, or 2 tablespoons salad dressing.
- *Limit sweets and added sugars.*
- *Limit your intake of foods that are high in calories from solid fats and added sugars*, such as cakes, cookies, candy, and ice cream; pizza; cheese; processed and fatty meats; and sweetened beverages.
- *Adopt heart-healthy cooking methods*, such as broiling, baking, steaming, and stir-frying.
- *Choose and prepare foods with little or no salt.* To lower blood pressure, aim to eat no more than 2,300 milligrams of sodium per day. Reducing daily intake to 1,500 mg is desirable because it can lower blood pressure even further.[50]

- *Consume alcohol only in moderation*, if at all. Have no more than one alcoholic drink per day if you're a woman and no more than two if you're a man. "One drink" means it has no more than ½ ounce of pure alcohol. Examples of one drink are 12 ounces of beer, 5 ounces of wine, 1½ ounces of 80-proof spirits, or 1 ounce of 100-proof spirits.[51]

Attention to emotional health is also important in reducing the risk of heart disease. Both love and affection seem to affect the heart. People with many social ties appear to develop less heart disease than do people with few or none. Similarly, pet owners, even owners of pet fish, have lower blood pressure than do people without pets. Clearly, the mystery of heart disease, like all the great human mysteries, involves the mind and spirit as well as the body. So nourish yourself in all ways—not just physically.

WHAT'S ONLINE

MINDTAP From Cengage

Visit www.cengagebrain.com to access MindTap, a complete digital course that includes Diet & Wellness Plus, interactive quizzes, videos, and more.

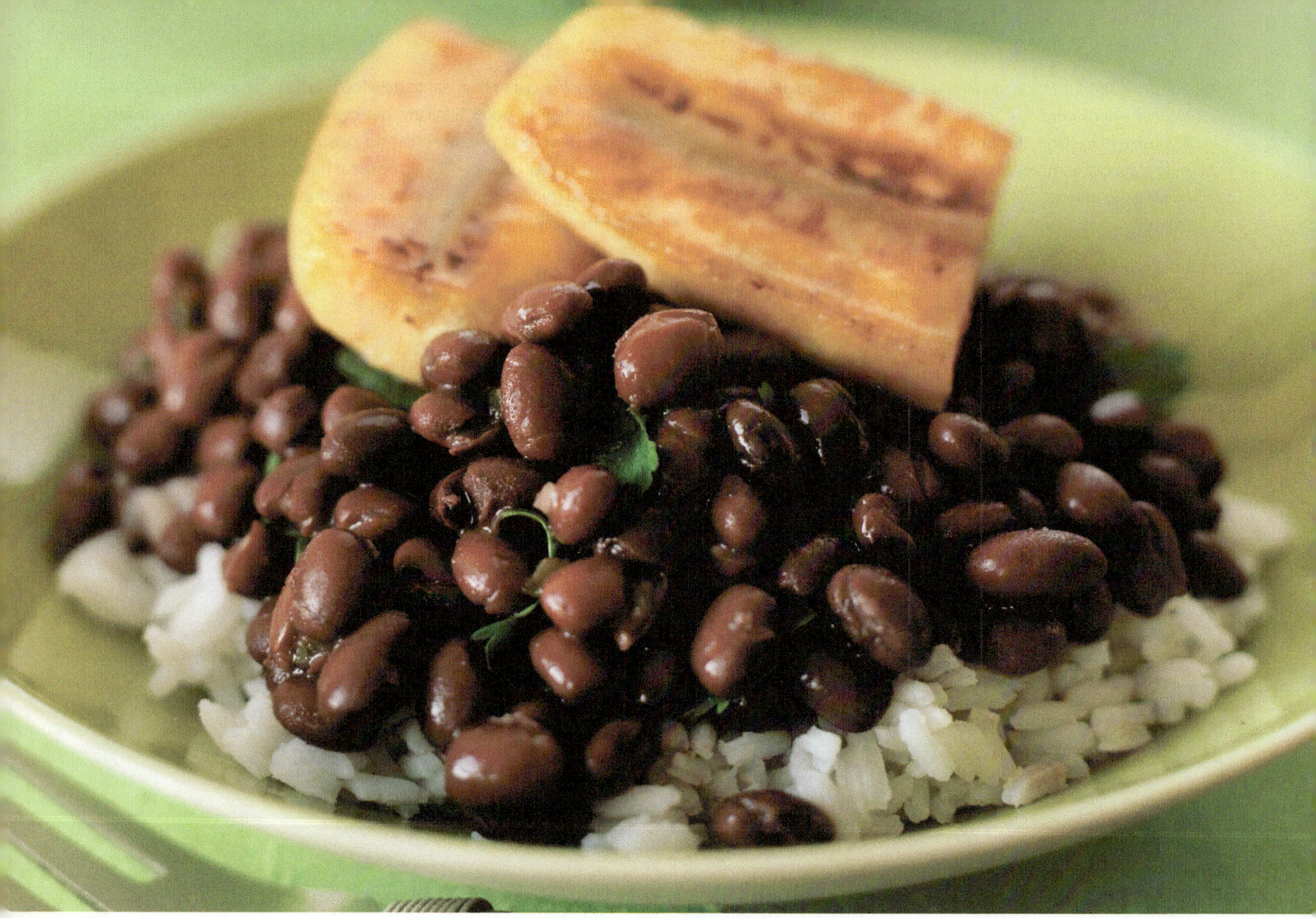

Quentin Bacon/StockFood Creative/Getty Images

AskYourself . . .

Which of the following statements about nutrition are true, and which are false? For each false statement, what is true?

1. When more protein is eaten than the body needs, it is stored intact in the body (the way fat is stored) so that it can be used when a person's diet falls short of supplying the day's need for essential proteins.
2. When a person doesn't eat enough food to meet the body's energy needs, the body devours its own protein tissue.
3. Milk protein is the standard against which the quality of other proteins is usually measured.
4. People who eat no meat need to eat a lot of special foods to get enough protein.

Answers found on page 158.

ChapterObjectives

6.1 Differentiate between essential amino acids and nonessential amino acids.

6.2 List the functions of protein in the body.

6.3 List the steps for protein digestion and absorption in the body.

6.4 Explain the differences between high-quality and low-quality proteins, including food sources of each.

6.5 Calculate the recommended protein intake for a given individual.

6.6 Develop a meal plan that incorporates protein-rich foods, including legumes.

6.7 Identify the most common allergenic foods for children and adults.

6.8 Describe the nutritional challenges of a vegan diet and methods for developing a vegetarian eating pattern that delivers nutritional adequacy.

The Proteins and Amino Acids

CHAPTER 6

The **proteins** are perhaps the most highly respected of the three energy nutrients, and the roles they play in the body are far more varied than those of carbohydrate or fat. First named 175 years ago after the Greek word *proteios* ("of prime importance"), proteins have revealed countless secrets about how living processes take place, and they account for many nutrition concerns. How do we grow? How do our bodies replace the materials they lose? How does blood clot? What makes us able to become immune to diseases we have been exposed to? To a great extent, the answers to these and many other such questions are found in an understanding of the nature of the proteins.

> The amino acids of proteins are the raw materials of heredity, the keys to life chemistry, handed from generation to generation.
>
> —R. M. Deutsch (1928–1988, Nutrition Author and Educator)

6.1 What Proteins Are Made Of

To appreciate the many vital functions of proteins, we must understand their structure. One key difference from carbohydrate and fat, which contain only carbon, hydrogen, and oxygen atoms, is that proteins contain nitrogen atoms. These nitrogen atoms give the name *amino* ("nitrogen containing") to the **amino acids** of which protein is made. Another key difference is that in contrast to the carbohydrates—whose repeating units, glucose molecules, are identical—the amino acids in a strand of protein are different from one another.

All amino acids have the same, simple chemical backbone, with an **amine group** (the nitrogen-containing part) at one end and an acid group at the other end (see Figure 6-1). The differences among the various amino acids are due to the varying structures of the chemical side chains that are attached to the backbone. Twenty amino acids with 20 different side chains make up most of the proteins of living tissue.

The side chains vary in complexity from a single hydrogen atom, like that on glycine, to a complex ring structure, like that on phenylalanine. Not only do these structures differ in composition, size, and shape, but they also differ in electrical charge. Some are negative, some are positive, and some have no charge. These side chains help to determine the shapes and behaviors of the larger protein molecules that the amino acids make up.

proteins Compounds composed of atoms of carbon, hydrogen, oxygen, and nitrogen and arranged as strands of amino acids. Some amino acids also contain atoms of sulfur.

amino (uh-MEEN-oh) acids Building blocks of protein; each is a compound with an amine group at one end, an acid group at the other, and a distinctive side chain.

amine (a-MEEN) group The nitrogen-containing portion of an amino acid.

essential amino acids Amino acids that cannot be synthesized by the body or that cannot be synthesized in amounts sufficient to meet physiological need.

FIGURE 6-1
Amino Acid Structure

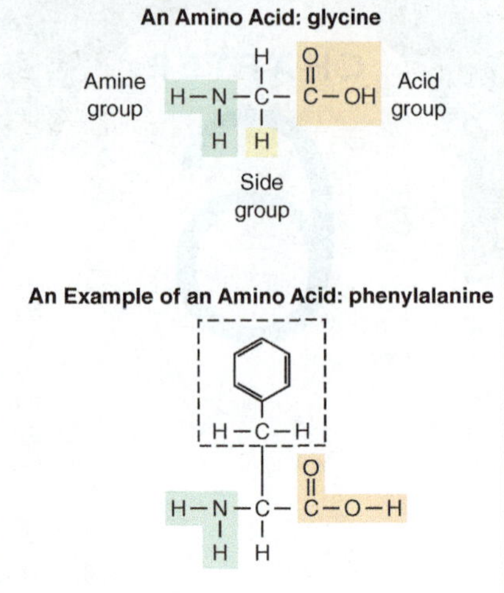

© Cengage

TABLE 6-1 Amino Acids[a]

Essential Amino Acids	
The essential amino acids that must be obtained from the diet:	
histidine	phenylalanine
isoleucine	threonine
leucine	tryptophan
lysine	valine
methionine	
Nonessential Amino Acids	
The nonessential amino acids—also important in nutrition:	
alanine	glutamine
arginine	glycine
asparagine	proline
aspartic acid	serine
cysteine	tyrosine
glutamic acid	

© Cengage

[a] The distinction between essential and nonessential amino acids is not quite as clear-cut as the list makes it appear. Some nonessential amino acids may become conditionally essential. For example, cysteine and tyrosine normally are not essential because the body makes them from methionine and phenylalanine. However, if there are not enough of these precursors from which to make cysteine and tyrosine, they must be supplied by the diet.

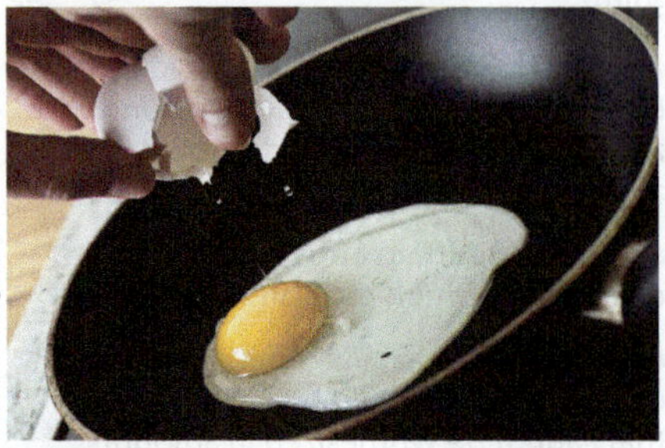

© iStock.com/gbrundin

Cooking an egg denatures its proteins.

Essential and Nonessential Amino Acids

The body can make about half of the amino acids (known as *nonessential amino acids*) for itself when it has the needed parts: nitrogen to form the amine group and backbone fragments, which are derived from carbohydrate or fat. But even a healthy body cannot make some amino acids. These are known as **essential amino acids** (see Table 6-1). If the diet does not supply them, the body cannot make the proteins it needs to do its work. The indispensability of the essential amino acids makes it necessary for people to eat protein food sources every day.

Proteins as the Source of Life's Variety

In the first step of **protein synthesis**, each amino acid is hooked to the next. A bond, called a **peptide bond**, is formed between the amino end of one and the acid end of the next. Proteins are made of many amino acid units, from several dozen to many hundred (see Figure 6-2).

A strand of protein is not straight; it is more like a tangled chain. The amino acids at different places along the strand are attracted to one another, and this attraction causes the strand to coil into a shape similar to that of a metal spring. Not only does the strand of amino acids form a long coil, but the coil also tangles, forming a globular structure.

The charged amino acids are attracted to water, and in the body fluids they orient themselves on the outside of the globular structure. The neutral amino acids are repelled by water and are attracted to one another; they tuck themselves into the center, away from the body fluids. All these interactions among the amino acids and the surrounding fluid result in the unique architecture of each type of protein. Additional steps may be needed for the protein to become functional. A mineral or a vitamin may be needed to complete and activate the unit, or several proteins may gather to form a functioning group.

The differing shapes of proteins enable them to perform different tasks in the body. In proteins that give strength and elasticity to body parts, several springs of amino acids coil together and form rope-like fibers. Other proteins, like those in the blood, do not have such structural strength but are water-soluble, with a globular shape like a ball of steel wool. Some are shaped like hollow balls that can carry and store minerals in their interiors. Still others provide support to tissues. Some—the enzymes—act on other substances to change them chemically.

Denaturation of Proteins

Proteins can undergo **denaturation**, resulting in distortion of shape by heat, alcohol, acids, bases, or the salts of heavy metals. The denaturation of a protein is the first step in breakdown of the protein. Denaturation is useful to the body in digestion. During the digestion of a food protein, an early step is denaturation by the stomach acid, which opens up the protein's structure, permitting digestive enzymes to break the peptide bonds (see Figure 6-6 later in this chapter). Denaturation can also occur during food preparation. For example, cooking an egg denatures the proteins of the egg and makes the egg firmer. Perhaps more important, cooking denatures two raw-egg proteins that bind the B vitamin biotin and the mineral iron, as well as a protein that slows the digestion of other proteins. Thus, cooking eggs liberates biotin and iron and aids in protein digestion.

ASK YOURSELF ANSWERS: **1.** False. When more protein is eaten than the body needs, it is *not* stored in the body (the way fat is stored), so it must be eaten every day to avoid protein depletion. **2.** True. **3.** False. Egg-white protein, not milk protein, is the standard against which the quality of other proteins is usually measured. **4.** False. People who eat no meat can easily get enough protein without eating a lot of special foods.

6.2 The Functions of Body Proteins

No new living tissue can be built without protein, for protein is part of every cell. About 20 percent of our total body weight is protein. Proteins come in many forms: enzymes, antibodies, hormones, transport vehicles, oxygen carriers, tendons and ligaments, scars, the cores of bones and teeth, the filaments of hair, the materials of nails, and more (see Table 6-2). A few of the many vital functions of proteins are described here to show why they have rightfully earned their position of importance in nutrition.

Growth and Maintenance One function of dietary protein is to ensure the availability of amino acids for building the proteins of new tissue. New tissue is needed in an embryo; in a growing child; in the blood that replaces that which has been lost in burns, hemorrhage, or surgery; in the scar tissue that heals wounds; and in new hair and nails. Not so obvious, but equally important, is the protein that helps replace worn-out cells. The cells that line the digestive tract live for only about three days, and they are constantly being shed and excreted. You have probably observed that the cells of your skin die, rub off, and are replaced from underneath. For this new growth, amino acids must constantly be resupplied by food.

Enzymes All enzymes are proteins, and they are among the most important proteins formed in living cells. Enzymes are *catalysts*—biological spark plugs—that help chemical reactions take place. There are thousands of enzymes inside a single cell, each type facilitating a specific chemical reaction. Enzymes are involved in such processes as the digestion of food, the release of energy from the body's stored energy supplies, and the growth and repair of tissue.

The mystery of how an enzyme can be specific for a particular reaction is only partially understood. Scientists believe that the surface of the enzyme is contoured so that it can recognize only the substances it works on, and ignore others. The surface provides a site that attracts one or more specific chemical compounds and promotes a specific chemical reaction. For example, two substances might first become attached

FIGURE 6-2

Peptide Bonds in a Molecule of Insulin

Amino acids are linked together with peptide bonds to form strands of protein. The sulfur groups (S) on two cysteine (cys) molecules can bond together, creating a "sulfur bridge" between the two protein strands.

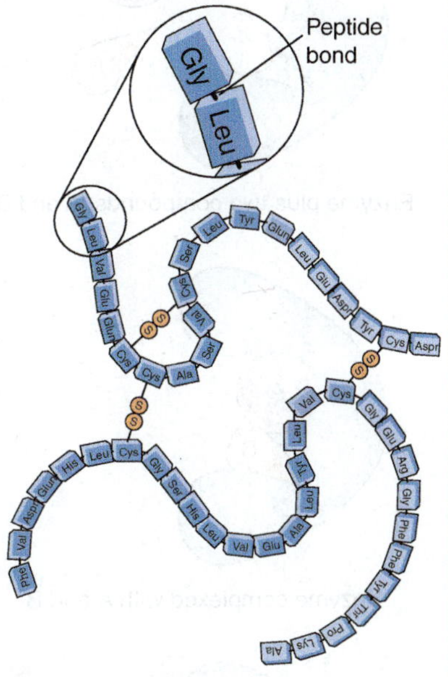

TABLE 6-2 The Functions of Body Proteins

1. Growth and Maintenance
- Proteins provide *building materials*—amino acids—for growth and repair of body tissues.
- *Body structures.* Proteins form vital parts of most body structures, such as skin, nails, hair, membranes, muscles, teeth, bones, organs, ligaments, and tendons.

2. Regulatory Roles
- *Enzymes.* Proteins facilitate numerous chemical reactions in the body; all enzymes are proteins.
- *Hormones.* Some proteins act as chemical messengers, regulating body processes; not all hormones are proteins. Examples include insulin, glucagon, and thyroid hormone.
- *Antibodies.* Proteins assist the body in maintaining its resistance to disease by acting against foreign disease-causing substances.
- *Fluid balance.* Proteins help regulate the quantity of fluids in body compartments.
- *Acid–base balance.* Proteins act as buffers to maintain the normal acid and base concentrations in body fluids.
- *Transportation.* Proteins move needed nutrients (e.g., minerals, lipids) and other substances, such as oxygen, into and out of cells and around the body.

3. Energy and Glucose Production
- *Energy.* Protein can be used to provide calories (4 calories per gram) to help meet the body's energy needs.
- *Glucose production.* Some amino acids can be converted to glucose as a fuel source for the brain and nervous system when carbohydrate intake is inadequate.

protein synthesis The process by which cells assemble amino acids into proteins. All individuals are unique because of minute differences in the ways their body proteins are made. The instructions for making all the proteins in our bodies are transmitted in the genetic information we receive at conception.

peptide bond A bond that connects one amino acid with another.

denaturation A change in the shape of a protein brought about by heat, alcohol, acids, bases, salts of heavy metals, or other agents.

FIGURE 6-3

Enzyme Action

Each enzyme facilitates a specific chemical reaction.

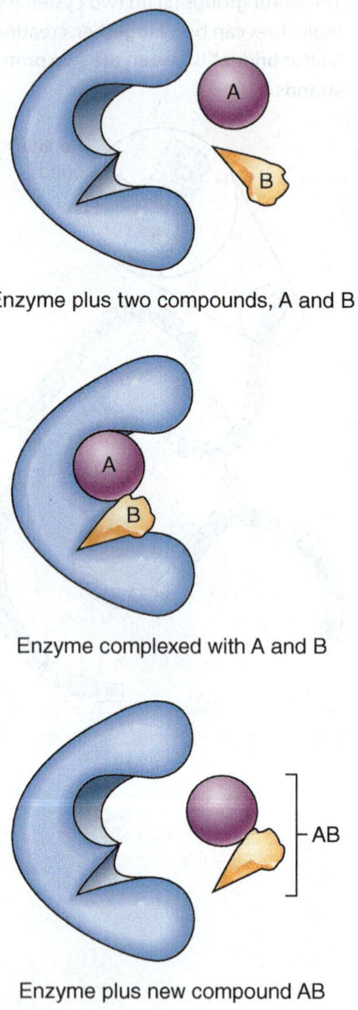

to the enzyme and then to each other. The newly formed product is then expelled by the enzyme into the fluid of the cell (see Figure 6-3). Enzymes are the hands-on workers in the production and processing of all substances needed by the body.

Hormones

Hormones are similar to enzymes in exerting profound effects. However, hormone molecules differ from enzyme molecules. For one thing, not all of them are made of protein. For another, hormones do not catalyze chemical reactions directly; rather, they act as messengers that elicit the appropriate responses to maintain a normal environment in the body. Hormones regulate overall body conditions, such as the blood glucose level (the hormones insulin and glucagon) and the metabolic rate (thyroid hormone).

Antibodies

Of all the great variety of proteins in living organisms, **antibodies** best demonstrate that proteins are specific to individual organisms. Antibodies form in response to the presence of *antigens* (foreign proteins or other large molecules) that invade the body. The foreign protein may be part of a bacterium, a virus, or a toxin, or it may be something present in food that causes a reaction we call an *allergy*. The Nutrition Action feature later in this chapter discusses the problem of protein-related food allergies in children and adults. The body, after recognizing that it has been invaded, manufactures antibodies that deactivate the foreign substance. Without sufficient protein to make antibodies, the body cannot maintain its resistance to disease.

One of the most fascinating aspects of the antibody response to foreign substances is that each antibody is uniquely designed to destroy a specific foreign substance. An antibody that has been manufactured to combat one strain of flu virus is of no help in protecting a person against another strain. Once the body has learned to make a particular antibody, it never forgets, and the next time it encounters that same foreign substance, it will be equipped to destroy it even more rapidly. In other words, the body develops an **immunity**. This is the principle underlying the effectiveness of the vaccines that have nearly eradicated most childhood diseases in the Western world.

Clearly, malnutrition injures the immune system. Without adequate protein in the diet, the immune system will not be able to make its specialized cells and the other tools required to function optimally. Often, protein deficiency and immune incompetence appear together. For this reason, measles can be fatal to a malnourished child.

Many nutrients other than proteins participate in conferring immunity, and many factors other than antibodies are involved.[1] Nevertheless, the immune system is extraordinarily sensitive to nutrition, and almost any nutrient deficit can impair its efficiency and reduce resistance to disease.

Fluid Balance

Proteins help regulate the quantity of fluids in the compartments of the body (see Figure 6-4). To remain alive, a cell must contain a constant amount of fluid; this is known as the **fluid balance**. Too much fluid might cause a cell to rupture, and too little would make it unable to function. Although water can diffuse freely into and out of the cell, proteins cannot—and proteins attract water. By maintaining a store of internal proteins, the cell retains the fluid it needs. (It also uses minerals this way.) Similarly, the cells secrete proteins (and minerals) into the spaces between them to keep the fluid volume constant in those spaces. Also, because the proteins secreted into the blood cannot cross the blood vessel walls, they help to maintain the blood volume in the same way.

hormones Chemical messengers. Hormones are secreted by a variety of glands in the body in response to altered conditions. Each affects one or more target tissues or organs and elicits specific responses to restore normal conditions.

antibodies Large proteins of the blood and body fluids that are produced by one type of immune cell in response to invasion of the body by unfamiliar molecules (mostly foreign proteins). Antibodies inactivate the foreign substances and so protect the body. The foreign substances are called *antigens*.

immunity Specific disease resistance derived from the immune system's memory of prior exposure to specific disease agents and its ability to mount a swift response against them.

fluid balance Distribution of fluid among body compartments.

Acid–Base Balance

Normal processes of the body continually produce **acids** and their opposite, **bases**, which must be carried by the blood to the organs of excretion. The blood must do this without allowing its own **acid–base balance** to be affected. To accomplish this, some proteins act as **buffers** to maintain the blood's normal **pH** between 7.35 and 7.45 (see the pH scale in Figure 6-5). They pick up hydrogen **ions** when there are too many in the blood (the more hydrogen, the more concentrated the acid). Likewise, protein buffers release hydrogens again when there are too few in the blood. The secret is that the negatively charged side chains of the amino acids can accommodate additional hydrogens (which are positively charged) when necessary.

FIGURE 6-4
Fluid Balance
Shown here are the fluids within and surrounding a cell. Body proteins help hold fluid within cells, tissues, and blood vessels.

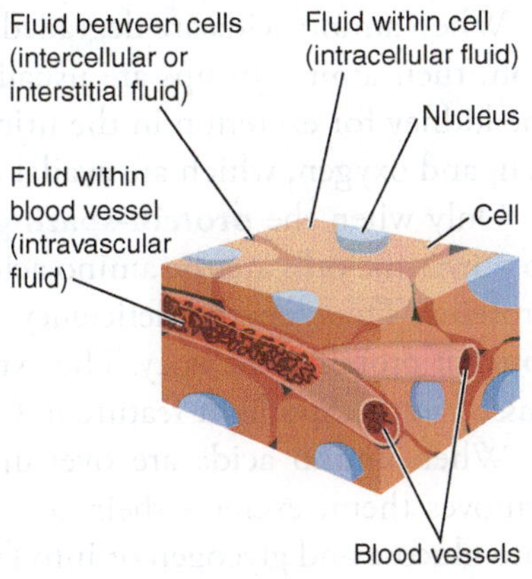

FIGURE 6-5
pH Values of Selected Fluids
A fluid's acidity or alkalinity is measured in pH units.

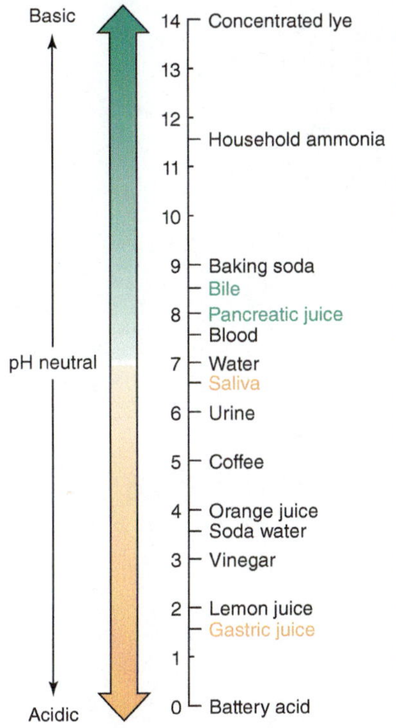

The acid–base balance of the blood is one of the most accurately controlled conditions in the body. If it changes too much, either the dangerous acidic condition called **acidosis** or the opposite basic condition, **alkalosis**, can cause coma or death. The hazards of these conditions are a result of their effect on proteins. When the proteins' buffering capacity is exceeded—for example, when proteins have taken on board or released all the acid hydrogens they can—additional acid or base deranges protein structures by pulling them out of shape; that is, it denatures the proteins—rendering them useless. Knowing how indispensable the structures of proteins are to their functions and how vital protein functions are to life, you can imagine how many body processes would be halted by such a disturbance.

Transport Proteins

A specific group of the body's proteins specializes in moving nutrients and other molecules into and out of cells. Some of these **transport proteins** act as pumps, picking up compounds on one side of the membrane and depositing them on the other, and thereby regulating what substances the cell will take up or release. One such pump is the "sodium–potassium pump," which resides in the cell membrane and acts as a revolving door, picking up potassium from outside the cell and depositing it inside the cell, and picking up sodium from within the cell and depositing it outside the cell as necessary. The protein machinery of cell membranes can be switched on or off in response to the body's needs. Often hormones do the switching with marvelous precision.

Other transport proteins move about in the body fluids, carrying nutrients and other molecules from one organ to another. Those that carry lipids in the lipoproteins are examples. Special proteins also can carry fat-soluble vitamins, water-soluble vitamins, and minerals. As a result, a protein deficiency can cause a deficiency of vitamin A or any other nutrient that needs a transport protein to reach its destination in the body.

This sampling of the major roles proteins play in the body illustrates their versatility, uniqueness, and importance. All the body's tissues and organs—muscles, bones, blood, skin, and nerves—are made largely of proteins. No wonder proteins are said to be the primary material of life.

acids Compounds that release hydrogens in a watery solution; acids have a low pH.

bases Compounds that accept hydrogens from a watery solution; bases have a high pH.

acid–base balance Equilibrium between acid and base concentrations in the body fluids.

buffers Compounds that help keep the acidity (amount of acid) or alkalinity (amount of base) of a solution constant.

pH The concentration of hydrogen ions. The lower the pH, the stronger the acid: pH 2 is a strong acid, pH 7 is neutral, and a pH above 7 is alkaline (a base).

ions (EYE-onz) Electrically charged particles, such as sodium (positively charged) and chloride (negatively charged).

acidosis (a-sih-DOSE-is) Blood acidity above normal, indicating excess acid.

alkalosis (al-kuh-LOW-sis) Blood alkalinity above normal.

transport proteins Proteins that either carry nutrients and other molecules in body fluids or reside in cell membranes and act as "pumps" by picking up compounds on one side of the membrane and releasing them on the other side as needed.

Protein as Energy Only protein can perform all the functions previously described, but it will be sacrificed to provide needed energy if insufficient fat and carbohydrate are available from the diet. The body's number one need is for energy. All other needs have a lower priority. Many amino acids can also be converted to glucose as a fuel source for the brain and nervous system during periods of starvation or when carbohydrate intake is inadequate.

When amino acids are degraded so they can be used for energy or glucose production, their amine groups are usually incorporated by the liver into **urea** and sent to the kidney for excretion in the urine. The remaining components are carbon, hydrogen, and oxygen, which are available for immediate energy use by the body.

Only when the **protein-sparing** calories from carbohydrate and fat are sufficient to power the cells are the amino acids used for their most important function: making proteins. Thus, energy deficiency (starvation) is always accompanied by the symptoms of protein deficiency. The extent and severity of malnutrition worldwide is discussed in the Spotlight feature in Chapter 13.

When amino acids are oversupplied, the body has no place to store them. It removes them, excretes their amine groups, and converts the remaining fragments into glucose and glycogen or into fat for energy storage. Amino acids are not stored in the body except in the sense that they are present in proteins in all the tissues. When there is a great shortage of amino acids, the body must break down such tissues as blood, muscle, and skin so that it can use their amino acids to maintain the heart, lungs, and brain.

6.3 How the Body Handles Protein

When a person eats a food protein, whether from cereals, vegetables, meats, or dairy products, the digestive system breaks down the protein and delivers the separated amino acids to the body cells. The cells then put the amino acids together in the order necessary to produce the particular proteins they need. (To review the digestive and absorptive systems relevant to the body's handling of protein, turn to Chapter 3.)

The stomach initiates protein digestion (see Figure 6-6). By the time proteins move into the small intestine, they are already broken into different-sized pieces: some single amino acids and many strands of two amino acids, **dipeptides**; some strands of three amino acids, **tripeptides**; and some longer chains. Digestion continues until almost all pieces of protein are broken into dipeptides, tripeptides, and free amino acids. Absorption of amino acids takes place all along the small intestine. Dipeptides and tripeptides are captured on the surface of the cells that line the small intestine. These cells split the peptides into amino acids, absorb them, and then release them into the bloodstream.

Once they are circulating in the bloodstream, the amino acids are available to be taken up by any cell of the body. The cells can use them to make proteins, either for the cell's own use or for secretion into the circulatory system for other uses.

If a *non*essential amino acid (that is, one the body can make for itself) is unavailable for a growing protein strand, the cell will make one and will continue attaching amino acids to the strand. If, however, an essential amino acid (one the body cannot make) is missing, the building of the protein will halt. The cell cannot hold partially completed proteins to complete them later, for example, the next day. Instead, it must dismantle the partial structures and return surplus amino acids to the circulation, making them available to other cells. If other cells do not

urea (yoo-REE-uh) The principal nitrogen excretion product of metabolism, generated mostly by the removal of amine groups from unneeded amino acids or from those amino acids being sacrificed to a need for energy.

protein-sparing A description of the effect of carbohydrate and fat, which, by being available to yield energy, allow amino acids to be used to build body proteins.

dipeptides (dye-PEP-tides) Protein fragments two amino acids long. A *peptide* is a strand of amino acids.

tripeptides (try-PEP-tides) Protein fragments three amino acids long.

FIGURE 6-6

A Summary of Protein Digestion and Absorption

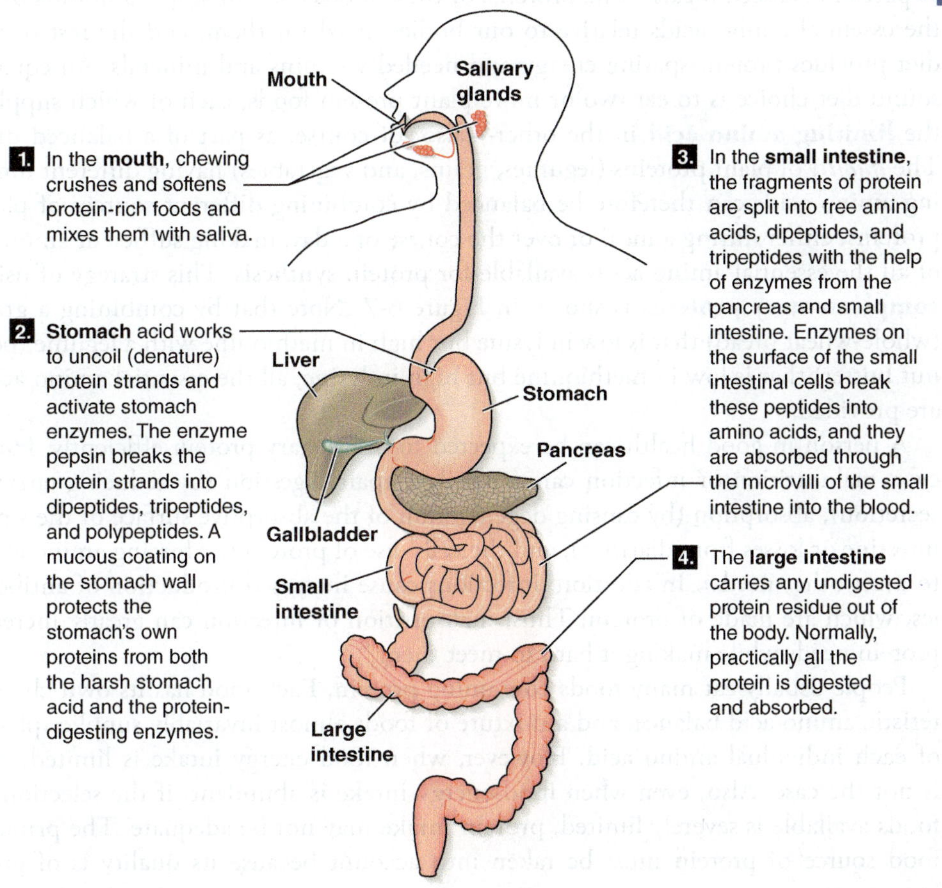

soon pick up these amino acids and insert them into protein, the liver will remove their amine groups for the kidney to excrete. Other cells will then use the remaining fragments for other purposes. The need for the production of that particular protein will not be met.

6.4 Protein Quality of Foods

The role of protein in food, as already mentioned, is not to provide body proteins directly but to supply the amino acids from which the body can make its own proteins. Because body cells cannot store amino acids for future use, it follows that all the essential amino acids must be eaten as part of a balanced diet. To manufacture body proteins, then, all the needed amino acids must be available to the cells. Three important characteristics of dietary protein, therefore, are (1) that it should supply at least the nine essential amino acids, (2) that it should supply enough other amino acids to make nitrogen available for the synthesis of whatever nonessential amino acids the cell may need to make, and (3) that it should be accompanied by enough food energy (preferably from carbohydrate and fat) to prevent sacrifice of its own amino acids for energy.

This presents no problem to people who regularly eat **high-quality proteins,** such as those of meat, fish, poultry, cheese, eggs, milk, or many soybean products,

high-quality proteins Proteins containing all the essential amino acids in the right proportion relative to need. The *quality* of a food protein is judged by the proportions of essential amino acids that it contains relative to our needs. Animal and soy proteins are the highest in quality.

FIGURE 6-7

How Two Plant Proteins Combine to Yield a Complete Protein

Two incomplete proteins (for example, legumes plus grains) can be combined to equal a complete protein (peanut butter sandwich). In this example, the peanut butter provides adequate amounts of the amino acid lysine but is lacking in methionine. The bread "complements" the peanut butter because it contains adequate methionine but is lacking in lysine. When these foods are combined as a sandwich, all essential amino acids are present.

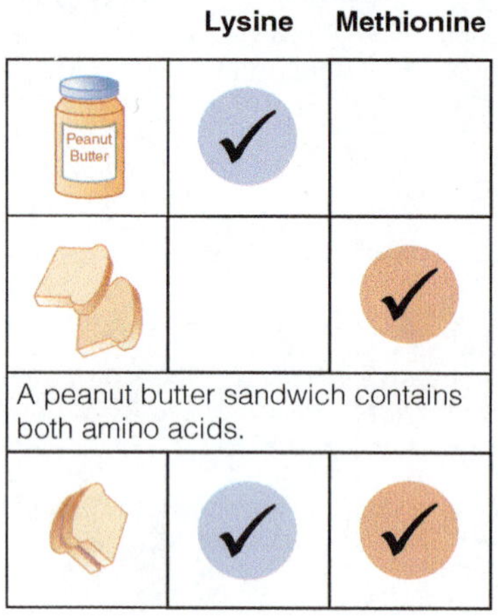

as part of balanced meals.[2] The proteins of these foods contain ample amounts of all the essential amino acids relative to our bodies' need for them, and the rest of the diet provides protein-sparing energy and needed vitamins and minerals. An equally sound diet choice is to eat two or more plant protein foods, each of which supplies the **limiting amino acid** in the other—also, of course, as part of a balanced diet. The *quality* of plant proteins (legumes, grains, and vegetables) having different limiting amino acids can therefore be balanced by combining different sources of plant proteins, either during a meal or over the course of a day, making sufficient amounts of all the essential amino acids available for protein synthesis. This strategy of using **complementary proteins** is shown in Figure 6-7. Note that by combining a grain (whole-wheat bread) that is low in lysine but high in methionine with a legume (peanut butter) that is low in methionine but high in lysine, all the essential amino acids are provided.

A person in good health can be expected to use dietary protein efficiently. However, malnutrition or infection can seriously impair digestion (by reducing enzyme secretion), absorption (by causing degeneration of the absorptive surface of the small intestine or losses from diarrhea), and the cells' use of protein (by forcing amino acids to meet other needs). In addition, infections cause increased production of antibodies, which are made of protein. Thus, malnutrition or infection can greatly increase protein needs while making it hard to meet them.[3]

People usually eat many foods containing protein. Each food has its own characteristic amino acid balance, and a mixture of foods almost invariably supplies plenty of each individual amino acid. However, when food energy intake is limited, this is not the case. Also, even when food-energy intake is abundant, if the selection of foods available is severely limited, protein intake may not be adequate. The primary food source of protein must be taken into account because its quality is of great importance.

Researchers have studied many different individual foods as protein sources and have developed many different methods of evaluating the **protein quality** of foods. Protein quality is determined by two factors—the protein's digestibility and its amino acid composition. One method of evaluating protein quality judges how easily the body can digest and absorb the protein. In general, amino acids from animal and soy proteins are the most easily digested and absorbed (90 to 99 percent). Amino acids from other legumes are next best (80 to 90 percent); the digestibility of grains and other plant foods vary (70 to 90 percent). The best guarantee of amino acid adequacy is to eat a variety of foods containing protein in the presence of adequate amounts of vitamins, minerals, and energy from carbohydrate and fat.

6.5 Recommended Protein Intakes

Recommended protein intakes can be stated in two ways: as a percentage of total calories, or as an absolute number (grams per day). The DRI committee recommends that protein provide 10 to 35 percent of total caloric intake.[4] The recommended protein allowance for a healthy adult is 0.8 gram per kilogram (or 2.2 pounds) of desirable body weight per day.

The recommendation for protein uses the desirable, not the actual, weight for a given height, because the desirable weight is proportional to the *lean* body mass of the average person. Lean body mass, not total weight, determines protein need. This is because fat tissue is composed largely of fat, which does not require much protein for maintenance.

limiting amino acid A term given to the essential amino acid in shortest supply (relative to the body's need) in a food protein; it therefore *limits* the body's ability to make its own proteins.

complementary proteins Two or more food proteins whose amino acid assortments complement each other in such a way that the essential amino acids limited in or missing from each are supplied by the others.

protein quality A measure of the essential amino acid content of a protein relative to the essential amino acid needs of the body.

The recommendations for protein intake are based on the assumption that the protein source will be a combination of plant and animal proteins, that it will be consumed with adequate calories from carbohydrate and fat, and that other nutrients in the diet will be adequate. These protein recommendations apply only to healthy individuals with no unusual metabolic need for protein. Chapter 11 discusses the protein needs of athletes, and the Spotlight in Chapter 11 presents the pros and cons of using popular amino acid and other supplements.

Although protein is essential to health, the body converts extra protein to energy (glucose), which is stored as body fat when energy needs are met. Despite the flood of new protein-packed snack bars and other products in the marketplace, there are no known benefits from consuming excess protein. The recommended upper range for protein intake applies *when calorie intake is adequate.* Note the qualification "when calorie intake is adequate" in the preceding statement. Remember that your recommended protein intake can be stated as a percentage of calories in the diet or as a specific number of grams of dietary protein. The recommended protein intake for a 150-pound person is roughly 55 grams, or about 12 percent of their daily caloric intake. Fifty-five grams of protein is equal to 220 calories and equals 11 percent of a 2,000-calorie intake, which is reasonable for a 150-pound active person. If this person were to drastically reduce his or her caloric intake to, say, 800 calories a day, then 220 calories from protein is suddenly 28 percent of the total. However, it is still this person's recommended intake for protein, and a reasonable intake. It is the caloric intake that is unreasonable in this example. Similarly, if the person eats too many calories—say, 4,000—this protein intake represents only 6 percent of the total caloric intake, yet it is still a reasonable intake. It is the caloric intake that may be unreasonable.

Thus, it is important to be careful when judging protein intakes as a percentage of calories. Always ask what the absolute number of grams is, too, and compare it with the recommended protein intake in grams. As calorie intake decreases, it is necessary to increase the percentage of calories from protein so as to consume the RDA for protein. Recommendations stated as a percentage of calories are useful only when food energy intakes (calories) are within reason. Calculate your own protein needs using the "Calculation Practice" in the margin.

6.6 Choosing Protein-Rich Foods

Misconceived notions abound regarding protein in the diet; the most obvious of these is that more is better. American women eat about 60 to 65 grams of protein a day, notably higher than the recommended 46 grams a day. Young men average about 100 grams a day and drop to about 75 to 85 grams as older adults, still considerably higher than their recommended intake of 56 grams. Moreover, more than 65 percent of this protein comes from animal and dairy products. Poultry and red meat have consistently provided the highest share of protein (see Figure 6-8), while average intakes of seafood are low for all age groups.

Protein foods are sorted into three subgroups—seafood (fish and shellfish); meats, poultry, and eggs; and unsalted nuts, seeds, and soy products (refer to Figure 2-12 on page 46). Protein-rich foods also include dairy foods and legumes. In addition to protein, these foods contribute B vitamins, vitamin D, vitamin E, iron, zinc, copper, selenium, phosphorus, choline, and magnesium to the diet. The fats in meat, poultry, and eggs are considered solid fats, while the fats in seafood, nuts, and seeds are considered oils.

Calculation Practice

To calculate the percentage of calories you derive from protein:

1. Use your total calories as the denominator (example: 1,900 cal).
2. Multiply your total protein intake in *grams* by 4 cal/g to obtain calories from protein as the numerator (example: 70 g protein × 4 cal/g = 280 cal).
3. Divide to obtain a decimal, multiply by 100, and round off (example: 280/1,900 × 100 = 15% cal from protein).

To calculate your recommended protein intake (RDA):

1. Find the desirable weight for a person your height (see Appendix A). Assume that this weight is appropriate for you.
2. Change pounds to kilograms (divide pounds by 2.2; 1 kilogram = 2.2 pounds).
3. Multiply kilograms by 0.8 g/kg.

Example (for a 5′8" male):

1. Desirable weight: about 150 lb.
2. 150 lb ÷ 2.2 lb = 68 kg (rounded off).
3. 68 kg × 0.8 g/kg = 54 g protein (rounded off).

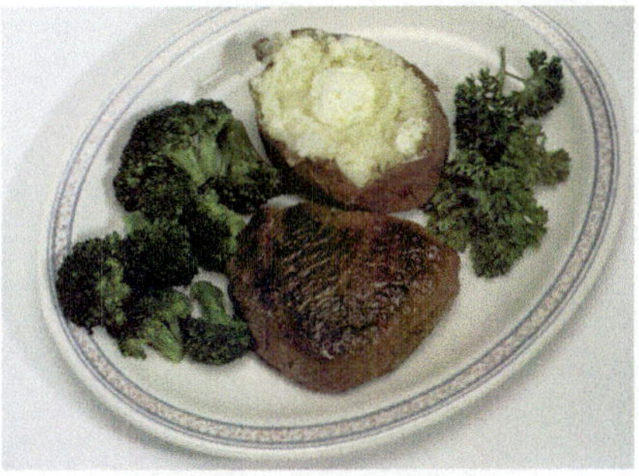
PhotoDisc/Getty Images

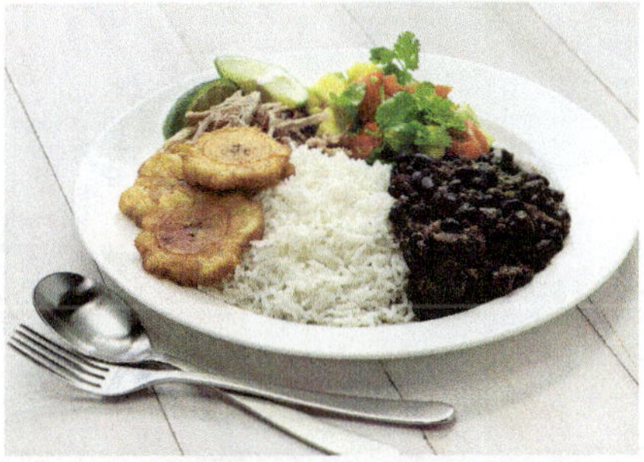
bonchan/Shutterstock.com

Both meals shown here supply an adequate assortment of amino acids needed for health.

FIGURE 6-8

Protein Contributed by Food Groups in the Average American Diet

Commonly consumed protein foods include beef (especially ground beef), chicken, pork, processed meats (e.g., hot dogs, sausages, ham, luncheon meats), and eggs. The most common seafood choices are shrimp, tuna, and salmon, and the most common nut choices are peanuts, peanut butter, almonds, and mixed nuts. Animal protein sources supply about 60 percent of the protein available in the U.S. food supply. Within the meats, poultry, and eggs subgroup, red meat and poultry (primarily chicken) have consistently provided the highest share of protein—about 35 percent. Seafood contributes about 4 percent. Grain products provide about 22 percent, while dairy products supply nearly one-fifth of the protein.

SOURCE: What We Eat in America, NHANES 2007–2010; U.S. Department of Health and Human Services and U.S. Department of Agriculture. *2015–2020 Dietary Guidelines for Americans*. 8th Edition. December 2015.

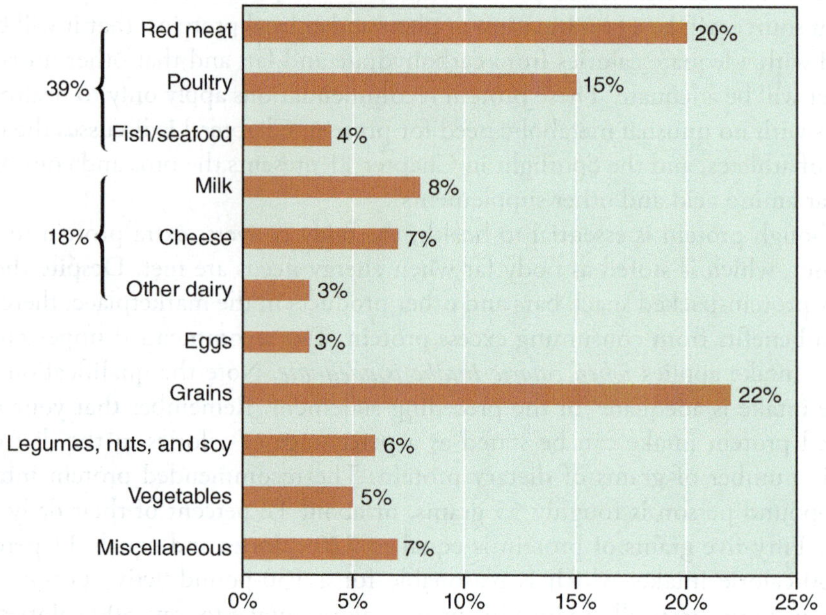

The *Dietary Guidelines for Americans* recommend including a *variety* of protein sources in nutrient-dense forms, because nutrients provided by various types of protein foods differ. For example, meats provide the most zinc, while poultry provides the most niacin. Seafood provides the most vitamin B_{12} and vitamin D, in addition to omega-3 fatty acids. Eggs provide the most choline, and nuts and seeds provide the most vitamin E. Soy products are a source of copper, manganese, and iron, as are legumes.[5]

The higher a person's intake of animal-protein sources such as meat, the more likely that fruits, vegetables, and whole grains will be crowded out of the diet, creating deficiencies of other nutrients. You can better balance your food choices by selecting one-third or less of your protein from animal sources and the rest from plants. (See the Eat Well Be Well feature later in this chapter.) To limit your intake of solid fat, consider the following tips when shopping for protein-rich foods:

- Dairy foods are excellent sources of protein, calcium, and other important nutrients. Look for fat-free and low-fat varieties for the recommended three servings each day. Look for low-fat cheeses that have less than 5 grams of

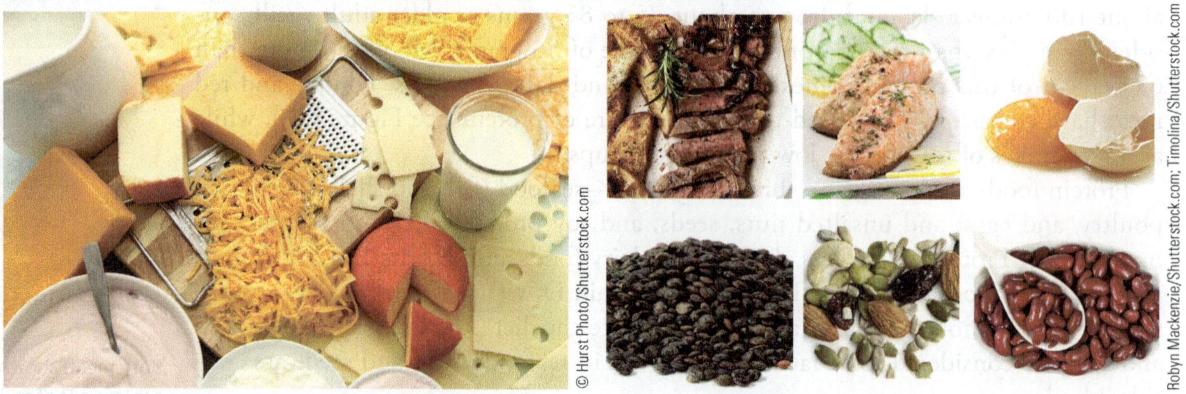

Foods that supply high-quality protein in abundance are shown here in the Dairy group (milk, yogurt, cheese) and the Protein Foods group (meat, poultry, seafood, beans and peas, soy products, eggs, nuts and seeds) of the MyPlate food guide.

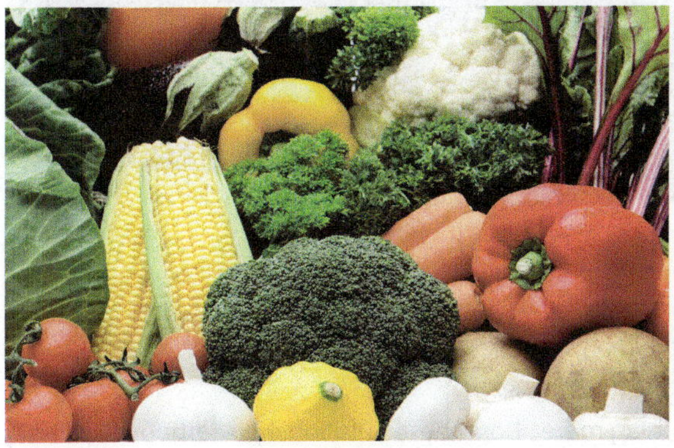
© Jill Chen/Shutterstock.com

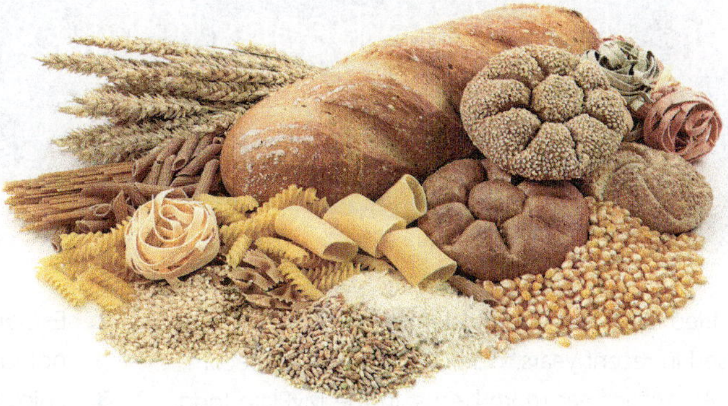
Elena Schweitzer/Shutterstock.com

Servings of foods from the Vegetable group and the Grains group can also contribute smaller amounts of protein to the diet.

fat per ounce, such as part-skim or fat-free ricotta or mozzarella, feta cheese, string cheese, or other reduced-calorie cheeses. These choices are lower in saturated fat and calories than their full-fat counterparts.

- Fish and shellfish—fresh, frozen, or canned in water—make excellent protein choices and are low in fat. Besides protein, seafood notably contributes the omega-3 fatty acids, eicosapentaenoic acid (EPA) and docosahexaenoic acid (DHA), which may lower risk for heart disease. Experts recommend that you eat at least two fish meals per week—a total of 8 or more ounces per week (less for young children) of a variety of seafood.
- Meat, chicken, and fish all provide excellent protein, as well as iron, zinc, and vitamin B_{12}. We are advised to choose meat and poultry in lean forms to decrease intake of solid fats. Look for the leanest meats:
    - Flank steak, round steak, sirloin, tenderloin, or extra lean ground beef
    - Lean ham, Canadian bacon, pork tenderloin, and center-loin pork chops
    - Chicken, turkey, or game hens without the skin; fresh ground turkey breast or chicken breast meat
- At the deli counter, select items with less than 1 gram of fat per ounce, such as lean ham, turkey, or chicken breast, and lean roast beef.
- Nuts, seeds, and nut butters are good sources of protein but are also high in calories. Look for nonhydrogenated varieties. A 1-tablespoon serving of peanut butter or ½ ounce of nuts or seeds counts as 1 ounce of meat in the MyPlate food guide.
- Eggs are another excellent source of protein. Also look for egg substitutes, and substitute ¼ cup for one whole egg in recipes. One egg counts as 1 ounce of meat.
- Many interesting sources of protein are available. Try adding **legumes** to your meals using the tips in the Savvy Diner feature that follows. A ¼-cup serving counts as 1 ounce of meat in the MyPlate food guide.

As vegetarians know, one can easily design a perfectly acceptable diet around plant foods alone by choosing an appropriate variety. This chapter's Spotlight discusses the benefits of vegetarian eating patterns and the use of soy products, an excellent source of protein in the diet.

Adequate protein in the diet is easy to obtain. A breakfast of one egg, two slices of wheat bread, and a glass of milk provide nearly 20 grams of protein. This meets about 35 percent of an average man's recommended protein intake of 56 grams and about 43 percent of a woman's recommended protein intake of 46 grams. The Scorecard feature in this chapter shows you how to estimate your own protein intake.

legumes (LEG-yoomz or leh-GYOOMZ) Plants of the bean and pea family having roots with nodules containing bacteria that can trap nitrogen from the air in the soil and make it into compounds that become part of the seed. The seeds are rich in high-quality protein compared with those of most other plant foods.

THE **SAVVY** Diner

Eat More Beans (Obj. 6.6)

Legumes—dried beans, peas, and lentils—have been very highly praised in recent years.[6] The *Dietary Guidelines* recommend that Americans eat more beans. In the MyPlate food guide, legumes are the only food featured in two different categories, the Vegetables group and the Protein Foods group. Legumes are rich in the B vitamins and fiber. They are good sources of protein, iron, and zinc and are naturally low in fat and are cholesterol free. The Food and Drug Administration approved a health claim for bean packages and cans: "Diets including beans may reduce your risk of heart disease and certain cancers."[7] However, Americans typically eat only about half the recommended amount of legumes: one cup instead of the recommended 1.5 to 2 cups per week for a 2,000-calorie diet (see bean recommendations for other calorie levels at www.ChooseMyPlate.gov).

Here are three simple ways to increase your intake of this low-cost, easy-to-include group of foods:

1. Enjoy adding more legumes to your weekly meals. Include legumes in entrees (tacos), side dishes (baked beans), soups (split pea or lentil), and salads (chickpeas from the salad bar, or three-bean combos). Recipes can be prepared from dried beans (soaked, rinsed, and cooked) or more quickly from canned beans (rinsed to remove excess sodium). Thorough rinsing is recommended to remove the gas-causing sugar, known as *raffinose*, found in beans.
2. Explore the many varieties of legumes used in cooking—as noted in the Miniglossary.
3. Enjoy learning more about these nutritional powerhouses online. The following three sites can help:
   - *American Dry Bean Board:* www.americanbean.org. Includes bean basics, photos, health tips, and 1,001 recipes.
   - *U.S. Dry Bean Council:* www.usdrybeans.com. A more global focus, with many links and a useful bibliography.
   - *USA Dry Pea & Lentil Council:* www.pea-lentil.com. Nutrition information, cooking instructions, and recipes.

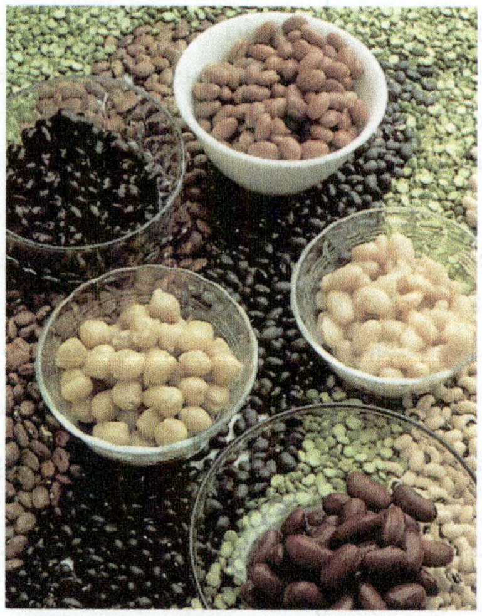

© Tom McCarthy Photography

Legumes include such plant foods as the soybean, kidney bean, garbanzo bean, black bean, lentil, garden pea, black-eyed pea, and lima bean.

Miniglossary of Legumes

black, Cuban, or turtle beans Medium-size, black-skinned oval beans that have a rich, sweet taste. They are best served in Mexican and Latin American dishes or thick soups and stews.

black-eyed peas Small, oval-shaped, creamy-white peas with a black spot. They have a vegetable flavor with mealy texture. Use in salads with rice and greens.

garbanzo beans or chickpeas Large, round, tan-colored legumes that have a nutty flavor and crunchy texture. Use in soups and stews and puréed for dips.

Great Northern beans A medium-white, kidney-shaped bean. Enjoy the delicate flavor and firm texture in salads, soups, and main dishes.

kidney beans These familiar beans are large, red, and kidney shaped (the white variety is called *cannellini*). They have a bland taste and soft texture but tough skins. Use in chili, bean stews, and Mexican dishes (for red) or Italian dishes (for white).

lentils Small, flat, and round legumes. Usually brown, lentils can also be green, pink, or red. They have a mild taste with firm texture. Best used when combined with grains or vegetables in salads, soups, or stews.

lima or butter beans Limas are soft and mealy in texture. They are flat, oval shaped, and white tinged with green. The smaller variety has a milder taste. Use in soups and stews.

pinto beans These medium-size, oval beans are mottled beige and brown and have an earthy flavor. They are most often used in Mexican dishes, such as refried beans, stews, or dips.

red beans These versatile beans are medium-size, dark-red oval. The taste and texture are similar to kidney beans. Use in soups and stews, and serve with rice.

soybeans You can find these creamy white ovals in numerous food products, such as tofu, flour, grits, and milk. They have a firm texture and bland flavor. See the Spotlight feature later in this chapter for a Miniglossary of the many readily available foods containing soy.

split peas Green or yellow, these small, halved peas supply an earthy flavor with a mealy texture. They are best used in soups and with rice or grains.

white navy beans These small, white, oval beans are best used in soups and stews and as baked beans.

SOURCE: Adapted from K. Mangum, *Life's Simple Pleasures: Fine Vegetarian Cooking for Sharing and Celebration* (Boise, ID: Pacific Press, 1990), 149.

Make Over Your Plate—Reshaping Your Protein Choices for Health (Obj. 6.6)

"The ancient inhabitants of South America liked to eat a kind of paste made from peanuts. But modern peanut butter came into being around 1890 as the bright idea of a St. Louis physician, who thought it would be a good health food for elderly people. It was not linked with jelly until the 1920s."[8]

Many health organizations now recommend a diet that emphasizes vegetables, fruits, legumes, and whole grains to protect against cancer, heart disease, stroke, diabetes, and obesity.[9] The key to getting enough, but not too much, protein seems to be to use a variety of plant-based foods and to de-emphasize meats.[10]

1 In the Kitchen.

- Small meat portions tend to work best when mixed into dishes with lots of vegetables and grains; try stir-fries, pastas, soups and stews, burritos, and main-dish salads. For example, cook a large pot of soup, stew, or chili. Minimize the amount of meat you use, and load up the pot with vegetables (fresh or frozen) and cooked beans.

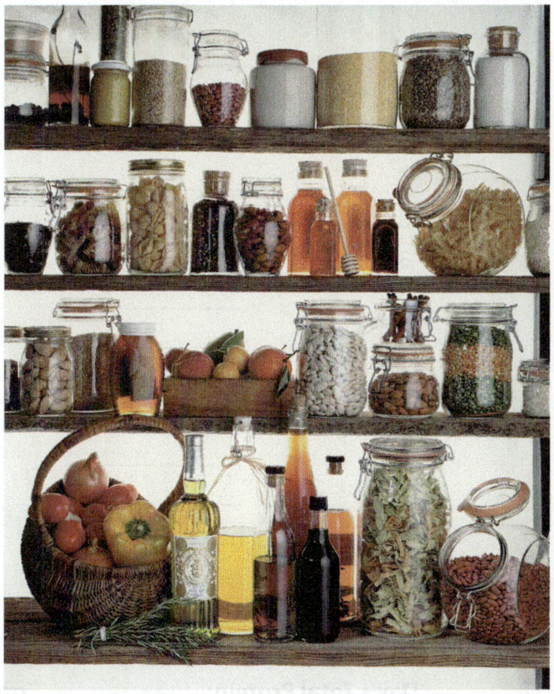

PhotoDisc/Getty Images

- Go meatless one or more days each week. Experiment with recipes from health-minded cookbooks and websites.
- Take a fresh look at your favorite recipes. Try to use less meat and add more vegetables. Instead of chicken and broccoli stir-fry, try stir-fried veggies with a little chicken.
- For quick, colorful, meals rich in nutrients and flavor, try various combinations of stir-fried vegetables on beds of steamed brown rice, whole-grain bulgur, quinoa, or couscous.

2 In the Lunch Box.

- Get out of the peanut butter and jelly rut by filling sandwiches with water-packed tuna mixed with mandarin oranges, bean sprouts, and a bit of plain low-fat yogurt; chopped, cooked, skinless chicken combined with raw sliced vegetables and a little French dressing; cooked, mashed dried beans seasoned with chopped onion, garlic powder, rosemary, thyme, and pepper; or low-fat cottage cheese flavored with drained, chopped pineapple.
- Take a thermos filled with chili, vegetable soup, or a milk-based soup, such as cream of tomato prepared with nonfat milk, instead of a sandwich. Try cold lunches such as low-fat yogurt and fruit, brown rice with cubes of skinless poultry, or cooked pasta tossed with raw vegetables, low-fat cheese, and a bit of Italian dressing.

3 At the Table.

- When dining out, choose an ethnic restaurant with plant-based entrées on the menu. Consider Spanish paella, Asian stir-fries, Moroccan stew, Indian curries, or French ratatouille as your entrée. Or try Chinese, Vietnamese, or Thai take-out with brown rice and lots of vegetables.
- Twice a week, make seafood the protein on your plate.
- Eat more legumes as well as red, orange, and dark green vegetables, such as tomatoes, sweet potatoes, and broccoli.
- Make whole grains, vegetables, and legumes the main event of your meals. At least two-thirds of your meal should come from these plant-based foods and one-third or less from lean meat, poultry, fish, or low-fat dairy products.

SCORE Card

Estimate Your Protein Intake (Obj. 6.6)

The average American consumes much more than his or her recommended protein intake. How do you compare? First, figure your recommended protein intake (divide your weight in pounds by 2.2 and then multiply by 0.8). Next, write down everything you ate and drank yesterday. Using the values given below, estimate the grams of protein you ate from both animal and plant sources. How close are you to your recommended protein intake? What percentage of your protein comes from animal versus plant sources?

Recommended Protein Intake: __________ grams

Protein Foods	Amount	Grams of Protein*	Grams of Protein in Your Typical Diet
Animal Sources			
Hard cheese (e.g., cheddar)	1 oz	7	______
Cottage cheese	1/2 c	14	______
Milk	1 c	8	______
Greek-style yogurt	6 oz	14	______
Traditional yogurt	6 oz	6	______
Egg	1 large	6	______
Fish	3 oz	21	______
Poultry	3 oz	21	______
Ground beef, lean	3 oz	21	______
Beef steak, lean	3 oz	21	______
Pork chop, lean	3 oz	21	______
Other	____	____	
		Animal Proteins Subtotal (grams):	______
Plant Sources			
Vegetables	1/2 c	2	______
Legumes, cooked	1/2 c	8	______
Tofu	3 oz	8	______
Cereals	1 c	2–6	______
Bread	1 slice	2	______
Tortilla	1	2	______
Rice, bulgur, couscous	1/2 c	3	______
Pasta	1/2 c	3	______
Peanut butter	1 tbsp	4	______
Nuts	1/2 oz	3	______
Seeds	2 tbsp	3	______
Other	____	____	
		Plant Proteins Subtotal (grams):	______
		Day's Total Protein:	______ **grams**

* Check the nutrition label for specific protein content.

Nutrition **ACTION**

6.7 Food Allergy—Nothing to Sneeze At

A mother of a 2-year-old discovered her son's food allergy the hard way when the young boy bit into a peanut candy. Within minutes, his face became red and swollen, then he started to vomit and showed trouble breathing. He was rushed to the emergency room, where the mother was told her son had anaphylaxis, a severe allergic reaction that can be life threatening. Follow-up testing confirmed that her son was highly allergic to peanuts.

The young boy in the story belongs to the estimated 3 percent of the population in the United States diagnosed with food allergies. Interestingly, although a relatively small percentage actually have food allergies, nearly 35 percent of people think they do.[11] What is the explanation? The answer may be in understanding the difference between **food allergy** and **food intolerance**. Although the physical responses to a food allergy and food intolerance may be very similar, the difference between the two is whether or not the immune system is involved in the reaction.

Food Intolerance versus Food Allergy

Food intolerance is far more common than food allergy. A food intolerance is an **adverse reaction** to food that *does not* involve the immune system. Lactose intolerance is one example of a food intolerance. A person with lactose intolerance lacks the enzyme needed to digest lactose. When that person eats milk products, symptoms such as gas, cramps, and bloating can occur. Some people may develop sensitivity to various other agents in a food. Tyramine, found in cheese or red wine, can induce a headache in some people. Others may have sensitivity to certain food additives, such as monosodium glutamate (MSG), sulfites, or coloring agents. The physical reactions to these agents can include hives, rashes, nasal congestion, or asthma.

A food allergy, in contrast, is an abnormal response to a food triggered by the immune system. The allergic reaction involves three main components: **food allergens**, immunoglobulin E (IgE), and mast cells. Food allergens are the fragments of food that are responsible for the allergic reaction. They consist of proteins from the food that are not broken down during the digestive process, which then cross the gastrointestinal lining to enter the bloodstream. IgE is a type of protein called an *antibody* that circulates through the blood. When allergic people eat certain foods, their immune system reacts to the food allergen by making IgE that is specific to that food. Once released, the IgE antibody attaches to a cell called the *mast cell.* Mast cells are specialized cells of the immune system that serve as the storehouse for various chemical substances, including **histamine**. Mast cells are found in all body tissues, but they are especially common in the areas of the body that are typical sites of allergic reaction: the nose and throat, lungs, skin, and gastrointestinal tract. When an allergic reaction occurs, the food allergen interacts with the IgE on the surface of the mast cells, which triggers those cells to release histamine. Depending on the tissue in which the histamine is released, these chemicals will cause a person to have various symptoms of a food allergy (see Figure 6-9). The most severe allergic reaction is **anaphylaxis**. This potentially fatal condition occurs when several parts of the body experience food allergy reactions at the same time. Signs of anaphylaxis include difficulty breathing, swelling of the mouth and throat, a drop in blood pressure, and loss of consciousness. The reaction can occur in a few seconds or minutes, and without immediate medical attention, death may result. The foods most associated with anaphylactic reactions include peanuts, tree nuts (for example, walnuts, cashews), eggs, and shellfish.

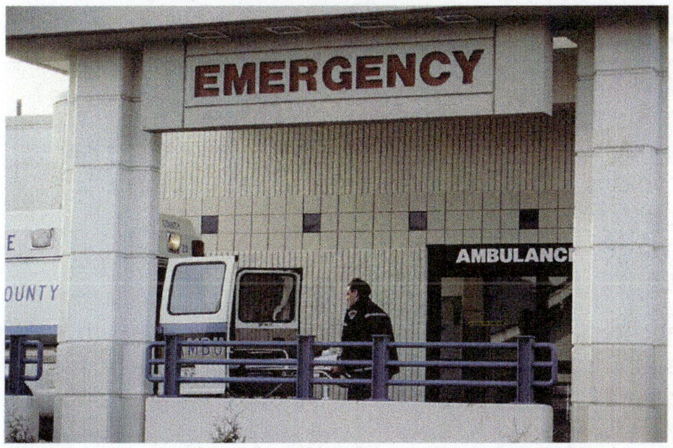

PhotoDisc/Getty Images

According to the Food Allergy Research and Education organization, eight foods cause 90 percent of all allergic reactions: egg, fish, milk, peanuts, shellfish, soy, tree nuts, and wheat.[12] In adults, the foods that most commonly cause allergic reactions include shellfish, peanuts, tree nuts, fish, and egg. In children, the problem foods are typically

food allergy An adverse reaction to an otherwise harmless substance that involves the body's immune system.

food intolerance A general term for any adverse reaction to a food or food component that does not involve the body's immune system.

adverse reaction An unusual response to food, including food allergies and food intolerances.

food allergen A substance in food (usually a protein) that is seen by the body as harmful and causes the immune system to mount an allergic reaction.

histamine A substance released by cells of the immune system during an allergic reaction to an antigen; causes inflammation, itching, hives, dilation of blood vessels, and a drop in blood pressure.

anaphylaxis (an-uh-fuh-LACKS-is) A potentially fatal reaction to a food allergen that causes reduced oxygen supply to the heart and other body tissues. Symptoms include difficulty breathing; low blood pressure; pale skin; a weak, rapid pulse; and loss of consciousness.

(Continued)

FIGURE 6-9

Common Sites for Allergic Reactions

SOURCE: U.S. Food and Drug Administration.

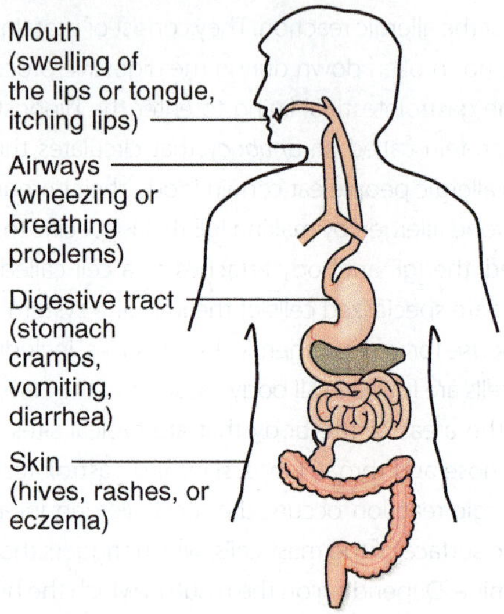

peanuts, milk, and shellfish.[13] **Cross-reaction** is a concern for someone diagnosed with a food allergy. For instance, if someone has a history of allergic reaction to shrimp, testing may show that person is also allergic to other shellfish, such as crab and lobster (see Table 6-3).

Children and Food Allergy

The prevalence of food allergy is greatest in the first few years of life, with 8 percent of children between 3 and 5 years old experiencing allergic responses.[14] Increased susceptibility of infants to food allergic reactions is believed to be the result of an immature immune system. The immature digestive system may also allow more intact allergenic proteins to enter the bloodstream. Cow's milk and soy are the most common allergens for infants, producing reactions such as hives, bloating, and diarrhea. Early exposure to certain foods can also play a role in the development of food allergy in children. The American Academy of Pediatrics recommends exclusive breastfeeding for 6 months and delaying the introduction of common allergenic foods until the baby is at least 6 months old to reduce the risk of allergy.[15] Young children with food allergies may lose their reaction to some foods such as milk, egg, and soy in a few years. Unfortunately, allergy to certain foods such as peanuts, tree nuts, fish, and shellfish can persist into adulthood.

Diagnosis and Management of Food Allergy

Because both food intolerance and food allergy present very similar symptoms, diagnosing a food allergy involves determining if the reaction is mediated by the immune system. A complete physical examination can rule out the possibility that an underlying physical condition may be causing the symptoms. The physician takes a detailed case history and considers the type and timing of symptoms as well as the suspected offending food. Individuals may be asked to keep a food diary and record all physical symptoms.

Once food allergy is identified as a likely cause of symptoms, confirmation of the diagnosis and positive identification of the allergen involve various tests. A prick skin test (PST) is a simple test done in the doctor's office. The doctor puts a drop of the substance being tested on the forearm of the patient and pricks it with a needle, which allows a tiny amount of the substance to enter the skin. If the patient is allergic, a small bump will occur at the site in approximately 15 minutes. The radioallergosorbent test (RAST) requires a blood sample. Laboratory tests are conducted using specific foods to find out if the patient has IgE antibodies to those foods. Also, the physician may recommend an elimination diet, in which the patient does not eat the food suspected of causing the allergy for a period of about 2 to 4 weeks. If the allergic symptoms improve, a diagnosis can be made.

The only treatment for food allergy is to avoid the offending food. People with food allergies must develop food label reading skills. The Food Allergen Labeling and Consumer Protection Act, which went into effect in January 2006, requires food labels to clearly state if food products include any ingredients that contain protein derived from the eight major allergenic foods.[16] Manufacturers are required to identify in plain English the presence of ingredients that contain protein derived from milk, eggs, fish, crustacean shellfish, tree nuts, peanuts, wheat, or soybeans in the list of ingredients or to say "contains" followed by name of the source of the food allergen after or adjacent to the list of ingredients.

The possibility of cross-contamination is also a problem for people with food allergies. When one food comes in contact with another

TABLE 6-3 Foods That Commonly Provoke Food Allergy

Food	Cross-Reacting Foods
Cows' milk	Goats' milk, ewes' milk
Hens' eggs	Eggs from other birds
Peanuts	Soybeans, green beans, green peas
Soybeans	Peanuts, green beans, green peas
Cod	Mackerel, herring
Shrimp	Other crustaceans
Wheat	Other grains, mostly rye

Patients allergic to pollen may have cross-reactions with hazelnuts, green apples, peaches, almonds, kiwis, tomatoes, and potatoes (birch pollen) or wheat, rye, and corn (grass pollen).

SOURCE: Adapted from C. Bindslev-Jensen, ABCs of allergies: Food allergy, *British Medical Journal* 316 (1998): 7140.

cross-reaction The reaction of one antigen with antibodies developed against another antigen.

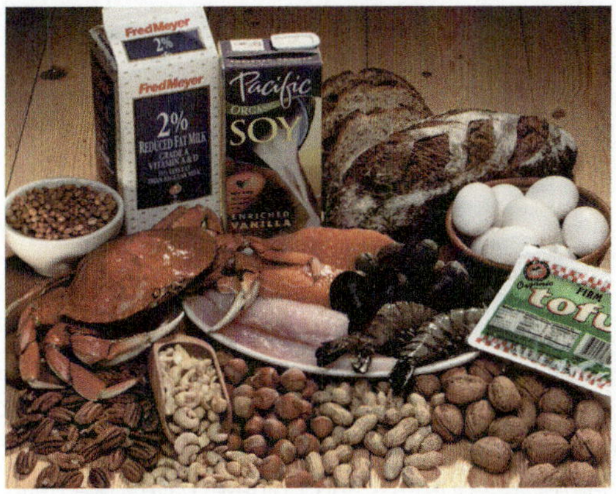

© Polara Studios, Inc.

The top eight foods causing adverse reactions in some individuals: milk, eggs, peanuts, nuts, fish, shellfish, soy, and wheat.

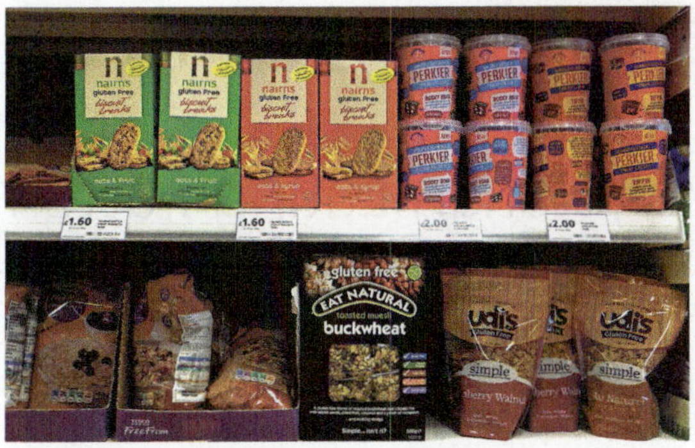

Kevin Britland/Alamy Stock Photo

More and more gluten-free products have entered the market in recent years.

food, trace amounts of each food mix with the other. Cross-contamination can occur in processing plants when different foods are processed on the same equipment. It can also occur at home—a knife inserted into the peanut butter jar and then used in the jelly will contaminate the jelly with peanut protein. The emerging field of biotechnology presents an additional challenge through genetic engineering (see Chapter 13). In genetic engineering, a gene from one species can be "spliced" into another species. The FDA requires that any food product of biotechnology that contains protein from a food known to be a common allergen must be properly labeled.

Currently, no drugs are available to cure food allergy. However, some medications, such as antihistamines and corticosteroids, are used to treat the symptoms. Individuals with a history of anaphylactic reactions to food allergens typically carry self-injecting syringes of epinephrine to use in case of accidental exposure.

Gluten-Related Disorders—Allergy or Sensitivity

There has been a recent increase in the number of people following a gluten-free diet. Global sales of gluten-free products were close to $4.6 billion in 2015.[17] Some market analysts in the United States have estimated that 15 to 25 percent of consumers have an interest in gluten-free foods.[18] What is behind this growing trend?

Gluten is a protein that is found in wheat, rye, and barley. Wheat, the most widely used gluten-containing grain, is commonly consumed as bread, pasta, noodles, and other baked goods. Gluten is also the compound linked to two disorders: wheat allergy and celiac disease. Although both conditions are considered immunologic responses, they differ in type.

Wheat allergy is a typical food allergy with presence of IgE antibodies that trigger the release of histamine from mast cells. The allergic response can affect the skin, gastrointestinal tract, respiratory tract, or sinuses. Diagnosis of wheat allergy is confirmed through a prick skin test or radioallergosorbent test (RAST) (a blood test). Celiac disease is an autoimmune condition affecting approximately one percent of the general population; individuals with a family history of celiac disease are at increased risk.[19] Ingestion of gluten causes the immune system to release autoantibodies (tTG and EMA), which leads to an inflammation of the gastrointestinal mucosa. Symptoms include chronic diarrhea, weight loss, and skin rash. Diagnosis is made through blood tests for the presence of specific autoantibodies. Biopsy of the small intestine will typically show a flattening of the villi.

In recent years, an emerging health care concern related to gluten has been examined. Non-celiac gluten sensitivity, or gluten sensitivity, is a reaction to gluten that results in symptoms that are similar to wheat allergy or celiac disease. The important difference is that gluten sensitivity does not involve allergic or autoimmune mechanisms.[20] Gluten sensitivity can be suspected if blood tests for wheat allergy and celiac disease are negative and symptoms of intolerance resolve with a gluten-free diet.[21] The diagnosis may be substantiated if a subsequent challenge of reintroducing gluten in the diet results in a return of symptoms.

The mechanism involved in gluten sensitivity is under investigation. It has been suggested that it may be related to a function of the body's **innate immunity**.[22] Possible risk factors under consideration include genetic modifications in wheat that result in increased gluten strength, increased exposure to gluten due to its use as a food additive, possible environmental toxins, and intestinal infections.[23] Health care providers and researchers acknowledge there are significant gaps in understanding gluten sensitivity. Specific diagnostic criteria and laboratory testing have yet to be identified. It is hoped that continued research will expand the current knowledge into all gluten-related disorders.

Many organizations offer additional information on food allergy and food intolerance:

Food Allergy Research & Education

www.foodallergy.org/about

Kids with Food Allergies Foundation

www.kidswithfoodallergies.org

Useful Resources on Food Allergies and Intolerances

www.nutrition.gov/nutrition-and-health-issues/food-allergies-and-intolerances
www.nlm.nih.gov/medlineplus/foodallergy.html

This government website provides information and links about food allergies.

innate immunity Type of immunity that is naturally existing and does not require prior sensitization to an antigen.

SPOTLight

6.8 Vegetarian Eating Patterns

Approximately 4 percent of U.S. adults are vegetarian; on the other hand, 47 percent of the population report eating at least one vegetarian meal a week.[24] The reasons for becoming vegetarian vary widely.[25] Some people have health reasons, whereas others have religious, philosophical, or ethical reasons. Some believe that vegetarianism is ecologically sound, and others believe that it is less costly than the meat-eating alternative. Vegetarians are traditionally described as individuals who do not consume meat; however, the eating patterns of some who consider themselves vegetarian may include consumption of seafood and/or poultry but not red meat (see Table 6-4). Whatever the particular reasons for choosing a vegetarian diet, vegetarians need to be aware of its implications for nutrition and health.

I've been thinking about becoming a vegetarian, but is this diet really healthy?

The plant-based eating pattern associated with vegetarianism is associated with a number of beneficial health effects. Vegetarians tend to consume foods that are higher in fiber, richer in certain vitamins and minerals, and lower in calories from fat than nonvegetarians.[26] Studies have found that people with vegetarian or near-vegetarian traditions, such as the Seventh-Day Adventists and Chinese, have lower rates of heart disease, cancer, diabetes, and obesity than those consuming the typical North American diet. Informed vegetarians are more likely to be at a healthy weight and to have lower blood cholesterol levels, lower blood pressure, lower rates of certain types of cancer, and better digestive function.[27] Several studies have reported that the rate of type 2 diabetes is lower among vegetarians compared with nonvegetarians.[28] Even compared with people who are health conscious, vegetarians experience fewer deaths from cardiovascular disease. It is unlikely that dietary practices alone account for the lower mortality rates found in vegetarians. Nondietary lifestyle factors such as not smoking, lower alcohol intake, and emphasis on supportive family also reduce one's risk for chronic diseases. These factors, together with a vegetarian-style eating pattern, appear to contribute to positive health outcomes.

TABLE 6-4 Vegetarian Eating Patterns

Type	Possible Limiting Nutrients	Poultry	Fish and Seafood	Eggs	Milk and Dairy Products	Grains, Legumes, Vegetables	Fruits, Nuts
Vegan • Includes only food from plant sources.	iron, vitamin D, calcium, riboflavin, vitamin B_{12}, omega-3 fatty acids, high-quality protein					✓	✓
OvoVegetarian • Includes plant foods and eggs.	iron, vitamin D, calcium, riboflavin			✓		✓	✓
Lacto-Vegetarian • Includes plant foods and milk and milk products.	iron				✓	✓	✓
Lacto-Ovovegetarian • Includes plant foods, milk and milk products, and eggs.	iron			✓	✓	✓	✓
Pesce-Vegetarian • Includes plant foods and seafood.			✓	✓	✓	✓	✓
Pollo-Vegetarian • Includes plant foods and poultry.		✓		✓	✓	✓	✓
Semi-Vegetarian • Includes some but not all groups of animal-derived products.		✓	✓	✓	✓	✓	✓

SOURCE: Adapted from D. Monti and L. Kehler, The vegetarian alternative? *International Journal of Childbirth Education* 16 (2001): 8–9.

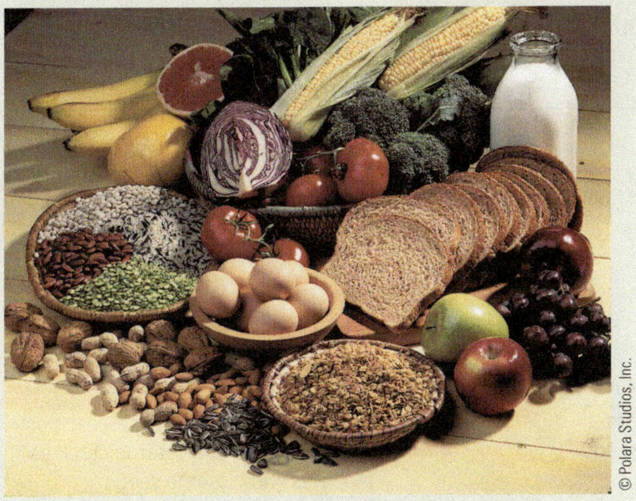

Well-planned, plant-based meals consisting of a variety of whole grains, legumes, nuts, vegetables, fruits—and for some vegetarians, eggs and dairy products—can offer sound nutrition and health benefits to vegetarians and nonvegetarians alike.

If I eliminate certain food groups from my diet, don't I have to worry about nutritional deficiencies?

The Academy of Nutrition and Dietetics affirms that vegetarian diets that include a wide variety of foods, consumed in the right amounts to meet calorie needs, are healthy and nutritionally adequate. This holds true for all stages of the life cycle. With careful planning, vegan or other types of vegetarian eating patterns can meet the dietary requirements during pregnancy, lactation, infancy, childhood, and adolescence.[29] The *Dietary Guidelines for Americans* provides adaptations in the protein and dairy foods groups to accommodate vegetarian food patterns (see Appendix A). The *Dietary Guidelines* recommend choosing foods that are nutrient dense, meaning they have minimal or no solid fats and added sugars. Individuals interested in following a vegetarian eating pattern can use these principles to develop a well-rounded meal plan that meets their nutrient needs (see Figure 6-10).

Proteins

Vegetarians need adequate amounts of all the essential amino acids. Because proteins from animals contain ample amounts of the essential amino acids, lacto-ovovegetarians can get a head start on meeting protein needs by drinking recommended amounts of milk daily or by consuming the equivalent in milk or egg products in the day's diet.

Adequate amounts of amino acids can be obtained from a plant-based diet when a varied diet is routinely consumed on a daily basis. Mixtures of proteins from whole grains, vegetables, beans, nuts, seeds, nut butters, peas, and soy products (tofu, tempeh, veggie burgers) eaten over the course of a day complement one another's amino acid profiles so that deficits in one are made up by the assets of another (see Table 6-5).

FIGURE 6-10

Vegetarian Food Patterns and MyPlate

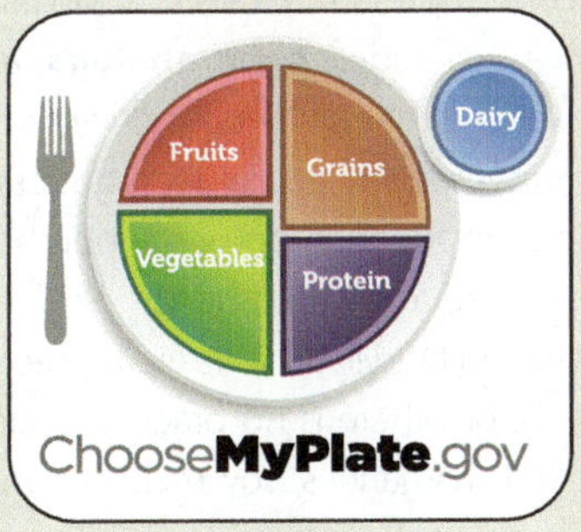

GRAINS	VEGETABLES	FRUITS	DAIRY	PROTEIN
amaranth barley bulgur[a] cereals[b] oats quinoa rice rye triticale wheat[a]	broccoli chard[a] collard greens kale potato red pepper[c] spinach[a] tomato[c] turnip greens[a]	apple berries cantaloupe dried apricot/prunes/raisins[a] grapefruit[c] kiwi[c] orange[c] papaya	calcium- and vitamin D-fortified beverages (soy, almond, or rice milk,[b] orange juice) soy cheeses soy yogurt **Additional choices for lacto-vegetarians:** milk yogurt low-fat cheeses	legumes (cooked beans, peas, lentils)[a] meat analogs[b] nuts nut butters seeds soy products (tofu, tempeh) veggie burgers **Additional choices for ovo-vegetarians:** eggs
In a 2,000-calorie eating pattern, you need the amounts below from each food group.* Also include a source of omega-3 fatty acids: ground flaxseed, flaxseed oil, soybean oil, walnuts, soy products, fortified margarine, fortified eggs.				
Eat 6 oz every day.	Eat 2 1/2 cups every day.	Eat 2 cups every day.	Eat 3 cups every day.	Eat 5 1/2 oz every day.

[a] Dietary source of iron
[b] Can be fortified with B_{12}
[c] Dietary source of vitamin C, increases iron absorption
* See Figure 2-12 on page 46 for tips and strategies for making the healthiest food choices from all food groups; see Appendix A for vegetarian eating patterns at 12 calorie levels.

SOURCE: Adapted from www.ChooseMyPlate.gov and USDA Dietary Guidelines for Americans, 2015.

TABLE 6-5 **Complementary Protein Combinations That Provide High-Quality Protein**

Combine			Examples
Cereal Grains Barley Bulgur Oats Rice Whole-grain breads Pasta Cornmeal	+	**Legumes** Dried beans Dried lentils Dried peas Peanuts	Bean taco Chili and corn bread Lentils or beans and rice Peanut butter sandwich
Legumes (or grains) Dried beans Dried lentils Dried peas Peanuts	+	**Seeds and Nuts** Sesame seeds Sunflower seeds Walnuts Cashews Nut butters	Hummus (chickpea and sesame paste) Split-pea soup and sesame crackers Noodles with sesame seeds

Examples

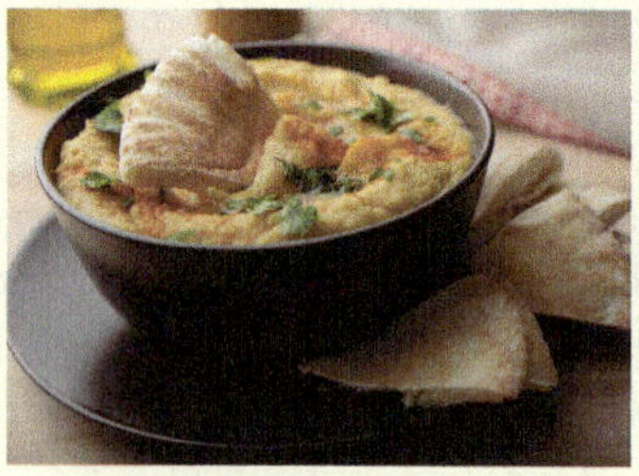
Lilyana Vynogradova/Shutterstock.com

Hummus and bread

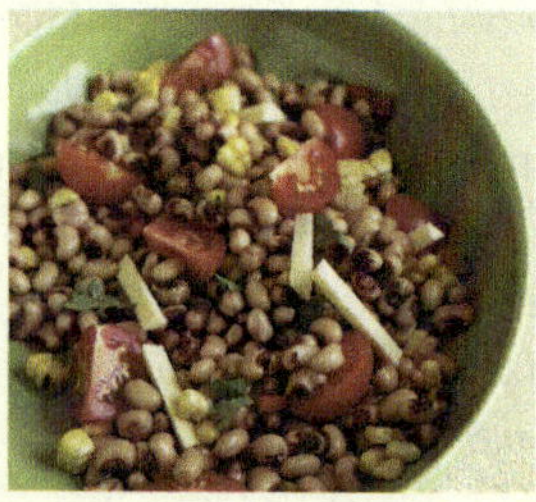
Rick Lew/Getty Images

Corn and black-eyed peas

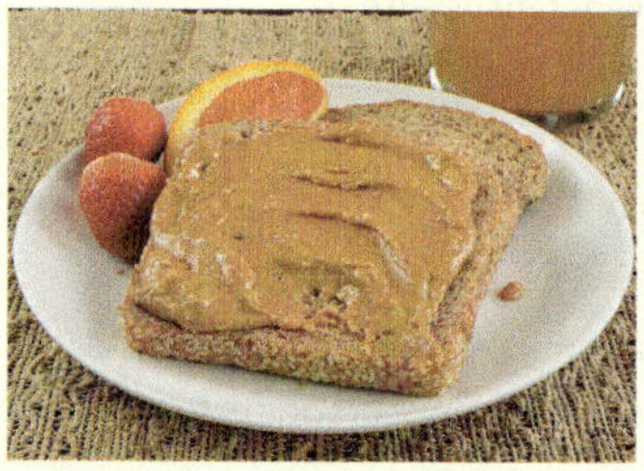
MSPhotographic/Shutterstock.com

Peanut butter and wheat bread

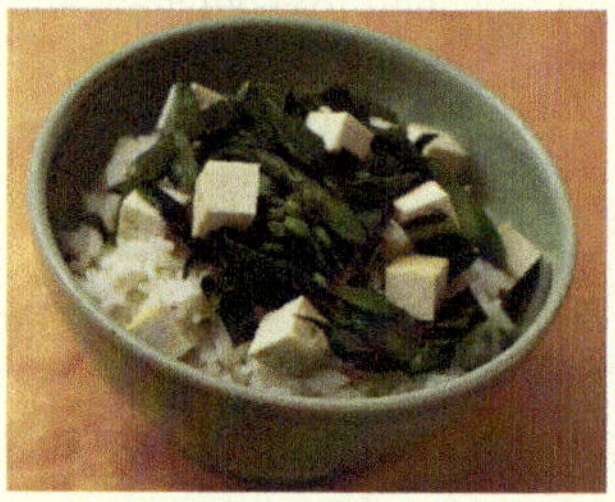
James And James/Getty Images

Tofu and rice

Fats

Vegetarian diets are typically adequate in omega-6 fatty acids. However, intake of omega-3 fatty acids may not meet the recommended amounts.[30] As discussed in Chapter 5, the omega-3 fatty acids that are most important nutritionally are alpha-linolenic acid (ALA), docosahexaenoic acid (DHA), and eicosapentaenoic acid (EPA). Fish, especially fatty fish, are good sources of DHA and EPA because the fish eat marine algae containing DHA and EPA. Additional sources include dairy products and DHA-fortified eggs. Vegetarian eating patterns that do not include consumption of these types of foods are especially lacking in these fatty acids. It is recommended that vegetarians include sources of omega-3 fats from ground flaxseed, flaxseed oil, canola oil, soy products, and walnuts. Incorporating foods that are fortified in omega-3 fatty acids, including algae-derived DHA, such as some brands of soy milk, orange juice, and breakfast bars is another option.

Vitamins

The lacto-ovovegetarian eating pattern can be adequate in all vitamins, but having adequate intake of some vitamins is a consideration in the vegan diet. One such vitamin is vitamin B_{12}, which does not occur naturally in plant foods. Regular consumption of vitamin B_{12}-fortified foods such as fortified soy and rice beverages, **meat analogs**, and **nutritional yeast** is important to reduce the risk for deficiency. Some vegans may consume seaweeds, fermented soy, and other products in the belief that they provide vitamin B_{12} in adequate amounts, but these products are not currently recommended as reliable sources.[31]

Another vitamin of concern is vitamin D. Milk drinkers are protected if the milk is fortified with vitamin D, but there is no practical source of vitamin D in plant foods. Fortified margarines, soy milk, rice milk, orange juice, and breakfast cereals can supply some vitamin D. Regular exposure to the sun can also help prevent a deficiency.

Riboflavin, another B vitamin obtained from milk, is present in the diet of vegans who eat ample servings of dark greens, whole and enriched grains, mushrooms, legumes, nuts, and seeds. Vegans who don't eat these foods, however, may not meet the body's riboflavin needs.

Minerals

Iron and zinc need special attention in the diets of all vegetarians.[32] Whole-grain products, soy foods, other legumes, dried fruit, nuts, and seeds are important sources of iron in the vegetarian diet. The iron in these foods, however, is not as easily absorbed by the body as that in meat. Because the vitamin C in fruits and vegetables can triple the absorption of the iron provided by other foods eaten at the same meal, vegetarian meals should be rich in foods offering vitamin C.

meat analogs Textured vegetable protein products formulated to look and taste like meat, fish, or poultry. Many of these are designed to match the known nutrient contents of animal protein foods.

nutritional yeast A fortified food supplement containing B vitamins, iron, and protein; can be used to improve the quality of a vegetarian diet.

Zinc is widespread in plant foods, but its availability may be reduced by the fibers and other binders found in fruits, vegetables, and whole grains. Vegetarians are advised to eat varied diets that include wheat germ, legumes, nuts, pumpkin seeds, and whole-grain products. Milk, yogurt, and cheese provide zinc to the lacto-vegetarian as well.

Having an adequate amount of calcium is also important. Whereas lacto-vegetarians will most likely meet their calcium needs through the consumption of dairy products, vegetarians and vegans must find other sources of calcium. Some good sources of calcium are *regular* servings of calcium-fortified breakfast cereals and juices; legumes; firm-style tofu made with calcium sulfate; other soy foods, including calcium-fortified soy milk; dried figs; some nuts, such as almonds; certain seeds, such as sesame seeds; and some vegetables, such as broccoli, collard greens, kale, mustard greens, turnip greens, okra, rutabaga, and Chinese cabbage (bok choy). The choices should be varied because the absorption of the calcium provided by some of these foods is hindered by binders in them. Strict vegetarians are urged to use calcium-fortified soy or rice beverages, juices, or cereals in ample quantities.[33]

You have mentioned things like soy products and meat analogs. What exactly are they?

Soybeans are legumes—members of the same plant family that includes other beans, peas, and lentils. Among edible legumes, the soybean is somewhat unusual because it is relatively low in carbohydrates. Soybeans are, however, high in fiber.

Among plant foods, legumes are high in protein. What distinguishes the soybean from its cousins, however, is the nature of the protein: Soybeans supply all of the essential amino acids needed for health. The amino acid pattern of soy protein is essentially the same quality as that found in meat, milk, and egg protein. Soybeans are the only vegetable food that contains high-quality protein. What emerges from this nutritional analysis of the soybean is the image of "balance." Soybeans as a food can basically stand alone, give or take a few vitamins and minerals.

The types of soy foods are incredibly varied and readily available in grocery and specialty food stores (see the Miniglossary that follows). Edamame are soybeans that are harvested early while they are still green and tender. They are available either in the pod or already shelled and can be served as a main vegetable dish. Tofu is a soft, cheese-like food that is available as firm or soft. Although somewhat bland tasting on its own, tofu readily absorbs the flavors of marinades or other foods it is cooked with. Whole soybeans can be fermented and then mixed with grains such as rice to form a chunky cake-like product known as tempeh. Both tofu and tempeh can be stir-fried, grilled, or cubed and added to soups or stews. Soy cheese is made from soy milk and comes in a variety of flavors that can be substituted for traditional cheeses. Soy milk is also available frozen as a nondairy dessert.

A meat analog is manufactured to look like meat products such as hamburger, steak, chicken, sausage, or hot dogs. Soy, wheat gluten, beans, mycoprotein, and/or nuts are used as the main protein source, with other ingredients used to provide texture and a meat-like taste. They are a good source of protein and can be broiled, baked,

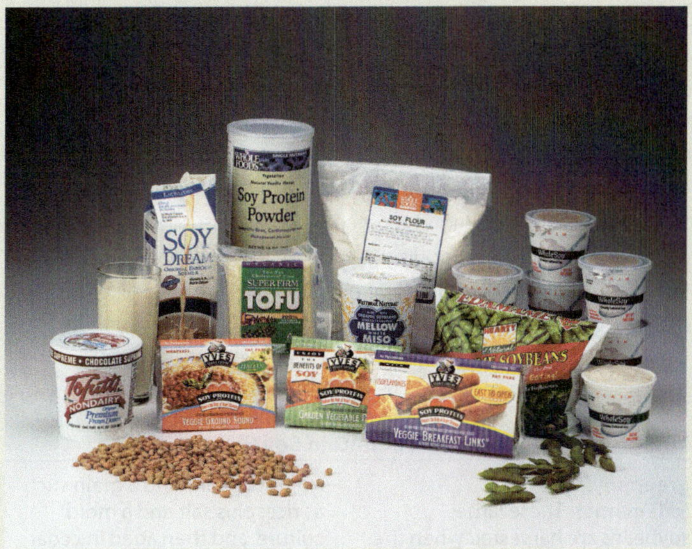

© Scott Hirko/Hespenheide Design

or roasted or added to stews, sauces, and soups. Meat analogs are generally low in fat and are cholesterol free and can be a convenient way to prepare a meat-free meal. As with any other prepared food product, it is important to read the label for the amount of added sugars and sodium.

I am just not sure I am ready to become a vegetarian overnight. Do you have any suggestions?

The Vegetarian Nutrition Dietetics Practice Group of the Academy of Nutrition and Dietetics provides several recommendations for eating a more plant-based eating pattern.[34] Explore the resources listed in Table 6-6 for many helpful tips. You can start by preparing at least one

TABLE 6-6 Vegetarian Resources

www.eatright.org
The Academy of Nutrition and Dietetics home page includes many nutrition resources and links.

http://fnic.nal.usda.gov
Select Diet and Health and click on Vegetarian Nutrition.

www.vrg.org
The Vegetarian Resource Group provides information on vegetarianism.

http://vegetariannutrition.net
Vegetarian Nutrition Dietetic Practice Group

www.choosemyplate.gov/healthy-eating-tips/tips-for-vegetarian.html
Healthy eating tips for vegetarians using the MyPlate Food Guide

https://www.nutrition.gov/smart-nutrition-101/healthy-eating/eating-vegetarian
Tips for creating a healthy vegetarian eating plan

www.soyfoods.com
This U.S. Soy Foods Directory website includes a searchable database, recipes, and research information about the health benefits of soy foods.

www.soyconnection.com
The United Soybean Board provides information and answers questions about soy foods.

© Cengage

vegetarian meal a week. Many of the dishes that typically contain meat can be prepared vegetarian: For example, vegetable lasagna, tofu-vegetable stir-fry, or bean burritos. If you already eat plant foods, eat a greater variety of them. Instead of a peanut butter and jelly sandwich, consider having oatmeal with nuts and raisins instead. Add more vegetables and beans to your soups and stews that contain animal products to slowly make them more vegetarian. Substitute soy food products or meat analogs for the poultry and beef in your current recipes. Add firm tofu chunks in place of meat or poultry in stir-fries, fajitas, or shish kebabs. Use soy milk to make hot chocolate. Make your own breakfast sandwich with a whole-grain English muffin, slice of soy cheese, and soy sausage-style patty. After a workout, whip up a chocolate banana soy smoothie made from vanilla soy yogurt, chocolate soy milk, and a frozen banana. Take time to visit health food or grocery stores that carry plant-based foods like nondairy beverages and frozen desserts and varieties of grains, fruits, nuts, and seeds. Even when dining out, be aware that many restaurants can make vegetarian modifications to menu items. Finally, share your newfound knowledge of vegetarian dining with friends or family by inviting them over for a vegetarian meal. Including them in the process can make it fun and more likely to last.

Miniglossary—What Foods Contain Soy?[35]

green soybeans (edamame) These large soybeans are harvested when the beans are still green and sweet and can be served as a snack or a main vegetable dish, after boiling in water for 15 to 20 minutes. They are high in protein and fiber and contain no cholesterol.

hydrolyzed vegetable protein (HVP) A protein obtained from any vegetable, including soybeans. The protein is broken down into amino acids by a chemical process called *acid hydrolysis*. HVP is a flavor enhancer that can be used in soups, broths, sauces, gravies, flavoring and spice blends, canned and frozen vegetables, and meats and poultry.

meat alternatives/analogs Meat alternatives made from soybeans contain soy protein or tofu and other ingredients mixed together to simulate various kinds of meat. These meat alternatives are sold as frozen, canned, dried, or refrigerated foods (e.g., Tofurkey products such as lunch "meat," hot dogs, etc.).

miso A rich, salty condiment that characterizes the essence of Japanese cooking. The Japanese make miso soup and use miso to flavor a variety of foods. A smooth paste, miso is made from soybeans and a grain such as rice, plus salt and a mold culture, and then aged in cedar vats for 1 to 3 years. Miso should be refrigerated. Use miso to flavor soups, sauces, dressings, marinades, and pâtés.

nondairy soy frozen dessert Nondairy frozen desserts are made from soy milk or soy yogurt. Soy ice cream is one of the most popular desserts made from soybeans and can be found in many grocery stores.

soy cheese Cheese made from soy milk. The standard soy cheese products (sandwich slices, shreds, blocks) have a firm texture and are substitutes for firm dairy cheese. Soy cream cheese and soy sour cream products are available as well.

soy flour Flour made from roasted soybeans ground into a fine powder. Soy flour gives a protein boost to recipes. Soy flour is gluten-free, so yeast-raised breads made with soy flour are denser in texture. Replace one-quarter to one-third wheat flour with soy flour in recipes for muffins, cakes, cookies, pancakes, and quick breads.

soy protein, texturized *Texturized soy protein* usually refers to products made from texturized soy flour. Texturized soy flour is made by running defatted soy flour through an extrusion cooker, which allows the creation of many different forms and sizes. When hydrated, it has a chewy texture. It is widely used as a meat extender.

soy yogurt Yogurt made from soy milk. Its creamy texture makes it an easy substitute for sour cream or cream cheese. Soy yogurt can be found in a variety of flavors in many food stores.

soybeans As soybeans mature in the pod, they ripen into a hard, dry bean. Most soybeans are yellow. However, brown and black varieties are also available. Whole soybeans can be cooked and used in sauces, stews, and soups.

soy milk, soy beverages Soybeans that are soaked, ground fine, and strained produce a fluid called *soybean milk*. Soy milk is an excellent source of high-quality protein and B vitamins. Look for calcium-fortified varieties.

soy-nut butter Made from roasted, whole soy nuts, which are then crushed and blended with soy oil and other ingredients. Soy-nut butter has a slightly nutty taste, contains significantly less fat than peanut butter, and provides many other nutritional benefits.

soy nuts Whole soybeans that have been soaked in water and then baked until browned. Soy nuts can be found in a variety of flavors, including chocolate covered. High in protein and isoflavones, soy nuts are similar in texture and flavor to peanuts. Try sprinkling some on salads.

tempeh A chunky, tender soybean cake; a traditional Indonesian food. Whole soybeans, sometimes mixed with another grain such as rice or millet, are fermented into a rich cake of soybeans with a smoky, nutty flavor. Tempeh can be marinated and grilled and added to soups, casseroles, or chili.

tofu and tofu products *Tofu*, also known as *soybean curd*, is a soft, cheese-like food made by curdling fresh, hot soy milk with a coagulant. Tofu is a bland product that easily absorbs the flavors of other ingredients with which it is cooked. Tofu is rich in high-quality protein and B vitamins and is low in sodium. Firm tofu is dense and solid and can be cubed and served in soups, stir-fried, or grilled. Firm tofu is higher in protein, fat, and calcium than other forms of tofu. Silken tofu is a creamy product and can be used as a replacement for sour cream in many dip recipes.

WHAT'S ONLINE

MINDTAP From Cengage

Visit www.cengagebrain.com to access MindTap, a complete digital course that includes Diet & Wellness Plus, interactive quizzes, videos, and more.

healthy eating for vegetarians

10 tips for vegetarians

A vegetarian eating pattern can be a healthy option. The key is to consume a variety of foods and the right amount of foods to meet your calorie and nutrient needs.

1 think about protein

Your protein needs can easily be met by eating a variety of plant foods. Sources of protein for vegetarians include beans and peas, nuts, and soy products (such as tofu, tempeh). Lacto-ovo vegetarians also get protein from eggs and dairy foods.

2 bone up on sources of calcium

Calcium is used for building bones and teeth. Some vegetarians consume dairy products, which are excellent sources of calcium. Other sources of calcium for vegetarians include calcium-fortified soymilk (soy beverage), tofu made with calcium sulfate, calcium-fortified breakfast cereals and orange juice, and some dark-green leafy vegetables (collard, turnip, and mustard greens; and bok choy).

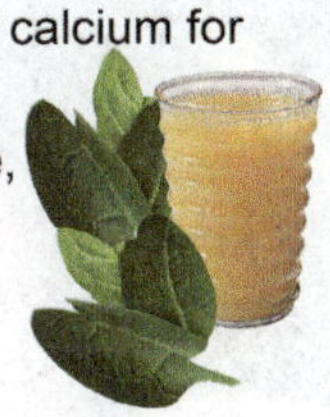

3 make simple changes

Many popular main dishes are or can be vegetarian—such as pasta primavera, pasta with marinara or pesto sauce, veggie pizza, vegetable lasagna, tofu-vegetable stir-fry, and bean burritos.

4 enjoy a cookout

For barbecues, try veggie or soy burgers, soy hot dogs, marinated tofu or tempeh, and fruit kabobs. Grilled veggies are great, too!

5 include beans and peas

Because of their high nutrient content, consuming beans and peas is recommended for everyone, vegetarians and non-vegetarians alike. Enjoy some vegetarian chili, three bean salad, or split pea soup. Make a hummus-filled pita sandwich.

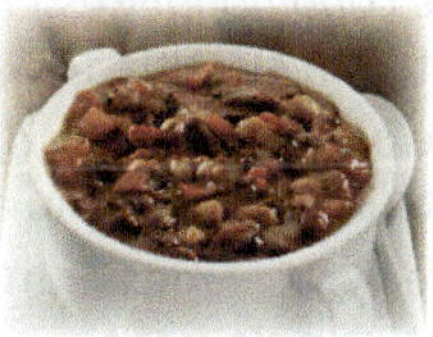

6 try different veggie versions

A variety of vegetarian products look—and may taste—like their non-vegetarian counterparts but are usually lower in saturated fat and contain no cholesterol. For breakfast, try soy-based sausage patties or links. For dinner, rather than hamburgers, try bean burgers or falafel (chickpea patties).

7 make some small changes at restaurants

Most restaurants can make vegetarian modifications to menu items by substituting meatless sauces or non-meat items, such as tofu and beans for meat, and adding vegetables or pasta in place of meat. Ask about available vegetarian options.

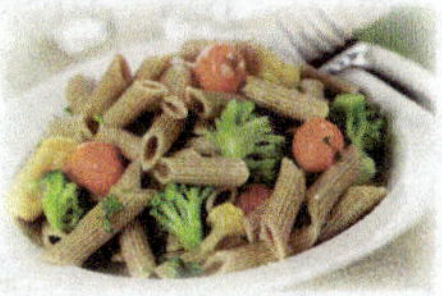

8 nuts make great snacks

Choose unsalted nuts as a snack and use them in salads or main dishes. Add almonds, walnuts, or pecans instead of cheese or meat to a green salad.

9 get your vitamin B_{12}

Vitamin B_{12} is naturally found only in animal products. Vegetarians should choose fortified foods such as cereals or soy products, or take a vitamin B_{12} supplement if they do not consume any animal products. Check the Nutrition Facts label for vitamin B_{12} in fortified products.

10 find a vegetarian pattern for you

Go to www.dietaryguidelines.gov and check appendices 8 and 9 of the *Dietary Guidelines for Americans, 2010* for vegetarian adaptations of the USDA food patterns at 12 calorie levels.

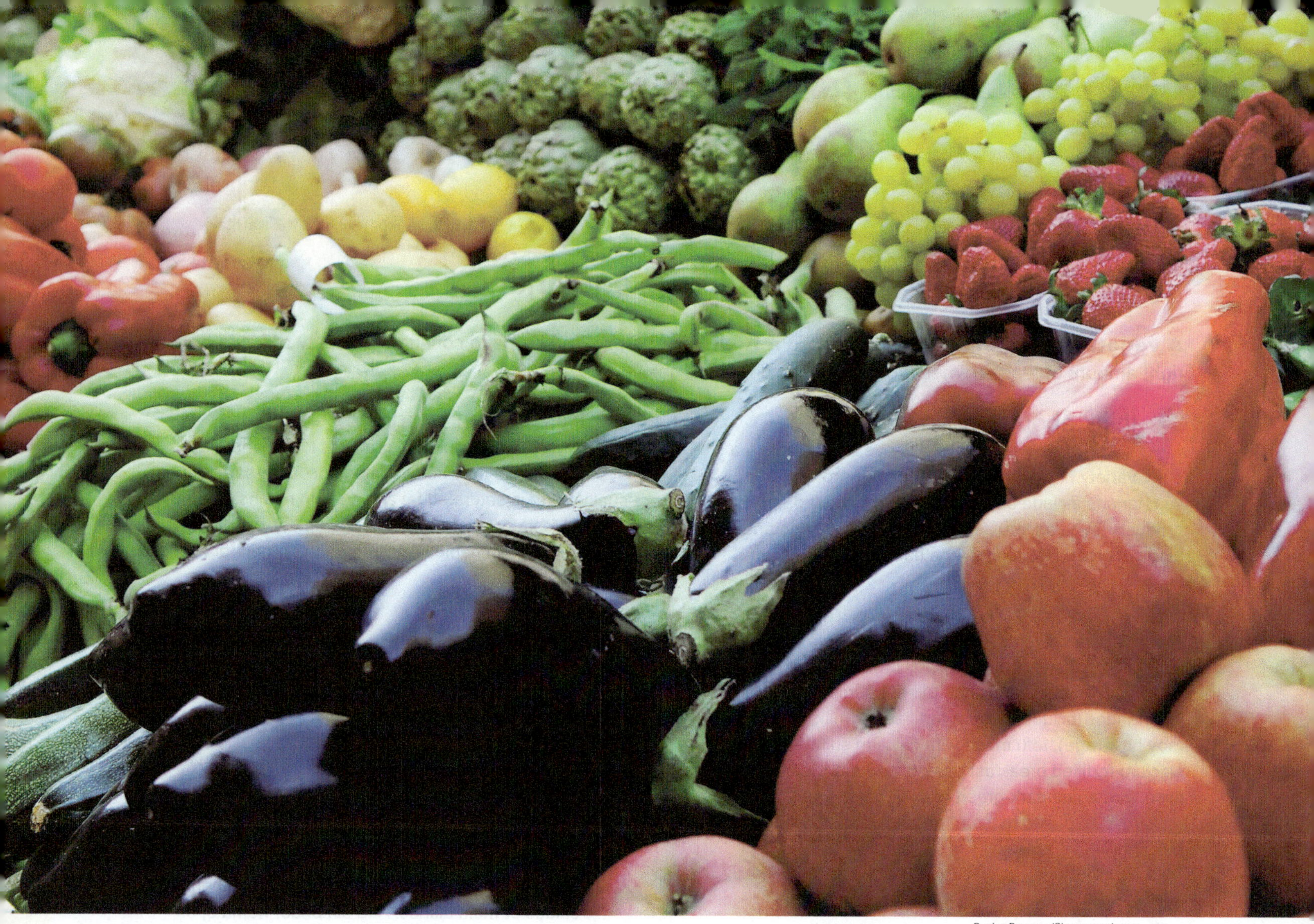

Regien Paassen/Shutterstock.com

AskYourself . . .

Which of the following statements about nutrition are true, and which are false? For each false statement, what is true?

1. The most important role that vitamins play is providing energy.
2. Serving for serving, fruits and vegetables tend to be the richest sources of vitamins.
3. Vitamin D is also known as the "sunshine vitamin" because the body can make vitamin D with the help of sunlight.
4. Maintaining a healthy weight may be one of the most important ways to protect against cancer.

Answers found on page 182.

ChapterObjectives

7.1 Differentiate between the water-soluble and fat-soluble vitamins.

7.2 Explain how antioxidants function within the body, and identify major food sources of these nutrients.

7.3 Identify the vitamins that work together to promote a healthy circulatory system, and name major food sources of these nutrients.

7.4 Describe the roles of vitamin D and vitamin K in promotion of bone health, and list major food sources of these nutrients.

7.5 Describe the roles of the B vitamins in energy metabolism, and list major food sources for each of the B vitamins.

7.6 Define *conditionally essential nutrient*, and give an example of a nonvitamin classified as such.

7.7 Define *phytochemicals*, discuss their relevance to health, and list ways to include them in a healthy diet.

7.8 List life cycle stages or medical conditions in which a vitamin-mineral supplement may be recommended.

7.9 List the key diet and physical activity guidelines for cancer prevention.

The Vitamins: A Functional Approach

CHAPTER 7

About a century ago, scientists ushered in a new era in the science of nutrition—the discovery of vitamins. They quickly realized that these substances, found in minute amounts in foods, were just as essential to health as fats, carbohydrates, and proteins. A diet lacking in one vitamin could cause a barrage of symptoms and, ultimately, death. Knowledge of the vital roles vitamins played quickly advanced, and today life-threatening vitamin deficiencies are rare in developed countries such as the United States and Canada.

Still, the vitamin research that has been conducted during the past decade or so has marked the beginning of yet another chapter in the annals of nutrition. Throughout the past 15 years, more and more scientists have investigated the possibility that certain vitamins will help stave off chronic diseases such as cancer and heart disease, which rank as major killers today. In fact, the study of vitamins, particularly a class known as the *antioxidant vitamins*, is one of the hottest, most widely publicized areas in current nutrition research. In addition, the pros and cons of taking vitamin supplements are the subject of heated debate within the scientific community. To help you sort through the steady stream of claims regarding vitamins, this chapter explores the history, roles, and current thrust of research on the various vitamins and offers practical advice on how to incorporate the information into decisions about your own lifestyle.

In France old Crainquebille sold leeks from a cart, leeks called "the asparagus of the poor." Now asparagus sells for the asking, almost, in California markets, and broccoli, that strong age-old green, leaps from its lowly pot to the Ritz's copper saucepan. Who determines, and for what strange reasons, the social status of a vegetable?

—M. F. K. Fisher (1908–1992, U.S. food writer)

7.1 Meet the Vitamins

Today, scientists recognize vitamins as potent compounds that perform many tasks in the body to promote growth and reproduction and maintain health and life. Vitamins constantly work to keep your nerves and skin healthy; build bone, teeth, and blood; and heal wounds, among many other things. Although they do not provide calories, vitamins are essential in helping the body make use of the calories consumed via foods.

Turning Back the Clock Many of the vitamin-deficiency diseases that have been virtually eliminated today were first recognized in Greek and Roman times, and ultimately led to the discovery of vitamins centuries later. One of the most prevalent was **scurvy**, a disease caused by lack of vitamin C and characterized by bleeding gums, tooth loss, and even death. The scourge of armies, sailors, and other travelers forced to do without vitamin C-rich foods for weeks on end, scurvy was recognized by Hippocrates, a Greek physician heralded today as the father of medicine.[1]

A cure for scurvy was not recorded until the 16th century, however, when a beverage made of spruce needles or oranges and lemons was recommended. In 1753, a British physician named James Lind published a famous report recommending consumption of herbs, lettuce, endive, watercress, and summer fruits to prevent scurvy. By the early 1800s, sailors in the British navy had been dubbed "limeys" because they were required to drink lemon or lime juice daily.[2] Although they still didn't know that vitamin C was the actual antidote, they did recognize that certain foods prevented and cured the illness.

Similarly, a deficiency disease called **rickets** dates back to Roman times, when children frequently suffered skeletal deformities as a result of a lack of vitamin D. By the 1600s, rickets was known as the "English disease" because it afflicted so many English children. Some 200 years later, cod liver oil was finally recognized as a cure for the disease; no one knew at the time, however, that the "magic" ingredient in the oil was vitamin D.

Another deficiency disease, called **pellagra**, was not recognized until 1730, when a Spanish physician named Gaspar Casal first described the crusty, dry, scabby, blackish patches of skin symptomatic of the disease (see Figure 7-1). In Italy, the disease was named pellagra, from the Italian *pelle agra*, meaning "sour skin." Called *mal de la rosa* in Spanish, pellagra was thought to be incurable until Dr. Casal noticed that the people who developed the disease were typically poor and had inadequate diets made up of mostly corn and little meat.

By the 19th century, physicians had recognized that certain foods prevented or cured pellagra and other deficiency diseases, although they still hadn't determined exactly what it was in these various foods that worked as remedies. By the middle of the 19th century, however, the science of chemistry had advanced to a point at which foods could be analyzed. Chemists had determined that foods consisted of fats, proteins, and carbohydrates, along with minerals and water, and they assumed that they had identified all the nutritionally significant compounds.

Then, in the early 20th century, scientists detected minute amounts of other substances that they found to be essential in preventing disease and maintaining health. The substances were dubbed *vitamines*, a term coined in 1912 by a scientist named Dr. Casimir Funk to indicate that these substances were *vital* for survival and that they contained nitrogen—that is, they were *amines*. (The *e* was later dropped when scientists discovered that some vitamins were not amines.)

Over the next few decades, scientists identified the various **vitamins**, established their chemical formulas, and determined their functions in the body. They also

FIGURE 7-1

Pellagra

The typical dry, crusty dermatitis of pellagra is found only on areas of the body exposed to sunlight.

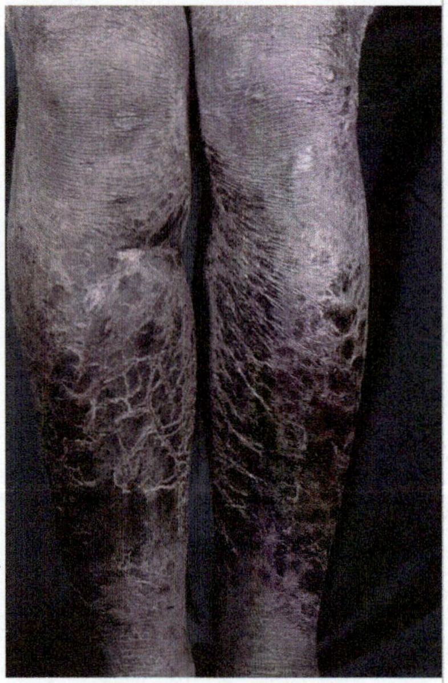

Dr. M. A. Ansary/Science Source

scurvy The vitamin C-deficiency disease characterized by bleeding gums, tooth loss, and, in severe cases, death.

rickets A disease that occurs in children as a result of vitamin D deficiency; characterized by abnormal growth of bone, which in turn leads to bowed legs and an outward-bowed chest.

pellagra (pell-AY-gruh) Niacin deficiency characterized by diarrhea, inflammation of the skin, and, in severe cases, mental disorders and death.

vitamin A potent, indispensable compound that performs various bodily functions that promote growth and reproduction and maintain health. Vitamins are *essential* nutrients required in minute amounts and *organic*, meaning that they contain or are related to carbon compounds. Contrary to popular belief, vitamins do not supply calories (energy).

ASK YOURSELF ANSWERS: **1.** False. Vitamins do not provide energy, though they do play roles in energy-yielding reactions in the body. **2.** True. **3.** True. **4.** True.

measured the amount of vitamins in various foods and determined human and animal requirements for the compounds. Knowledge of vitamins constantly evolves as scientists continue to study the actions of these substances in the human body.

TABLE 7-1 The Vitamins

Water-Soluble Vitamins include:

- B vitamins
  - Thiamin
  - Riboflavin
  - Niacin
  - Vitamin B_6
  - Folate
  - Vitamin B_{12}
  - Pantothenic acid
  - Biotin
- Vitamin C

Fat-Soluble Vitamins include:

- Vitamin A
- Vitamin D
- Vitamin E
- Vitamin K

The Two Classifications of Vitamins

Vitamins fall into two categories: those that dissolve in water (water-soluble vitamins) and those that dissolve in fat (fat-soluble vitamins). To date, scientists have identified 13 vitamins, each with its own special roles to play (see Table 7-1). As Figure 7-2 shows, each of the food groups in the MyPlate food guide supplies a number of vitamins. Eating plans that exclude entire food groups or fail to include the minimum amounts of food from each group may lead to vitamin deficiencies over time.

The nine water-soluble vitamins—eight B vitamins and vitamin C—are found in the watery components of foods, such as the juice of an orange. Table 7-2 identifies major functions and good food sources of the water-soluble vitamins. These vitamins are distributed into water-filled compartments of the body, including the fluid that surrounds the spinal cord. The body excretes excess water-soluble vitamins if blood levels rise too high. As a result, these vitamins rarely reach toxic levels in the body. This is not to say, however, that excess levels cannot cause problems, at least in some people.

In contrast, the four fat-soluble vitamins—A, D, E, and K—are generally found in the fats and oils of foods. Table 7-3 identifies major functions and good food sources of the fat-soluble vitamins. Because they are stored in the liver and in body fat, it is possible for megadoses of fat-soluble vitamins to build up to toxic levels in the body and cause undesirable side effects. Table 7-4 shows the contrasts between the two classes of vitamins.

Water-Soluble Vitamins In the body, water-soluble vitamins act as **coenzymes**—that is, they assist enzymes in doing their metabolic work within the body (see Figure 7-3 on page 186). You may recall from Chapter 6 that enzymes are proteins that act as catalysts to help boost chemical reactions in the body.

In foods, the water-soluble vitamins are relatively fragile. Although large amounts of them are naturally present in many foods, they can be washed out or destroyed during food storage, processing, and preparation. These effects are described in detail in The Savvy Diner feature in this chapter.

coenzymes Enzyme helpers; small molecules that interact with enzymes and enable them to do their work. Many coenzymes are made from water-soluble vitamins.

Fat-Soluble Vitamins The four fat-soluble vitamins—A, D, E, and K—are absorbed from the digestive tract with the aid of fats in the diet and bile produced by the liver. Any disorder that interferes with fat digestion or absorption can precipitate a deficiency of the fat-soluble vitamins. Once in the bloodstream, these vitamins

FIGURE 7-2

Good Sources of Vitamins in the USDA MyPlate Food Guide*

*Serving sizes shown here are based on a 2,000-calorie diet. Go to www.ChooseMyPlate.gov for a quick estimate of how much food you should eat from the different food groups based on your age, gender, height, weight, and activity level.

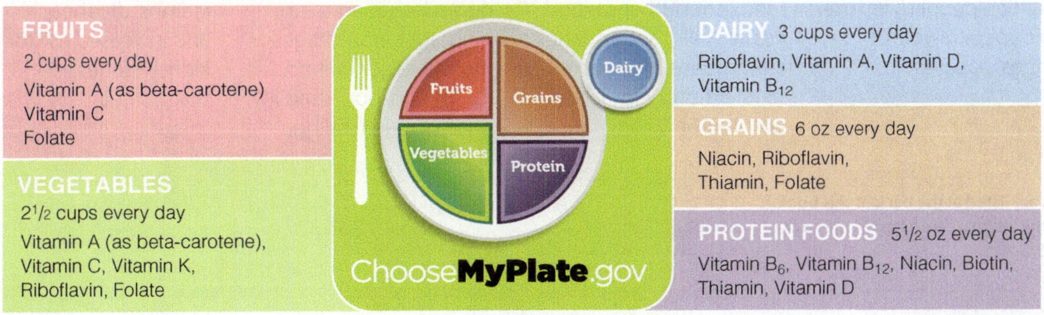

TABLE 7-2 A Guide to the Water-Soluble Vitamins

Vitamin (Chemical Name)	Best Sources[a]	Chief Roles	Deficiency Symptoms	Toxicity Symptoms[b]
Thiamin	Meat, pork, liver, fish, poultry; whole-grain and enriched breads, cereals, and grain products; nuts, legumes	Helps enzymes release energy from carbohydrate; supports normal appetite and nervous system function	Beriberi: edema, heart irregularity, mental confusion, muscle weakness, apathy, impaired growth	None reported
Riboflavin	Milk, leafy green vegetables, yogurt, cottage cheese, liver, meat; whole-grain or enriched breads, cereals, and grain products	Helps enzymes release energy from carbohydrate, fat, and protein; promotes healthy skin and normal vision	Eye problems, skin disorders around nose and mouth, magenta tongue, hypersensitivity to light	None reported
Niacin	Meat, eggs, poultry, fish, milk; whole-grain and enriched breads, cereals, and grain products; nuts, legumes, peanuts	Helps enzymes release energy from energy nutrients; promotes health of skin, nerves, and digestive system	Pellagra: flaky skin rash on parts exposed to sun, loss of appetite, dizziness, weakness, irritability, fatigue, mental confusion, indigestion, delirium	Flushing, nausea, headaches, cramps, ulcer irritation, heartburn, abnormal liver function, rapid heartbeat with doses above 500 mg per day
Vitamin B_6 (pyridoxine)	Meat, poultry, fish, shellfish, legumes, fruits, soy products, whole-grain products, green leafy vegetables	Protein and fat metabolism; formation of antibodies and red blood cells; helps convert tryptophan to niacin	Nervous disorders, skin rash, muscle weakness, anemia, convulsions, kidney stones	Depression, fatigue, irritability, headaches, numbness, damage to nerves, difficulty walking
Folate (folacin, folic acid)	Green leafy vegetables, liver, legumes, seeds, citrus fruits, melons; enriched breads, cereals, and grain products	Red blood cell formation; protein metabolism; new cell division	Anemia, heartburn, diarrhea, smooth red tongue, depression, poor growth, neural tube defects, increased risk of heart disease, stroke, and certain cancers	Diarrhea, insomnia, irritability, may mask a vitamin B_{12} deficiency
Vitamin B_{12} (cobalamin)	Animal products: meat, fish, poultry, shellfish, milk, cheese, eggs; fortified cereals	Helps maintain nerve cells; red blood cell formation; synthesis of genetic material	Anemia, smooth red tongue, fatigue, nerve degeneration progressing to paralysis	None reported
Pantothenic acid	Widespread in foods	Coenzyme in energy metabolism	Rare; sleep disturbances, nausea, fatigue	None reported
Biotin	Widespread in foods	Coenzyme in energy metabolism; fat synthesis	Loss of appetite, nausea, depression, muscle pain	None reported
Vitamin C (ascorbic acid)	Citrus fruits, cabbage-type vegetables, tomatoes, potatoes, dark green vegetables, peppers, lettuce, cantaloupe, strawberries, mangoes, papayas	Synthesis of collagen (helps heal wounds, maintains bone and teeth, strengthens blood vessel walls); antioxidant; strengthens resistance to infection; helps body absorb iron	Scurvy: anemia, depression, frequent infections, bleeding gums, loosened teeth, pinpoint hemorrhages, muscle degeneration, rough skin, bone fragility, poor wound healing, hysteria	Intakes of more than 1 g per day may cause nausea, abdominal cramps, diarrhea, and increased risk for kidney stones

[a]The recommended intakes for the vitamins are listed at the back of this book.
[b]The Tolerable Upper Intake Levels (UL) for the vitamins are listed at the back of this book.

TABLE 7-3 A Guide to the Fat-Soluble Vitamins

Vitamin (Chemical Name)	Best Sources[a]	Chief Roles	Deficiency Symptoms	Toxicity Symptoms[b]
Vitamin A	*Retinol:* fortified milk and margarine, cream, cheese, butter, eggs, liver *Beta-carotene:* Spinach and other dark leafy greens, broccoli, deep orange fruits (apricots, peaches, cantaloupe) and vegetables (squash, carrots, sweet potatoes, pumpkin)	Vision; growth and repair of body tissues; maintenance of mucous membranes; reproduction; bone and tooth formation; immunity; hormone synthesis; antioxidant (in the form of beta-carotene only)	Night blindness, rough skin, susceptibility to infection, impaired bone growth, abnormal tooth and jaw alignment, eye problems leading to blindness, impaired growth	Red blood cell breakage, nosebleeds, abdominal cramps, nausea, diarrhea, weight loss, blurred vision, irritability, loss of appetite, bone pain, dry skin, rashes, hair loss, cessation of menstruation, liver disease, birth defects
Vitamin D (cholecalciferol)	Self-synthesis with sunlight; fortified milk, fortified margarine, eggs, liver, fish	Calcium and phosphorus metabolism (bone and tooth formation); aids body's absorption of calcium	Rickets in children; osteomalacia in adults; abnormal growth, joint pain, soft bones	Deposits of calcium in organs such as the kidneys, liver, or heart, mental retardation, abnormal bone growth
Vitamin E	Vegetable oils, green leafy vegetables, wheat germ, whole-grain products, liver, egg yolk, salad dressings, mayonnaise, margarine, nuts, seeds	Protects red blood cells; antioxidant (protects fat-soluble vitamins); stabilization of cell membranes	Muscle wasting, weakness, red blood cell breakage, anemia, hemorrhaging	Doses over 800 IU/day may increase bleeding (blood clotting time)
Vitamin K	Bacterial synthesis in digestive tract, liver, green leafy and cabbage-type vegetables, soybeans, milk, vegetable oils	Synthesis of blood-clotting proteins and a blood protein that regulates blood calcium	Hemorrhaging, decreased calcium in bones	Interference with anticlotting medication; synthetic forms may cause jaundice

[a]The recommended intakes for the vitamins are listed at the back of this book.
[b]The Tolerable Upper Intake Levels (UL) for the vitamins are listed at the back of this book.

TABLE 7-4 General Characteristics of Water-Soluble and Fat-Soluble Vitamins

Characteristic	Water-Soluble Vitamins (B vitamins and vitamin C)	Fat-Soluble Vitamins (A, D, E, and K)
Dietary intake	Excess intake usually detected and excreted by the kidneys	Excess intake tends to be stored in fat-storage sites
Body stores	Only a short-term supply available, with little storage; daily intake recommended	Long-term storage available in body tissues; regular intake recommended
Deficiency	Deficiency symptoms appear relatively quickly	Deficiency symptoms are slow to develop
Toxicity	Lower risk of toxicity	Higher risk of toxicity
Absorption and transport	Easily absorbed into blood; travel freely in blood	Like lipids, absorbed into lymph; many require protein carriers if they are to travel in the blood
Solubility	Dissolves in water	Dissolves in lipid
Stability in food handling and processing	Less stable	Stable
Role(s) in the body	Most B vitamins share similar roles; vitamin C serves many different roles in the body	Each has unique roles in the body

are escorted by protein carriers because they are *insoluble* in water. Because they are stored in the liver and in body fat, you need not consume them daily unless your intakes are usually marginal.

This chapter discusses the vitamins known to be important in human nutrition and provides information about food sources and human requirements. The discussions

FIGURE 7-3

How a Coenzyme Works

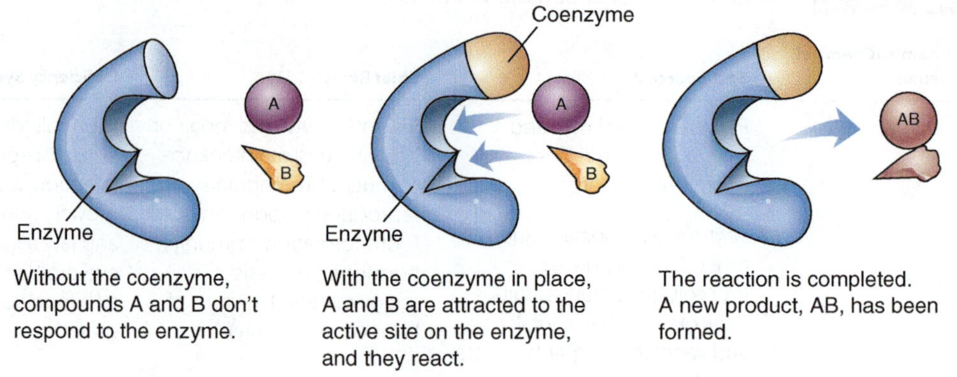

TABLE 7-5 Antioxidant Vitamins
• Enhance the immune system. • Limit free-radical formation. • Destroy free radicals and prevent oxidative damage to cells. • Reduce inflammation in blood vessel walls. • Vitamin C defends body cells and tissues such as skin, lungs, and blood. • Vitamin E and beta-carotene defend the body's lipids such as cell membranes and lipoproteins.

about the vitamins are organized according to the biological roles these substances play in the body.

7.2 The Antioxidant Vitamins

As their name suggests, **antioxidants** are "antioxygen": they fight oxygen, in a manner of speaking. Some chemical reactions that occur in the body involve the use of oxygen. Although these reactions are essential to the body's ability to function, they also lead to the creation of highly toxic compounds called **free radicals** (see Figure 7-4). Environmental pollutants such as cigarette smoke and ozone also prompt the formation of free radicals. Left unchecked, these compounds can cause severe cell injury and ultimately may contribute to the development of chronic diseases such as cancer and heart disease.

Fortunately, the body has a built-in defense system to protect against potential damage from free radicals. That defense system makes use of the antioxidant nutrients: vitamin C, vitamin E, and the carotenoid called **beta-carotene** (see Table 7-5). In addition, the body manufactures certain enzymes, one of which contains the mineral selenium—discussed in Chapter 8—that help fight free radicals.

Vitamin C

The antioxidants work to squelch free radicals before they injure the body, as explained in Figure 7-4. Vitamin C helps stop free radicals in their tracks, working with vitamin E to block damaging chain reactions that appear to promote heart disease and cancer. In addition, vitamin C is a powerful scavenger of environmental air pollutants. In fact, the National Academy of Sciences advises smokers to consume an additional 35 milligrams of vitamin C a day as compared to nonsmokers. The more smoke a person inhales, the more free radicals are produced, and the more vitamin C is needed to fight them.

Other Important Roles for Vitamin C

Vitamin C is required for the production and maintenance of **collagen**, the proteinaceous foundation material for the body's connective tissue, including bones, teeth, skin, and tendons. Vitamin C has also been touted as a nutrient that can help fight stress. In times of stress, the body does use more vitamin C than usual because the vitamin is involved in the release of stress hormones. However, the amount of extra vitamin C used as a result of, say, work-related stress or the stress of ending a significant relationship is minuscule and

antioxidants Substances, such as vitamins, that are "antioxygen"; that is, they help prevent damage done to the body as a result of chemical reactions involving oxygen.

free radicals Highly toxic compounds created in the body as a result of chemical reactions that involve oxygen. Environmental pollutants such as cigarette smoke and ozone also prompt the formation of free radicals.

beta-carotene An orange pigment found in plants that is converted into vitamin A inside the body. Beta-carotene is also an antioxidant.

collagen (KAHL-uh-jen) The characteristic protein of connective tissue (*kolla* = glue; *gennan* = to produce).

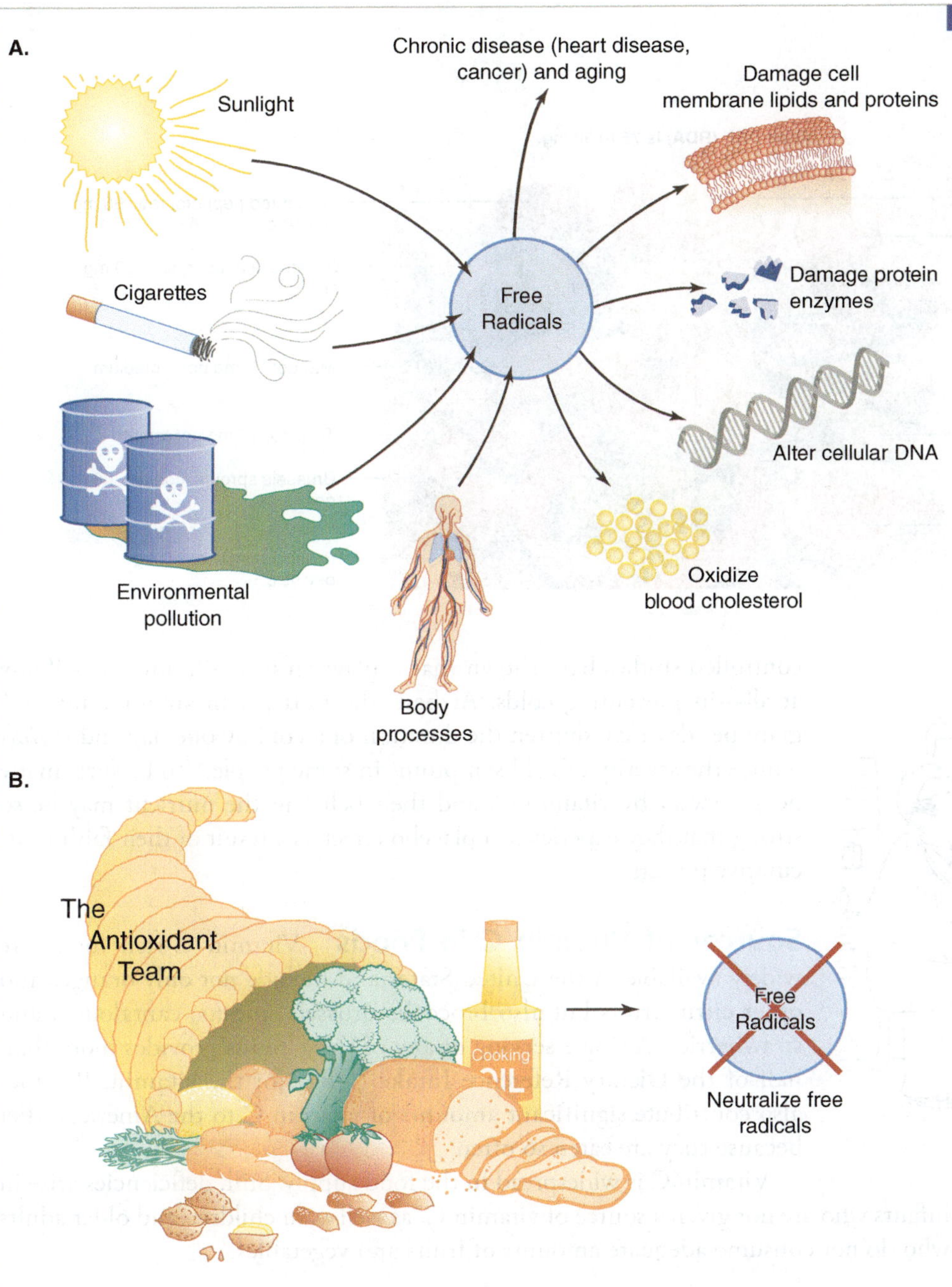

FIGURE 7-4

The Antioxidants versus Free Radicals in the Body

A. Free radicals—unstable oxygen molecules—can be formed from sunlight, in cigarette smoke and environmental pollution, and as a result of many normal chemical reactions involving oxygen in the body. These free radicals attack healthy molecules in the body in hopes of stealing an electron to help stabilize themselves, which in turn can cause cell and tissue damage to the body. Free-radical activity can cause damage to the body's enzymes, cell membranes, and nuclear DNA, or it can result in the formation of oxidized LDL-cholesterol in the arteries.

B. The antioxidant team includes vitamin C, vitamin E, the carotenoids (for example, beta-carotene, lutein, zeaxanthin, lycopene), selenium (a trace mineral), and many naturally occurring nonnutrients—called phytochemicals—found in fruits, vegetables, legumes, and whole grains. The antioxidants prevent free radicals from attacking cells and causing damage by neutralizing the free radicals and converting them back into stable oxygen molecules.

SOURCE: Adapted from *Antioxidant Nutrients* (Mount Olive, NJ: BASF Corporation, 1997).

is more than accounted for by a diet that regularly includes vitamin C-rich foods such as oranges and broccoli (see Table 7-6 and Figure 7-5).

Vitamin C also boosts the body's ability to fight infection, and a growing body of research suggests that it may protect against heart disease and certain types of cancer. Vitamin C's potential role as a chronic disease fighter stems from its function as an antioxidant.[3]

Of course, vitamin C is most famous for its long-standing notoriety as a cure for the common cold. Ever since the publication of the controversial book *Vitamin C and the Common Cold*, by the award-winning scientist Linus Pauling, millions of Americans have followed Dr. Pauling's advice and swallowed megadoses of vitamin C. Despite the popularity of vitamin C as a cold remedy, however, many carefully

For additional perspectives on the use of vitamin and mineral supplements, see the Nutrition Action feature later in this chapter.

FIGURE 7-5

Sources of Vitamin C

***Dietary Reference Intakes (DRI) for all age groups are listed at the back of the book.**

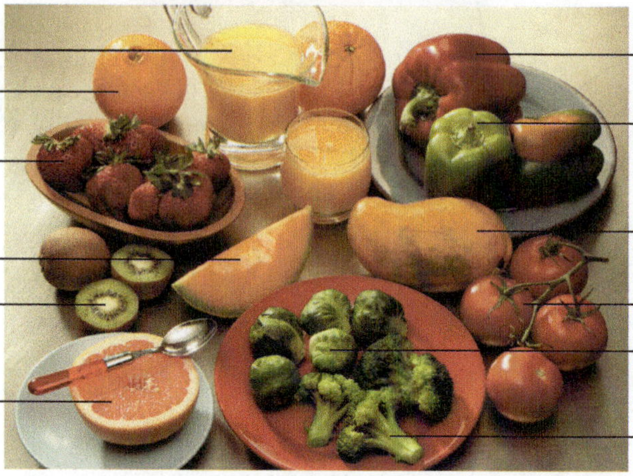

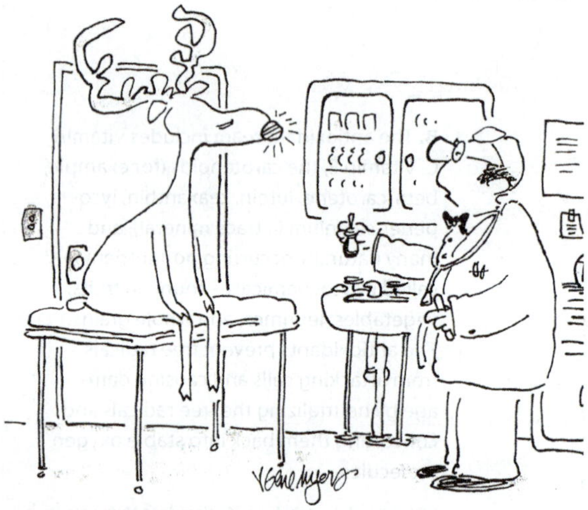

"A little vitamin C ought to clear that up in no time."

controlled studies have shown that it plays an insignificant role—if any at all—in preventing colds. At best, the nutrient in amounts up to 1 gram per day may shorten the duration of a cold by one day and *slightly* reduce the severity of cold symptoms in some people.[4] To be sure, many people swear by vitamin C, and their belief in the nutrient may be so strong that they experience a placebo effect as a result of their faith in its curative powers.

Sources of Vitamin C in Foods

Vitamin C-rich foods are widely available in the United States and include not only oranges and other citrus fruits but also broccoli, Brussels sprouts, cantaloupe, and strawberries. A single serving of any of those foods provides more than half of the Dietary Reference Intake (DRI) for the vitamin. Potatoes also contribute significant amounts of vitamin C to the American diet because they are eaten so often.

Vitamin C is widespread in the food supply. Still, deficiencies arise in infants who are not given a source of vitamin C, as well as in children and older adults who do not consume adequate amounts of fruits and vegetables.

TABLE 7-6 Vitamin C in Foods

(mg)*	Sources
341	Yellow bell pepper (1)
71	Kiwi (1)
70	Orange (1)
62	Orange juice, fresh (½ c)
60	Green bell pepper (½ c)
58	Cantaloupe (1 c)
57	Mango (1)
56	Cabbage, raw (1 c)
51	Broccoli, cooked (½ c)
48	Brussels sprouts, cooked (½ c)
47	Grapefruit juice (½ c)
44	Bok choy, cooked (1 c)
43	Pink/red grapefruit (½ c)
42	Strawberries (½ c)
40	Sweet potato, baked (1 c)

*DRI, adult: men, 90 mg/day; women, 75 mg/day.

Vitamin E

Vitamin E performs a key role as a fat-soluble antioxidant in the body. Vitamin E is involved in protecting red blood cells, nerve cells, and the membranes of the lungs, brain, and other organs against damage from pollutants and other environmental hazards. Vitamin E may also protect against heart disease because it can neutralize the free radicals that might otherwise damage the walls of blood vessels and contribute to coronary artery disease.[5] Scientists believe that the vitamin E residing in the fatty cell membranes that surround cells acts as a scavenger of free radicals that enter the area.[6] When vitamin E is absent, the free radicals can attack the vulnerable polyunsaturated fatty acids found within the cell membrane and start a chemical chain reaction that damages the cell membrane and ultimately causes it to break down completely.

Vitamin E helps maintain a healthy immune system by protecting white blood cells. Vitamin E also protects other lipids, such as low-density lipoproteins (LDLs), throughout the body and fat-soluble compounds, including vitamin A. Additionally, vitamin E is important throughout life for normal neuromuscular function.

FIGURE 7-6

Sources of Vitamin E

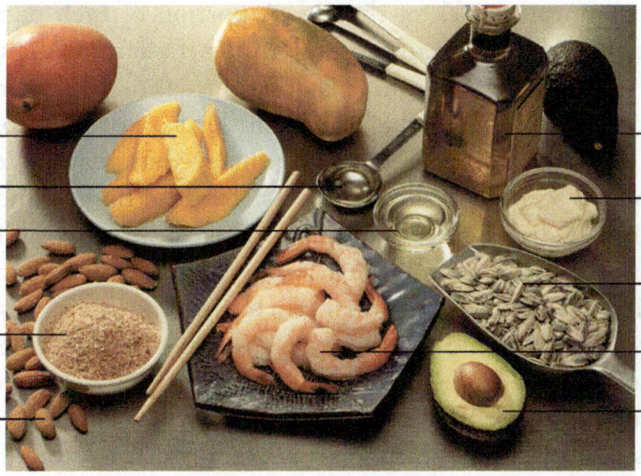

The cell membranes harbor vitamin E, and a deficiency of the nutrient causes those membranes, particularly those in red blood cells, to rupture, causing a type of anemia. Although extremely rare in healthy adults, this problem sometimes occurs in premature infants who are born before enough vitamin E is transferred to them from their mothers in the last few weeks of pregnancy. Other groups of people who run the risk of deficiency include those who cannot absorb fats as a result of diseases and those with certain blood disorders.

Vitamin E toxicity appears to be rare, occurring only in people who take extremely high doses. Suspected symptoms include alteration of the body's blood-clotting mechanisms and interference with the function of vitamin K.

TABLE 7-7 Vitamin E in Foods

(mg)*	Sources
8.6	Almonds (¼ c)
4.5	Wheat germ (1 oz)
4.0	Sunflower seeds (2 tbsp)
3.0	Peanut butter (2 tbsp)
3.0	Peanuts (1 oz)
3.0	Avocado (1)
1.9	Shrimp (3 oz)
1.7	Sardines (3 oz)
1.5	Mango (1 c)
1.4	Apricots, dried (¼ c)
1.2	Salmon (3 oz)
Fats & Oils	
4.6	Safflower oil (1 tbsp)
2.4	Canola oil (1 tbsp)
2.1	Peanut oil (1 tbsp)
2.0	Corn oil (1 tbsp)
2.0	Olive oil (1 tbsp)
0.9	Mayonnaise (1 tbsp)

*DRI, adult: 15 mg/day.

Sources of Vitamin E in Foods

Vitamin E is widespread in plant foods. The great majority of vitamin E in the diet comes from vegetable oils and products made from them, such as margarine and salad dressings. Soybean, sunflower, canola, and safflower oils contain generous amounts of vitamin E, as do nuts, seeds, and wheat germ. Smaller amounts come from fruits and vegetables. Table 7-7 and Figure 7-6 provide sources of vitamin E.

The Vitamin A Precursor: Beta-Carotene

Beta-carotene is a member of the **carotenoid** family of pigments. The carotenoids possess antioxidant properties and work with vitamins C and E in the body to protect against free-radical damage that leads to chronic diseases of the respiratory tract. Certain carotenoids with antioxidant properties, found in dark-green leafy vegetables such as spinach, kale, collard greens, and Swiss chard, may help prevent **age-related macular degeneration**, as well as lower the risk of cataracts.[7] These carotenoids work by filtering out harmful light rays that could cause free-radical damage to the eye. See this chapter's Spotlight feature for more information about the role of the carotenoids in disease prevention.

Beta-carotene is an orange plant pigment that is a vitamin A **precursor**. Inside the body, beta-carotene is converted into vitamin A; however, this happens so slowly that excess amounts are not stored as vitamin A, but are stored in fat deposits instead.

Other Roles for Vitamin A

Vitamin A is one of the most versatile vitamins, playing roles in several important body processes. The best-known function of vitamin A relates to vision. For a person to see, light reaching the eye must be

carotenoids (kah-ROW-teh-noyds) A group of pigments (yellow, orange, and red) found in foods.

age-related macular degeneration (AMD) Oxidative damage to the central portion of the eye (the *macula*) that allows you to focus and see details clearly (peripheral vision remains unimpaired). The carotenoids lutein and zeaxanthin (found in broccoli, Brussels sprouts, kale, spinach, corn, lettuce, and peas) may protect normal macular function.

precursor A compound that can be converted into another compound. For example, beta-carotene is a precursor of vitamin A (*pre* = before; *cursor* = runner, forerunner).

transformed into nerve impulses that the brain interprets to produce visual images. The *transformers* are molecules of **pigment** in the cells of the **retina**, a paper-thin tissue lining the back of the eye. A portion of each pigment molecule is **retinal**, a compound the body can synthesize only if vitamin A is supplied by the diet in some form. Thus, when vitamin A is deficient, vision is impaired. Specifically, the eye has difficulty adapting to changing light levels. For a person deficient in vitamin A, a flash of bright light at night (after the eye has adapted to darkness) is followed by a prolonged spell of **night blindness**. Because night blindness is easy to diagnose, it aids in the diagnosis of vitamin A deficiency. (Night blindness is only a symptom, however, and it may indicate a condition other than vitamin A deficiency.)

Vitamin A also helps to maintain healthy **epithelial tissue**: skin and the cells (called *epithelial cells*) lining such body cavities as the small intestine and lungs. Vitamin A is also involved in the production of sperm, the normal development of fetuses, the immune response, hearing, taste, and growth.

As much as a year's supply of vitamin A can be stored in the body—90 percent of it in the liver. If you stop eating good food sources of vitamin A, deficiency symptoms will not begin to appear until your stores are depleted. Then, however, the consequences are profound and include blindness and reduced resistance to infection. Although vitamin A deficiency is rarely seen in developed countries such as the United States and Canada, it is a serious public health problem in developing countries, where millions of children suffer from blindness, infections, and the other consequences of vitamin A deficiencies.

Vitamin A toxicity, in contrast, is not nearly as widespread as deficiency. Nevertheless, it can also lead to severe health consequences, including joint pain, dryness of skin, hair loss, irritability, fatigue, headaches, weakness, nausea, and liver damage. Thus, it's especially important not to take megadoses of this nutrient.

Although toxicity poses a hazard to people who take supplements of **preformed vitamin A**, toxicity poses virtually no risk to people who obtain vitamin A from foods in the form of beta-carotene.

Sources of Vitamin A and Beta-Carotene in Foods Because the body uses both the preformed vitamin A and the beta-carotene in foods to make **retinol**, the amount of vitamin A that comes from foods is usually expressed in **retinol activity equivalents (RAE)**—a measure of the amount of retinol the body will derive from the food. Figure 7-7 and Table 7-8 show the amount of vitamin A, expressed in RAE, that comes from various foods.

The major sources of vitamin A (in the form of beta-carotene) are almost all brightly colored, in hues of green, yellow, orange, and red. Any plant food with significant vitamin A activity must have some color, because beta-carotene is a rich, deep-yellow, almost orange color. (Preformed vitamin A is pale yellow.) The dark-green leafy vegetables contain large amounts of the green pigment **chlorophyll**, which masks the carotene in them.

In the United States, about half of the vitamin A consumed in foods comes from fruits and vegetables, and about half of that comes from *dark* leafy greens, such as broccoli and spinach and *rich* yellow or *deep*-orange vegetables, such as winter squash, carrots, and sweet potatoes. The other half of the vitamin A comes from milk, cheese, butter, and other dairy products, eggs, and a few meats, such as liver. When whole milk is processed to produce fat-free milk, the vitamin is lost along with the fat that is skimmed. (Remember that vitamin A is found in the fat.) In the United States and Canada, fat-free milk is fortified with vitamin A to compensate for this loss. Likewise, margarine is fortified to provide the amount of vitamin A typically found in butter. (Milk and margarine are also fortified with vitamin D.)

pigment A molecule capable of absorbing certain wavelengths of light. Pigments in the eye permit us to perceive different colors.

retina (RET-in-uh) The paper-thin layer of light-sensitive cells lining the back of the inside of the eye.

retinal (RET-in-al) One of the active forms of vitamin A that functions in the pigments of the eye. Other active forms of vitamin A include retinol and retinoic acid.

night blindness Slow recovery of vision following flashes of bright light at night; an early symptom of vitamin A deficiency.

epithelial (ep-ih-THEE-lee-ul) tissue The cells that form the outer surface of the body and line the body cavities and the principal passageways leading to the exterior. Examples include the cornea, digestive tract lining, respiratory tract lining, and skin. The epithelial cells produce mucus to protect these tissues from bacteria and other potentially harmful substances. Without this mucus, infections become more likely.

preformed vitamin A Vitamin A in its active form.

retinol One of the active forms of vitamin A.

retinol activity equivalents (RAE) A measure of the amount of retinol the body will derive from a food containing preformed vitamin A or beta-carotene and other vitamin A precursors. Note that some tables list vitamin A in terms of *international units (IU)*. (See Appendix A for methods of converting from one measure to another.)

chlorophyll The green pigment of plants that traps energy from sunlight and uses this energy in photosynthesis (the synthesis of carbohydrate by green plants).

FIGURE 7-7

Sources of Vitamin A and Beta-Carotene

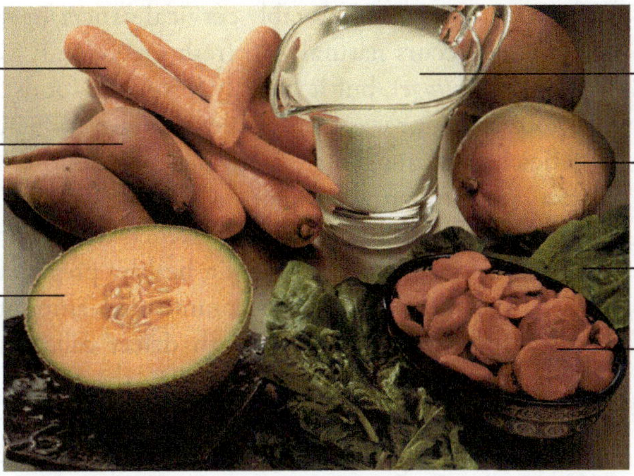

TABLE 7-8 Vitamin A in Foods

(μg RAE)[a]	Sources	(μg RAE)[a]	Sources
6,586	Beef liver (3 oz)[b]	150	Fortified milk (1 c)[b]
961	Sweet potato (½ c)	85	Egg, boiled (1)[b]
510	Carrot, raw (½ c)	78	Mango (1)
472	Spinach, cooked (½ c)	66	Grapefruit, red (½ c)
274	Turnip greens, cooked (½ c)	60	Apricot halves, dried (¼ c)
270	Cantaloupe (1 c)	60	Broccoli, cooked (½ c)
203	Butternut squash (½ c)	52	Tomato, fresh (1)
180	Bok choy, cooked (½ c)	42	Watermelon (1 c)
162	Romaine lettuce (1 c)	35	Plantain, cooked (½ c)

[a] DRI, adult: men, 900 μg RAE/day; women, 700 μg RAE/day.
[b] Preformed vitamin A. The rest of the items on the chart derive vitamin A from beta-carotene.

7.3 Vitamins for Healthy Blood

Every cell in the body needs a continuous supply of water, oxygen, energy, and building materials. As the blood, pumped by the heart, travels through the circulatory system, it picks up and delivers materials as needed. Every cell continuously uses up oxygen (producing carbon dioxide) and nutrients (producing waste products). The blood transports oxygen and nutrients to the cells and carries carbon dioxide and waste away from them.

Many vitamins serve blood-related functions in the body (see Table 7-9). Folate and vitamin B_{12} assist with the formation of new blood cells. Vitamin B_6 is associated with hemoglobin, the compound that carries oxygen in the blood. Vitamin K is needed for blood clotting.

TABLE 7-9 Vitamins Essential for Healthy Blood

- Folate is needed for formation and maintenance of healthy red blood cells.
- Vitamin B_{12} is needed for formation of healthy red blood cells.
- Vitamin B_6 is needed for synthesis of hemoglobin, which carries oxygen in the blood.
- Vitamin K is needed for blood clotting.

Folate

Folate (also called *folic acid* or *folacin*) is a coenzyme with many functions in the body. It is particularly important in the synthesis of DNA and the formation of red blood cells. A folate deficiency creates misshapen red blood cells that are unable to carry sufficient oxygen to the body's other cells, thereby causing a certain kind of **anemia**. Thus, folate deficiency results in a generalized malaise with many

anemia Any condition in which the blood is unable to deliver oxygen to the cells of the body. Examples include a shortage or abnormality of the red blood cells. Many nutrient deficiencies and diseases can cause anemia.

FIGURE 7-8

Neural Tube Defect

This child has spina bifida—a birth defect characterized by the incomplete closing of the casing around the spinal cord. Afflicting some 3,000 U.S. infants born each year, the problem causes partial paralysis.

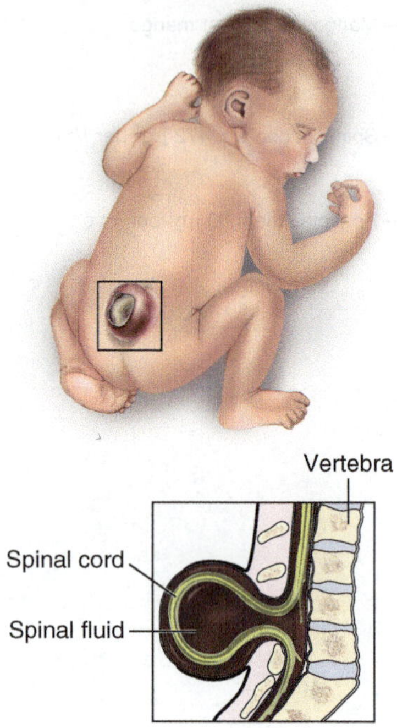

© Cengage

symptoms, including fatigue, diarrhea, irritability, forgetfulness, lack of appetite, and headache. Folate deficiency can easily be confused with general ill health, depressed mood, and dementia in older adults. Folate deficiency may also elevate a person's risk for certain cancers—notably cervical cancer in women and colon cancer.[8]

Folate occurs naturally in fresh green, leafy vegetables (hence its derivation from the word *foliage*), but it is easily lost when foods are overcooked, canned, dehydrated, or otherwise processed. People who are growing rapidly run a high risk of folate deficiency because folate is needed to promote the rapid multiplication of cells that occurs during growth. That's why, for example, the need for folate increases during pregnancy, when the vitamin is needed to support the growth of the fetus.

Folate plays a crucial role in a healthy pregnancy. A growing body of evidence indicates that consuming the recommended amount of folate reduces the risk of bearing a baby with a type of birth defect called **neural tube defect** (see Figure 7-8). Afflicting some 3,000 infants born in the United States each year, neural tube defects include *spina bifida*—the incomplete closing of the bony casing around the spinal cord that causes partial paralysis—and *anencephaly*—a condition in which major parts of the brain are missing. All women of childbearing age are advised to consume the recommended amount of folate, because adequate levels of the nutrient must be ingested before and during the first few weeks of pregnancy—the period during which the neural tube of the embryo is closing, but when most women are not even aware that they are pregnant.

neural tube defects Malformations of the brain and/or spinal cord during embryonic development.

Sources of Folate in Foods

Although folate is abundant in vegetables, legumes, and seeds, as shown in Figure 7-9 and Table 7-10, most women typically consume foods that provide only about half the 400-microgram amount recommended. For this reason, the Food and Drug Administration has mandated that all enriched grain products be fortified with folic acid, an easily absorbed synthetic form of folate, to improve intakes in the United States.[9] As a result, the United States has recorded significant declines in neural tube defects since folic acid fortification of all enriched cereal-grain products began. Labels on fortified products may make the health claim "adequate intake of folate has been shown to reduce the risk of neural tube defects." A person can obtain the recommended 400 micrograms of folate by increasing consumption of foods naturally rich in folate (orange juice and green vegetables) and foods fortified with folic acid (breakfast cereals, breads, rice, or pasta), or

FIGURE 7-9

Sources of Folate

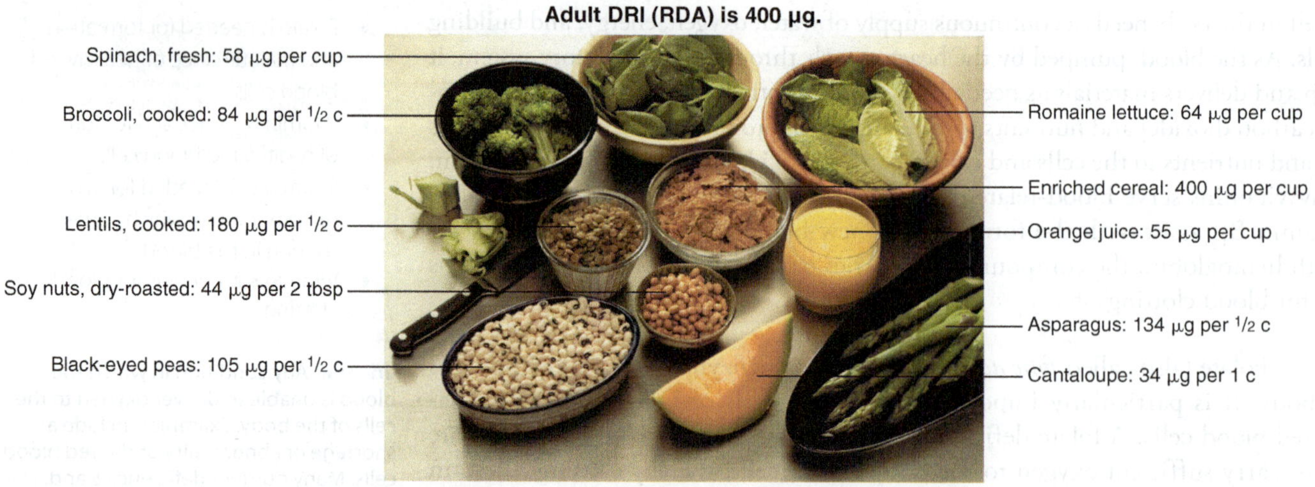

© Matthew Farruggio Photography

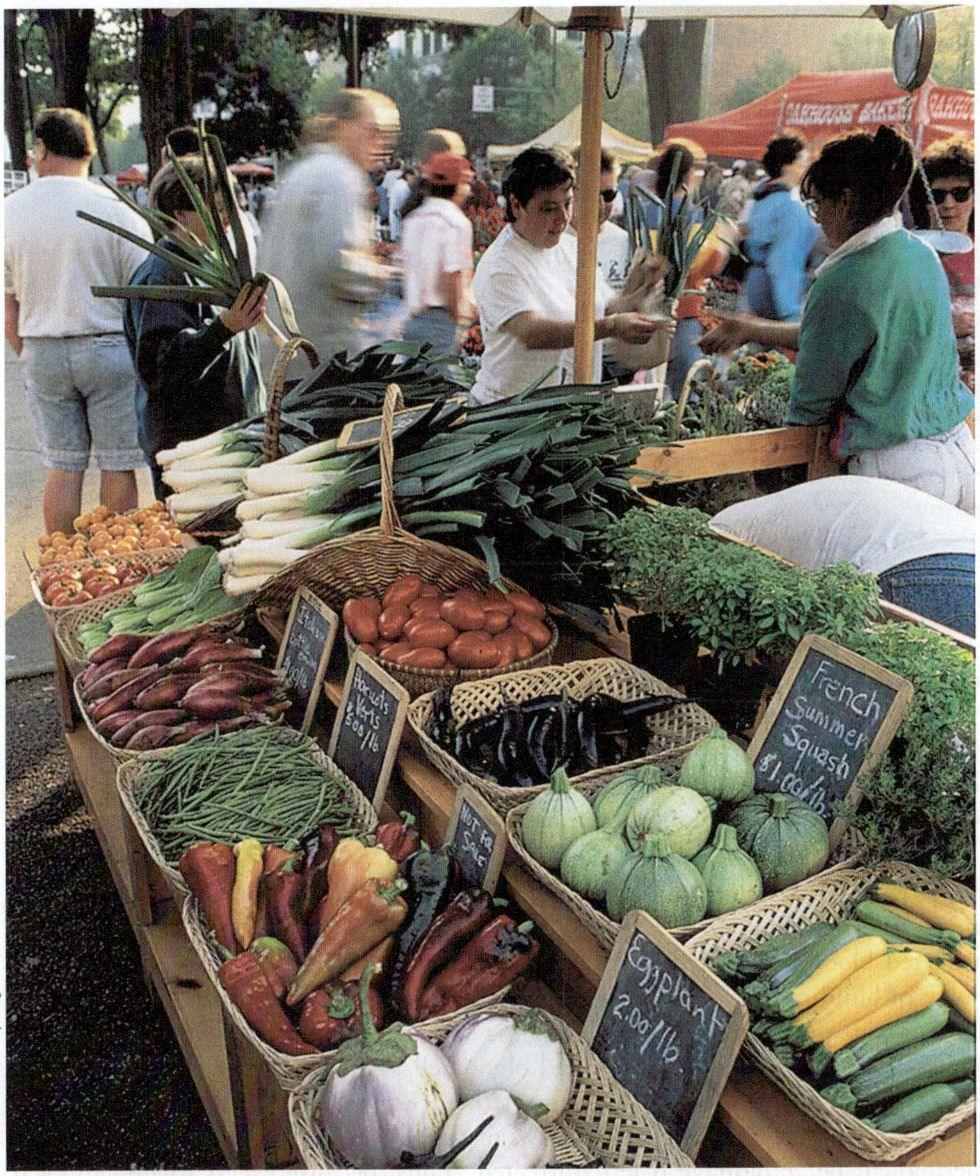

© Zane Williams/Getty Images

When you think of the B vitamin folate, think of fresh produce. Folate derives its name from the word *foliage*, and it is naturally abundant in fresh dark-green vegetables (such as spinach and broccoli), some fresh fruits (oranges and melons), and legumes (lentils and black-eyed peas). Other sources include foods made from grains enriched with folic acid such as breakfast cereals, breads, rice, or pasta.

TABLE 7-10 **Folate in Foods**

(μg)*	Sources
400	Fortified cereal (1 c)
180	Lentils, cooked (½ c)
134	Asparagus, cooked (½ c)
128	Black beans (½ c)
127	Navy beans (½ c)
115	Spinach, cooked (½ c)
107	Pomegranate (1)
105	Black-eyed peas (½ c)
102	Avocado (½ c)
100	Soybeans, green, cooked (½ c)
85	Turnip greens, cooked (½ c)
84	Broccoli, cooked (½ c)
64	Romaine lettuce (1 c)
58	Spinach, fresh (1 c)
57	Oatmeal, instant (½ c)
53	Peanuts (¼ c)
40	Orange (1)
40	Sunflower seeds (2 tbsp)
37	Tofu (soybean curd) (3 oz)
36	Whole-wheat bread (1 slice)
34	Cantaloupe (1 c)
12	Fat-free milk (1 c)

*DRI, adult: 400 μg/day.

by taking a folic acid supplement daily.[10]* Because high levels of blood folate can mask a true vitamin B_{12} deficiency, total folate intake should not exceed 1 milligram daily.[11]

B Vitamins and Heart Disease Low intakes of three B vitamins—folate, vitamin B_{12}, and vitamin B_6—may be linked with increased risk of fatal heart disease in both men and women.[12] People with low blood levels of these B vitamins tend to have high blood levels of the protein-related compound **homocysteine**.[13] High levels of homocysteine may enhance blood clot formation and damage to arterial walls. However, scientists

*All enriched cereal-grain products are fortified with 1.4 milligrams of folic acid per 100 grams of food. Recommended folate intakes are stated in micrograms (μg) DFE. A microgram is a thousandth of a milligram. *DFE* stands for dietary folate equivalent, a unit of measure expressing the amount of folate available to the body from naturally occurring food sources. The measure accounts for the differences in absorption between food folate and the more absorbable synthetic folic acid added to foods and supplements. Appendix A offers a conversion factor for calculating DFE.

homocysteine (hoe-moe-SIS-teen) A chemical that appears to be toxic to the blood vessels of the heart. High blood levels of homocysteine have been associated with low blood levels of vitamin B_{12}, vitamin B_6, and folate.

FIGURE 7-10

Sources of Vitamin B_{12}

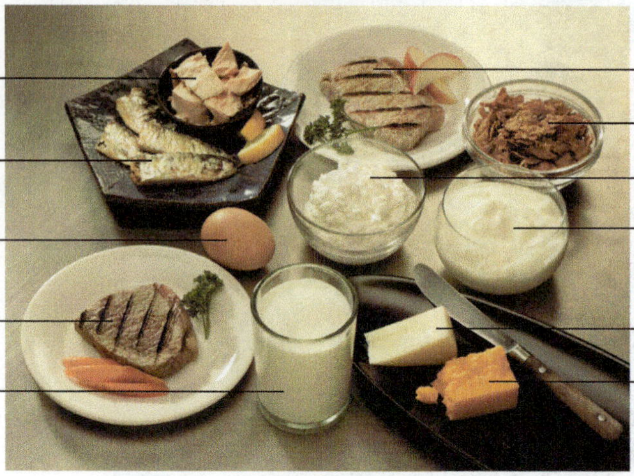

TABLE 7-11 Vitamin B_{12} in Foods

(μg)*	Sources
7.60	Sardines (3 oz)
4.20	Tuna (3 oz)
2.50	Ground beef (3 oz)
2.00	Fortified cereal (1 c)
1.80	Salmon (3 oz)
1.50	Plain nonfat yogurt (1 c)
1.40	Cottage cheese (1 c)
1.40	Shrimp (3 oz)
1.20	Haddock (3 oz)
0.90	Fat-free milk (1 c)
0.60	Egg (1)
0.30	Cheddar cheese (1.5 oz)

*DRI, adult: 2.4 μg/day.

conclude that homocysteine-lowering interventions have thus far been ineffective in preventing heart attacks.[14] In addition, some evidence suggests that high homocysteine levels may also be toxic for brain tissue and impair cognitive ability.[15] The B vitamins clear homocysteine from the blood and prevent its toxic buildup. More research is needed to clarify the associations linking a vitamin B-poor diet with increased homocysteine levels.

Vitamin B_{12}

Vitamin B_{12} maintains the sheaths that surround and protect nerve fibers. The nutrient also works closely with folate, enabling it to manufacture red blood cells. When a B_{12} deficiency is present, folate is unable to do its work of building red blood cells. As a result, a person suffering a lack of vitamin B_{12} ends up with the same sort of anemia seen in people with a folate deficiency, characterized by large, immature red blood cells. Although extra folate will clear up the anemia, it does not take care of the other problems resulting from a B_{12} deficiency: namely, a creeping paralysis of the nerves and muscles that can cause permanent nerve damage if left untreated. Thus, because excess folate can clear up the blood problems that signal an otherwise hard-to-diagnose vitamin B_{12} deficiency, the amount of folate that can be added to enriched foods is limited by law.

To be sure, dietary deficiencies of vitamin B_{12} are unlikely for people who eat animal foods such as meat, milk, cheese, and eggs, all of which supply generous amounts of the nutrient (see Table 7-11 and Figure 7-10). Strict vegetarians who avoid meat, eggs, and dairy products, however, need to find alternative sources of the nutrient, such as vitamin B_{12}-fortified soy beverages, fortified cereals, or B_{12} supplements.

Several other groups of people are also at high risk for vitamin B_{12} deficiency, not because of a lack of the vitamin in their diets, but because of physical conditions that hamper the body's ability to make use of the nutrient. One such group is people who inherit a genetic defect that leaves the body unable to make a compound known as **intrinsic factor**. Produced in the stomach, intrinsic factor enables the body to absorb and make use of vitamin B_{12}; without the compound, vitamin B_{12} deficiency develops. In this instance, or in the case of stomach damage that interferes with the production of intrinsic factor, people must get vitamin B_{12} injections.

Older adults are also likely to experience vitamin B_{12} deficiencies. An estimated 20 percent of older adults in their 60s and 40 percent of those in their 80s develop **atrophic gastritis**, an age-related condition characterized by the stomach's inability

intrinsic factor A compound made in the stomach that is necessary for the body's absorption of vitamin B_{12}.

atrophic gastritis An age-related condition characterized by the stomach's inability to produce enough acid, which in turn leads to vitamin B_{12} deficiencies.

FIGURE 7-11

Sources of Vitamin B_6

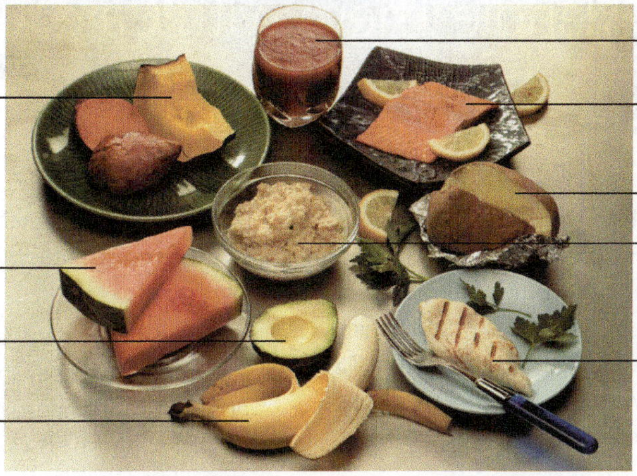

to produce enough acid, which in turn hampers the body's ability to use vitamin B_{12}. In severe cases, the condition also limits the stomach's ability to make intrinsic factor. Vitamin B_{12} deficiencies resulting from atrophic gastritis appear to be easily treated with vitamin B_{12} supplements or injections.[16]

Vitamin B_6 Like the other B vitamins, vitamin B_6 functions as an indispensable coenzyme. For example, vitamin B_6 helps make **hemoglobin** for red blood cells. Vitamin B_6 also plays many roles in protein metabolism. In fact, a person's requirement for vitamin B_6 is proportional to protein intakes. Because vitamin B_6 performs this and so many other tasks, a deficiency causes a multitude of symptoms, including weakness, irritability, and insomnia. Low levels of vitamin B_6 may also weaken the body's immune response and increase a person's risk of heart disease. Vitamin B_6 is found in meats, vegetables, and whole-grain cereals, and true vitamin B_6 deficiencies are rare—occurring in some people who eat inadequate diets and whose nutrient needs are higher than usual because of pregnancy, alcohol abuse, some diseases, use of certain prescription drugs, and other unusual circumstances. Figure 7-11 and Table 7-12 show the vitamin B_6 content of various foods.

Vitamin K The *K* in vitamin K stands for the Danish word *koagulation* (coagulation or clotting). The key function of vitamin K is its role in the blood-clotting system of the body, where its presence can mean the difference between life and death. It is essential for the synthesis of at least 4 of the 13 proteins involved, along with

TABLE 7-12 **Vitamin B_6 in Foods**

(mg)*	Sources	(mg)*	Sources
0.69	Turkey (3 oz)	0.25	Salmon (3.5 oz)
0.63	Baked potato (1)	0.23	Ground beef (3 oz)
0.46	Chicken breast (3.5 oz)	0.22	Spinach, cooked (½ c)
0.45	Pork chop (3 oz)	0.21	Pomegranate (1)
0.43	Banana (1)	0.20	Flounder/sole (3 oz)
0.30	Tuna (3 oz)	0.20	Soybeans (½ c)
0.29	Sweet potato (½ c)	0.10	Fat-free milk (1 c)

*DRI, adult (19–50 years): 1.3 mg/day.

hemoglobin (HEEM-uh-glow-bin) The oxygen-carrying protein of the blood; found in the red blood cells.

THE SAVVY Diner Color Your Plate with Vitamin-Rich Foods—And Handle Them with Care (Obj. 7.3)

Buying a variety of vitamin-rich fruits and vegetables at the market is one of the first steps to obtaining plenty of those all-important nutrients in your diet. The next step is storing and cooking those foods in ways that minimize the loss of vitamins that can occur as a result of improper storage and preparation. To help get the most from the produce you buy, use the following tips on fruit and vegetable storage and preparation:

- Shop for produce at least once a week. The longer fruits and vegetables stay in your refrigerator before being eaten, the more nutrients are likely to be lost.
- Store fruits and vegetables (other than bananas, tomatoes, and potatoes) in your refrigerator rather than in a fruit bowl or on the kitchen counter. Chilling slows the metabolic rate of the cells of a fruit or vegetable, which in turn causes the cells to use less of their own nutrients. Thus, chilling prevents nutrient depletion.
- Store fruits and vegetables whole, peeling and cutting only what you need immediately before cooking or eating. Once you cut into the skin of an item and expose it to air, vitamin loss begins. After slicing, the vitamin C content of oranges, grapefruits, tomatoes, and strawberries begins to decline. If you do have leftover cut produce, wrap it tightly in airtight plastic or store it in an airtight container inside the refrigerator.
- Try to eat frozen vegetables within a month or two of purchase, because nutrient losses occur over time in stored vegetables.
- Cook vegetables in the least amount of water and for the shortest period of time possible. Water-soluble vitamins readily dissolve into cooking water, and heat destroys some as well. To minimize such losses, steam vegetables over water, or cook vegetables in a microwave oven.

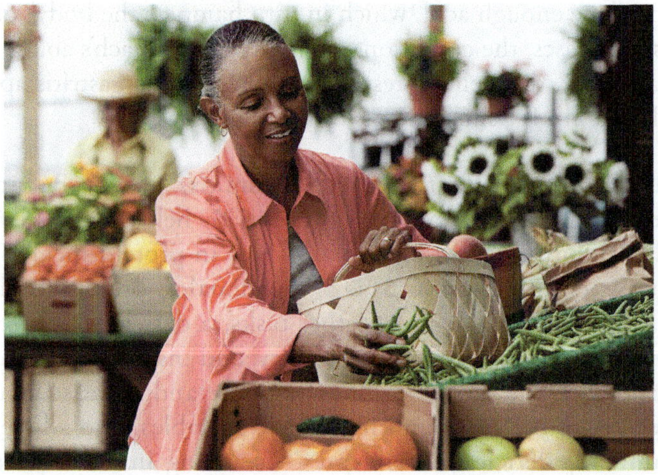

Ariel Skelley/Blend Images/Alamy Stock Photo

Once you've taken the time to select fresh, vitamin-rich fruits and vegetables, be sure to handle them with care when you get them home.

calcium, in making the blood clot. When *any* of these blood-clotting factors is absent, blood cannot clot, leaving a person vulnerable to excessive bleeding upon injury.

Vitamin K can be synthesized by the **intestinal microflora**—the bacteria that reside in the digestive tract. In addition, as Figure 7-12 and Table 7-13 show, many foods supply ample amounts of the vitamin; particular standouts are green leafy vegetables and members of the cabbage family.

Because vitamin K is obtained both in the diet and via the intestinal bacteria, deficiencies are rare and occur only under unusual circumstances. Taking antibiotics for an extended period of time, for instance, could kill some of the intestinal bacteria and thereby prompt a deficiency.

Newborn babies are the one group that is commonly susceptible to vitamin K deficiency, because a baby's digestive tract contains no bacteria before birth. After birth, the infant's intestinal tract gradually becomes populated with bacteria, but this happens over time. What's more, baby formula or breast milk generally doesn't contain adequate amounts of vitamin K. Thus, newborns are given a dose of vitamin K to prevent the possibility of a life-threatening hemorrhage in the case of injury.

intestinal microflora The normal bacterial inhabitants of the digestive tract (*flora* = plant inhabitants).

FIGURE 7-12

Sources of Vitamin K

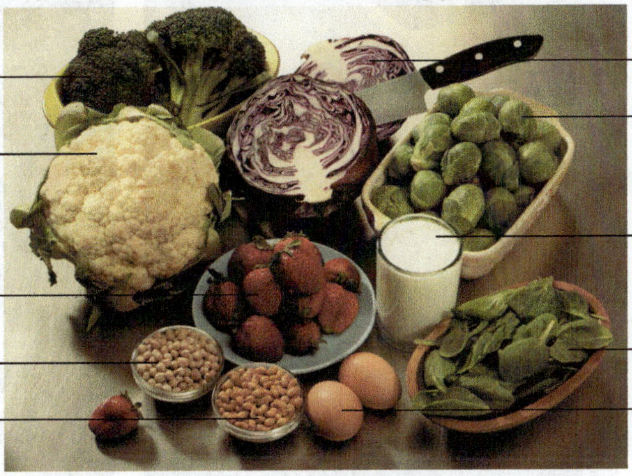

TABLE 7-13 Vitamin K in Foods

(µg)*	Sources	(µg)*	Sources
520	Kale, cooked (½ c)	58	Broccoli, raw (½ c)
460	Brussels sprouts (½ c)	52	Chickpeas (½ c)
380	Spinach, cooked (½ c)	30	Sauerkraut (½ c)
364	Turnip greens, cooked (½ c)	29	Berries, blue or black (1 c)
248	Broccoli, cooked (½ c)	25	Soybean oil (1 tbsp)
140	Spinach, raw (1 c)	25	Egg (1)
104	Cabbage, raw (1 c)	20	Soybeans, dry roasted (¼ c)
96	Cauliflower, raw (½ c)	19	Canola oil (1 tbsp)
72	Asparagus, cooked (½ c)	10	Strawberries (½ c)
60	Lettuce (1 c)	10	Milk, whole (1 c)

*DRI, adult: 90 to 120 µg/day.

Vitamin K toxicity is rare, but it can occur when supplemental doses are taken. In particular, adults who must pay attention to the amount of vitamin K in their diet are those who take anticoagulant drugs designed to prevent the blood from clotting and possibly causing a stroke or heart attack. People taking such medications are advised to keep their consumption of vitamin K fairly constant from day to day, because large fluctuations can limit the effectiveness of the anticlotting drugs.[17]

7.4 Vitamins for Healthy Bones

Bones are made up of a complex matrix of living tissue based on the protein collagen, into which the crystals of the bone minerals discussed in the next chapter—principally calcium and phosphorus—are deposited. When calcium intakes are low, vitamin D, acting as a hormone, calls upon the bones to release calcium into the

FIGURE 7-13

Healthy Bone versus Bone Loss

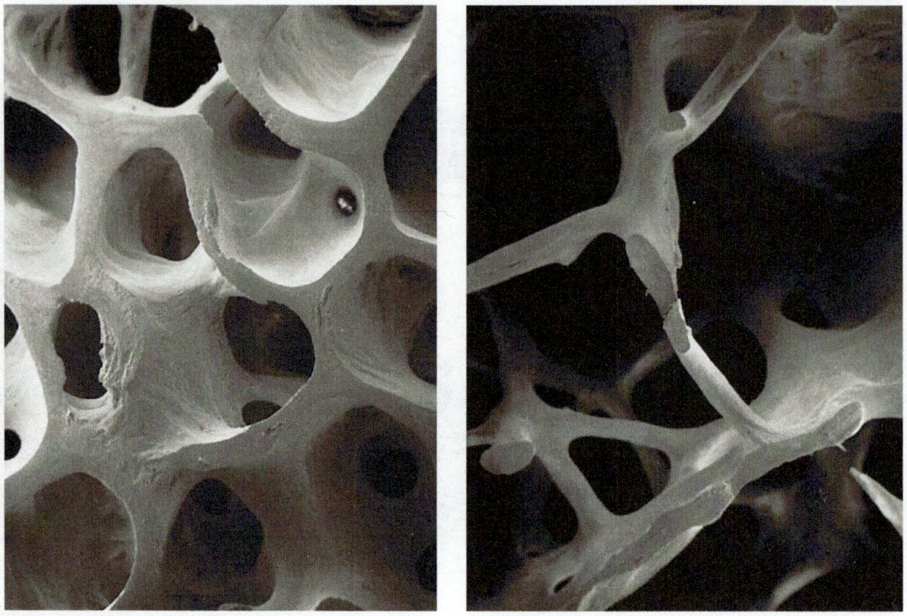

From *Journal of Bone and Mineral Research* 1 (1986): 15–21 with permission of the American Society for Bone and Mineral Research.

Electron micrograph of healthy, dense trabecular bone.

From *Journal of Bone and Mineral Research* 1 (1986): 15–21 with permission of the American Society for Bone and Mineral Research/American Society for Bone and Mineral Research

Electron micrograph of thin and weakened trabecular bone affected by osteoporosis.

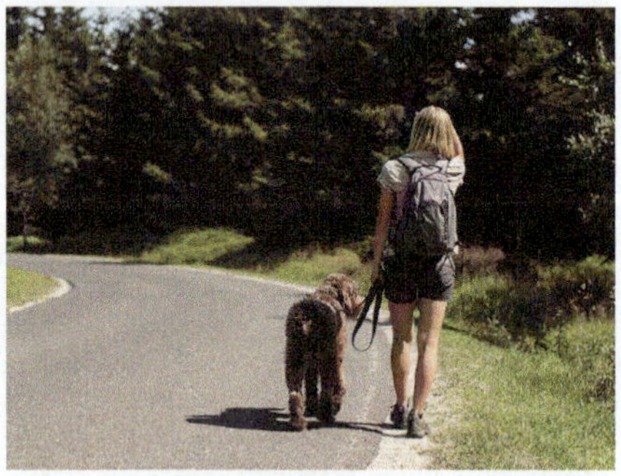

Kamila Starzycka/Shutterstock.com

Vitamin D is the sunshine vitamin. A 15-minute walk, on a clear summer day, two to three times per week, can help supply much of your needed vitamin D. Note that although many people can meet at least some of their vitamin D needs through exposure to sunlight, factors such as season, time of day, cloud cover, smog, skin melanin content, and sunscreen can affect ultraviolet radiation exposure and vitamin D synthesis.

blood for use by the rest of the body whenever levels fall too low.* Over time, the lacy network of bones becomes less dense and more fragile as calcium deposits are withdrawn (see Figure 7-13).

Several vitamins are needed for the growth and maintenance of a healthy skeleton (see Table 7-14). Vitamin D directs a large bone-making and bone-maintenance team composed of several nutrients and other compounds, including vitamin C and vitamin K; hormones; the protein collagen; and several minerals.

Vitamin D Vitamin D's special role in bone health involves assisting in the absorption of dietary calcium and helping to make calcium and phosphorus available in the blood that bathes the bones, so that these minerals can be deposited as

TABLE 7-14 Vitamins Essential for Healthy Bones

Vitamin D	Assists in the absorption of dietary calcium and phosphorus and helps to maintain calcium and phosphorus concentrations in the blood, so that these minerals can be deposited as the bones harden.
Vitamin K	Vitamin K works in conjunction with vitamin D to synthesize a bone protein (osteocalcin) that binds to the minerals that form bones and helps regulate bone density.
Vitamin C	Vitamin C is required for the production and maintenance of collagen, the protein foundation material for the body's connective tissue, including bones and teeth.

*Vitamin D and parathyroid hormone circulate in the blood whenever the calcium concentration in the blood falls too low. These hormones cause the release of calcium from the bones and decreased excretion of calcium by the kidneys. Vitamin D also acts to increase absorption of dietary calcium by the intestines. The hormone calcitonin is released from the thyroid gland when levels of blood calcium get too high; it acts to stop the release of calcium from bone and to slow intestinal absorption of the mineral.

the bones harden. In addition, vitamin D acts as a hormone—a compound manufactured by one organ of the body that affects another. Indeed, vitamin D exerts an influence on a number of organs, including the kidneys and the intestines.

Another unique feature of vitamin D is that the body can synthesize it with the help of sunlight, regardless of dietary consumption. Vitamin D is commonly called the "sunshine vitamin" because sunlight can transform a cholesterol compound in skin into a vitamin D precursor, which is absorbed directly into the blood. The liver alters the molecule, and the kidney alters it further to produce the active form of the vitamin. This is why diseases affecting either the liver or the kidneys, which in turn upset vitamin production, may ultimately lead to bone deterioration.

Because the body can make vitamin D with the help of sunlight, you can meet your needs for the nutrient either via sun exposure or through diet.* However, significant amounts of the nutrient come from only a few animal foods—notably eggs, liver, and some fish (see Table 7-15 and Figure 7-14). And, even in these foods, the vitamin D content varies greatly.

Although vitamin D is not prevalent in the diet, adults living in sunny, southern regions may not need to worry about the vitamin D content of the foods they eat, because their bodies are getting plenty of the nutrient as a result of sun exposure. Sun exposure of the face, hands, and arms for just 5 to 15 minutes several times a week is usually all it takes to meet vitamin D needs. However, during the winter (from November through February) people who live in most parts of the country, north of an imaginary line drawn at latitudes above 35 degrees (above northern borders of Alabama and Georgia), are not exposed to enough ultraviolet rays from the sun to synthesize vitamin D. The same holds true for those with very dark skin and housebound or institutionalized older adults—who not only get outside less often than younger people but also tend to be much less efficient at producing vitamin D via the skin/sun synthesis pathway. Others at risk for vitamin D deficiency include people with **osteoporosis** or conditions that interfere with vitamin D absorption.

The *2015–2020 Dietary Guidelines for Americans* report lists vitamin D as a nutrient of public health concern because low intakes are associated with health concerns. Eating vitamin D-rich foods, such as seafood with higher amounts of vitamin D

TABLE 7-15 Vitamin D in Foods

(µg)*	Sources
16.2	Trout, rainbow, farmed, cooked (3 oz)
12.3	Salmon, pink, canned
11.1	Salmon, cooked (3 oz)
5.7	Tuna, light, canned in oil (3 oz)
4.1	Sardines (3 oz)
3.0	Shrimp (3 oz)
3.0	Fortified milk (1 c)
2.5	Fortified cereals (1 c)
1.1	Egg (1)
0.5	Fortified margarine (1 tsp)

*DRI, adult, 18–70 years: 15 µg/day; ≥ 70 years: 20 µg/day.

osteoporosis (OSS-tee-oh-pore-OH-sis) Also known as *adult bone loss*; a disease in which the bones become porous and fragile (*osteo* = bones; *poros* = porous).

FIGURE 7-14

Sources of Vitamin D

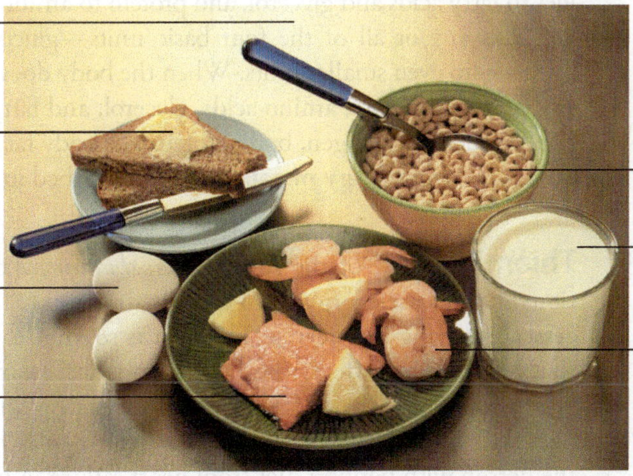

*To protect against skin cancer, avoid prolonged exposure to the sun.

FIGURE 7-15

Rickets

This child has the bowed legs characteristic of rickets. Worldwide, rickets affects many children who live in poverty and do not have access to sunlight or adequate foods containing vitamin D.

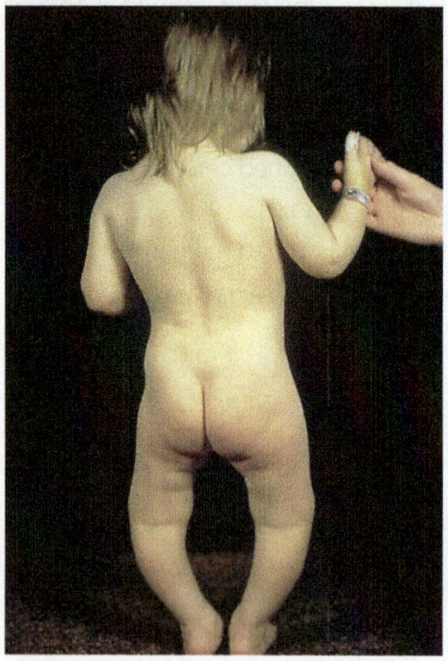

(including salmon, sardines, herring, mackerel, trout, and light tuna), and consuming more foods fortified with vitamin D, especially milk, yogurt, soy milk, almond milk, rice milk, orange juice, and breakfast cereals, is particularly important.

Some evidence suggests an association between low blood levels of vitamin D and increased risk for certain cancers, inflammation, high blood pressure, and other conditions, but thus far the evidence is limited.[18] However, in an effort to improve bone health, the Institute of Medicine now recommends 15 micrograms for adults between ages 18 and 70, and 20 micrograms for adults age 71 or older (the earlier DRIs ranged from 5 to 15 micrograms).[19]

Children who fail to get enough vitamin D characteristically develop bowed legs, which are often the most obvious sign of the deficiency disease rickets (see Figure 7-15). In adults, vitamin D deficiency causes **osteomalacia**, most often in women whose diets lack calcium, who get little exposure to the sun, and who go through several closely spaced pregnancies and prolonged periods of breastfeeding. Osteomalacia causes the bones, particularly the leg bones and spine, to become soft, porous, and weak.

Although vitamin D deficiency depresses calcium absorption, resulting in low blood calcium levels and abnormal bone development, an excess of vitamin D does just the opposite. It increases calcium absorption, causing abnormally high concentration of the mineral in the blood, which then tends to be deposited in the soft tissues. This is especially likely to happen in the kidneys, resulting in the formation of calcium-containing stones called *kidney stones*. The Tolerable Upper Intake Level for vitamin D is set at 50 micrograms per day.

Vitamin K

Accumulating evidence also supports an active role for vitamin K in the maintenance of bone health. Vitamin K works in conjunction with vitamin D to synthesize a bone protein that helps regulate the calcium levels in the blood. Low levels of vitamin K in the blood have been associated with low bone mineral density, and researchers have noted a lower risk of hip fracture in older women who have optimal intakes of vitamin K than in those who have low intakes of the vitamin (see Table 7-13).[20]

TABLE 7-16 Vitamins Essential for Producing Energy

- Thiamin
- Riboflavin
- Niacin
- Folate
- Vitamin B_6
- Vitamin B_{12}
- Pantothenic acid
- Biotin

7.5 Vitamins and Energy Metabolism

As described in Chapter 3, glycogen can be broken down in the body to glucose, triglycerides to fatty acids and glycerol, and protein to amino acids. When the body needs energy, it breaks any or all of the four basic units—glucose, fatty acids, glycerol, and amino acids—into even smaller units. When the body does not require energy, the end products of digestion (glucose, amino acids, glycerol, and fatty acids) are used to build body compounds such as glycogen, body proteins, or body fat. Many vitamins (as well as minerals) are essential for **energy metabolism**, as described in the following sections (Table 7-16).

Thiamin

One of the B vitamins, *thiamin*, acts primarily as a coenzyme in reactions that release energy from carbohydrates. Thiamin also plays a crucial role in processes involving the nerves. Thiamin is so vital to the functioning of the entire body that a deficiency affects the nerves, muscles, heart, and other organs. A severe deficiency, called **beriberi**, causes extreme wasting and loss of muscle tissue, swelling all over the body, enlargement of the heart, irregular heartbeat, and paralysis. Ultimately, the person with beriberi dies from heart failure. A mild thiamin deficiency, in contrast, often mimics other conditions and typically manifests itself as vague, general symptoms such as stomachaches, headaches, fatigue, restlessness, sleep disturbances, chest pains, fevers, personality changes (aggressiveness and hostility), and neurosis.

osteomalacia (os-tee-oh-muh-LAY-shuh) The disease resulting from vitamin D deficiency in adults and characterized by softening of the bones. (Its counterpart in children is called rickets.) Symptoms include bowed legs and a curved spine.

energy metabolism All the reactions by which the body obtains and expends the energy from food.

beriberi The thiamin deficiency disease, characterized by irregular heartbeat, paralysis, and extreme wasting of muscle tissue.

FIGURE 7-16

Sources of Thiamin

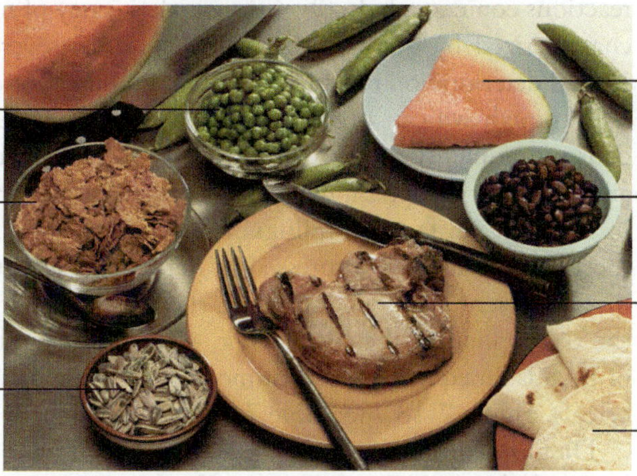

Thiamin is found in a wide variety of foods, and virtually no single food will supply your daily needs in a single serving (in the same way that, say, an orange provides a plentiful supply of vitamin C). However, people who eat a balanced diet following the framework of the MyPlate food guide typically consume plenty of thiamin. As Figure 7-16 and Table 7-17 show, thiamin is found in a variety of meats, legumes, fruits, and vegetables, as well as in all enriched and whole-grain products.

Riboflavin

Like thiamin, the B vitamin *riboflavin* acts as a coenzyme in energy-releasing reactions in the body. In addition, riboflavin helps to prepare fatty acids and amino acids for breakdown. Deficiencies of the vitamin, which are rare, are characterized by severe skin problems, including painful cracks at the corners of the mouth; a red, swollen tongue; and teary or bloodshot eyes.

Table 7-18 and Figure 7-17 show the riboflavin content of foods. Milk and dairy products contribute a good deal of the riboflavin in many people's diets. Meats are another good source, as are dark-green vegetables such as broccoli. Leafy green vegetables and whole-grain or enriched bread and cereal products also supply a generous amount of riboflavin in most people's diets. Because riboflavin can be destroyed by the ultraviolet rays of the sun or by fluorescent lamps, milk is usually sold in protective cardboard or opaque plastic containers rather than in transparent glass bottles.

TABLE 7-17 Thiamin in Foods

(mg)*	Sources
0.46	Pork chop (3 oz)
>0.38	Fortified cereal (1 c)
0.23	Watermelon (1 slice)
0.23	Green peas (½ c)
0.22	Enriched pasta (½ c)
0.21	Black beans (½ c)
0.21	Pistachios (¼ c)
0.18	Oatmeal, cooked (½ c)
0.17	Black-eyed peas (½ c)
0.16	Peanuts (⅓ c)
0.14	Salmon (3 oz)
0.14	Wheat bread (1 slice)
0.13	Baked potato (1)
0.11	Sirloin steak (3 oz)
0.11	Orange (1)
0.10	Milk, fat-free (1 c)

*DRI, adult: men, 1.2 mg/day; women, 1.1 mg/day.

FIGURE 7-17

Sources of Riboflavin

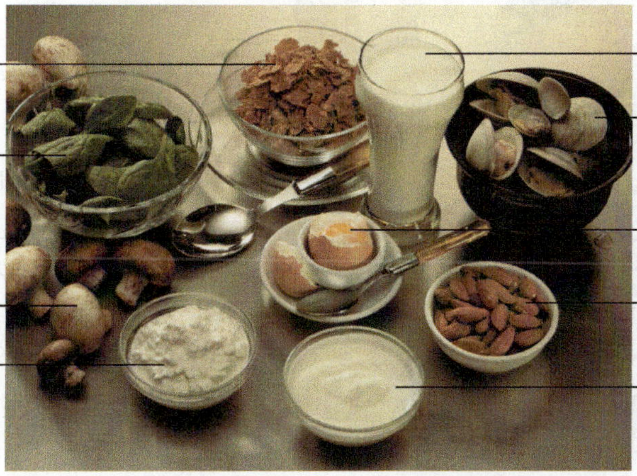

TABLE 7-18 Riboflavin in Foods

(mg)*	Sources
0.57	Low-fat yogurt (1 c)
0.51	Soymilk (1 c)
0.45	Fat-free milk (1 c)
>0.35	Fortified cereal (1 c)
0.33	Almonds (⅓ c)
0.27	Tofu, firm (3 oz)
0.26	Egg, cooked (1)
0.24	Feta cheese (1 oz)
0.24	Pork chop (3 oz)
0.23	Ground beef (3 oz)
0.23	Ricotta cheese (½ c)
0.21	Beet greens, cooked (½ c)
0.17	Cheddar cheese (1.5 oz)

*DRI, adult: men, 1.3 mg/day; women; 1.1 mg/day.

TABLE 7-19 Niacin in Foods

(mg NE)*	Sources
11.30	Tuna (3 oz)
8.90	Chicken breast (½)
6.70	Halibut (3 oz)
6.37	Turkey (3 oz)
5.08	Ground beef (3 oz)
4.29	Peanut butter (2 tbsp)
>4.00	Fortified cereal (1 c)
3.30	Baked potato (1)
3.29	Sirloin steak (3 oz)
2.00	Flounder/sole (3 oz)
1.49	Brown rice, cooked (½ c)
1.24	Wheat bread (1 slice)
1.21	Peach (1)
1.20	Cantaloupe (1 c)
0.89	Broccoli, cooked (½ c)

*DRI, adult: men, 16 mg NE/day; women, 14 mg NE/day.

Niacin

Like thiamin and riboflavin, the B vitamin *niacin* is part of a coenzyme that is vital to producing energy. Without niacin to form this coenzyme, energy-yielding reactions come to a halt. Over time, a deficiency of niacin leads to the disease pellagra, characterized by diarrhea, dermatitis, and, in severe cases, dementia—a progressive mental deterioration resulting in delirium, mania or depression, and eventually death.

Although we can prevent niacin deficiency by eating a diet rich in niacin itself, consuming plenty of protein also staves off the problem. That's because the essential amino acid tryptophan, which is a component of protein, can be converted to niacin in the body. In fact, 60 milligrams of tryptophan yield 1 milligram of niacin. Thus, the DRI for niacin is expressed in niacin equivalents (NEs)—that is, the amount of niacin present in food, including the amount that can theoretically be made from the tryptophan in the food. Milk, eggs, meat, poultry, and fish contribute the bulk of the niacin equivalents consumed by most people, followed by enriched breads and cereals. Figure 7-18 and Table 7-19 show the niacin content of some common foods.

Diet aside, for many years, niacin has been used as a druglike supplement to help lower cholesterol. Doses ranging from 10 to 15 times the Recommended Dietary Allowance (RDA) have been shown to raise "good" HDL-cholesterol.[21] The hitch, however, is that such high doses of niacin can lead to side effects such as nausea, flushing of the skin, rash, fatigue, and liver damage and are no longer recommended.

Pantothenic Acid and Biotin

Two other B vitamins—*pantothenic acid* and *biotin*—are needed to synthesize coenzymes that are active in energy metabolism and in a multitude of body systems. Biotin is also required for cell growth, synthesis of DNA (the genetic "blueprint" present in every cell), and maintenance of blood glucose levels. Because both pantothenic acid and biotin are widespread in foods (see Figure 7-19), people who eat a varied diet are not at risk for deficiencies.

7.6 Vitamin-Like Compounds

In addition to B vitamins, **choline**—a vitamin-like substance—is needed by the body to metabolize homocysteine. Choline is also needed to make lecithin and other molecules—and is considered a "conditionally" essential nutrient because the body becomes unable to make sufficient amounts of choline when fed a choline-free diet.[22] However, because choline is found in milk, eggs, peanuts, and many other foods, deficiencies are rare. The recommended intake for choline is listed in the DRI Table at the back of this book.

FIGURE 7-18
Sources of Niacin

Adult DRI (RDA) is 14 to 16 mg NE.

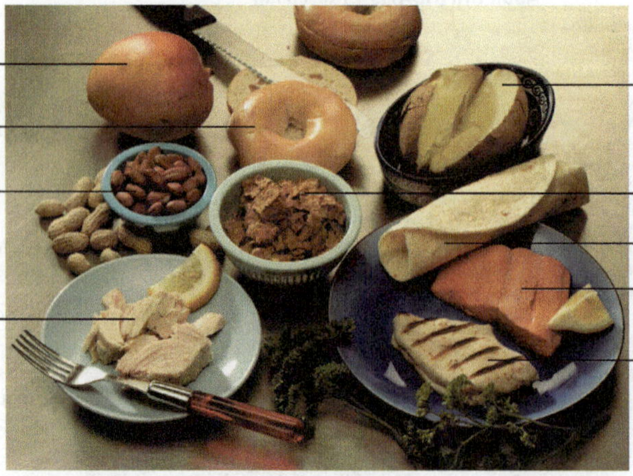

FIGURE 7-19

Sources of Biotin and Pantothenic Acid*

*Information concerning biotin and pantothenic acid in foods is incomplete: Deficiencies are rare.

Adult DRI (AI): **Biotin: 30 μg**
Pantothenic acid: 5 mg

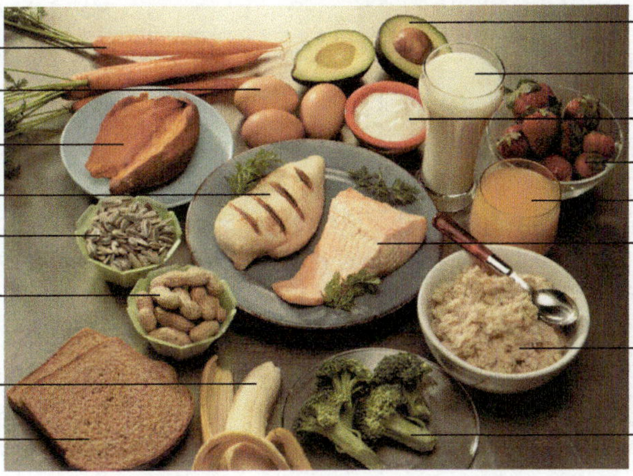

Nonvitamins Various other substances have been mistaken as essential nutrients for humans because bacteria or animals need them to live. Sometimes called nonvitamins, some of these substances are important to cell membranes (inositol) and cellular activities (carnitine) but are not essential in human diets because our bodies can make these compounds as needed. Moreover, these substances are abundant in common foods. Research about the role of these substances for humans is ongoing.

Other substances that are sometimes added to vitamin supplements because they are essential for growth in certain nonhuman species are truly nonessential in human diets. These include PABA (para-aminobenzoic acid), the bioflavonoids ("vitamin P" or hesperidin) and ubiquinone (coenzyme Q_{10}), vitamin B_{15} (a hoax), and vitamin B_{17} (laetrile, a falsely touted cancer cure).

7.7 Phytonutrients in Foods: The Phytochemical Superstars

One of the most exciting areas of nutrition research today focuses on a class of substances in plant foods called **phytochemicals**, nonnutritive substances in plants that possess health-protective benefits. Phytochemicals are the compounds that give plants their brilliant colors (e.g., lycopene, a pigment that makes tomatoes red and watermelon pink) and distinctive aromas (e.g., the allium compounds that give us "garlic breath"). These natural compounds also protect plants from the ravages of overexposure to sunlight and other environmental threats and insects.

The term *phytochemicals* has been popularized to refer in particular to plant chemicals that may affect health and prevent disease. Of particular interest are phytochemicals in edible plants, including fruits and vegetables, whole grains, legumes, herbs, and seeds. See Table 7-20 for a sampling of the phytochemicals that have been identified to date, as well as common food sources and beneficial effects and attributes of each phytochemical group. In the classic sense, the naturally occurring phytochemicals are not nutrients, for they do not provide energy or building materials. However, ongoing research shows that phytochemicals might perform important functions by acting as powerful antioxidants, decreasing blood pressure and cholesterol, preventing cataracts, reducing menopause symptoms and risk for osteoporosis, and slowing or even reversing certain cancers.

choline A nonessential nutrient used by the body to synthesize various compounds, including the phospholipid lecithin; the body can make choline from the amino acid methionine.

phytochemicals (FIGHT-oh-KEM-ih-kulz) Physiologically active compounds found in plants that are not essential nutrients but appear to help promote health and reduce risk for cancer, heart disease, and other conditions. Also called *phytonutrients* (*phyto* = plant).

TABLE 7-20 A Sampling of Phytochemicals: Classifications, Food Sources, and Possible Health Benefits

Phytochemical	Food Sources	Possible Health Benefits
Beta-glucan	Oat bran, rolled oats, oat flour	May reduce risk of coronary heart disease
Capsaicin	Hot peppers	May reduce risk of fatal clotting in heart disease
Carotenoids	Deeply colored fruits and vegetables	Act as antioxidants
Beta-carotene	Orange fruits and vegetables (apricots, cantaloupe, carrots, mango, pumpkin, sweet potato, winter squash); dark-green vegetables (spinach, kale, turnip greens)	May help reduce risk of many cancers and strengthen the immune system
Lutein and zeaxanthin	Pumpkin, summer squash, corn, eggs, broccoli; dark-green leafy vegetables, such as kale, collard greens, and spinach	May reduce risk of age-related eye disorders by protecting the retina from harmful ultraviolet radiation and by neutralizing free radicals[a]
Lycopene	Tomatoes, tomato products, watermelon, red grapefruit, red peppers	May help reduce risk of prostate and other cancers
Curcumin	Turmeric, a spice	May inhibit enzymes that activate carcinogens
Flavonoids and other phenols[b]		
Anthocyanin Ellagic acid Resveratrol	Fruits (apples, berries, cherries, citrus, grapes, pears, pomegranates, prunes); whole grains, nuts, chocolate, black or green tea, eggplant, potato peel, red cabbage, beets, celery, peppers, onions, soy, red wine	May act as antioxidants, decrease inflammation, reduce plaque buildup in arteries, increase HDL-cholesterol levels, deactivate carcinogens, and inhibit cancer development
Indoles	Cruciferous vegetables such as broccoli, kale, cauliflower, cabbage, turnip, and Brussels sprouts	May stimulate enzymes that make the hormone estrogen less effective, possibly reducing breast cancer risk
Isothiocyanates (most notably, sulforaphane)	Broccoli, kale, cabbages, and other cruciferous vegetables; horseradish	May help stimulate protective enzymes that detoxify carcinogens, bolstering the body's natural ability to ward off cancer
Monoterpenes (such as limonene)	Citrus (fruits, juices, peels, oils)	May act as antioxidants and increase production of enzymes that may help the body dispose of carcinogens
Organosulfur compounds (such as allicin)	Onions, garlic, chives, leeks	May block the action of cancer-causing chemicals; may offer heart protection by decreasing production of cholesterol by the liver
Phytic acid	Whole grains	May prevent free-radical formation by binding to minerals and thereby reduce cancer risk
Phytoestrogens (part of flavonoid family)		
Isoflavones (genistein and daidzein)	Soybeans, soy foods, and other legumes	May protect against heart disease by lowering blood cholesterol; may lower risk of breast, ovarian, and other cancers by blocking the action of the hormone estrogen
Lignans	Flaxseed, whole grains	Exhibits estrogen-blocking activity and may lower risk of breast, ovarian, colon, and prostate cancer
Saponins	Sprouts, potatoes, green vegetables, tomatoes, nuts, whole grains, soy foods, legumes	May strengthen the immune system and interfere with DNA replication, preventing cancer cells from multiplying
Tannins	Grapes, black-eyed peas, lentils, red and white wine, tea	Act as antioxidants; may inhibit enzymes that activate carcinogens

[a] Disorders causing vision loss in older adults, including age-related macular degeneration (AMD) and cataracts.

[b] Flavonoids are a subset of phenols. Flavonoids of interest include anthocyanins, catechins, ferulic acid, flavones, glycosides, quercetin, resveratrol, rutin, tangeretin, and nobiletin. The larger class of phenolic phytochemicals includes phenols, ellagic acid, capsaicin (in chili peppers), coumarin, curcumin, and others.

An individual fruit or vegetable may contain many (50 or more) of the thousands of known phytochemicals, but one, or only a select few, are usually present in a large amount. For example, garlic contains more than 160 identified compounds. When a clove of garlic is cut or crushed, it produces sulfur compounds, such as *allicin*, which scientists believe is partly responsible for the health benefits attributed to garlic. Finding the specific chemical in a food that offers the disease-protecting potential is not easy, however. Clinical studies in which people eat foods rich in certain phytochemicals are currently under way. If health benefits, such as protection against cancer, are observed, then the active ingredient in the food must be determined. Is the phytochemical, a vitamin, fiber, or the overall content of the increased fruit or vegetable diet responsible for the benefit? Based on current research, any one or a combination of these factors might be responsible.

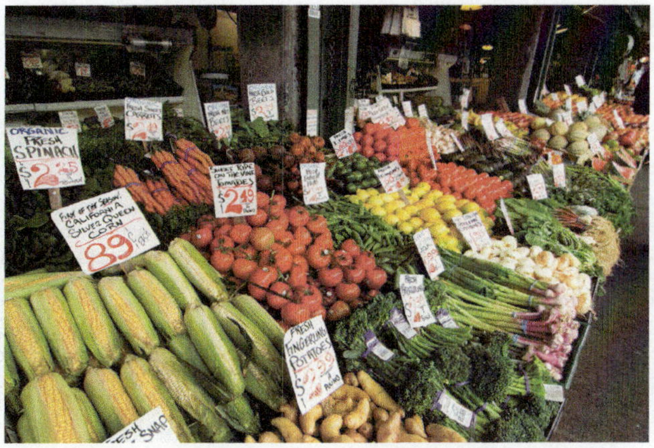

Visit your local farmers' market or grocery store produce aisle for a cornucopia of health-promoting compounds: carotenoids in carrots, spinach, and tomatoes; sulforaphane in broccoli and bok choy, capsaicin in chili peppers. To find the farmers' market nearest you, log on to the USDA website at www.ams.usda.gov/local-food-directories/farmersmarkets.

Jeffrey M. Frank/Shutterstock.com

Mechanisms of Actions of Phytochemicals

Many foods contain numerous phytochemicals, each one acting with or through one or several mechanisms. Some have antioxidant properties (protecting against harmful cell damage), others have anticancer properties (preventing initiation and promotion of cancer), and some have anti-estrogen properties (blocking the action of estrogen and lowering the risk of some cancers).

Different phytochemicals have different modes of action, and one individual phytochemical may exhibit more than one mechanism of action. A phytochemical may influence one or more stages of cancer, from initiation to promotion and progression to a malignant tumor. Phytochemicals act by both *direct* and *indirect* mechanisms. They may act directly to *inhibit* enzymes that activate carcinogens or to *induce* enzymes that detoxify carcinogens. They may act indirectly by stimulating the immune response or scavenging free radicals to prevent DNA damage. See the Spotlight feature in this chapter for a discussion of the role of nutrition in cancer.

Although many phytochemicals act on cells to suppress cancer development, they may also help protect against other diseases, notably heart disease. Some phytochemicals may influence blood pressure and blood clotting, whereas others reduce the synthesis and absorption of cholesterol. Certain pigments (especially carotenoids) in plant foods may protect the eye against free-radical damage and thus prevent or postpone macular degeneration, which can lead to blindness in older adults. One of the most widely studied groups of phytochemicals, the isoflavones found in soy products, is currently being researched for its potential role in preventing diseases such as osteoporosis, heart disease, and various cancers (mainly prostate, breast, and ovarian), and for alleviating symptoms associated with menopause.

Functional Foods: Let Food Be Your Medicine

Nutritionists, food scientists, food marketers, and others are exploring how today's traditional foods, and perhaps new formulations, may open doors to a healthier tomorrow.[23] The fact that food is intimately linked to optimal health is not a novel concept. "Let food be your medicine and medicine be your food" was a tenet Hippocrates espoused in approximately 400 B.C.E.[24] Almost 2,500 years later, this philosophy is still important because the "food as medicine" philosophy underpins the paradigm of functional foods. In this section, we look at the promising benefits of

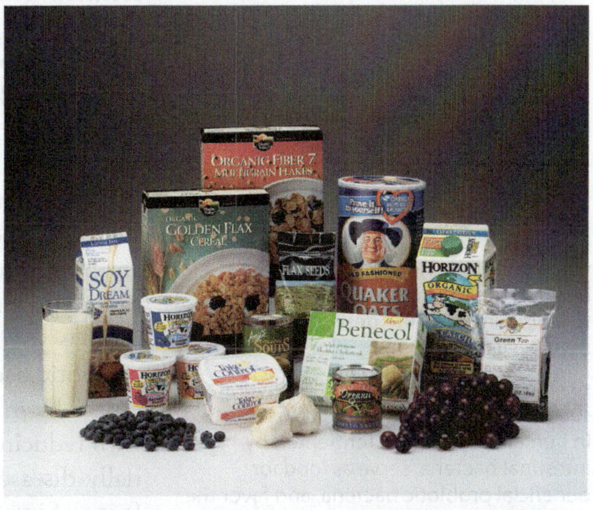

You can visit your grocery store for a wide assortment of functional foods.

© Scott Hirko/Hespenheide Design

FIGURE 7-20

Functional Food Guide

SOURCE: Adapted from University of Illinois, Functional Foods for Health.

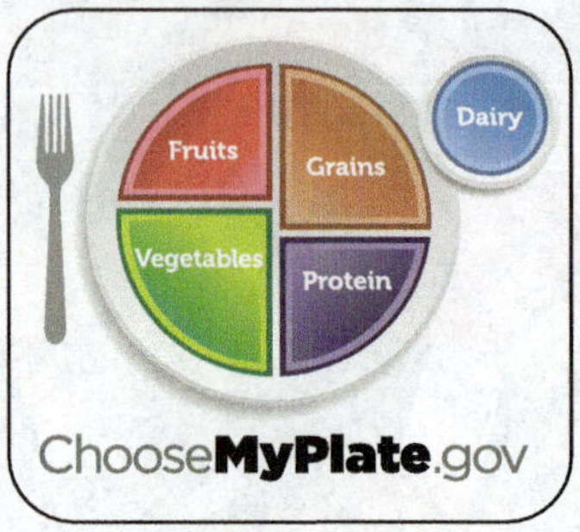

GRAINS	VEGETABLES	FRUITS	DAIRY	PROTEIN FOODS
Psyllium-containing bread and cereal, Corn products, Flaxseed, Oat products, Rye products, Wheat bran products	Broccoli, Brussels sprouts, Cabbage, Carrots, Cauliflower, Celery, Garlic, Horseradish, Jerusalem artichokes, Leeks, Onions, Scallions/Shallots, Soybeans, Tomatoes, Watercress	Apples, Bananas, Blueberries, Cranberries, Grapefruit, Grapes/Juice, Lemons, Limes, Oranges, Raspberries	Cheese, Milk, Milk products, Soy milk products, Yogurt	Beans, Beef, Eggs, Mackerel, Salmon, Soy nuts, Soy protein, Sardines, Tuna, Walnuts

Here are examples of some foods that are potentially associated with maintaining health.

Antioxidant
Broccoli family
Carrots
Citrus fruit
Cocoa/chocolate
Flaxseed
Grapes/juice
Honey
Horseradish
Raspberries
Tomatoes

Maintains Vision
Blueberries
Broccoli
Carrots
Corn products
Eggs
Leafy greens

Improves Gastrointestinal Health
Bananas
Honey
Horseradish
Jerusalem artichokes
Milk
Onion family
Yogurt

Reduces Cancer Risk
Apples
Beans
Berries
Broccoli family
Citrus fruit
Corn products
Flaxseed
Garlic
Grapes/juice
Green or black tea
Milk products
Onion family
Rye products
Salmon
Soy products
Tomatoes
Wheat bran products

Improves Heart Health
Apples
Beans
Berries
Fish (salmon, tuna, mackerel, sardines)
Flaxseed
Garlic
Grapes/juice
Green or black tea
Milk products
Oat products
Onion family
Psyllium-containing bread and cereals
Soy products
Walnuts

Maintains Urinary Tract Health
Blueberries
Cranberries

Reduces Blood Pressure
Bananas
Celery
Cheese
Garlic
Milk
Soy products

Improves Bone Health
Cheese
Milk
Milk products
Soy milk products
Soy nuts

functional foods in disease prevention, as well as how we can incorporate phytochemicals and functional foods into our daily eating plan so we can reap their benefits.

Functional foods are not really a new concept; grocery stores are already filled with numerous items that meet the definition of functional foods (see Figure 7-20).[25] One of the first to appear was calcium-fortified orange juice, which gave people who don't like milk as much bone-healthy calcium per glass as milk. We now have grain products fortified with folate to prevent birth defects and possibly heart disease. Many cereal grains, fruits, vegetables, nuts, and dairy products are touted for their potential cancer prevention benefits as well as cardiovascular protection.

The Quaker Oats man continues to smile as the cholesterol-lowering effects of the soluble fiber beta-glucan in oats are well documented. Omega-3 fatty acids in flaxseed oil and fatty fish such as salmon and halibut appear to reduce the risk of heart disease, as well as having anti-inflammatory properties. Research indicates that the organosulfur compounds in garlic may have it all—cancer fighting, cholesterol-lowering, antibiotic, and antihypertensive properties—which far outweigh the herb's ability to cause bad breath. **Probiotics** (friendly living bacteria) in fermented milk products such as yogurt and **prebiotics** (fermentable dietary fiber that can serve as food for probiotic bacteria) in oatmeal, flax, and legumes also appear to have multiple effects, especially in promoting a healthy gastrointestinal tract. Probiotics are also associated with reducing the risk of colon cancer, lowering cholesterol, and outcompeting potentially disease-causing bacteria in the gastrointestinal tract. Soy protein has been the focus of intense research efforts because of its ability to lower cholesterol and possibly reduce the risk of cancer, osteoporosis, and symptoms associated with menopause.[26]

probiotics Living microorganisms that when consumed are intended to have health benefits for the host, such as helping to maintain or restore desirable numbers of beneficial bacteria in the digestive tract.

prebiotics Nondigestible carbohydrates, such as fiber, that are resistant to digestion in humans, but can be fermented by intestinal bacteria, serve as food for beneficial probiotic bacteria, and favor the growth of beneficial bacteria over harmful bacteria.

Scientists are investigating a certain type of fat called conjugated linoleic acid (CLA), found primarily in dairy products, for numerous potential health benefits, including improvements in immune function, body composition, and bone mineralization. Identification of CLA underscores the importance of meeting nutrient needs through consumption of foods from all the major food groups.[27]

Follow the Research: Future Foods So much is still unknown when it comes to functional foods that additional research is needed to clarify the role of phytochemicals in health promotion. Such research will also provide plant physiologists and human nutritionists with the vital information they need to develop an enhanced food supply and better target dietary recommendations for the general public.[28] For years, the food industry focused on "taking out the bad stuff" (fat, sodium, cholesterol, calories) and restoring or enhancing favorable nutrients (calcium, folate, fiber). We may soon see the day where we have tomatoes with extra lycopene, sulforaphane-enriched broccoli, and sweet potatoes with extra carotene.

How to Optimize Phytochemicals and Functional Foods in a Daily Eating Plan Research indicates that pure extracts of phytochemicals in supplements are less effective than phytochemicals in whole foods. Some phytochemicals might not be metabolized in pure form, and some might not function by themselves. Thus, phytochemicals have less protective power when ingested as concentrated extracts, such as in pills.

We know that the absorption, metabolism, and distribution of some nutrients are dependent upon the presence of other nutrients. Likewise, it appears that the absorption, metabolism, distribution, and function of phytochemicals also depend on the combination of one phytochemical with other phytochemicals or other substances that occur naturally in food. An individual phytochemical does not necessarily provide protection against disease; rather, the combination of the phytochemical with other phytochemicals or food components provides the protection.

Until more is known about phytochemicals and how they function, it is best to incorporate the MyPlate food guide into your daily food planning if you are not already using it (see Figure 7-20 and Table 7-21). Begin with the Grains group, and consume the recommended amount of whole-grain breads and cereals, especially oatmeal. Grind flaxseed in a coffee grinder and add it to your cereal.

Consume at least nine half-cup servings of vegetables and fruits daily. Be sure to include a variety of vegetables and fruits, including orange vegetables and fruits such as sweet potatoes, carrots, winter squash, apricots, cantaloupe, and peaches. Add dark-green leafy vegetables such as kale, mustard greens, collards, and spinach, along with broccoli and Brussels sprouts. Include tomatoes as often as possible, and also add garlic and onions to your diet. Eat plenty of purple vegetables such as eggplant and red cabbage. Use the Scorecard feature on page 214 to evaluate your current intake of fruits and vegetables.

Try experimenting with soy milk, tofu, miso, and tempeh, and include them regularly in your diet. Salmon and other fatty fish (sardines, mackerel, herring, tuna) contain omega-3 fatty acids, which are shown to offer heart protection. Try selecting two fish meals per week. Yogurt, cheese, and milk products go a long way toward providing the calcium needed for healthy bones; be sure to have at least three one-cup equivalents daily. Many dairy products are functional foods. The live bacteria used to ferment milk products such as yogurts and yogurt-based drinks enhance intestinal flora.

Last but not least, top off your meal with a cup of green or black tea, a source of phenolic compounds, which many researchers are convinced protect against cancer, heart disease, and stroke. As you can see, the best advice is to consume a variety of foods that contain both known beneficial compounds and those still awaiting discovery.

TABLE 7-21 Tips for Adding Phytochemicals and Functional Foods to Your Daily Diet

At breakfast:
- Add blueberries to oatmeal.
- Add fresh fruits and berries and/or whole-grain cereal to yogurt.
- Spread soy nut butter on whole-grain toast.
- Blend soy milk with frozen berries.

Healthy meal ideas:
- Mix tuna salad with grated carrots, red peppers, onions, and garlic.
- Serve whole-grain pasta with tomato sauce and fresh herbs.
- Grill salmon and serve with fresh greens and yogurt salad dressing.
- Enjoy a cup of green tea with a meal.

Snacks on the go:
- Grab a piece of fresh fruit.
- Mix soy nuts, whole-grain cereal, and dried fruit together and hit the trail.
- Grab a glass of tomato, cranberry, or orange juice.
- Try fresh broccoli, cauliflower, and carrots with tofu dip.

Nutrition **ACTION**

7.8 Choosing a Vitamin-Mineral Supplement or Herbal Remedy

For years, health experts have been saying that most healthy people can meet their vitamin and mineral needs with a balanced diet. Nevertheless, almost half of the U.S. population, including about half of young adults and college students, pop vitamin and mineral pills. Americans spend billions of dollars annually on pills, powders, liquids, herbal remedies, and vitamin and mineral supplements, often in the mistaken belief that such preparations will ensure proper nutrition, help reduce stress, decrease fatigue, and increase pep and energy. Figure 7-21 reveals frequently cited reasons for using dietary supplements.

FIGURE 7-21

Most Common Reasons Reported by U.S. Adults for using Dietary Supplements and the Most Frequently Used Dietary Supplements, NHANES 2007–2010

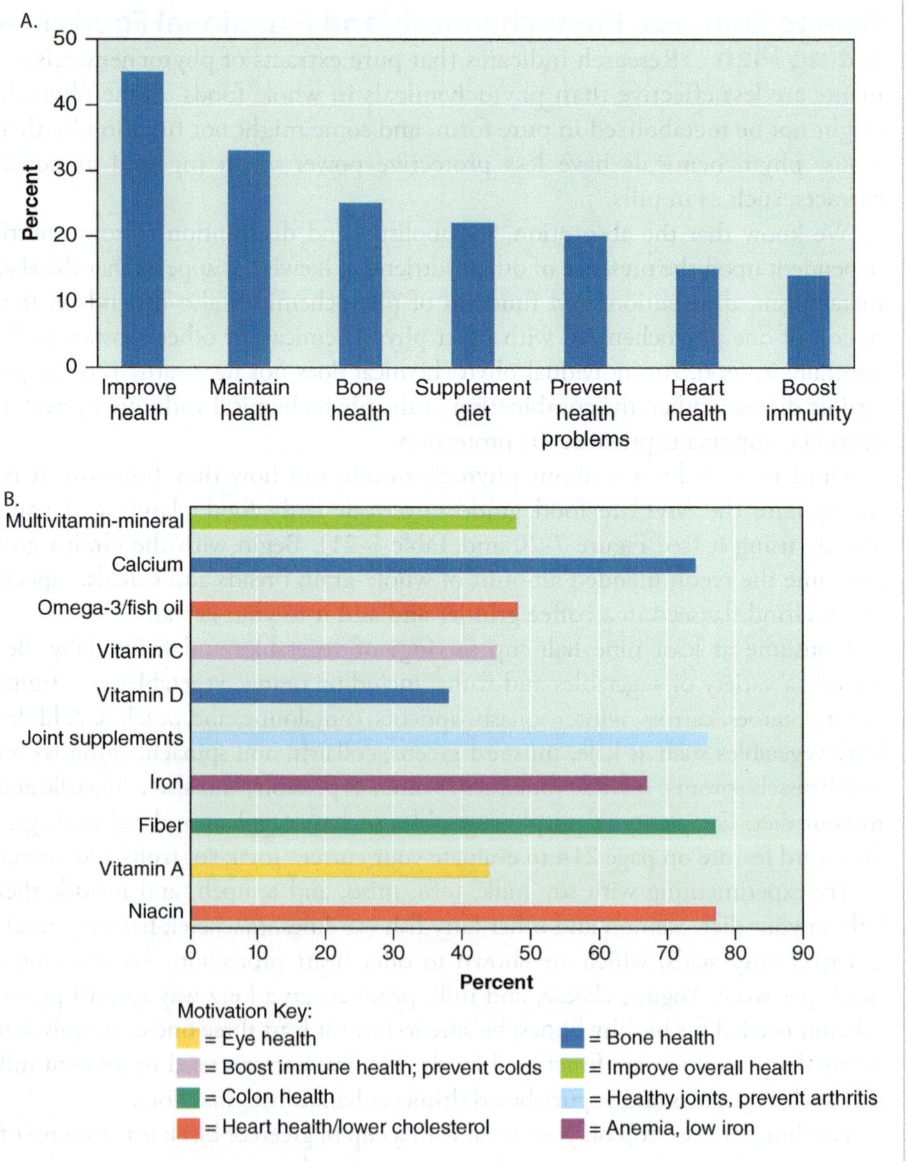

A. The top three reasons reported by adults for using dietary supplements were to improve overall health (45%), maintain health/stay healthy (33%), and for bone health (25%).

B. The graph shows the most frequently cited motivations (e.g., eye health, bone health, colon health, etc.) reported by adults using the specific type of supplement. For example, 77% of adults using fiber supplements cited colon health as their motivation for doing so. The supplements are listed in descending order by frequency of reported use. The top three dietary supplements used by adults were: Multivitamin-minerals (32% of supplement users)—used primarily to maintain health or to supplement the diet; calcium supplements (12% of supplement users)—used for bone health; and omega-3 fatty acids and fish oils (10% of supplement users)—used most commonly for heart health or to lower cholesterol.

SOURCE: Adapted from R. L. Bailey and coauthors, Why US Adults Use Dietary Supplements, *JAMA Internal Medicine* 173 (2013): 355–361.

Vitamin-Mineral Supplements

Before you buy a supplement, remember that most major health organizations—from the Academy of Nutrition and Dietetics to the American Medical Association to the American Academy of Pediatrics—essentially agree that healthy children and adults should be able to get all the nutrients they need by eating a variety of foods.[29] However, those organizations and other experts say that taking a multivitamin-mineral supplement, under the guidance of a physician or dietitian, may be in order for these particular groups of people:

- People restricting energy intake for weight loss
- People with certain diseases or those taking medications that interfere with appetite, absorption, or excretion of nutrients
- Strict vegetarians, whose diets may fall short in vitamin B_{12}, vitamin D, calcium, iron, and zinc
- Women who are pregnant or breastfeeding, phases that bolster the need for nutrients, including iron and folate
- Women with excessive menstrual bleeding, who may need iron supplements
- Women during their childbearing years who do not consume folate-rich foods or foods fortified with folic acid; they may need more folate in their diets to prevent neural tube defects in infants
- People with a specific nutrient gap that cannot or is not otherwise being filled by the individual's food intake. For example, people with lactose intolerance, or who do not consume milk or other dairy products—they need a source of calcium; those with inadequate exposure to sunlight may also need vitamin D
- Older adults, who may have difficulty choosing an adequate diet, chewing problems, or a reduced ability to absorb and metabolize certain nutrients
- People who are recovering from surgery, burn injuries, or other illnesses that increase nutrient needs
- People with chronic diseases of the digestive tract or other conditions that lead to poor intake or depleted nutrient stores
- People with alcohol or other drug addictions, who are likely to have a shortage of vitamins and minerals in their diets

If you decide to start taking a supplement, keep the following points in mind when choosing one.

This symbol on a dietary supplement label helps you know that the supplement actually contains the listed ingredients in the declared amount, does not contain harmful levels of contaminants, will break down and release its ingredients in the body, and has been made under good manufacturing practices. See also www.uspverified.org.

1. Remember that price is not an indication of quality. Many products sold at major retail chains and drugstores are just as high in quality as pricier versions sold in health food stores. Look for a product that meets high standards for manufacturing. One way to do this is to check the label to see whether the product meets USP standards—manufacturing practices set forth by the U.S. Pharmacopeia, the organization that establishes drug standards. The organization's standards require that a supplement be able to disintegrate and dissolve thoroughly in the stomach within a certain period of time, thereby increasing the chances that the nutrients inside will be absorbed and used by the body. Also look for a bottle or package that carries an expiration date. If it doesn't, you run the risk of buying a product that has been sitting on a shelf for a long time. After a while, the product may lose its potency.
2. Look for a supplement that contains both vitamins and minerals, with no more than 100 percent to 150 percent of the recommended Daily Values for each. For the most part, nutrients work in concert with one another, promoting the body's ability to make use of them. Products that include a balanced mix of vitamins and minerals are the best bet for most people. Steer clear of products containing extraneous substances such as PABA, hesperidin, inositol, and bee pollen. These nonvitamin substances have never been proved essential to humans and only add to the price of the supplement. Be wary of taking multivitamins that also contain herbs. Although herbal products are considered to be dietary supplements, the unregulated herbal industry of today is a buyer-beware market.
3. Buy products sold in childproof bottles or packages if you have children around. Vitamins and minerals, especially iron, can be highly toxic to children. Every year, tens of thousands of children swallow excess vitamin-mineral supplements, and iron-tablet overdoses alone are one of the top causes of accidental death in youngsters.

(Continued)

Medicinal Herbs

Throughout human history, people have relied on herbal medicines, and the use of herbs and medicinal plants for any number of ailments is a universal phenomenon. Many of the world's populations depend on traditional herbal medicine for primary health care.[30] Only with the development of 20th-century Western medicine have synthetic chemicals found their place in the medical system. Yet, even in a modern pharmacy in the United States, more than 25 percent of medicines are extracted from plants or are synthetic copies or derivatives of plant chemicals.[31]

In the United States, plant medicines composed of whole plants (crude drugs) or complex extracts are sold as dietary supplements because natural (or herbal) medicines are not economically viable candidates for drug research and development. Most botanicals contain one or several relatively dilute compounds, and thus they tend to have milder actions than the more concentrated chemicals found in most drugs. Therefore, herbal medicines usually take longer to act than regular medicinal products, and few herbs have the potency of a prescription drug.

Pharmaceutical companies are less willing to spend the millions of dollars needed to fund research on plants that grow in the wild (and therefore cannot be patented), and most herb manufacturers don't have the funds to support large research studies. Despite this, herbal products are increasingly popular in the United States.[32] See Table 7-22 for a list of herbs thought to be effective and those that should be avoided.

What is driving this trend toward increased use of herbal products? Primarily, the growth is consumer driven. Most consumers learn of herbal products through the media, either in magazines, television, or radio commercials, or by word of mouth from others. Other factors responsible for this trend are an interest in returning to a more natural lifestyle; dissatisfaction with the current state of Western health care; the unwanted side effects of prescription drugs; the spiraling cost and disarray of managed health care; aging baby boomers who want a better quality of health; a strong interest in alternative and complementary therapies; and, finally, a large arena of sales and marketing campaigns, often making use of famous personalities to market herbal products to consumers.

Many herbal product users believe that herbal medicines are the "natural" way to good health. However, *natural* is not always synonymous with *safe*—there are no regulations or oversight agencies for the manufacture and marketing of herbal supplements. Also, when it comes to botanicals, several plant species may look identical, but one may in fact be toxic. If the person collecting the herbs is not entirely knowledgeable, there is a danger that the toxic herb may be mixed with the medicinal herb; such mistakes have been made.

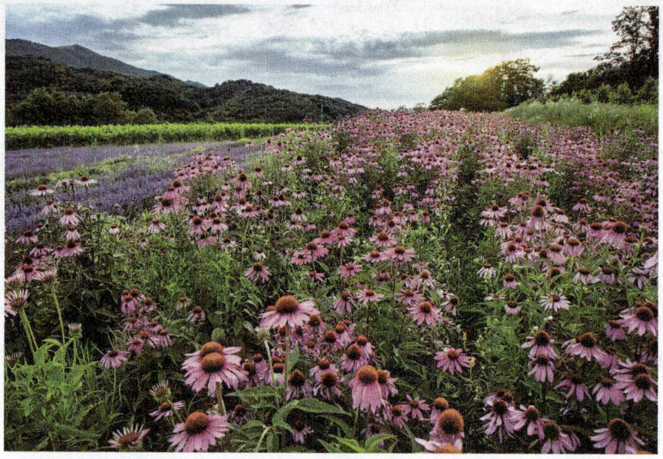

JRP Studio/Shutterstock.com

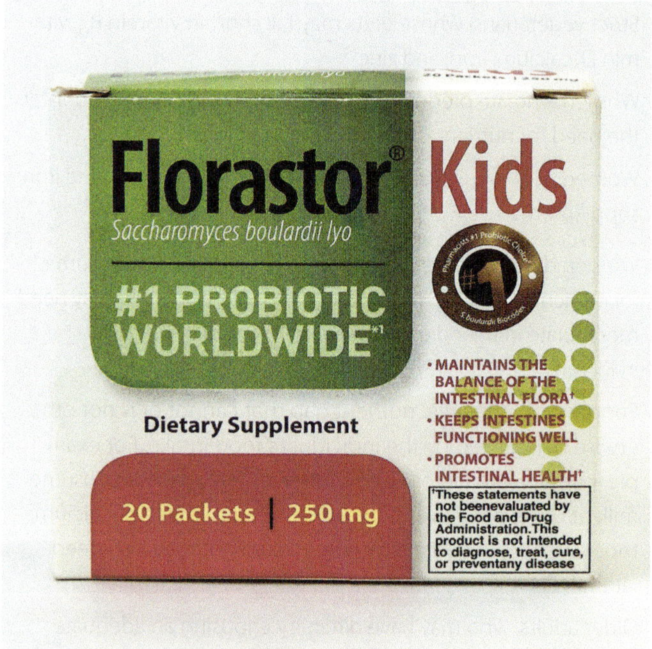

Roman Tiraspolsky/Shutterstock.com

Like foods, dietary supplements cannot claim to treat, cure, or prevent a "disease," but can claim to "affect the structure or any function of the body of man or other animals." Unlike foods, dietary supplements making structure/function claims must bear a mandatory disclaimer that reads: "This statement has not been evaluated by the FDA. This product is not intended to diagnose, treat, cure, or prevent any disease." Examples of structure/function claims include:

- Supports digestive health (probiotic)
- Helps promote restful sleep (valerian or melatonin)
- Supports a healthy immune system (echinacea or vitamin C)

A further concern is that consumers have no way of knowing if the product they purchase has an "effective" amount of the active compound.

In 1994, Congress passed the Dietary Supplement Health and Education Act (DSHEA), which severely restricted the FDA's authority over virtually any product labeled "supplement" as long as the product made no claim to affect a disease. The DSHEA allowed herbal medicines to be marketed without prior approval from the FDA. What the DSHEA does allow manufacturers to state on a label is how the product affects a structure or function of the body, such as the claim that the herbal product can "support," "promote," or "maintain" health. The DSHEA states that a product cannot claim that it affects disease, and a manufacturer cannot state on the label that the herbal product will "prevent," "treat," "diagnose," "mitigate," or "cure" disease. A disclaimer must always be included on the label, stating: "This product has not been evaluated by the Food and Drug Administration. This product is not intended to diagnose, treat, cure, or prevent any disease." Therefore, herbal products are not obliged to meet any standards of effectiveness or safety that have been established for other medicines, which require extensive laboratory and clinical trials before the FDA grants approval. Today, a supplement is presumed safe until the FDA receives well-documented reports of adverse reactions.

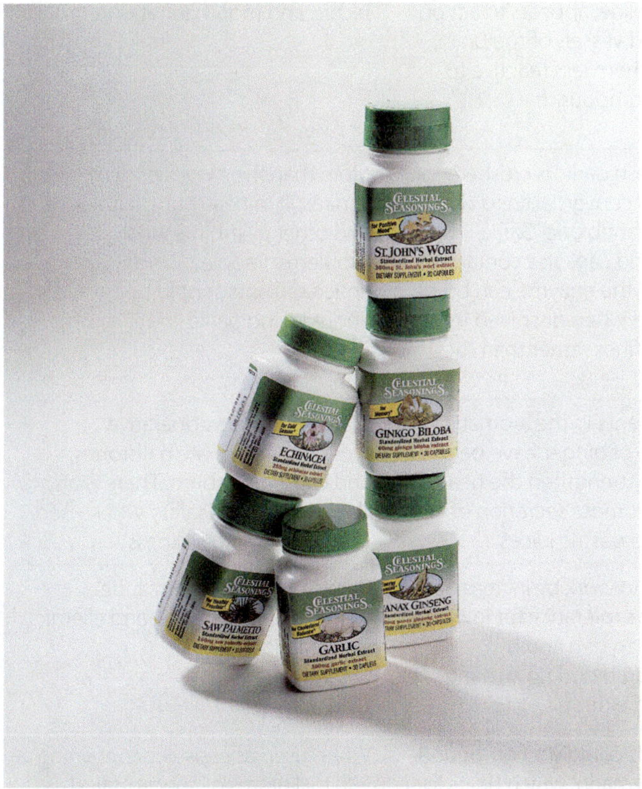

Jessica Wecker/Science Source

Research is currently under way in the United States to test the safety and efficacy of a few of the most popular herbs on the market today.

In October 1998, Congress established the National Center for Complementary and Alternative Medicine (NCCAM), a division of the National Institutes of Health. The center is devoted to conducting and supporting basic and applied research and training, and it disseminates information on complementary and alternative medicine to practitioners and the public. Some of the herbs that are currently undergoing research here in the United States are garlic, St. John's wort, ginkgo biloba, saw palmetto, echinacea, hawthorn, and cranberry.

Until we have further research studies with which to evaluate the safety and efficacy of herbal medicines, physicians, health professionals, and consumers must continue to seek valid information and further education from reliable sources. Use the following guidelines for choosing and using herbal medicines:

- Be informed; seek out unbiased, scientific sources. Inform your physician, especially if taking prescribed medications.
- Do not exceed recommended doses or use herbal medicines for prolonged periods. Call your physician or the FDA Med Alert hotline at 800-332-1088 if you experience adverse effects.
- To find out more about herbal medicines, try the following recommended publications and websites:
  - American Botanical Council, *The Complete German Commission E Monographs: Therapeutic Guide to Herbal Medicines*
  - Tyler's *Herbs of Choice: The Therapeutic Use of Phytomedicinals*, 3rd ed., 2009
  - American Botanical Council, *HerbalGram*, a peer-reviewed journal
  - American Botanical Council: www.herbalgram.org
  - Herb Research Foundation: www.herbs.org
  - U.S. Food and Drug Administration: www.fda.gov
  - National Institutes of Health/National Center for Complementary and Integrative Health (NCCIH): http://nccih.nih.gov
  - U.S. Pharmacopeia: www.usp.org
  - Herbs at a Glance: http://nccih.nih.gov/health/herbsataglance.htm
  - Search Dietary Supplements on PubMed: https://ods.od.nih.gov/Research/PubMed_Dietary_Supplement_Subset.aspx
  - The Food and Nutrition Information Center—Go to Browse by Subject and click on Dietary Supplements: http://fnic.nal.usda.gov

(Continued)

TABLE 7-22 **The Garden of Herbal Remedies**

These herbs are thought to be effective:*

Herb	Why It Is Used	How It Works	Cautions
Black cohosh 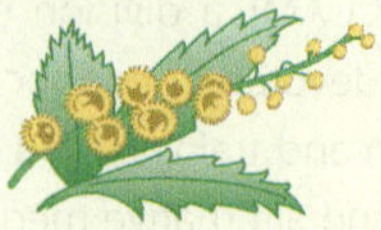	Reduces symptoms of premenstrual syndrome, painful menstruation, and the hot flashes associated with menopause.	Appears to function as an estrogen substitute and a suppressor of luteinizing hormone.	Occasional stomach pain or intestinal discomfort. Because no long-term studies have been done, use of black cohosh should be limited to 6 months.
Capsicum 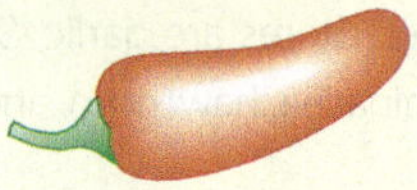	Best known as the hot red peppers cayenne and chili. Applied topically for chronic pain from conditions such as shingles and trigeminal neuralgia.	The active ingredient, capsaicin, works as a counterirritant and decreases sensitivity to pain by depleting substance P, a neurotransmitter that facilitates the transmission of pain impulses to the spinal cord.	Overuse can result in a prolonged insensitivity to pain. More concentrated products can cause a burning sensation. Users must avoid contact with eyes, genitals, and other mucous membranes.
Echinacea 	These species of purple coneflower may have a modest effect on the intensity and duration of colds and flus; may help to control urinary tract infections; when applied topically, may speed the healing of wounds.	Though echinacea lacks direct antibiotic activity, it helps the body muster its own defenses against invading microorganisms.	May cause nausea, dizziness, and headaches.
Feverfew 	The dried leaves of this plant have been shown to reduce the frequency and severity of migraine, as well as its frequently associated symptoms of nausea and vomiting.	The active ingredient, parthenolide, appears to act on the blood vessels of the brain, making them less reactive to certain compounds.	May cause gastrointestinal distress, ulcers, and mouth irritation.
Garlic 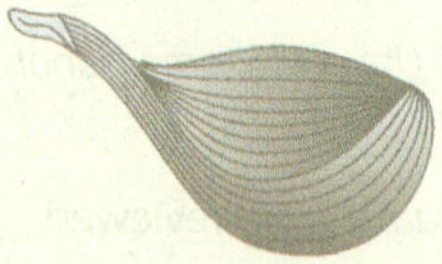	Active against viruses, fungi, and parasites. It may also lower cholesterol and inhibit the formation of blood clots, actions that might help to prevent heart attacks.	When fresh garlic is crushed, enzymes convert alliin to allicin, a potent antibiotic. Garlic tablets and capsules containing alliin and the enzyme can be absorbed when dissolved in the intestines rather than the stomach.	More than five cloves of garlic a day can result in heartburn, flatulence, and other gastrointestinal problems. People taking anticoagulants should be cautious about taking garlic.
Ginger 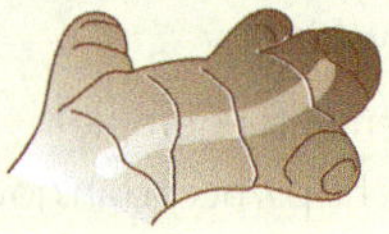	A time-honored remedy for settling an upset stomach, ginger has been shown in clinical studies to prevent motion sickness and nausea following surgery.	Components in the aromatic oil and resin of ginger have been found to strengthen the heart and to promote secretion of saliva and gastric juices.	May prolong postoperative bleeding, aggravate gallstones, and cause heartburn. There is also debate about its safety when used to treat morning sickness.
Ginkgo 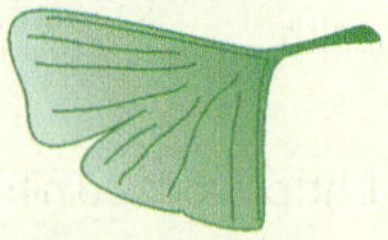	Used medicinally in China for hundreds of years, ginkgo biloba is touted to improve short-term memory and relieve vertigo, but little evidence is available.	Appears to work by increasing the brain's tolerance for low levels of oxygen and by enhancing blood flow to the brain and extremities.	Possible side effects include indigestion, headache, and allergic skin reactions.
Milk thistle 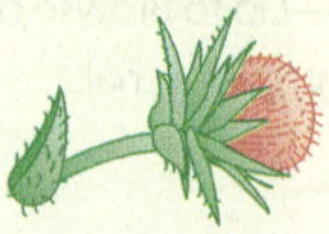	May benefit the liver by protecting and promoting the growth of liver cells, fighting oxidation, and inhibiting inflammation. However, results from clinical trials are mixed.	The seeds contain a compound called silymarin, which helps liver cells keep out toxins and may promote formation of new liver cells.	When used as capsules containing 200 milligrams of concentrated extract (140 milligrams of silymarin), no harmful effects have been reported.

Herb	Why It Is Used	How It Works	Cautions
Psyllium 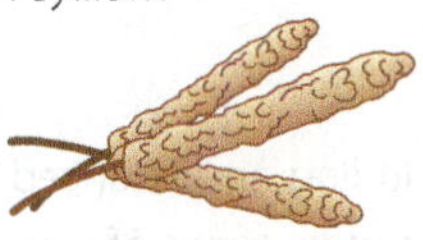	A laxative that doesn't undermine the natural action of the gut. It may reduce the risk of colorectal cancer and reduce blood levels of cholesterol.	The seeds of this herb have husks that are filled with mucilage, a fiber that swells with water in the intestines to add bulk and lubrication to the stool.	Increase in flatulence in some people, especially if a great deal is consumed.
Saw palmetto 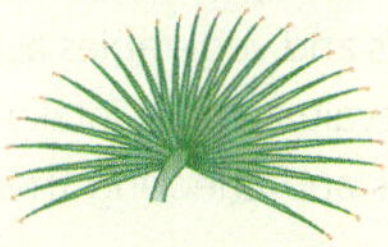	Studies on patients with an enlarged prostate have shown that extracts of this palm tree can reduce urinary symptoms even though the gland may not shrink.	Nonhormonal chemicals in saw palmetto appear to work through antiandrogenic and anti-inflammatory activity.	Some experts are concerned that those taking the herb may have inaccurate PSA readings, used as an early warning sign of prostate cancer.
St. John's wort 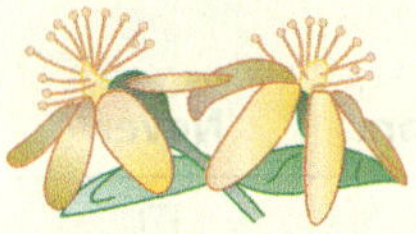	Some reports attest to this herb's ability to relieve mild depression. It may also have sedating and antianxiety activity.	Inhibits uptake of serotonin by nerve cells.	May cause gastrointestinal distress and increased sensitivity to bright sunlight.
Valerian 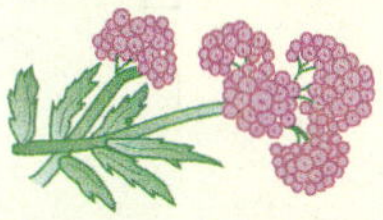	Perhaps best characterized as a mild tranquilizer.	Parts of this plant have antianxiety effects, making it potentially useful in treating nervousness and insomnia.	Long-term use is associated with liver damage.

These herbs should be avoided:

Herb	Why It Is Used	Reasons for Caution
Aconite	Pain, rheumatism, headaches	Numerous poisonings in China
Belladonna	Spasms, gastrointestinal pain	Contains three toxic alkaloids, including atropine
Blue cohosh	Menstrual ailments, worms	Can induce labor
Borage	Coughs, diuretic, mood booster	May contain liver toxins and carcinogens
Broom	Intoxicant, diuretic, heart problems	May slow heart rhythm; contains toxic alkaloids
Chaparral	Arthritis, cancer, pain, colds	Can cause severe hepatitis and liver failure
Comfrey	Cuts, bruises, ulcers	Contains toxins linked to liver disease and death
Ephedra	Stimulant, decongestant	Contains cardiac toxins that have resulted in dozens of deaths
Germander	Digestion, fever	Stimulant can cause heart problem
Kava	Sedative, anxiety, insomnia, restlessness	Possible liver damage; should not be used with alcohol or other depressants, or by pregnant women
Kombucha tea	AIDS, insomnia, acne	Can cause liver damage, intestinal problems, and death
Lobelia	Mood booster	Can cause rapid heartbeat, coma, and death
Pennyroyal	Stimulant, gastric distress	Liver damage, convulsions, and deaths
Poke root	Emetic, rheumatism	Extremely toxic; can cause low blood pressure, respiratory depression
Sassafras	Stimulant, sweat producer, syphilis	Contains the carcinogen safrole; banned from use in food
Skullcap	Tranquilizer	Can cause liver damage
Wormwood	Tonic, digestion	Can cause convulsions, loss of consciousness, and hallucinations

***In general, much more controlled research is needed to examine the potential active components, efficacy, and long-term safety of the herbs listed here.**

SOURCES: *The Physician's Desk Reference for Herbal Medicines*; Tyler's *Herbs of Choice: The Therapeutic Use of Phytomedicinals*, 3rd ed., 2009; Herbs at a Glance, nccam.nih .gov/health/herbsataglance.htm.

SCORE Card

Are You Reaping the Power of Produce? (Obj. 7.7)

Overwhelming evidence points to the health benefits derived from diets rich in fruits and vegetables, including an enhanced immune system and reduced risk of many chronic conditions, such as heart disease, high blood pressure, certain types of cancer, and age-related vision loss. To achieve the maximum benefits from the vitamins, minerals, antioxidants, and phytochemicals available in produce, aim for a *minimum* of five servings every day. Be adventurous! Select from as wide a variety of fruits and vegetables as possible. Be sure to frequently include members of the "superstar" categories of fruits and vegetables listed here. To evaluate your intake of fruits and vegetables, take the "Fruits and Veggies: More Matters" challenge by answering the following questions and checking the appropriate boxes.

A. Evaluate Your Intake of the Superstar Fruits and Vegetables

	Daily	Occasionally	Seldom	Never
I eat citrus fruits (oranges, grapefruits, etc.).	☐	☐	☐	☐
I eat berries (strawberries, blueberries, etc.), kiwi, or grapes.	☐	☐	☐	☐
I eat cruciferous vegetables such as cabbage, broccoli, cauliflower, Brussels sprouts, and kale.	☐	☐	☐	☐
I eat dark-green leafy vegetables such as spinach, turnip greens, collard greens, mustard greens, or beet greens.	☐	☐	☐	☐
I eat deep-yellow, orange, and red fruits and vegetables such as sweet potatoes, carrots, winter squash, pumpkin, cantaloupe, nectarines, peaches, apricots, mangos, papayas, tomatoes, red peppers, and watermelon.	☐	☐	☐	☐

B. Take the "Fruits and Veggies: More Matters" Challenge

	Number of Servings (each box represents one serving)*			
I start the day with a serving of fruit at breakfast.	☐	☐	☐	☐
I snack on fruits or vegetables during the day.	☐	☐	☐	☐
I include a serving of fruit or a vegetable at lunch.	☐	☐	☐	☐
I eat one or more vegetable servings at dinner.	☐	☐	☐	☐
I choose berries, melon, pears, apples, or other fruit for a sweet dessert.	☐	☐	☐	☐

Total Boxes Checked: ______________________

Scoring for the "Fruits and Veggies: More Matters" Challenge

Fewer than five boxes checked:

Ouch! You're missing out on the health benefits from produce. Visit the *Fruits and Veggies—More Matters* campaign at www.fruitsandveggiesmorematters.org to get tools and information to help you eat more fruits and vegetables each day!

At least five boxes checked:

Good! You're getting the *minimum* number of servings of fruits and vegetables for a healthy diet. Be sure to select a variety of fruits and vegetables and to include servings from the superstar groups as well.

Nine boxes or more checked:

Excellent! You're getting the recommended number of servings for fruits and vegetables in a healthy diet. Be sure to select a variety of fruits and vegetables and to include servings from the superstar groups as well.

*A serving of fruit equals one medium piece of fruit, ½ cup cut or cooked fruit, ¼ cup dried fruit, or ½ cup fruit juice. A serving of vegetables equals 1 cup leafy vegetables, ½ cup cooked or cut vegetables, or ½ cup vegetable juice.

SPOTLight

7.9 Nutrition and Cancer Prevention

You probably know someone who has cancer, who has recovered from it, or who has died of it. After heart disease, cancer is our most prevalent disease and can be expected, in one form or another, to affect one out of every three Americans living today. In fact, cancer is the primary cause of death for men and women ages 40 to 79.[33]

Eating pattern is only one of many factors that contribute to the development of cancer (see Figure 7-22), but unlike so many factors in our environment, the food you choose to eat is a factor you can control to a great extent. This discussion attempts to answer questions about the connection between diet and cancer. See the accompanying box for links to additional resources.

Nutrition and Cancer Resources on the Web

http://fnic.nal.usda.gov
The Food and Nutrition Information Center (FNIC) provides credible information about cancer. Go to Browse by Subject and click on Diet and Health and then select Cancer.

www.cancer.gov
Information about cancer, research, and statistics is found at this government website.

www.cancer.org
The American Cancer Society provides information on this website.

www.aicr.org
The American Institute for Cancer Research (AICR) provides information about cancer.

How is diet associated with cancer?

Mounting evidence continues to show that many connections exist between diet and cancer. Constituents in foods may be responsible for starting the cancer (a process called *initiation*) or for speeding its development (a two-step process that includes tumor *promotion* and *progression*)—or they may protect against cancer (see Figure 7-23). Also, for the person who has cancer, diet can make a crucial difference in recovery by helping to restore body weight and improve nutritional status.

Our diets are complex and diverse, making it difficult to separate the effect of a single dietary component from the hundreds of other constituents in foods. In addition, the difficulty of evaluating the diet–cancer link is compounded by the fact that many cancers take up to 20 years to develop. Thus, assessing a cancer patient's diet today is not as helpful as knowing how that patient ate 10, 20, or even 30 years before the cancer was diagnosed.

Is nutrition related to causing cancer the way other environmental factors are, such as smoking or air pollution?

Yes. The National Cancer Institute estimates that more than 85 percent of all cancers are associated with lifestyle and environmental factors, including nutrition. Lifestyle factors include tobacco use, diet, lack of physical activity, alcohol consumption, exposure to sunlight, patterns of

FIGURE 7-22
The Impact of Genetic, Environmental, and Lifestyle Risk Factors on Cancer

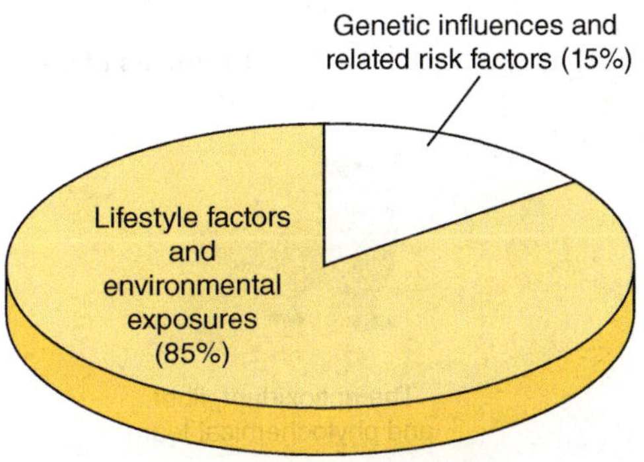

Lifestyle: Tobacco use, diet, obesity, physical inactivity, occupation/job-related factors, alcohol, salt/food additives, and other preservatives/contaminants

Environment: Viruses/other biologic agents, pollution, ionizing/ultraviolet radiation

FIGURE 7-23

How Cancer Develops

A. *Cancer initiation*. Initiation by a carcinogen causes cancerous alterations in previously healthy body cells.

B. *Cancer promotion*. Cancer promoters enhance the growth of abnormal cancerous cells.

C. *Cellular repair*. Cancer antipromoters squelch free radical damage and enhance the body's ability to repair damaged DNA strands.

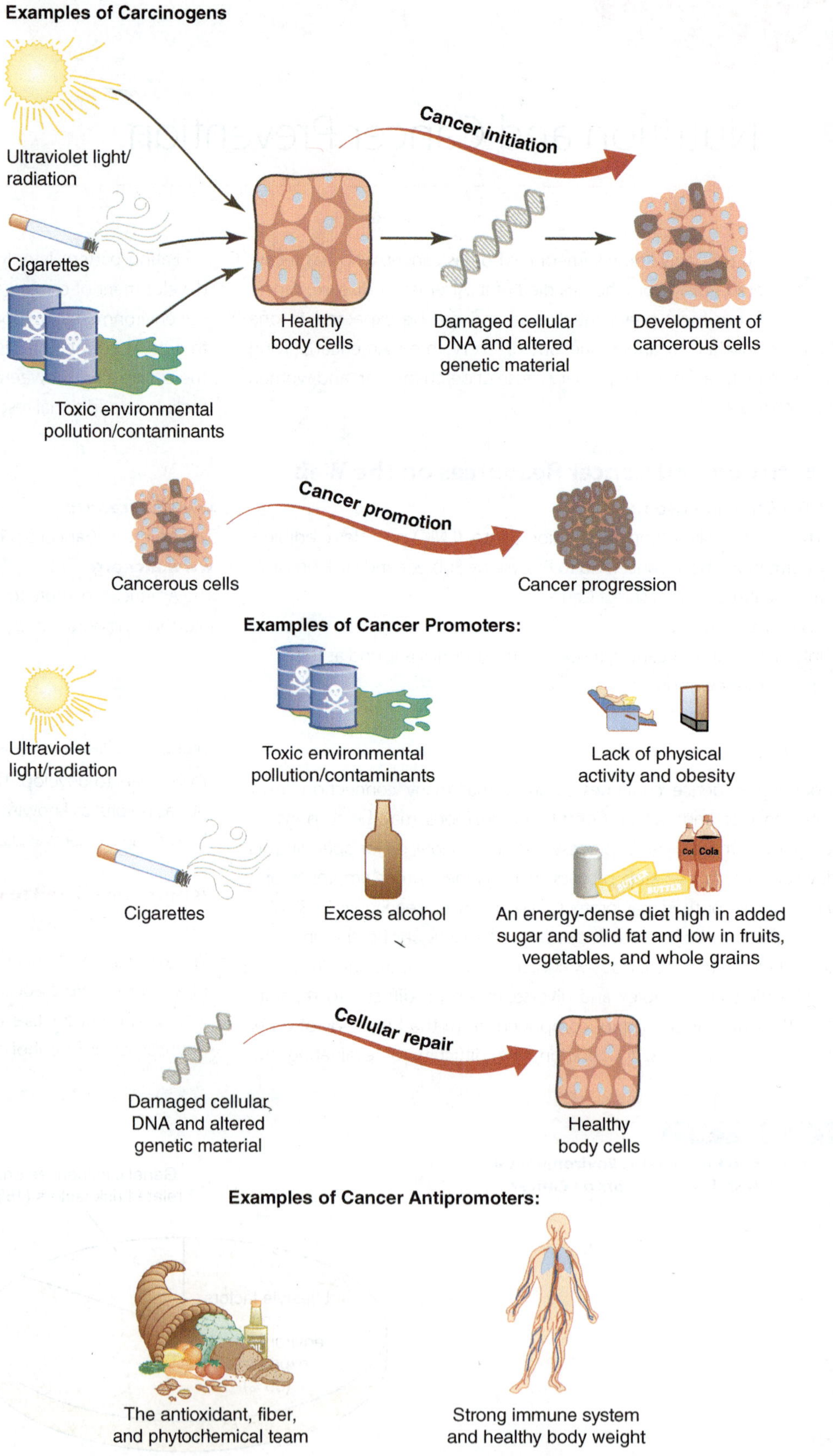

sexual behavior, and personal hygiene; these can usually be controlled by the individual. In contrast, individuals typically have little control over environmental factors, such as exposure to carcinogens in the workplace, radiation during medical and dental procedures, and contaminants (either naturally occurring or artificially created) present in the soil, air, and water. We also have no control over the genetic factors that contribute to the development of cancer.

Diet and physical activity habits, as well as overweight and obesity, are lifestyle factors that may account for as much as one-third of the more than 595,000 cancer deaths that occur in the United States each year; another one-third is caused by exposure to tobacco products.[34] Thus, researchers take the study of nutrition and cancer seriously. Scientists have identified various dietary factors that may contribute to or protect against many different types of cancer. As noted in Table 7-23, practicing healthy behaviors such as not smoking, maintaining a healthy weight, being physically active, and consuming a healthy diet can greatly reduce the risk of developing or dying from cancer.[35]

What is some of the evidence linking diet and cancer?

Studies of the eating habits of different population groups provide some of the knowledge we already have about the diet–cancer connection. Research involving Seventh-Day Adventists, a group of people with a remarkably low death rate from cancers of all kinds, is particularly telling. This religious group has rules against smoking and using alcohol, discourages the use of hot condiments and spices, and encourages a meatless diet. After cancers linked to smoking and alcohol are discounted, these people still have a cancer mortality rate about one-half to two-thirds that of the rest of the population. This may be due to a low consumption of meat and to a high consumption of fruits, vegetables, and cereal grains.

Does the type of cancer matter, in terms of nutrition-related risk factors and recommendations?

Yes. Although many risk factors overlap, certain behaviors increase the likelihood of specific cancers (see Table 7-23). There are also dietary components associated with preventing certain types of cancers. When it comes to colon cancer, the best nutrition and physical activity-related advice to reduce the risk of colon cancer is to:[36]

- Increase the intensity and duration of physical activity.
- Limit intake of red and processed meat.
- Consume recommended levels of calcium and vitamin D.
- Eat more vegetables and fruits.
- Avoid obesity (especially weight gain around the abdomen).
- Avoid excess alcohol consumption.

What about breast cancer?

The case of the connection between diet and breast cancer is a good example of the difficulty of interpreting study results. A group of researchers in Athens, Greece, who studied 120 women with breast cancer and 120 women without cancer, reported no association between breast cancer and the consumption of fats and oils.[37] By comparison, a research group in China reported that women with a high intake of fat and calories and a low intake of vegetables and dietary fiber had an increased risk of breast cancer.[38] As you can see from these apparently conflicting results, the role of dietary fat in breast cancer development has been controversial for decades and remains unclear. Most studies of human populations fail to confirm an association between dietary fat and breast cancer. Laboratory studies, however, show that eating a low-fat diet can reduce estrogen levels and, theoretically, may reduce

TABLE 7-23 Diet and Cancer

Cancer Site	Associated with These Diet and Physical Activity Risk Factors
Breast	Alcohol; adult weight gain; excess body fatness, abdominal fatness; low fruit and vegetable intake; low level of physical activity
Colon or Rectum	Red meat and processed meat intake; alcohol; low-fiber diets; low calcium intake; excess body fatness; abdominal fatness; low level of physical activity
Mouth, Throat, and Esophagus	Alcohol; low intakes of vitamins and minerals from fruits and nonstarchy vegetables; low intake of foods containing carotenoids; excess body fatness
Lung	Low fruit and vegetable intake; low level of physical activity; arsenic in drinking water; low intake of foods containing carotenoids
Ovary and Endometrium	Excess body fatness; abdominal fatness; low fruit and vegetable intake; low level of physical activity
Prostate	Diets high in calcium; low intake of foods containing lycopene; low intake of foods containing selenium
Pancreas	Low fruit and vegetable intake; excess body fatness, abdominal fatness
Stomach	Regular consumption of smoked foods and foods cured with salt or nitrite compounds; low fruit and vegetable intake; low intake of allium vegetables (garlic, leeks, onions, shallots)
Liver	Ingestion of aflatoxin-contaminated grains; regular consumption of smoked foods and foods cured with salt or nitrite compounds; alcohol abuse

SOURCE: Adapted from Nutrition and Physical Activity for Cancer Prevention: Reducing the Risk of Cancer with Healthy Food Choices and Physical Activity, *CA: A Cancer Journal for Clinicians*, 62 (2012): 30–67.

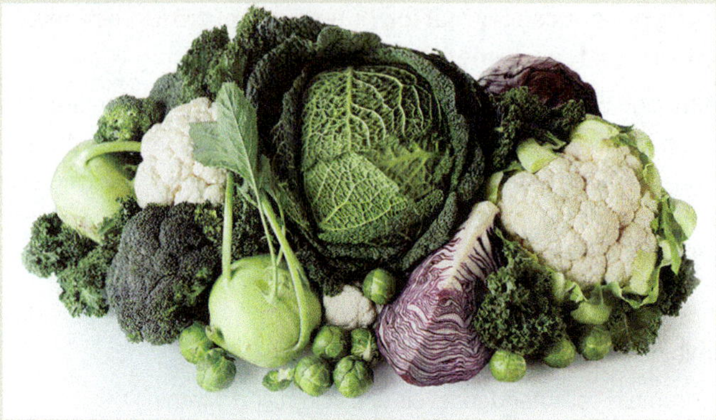

Cruciferous vegetables, a group of cabbage-family vegetables named for their cross-shaped blossoms, such as cauliflower, broccoli, cabbages, kale, kohlrabi, rutabaga, turnip root, and Brussels sprouts, contain nutrients and nonnutrients that protect against cancer.

the risk of breast cancer. Many ongoing studies continue to examine the possible role of dietary fat in breast cancer.

Of course, excess fat in the diet can contribute to overweight, and recent studies have indicated that women who gain excess weight as adults may have an increased risk of breast cancer.[39] Health experts advise us to limit weight gain during adulthood to no more than 10 pounds and to get regular physical activity. In fact, regular physical activity throughout the reproductive years may significantly lower breast cancer risk. Body fat is involved in the production of estrogen. Therefore, by discouraging the accumulation of excess body fat (especially around the abdomen), exercise may decrease the total amount of estrogen a woman is exposed to over her lifetime.

What should consumers do?

The American Cancer Society and the National Cancer Institute have reviewed the evidence independently and have identified the following specific concerns:[40]

- *Total calorie intake.* Studies on animals show that reduced food intake reduces cancer incidence at any age, but the evidence is less clear for human beings. Obesity, however, does increase risks for several types of cancers including breast (in postmenopausal women), colon and rectum, endometrium, esophagus, kidney, and pancreas. Being overweight or obese may also raise the risk for gallbladder and liver cancer.[41]
- *Fat.* Both animal studies and population studies support the view that high fat intake increases the incidence of cancers of the ovaries, colon, and prostate.
- *Protein.* High protein intake may be associated with increased risks of certain kinds of cancer, but the evidence is not yet firm enough to permit a definitive statement.
- *Beta-carotene.* Inadequate intakes of beta-carotene correlate with a high incidence of cancers of the lung, bladder, and larynx; by inference, adequate intakes may help protect against these cancers.[42]
- *Vitamin C.* Vitamin C may help prevent the formation of cancer-causing agents and thereby protect against cancers of the esophagus and stomach.[43]

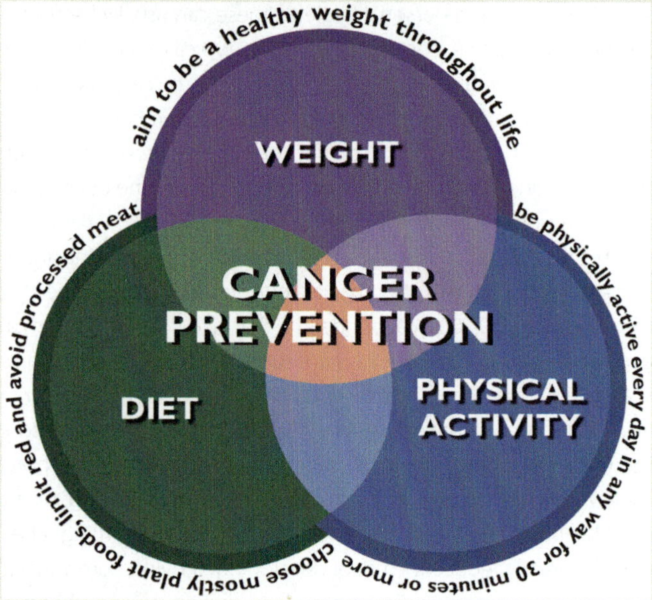

- *Cruciferous vegetables.* The consumption of cauliflower, cabbage, and broccoli is associated with a reduced incidence of cancer at several sites.[44]
- *Other vitamins and minerals.* The effect of the antioxidant nutrients—vitamin C, beta-carotene, vitamin E, and selenium—on cancer risk is an area of active research.[45] The trace mineral selenium, used in the body's production of its own antioxidants, is believed to protect against cancer of the esophagus, stomach, colon, and rectum.[46] Likewise, vitamin E may protect against cancer, particularly cancer of the gastrointestinal tract.[47]
- Calcium. Low calcium intake has been associated with increased incidence of colon cancer. Conversely, people who consume adequate calcium and vitamin D tend to develop less colon cancer.[48]
- *Fiber.* Fiber may help protect against some cancers by, for example, speeding up the passage of all materials through the colon so that its walls are not exposed for long to cancer-causing substances.

Do vegetarians have a lower incidence of cancer?

Yes, they do. The Seventh-Day Adventists have already been mentioned. Vegetarian women also have less breast cancer than do women who eat meat.

A number of studies have examined the relationship between cancer and vegetable consumption. Many of them have shown that people with colon cancer eat vegetables less frequently than do others. One study revealed that people with colon cancer specifically consumed less cabbage, broccoli, and Brussels sprouts than did people free of cancer. Similarly, comparisons of the diets of people who have stomach cancer with those of carefully matched people without cancer showed lower consumption of vegetables in the cancer group: in one case, vegetables in general; in another case, fresh vegetables; in still others, lettuce and other fresh greens or vegetables containing vitamin C. Some of the suspects for causing stomach cancer are chemicals known as nitrosamines, which are produced in the stomach and

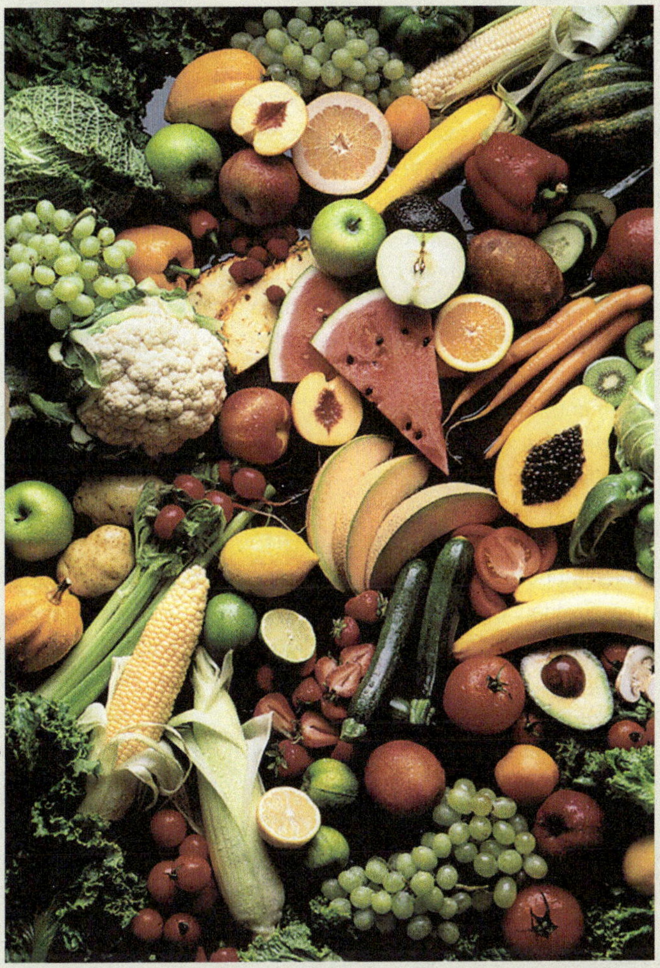

Thomas Del Brase/Stone/The Image Bank/Getty Images

The more varied the kinds of fruits and vegetables you eat, the better nourished you are likely to be. The National Cancer Institute's National Fruit and Vegetable program urges consumers to eat five to nine servings (or more) of fruits and vegetables rich in fiber, vitamins, minerals, antioxidants, and phytochemicals every day to help protect against cancer.

intestines from nitrites found in foods. Vegetables may help in cancer prevention by contributing vitamin C, which inhibits the conversion of nitrites to nitrosamines.[49]

Another healthy aspect of many plant-based diets is the use of soy foods. A number of studies conducted in China and Japan have shown that consumers of soy foods have lower cancer rates than those who rarely consume these foods. The data suggest that consuming one or two servings of soy a day (e.g., 1 cup of soy milk or 4 ounces of tofu) may reduce risk of breast, prostate, endometrium, and possibly other cancers.[50]

What about alcohol? Is it connected with cancer?

Yes. Environmental causes of head, neck, and esophageal cancer have been studied, and the major factor appears to be the combination of alcohol and tobacco use. However, dietary factors have turned up, pointing to a low intake of fruits and raw vegetables, specifically of the fruits and vegetables that contribute the orange pigment beta-carotene (which converts to vitamin A in the body) and the vitamin riboflavin. Beta-carotene—noted for giving carrots, winter squash, sweet potatoes, apricots, cantaloupe, and other fruits and vegetables their familiar colors—and its relatives may also be important in reducing the risk of skin cancer.

Researchers are probing the association of alcohol consumption with increased risk of breast cancer.[51] Some studies have shown a modest but significant increase in risk of breast cancer for women who were classified as heavy drinkers (more than four drinks per day). Other studies have found that even low levels of alcohol intake increase the risk.[52]

What is the association between beta-carotene and other carotenoids and cancer?

Among the known actions of vitamin A (beta-carotene) are its important roles in maintaining immune function. A strong immune system may be able to prevent cancers from gaining control even after they have been initiated in the body.

The carotenoids are a family of powerful antioxidants found in dark-yellow, orange, and red fruits and vegetables and in dark-green vegetables. They are potent free-radical fighters that may play important roles in preventing cancer. The family includes alpha- and beta-carotene, lycopene, lutein, zeaxanthin, and others. Alpha- and beta-carotene appear to protect against the progression of cancer, whereas other carotenoids may offer more protection at earlier stages of cancer development. Carotenoids may work against cancer by boosting the immune system and supporting the enzymes that detoxify carcinogens. Beta-carotene and lycopene may be effective in preventing damaged cells from proliferating and becoming malignant. Scientists now believe that lycopene, which is found in red fruits and vegetables such as tomatoes, tomato products, red peppers, and watermelon, is the most powerful of the antioxidant carotenoids. Research is currently under way to examine a link between lycopene and lowered risk of prostate and other cancers.[53] Meanwhile, we are advised to consume a *minimum* of 2½ cups of a variety of fruits and vegetables each day. Be sure to include deep-green and brightly colored fruits and vegetables every day. By doing so, your ability to repair free-radical damage in the body is likely to be enhanced by the carotenoids (or possibly by something else) in these plant foods.

Would that "something" in the vegetables be a vitamin?

Not necessarily. Both fruits and vegetables appear to have a protective effect beyond those already discussed for beta-carotene, vitamin C, and fiber. Researchers have identified substances known as *phytochemicals*—naturally occurring plant compounds—in fruits and vegetables that may play a role in decreasing cancer risk and strengthening the immune system.[54] (Refer to Table 7-20 for a sampling of these compounds.) These vegetables also contain folate, a vitamin, which is involved in cell multiplication, and may prove to play an important role in prevention of colon and other cancers.[55] The effects of the members of the cabbage family may be due to substances known as *indoles*, a type of phytochemical, which may act by inducing an enzyme in the host that destroys cancer-causing agents.

Do these findings have any implications for the way a person should eat right now, today?

Although clearly there is still much to learn, many experts believe that enough is known to take preventive steps. An exhaustive review of some 7,000 previous studies on cancer has led scientists at the American Institute for Cancer Research to release a comprehensive set of recommendations for cancer prevention.[56] To put these recommendations into action, consider these simple steps:

1. *Body fatness.* Be as lean as possible without becoming underweight. Maintaining a healthy weight is one of the most important things you can do to reduce your risk of cancer. Aim to be at the lower end of the healthy weight range (see Chapter 10).
2. *Physical activity.* Be physically active for at least 30 minutes every day. Physical activity in any form helps lower cancer risk. Aim to build more activity, like brisk walking, into your daily routine.
3. *Foods and drinks that promote weight gain.* Avoid sugary drinks. Limit consumption of energy-dense foods (particularly processed foods high in added sugar, low in fiber, or high in solid fat). Choosing healthy foods and drinks instead of those that are high in refined carbohydrates and often in added sugar and fat (energy-dense foods) can help us avoid overweight and obesity and thereby reduce our cancer risk.
4. *Plant foods.* Eat more of a variety of vegetables, fruits, whole grains, and legumes such as beans. Basing our diets on plant foods, which contain fiber and other nutrients, can reduce our risk of cancer. Go to www.fruitsandveggiesmorematters.org to find the amount of fruits and vegetables that is right for you each day!
5. *Animal foods.* Limit consumption of red meats (such as beef, pork, and lamb) and avoid processed meats. To reduce your cancer risk, eat no more than 18 ounces (cooked weight) per week of red meats, like beef, pork, and lamb, and avoid processed meat such as ham, bacon, salami, hot dogs, and sausages.
6. *Alcoholic drinks.* If you do drink alcohol, limit your consumption to no more than two drinks a day for men and one drink a day for women.
7. *Preservation, processing, preparation.* Avoid salt-preserved, salted, or salty foods. Throw away moldy grains or legumes. Limit consumption of salty foods and foods processed with salt (sodium). Consuming too much salt can be harmful to our health, increasing our risk of stomach cancer as well as high blood pressure.
8. *Dietary supplements.* Don't use supplements to protect against cancer. To reduce your risk of cancer, aim to meet your nutritional needs with a variety of foods rather than taking supplements.
9. And always remember—avoid exposure to tobacco products.

Your lifestyle choices regarding diet, physical activity, and smoking can be powerful tools in reducing your risk for cancer (see Figure 7-24). Taken together, this advice agrees with most recommendations made to the public for helping prevent heart disease, diabetes, and many other ills, as well as cancer.

Does it make a difference if I choose to take supplements instead of eating vegetables?

Yes. Fiber, vitamin C, beta-carotene, riboflavin, indoles, and other phytochemicals found in *foods* appear to have preventive effects on cancer development. And because it is obvious that researchers do not have "the answer"—just many partial answers—it is best to stick with foods. Supplements may not contain some as yet unidentified components found in foods that may help to protect against cancer. Also, with vitamin-mineral supplementation, there is always the risk of an excessively high intake. (Recall that vitamin A and other vitamins and minerals can be toxic at high doses.) In fact, there is evidence that some high-dose supplements can increase cancer risk.[57] *It is best to rely on foods.* Fruits and vegetables add vitamins, minerals, and fiber to your diet—as well as color and flavor.

What about adding probiotics and prebiotics to the diet?

Research is under way to find out whether probiotics may help prevent or treat a variety of health problems, including digestive disorders. As mentioned earlier in the chapter, probiotics are friendly bacteria found in fermented products such as yogurt, kefir, miso, tempeh, and some soy beverages. In the digestive tract, probiotics may improve digestive health. Prebiotics are nondigestible carbohydrates (such as the oligosaccharides inulin and lactulose) resistant to digestion in humans. When the nondigested carbohydrate enters the colon, it is fermented by colonic bacteria. Prebiotics can play a role in stimulating the growth of the beneficial microflora.[58] Prebiotics are found in such foods as bananas, barley, chicory, garlic, leeks, onions, wheat, soy, and peas and beans.

Although the utilization of synbiotics—products that combine probiotics and prebiotics—is still being studied in regard to cancer prevention, some evidence suggests that intestinal microflora are important for reducing damage that can lead to cancer. In studies with mice, those mice without intestinal bacteria were unable to heal colon injuries, which led to inflammation and the development of tumors, unlike the mice with normal intestinal bacteria who were less likely to develop tumors. Furthermore, supplementing the germ-free mice with bacteria strains also suppressed tumor growth. This suggests that intestinal bacteria may protect against colon cancer. Limited research in humans also supports an association between the use of synbiotics and both preventative effects as well as decreased recurrence of bladder cancer.[59] Additional research is needed to better understand the benefits versus risks in using probiotics and prebiotics, particularly in supplement form.

Are any anticancer benefits derived from drinking tea?

Scientists note that people in Asia, where large quantities of tea—both green and black—are consumed, have a lower incidence of esophageal, colon, stomach, and other cancers. Laboratory studies suggest that *polyphenols*—phytochemicals having potent antioxidant properties—found in tea may help protect against these cancers by blocking the formation of carcinogenic compounds in the body. However, the implications for humans remain inconclusive.

Does cooking food at high temperatures increase the risk of cancer?

Some research suggests that frying or charcoal-broiling meats—especially fatty meats—at very high temperatures creates chemicals on the surface of the food that may increase cancer risk. Preserving meats by methods involving smoke also increases their content of potentially carcinogenic chemicals. We are advised to eat grilled, smoked, or cured foods only occasionally. When you do, consume them with fruits and vegetables that contain protective antioxidant and phytochemical factors. Choose techniques such as braising, poaching, stewing, baking, or roasting instead.

Why should I vary my diet?

The recommendation to eat a varied diet is based on an important cancer-prevention strategy: dilution. The standard advice to eat a variety of foods takes on new meaning in this quote: "The wider the variety of food intake, the greater the number of different chemical substances consumed, and the less is the chance that any one chemical will reach a hazardous level in the diet."[60] In other words, when you add new foods to the diet, you dilute what is in one food with what is in another.

The variety principle traditionally means to eat foods from each of the various food groups. This principle must also be applied within each of the food groups. Don't alternate just between corn and potatoes. Select different vegetables each time you go to the store—broccoli, kale, green beans, carrots, squash, and many others.

Although you cannot control many cancer-causing factors, you can decide which food habits you will keep and which ones you will change. By using these guidelines in making your choices, you will have every reason to feel confident that you are providing your body with the best nutrition at the lowest possible risk. Remember that in the final analysis, your risk of developing cancer can be reduced significantly by not smoking, by consuming alcohol in moderation if at all, and by adopting healthful eating and physical activity habits.

FIGURE 7-24

Factors That Decrease or Increase Cancer Risk

SOURCE: Adapted from *Food, Nutrition, Physical Activity, and the Prevention of Cancer: A Global Perspective* (Washington, DC: World Cancer Research Fund/American Institute for Cancer Research).

Cancer Type	Estimated Annual Deaths (2017)*	Vegetables	Fruits	Fiber	Physical activity	Alcohol	Salt and salting	Red meat	Grilled or barbecued (animal foods)	Total and saturated animal fats	Obesity	Smoking tobacco
Lung	155,870	Decreases risk possible	Decreases risk probable		Decreases risk possible			Increases risk possible		Increases risk possible		Increases risk convincingly
Colon and rectum	50,260	Decreases risk possible	Decreases risk possible	Decreases risk probable	Decreases risk convincingly	Increases risk convincingly		Increases risk convincingly		Increases risk possible	Increases risk convincingly	Increases risk possible
Breast	41,070				Decreases risk probable	Increases risk convincingly				Increases risk possible	Increases risk convincingly	
Pancreas	43,090										Increases risk convincingly	Increases risk convincingly
Prostate	26,730	Decreases risk possible	Decreases risk possible					Increases risk possible				
Liver	28,920		Decreases risk possible			Increases risk probable					Increases risk possible	
Esophagus	15,690	Decreases risk convincingly	Decreases risk convincingly	Decreases risk possible		Increases risk convincingly		Increases risk possible			Increases risk convincingly	Increases risk convincingly
Kidney	14,400										Increases risk convincingly	Increases risk possible
Stomach	10,960	Decreases risk probable	Decreases risk probable				Increases risk probable		Increases risk possible			
Oral cavity and pharynx	9,700	Decreases risk probable	Decreases risk probable			Increases risk convincingly						Increases risk convincingly
Uterus (endometrium)	10,920	Decreases risk possible			Decreases risk probable			Increases risk possible			Increases risk convincingly	

Decreases risk convincingly — Decreases risk probable — Decreases risk possible — Increases risk convincingly — Increases risk probable — Increases risk possible

*From: Cancer Facts and Figures, 2017; available at www.cancer.org.

WHAT'S ONLINE

MINDTAP From Cengage

Visit www.cengagebrain.com to access MindTap, a complete digital course that includes Diet & Wellness Plus, interactive quizzes, videos, and more.

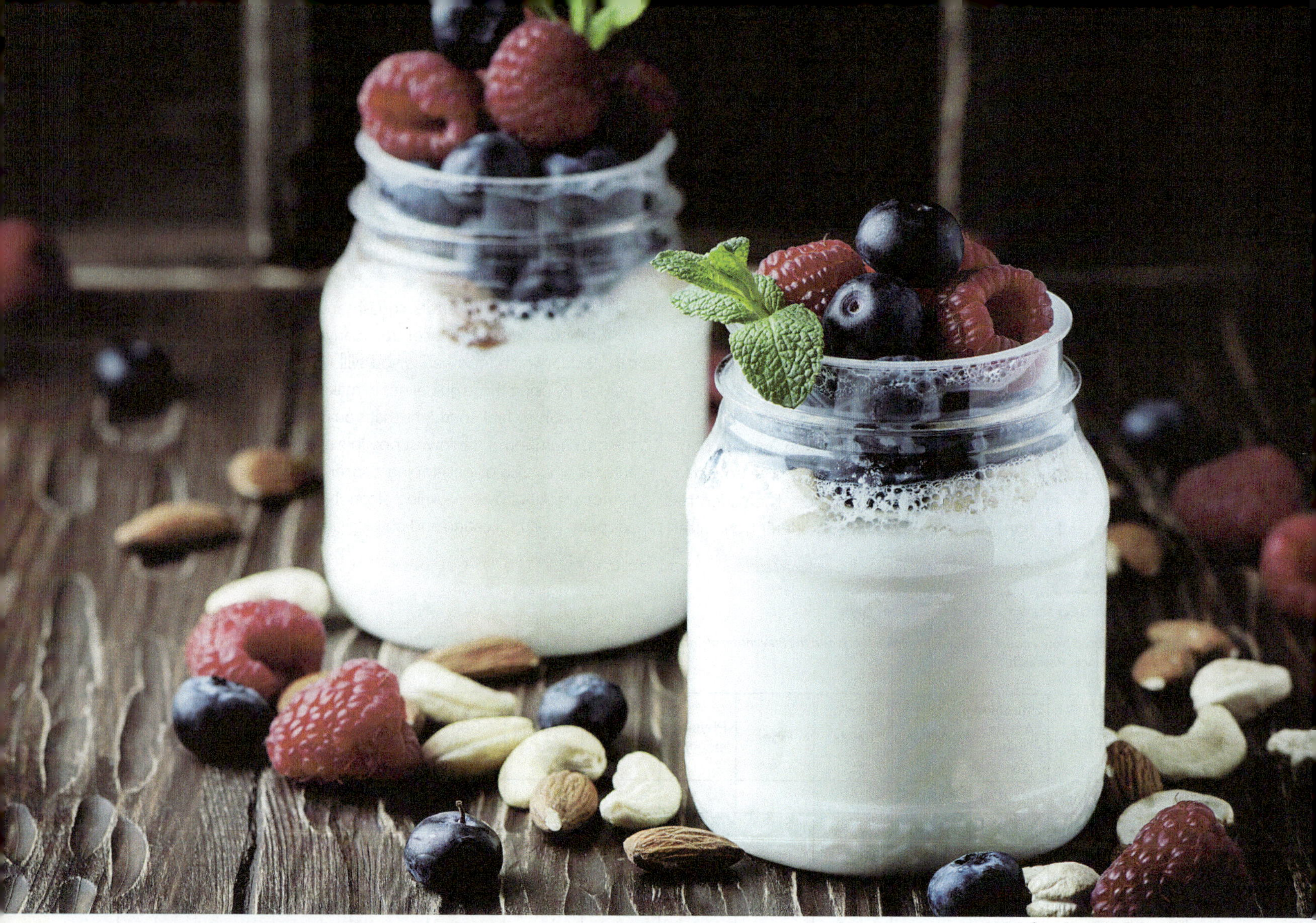

Oxana Denezhkina/Shutterstock.com

AskYourself . . .

Which of the following statements about nutrition are true, and which are false? For each false statement, what is true?

1. Water accounts for about 60 percent of an adult's body weight.
2. Sodium is bad for the body and should be avoided.
3. When a person becomes deficient in iron, the very first symptom to appear is anemia.
4. Osteoporosis is a disease that can affect men and women at any age.

Answers found on page 224

ChapterObjectives

8.1 Differentiate between the two classifications of minerals.

8.2 Identify the major roles, deficiency symptoms, and food sources for the minerals needed for maintaining healthy bones.

8.3 Identify the major roles, deficiency symptoms, and food sources for the trace minerals iron and zinc.

8.4 Identify the minerals essential for energy metabolism, and list food sources for each.

8.5 Identify other major roles, deficiency symptoms, and food sources of the minerals that function as electrolytes in the body.

8.6 Describe factors associated with the development of osteoporosis, and list strategies for prevention.

The Minerals and Water: A Functional Approach

CHAPTER 8

For hundreds, if not thousands, of years, the physical and chemical properties of minerals such as gold, silver, lead, and copper have been known to metallurgists and alchemists. Even so, the role of some minerals in biological processes has been recognized only within the past few hundred years. The discovery of iron in blood, for example, occurred in 1713. The identification of calcium in bone was made in 1771.[1] The role of minerals in human nutrition was not fully appreciated until the late 19th century.

The previous chapter described the water-soluble and fat-soluble vitamins, their biological roles, food sources, and human requirements. This chapter discusses the minerals known to be important in human nutrition. In some respects, minerals are similar to vitamins. Like the vitamins, minerals themselves do not contribute energy (calories) to the diet. Of the minerals important in human nutrition, most have diverse functions within the body and work with enzymes to facilitate chemical reactions. Also like the vitamins, most minerals are required in the diet in very small amounts.

Unlike vitamins, some minerals (such as calcium) contribute directly to the building of body structures (such as bone). In other respects, minerals are different from vitamins. Whereas vitamins are organic compounds, minerals are **inorganic** compounds that occur naturally in the Earth's crust.

As with other areas of research in human nutrition, many questions related to mineral metabolism remain unanswered. Scientists continue to study the biochemical functions of minerals, the mechanisms by which they activate enzymes, the factors that control their levels in blood and tissues, and the ways in which the composition of the diet

> The pleasure of eating . . . is of all times, all ages, all conditions. . . . Because it may be enjoyed with other enjoyments, and even console us for their absence. . . . Because its impressions are more durable and more dependent on our will. . . . Because in eating we experience a certain indescribably keen sensation of pleasure, by what we eat we repair the losses we have sustained, and prolong life.
>
> —Anthelme Brillat-Savarin (1755–1826, French politician and gourmet; author of *Physiology of Taste*)

TABLE 8-1 A Guide to the Minerals

Mineral	Best Sources	Chief Roles	Deficiency Symptoms	Toxicity Symptoms
Major Minerals				
Calcium	Milk and milk products, small fish (with bones), calcium-set tofu, certain green vegetables (broccoli, kale, bok choy, turnip greens), legumes, fortified juices	Mineralization of bones and teeth; involved in muscle contraction and relaxation, nerve function, immune function, blood clotting, blood pressure	Stunted growth in children; bone loss (osteoporosis) in adults	Calcification of soft tissue (kidneys), kidney stones, constipation, abnormal heart rhythm
Phosphorus	Meat, poultry, fish, eggs, dairy products, soft drinks, legumes	Part of every cell; involved in acid–base balance and energy transfer; mineralization of bones and teeth	Muscle weakness and bone pain (rarely seen)	Calcification of soft tissue (kidneys)
Magnesium	Nuts, legumes, whole grains, dark green vegetables, seafood, chocolate, cocoa	Involved in bone mineralization, protein synthesis, enzyme action, normal muscular contraction, nerve transmission, immune function	Weakness, confusion, depressed pancreatic hormone secretion, growth failure, hallucinations, muscle spasms	Excess intakes (from overuse of laxatives) have caused alkalosis, low blood pressure, lack of coordination, coma, and death
Sodium	Salt, soy sauce, processed foods such as cured, canned, pickled, and many boxed foods and fast foods	Helps maintain normal fluid and acid–base balance; nerve impulse transmission	Muscle cramps, mental apathy, loss of appetite	High blood pressure
Chloride	Salt, soy sauce, processed foods	Part of hydrochloric acid found in the stomach, necessary for proper digestion, fluid balance	Growth failure in children, muscle cramps, mental apathy, loss of appetite	Normally harmless (the gas chlorine is a poison but evaporates from water); vomiting
Potassium	All whole foods: meats, milk, fruits, vegetables, grains, legumes	Facilitates many reactions, including those of protein synthesis, fluid balance, nerve transmission, and contraction of muscles	Muscle weakness, paralysis, confusion; can cause death; accompanies dehydration	Causes muscular weakness; triggers vomiting; if given into a vein, can stop the heart
Sulfur	All protein-containing foods	Component of certain amino acids; part of biotin, thiamin, and insulin	None known; protein deficiency would occur first	Would occur only if sulfur amino acids were eaten in excess; this (in animals) depresses growth

affects the body's ability to make use of these dietary components. The many complex metabolic interactions of minerals make this a challenging area of research. The discussions about the minerals that follow are organized according to the biological roles these substances play in the body.

8.1 The Two Classifications of Minerals

Nutritionists traditionally divide **minerals** into two large classes: the **major minerals** and the **trace minerals**. The distinction between them is that the major minerals occur in relatively larger quantities in the body and are needed in the daily diet in relatively larger amounts. The trace minerals occur in the body in minute quantities and are needed in smaller amounts in the daily diet. Table 8-1 lists the minerals known to be essential in human nutrition, and Figure 8-1 offers tips for locating the minerals in the MyPlate food guide.

inorganic Being or composed of matter other than plant or animal.

minerals Naturally occurring, inorganic, chemical elements; serve as structural components of the body and are used in many vital body processes.

major mineral An essential mineral nutrient found in the human body in amounts greater than 5 grams.

trace mineral An essential mineral nutrient found in the human body in amounts less than 5 grams.

ASK YOURSELF ANSWERS: **1.** True. **2.** False. Sodium is an essential nutrient, but excess sodium should be avoided. **3.** False. When a person becomes deficient in iron, one of the last symptoms to appear is anemia; fatigue and weakness appear first. **4.** True.

TABLE 8-1 A Guide to the Minerals *(continued)*

Mineral	Best Sources	Chief Roles	Deficiency Symptoms	Toxicity Symptoms
Trace Minerals				
Iodine	Iodized salt, seafood, bread	Part of thyroid hormone (thyroxine), which regulates growth and metabolic rate	Underactive thyroid gland, goiter, cretinism	Depressed thyroid activity
Iron	Red meats, fish, poultry, shellfish, eggs, legumes, dried fruits, green leafy vegetables, fortified cereals	Hemoglobin formation; part of myoglobin; energy utilization	Anemia: weakness, pallor, headaches, reduced immunity, inability to concentrate, cold intolerance	Iron overload: infections, liver injury, acidosis, shock
Zinc	Protein-containing foods: yogurt, meats, fish, shellfish, poultry, whole grains, fortified cereals	Part of insulin and many enzymes; involved in making genetic material and proteins, immunity, vitamin A transport, taste, wound healing, making sperm, fetal development	Growth failure in children, delayed development of sexual organs, loss of taste, poor wound healing	Fever, nausea, vomiting, loss of appetite, diarrhea, kidney failure
Copper	Meats, seafood, legumes, nuts, seeds, drinking water	Helps make hemoglobin and collagen; part of several enzymes	Anemia, bone abnormalities, impaired immunity	Nausea, vomiting, diarrhea
Fluoride	Drinking water (if fluoride containing or fluoridated), tea, seafood	Formation of bones and teeth; helps make teeth resistant to decay	Susceptibility to tooth decay	Fluorosis (discoloration of teeth); nausea, vomiting, diarrhea
Selenium	Seafood, meats, grains, vegetables (depending on soil conditions)	Helps protect body compounds from oxidation; works with vitamin E	Fragile red blood cells, cataracts, growth failure, heart damage (Keshan disease)	Nausea, abdominal pain; nail and hair brittleness, fatigue; liver and nerve damage
Chromium	Meats, whole grains vegetable oils	Associated with insulin; needed for release of energy from glucose	Abnormal glucose metabolism	Occupational exposures damage skin and kidneys
Molybdenum	Legumes, nuts, cereals	Facilitates, with enzymes, many cell processes	Unknown	Enzyme inhibition; kidney damage and reproductive abnormalities in animals
Manganese	Nuts, leafy green vegetables, whole grains, tea	Facilitates, with enzymes, many cell processes	In animals: poor growth, nervous system disorders, abnormal reproduction	Poisoning, nervous system disorders

FIGURE 8-1

Good Sources of Minerals in the USDA MyPlate Food Guide[a]

[a] Recommended intakes shown here are based on a 2,000-calorie diet. Go to www.ChooseMyPlate.gov for a quick estimate of how much food you should eat from the different food groups based on your age, gender, height, weight, and activity level.
[b] In whole-grain choices.

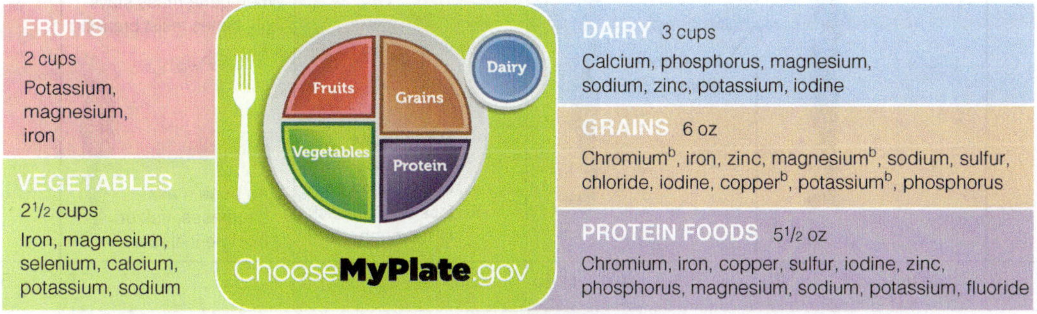

If you could extract all of the trace minerals from the body, you would obtain only a bit of dust, hardly enough to fill a teaspoon. As tiny as their quantities are, though, each of the trace minerals performs several vital roles for which no substitute will do. A deficiency of any of them may be fatal, and an excess of many can be equally deadly.

trabecular (tra-BECK-you-lar) bone The lacy inner network of calcium-containing crystals; spongelike in appearance, it supports the bone's structure.

cortical bone The dense outer ivory-like layer of bone that provides an exterior shell over trabecular bone.

cofactor A mineral element that, like a coenzyme, works with an enzyme to facilitate a chemical reaction.

osteoporosis (OSS-tee-oh-pore-OH-sis) Also known as *adult bone loss*; a disease in which the bones become porous and fragile *(osteo* = bones; *poros* = porous).

8.2 Minerals for Healthy Bones

Bones are made up of a complex matrix of living tissue based on the protein collagen, into which the crystals of the bone minerals—principally calcium and phosphorus—are deposited. Bone tissue has two forms: **trabecular bone** and **cortical bone**. The thick, ivory-like outer portion of a bone is the cortical bone. Cortical bone provides a covering for the inner trabecular bone, which is a lacy network of calcium-containing crystals that are almost spongelike in appearance (see Figure 8-2). When calcium intakes are low, hormones and vitamin D call first upon the trabecular bone to release calcium into the blood for use by the rest of the body whenever levels fall

FIGURE 8-2

A Bone's Life

A. Bone is living tissue that continuously remodels itself. Bone contains cells embedded in a hard, mineralized matrix. The osteoblast cells make new bone; the osteoclast cells break down old or damaged bone.

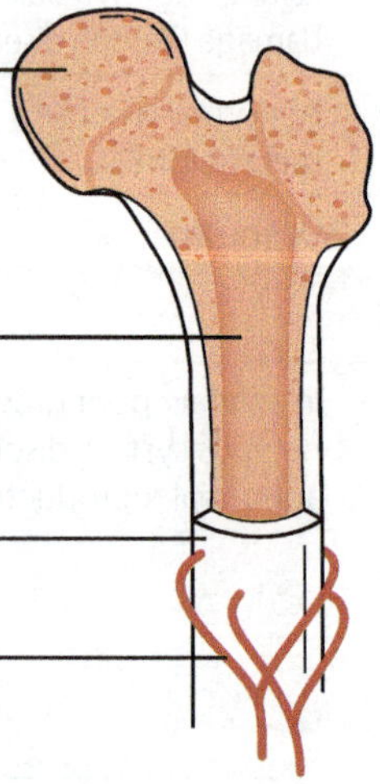

Cross section of bone. The lacy structural elements are trabeculae (tra-BECK-you-le), which can be drawn on to replenish blood calcium.

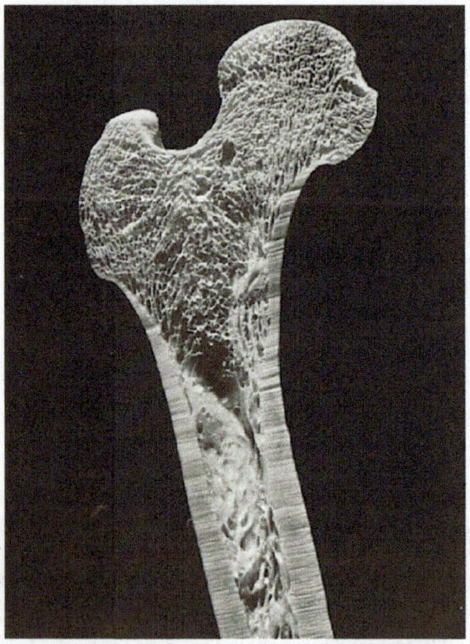

Courtesy of Gjon Mills

B. Peak bone mass occurs at approximately 30 years of age. Afterward, bone loss starts to outpace bone deposition; at menopause there is a surge of calcium out of the bones.

SOURCE: Adapted from The Stay Well Company, San Bruno, CA. © 1998.

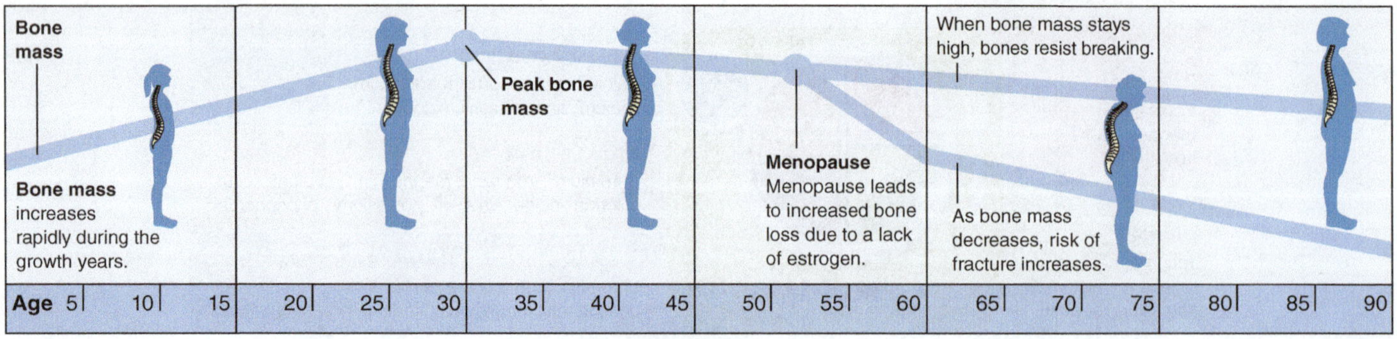

© Cengage

too low.* Over time, the lacy network of bones becomes less dense and more fragile as calcium deposits are withdrawn (see Figure 7-13 on page 198).

Although bones undergo remodeling throughout life—adding and losing bone minerals—the total amount of bone mass in the human body reaches a peak by about age 30.[2] Afterward, bones lose strength and density as bone minerals are lost. The principal determinant of bone health is *peak bone mass.* Think of bone mass as money in the bank: The larger the savings account, the easier it will be to withstand some loss of bone as one ages. To attain a healthful peak bone mass, it is necessary to have an optimal intake of calcium during the years of bone growth, all through the growing years and on into the years of young adulthood.

Besides calcium, several other vitamins and minerals are needed for the growth and maintenance of a healthy skeleton (see Table 8-2). As discussed in Chapter 7, vitamin D directs a large bone-making and bone-maintenance team composed of several nutrients and other compounds, including vitamin C and vitamin K; hormones; the protein collagen; and the minerals calcium, phosphorus, magnesium, and fluoride.

TABLE 8-2 Minerals for Healthy Bones

Minerals involved in bone mineralization and maintenance of teeth include:

- Calcium: the chief mineral of bones and teeth
- Phosphorus: combines with calcium in the hard crystals of bones and teeth
- Magnesium: a factor in bone mineralization; helps make teeth resistant to decay
- Fluoride: strengthens tooth enamel and helps make teeth resistant to decay

Calcium

Calcium is the most abundant mineral in the body. Ninety-nine percent of the body's calcium is found in the bones, which play two important roles. First, the bones support and protect the body's soft tissues. Second, they serve as a calcium bank, providing calcium to the body fluids whenever the supply runs low.

Although only a small part (about one percent) of the body's calcium is in its fluids, circulating calcium is vital to life. Calcium is required for the transmission of nerve impulses. It is essential for muscle contraction and thus helps maintain the heartbeat. It appears to be essential for the integrity of cell membranes and for the maintenance of normal blood pressure. Calcium must also be present if blood clotting is to occur, and it is a **cofactor** for several enzymes. Current research is investigating the role of calcium in the prevention of a number of chronic diseases. Some studies suggest that an adequate intake of calcium may provide a protective role in hypertension, heart disease, diabetes, colon cancer, and the maintenance of a healthy body weight, but more research is needed to fully explore these roles for calcium.[3]

Everyone knows that children need calcium daily to support the growth of their bones and teeth, but not everyone is aware of adults' needs for daily intakes of calcium. Abundant evidence now supports the importance of calcium for adults, especially women, who need about as much calcium in their later years as they did when they were adolescents.[4] A calcium deficit during the growing years and in adulthood contributes to gradual bone loss—**osteoporosis**, which can totally cripple a person in later life. This chapter's Spotlight feature describes the many factors that lead to osteoporosis.

Other nutrients are also important to bone growth and maintenance. Fluoride and vitamin D deficiencies, like calcium deficiencies, can cause loss of bone density. So can heredity, abnormal hormone levels, alcohol, prescription medications, other drugs, and lack of exercise (especially weight-bearing exercises)—but dietary calcium is one of the most important factors.

Table 8-3 shows that calcium appears almost exclusively in three classes of foods: milk and milk products; green vegetables such as broccoli, kale, bok choy, Brussels sprouts, green cabbage, mustard greens, collard greens, and turnip greens; and a few

TABLE 8-3 Calcium in Foods

(mg)[a]	Sources
452	Yogurt, plain, nonfat (8 oz)
451	Almond milk, calcium-fortified (1 c)
434[b]	Tofu, regular (calcium-set) (½ c)
380	Swiss cheese (1½ oz)
383	Fruit yogurt, low-fat (8 oz)
350	Orange juice, calcium-fortified (1 c)
340	Soymilk, calcium-fortified (1 c)
337	Ricotta cheese, part skim (½ c)
325	Sardines (with bones) (3 oz)
304	Mozzarella cheese (1½ oz)
300	Nonfat or Low-fat milk (1 c)
287	Cheddar cheese (1½ oz)
275	Shrimp (3 oz)
250	Turnip greens, cooked (1 c)
241	Salmon (with bones) (3 oz)
240	Pizza (1 slice)
>200	Cereal and snack bars, calcium-fortified (1 c or 1 bar)
193	American cheese (1 oz)
196	Waffle, whole-grain (1)
186	Cream soup (1 c)
180	Kale, cooked (1 c)
160	Bok choy (1 c)
150	Pudding, chocolate (½ c)
134	Collard greens, cooked (½ c)
117	Frozen yogurt (½ c)
111	Almond butter (2 tbsp)
110	Parmesan cheese (2 tbsp)
109	Instant oatmeal (1 packet)
103	Cottage cheese (½ c)
100	Almonds (⅓ c)
92	Ice cream (½ c)
80	Kidney beans, cooked (½ c)
60	Broccoli (1 c)

[a] DRI, ADULT: 1,000 mg/day; > 50 years (women): 1,200 mg/day; > 70 years: 1,200 mg/day.
[b] The calcium content of tofu varies depending on processing methods. Look for tofu processed with calcium sulfate.

*As mentioned in Chapter 7, vitamin D and parathyroid hormone circulate in the blood whenever the calcium concentration in the blood falls too low. These hormones cause the release of calcium from the bones and decreased excretion of calcium by the kidneys. Vitamin D also acts to increase absorption of dietary calcium by the intestines. The hormone calcitonin is released from the thyroid gland when levels of blood calcium get too high; it acts to stop the release of calcium from bone and to slow intestinal absorption of the mineral.

FIGURE 8-3

Calcium Recommendations*

* In general, 1 cup milk or yogurt, 1½ ounces natural cheese, or 2 ounces processed cheese can be considered as 1 cup from the milk group. Equivalent choices include nondairy beverages or foods such as calcium-fortified juices that provide a similar amount of calcium as found in 1 cup milk.

†The USDA MyPlate food guide sets a minimum of 3 cups milk each day for a 2,000-calorie diet and 2 cups per day for children under 4 years of age.

Age (years)	Calcium needed (mg) per day
1–3	700
4–8	1,000
9–18	1,300
19–50 51–70 (men)	1,000
51+ (women) > 70	1,200

Cups of milk or milk products per day (or the equivalent)†

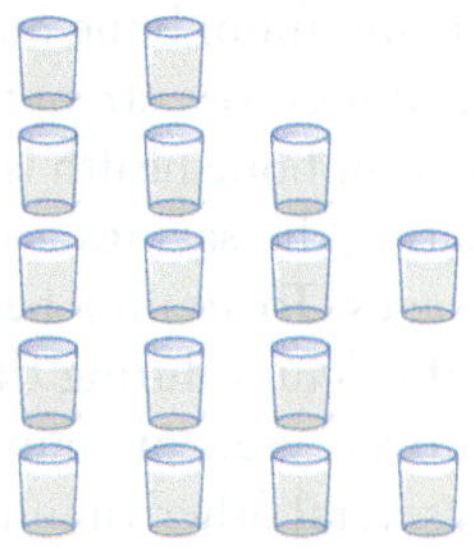

© Cengage

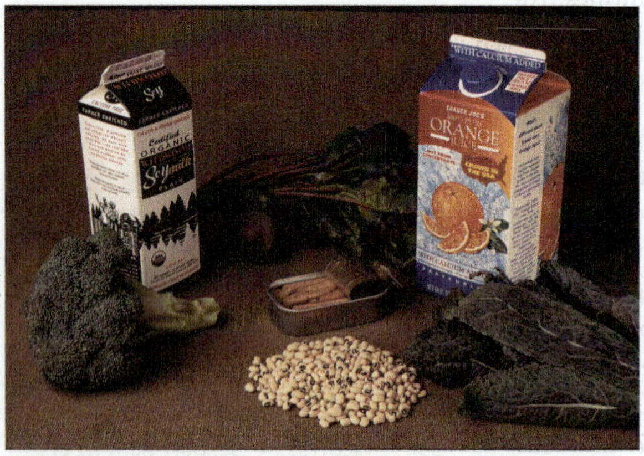

Felicia Martinez Photography/PhotoEdit

A number of foods are available as acceptable substitutes for regular milk, including calcium-fortified juices and soy products (soy milk, yogurt, calcium-set tofu). Small fish, such as sardines or canned salmon; dark-green vegetables such as kale, bok choy, and broccoli; and legumes such as black-eyed peas are also rich in calcium.

fish and shellfish. Milk and milk products typically contain the most calcium per serving. Many greens are also good choices, but a complication enters in—absorption. Calcium is not well absorbed from certain green vegetables (notably, spinach and Swiss chard), whereas calcium is better absorbed from milk and calcium-fortified foods and beverages. Milk contains both vitamin D and lactose, both of which enhance calcium absorption and promote bone health. Milk and milk products also normally supply about 40 percent of people's intake of riboflavin. Figure 8-3 shows the Dietary Reference Intakes (DRI) committee's current recommendations for calcium intakes.

Some food components interfere with calcium absorption. Phytate is one example; it occurs in some fruits, vegetables, and whole grains, as well as in nonherbal tea. Oxalate is found in beet greens, rhubarb, and spinach, among other foods. These **binders** seem to depress absorption of the calcium present in the *same* food as the binder but do not depress the absorption of calcium from other foods consumed at the same time. This fact doesn't detract from the overall value of high-fiber foods, which are important and nutritious for many reasons.

binders In foods, compounds that can combine with nutrients to form complexes the body cannot absorb. For example, *phytates* (FYE-tates) in whole grains and *oxalates* (in vegetables) may bind iron and calcium and interfere with their absorption to a minor extent.

Alternative Sources of Calcium

Milk need not be your only source of calcium (see Figure 8-4). Yogurt is an acceptable substitute for regular milk, and puddings, custards, and baked goods can be prepared in such a way that they also contain appreciable amounts of calcium. Fat-free powdered milk, which is an excellent and inexpensive source of protein, calcium, and other nutrients, can be added to many foods (such as cookies, soups, casseroles, and meatloaf) during preparation. Milk or yogurt fortified with extra calcium are other excellent calcium sources. Also, small fish, such as Atlantic sardines or canned pink salmon with soft edible bones, are similar to milk and milk products in calcium richness.

A number of calcium-fortified foods are available, including calcium-fortified juices, mineral water, soymilk, breads, cereals, snack bars, and hot cocoa mixes. Many times, these foods are fortified to match or exceed the amount of calcium in a cup of milk. For example, an 8-ounce serving of fortified orange juice provides about 350 milligrams of calcium. Remember to check the Nutrition Facts panel on food labels for the amount of calcium contained in the foods you eat.

The word *daily* must be stressed with respect to calcium intake. Because of the body's limited ability to absorb calcium, it cannot handle massive doses periodically; it needs frequent opportunities to take in small amounts.

Phosphorus

Phosphorus is second to calcium in mineral abundance in the body. About 85 percent of it is found combined with calcium in the crystals of the

FIGURE 8-4

Sources of Calcium

Adult DRI (RDA): Men: 19 to 70 years, 1,000 mg; 70 years and older, 1,200 mg
Women: 19 to 50 years, 1,000 mg; 51 years and older, 1,200 mg

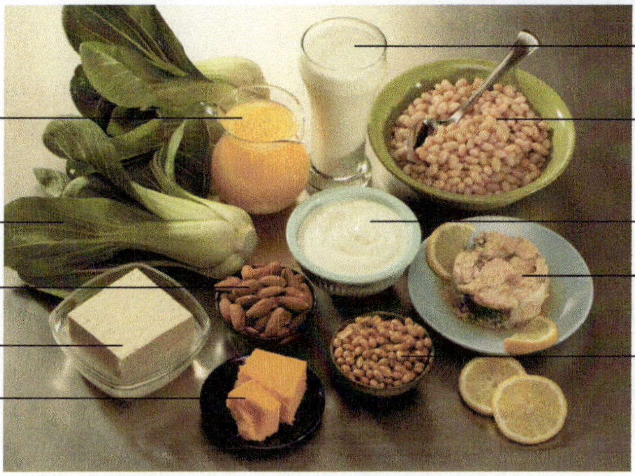

© Matthew Farruggio Photography

bones and teeth as calcium phosphate, the chief compound that gives them strength and rigidity. Phosphorus is also a part of DNA and RNA, the genetic code material present in every cell. Phosphorus is thus necessary for all growth, because DNA and RNA provide the instructions for new cells to be formed.

Phosphorus plays many key roles in the cells' use of energy nutrients. Many enzymes and the B vitamins become active only when a phosphate group is attached. Phosphorus is critical in energy exchange and in maintaining fluid balance in the body.

Some lipids (phospholipids) contain phosphorus as part of their structure. They help transport other lipids in the blood; they also form part of the structure of cell membranes, where they affect the transport of nutrients and wastes into and out of the cells.

Animal protein is the best source of phosphorus, because phosphorus is so abundant in the energetic cells of animals. People who eat large amounts of animal protein have high phosphorus intakes. People who regularly consume carbonated beverages also have higher phosphorus intakes, because those drinks contain phosphoric acid. When soft drinks replace milk in the diet, bone density is limited and fracture risks increase, especially for girls and women due to a lower calcium intake.[5]

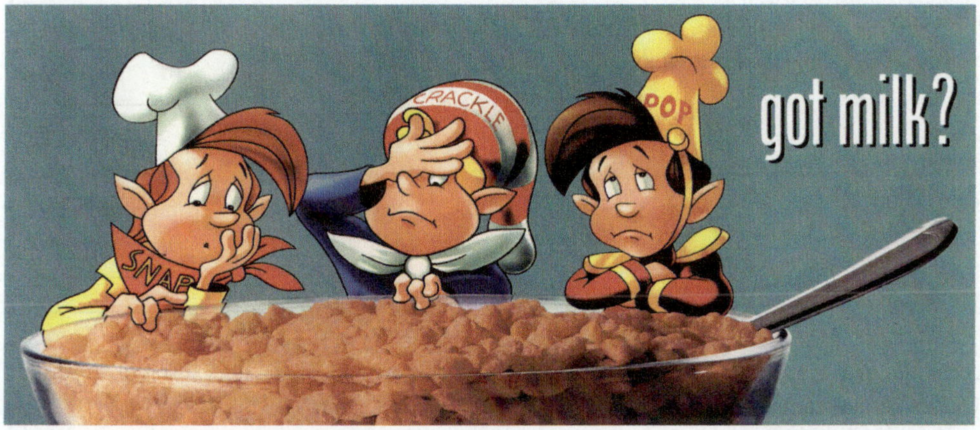

Advertising Archives

Got milk? If not, be sure to consume the recommended amount of calcium—the amount found in three to four glasses of milk—from the many alternate sources of calcium available on the market today (see Table 8-3).

SCORE Card Calcium Sources (Obj. 8.2)

Adults need between 1,000 and 1,200 milligrams of calcium daily—the amount found in 3 to 4 cups of milk or the equivalent. To estimate your calcium intake, answer these questions by considering what you ate yesterday.

1. Did you eat plain yogurt (low-fat or fat-free)? Give yourself *4 points* for each 1-cup serving. ________

2. Did you eat or drink any of these items? If so, give yourself *3 points* for each serving.

- Calcium-fortified juice, 1 cup ________
- Calcium-fortified soy or rice beverage, 1 cup ________
- Firm cheese (cheddar, Swiss, mozzarella), 1½ ounces ________
- Fruit-flavored or blended regular or Greek-style low-fat yogurt, 1 cup ________
- Milk (non-fat, 1%, 2%, whole, chocolate), 1 cup ________
- Nonfat milk powder, ⅓ cup ________
- Ricotta cheese, part skim, ½ cup ________
- Yogurt beverage or yogurt smoothie, 1 cup ________

3. Did you eat or drink any of these items? If so, give yourself 2.5 points for each serving.

- Calcium-fortified cereal (1 cup) with ½ cup of milk ________
- Canned fish with soft bones (salmon, mackerel), 4 ounces ________
- Lattes or mochas, made with milk, 12 ounces (1½ cup) ________
- Milkshake, any flavor, 8 ounces (1 cup) ________
- Sardines, 3 ounces (½ can) ________

4. Did you eat any of these items? If so, give yourself 1.5 points for each serving.

- Baked beans, white beans, soybeans, 1 cup ________
- Bok choy Chinese cabbage, cooked, 1 cup ________
- Cereal (1 cup) with ½ cup milk ________
- Collard greens, kale, spinach, ½ cup, cooked ________
- Custard, flan, pudding made with milk, ½ cup ________
- Processed cheese, string cheese, 1 ounce ________
- Soft cheeses (feta, Brie, Camembert), 1½ ounces ________
- Soup made with milk, 1 cup ________
- Tofu processed with calcium, 3 ounces ________

5. Did you eat any of these items? If so, give yourself 1 point for each serving.

- Cottage cheese, 1% or 2%, ¾ cup ________
- Ice cream, ice milk, or frozen yogurt, ½ cup ________

6. Did you eat any of these items? If so, give yourself ½ point for each serving.

- Almonds, ¼ cup ________
- Broccoli or kale, 1 cup ________
- Hummus, ½ cup ________
- Kidney beans, black beans, lima beans, 1 cup ________
- Orange, 1 ________
- Parmesan cheese, 1 tablespoon ________
- Soy nuts, ¼ cup ________

Now add up all your points. *Total Points:* ____________________ Multiply your total points × 100: __________ This gives you an idea of how many milligrams of calcium you are getting each day.

SOURCE: Adapted from Dairy Council of California, Online Calcium Quiz, 2009, available at www.dairycouncilofca.org/Tools/CalciumQuiz/Default.aspx.

FIGURE 8-5

Sources of Phosphorus

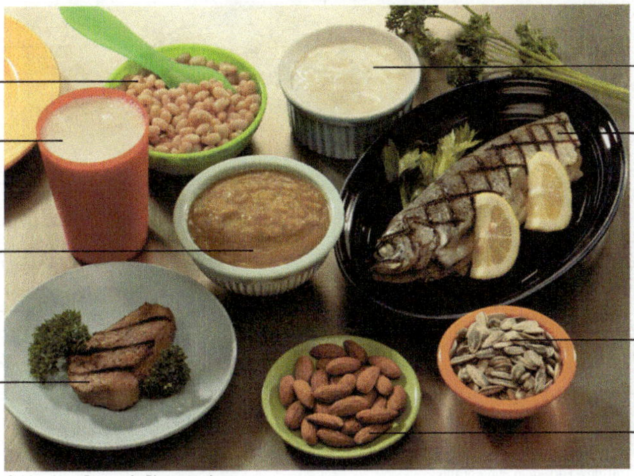

The recommended intake of phosphorus is lower than that for calcium. It is believed to provide sufficient phosphorus to ensure adequate absorption and retention of calcium. Higher intakes of phosphorus may interfere with calcium absorption. The good news is that people do not need to make a special effort to eat foods containing phosphorus, because it is present in virtually all foods (see Figure 8-5 and Table 8-4).

Magnesium In addition to maintaining bone health, magnesium helps relax muscles after contraction and promotes resistance to tooth decay by helping to hold calcium in tooth enamel. Bone magnesium seems to be a reservoir to ensure that some of this mineral will be on hand for vital reactions regardless of recent dietary intake. Magnesium also acts in all the cells of the muscles, heart, liver, and other soft tissues, where it forms part of the protein-making machinery and is necessary for the release of energy. Areas of the country that have hard water—higher in magnesium and calcium—have lower rates of death from cardiovascular disease. A deficiency of magnesium may be related to sudden death from heart failure and to high blood pressure.[6] Average dietary intakes fall below current recommendations. A dietary deficiency may also occur as a result of vomiting, diarrhea, alcohol abuse, or protein malnutrition. Good food sources of magnesium include nuts, seeds, legumes, cereal grains, dark-green vegetables, seafoods, chocolate, and cocoa (see Table 8-5 and Figure 8-6).

TABLE 8-4 Phosphorus in Foods

(mg)*	Sources
422	American cheese (2 oz)
341	Cottage cheese (1 c)
325	Yogurt (1 c)
280	Salmon (canned) (3 oz)
242	Pork (3 oz)
235	Fat-free milk (1 c)
200	Sirloin steak (3 oz)
189	Sunflower seeds (2 tbsp)
186	Turkey (3 oz)
174	Peanuts (⅓ c)
161	Hamburger (3 oz)
149	Shredded wheat (1 c)
143	Navy beans (½ c)
139	Tuna (3 oz)
115	Potato (1)
104	Peanut butter (2 tbsp)
67	Corn (½ c)
51	Cola (12 oz)
46	Broccoli (½ c)
46	Wheat bread (1 slice)
45	Diet cola (12 oz)

* DRI, adult: 700 mg/day.

TABLE 8-5 Magnesium in Foods

(mg)*	Sources
100	Raisin bran (1 c)
97	Almonds (¼ c)
89	Cashews (¼ c)
78	Spinach, cooked (½ c)
64	Peanuts (¼ c)
63	Lima beans (½ c)
60	Black beans (½ c)
51	Tofu (3 oz)
47	Yogurt, plain (1 c)
43	Black-eyed peas (½ c)
43	Brown rice, cooked (½ c)
40	Soy milk (1 c)
37	Oysters (steamed) (3 oz)
33	Avocado (½ c)
28	Fat-free milk (1 c)
27	Chicken (3 oz)
25	Baked potato (1)
21	Sunflower seeds (2 tbsp)
21	Hamburger (3 oz)
21	Milk chocolate (1 oz)

* DRI, adult: men (19–30 years), 400 mg/day; men (> 31 years), 420 mg/day; women (19–30 years), 310 mg/day; women (> 31 years), 320 mg/day.

FIGURE 8-6

Sources of Magnesium

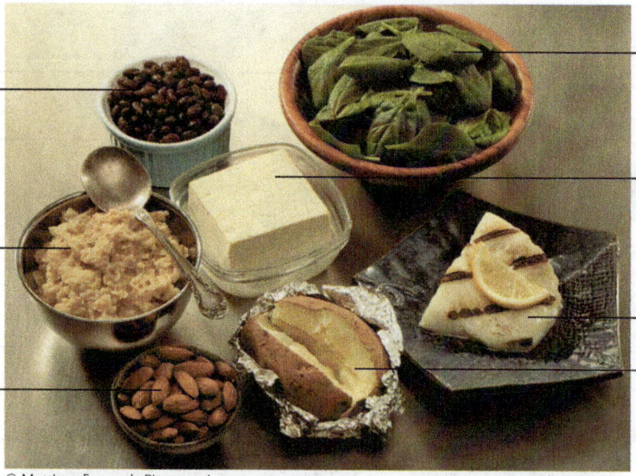

© Matthew Farruggio Photography

Fluoride Only a trace of fluoride occurs in the human body, but studies have demonstrated that the crystalline deposits in the bones and teeth of people who live where diets are high in fluoride are larger and more perfectly formed than in people who live where diets are low in fluoride. The trace mineral fluoride not only protects children's teeth from decay but also makes the bones of older people resistant to adult bone loss (osteoporosis). Thus, its continuous presence in body fluids is desirable.

Drinking water is the usual source of fluoride. Where fluoride is lacking in the water supply, the incidence of dental decay is very high. Fluoridation of community water, where needed to raise its fluoride concentration to one part per million (ppm), is thus an important public health measure (see Figure 8-7).

In some communities, the natural fluoride concentration in water is high (2 to 8 ppm), and children's teeth develop with mottled enamel—a condition called **fluorosis**. True toxicity from fluoride overdoses can occur, but usually only after years of chronic daily intakes of 20 to 80 times the amounts normally consumed from fluoridated water.

FIGURE 8-7

Current U.S. Population with Access to Community Water Fluoridation

Alternatives to water fluoridation:

- Fluoride toothpastes
- Fluoride treatments for teeth
- Fluoride tablets and drops

SOURCE: Centers for Disease Control and Prevention

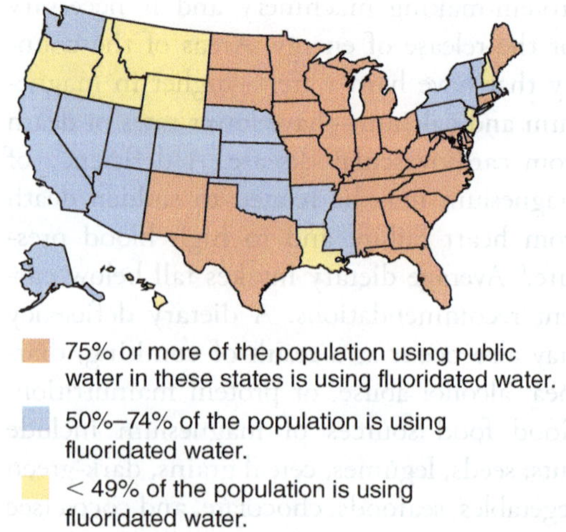

fluorosis (floor-OH-sis) Discoloration of the teeth from ingestion of too much fluoride during tooth development.

8.3 Minerals for Healthy Blood

All body cells require a continuous supply of water, oxygen, energy, and building materials. As the blood circulates through the body, it picks up and delivers materials as needed. The blood transports oxygen and nutrients to the cells and carries cellular wastes away from them. Along with the vitamins discussed in Chapter 7, three of the trace minerals serve blood-related functions in the body (see Table 8-6). Iron, zinc, and copper are associated with **hemoglobin**, the compound that carries oxygen in the blood.

TABLE 8-6 Minerals for Healthy Blood

- **Iron**: hemoglobin, the iron-containing protein in red blood cells, carries oxygen from the lungs to body tissues; iron in myoglobin holds oxygen for muscle use.
- **Zinc**: needed to make hemoglobin
- **Copper**: needed to make hemoglobin

Iron

Every living cell contains iron. Bound into the protein hemoglobin in the red blood cells, it helps transport oxygen from lungs to tissues and thus permits the release of energy from fuels to do the cells' work. Iron is also part of the protein **myoglobin** in muscles, which makes oxygen available for the work of muscles. When the iron supply is too low, **iron-deficiency anemia** occurs, characterized by weakness, tiredness, apathy, headaches, increased sensitivity to cold, and a paleness that reflects the reduction in the number and size of the red blood cells. A person with this **anemia** can do very little muscular work without disabling fatigue, but can replenish iron status by eating iron-rich foods (see Table 8-7 and Figure 8-8).

Iron deficiency is the most common and widespread nutritional disorder in the world and the most common cause of anemia.[7] People begin to feel the impact of iron deficiency, without knowing it, long before anemia is diagnosed. They don't appear to have an obvious deficiency disease; they just appear unmotivated and apathetic. Because they work and play less, they are less physically fit. In the United States, iron deficiency remains relatively prevalent among toddlers, adolescent girls, and women of childbearing age.[8]

The cause of iron deficiency is usually malnutrition—that is, inadequate intake, either from limited access to food or from high consumption of foods low in iron. Among causes other than malnutrition, blood loss is the primary one, caused in many countries by parasitic infections of the digestive tract.

The typical Western mixed diet provides only about 5 to 6 milligrams of iron in every 1,000 calories. The recommended daily intake for an adult man is 8 milligrams. Because most men easily eat more than 2,000 calories, they can meet their iron needs without special effort.

The situation for women is different. Women may have normal blood cell counts or hemoglobin levels and yet may need more iron because their body stores are depleted, a factor that doesn't show up in standard tests. Because most women typically eat less food than men, their iron intakes are lower. Also, because women menstruate, their iron losses are greater. These two factors may put women much closer to the borderline of deficiency.

The recommended intake for a woman before menopause is 18 milligrams per day; women age 51 and older need 8 milligrams; pregnant women need 30 milligrams daily. Because women typically consume fewer than 2,000 calories per day, many women understandably have trouble achieving adequate iron intakes. Before menopause, a woman who wants to meet her iron needs from foods must increase the iron-to-calorie ratio of her diet so that she will receive about double the average amount of iron: about 10 milligrams per 1,000 calories. This means she must emphasize iron-rich foods in her daily diet.

Table 8-7 shows the amounts of iron in foods. Meats, fish, and poultry are superior sources on a per serving basis. People must select foods carefully to obtain enough iron, because it is present in such small quantities in most foods. The best meat sources are liver, red meats, poultry, fish, oysters, and clams. Among the grains, whole grains and enriched and fortified breads and cereals are best, and dried beans are

TABLE 8-7 Iron in Foods

(mg)*	Sources
23.80	Clams, steamed (3 oz)
8.00	Enriched cereal (1 c)
6.00	Instant Cream of Wheat (½ c)
4.79	Oatmeal, cooked (1 packet)
3.30	Lentils (½ c)
3.20	Spinach, cooked (½ c)
3.13	Beef pot roast (3 oz)
3.00	Prune juice (1 c)
2.56	Sirloin steak (3 oz)
2.48	Sardines (3 oz)
2.30	Hamburger (3 oz)
2.18	Baked potato (1)
2.15	Navy beans (½ c)
1.80	Black beans (½ c)
1.44	Veggie burger (1)
1.40	Whole-wheat bread (1 slice)
1.40	Tofu (3 oz)
1.07	Shrimp (3 oz)
1.07	Raisins (¼ c)
1.04	Broccoli, cooked (1 c)
0.92	Tuna, light (3 oz)
0.87	Apricot halves, dried (¼ c)
0.85	Pomegranate (1)

* DRI, adult: men, 8 mg/day; women (19–50 years), 18 mg/day; women (> 50 years), 8 mg/day.

hemoglobin (HEEM-uh-glow-bin) The oxygen-carrying protein of the blood; found in the red blood cells.

myoglobin The heme-containing protein in muscles that carries and holds oxygen for use by muscles.

iron-deficiency anemia A reduction of the number and size of red blood cells and a loss of their color because of iron deficiency.

anemia Any condition in which the blood is unable to deliver oxygen to the cells of the body. Examples include a shortage or abnormality of the red blood cells. Many nutrient deficiencies and diseases can cause anemia.

FIGURE 8-8

Sources of Iron

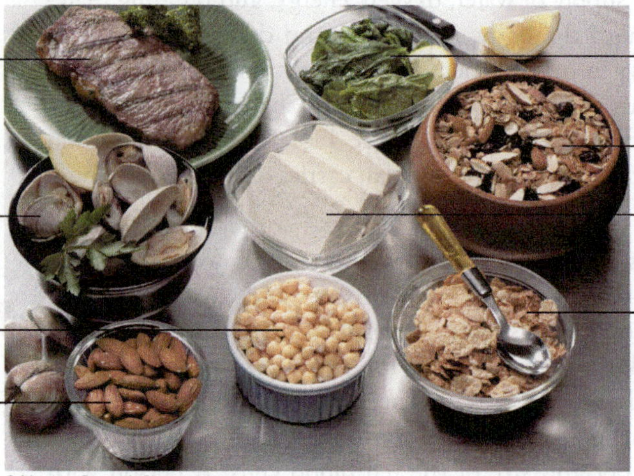

© Matthew Farruggio Photography

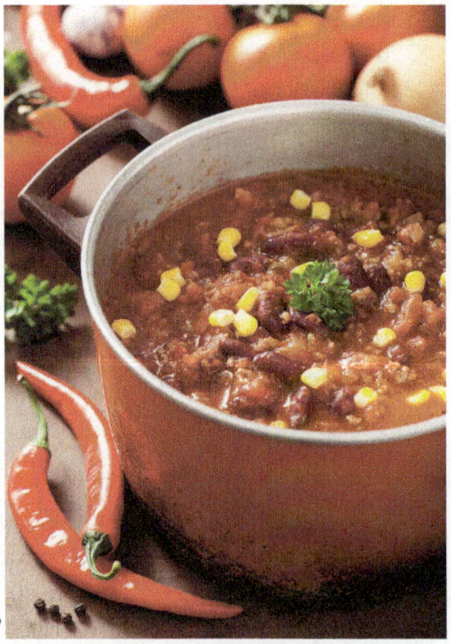

Olga Miltsova/Shutterstock.com

You can combine foods to achieve maximum iron absorption—the heme iron in the meat and the vitamin C in the tomatoes in this chili help you absorb the nonheme iron from the beans.

heme (HEEM) iron The iron-holding part of the hemoglobin protein, found in meat, fish, and poultry. About 40 percent of the iron in meat, fish, and poultry is bound into heme. Meat, fish, and poultry also contain a factor (MFP factor) other than heme that promotes the absorption of iron, even of the iron from other foods eaten at the same time as the meat.

nonheme iron The iron found in plant foods.

iron overload A condition in which the body contains more iron than it needs or can handle; excess iron is toxic and can damage the liver. The most common cause of iron overload is the genetic disorder hemochromatosis.

a good source. Some fruits and vegetables contain appreciable amounts of iron, as shown in the table. Foods in the milk group are notoriously poor iron sources.

Ways to Enhance Iron Absorption

Iron occurs in two forms in foods: as **heme iron**, bound into the iron-carrying proteins such as hemoglobin in meats, poultry, and fish; and as **nonheme iron**, in both plant and animal foods. Heme iron is much more reliably absorbed than is nonheme iron. Absorption of nonheme iron is affected by many factors, including the amount of vitamin C consumed with meals.[9] Vitamin C promotes iron absorption and can triple the amount of nonheme iron absorbed from foods eaten at the same meal.

Consumers who cook their foods in iron cookware thereby contribute to their iron intake.[10] For example, the iron content of a half-cup of spaghetti sauce simmered in a glass dish is 3 milligrams, but it is 87 milligrams when the sauce is cooked in an iron skillet. Similarly, dried apricots and raisins contain more iron than the fresh fruit because they are dried in iron pans. Admittedly, this form of iron is not as well absorbed as the iron from meat, but every little bit helps.

As mentioned earlier, some foods contain binders that combine chemically with iron and other minerals, such as calcium and zinc, thus preventing absorption of those substances and carrying them out of the body with other wastes. For example, *phytates* render the iron, calcium, zinc, and magnesium in certain foods less available than they might otherwise be; *oxalate* binds iron and calcium. Phytate is found in oatmeal and other whole grains. Other binders are the tannins, which occur in black teas, coffee, cola drinks, chocolate, and red wines. Fiber also can reduce iron absorption because it speeds up the transit of materials through the intestines.

Iron Toxicity

Large amounts of iron can be toxic to the body.[11] **Iron overload** is a condition in which the body absorbs excessive amounts of iron. As a result, tissue damage occurs, especially in organs such as the liver that store iron. Infections are more likely to occur with iron overload, because bacteria thrive on iron-rich blood. This condition is more common in men than in women.

Although iron is an important essential nutrient in the body, it can also act as a powerful oxidizing agent in reactions that produce free radicals in the body. Therefore, avoid taking extra supplemental iron unless you have been diagnosed as deficient.

Be sure to keep iron supplements out of the reach of children, too—they can fatally overdose on such tablets.

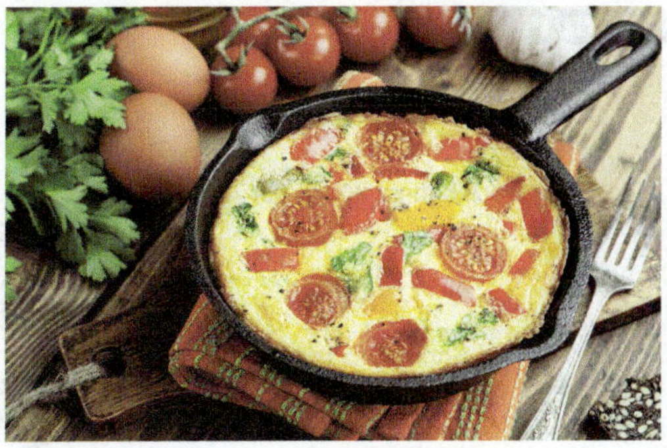

minadezhda/Shutterstock.com

Iron cookware adds supplemental iron to foods.

Zinc Zinc is found in every cell of the body and plays a major role along with more than 50 enzymes that regulate cell multiplication and growth; normal metabolism of protein, carbohydrate, fat, and alcohol; and disposal of damaging free radicals. Zinc is associated with the hormone insulin, which regulates the body's fuel supply. It is involved in the formation of proteins, including hemoglobin, utilization of vitamin A, taste perception, thyroid function, wound healing, the synthesis of sperm, and the development of sexual organs and bone.

Zinc is also known for its role in promoting a healthy immune system.[12] A flurry of zinc lozenges has appeared on the market following the results of a study seeking an antidote for the common cold.[13] People who used zinc gluconate lozenges every 2 hours, starting within 24 hours of the onset of a cold, reduced the length of their colds by three days. However, other studies have not reported similar results, and whether zinc lozenges are any more effective than placebos remains to be determined. Furthermore, the long-term effects of such supplemental use of zinc are unknown.

Zinc deficiencies were first reported in the 1960s in the Middle East, where studies on adolescent boys revealed severe growth retardation and delayed sexual maturation—symptoms responsive to zinc supplementation (see Figure 8-9). The native diets were typically low in animal protein and zinc, but they were high in fiber and other compounds that bind minerals. The researchers learned that the binders were carrying zinc out of the boys' bodies, thus causing the deficiency.

Zinc deficiency can cause night blindness, hair loss, poor appetite, susceptibility to infection, delayed healings of cuts or abrasions, decreased taste and smell sensitivity, and poor growth in children.[14] Because zinc is lost from the body daily in much the same way as protein is, it must be replenished daily.

The highest zinc needs are those for people who are building new tissue: infants, children, teenagers, and pregnant women. A pregnant teenager is at particular risk because she needs zinc for her own growth as well as her fetus's growth. Pregnant vegetarians are at risk, too, because their diets are high in fiber and zinc-binding factors. Dieters also need to be reminded that very low-calorie diets cause not only low zinc intake but also a loss of zinc from body tissues as they break down to release fuel.

Zinc is a relatively nontoxic element. However, it can be toxic if consumed in large enough quantities. Consumption of high levels of zinc can cause a host of symptoms, including vomiting, diarrhea, fever, and exhaustion.[15] The hazards of overconsumption are greatest when consumers dose themselves with supplements. Excess supplemental zinc can cause imbalances of both copper and iron in the body. Chronic consumption of zinc exceeding 15 milligrams per day is not recommended without close medical supervision.

Table 8-8 shows the zinc amounts in foods. An average 1,500-calorie diet provides

TABLE 8-8 Zinc in Foods

(mg)*	Sources
31.00	Oysters, cooked (3 oz)
5.90	Beef pot roast (3 oz)
5.80	Ground beef (3 oz)
4.70	Crabmeat (3 oz)
4.40	Sirloin steak (3 oz)
4.00	Soybeans, dry-roasted (½ c)
3.10	Enriched cereal (1 c)
2.40	Yogurt (1 c)
1.48	Turkey (3 oz)
1.40	Shrimp (3 oz)
1.24	Swiss cheese (1 oz)
1.21	Peanuts (¼ c)
1.00	Black beans (½ c)
1.00	Tofu (4 oz)
1.00	Fat-free milk (1 c)
0.87	Cheddar cheese (1 oz)
0.85	Black-eyed peas (½ c)
0.79	Kidney beans (½ c)
0.73	Baked potato (1)
0.69	Whole-wheat bread (1 slice)
0.68	Spinach, cooked (½ c)

* DRI, adult: men, 11mg/day; women, 8 mg/day.

© Cengage

FIGURE 8-9

Zinc Deficiency

The Egyptian boy in this picture is 17 years old but is only 4 feet tall, the height of an average 7-year-old in the United States. His genitalia are like those of a 6-year-old. The retardation, known as dwarfism, is rightly ascribed to zinc deficiency because it is partially reversible when zinc is restored to the diet.

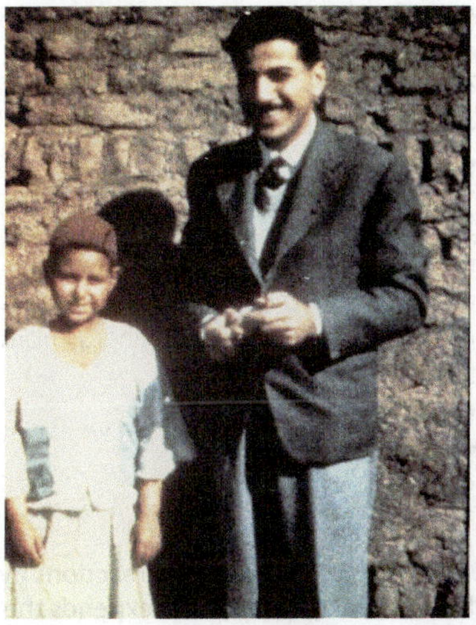

Harold Sanstead

FIGURE 8-10

Sources of Zinc

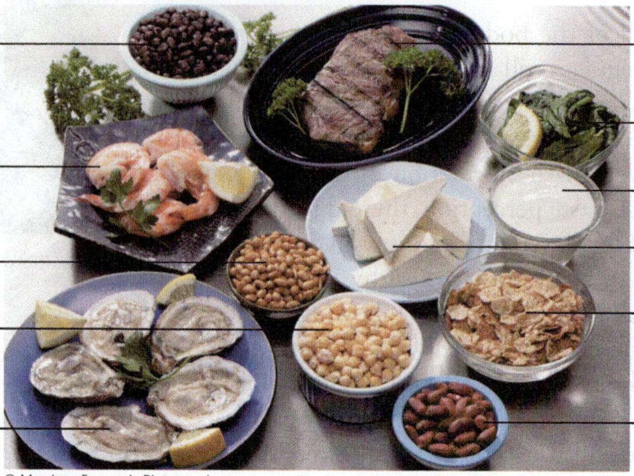

about 6.3 milligrams of zinc per day, or about 60 to 80 percent of the recommended intake. Zinc is highest in foods of high protein content, such as shellfish (especially oysters), meats, and liver (see Figure 8-10). As a rule of thumb, two servings a day of animal protein will provide most of the zinc a healthy person needs. Whole-grain products are good sources of zinc if large quantities are eaten (the phytate in grains does not inhibit the absorption of zinc in people consuming ordinary diets). Cow's milk protein (casein) binds zinc avidly and seems to prevent its absorption somewhat; infants absorb zinc better from human breast milk. Fresh and canned vegetables vary in zinc content, depending on the soil in which they are grown. The zinc content of cooking water varies from region to region as well.

Copper Copper is a trace mineral and a component of several enzymes with important roles in a variety of metabolic and physiological processes. For example, copper is involved in making hemoglobin, manufacturing collagen, healing wounds, and maintaining the sheaths around nerve fibers. Good food sources of copper include whole grains, nuts, seeds, legumes, and shellfish.

TABLE 8-9 **Minerals for Energy Metabolism**

Some minerals assist enzymes and vitamins needed for the release and use of energy from the energy nutrients: • Phosphorus • Magnesium • Iron • Zinc • Copper • Chromium • Sulfur
Some minerals are essential for normal metabolic rate, which regulates energy metabolism—the reactions by which the body obtains and uses energy from foods: • Iodine • Zinc • Selenium

8.4 Minerals and Energy Metabolism

As described in Chapter 3, the carbohydrate glycogen can be broken down in the body to glucose, triglycerides to fatty acids and glycerol, and protein to amino acids. When the body needs energy, it breaks any or all of the four basic units—glucose, fatty acids, glycerol, and amino acids—into even smaller units. When the body does not require energy, the end products of digestion (glucose, amino acids, glycerol, and fatty acids) are used to build body compounds such as glycogen, body proteins, or body fat. Along with several vitamins (discussed in the previous chapter), several minerals are essential for **energy metabolism**, as described in the following sections (see Table 8-9).

energy metabolism All the reactions by which the body obtains and expends the energy from food.

Chromium *Chromium* is a trace mineral involved in carbohydrate and lipid metabolism. Chromium works closely with the hormone insulin by enhancing its ability to help the cells take up glucose and break it down for energy.[16] Chromium is found in a wide variety of unrefined foods. Good sources include nuts, mushrooms, asparagus, prunes, meats (especially liver), brewer's yeast, dark chocolate, and whole grains.

FIGURE 8-11

Goiter

In iodine deficiency, the thyroid gland enlarges—a condition known as goiter.

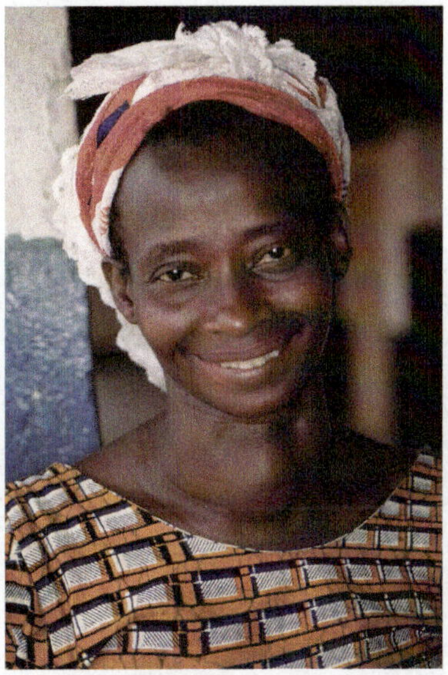

Scott Camazine/Science Source

Sulfur

Sulfur is a major mineral and a component of the hormone insulin. It is also a part of the B vitamins—thiamin and biotin—which have important roles in helping enzymes convert nutrients into energy for the body's use. Sulfur is present in some amino acids and in all dietary proteins. It helps strands of protein assume and hold a particular shape, thus enabling them to do their specific jobs, such as enzyme work. Skin, hair, and nails contain some of the body's more rigid proteins, and they have a high sulfur content. There is no recommended intake for sulfur, and no deficiencies are known. Only a person who lacks dietary protein to the point of severe protein deficiency will lack the sulfur-containing amino acids.

Iodine

Iodine is a trace mineral that occurs in the body in an infinitesimal quantity, but its principal role in human nutrition is well known. It is an integral part of the thyroid hormones, which regulate body temperature, metabolic rate, reproduction, and growth. The hormones enter every cell of the body to control the rate at which the cells use oxygen and release energy.

When the iodine level of the blood is low, the thyroid gland may enlarge in an attempt to trap more iodine, until it causes swelling in the throat area—a condition called **goiter** (see Figure 8-11). Goiter is estimated to affect about 200 million people worldwide.

In addition to causing sluggishness and weight gain, an iodine deficiency can have serious effects on fetal development. Severe thyroid undersecretion by a woman during pregnancy causes extreme and irreversible mental impairment and growth retardation of the child; this condition is known as **cretinism**. A person with cretinism has a face and body with many abnormalities. Much of the mental impairment associated with cretinism can be averted by early diagnosis and treatment of the mother's iodine deficiency.

The amount of iodine in foods reflects the amount present in the soil in which plants are grown or on which animals graze. Soil iodine is greatest along the coastal regions. In the inland areas of the United States, where the soil is low in iodine, widespread goiter appeared in the local inhabitants during the 1930s. Iodized salt was introduced as a preventive measure, and iodine deficiency disappeared.

The average American dietary iodine intake is above the recommended intake, but falls below toxic levels. Excessive intakes of iodine can cause an enlargement of the thyroid gland resembling a goiter; in infants, the enlargement can be so severe as to block the airways and cause suffocation. Some of the excess iodine may come from salted fast foods, bakery products, and from milk. Iodates (iodine salts) are used as dough conditioners in the baking industry; and many dairy producers give cows iodized grain, and use iodine-containing antiseptics during the milk treatment process. Today, the baking and dairy industries have reduced their use of iodine-containing compounds, and there is an increasing use of noniodized salt in manufactured foods.[17]

People sometimes ask if they should be sure to buy *iodized* salt in the grocery store to ensure adequate iodine intake. Although most consumers now have access to fruits and vegetables grown in coastal areas rich in iodine, health experts state the importance of using iodized salt to maintain an adequate iodine intake. Check the label, because only "iodized salt" has iodine added. Less than a half-teaspoon of iodized salt

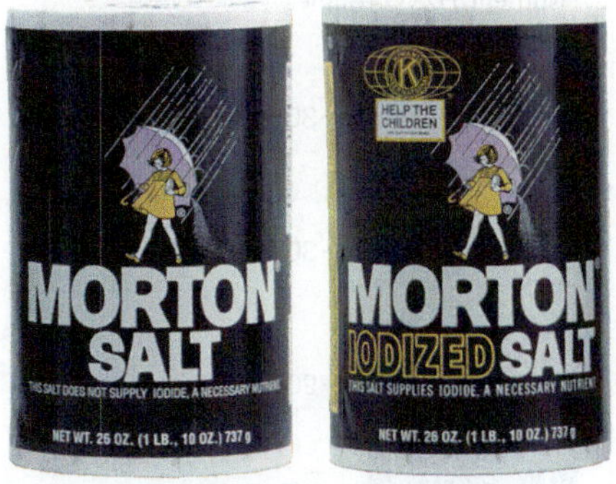

© Craig M. Moore

Only the *iodized* salt contains iodine.

goiter (GOY-tur) Enlargement of the thyroid gland caused by iodine deficiency.

cretinism (CREE-tin-izm) Severe mental and physical retardation of an infant caused by iodine deficiency during pregnancy.

TABLE 8-10 Antioxidant Nutrients
• Vitamin C
• Vitamin E
• Beta-carotene/other carotenoids
• Selenium

© Cengage

meets the entire adult RDA for iodine. However, seafood, bread, dairy products, and fruits and vegetables grown in iodine-rich soil can also provide significant amounts of iodine to the diet.

Selenium *Selenium* is a trace mineral found in the soil in varying amounts. Like iodine, selenium is necessary for the synthesis of the active form of the thyroid hormone that regulates the body's metabolic processes. Selenium is also an antioxidant nutrient (see Table 8-10); it functions as part of an antioxidant enzyme system that defends the body by preventing the formation of free radicals. See Chapter 7 for more details regarding the antioxidant nutrients. Limited research suggests a possible role for selenium in protecting against the development of some forms of cancer due to its antioxidant properties. However, selenium supplements are not recommended as they can cause harm in adequately nourished people.[18] A deficiency of selenium is associated with a form of heart disease prevalent in some areas of China with selenium-poor soil.* Good sources of selenium include whole grains, meat, seafood, and fruits or vegetables (depending on the soil content).

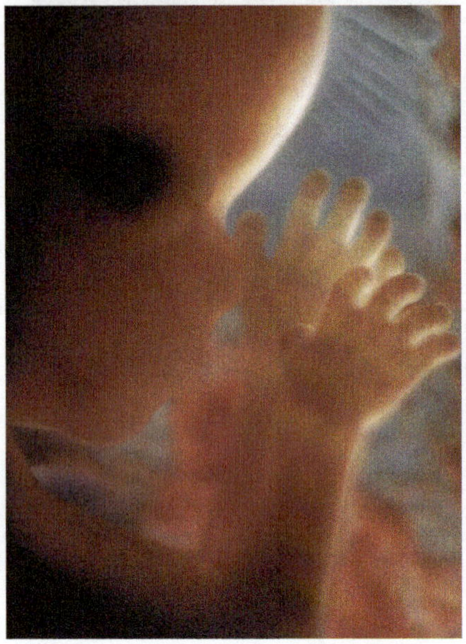

Petit Format/Science Source

Life begins in water.

8.5 Water, Minerals, and Fluid Balance

Throughout history, humans have known that water is indispensable to life itself as well as essential for health. Although we often take it for granted, water is by far the nutrient most needed by the body. Consisting entirely of a combination of hydrogen and oxygen atoms, water makes up part of every cell, tissue, and organ in the body and accounts for about 60 percent of body weight (see Figure 8-12), even contributing to body parts thought of as "dry." For example, bone is more than 20 percent water, muscle is 75 percent water, and teeth are about 10 percent water. See Chapter 9 for a discussion of water balance in the body and the sources of water in our diet.

Inside the body, water performs many tasks vital to life (see Table 8-11), such as helping to transport the nutrients needed to nourish the cells. The blood is a river of water that flows through the arteries, capillaries, and veins, bringing each cell the exact substances and particles it requires. This same river carries away waste products formed during the reactions that take place in the cells. In addition, water acts as a shock absorber in joints and around the spinal cord; lubricates the digestive tract, as well as all the tissues moistened with mucus; surrounds and cushions an unborn child; and plays a key role in maintaining body temperature.

About 40 percent of the body's water weight is inside the cells, and about 15 percent bathes the outsides of the cells. The remainder is in the blood vessels. Special conditions are needed to regulate the amount of water inside and outside the cells, so that the cells do not collapse from water leaving them or swell up under the stress of too much water entering them. The cells cannot manage this by pumping water across their membranes, because water slips back and forth freely. However, they can pump minerals across their membranes, and these minerals attract the water to come along with them. This is how the cells maintain water balance. Minerals used for this purpose take the special form of **ions** or **electrolytes** (see Table 8-12). In this form, as single, electrically charged particles, the minerals play many roles, including helping to maintain water balance and acid–base balance.

FIGURE 8-12

Water—The Number One Nutrient

SOURCE: C. Lecos, Water: The Number One Nutrient, FDA Consumer.

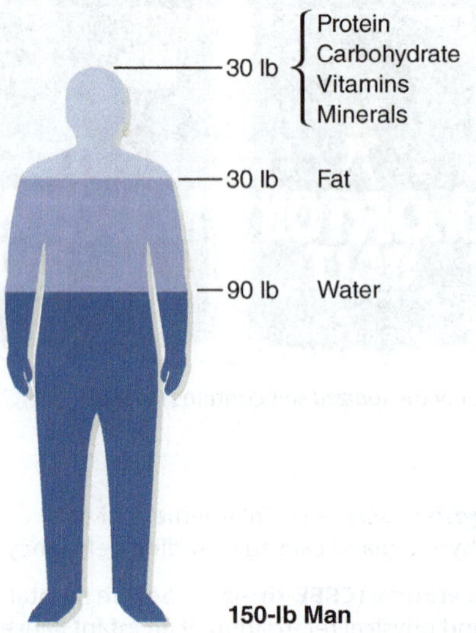

© Cengage

*Keshan (KEE-shan) disease is a form of heart disease associated with selenium deficiency and is named after the province in China where it was studied. This form of heart disease is characterized by enlargement of the heart with fibrous tissue.

TABLE 8-11 The Functions of Water in the Body

- Transports nutrients throughout the body
- Serves as a solvent for water-soluble nutrients needed by the cells
- Carries away waste from the blood and body tissues
- Moistens eyes, mouth, and nose
- Hydrates skin
- Ensures adequate blood volume
- Forms main component of body fluids
- Participates in many chemical reactions
- Helps maintain normal body temperature
- Acts as a lubricant around joints
- Serves as a shock absorber inside the eyes, joints, spinal cord and in the amniotic sac surrounding a fetus

FIGURE 8-13

Electrolytes

Sodium, potassium, and chloride are examples of body electrolytes. Potassium, which is usually found in the fluids inside the cells, carries a positive charge. Sodium and chloride are usually found in the fluids outside the cells. Sodium carries a positive charge, whereas chloride carries a negative charge.

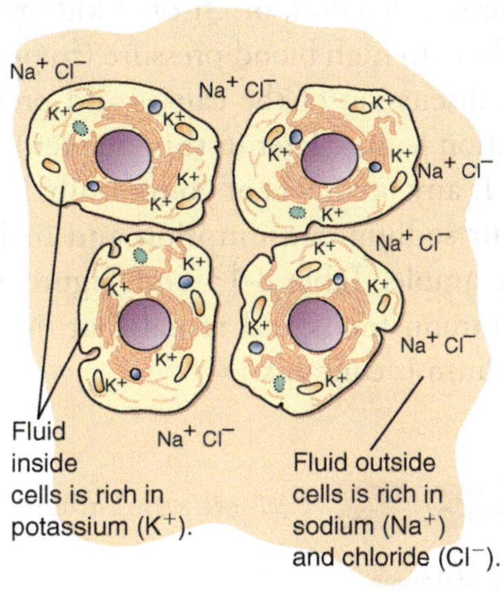

Electrolytes

Sodium, potassium, phosphorus, and chloride are examples of *electrolytes*—dissolved substances in blood and body fluids that carry electric charges (see Figure 8-13). Sodium is the chief positively charged ion needed to maintain the volume of fluid outside cells; potassium is the chief positively charged ion inside the cells. Chloride is the major negatively charged ion in the fluids outside the cells, where it is found mostly in association with sodium. Phosphorus is the major negatively charged ion found inside cells.

Electrolytes influence the distribution of fluids among the various body compartments. Specifically, when present in healthful amounts, electrolytes serve to keep the fluids inside and outside the cells in balance so that the cells can function properly and allow body fluids to bring cells the needed nutrients and remove waste products from the cells. With a normal diet, many factors in addition to the intake of sodium and chloride found in salt work together to keep the fluid volume fairly constant inside and outside of cells.

Electrolytes also help create the environment in which the cells' work takes place—work such as nerve-to-nerve communication, heartbeats, and contraction of muscles. When a person's body loses fluid, whether as sweat, blood, or urine, the person also loses electrolytes. Maintaining healthful concentrations of electrolytes is crucial to the life-sustaining activities of the vital organs. When large amounts of body fluid are lost, as in **heat stroke**, infant diarrhea, or injury, replacing them is a critical medical task.

People who exercise also lose fluids, and they must replace those fluids to avoid dehydration. Chapter 11 discusses fluid needs during and after exercise, as well as popular sports drinks that can help replace electrolytes that may have been lost along with the fluids.

TABLE 8-12 Minerals for Fluid and Electrolyte Balance

The body maintains fluid balance inside and outside of cells by using the major minerals. Electrolytes located primarily outside the cells:

- Sodium
- Chloride
- Calcium

Electrolytes located primarily inside the cells:

- Potassium
- Phosphorus
- Magnesium
- Sulfur

ions (EYE-onz) Electrically charged particles, such as sodium (positively charged) and chloride (negatively charged).

electrolytes Compounds that partially dissociate in water to form ions; examples are sodium, potassium, and chloride.

heat stroke An acute and dangerous reaction to heat buildup in the body, requiring emergency medical attention; also called *sun stroke*.

Sodium Sodium is part of sodium chloride, ordinary table **salt**, a food seasoning and preservative. The recommended Adequate Intake (AI) for sodium is set at 1,500 milligrams for young adults, 1,300 milligrams for adults aged 51 through 70, and 1,200 milligrams for older adults. Because average sodium intakes are about 3,440 milligrams per day, substantially higher than recommended, the *Dietary Guidelines for Americans* recommends limiting sodium to less than the upper limit of 2,300 milligrams of sodium per day (approximately 1 teaspoon of salt). Reducing sodium intake to 1,500 milligrams is recommended for adults who are 51 and older, and for those of any age who are African American or have prehypertension or hypertension, diabetes, or chronic kidney disease. The use of highly salted foods can contribute to high blood pressure (**hypertension**) in those who are genetically susceptible. (A discussion of the causes and prevention of hypertension appears in the Nutrition Action feature later in this chapter.)

If any members of your family have high blood pressure, you are advised to curtail your sodium consumption and make sure that your potassium and calcium intakes are ample. Table 8-13 and Figure 8-14 show a sampling of the sodium content of common foods and reveal that, in general, the more processed a food is, the more sodium it contains.

TABLE 8-13 **Where's the Sodium?**

Food Groups	Sodium (mg)
Grains and Grain Products	
Cooked cereal, rice, pasta, unsalted, ½ c	0–5
Ready-to-eat cereal, 1 c	0–360
Bread, 1 slice	110–175
Vegetables	
Fresh or frozen, cooked without salt, ½ c	1–70
Canned or frozen with sauce, ½ c	140–460
Tomato juice, canned, ½ c	330
Fruit	
Fresh, frozen, canned, ½ c	0–5
Low-Fat or Fat-Free Dairy Foods	
Milk, 1 c	107
Yogurt, 1 c	75–150
Natural cheeses, 1½ oz	110–450
Processed cheeses, 2 oz	600
Nuts, Seeds, and Legumes	
Peanuts, unsalted, ⅓ c	0–5
Peanuts, salted, ⅓ c	120
Beans, cooked from dried or frozen, without salt, ½ c	0–5
Beans, canned, ½ c	400
Meats, Fish, and Poultry	
Fresh meat, fish, poultry, 3 oz	30–90
Tuna, canned, water pack, no salt added, 3 oz	35–45
Tuna, canned, water pack, 3 oz	250–350
Ham, lean, roasted, 3 oz	1,020

SOURCE: Adapted from the National Heart, Lung, and Blood Institute, The DASH Eating Plan.

salt A pair of charged mineral particles, such as sodium (Na^+) and chloride (Cl^-), that associate together. In water, they dissociate and help carry electric current; that is, they become *electrolytes*.

hypertension Sustained high blood pressure (*hyper* = too much; *tension* = pressure).

People who wish to choose and prepare foods with less salt need to know that what they pour from the salt shaker may be only a sixth of the total salt they consume (see Figure 8-15). Up to 75 percent of the salt in the diet has been added to foods by food processors. Because processed foods don't always taste salty, eating can sometimes be a guessing game. Remember to check food labels for sodium content. See The Savvy Diner feature on page 248 for suggested ways to reduce sodium intake.

FIGURE 8-14

Sources of Sodium

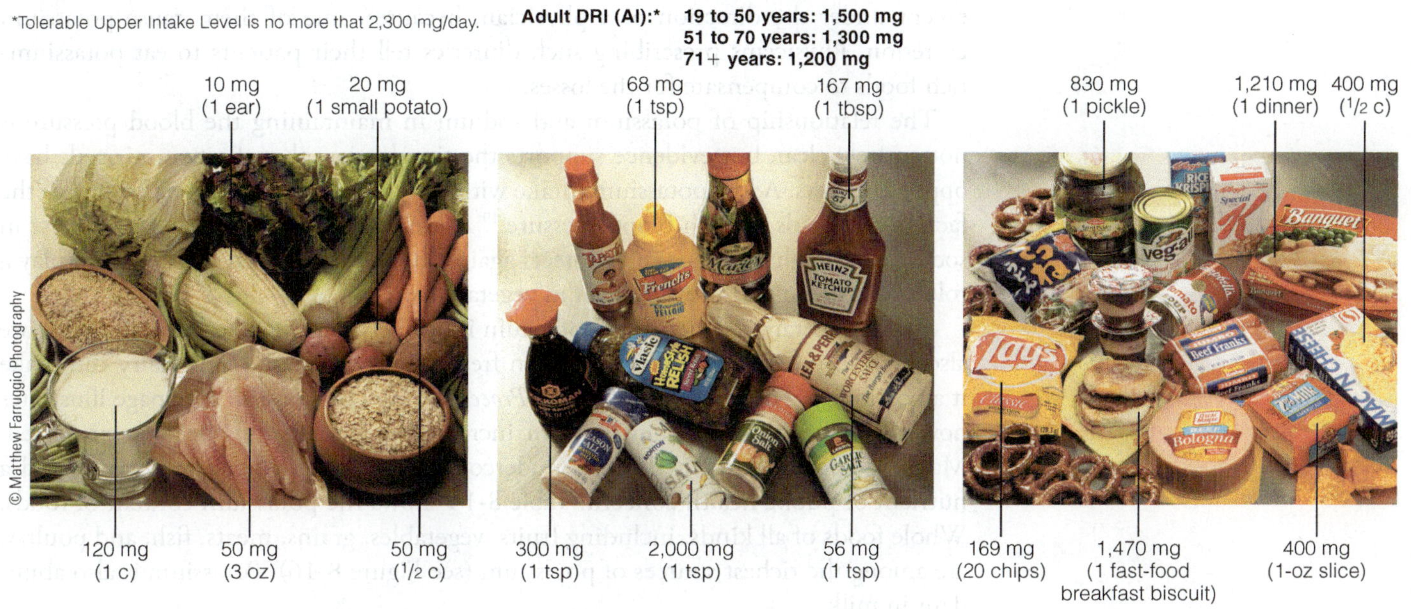

FIGURE 8-15

Common Sources of Sodium in the U.S. Diet, Ages Two Years and Older

Most sodium consumed in the United States comes from salts added during commercial food processing and preparation. Mixed dishes—including burgers, sandwiches, and tacos; rice, pasta, and grain dishes; pizza; meat, poultry, and seafood dishes; and soups—account for almost half of the sodium consumed in the United States. Most consumers have sodium intakes above the Tolerable Upper Intake Level (2,300 milligrams). The average daily intake of sodium is 4,240 milligrams for men and 2,980 milligrams for women.

Data from What We Eat in America (WWEIA) Food Category analyses for the 2015 Dietary Guidelines Advisory Committee. Estimates based on dietary recalls from WWEIA, NHANES 2009–2010.

SOURCE: U.S. Department of Health and Human Services and U.S. Department of Agriculture, *2015–2020 Dietary Guidelines for Americans*, 8th edition, December 2015.

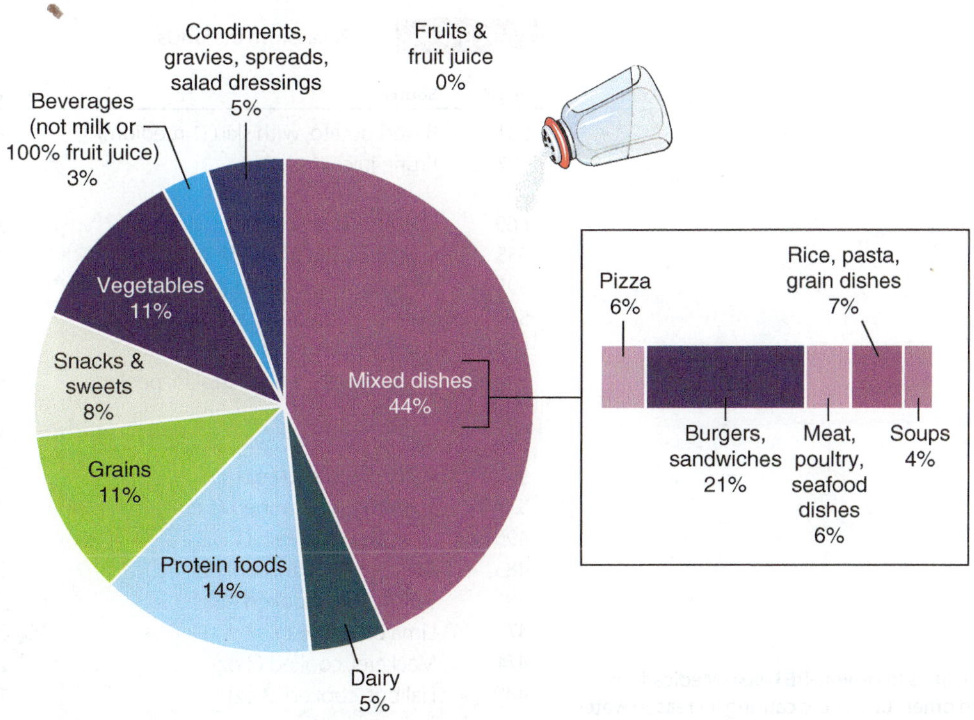

Potassium Potassium is critical to maintaining the heartbeat. The sudden deaths that occur during fasting, severe diarrhea, or severe vomiting are thought to be due to heart failure caused by potassium loss. As the principal positively charged ion inside body cells, potassium plays a major role in maintaining water balance and cell integrity.

In dehydration, sodium is lost along with water that is lost from the body, but more critical damage comes because potassium is lost from inside cells at the same time. Potassium deficiency is especially dangerous because it affects the brain cells, making a person unaware of the need for water. Adults are warned not to take **diuretics** except under the direction of a physician, because some of them cause potassium excretion. Physicians prescribing such diuretics tell their patients to eat potassium-rich foods to compensate for the losses.

The relationship of potassium and sodium in maintaining the blood pressure is not entirely clear, but evidence supports the simple view that the two minerals have opposite effects. A low potassium intake with a high sodium intake may be one of the factors that leads to high blood pressure.[19] A lifelong intake of foods that are low in sodium and high in potassium protects against hypertension and is thought to play a role in the low blood pressure seen in vegetarians.[20]

A severe dietary deficiency of potassium is unlikely, but high-sodium diets that are also high in processed foods and low in fresh fruits, vegetables, and dairy can make it a possibility. The *Whole Foods versus Processed Foods* box on the next page illustrates how potassium decreases and sodium increases as whole foods become processed. Many people in the United States underconsume potassium, and it is considered a nutrient of public health concern. Table 8-14 shows the potassium content of foods. Whole foods of all kinds, including fruits, vegetables, grains, meats, fish, and poultry, are among the richest sources of potassium (see Figure 8-16). Potassium is also abundant in milk.

Toxicity from potassium in supplement form is a greater concern than potassium deficiency. The body protects itself from this eventuality as best it can. If you

TABLE 8-14 Potassium in Foods

(mg)*	Sources	(mg)*	Sources
941	Baked potato, with skin (1 medium)	422	Banana (1 medium)
707	Prune juice (1 c)	419	Spinach, cooked from fresh or canned (½ c)
669	Tomato paste, canned (¼ c)	382	Fat-free milk (1 c)
655	Beet greens, cooked from fresh (½ c)	378	Apricots, dried (¼ c)
595	White beans, canned (½ c)	373	Pinto beans (½ c)
582	Butternut squash, baked (1 c)	365	Lentils, cooked (½ c)
579	Yogurt, plain, nonfat (1 c)	364	Avocado (½ c)
542	Sweet potato, baked in skin, peeled (1 medium)	358	Plantain, slices, cooked (½ c)
534	Salmon, Atlantic, wild, cooked (3 oz)	357	Kidney beans (½ c)
533	Pomegranate juice (1 c)	340	Raisins (¼ c)
527	Tomato juice, canned (1 c)	329	Kale, cooked (½ c)
496	Orange juice, fresh (1 c)	310	Raisin bran (1 c)
485	Soybeans, green, cooked (½ c)	300	Pork (3 oz)
481	Swiss chard, cooked (½ c)	292	Tomato (1 medium)
478	Lima beans (½ c)	250	Hamburger (3 oz)
474	Mackerel, cooked (3 oz)	229	Broccoli (½ c)
449	Halibut, cooked (3 oz)	213	Cantaloupe (½ c)

* DRI, adult: 4,700 mg/day.

diuretics (dye-you-RET-iks) Medications and other substances causing increased water excretion (*dia* = through; *ouron* = urine).

FIGURE 8-16

Sources of Potassium

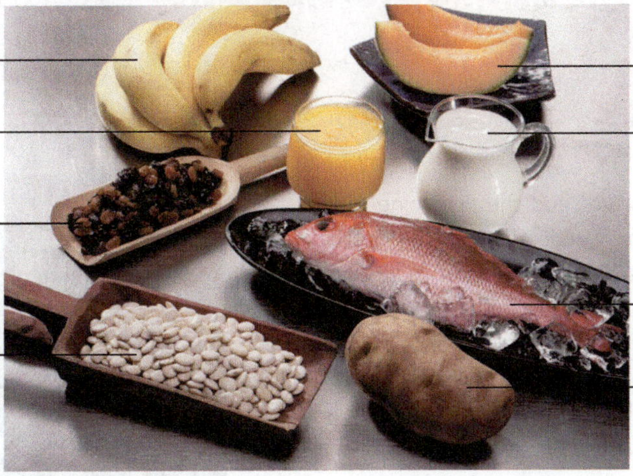

Whole Foods versus Processed Foods

Note the effects of processing: The potassium-to-sodium ratio falls with processing.

Food	Potassium (mg)	Sodium (mg)	Potassium-to-Sodium Ratio
Cucumber, raw, ¼ item	112	2	56 to 1
Cucumber, dill pickled, ¼ c	40	360	1 to 9
Cucumber, dill pickled, ¼ c, low-sodium	45	7	6 to 1
Potato, baked, 1	1080	20	54 to 1
Au gratin potatoes, mix, ½ c	267	536	1 to 2
Apple, raw, 1 medium	190	2	95 to 1
Apple pie, 1 slice	110	330	1 to 3
Milk, 1 c	360	107	3 to 1
Instant pudding, ½ c	190	380	1 to 2

consume more than you need, the kidneys accelerate their excretion and so maintain control. Should their limit be exceeded (if you ingest too much potassium too fast), a vomiting reflex is triggered. However, if the digestive tract is bypassed and potassium is injected into a vein, the heart can stop.

Chloride The negative ion chloride accompanies sodium in the fluids outside the cells, where it helps to maintain fluid and electrolyte balance. Because chloride can move freely across membranes, it is also found inside the cells in association with potassium. In the blood, chloride helps in maintaining the acid–base balance. In the stomach, the chloride ion is part of hydrochloric acid, which maintains the strong acidity of the stomach needed for protein digestion. Nearly all dietary chloride comes from sodium chloride or salt, found naturally occurring in foods, added from the salt shaker, or found abundantly in processed foods. The recommended intakes for chloride are listed in the DRI Table at the back of this book..

Nutrition **ACTION**

Diet and Blood Pressure—Beyond Just the Salt Shaker (Obj. 8.5)

Think "diet" and "blood pressure," and the first thing that comes to mind is salt. Small wonder, given that experts have long emphasized that a diet high in salt or, more specifically, the sodium it contains, contributes to a public health problem known as *hypertension* (or high blood pressure), as shown in Figure 8-17.[21] Nevertheless, a number of other, albeit less notorious, dietary factors play a role in the unhealthful rise in blood pressure that afflicts some 78 million Americans.

Obesity, for instance, inarguably ranks as the number one dietary culprit linked to hypertension.[22] That's because excess weight forces the heart to work harder to supply blood to the extra pounds of fat tissue. High blood pressure occurs about twice as often among people with obesity as among thinner people. Fortunately, losing as little as 5 percent of the excess weight has been shown, in some cases, to lower blood pressure to the point that antihypertensive medications may become unnecessary.[23] In other words, a little weight loss, regardless of sodium intake, can be enough to get high blood pressure back under control. With increasing obesity, age, and blood pressure levels

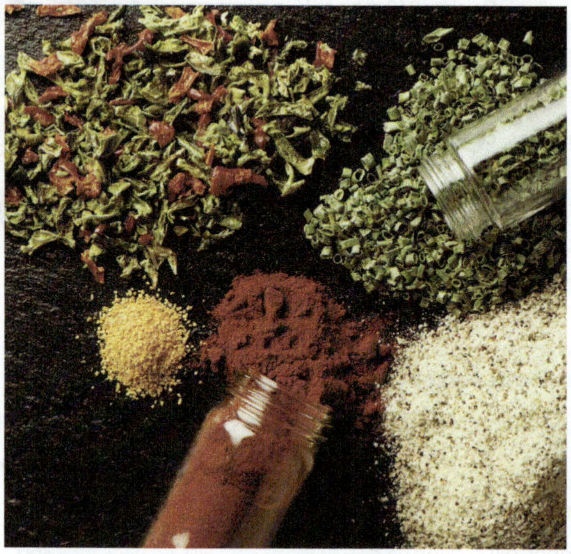

PhotoDisk/Getty Images

FIGURE 8-17

Are Your Numbers Up?

Hypertension has been called a "silent killer" that cannot be felt and may go undetected for years. That's why it is crucial to have your blood pressure checked regularly. Diagnosis of hypertension requires at least two elevated readings. The first of the two numbers in a blood pressure reading, systolic pressure, represents the force exerted by the heart as it contracts to pump blood throughout the body, as measured by the number of millimeters that the pressure pushes a column of mercury up a tube. The second number, diastolic pressure, is a measure of the pressure the blood exerts on artery walls between heartbeats. A reading of below 120 over 80 millimeters of mercury is considered "optimal" for adults 18 years and older. Measurements between 120 over 80 and 139 over 89 are classified as prehypertension. Individuals with prehypertension are at increased risk for progression to hypertension and are encouraged to make lifestyle changes to prevent hypertension. Individuals in the 130 over 80 to 139 over 89 range are at twice the risk to develop hypertension as those with lower values. Beyond those levels, the risks of heart attacks and strokes rise in direct proportion to increasing blood pressure.*

* The categories are for adults not taking high blood pressure medications. If your systolic and diastolic numbers fall into different categories, your overall status depends on the higher category.

SOURCE: National Institutes of Health, National Heart, Lung, and Blood Institute, *The Eighth Report of the Joint National Committee on Prevention, Detection, Evaluation, and Treatment of High Blood Pressure* (Washington, DC: U.S. Department of Health and Human Services, 2014).

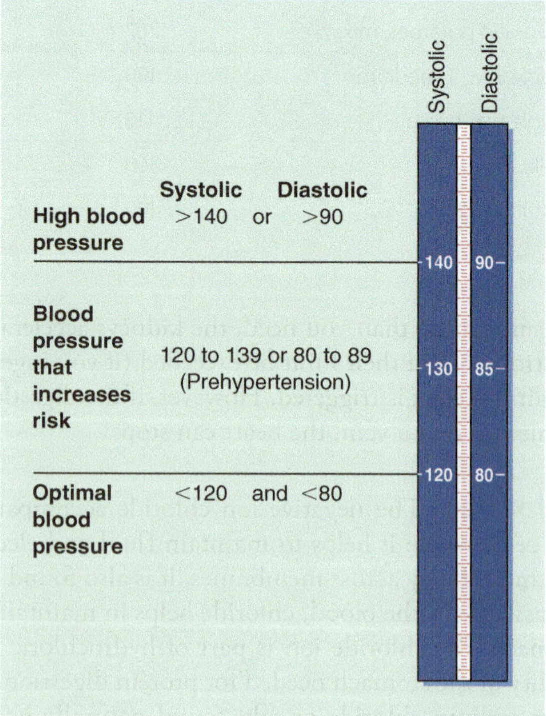

© Cengage

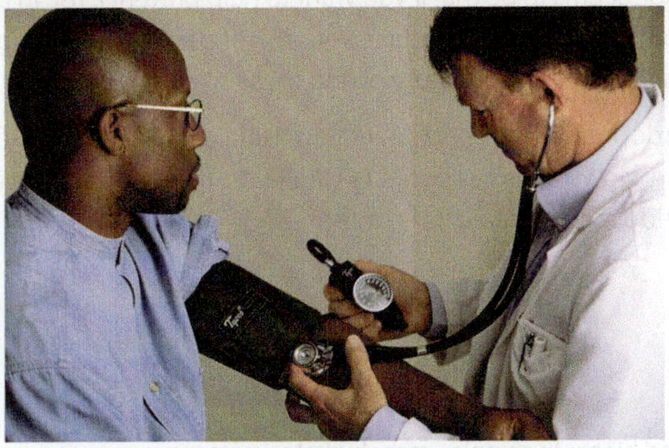

Will & Deni McIntyre/Science Source

The most effective single measure you can take to protect yourself against high blood pressure is to know what your blood pressure is. Risk factors for high blood pressure:

- Obesity
- Family history of high blood pressure
- Race (African Americans are more likely than whites to develop hypertension.)
- Age (In the United States, blood pressure tends to rise with age.)
- Excess alcohol consumption
- Sedentary lifestyle

comes an increasing probability that a person will become *salt sensitive*, meaning that the blood pressure rises in proportion to the amount of sodium the person consumes.[24] For these people, of course, keeping dietary sodium to a minimum can help lower blood pressure.

Drinking excessive amounts of alcohol is another dietary factor that may lead to high blood pressure (not to mention poor compliance with drug regimens and other treatments for the problem). In fact, consuming more than a couple of ounces of alcohol daily has been blamed for leading to 5 to 11 percent of cases of hypertension among men.[25] The National High Blood Pressure Education Program thus recommends that to control high blood pressure, those who drink should do so only in moderation.[26]

In addition to recommending that people with hypertension lose weight and drink alcohol in moderation, it is clear that modest changes in lifestyle can add up to significant gains in controlling high blood pressure. It appears that attention to a healthful lifestyle can also help prevent the problem from arising in the first place. For example, researchers at Northwestern University Medical School in Chicago put one group of adults prone to high blood pressure on a preventive program that included losing weight, lowering sodium intake, cutting down on alcohol, and exercising more. They then compared them to a similar group whose members were left to their own devices. The researchers found that over the course of five years, only 1 in 11 people who changed their lifestyle ended up with hypertension. Of those who didn't alter their habits, though, one in five became hypertensive.[27]

Along with the factors just explained, scientists are exploring other nutrients that may influence blood pressure.[28] Some researchers believe, for instance, that it is not dietary sodium per se that alters blood pressure, but rather the ratio between it and potassium, sodium's partner in regulating the body's water balance. In other words, the more potassium and less sodium in the diet, the greater the likelihood that the body will maintain a normal blood pressure. Diets rich in high-potassium foods such as fresh fruits and vegetables tend to go hand in hand with low sodium consumption.[29]

In addition, some studies indicate that people who eat high-calcium diets are less likely to have high blood pressure; conversely, people with inadequate calcium intakes are more likely to have hypertension.[30] It is recommended, therefore, that people eat a diet including two to three servings daily of calcium-rich foods, such as milk or calcium-fortified orange juice.

Finally, some evidence suggests that eating a diet that includes monounsaturated fat and is low in saturated fat helps lower blood pressure. It certainly makes sense for those with high blood pressure to eat such a diet, if for no other reason than to help prevent heart disease, a condition that people with hypertension run a high risk of developing (refer to the Spotlight feature in Chapter 5).[31]

An Eating Plan to Reduce High Blood Pressure

Researchers have shown that following a particular eating plan—called the *DASH diet*—and reducing sodium intake lowers blood pressure. The Dietary Approaches to Stop Hypertension (DASH) study examined the effects of overall diet on 459 adult participants with normal to high blood pressures. After just eight weeks, those people with mild hypertension who were on the DASH diet—a diet high in fruits, vegetables, whole grains, and low-fat dairy products and low in total fat, saturated fat, and cholesterol—saw their blood pressures decrease.[32]

A second landmark study, DASH-Sodium, has shown that a combination of the DASH diet and sodium reduction can lower blood pressure even more. The DASH-Sodium study looked at the effect on blood pressure of a reduced dietary sodium intake as 412 participants followed *either* the DASH diet or an eating pattern resembling the typical American diet. Participants were followed for a month at each of three sodium levels: 3,300 milligrams per day (a level consumed by many Americans), 2,300 milligrams per day, and the lower-intake DASH diet of 1,500 milligrams per day. Results showed that reducing dietary sodium reduced blood pressure in participants following the DASH diet and those on the typical American diet, but the biggest reductions in blood pressure were seen for those following the DASH diet. Although those with hypertension saw the biggest reductions, those without the disease also saw declines in blood pressure.

(Continued)

Figure 8-18 illustrates the DASH diet. The Savvy Diner feature that follows offers tips for seasoning foods without excess salt.

Overall, the results of the DASH studies echo the recommendations for an overall healthful diet: Choose low-fat dairy products, smaller portions of meat, plenty of fruits and vegetables, and ample servings of high-fiber, whole-grain products. This eating pattern may reduce the risk not only for hypertension, but also for heart disease (low in saturated fat and cholesterol), diabetes (high in complex carbohydrates and fiber), osteoporosis (adequate in calcium), and cancer (lots of fruits and vegetables). The take-home message seems to be that if you want to help prevent a rise in blood pressure as you age and reduce your risk of developing high blood pressure, you can do so by following these six tips:

1. Adopt an eating pattern rich in fruits, vegetables, legumes, and low-fat dairy products (similar to the DASH diet) with reduced saturated-fat content.

FIGURE 8-18

The DASH Diet Eating Pattern

The DASH eating pattern is lower in fat, saturated fat, cholesterol, and sodium, and higher in complex carbohydrates, potassium, magnesium, and calcium than the typical American diet.

SOURCE: NHLBI, *DASH Eating Plan*; available at www.nhlbi.nih.gov.

Following the DASH Eating Plan

Use this chart to help you plan your menus—or take it with you when you go to the grocery store.

Food Group	Servings Per Day: 1,600 Calories	2,000 Calories	2,600 Calories	Serving Sizes	Examples and Notes	Significance of Each Food Group to the DASH Eating Plan
Grains[a] 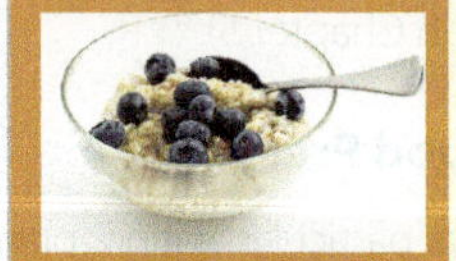 photogal/Shutterstock.com	6	6–8	10–11	1 slice bread 1 oz dry cereal[b] ½ cup cooked rice, pasta, or cereal	Whole wheat bread and rolls, whole wheat pasta, English muffin, pita bread, bagel, cereals, grits, oatmeal, brown rice, unsalted pretzels and popcorn	Major sources of energy and fiber
Vegetables 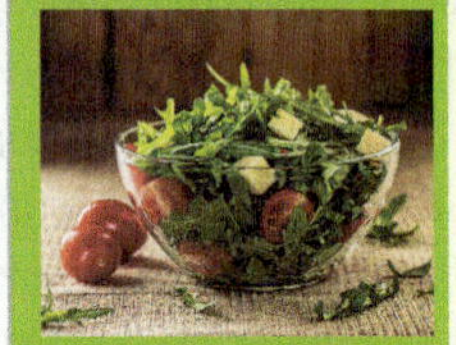 OnlyFOOD/Shutterstock.com	3–4	4–5	5–6	1 cup raw leafy vegetable ½ cup cut-up raw or cooked vegetable ½ cup vegetable juice	Broccoli, carrots, collards, green beans, green peas, kale, lima beans, potatoes, spinach, squash, sweet potatoes, tomatoes	Rich sources of potassium, magnesium, and fiber
Fruits 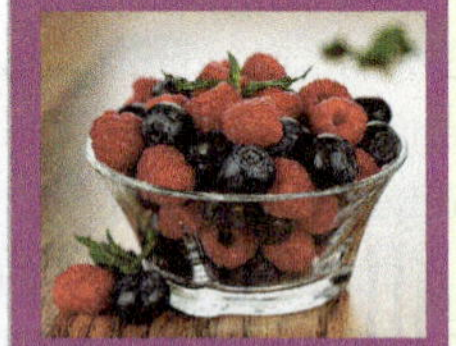 Olyina/Shutterstock.com	4	4–5	5–6	1 medium fruit ¼ cup dried fruit ½ cup fresh, frozen, or canned fruit ½ cup fruit juice	Apples, apricots, bananas, dates, grapes, oranges, grapefruit, grapefruit juice, mangoes, melons, peaches, pineapples, raisins, strawberries, tangerines	Important sources of potassium, magnesium, and fiber
Fat-free or low-fat milk and milk products 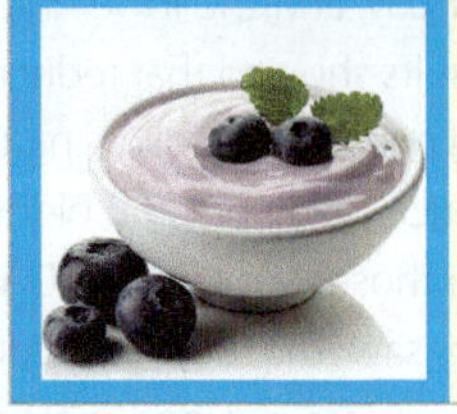 baibaz/Shutterstock.com	2–3	2–3	3	1 cup milk or yogurt 1½ oz cheese	Fat-free (skim) or low-fat (1%) milk or buttermilk; fat-free, low-fat, or reduced-fat cheese; fat-free or low-fat regular or frozen yogurt	Major sources of calcium and protein

Food Group	Servings Per Day: 1,600 Calories	Servings Per Day: 2,000 Calories	Servings Per Day: 2,600 Calories	Serving Sizes	Examples and Notes	Significance of Each Food Group to the DASH Eating Plan
Lean meats, poultry, and fish 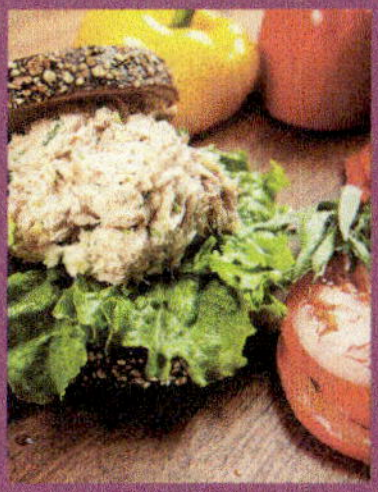 msheldrake/Shutterstock.com	3–6	6 or less	6	1 oz cooked meats, poultry, or fish 1 egg[c]	Select only lean meats; trim away visible fat; broil, roast, or poach; remove skin from poultry	Rich sources of protein and magnesium
Nuts, seeds, and legumes 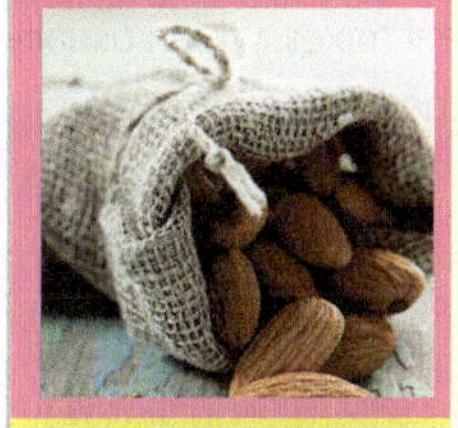 Sea Wave/Shutterstock.com	3 per week	4–5 per week	1	⅓ cup or 1½ oz nuts 2 Tbsp peanut butter 2 Tbsp or ½ oz seeds ½ cup cooked legumes (dry beans and peas)	Almonds, hazelnuts, mixed nuts, peanuts, walnuts, sunflower seeds, peanut butter, kidney beans, lentils, split peas	Rich sources of energy, magnesium, protein, and fiber
Fats and oils[d] 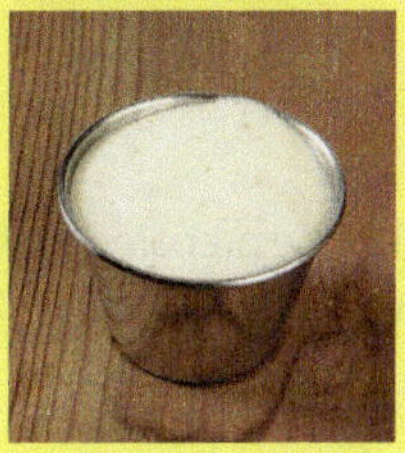 MSPhotographic/Shutterstock.com	2	2–3	3	1 tsp soft margarine 1 tsp vegetable oil 1 Tbsp mayonnaise 2 Tbsp salad dressing	Soft margarine, vegetable oil (such as canola, corn, olive, or safflower), low-fat mayonnaise, light salad dressing	The DASH study had 27 percent of calories as fat, including fat in or added to foods
Sweets and added sugars 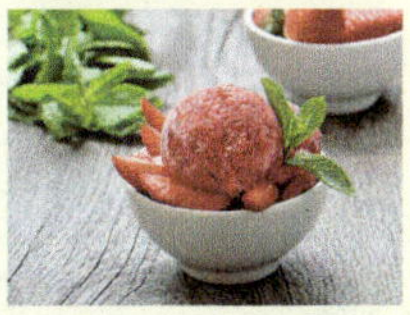 Nadezhda Nesterova/Shutterstock.com	0	5 or less per week	≤2	1 Tbsp sugar 1 Tbsp jelly or jam ½ cup sorbet, gelatin 1 cup lemonade	Fruit-flavored gelatin, fruit punch, hard candy, jelly, maple syrup, sorbet and ices, sugar	Sweets should be low in fat

[a]Whole grains are recommended for most grain servings as a good source of fiber and nutrients.
[b]Serving sizes vary between ½ cup and 1¼ cups, depending on cereal type. Check the product's Nutrition Facts label.
[c]Since eggs are high in cholesterol, limit egg yolk intake to no more than four per week; two egg whites have the same protein content as 1 oz of meat.
[d]Fat content changes serving amount for fats and oils. For example, 1 Tbsp of regular salad dressing equals one serving; 1 Tbsp of a low-fat dressing equals one-half serving; 1 Tbsp of a fat-free dressing equals zero servings.

2. Maintain a normal weight. Lose weight if you're overweight; even losing just a few pounds can reduce blood pressure if you're overweight.
3. Keep your sodium intake at *or below* recommended levels: not more than 2,300 milligrams a day, or not more than 1,500 milligrams a day if you are age 51 or older, or African American, have diabetes, high blood pressure, or chronic kidney disease.
4. Pursue an active lifestyle: Walk briskly, swim, jog, cycle, or do other moderately paced aerobic activities. Aim for at least 30 minutes of activities daily.
5. If you drink, do so in moderation: no more than one drink a day for women, and no more than two drinks a day for men.
6. Don't smoke. Cigarette smoking raises blood pressure and seriously increases risk for heart disease.

THE SAVVY Diner

Choose and Prepare Foods with Less Salt (Obj. 8.5)

You've decided to cut your salt intake. How do you know which foods to buy? How can you cook foods with less salt and good flavor? Fortunately, cutting some of the salt out of your diet isn't difficult. Here are a few basic principles.

At the Supermarket

- Read the Nutrition Facts label to compare the amount of sodium in processed foods, such as frozen dinners, cereals, soups, salad dressings, and sauces. The amount in different types and brands often varies widely. Look for labels that say "low sodium." They contain 140 mg (about 5 percent of the Daily Value) or less sodium per serving. Look for the key words *salt* and *sodium* in the ingredients list.
- Limit your intake of cured foods (such as bacon and ham), foods packed in brine (such as pickles, pickled vegetables, olives, and sauerkraut), and condiments (such as MSG, mustard, horseradish, ketchup, soy sauce, and barbecue sauce).
- Cut back on your intake of frozen dinners, mixed dishes such as pizza, packaged mixes, canned soups or broths, and salad dressings; these products often contain a lot of sodium. Choose reduced-sodium or no-salt-added products when possible. Many commercially prepared products are available in sodium-reduced versions. For example, most supermarkets carry reduced-sodium soy sauce, ketchup, canned tuna, soups, tomato sauce, nuts, canned vegetables, crackers, and pretzels.
- Buy fresh, natural foods more frequently than processed foods, which tend to be high in salt.

At Home

- Explore what herbs and spices complement specific foods. Add flavor with herbs, spices, lemon, lime, vinegar, or salt-free seasoning blends.
- Cook rice, pasta, and hot cereals without salt. Cut back on instant or flavored rice, pasta, and cereal mixes, which usually have added salt, and use only half of the seasoning packet provided.
- Rinse canned foods, such as black beans or tuna, to remove some sodium.
- Consult the *DASH Eating Plan* for more sodium-reducing tips at www.nhlbi.nih.gov.

When Eating Out

- Ask how foods are prepared. Ask that they be prepared without added salt or salt-containing ingredients.
- Move the salt shaker away.
- Limit condiments, such as mustard, ketchup, and pickles.
- Choose fruit or vegetables, instead of salty snack foods.

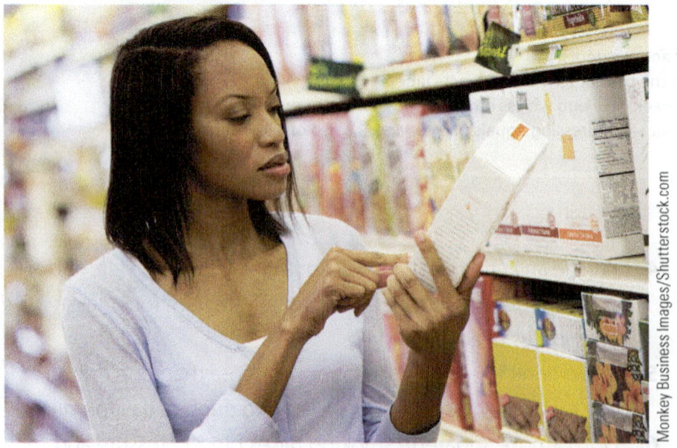

Read the Nutrition Facts label to compare the amount of sodium in processed foods.

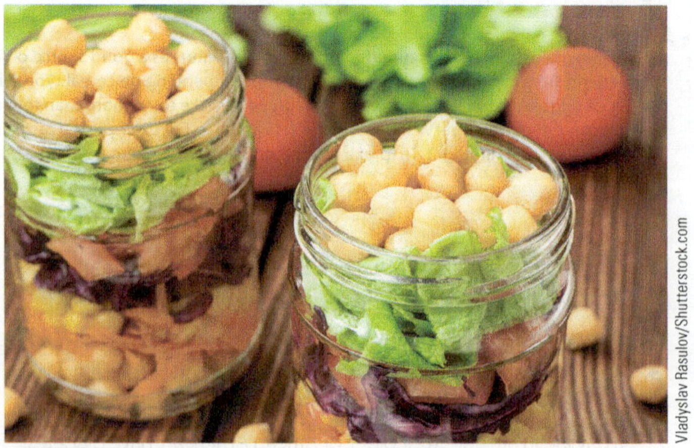

Rinse canned foods, such as chickpeas, to remove some sodium.

SPOTLight

8.6 Osteoporosis—The Silent Stalker of the Bones

- As she waited in a grocery checkout line, Nancy felt a stab of pain in her left hip. The 40-year-old woman had always been healthy and active—suddenly she could barely stand. When she went to her family doctor, she learned that several of her vertebrae had fractured. The radiologist studying her X-rays thought he was looking at the bones of a 70-year-old woman.
- Lila had just teed off at her local golf course. Putting down her club, the robust 63-year-old felt a searing back pain. When Lila met with her orthopedic surgeon, she was told she'd suffered a serious compression fracture.
- Debra wasn't worried when her physician diagnosed a mild curvature of her upper spine 7 years ago. She was only 31 and in otherwise excellent health. Then last year, her right wrist began aching and her back tired easily. After tests, she learned that at age 37, she had the brittle bones of a woman twice her age.

The three women just described share the potentially crippling and sometimes deadly condition *osteoporosis*.[33] Osteoporosis threatens the integrity of the skeleton in some 53 million adults in the United States. More than 10 million Americans have osteoporosis, and an additional 43 million have low bone density.[34] One out of two women and one out of five men over the age of 50 will suffer an osteoporosis-related fracture in their lifetime. Osteoporosis is more prevalent in women than in men after age 50, for several reasons:

- Women generally have less bone mass than men.
- Women typically have lower calcium intakes than men.
- Women more often use weight-loss diets, which tend to be low in calcium and lead to bone loss.[35]
- Bone loss begins earlier in women because of women's different hormonal makeup, and the loss is accelerated at **menopause**, when their protective **estrogen** secretion declines.
- Pregnancy and lactation decrease the calcium reserves in bones whenever calcium intake is inadequate.
- Women live longer than men, and bone loss continues with aging.

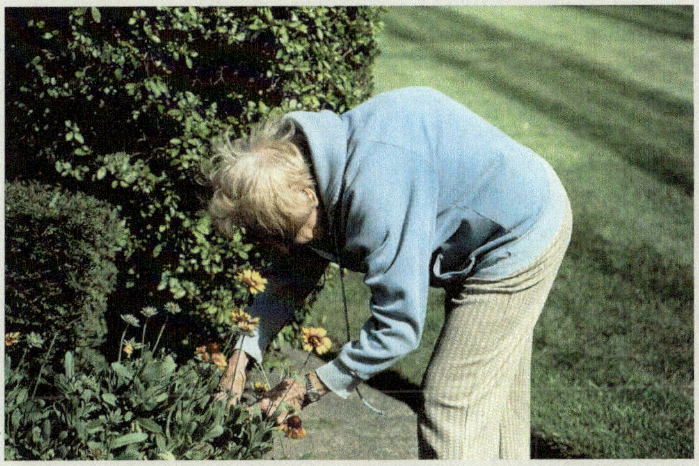
Larry Mulvehill/Science Source

Osteoporosis strikes the bones. This 75-year-old woman has lost height—not because her legs have grown shorter, but because vertebrae in her back have collapsed. These fractures occur on the front side of the spinal bones, resulting in a hunched-over posture.

What is bone loss?

Adult bone loss affects the entire skeleton, but it occurs first in the pelvis and the spine. Unfortunately, osteoporosis establishes itself silently in its victims' lives. Symptoms do not usually occur until late in life. The disease often results in fractures of the hip, spine, and wrists—and more than 2.0 million such fractures a year—that occur with very little or no stress or pressure (see Figure 8-19).[36] Often, osteoporosis first becomes apparent when someone's hip suddenly gives way. Fewer than 40 percent of all women with hip fractures return to previous activity levels, and many are confined to wheelchairs for the remainder of their lives. Approximately 20 percent of these women die of complications within the first year after hip fracture.

Can osteoporosis be prevented?

Although there is no cure for osteoporosis, the good news is that you can take steps to minimize your risk. First, determine your risk by considering the following list of factors that play a role in osteoporosis:

- *Age.* During childhood, adolescence, and the young adult years, the cells that build bone (**osteoblasts**) form more bone than the bone-dismantling cells (**osteoclasts**) take away. With aging, the bone-building cells become less active, but the bone dismantlers continue to work, causing bone tissue and strength to decline.
- *Gender.* Osteoporosis is four times more common in women. Men achieve a higher **peak bone mass** than women do, and the rate of age-related bone loss is lower in men than in women (see Figure 8-20).

FIGURE 8-19

Bone Loss and Most Common Types of Bone Fractures in Women

More than 2.0 million fractures occur each year, including nearly 1.5 million fractures in women and 590,000 fractures in men, including fractures of the pelvis and other sites not shown here.

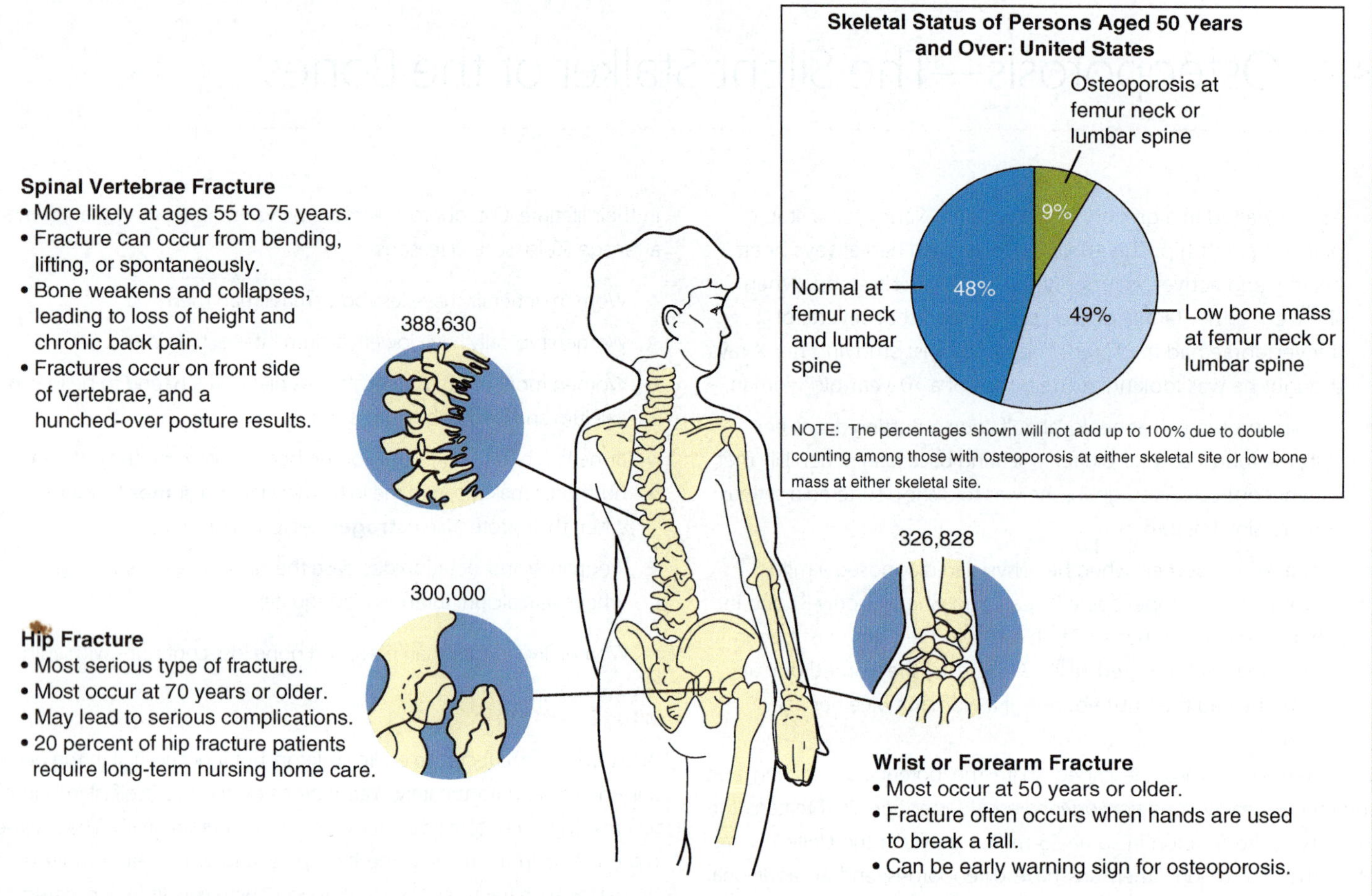

FIGURE 8-20

Bone Loss That Occurs with Age

SOURCE: Data from National Osteoporosis Foundation; www.nof.org.

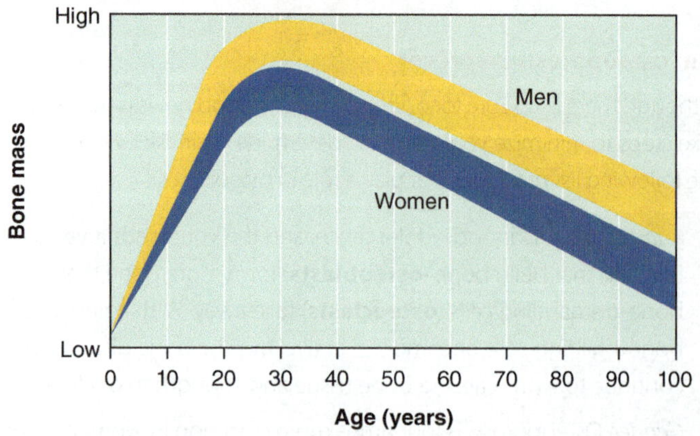

- *Age-related decline in hormones.* Hormones are important in bone health for both men and women. Menopause deprives women of the protective effects of estrogen. Estrogen improves calcium absorption from the intestines and reduces excretion of the mineral by the kidneys.[37] Bone loss accelerates in women for the 5 to 10 years following menopause. The earlier menopause occurs, the greater a woman's risk of osteoporosis. Women who have ceased menstruating (a reliable indicator of reduced estrogen levels) comprise the largest segment of people with osteoporosis. Menopause occurs naturally in women typically between the ages of 45 and 55, but it can occur earlier in life with the removal of diseased ovaries. Risk of osteoporosis increases in men with the age-related decline in testosterone, as low testosterone levels increase the risk of fractures in men.[38]
- *Abnormal absence of menstrual periods (estrogen deficiency).* Menstruation can also cease in women who overexercise and are underweight, a condition called *athletic amenorrhea* (discussed in Chapter 11). For the same reason, eating disorders (anorexia nervosa and bulimia) increase the risk of osteoporosis later in life.[39]

- *Family history.* The greater the history of skeletal fractures of the hips and vertebrae among older relatives, the greater your risk for osteoporosis.
- *Race and ethnic background.* Those of British, northern European, Chinese, Japanese, or Mexican American background, or Hispanic people from Central and South America are at the highest risk. African American women tend to have denser bones and are at lower risk.[40] Undoubtedly, environmental factors—such as calcium and vitamin D intakes, physical activity, smoking, body weight, and alcohol intake—can influence the ultimate outcome of one's bone health over genetic heritage. In fact, these environmental factors can impact bone mass by 40 to 60 percent.[41]

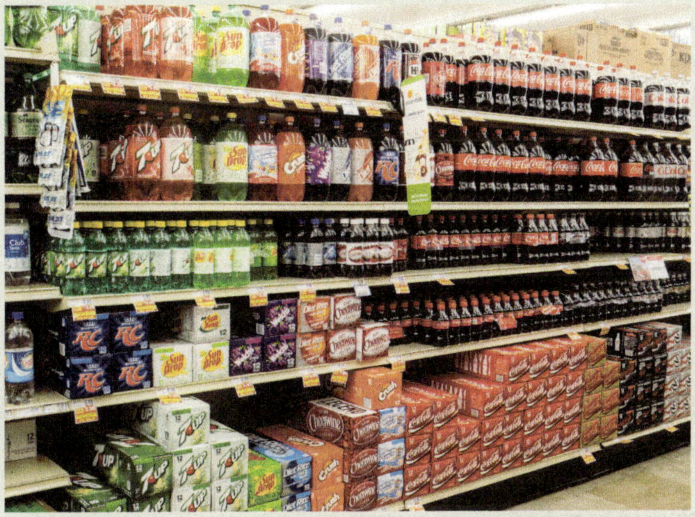

Patti McConville/Alamy Stock Photo

Soft drinks often replace milk as a beverage in the diet of teenagers, accounting for about 10 percent of their caloric intake.

- *Body build.* The smaller the frame and the thinner the person (under 127 pounds), the greater the risk. Petite women have less bone to lose than larger-boned women.
- *Sedentary lifestyle.* Inactivity leads to bone loss.[42]
- *Smoking and alcohol.* There are multiple mechanisms through which smoking and excessive alcohol intake increase the risk. People who smoke tend to have lower body weights than nonsmokers. In addition, some women smokers have lower levels of estrogen in their blood and experience an earlier onset of menopause compared to nonsmokers.[43] Alcohol decreases the activity of the bone-building cells, interferes with the absorption of calcium, and may increase excretion of calcium from the kidneys. In general, people who abuse alcohol also tend to have poor nutrition status, including low intakes of calcium.
- *Medical conditions.* Certain medical conditions, including type 1 diabetes, thyroid disorders, rheumatoid arthritis, asthma, seizures, and organ transplants, are associated with increased risk, primarily because of the drugs used to treat them. Prolonged use of medications such as thyroid hormone, antiseizure drugs, and the anti-inflammatory drugs (such as prednisone) used to treat asthma, arthritis, and some cancers may reduce calcium absorption, impair bone formation, and accelerate bone loss.
- *A bone-healthy diet that includes calcium, vitamin D, and other nutrients.* Calcium intake early in life affects the attainment of peak bone mass, achieved by about age 30, which may be the most important determinant of the risk of a fracture in later life.[44] Hence, ensuring an adequate calcium intake throughout life appears to be a sensible strategy. Adequate intake of vitamin D is required for the absorption of calcium. Many older adults, who typically have lower intakes of vitamin D and reduced ability to synthesize the vitamin from sunshine, absorb less calcium as they age.

The calcium intake of a sizeable portion of the U.S. population, especially female adolescents and female adults, is estimated to be below the recommended intake (see Figure 8-21).[45] Between the ages of 18 and 30 years, the time of the attainment of peak bone mass, more than

FIGURE 8-21

The Calcium Gap: Daily Calcium Intakes in the United States Compared to Recommended Intakes

Maintaining adequate calcium intake during childhood and adolescence is necessary for the attainment of peak bone mass, which may be important in reducing the risk of fractures and osteoporosis later in life. For the most part, very young children—less than age 3—meet their recommended calcium intakes. In contrast, according to national survey data, most older children fail to achieve the recommended intake of calcium. Likewise, most adult women of any age and adult men after age 50 do not meet their recommended calcium intakes.

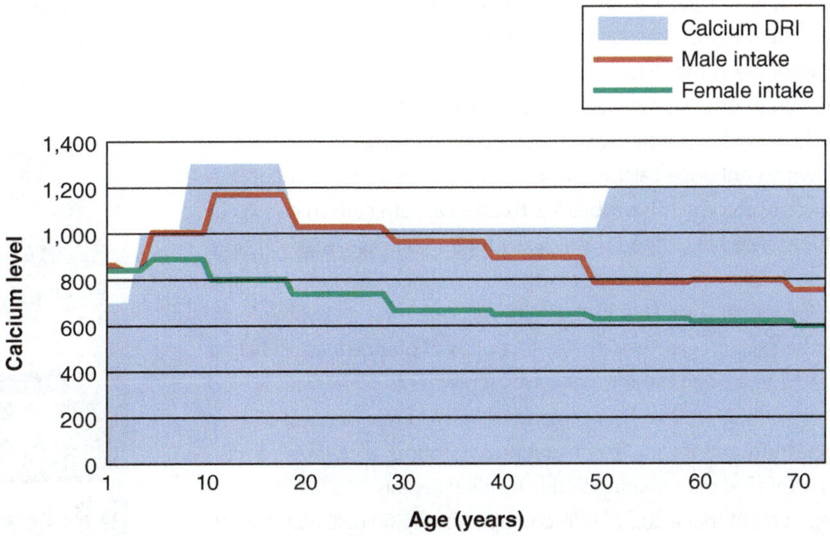

two-thirds of all American women consume less calcium than they need. One explanation is the obsession (especially among adolescent girls) with dieting. Another explanation is the dramatic increase in consumption of diet sodas over the past three decades, often displacing milk as an accompanying beverage to meals.[46] The reduction in dairy consumption correlates with lower calcium intake; however. researchers question whether cola itself is associated with decreased bone mineral density. Studies have shown that excessive caffeine and cola intake may reduce bone mineral density, more so in females than in males.[47] Some evidence also suggests that cola drinks may lead to kidney damage and a disruption of the normal mineral balance of the body, resulting in a decrease in bone mineral density.[48]

Other nutrients also play a role in bone health.[49] For example, high intakes of phosphorus, vitamin A (as retinol), and sodium may adversely affect calcium in the body.[50] Adequate intakes of protein and vitamins C and K are needed to maintain healthy bone. Low vitamin K intakes have recently been associated with increased risk of hip fractures in older adults.[51] Potassium, magnesium, and fruit and vegetable intakes are also associated with greater bone density in older adults.[52] The many phytochemicals found in fruits, vegetables, and legumes also offer protective benefits to bone (as discussed in Chapter 7).

Should I consider taking calcium supplements if I am unable to meet the recommended intake for calcium using foods? If so, what should I consider when choosing a supplement?

Although it is preferable to meet calcium needs by consuming calcium-rich foods, calcium supplements are an alternate way to obtain calcium and reduce risk of fracture.[53] In populations at risk for osteoporotic fractures, supplementation of calcium with vitamin D can decrease this risk by 15 to 30 percent.[54] Supplementation may be needed by those who either cannot or will not adjust their diets to get enough calcium from food. Supplements have the advantage of being easy to take, but they have the disadvantage of not offering other nutrients, such as the thiamin, riboflavin, niacin, potassium, phosphorus, magnesium, zinc, vitamin A, vitamin D, and protein found naturally in milk products.

Choosing a calcium supplement can be confusing. The organic salts include calcium citrate, calcium citrate-malate, and calcium lactate; the inorganic salts include calcium carbonate and calcium phosphate. Calcium carbonate is the least expensive and contains the most calcium per pill, but an organic salt, such as calcium citrate, is better absorbed, especially by older people whose secretion of stomach acid—a factor known to enhance calcium absorption—tends to be reduced.[55] A strategy to overcome this problem is to take calcium carbonate two or three times a day in divided doses, with meals, to improve absorption. Choosing a calcium supplement with vitamin D can also improve the absorption of calcium. Need other alternatives? Try a chewable form, or take the calcium carbonate pill with a glass of orange juice to help it dissolve. Note, too, that many calcium supplements come with added nutrients, such as vitamin D and magnesium. You may not need these additional nutrients if you are consuming a nutritious diet, taking a multivitamin-mineral pill, or eating highly fortified cereals.

Keep in mind that a cup of milk contains about 300 milligrams of calcium. If you are using supplements to replace the calcium found in milk, choose a supplement that contains at least 300 milligrams of calcium. Also, because calcium is best absorbed in doses of 500 milligrams or less, consuming supplements with more than 500 milligrams of calcium per pill is not advantageous. For example, if you need to take 1,000 milligrams of calcium in supplement form, choose a 500-milligram tablet and take one in the morning and one in the evening. A generic brand is fine to use—just be sure to check the label to see how much elemental calcium and which form of calcium it contains. Avoid calcium supplements derived from dolomite, oyster shell, or bone meal, because some have been found to be contaminated with lead.[56] See the Nutrition Action feature in Chapter 7 for more about choosing a vitamin-mineral supplement.

Is there a way to detect bone loss before a fracture occurs?

A test for **bone density** (Figure 8-22) can detect low bone density before a fracture occurs, and it can predict your chances of fracturing a bone in the future. The National Osteoporosis Foundation encourages women to discuss with their physician the possibility of having their bone density measured at the onset of menopause, when bone loss sharply accelerates, or if they have other medical conditions that increase their risk for osteoporosis. The more risk factors you have for osteoporosis, the more you need to evaluate your bone density as you age.

Are any drug treatments available to reverse bone loss?

Yes. Among the bone-conserving drugs currently approved by the Food and Drug Administration (FDA) are **estrogen/hormone therapy**, **designer estrogens**, **bisphosphonates**, and **denosumab** for osteoporosis prevention. These options and the hormones **calcitonin** and **parathyroid hormone** are also available for the treatment of osteoporosis.[57] These drugs work by slowing bone loss, allowing bones to slowly rebuild and increase bone density, and by reducing the risk of fractures by 50 percent or more. To be effective, these treatments should be accompanied by the recommended intakes of calcium (1,200 mg for women over 50 years of age) and vitamin D (15 micrograms for adults 51 to 70 years; 20 micrograms for adults 71 years and older), as well as regular weight-bearing exercise.[58]

FIGURE 8-22

Bone Density

Duel-energy X-ray absorptiometry (DEXA) can be used to measure bone density.

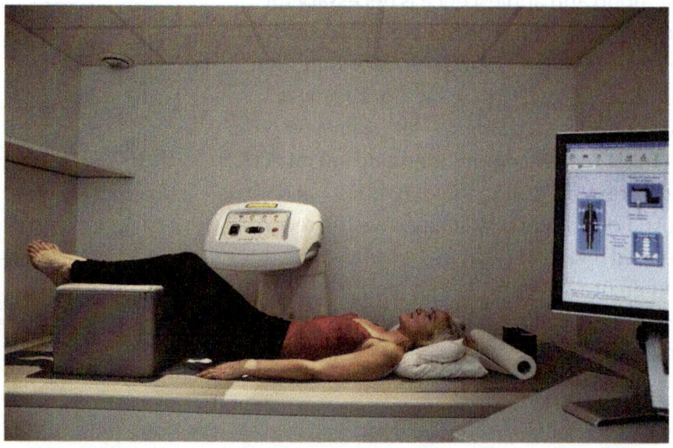

B. Boissonnet/ BSIP/AGE Fotostock

What can be done to prevent the debilitating effects of osteoporosis?

Not surprisingly, the same recommendations have been made before for lowering risks for other chronic diseases. Eat a nutritious diet and exercise *throughout life*. Consider the following steps for building bone mass and lowering your risk for osteoporosis:[59]

- Maximize peak bone mass and be vigilant about keeping the bones well supplied with calcium. Consume the recommended amount of calcium (and vitamin D) for your age group (refer to Figure 8-3). According to researcher Robert Heaney, only a few simple changes can add an extra 1,000 milligrams of calcium to an ordinary diet. Put a couple of heaping teaspoons of nonfat dried milk powder in each cup of coffee or tea, drink calcium-fortified orange juice, and eat 1 cup low-fat yogurt, a dark-green leafy vegetable, and a 1-inch cube of hard cheese.[60]
- Consume alcohol only in moderation, if at all, and avoid cigarettes altogether.
- Keep caffeine intake to a moderate level, and consider avoiding daily consumption of cola beverages.
- Exercise regularly, because exercise can reduce the risk of developing osteoporosis by making bones stronger and increasing their ability to absorb calcium.[61] Incorporate regular sessions of weight-bearing exercise, such as brisk walking, weight training, stair climbing, rope jumping, dancing, hiking, tennis, or aerobic dance classes, into your weekly schedule to slow and possibly even prevent bone loss.[62] Exercises designed to strengthen the back muscles and improve posture are also recommended, because they help the skeleton bear its burden of weight. Increased muscle strength and flexibility improve balance and help prevent debilitating falls.[63]
- For women at or nearing menopause, talk to your health care provider about the need for bone-density testing, medications, and nondrug treatments to slow bone loss after menopause.

Taking these steps to lower your risk of osteoporosis or to treat it if you already have it improves the chances of enjoying a quality life in your later years. Determine your own risk for osteoporosis by taking the quiz on the following page, which examines your current lifestyle for osteoporosis risk factors. The Box that follows offers additional resources regarding minerals and health.

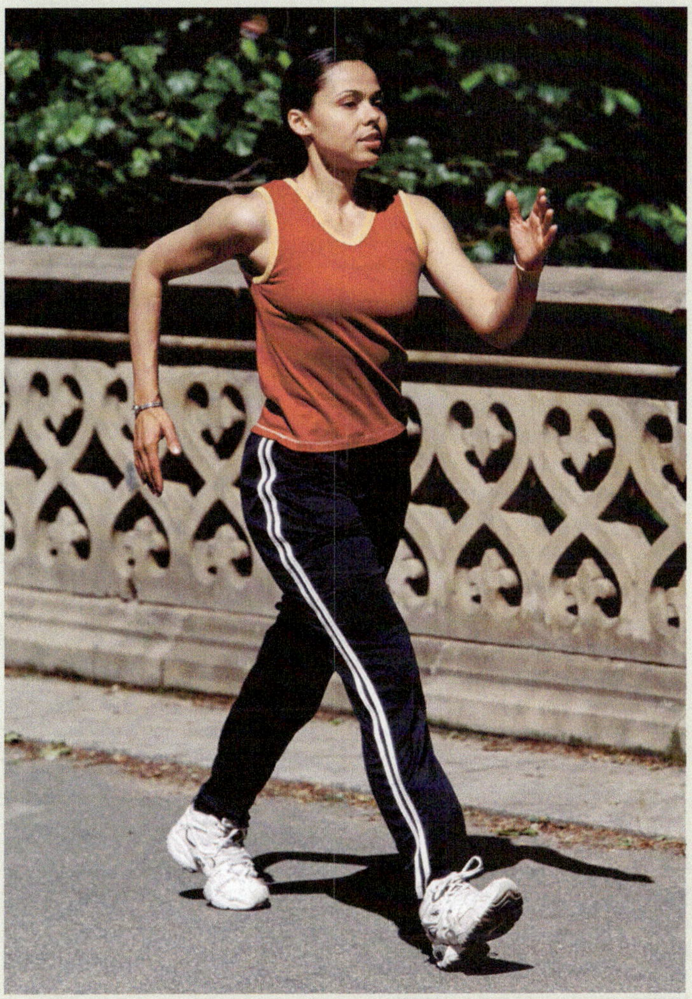
PCN Photography/Alamy Stock Photo

Incorporate regular sessions of weight-bearing exercise, such as brisk walking, into your weekly schedule to slow and possibly even prevent bone loss (for more about exercise, see Chapter 11).

Nutrition on the Web

http://fnic.nal.usda.gov

The Food and Nutrition Information Center (FNIC) provides credible and accurate information about vitamins and minerals. Browse by Subject to access links:

- Click on Dietary Guidance and then select Dietary Reference Intakes (DRIs).
- Click on Food Composition and then select Vitamins and Minerals.
- Click on Diet and Health and then select Osteoporosis.

www.eatright.org

The Academy of Nutrition and Dietetics home page includes many nutrition resources and links.

www.nationaldairycouncil.org

Search here for the latest in calcium and nutrition research.

www.nhlbi.nih.gov

The National Heart Lung and Blood Institute (NHLBI) provides up-to-date and practical information for preventing and controlling high blood pressure. Go to Health Topics, click on See All Health Topics, and scroll to high blood pressure.

www.nhlbi.nih.gov/health/health-topics/topics/dash

Access the DASH Eating Plan—"Lowering Your Blood Pressure with DASH"—from this government website.

www.niams.nih.gov/Health_Info/Bone

Search for information about bone health at this government website.

www.womenshealth.gov

Search the National Women's Health Information Center for information about bone health.

Do You Have a Bone-Healthy Lifestyle?

No matter what your age, your food and lifestyle choices make a difference to your bone health. How are you "banking" on bones? Give yourself 10 points for each "always," 5 points for each "sometimes," and zero for each "never."

Do You . . .	Always	Sometimes	Never
1. Eat three or more servings of milk, yogurt, cheese, or other calcium-rich foods?	☐	☐	☐
2. Drink vitamin D-fortified milk or get moderate exposure to sunlight?	☐	☐	☐
3. Keep your body moving—with at least 30 minutes of weight-bearing activity, at least 3 times weekly?	☐	☐	☐
4. Consume enough calories to maintain a healthy weight (not too thin)?	☐	☐	☐
5. Avoid cigarettes?	☐	☐	☐
6. Drink alcohol in moderation, if at all?[a]	☐	☐	☐
Score	_______ +	_______ +	_____ = _______

Scoring

A perfect 60: You are banking on beautiful bones as a lifelong investment. Toast to a perfect score with an ice-cold glass of milk!

35–55 points: For healthier bones, you'd be wise to improve your investment strategies. Otherwise, there may be future penalties.

30 or less points: Your calcium withdrawals may exceed your deposits. Make changes now before your window of opportunity closes.

[a] *Moderation* is defined as: Men: no more than two drinks per day (e.g., 12 ounces of beer or 5 ounces of wine); Women: no more than one drink per day.

SOURCE: *Banking on Beautiful Bones: A Lifelong Commitment to Calcium* (Rosemont, IL: National Dairy Council, 1998). Reprinted by permission.

Miniglossary

bisphosphonates Drugs that decrease the risk of fractures by acting on the bone-dismantling cells (osteoclasts) and inhibiting their resorption of bone tissue; examples are Fosamax, Actonel, Boniva, and Reclast.

bone density A measure of bone strength that reflects the degree of bone mineralization. The DEXA (dual-energy X-ray absorptiometry) bone-density test compares your bone density to that of a healthy young adult. Bone-density tests—using a dual beam of low-level X-rays—take a snapshot of bone density in the spine, wrist, and hip.

calcitonin A hormone used as a drug to decrease the rate of bone loss in osteoporosis. Administered as a nasal spray (Miacalcin) or by injection, calcitonin works by inhibiting the bone resorption activity of osteoclasts.

denosumab A drug (brand name Prolia™) in a class of medications called RANK ligand (RANKL) inhibitors. Administered by injection every 6 months, denosumab works by stopping the development of osteoclasts and thereby inhibiting their ability to damage bone.

designer estrogens Drugs that act like estrogen on *estrogen receptors* in osteoblasts to promote an increase in bone mass; an example is raloxifene (Evista). *Estrogen receptors* are cellular molecules that bind to estrogen, estrogen agonists/antagonists, or phytoestrogens and deliver these compounds to the nucleus of the cell.

estrogen A hormone; important in connection with nutrition because it maintains calcium balance and because its secretion abruptly declines at menopause.

estrogen/hormone therapy (ET/HT) Administration of estrogen to replace the natural hormone that declines with menopause. Because ET may increase the risk of uterine and breast cancer, *hormone replacement therapy* (the administration of a combination of estrogen with the hormone progesterone) is often used. However, the FDA recommends that HT and ET be considered only for women with significant risk of osteoporosis that outweighs the risk of the drugs (possible increased risk for breast cancer, stroke, and heart disease).

menopause The time of life at which a woman's menstrual cycle ceases, usually at about 45 to 50 years of age.

osteoblast A bone-building cell; responsible for formation of bone.

osteoclast A bone-destroying cell; responsible for resorption and removal of bone.

parathyroid hormone A hormone used as a drug to stimulate new bone formation; administered by injection once a day. Daily injections of teriparatide (brand name Forteo) lead to increased bone mineral density.

peak bone mass The highest bone density achieved for an individual; accumulated over the first three decades of life; typically occurs by 30 years of age. After age 30, bone resorption slowly begins to exceed bone formation.

WHAT'S ONLINE

MINDTAP From Cengage

Visit www.cengagebrain.com to access MindTap, a complete digital course that includes Diet & Wellness Plus, interactive quizzes, videos, and more.

USDA

United States Department of Agriculture

10 tips
Nutrition Education Series

MyPlate MyWins

Based on the **Dietary Guidelines for Americans**

Got your dairy today?

The Dairy Group includes milk, yogurt, cheese, and fortified soymilk. They provide calcium, vitamin D, potassium, protein, and other nutrients needed for good health throughout life. Choices should be low-fat or fat-free—to cut calories and saturated fat. How much is needed? Older children, teens, and adults need 3 cups* a day, while children 4 to 8 years old need 2½ cups, and children 2 to 3 years old need 2 cups.

1 "Skim" the fat

Drink fat-free (skim) or low-fat (1%) milk. If you currently drink whole milk, gradually switch to lower fat versions. This change cuts saturated fat and calories but doesn't reduce calcium or other essential nutrients.

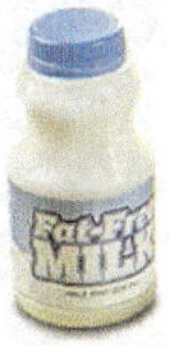

2 Boost potassium and vitamin D, and cut sodium

Choose fat-free or low-fat milk or yogurt more often than cheese. Milk and yogurt have more potassium and less sodium than most cheeses. Also, almost all milk and many yogurts are fortified with vitamin D.

3 Top off your meals

Use fat-free or low-fat milk on cereal and oatmeal. Top fruit salads and baked potatoes with low-fat yogurt instead of higher fat toppings such as sour cream.

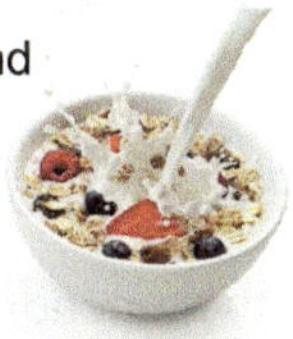

4 Choose cheeses with less fat

Many cheeses are high in saturated fat. Look for "reduced-fat" or "low-fat" on the label. Try different brands or types to find the one that you like.

5 What about cream cheese?

Cream cheese, cream, and butter are not part of the dairy food group. They are high in saturated fat and have little or no calcium.

6 Switch ingredients

When recipes such as dips call for sour cream, substitute plain yogurt. Use fat-free evaporated milk instead of cream, and try low-fat or fat-free ricotta cheese as a substitute for cream cheese.

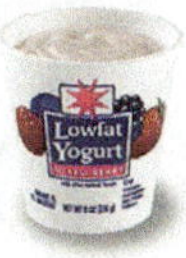

7 Limit added sugars

Flavored milks and yogurts, frozen yogurt, and puddings can contain a lot of added sugars. Get your nutrients from dairy foods with fewer or no added sugars.

8 Caffeinating?

If so, get your calcium along with your morning caffeine boost. Make or order coffee, a latte, or cappuccino with fat-free or low-fat milk.

9 Can't drink milk?

If you are lactose intolerant, try yogurt, lactose-free milk, or soymilk (soy beverage) to get your calcium. Calcium in some leafy greens is well absorbed, but eating several cups each day to meet calcium needs may be unrealistic.

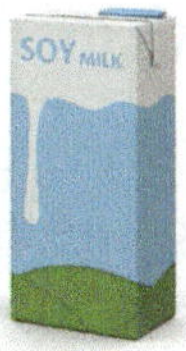

10 Take care of yourself and your family

Parents who drink milk and eat dairy foods show their kids that it is important for their health. Dairy foods are important to build the growing bones of kids and teens and to maintain bone health in adulthood.

* What counts as a cup in the Dairy Group? 1 cup of milk, yogurt, or soy beverage; 1½ ounces of natural cheese; or 2 ounces of processed cheese.

Center for Nutrition Policy and Promotion
USDA is an equal opportunity provider, employer, and lender.

Go to ChooseMyPlate.gov for more information.

DG TipSheet No. 5
June 2011
Revised October 2016

USDA

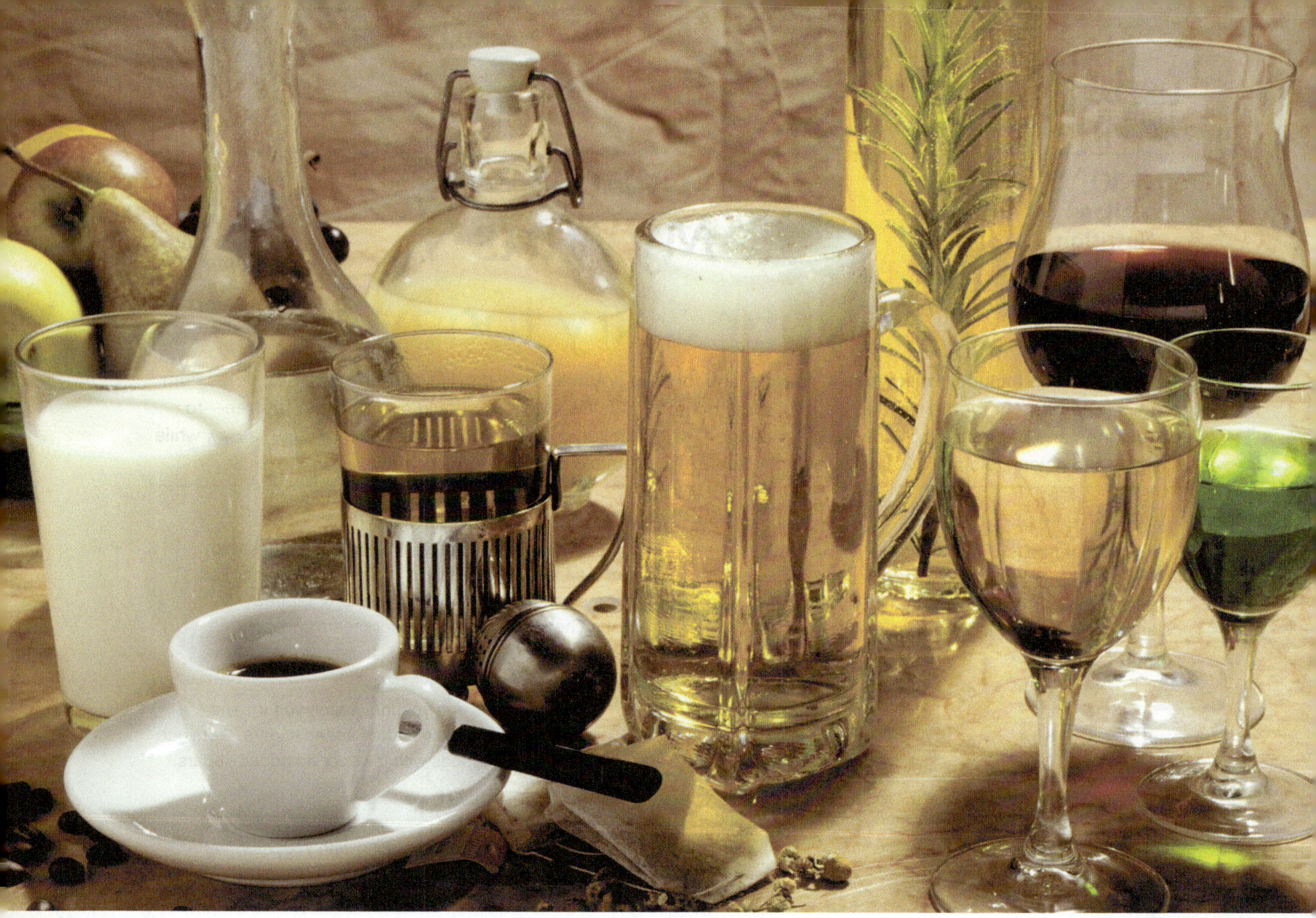

Bon Appetit/Alamy Stock Photo

Ask Yourself . . .

Which of the following statements about nutrition are true, and which are false? For each false statement, what is true?

1. Bottled water sold in the United States is always cleaner and safer than most tap water.
2. Caffeine can cross the placenta and enter the fetus.
3. Energy drinks are regulated and therefore always safe to consume.
4. Drinking alcohol may be associated with an increased risk of breast cancer.

Answers found on page 258.

Chapter Objectives

9.1 Describe the functions of water (fluid) in the body.

9.2 Identify strategies for selecting juices with maximum nutritional benefits.

9.3 List nutritional benefits derived from milk consumption.

9.4 Identify benefits and risks associated with consumption of caffeinated beverages.

9.5 List health concerns associated with functional beverages.

9.6 Identify factors that influence absorption and metabolism of alcohol.

9.7 Describe the effects of fetal exposure to alcohol.

Impact of Fluids and Beverages on Nutritional Health

CHAPTER 9

From the time humans first appeared on Earth, we have consumed a plethora of various beverages: breast milk, water, plant juices, animal fluids, fermented plant and animal products, and various mixtures. Beverages are used to quench thirst or provide recreation. Some beverages, such as wine, possess cultural and religious significance, whereas others are consumed for medicinal value. Beverages have even been specially formulated for use in outer space.[1]

> In wine there is wisdom, in beer there is strength, in water there is bacteria.
>
> —David Auerback, 2002

What do Americans drink now? This chapter discusses selected beverages and evaluates their impact on nutrition and health.

An individual's beverage choices can substantially affect the healthfulness of the overall diet. Plain water, coffee, and soft drinks are the beverages reported by the largest percentages of adults age 20 years and over. Men drink a combined total of about 11 cups of beverages per day, and women drink about 10 cups. Beverage groups consumed include:

- *100% juice:* Includes all fruit and vegetable juices that are 100 percent juice.
- *Alcoholic beverages:* Includes wine, beer, liquor, and mixed drinks.
- *Coffee:* Includes coffee and coffee-based drinks, such as latte and coffee made from presweetened mix.
- *Diet soft/other drinks:* Includes low-calorie versions of soft drinks (pop, soda), fruit drinks (fruit flavored or containing less than 100 percent juice), sports drinks, and energy drinks. Also includes carbonated water.
- *Milk and milk drinks:* Includes plain milk (whole, reduced-fat, low-fat, skim) and milk-based drinks such as chocolate milk, milk shakes, and hot cocoa.
- *Plain water:* Includes tap and noncarbonated bottled water without caloric sweeteners or additions.

FIGURE 9-1

Liquid Calories Consumed from Beverages

SOURCE: Adapted from R. P. LaComb and coauthors, Beverage choices of U.S. adults: What We Eat in America, USDA Dietary Surveys Research Group, Dietary Data Brief; available at www.ars.usda.gov.

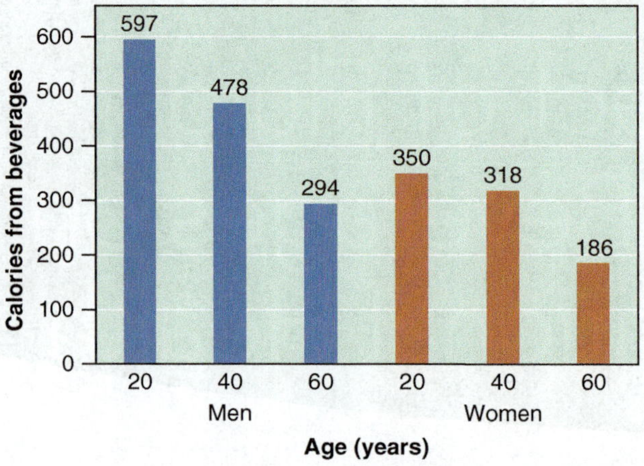

- *Regular soft/other drinks:* Includes regular (i.e., calorically sweetened) versions of soft drinks (pop, soda), fruit drinks (fruit flavored or containing less than 100 percent juice), sports drinks, and energy drinks.
- *Tea:* Includes tea and tea-based drinks, such as ready-to-drink sweet tea and tea made from presweetened mix.[2]

Overall, beverages provide 18 percent (385 calories/day) of total calories for adults, but the intake of calories from beverages varies by age, with young men consuming the largest amounts (see Figure 9-1). Sweetened beverages also provide high proportions of adults' daily intakes of added sugars. Table 9-1 offers tips for making beverage choices.

TABLE 9-1 **Rethink Your Drink**

As you can see below, calories from drinks can really add up. But there is good news: you have plenty of options for reducing the number of calories in what you drink. Substituting no- or low-calorie drinks for sugar-sweetened beverages cuts about 650 calories in the example below.

Occasion	Instead of...	Calories	Try...	Calories
Morning coffee shop run	Medium café latte (16 ounces) made with whole milk	265	Small café latte (12 ounces) made with fat-free milk	125
Lunchtime combo meal	20-oz. bottle of nondiet cola with your lunch	227	Bottle of water or diet soda	0
Afternoon break	Sweetened lemon iced tea from the vending machine (16 ounces)	180	Sparkling water with natural lemon flavor (not sweetened)	0
Dinnertime	A glass of nondiet ginger ale with your meal (12 ounces)	124	Water with a slice of lemon or lime, or seltzer water with a splash of 100% fruit juice	0 calories for the water with fruit slice, or about 30 calories for seltzer water with 2 ounces of 100% orange juice.
Total beverage calories:		796		125–155

SOURCE: Department of Health and Human Services, Centers for Disease Control and Prevention; USDA National Nutrient Database for Standard Reference.

ASK YOURSELF ANSWERS: **1.** False. Depending on the brand, bottled water may itself be tap water. **2.** True. **3.** False. Energy drinks are not regulated; therefore, manufacturers do not have to prove the safety or efficacy of these products. **4.** True.

9.1 Water

Adults consume and excrete some 1½ to 3 quarts of water a day (see Figure 9-2). Although most of the water we take in comes from juice, milk, soft drinks, and other beverages, including tap water, foods also add considerable amounts of water to the diet. For example, water makes up as much as 85 to 95 percent of fruits and vegetables. Adults are advised to consume 1.0 to 1.5 milliliters of water from all sources for each calorie expended. For instance, if you expend 2,000 calories a day, you need approximately 2 quarts of fluid.[3]

Just as the sources of water in our diet vary, so too does the water we drink "straight." The makeup of water differs depending on where it comes from and how it is processed—variations that can have significant health implications. One of the most basic distinctions, hard versus soft water, is based on concentrations of three minerals: calcium, magnesium, and sodium. **Hard water** usually comes from shallow ground and contains relatively high levels of minerals, primarily calcium and magnesium. **Soft water**, in contrast, generally flows from deep in the earth and has a higher concentration of sodium.

Although your water utility company can tell you whether your water is soft or hard, you can probably distinguish between the two based on your own experience. Soft water helps soap lather better than hard water and leaves less of a ring on the bathtub. Hard water, to the contrary, doesn't clean clothes as thoroughly as soft water and leaves a residue of rocklike crystals on the inside of the teakettle over time. That's why many consumers prefer soft water.

hard water Water that has a high mineral (calcium and magnesium) content.

soft water Water containing a high sodium concentration and little or no calcium or magnesium.

From a health standpoint, however, hard water seems to be the better alternative.[4] One reason is that the excess sodium carried in soft water, even in small amounts, adds more of that mineral to our already sodium-laden diets. More important, soft water dissolves potentially toxic substances, such as lead, from pipes. Therefore, people who install water softeners in their homes for the purpose of getting cleaner laundry and better mileage from soap would do well to connect them only to their hot-water lines. That way, they can use hot, soft water for washing and bathing and use cold, hard water for drinking and cooking.

FIGURE 9-2

Water Balance in the Body

Water enters the body in liquids and foods, and some water is created in the body as a by-product of metabolic processes. Water leaves the body through the evaporation of sweat, in the moisture of exhaled breath, in urine, and in feces.

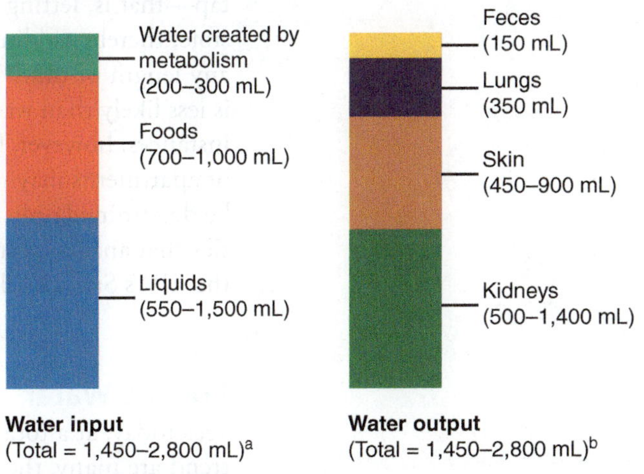

[a]This amount equals 1½ to 3 quarts (1 oz equals approximately 30 mL).

[b]Adults are advised to consume 1.0 to 1.5 mL of water from all sources for each calorie expended. For instance, if you require 2,000 calories a day, you need approximately 2 quarts of fluid.

$$2{,}000 \text{ cal} \times 1 \text{ mL/cal} = 2{,}000 \text{ mL}$$
$$2{,}000 \text{ mL} \div 30 \text{ mL/1 oz} = 67 \text{ oz}$$
$$67 \text{ oz} \div 32 \text{ oz/qt} = 2 \text{ qt}$$

SOURCE: Adapted from F. Sizer and E. Whitney, *Nutrition: Concepts and Controversies*, 11th ed. (Belmont, CA: Thomson Wadsworth, 2008), 273. Information on fluid requirements from S. Kleiner, Water: An essential but overlooked nutrient, *Journal of the American Dietetic Association* 99 (1999): 200.

Keeping Water Safe

In addition to having varying concentrations of minerals, water taken from the earth contains different levels of bacteria, microorganisms, and heavy metals such as lead. To ensure that water flowing from the tap is safe to drink, the Environmental Protection Agency (EPA), the arm of the U.S. government responsible for monitoring municipal water supplies, sets limits for potential contaminants such as mercury, nitrate, and silver in drinking water. By law, the public must be notified by a water utility company within 24 hours of the discovery of any potentially dangerous contaminants in drinking water. The EPA also mandates that tap water be disinfected if bacteria levels run high, to prevent the spread of waterborne diseases such as typhoid and dysentery. Such precautionary measures go a long way toward keeping the U.S. water supply one of the safest in the world.

One potential contaminant is a parasite called *Cryptosporidium*. Found in lakes and rivers that have come into contact with sewage or animal waste, *Cryptosporidium* has emerged as a health threat to vulnerable people because it is highly resistant to the chlorine and other disinfectants used in municipal water supplies. In healthy people, the parasite can cause diarrhea and other flu-like symptoms that typically subside within a week to 10 days. In people with weak immune systems, however, this parasite can lead to severe, long-lasting gastrointestinal problems that can even cause death.

Because of the *Cryptosporidium* hazard, the EPA and the Centers for Disease Control and Prevention recommend special precautions for people with severely weakened immune systems (those with HIV infection, cancer, transplant patients taking immunosuppressive drugs, and people born with a weakened immune system). Public health groups advise such individuals to talk to a health care provider about boiling tap water for 1 minute (if it is meant to be used for drinking water) to destroy any *Cryptosporidium* present, or about buying a special water filter system.[5]

Another potential health threat over which the EPA has little control is the level of lead that comes out of your faucet. Although the EPA has put a ceiling on the concentration of lead that may be present in public water supplies, once the water leaves the reservoir, unhealthy levels of the metal may dissolve into it. Before the water comes out of your faucet, it may flow through pipes made of lead or joined by lead solder; the metal can leach into the water as it passes through. Even though the U.S. government banned the use of lead-containing plumbing systems back in 1986, dwellings (and portions of public water systems) built before that time may not have lead-free pipes.

The issue of possible lead contamination in water has generated a good deal of publicity and concern. Certainly, the attention is warranted, given that when lead accumulates in the body, it begins to damage the nerves, kidneys, and liver along with the cardiovascular, reproductive, immunologic, and gastrointestinal systems. Lead is especially toxic to children and fetuses, in whom it can cause neurologic problems as severe as brain damage.[6]

Luckily, lead levels can usually be kept to a minimum simply by "flushing" the tap—that is, letting the water run for about a minute until it becomes as cold as possible, thereby ridding it of water that has been sitting in pipes and dissolving lead for any length of time. Pipes should be flushed with cold water only, because cold water is less likely than warm or hot water to pick up lead as it flows through them. In some instances, however, flushing is not enough to reduce harmful lead levels. Some homes or apartments may require special water treatment systems, the necessity of which can be determined only by subjecting tap water to a lead test. Names of certified laboratories that analyze water can be obtained from a local branch of the EPA, or by calling the EPA's Safe Drinking Water Hotline (800-426-4791).

Bottled Water Bottled water has become one of America's most popular beverages today, at a total cost of more than $12 billion a year.[7] Although reasons for this trend are many, the perceived health benefits of bottled water fall near the top of the list. Surveys have found that about 25 percent of bottled-water drinkers choose the beverage for health and safety reasons, and another 25 percent believe that bottled water is pure and free of contaminants.[8]

Regardless of its pristine image, bottled water is not necessarily any more pure or healthful than water that flows out of the tap. The Food and Drug Administration (FDA), the watchdog of the bottled-water industry, does not require that bottled water meet higher standards for quality, such as the maximum level of contaminants, than public water supplies regulated by the EPA. For the most part, the FDA simply follows EPA's regulatory lead. Typically, bottled water is filtered to remove chemicals such as chlorine that may impart a certain taste, but that doesn't make it any safer. In fact, some bottled water comes from the same municipal water supplies as tap water.[9] Furthermore, some bottled waters do not contain any or enough of the

Miniglossary for Bottled Water

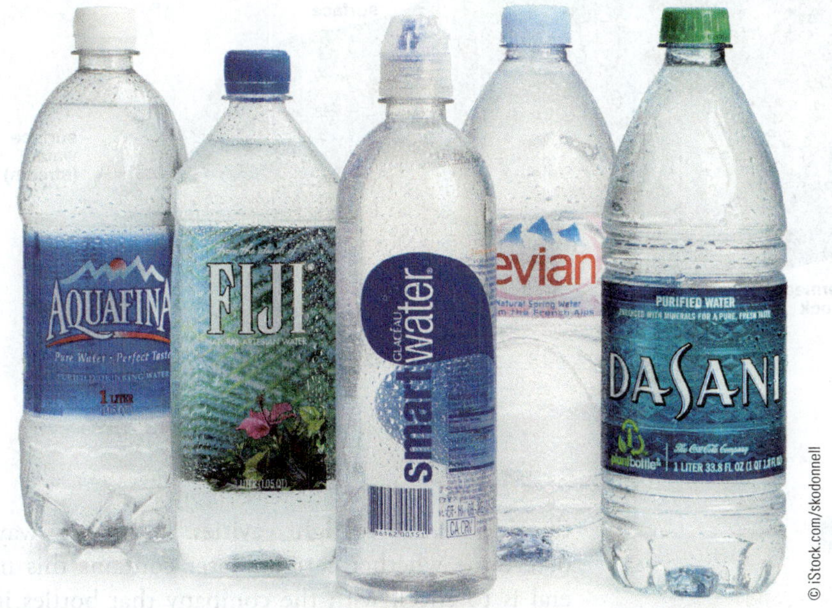

© iStock.com/skodonnell

The Food and Drug Administration classifies some bottled water according to its origin (Figure 9-3).

artesian water or artesian well water Water drawn from a well that taps a confined water-bearing rock or rock formation.

ground water Water that comes from an underground body of water that does not come into contact with any surface water.

mineral water Water that is drawn from an underground source and contains at least 250 parts per million of dissolved solids. If the water contains between 250 and 500 parts per million total dissolved solids, the statement "low mineral content" must appear. If it contains more than 1,500 parts per million, the statement "high mineral content" must appear. If a cup of the water contains at least 20 milligrams of calcium, 0.36 milligram of iron, or 5 milligrams of sodium, the product must carry nutrition labeling.

purified water (also known as demineralized water, distilled water, deionized water, or reverse osmosis water) Water from which all minerals have been removed, thereby eliminating the possibility that the minerals might corrode pipes or appliances (such as a steam iron).

sparkling bottled water Water in which carbon dioxide (the ingredient that makes soda pop bubbly) is naturally present; that is, carbonation is not added from an outside source.

spring water Water derived from an underground formation from which water flows naturally to the surface of the earth and to which minerals have not been added or taken away. It may be collected either at the spring itself or through a hole tapping the underground formation feeding the spring.

well water Ground water derived from a rock formation by way of a hole bored, drilled, or otherwise constructed in the ground.

from a community water system or from a municipal source Statement that must appear on bottles containing water derived from a municipal water supply. The phrase must conspicuously precede or follow the name of the brand.

seltzer* Tap water injected with carbon dioxide and containing no added salts.

club soda* Artificially carbonated water containing added salts and minerals.

tonic water* Artificially carbonated water with added sugar and/or high-fructose corn syrup, sodium, and quinine.

---

*These items are not considered bottled water in government parlance. The FDA defines *bottled water* as water that is sealed in bottles or other containers and is intended for human consumption, excluding soda, seltzer, flavored, and vended water products.

FIGURE 9-3

Origins of Bottled Water

SOURCE: A. C. Bullers, "Bottled water: Better Than the Tap?" *FDA Consumer Magazine*, July–August 2002.

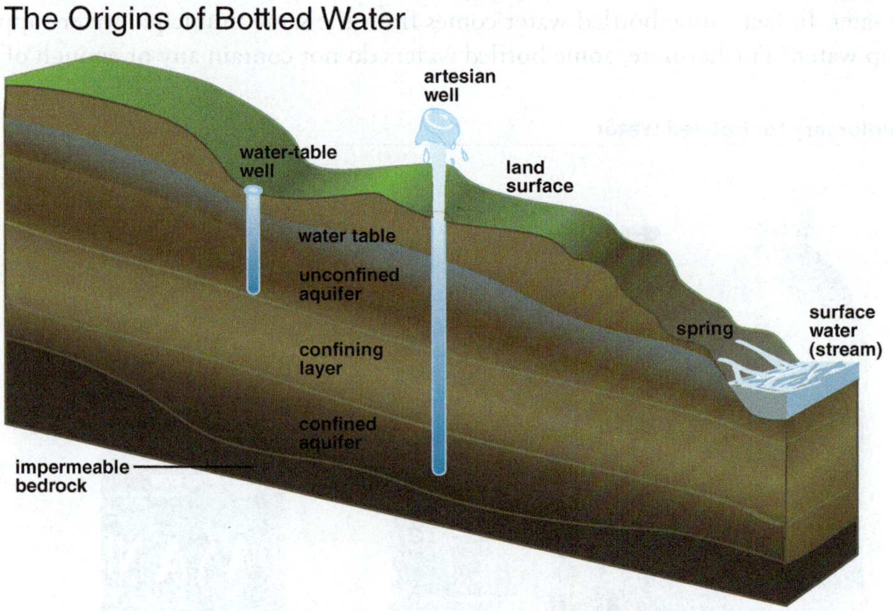

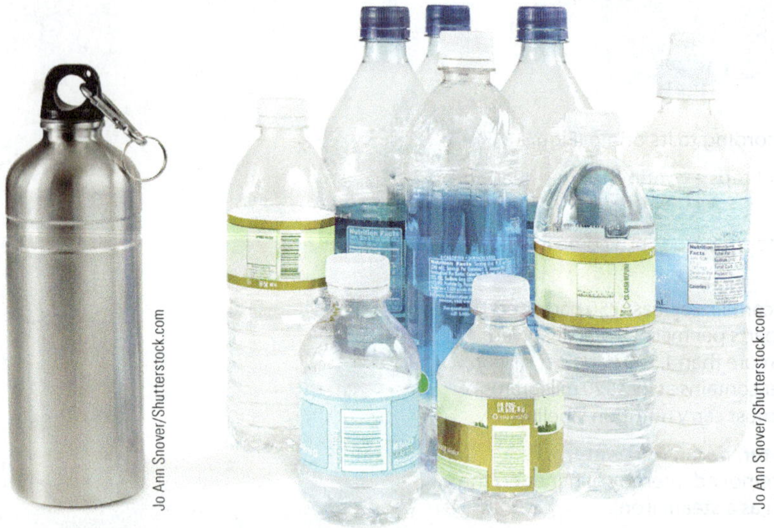

Consider using a refillable water bottle to save money and help the environment. Millions of barrels of oil are used to produce and transport disposable plastic water bottles to consumers, and the majority of these bottles end up in landfills or waterways.

fluoride needed to fight cavities.[10] The only way to determine whether certain water contains this mineral is to check with the company that bottles it. If you use bottled water, look for the trademark of the International Bottled Water Association (IBWA)—a trade organization that supports the FDA regulations.

This is not to say that bottled water is necessarily any better or worse, from a health standpoint, than tap water. It's certainly preferable to tap water for those who like its taste. The problem is that the demand for bottled water increases the use of nonrenewable resources to make the plastic bottles, which in turn creates an energy demand for recycling the used bottles. Additionally, many consumers pay 250 to 10,000 times more per gallon for bottled water than for tap water because they think bottled water is more healthful. Bottlers add to the confusion by sprinkling terms such as *pure*, *crystal pure*, and *premium* on labels illustrated with pictures of glaciers, mountain streams, and waterfalls, even when the water inside comes from a public reservoir. However, the FDA has set forth regulations mandating clear labeling of bottled waters. The Miniglossary for bottled water explains what some of the terms used on bottles actually mean.

9.2 Juices

It is hard to believe that once upon a time, the only choices of juice in supermarkets were orange, grapefruit, grape, and cranberry. Now there is an apparently infinite assortment of not only juices, but also blended fruit and vegetable juices. You've already learned that fruit and vegetable juices are great sources of antioxidants and phytochemicals that help fight diseases like heart disease, cancer, and diabetes. You've also learned that any fruit or vegetable juice you enjoy can count toward the MyPlate recommendations for these food groups.

Is there a downside to fruit and vegetable juices? There can be. It is very important to be a conscientious label reader when selecting juices. Juices can add extra calories, and not all juices are uniformly beneficial. The best nutritional choice is 100 percent fruit/vegetable juice. "Juice drinks," "fruit-flavored drinks," or "juice blends" contain little real juice, but serve up quite a bit of added sugar. Remember, too, that even 100 percent fruit/vegetable juice lacks the fiber of the whole fruit or vegetable. Additionally, some juices use concentrated white grape juice as a sweetener, making the beverage higher in simple sugar and calories even though the label can truthfully claim that the beverage is 100 percent fruit juice.[11]

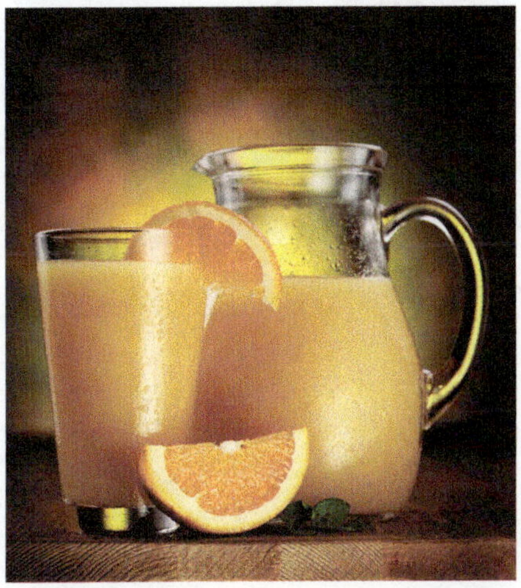

Valentyn Volkov/Shutterstock.com

Juices with Benefits After making sure your juice is 100 percent pure juice, look at the color of the juice. As a general rule, the more colorful the juice is, or the darker its color, the more nutritious the juice is. One example is pink grapefruit juice, which contains two phytochemicals not found in regular grapefruit juice that function as antioxidants: lycopene and beta-carotene. Cranberry juice products available commercially vary extensively, but 10 to 12 ounces of 27 percent cranberry juice per day may be protective against urinary tract infections in people at risk for recurring infections, according to limited evidence.[12] Cranberry juice also contains phytochemicals that are believed to protect against heart disease and cancer.[13]

Citrus fruits and juices are rich in vitamins (vitamin C, folate) and flavonoids (phytochemicals) that help reduce overall rate of cancer occurrence. Ounce for ounce, orange juice is the most nutrient-dense juice consumed in the United States. Additionally, citrus juices are rich in potassium and low in sodium content, which may reduce risk of high blood pressure and stroke.[14] The best orange juice, of course, is freshly squeezed; the packaged orange juice you purchase in stores loses vitamin C content daily. Compared to orange juice purchased in gable-top cartons, orange juice sold in plastic jugs retains vitamin C content the best, losing only 2 percent of its vitamin C daily. Orange juice stored in gable-top cartons will have lost most of its vitamin C content by its expiration date.[15]

Orange juice fortified with calcium is also available. Each ounce of calcium-fortified orange juice provides the same amount of absorbable calcium as an ounce of milk. This is an easy way to get calcium or increase calcium intake if you don't like or cannot consume dairy foods.

Tomatoes and tomato products are rich in nutrients and the phytochemical lycopene. Lycopene has been found to be protective against prostate cancer and cardiovascular disease. One word of caution: Salt is often added to tomato products, especially tomato juice. Those with high blood pressure or at risk for high blood pressure may prefer to use low-sodium versions of these products.[16]

9.3 Milk

"Drink milk, for it wipes away heat from the heart, strengthens the back, increases the brain, augments the intelligence, renews vision, and drives away forgetfulness."[17] Humans are the only mammals that consume milk past infancy. Milk is a white, opaque liquid made by mammary glands, but the term *milk* is also applied to non-animal beverages such as soy milk. Milk is the infant's principal source of nutrition before maturation of the gastrointestinal tract and ability to digest other types of foods. Nutritional composition of milk differs widely among mammal species. For example, cow's milk contains a relatively high percentage of protein compared to human milk due to the much larger size of calves as compared to human infants. This and other differences make human milk an unsuitable substitute for cow's milk for the calf since it would not support the growth of such a large animal. Likewise, cow's milk is an unsuitable substitute for human infants because the high protein

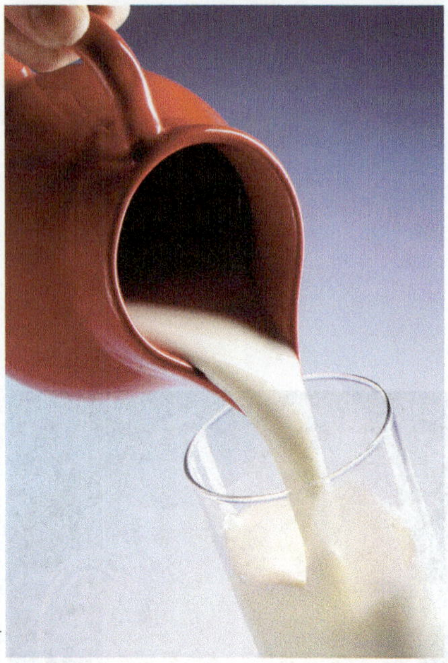
Chepko Danil Vitalevich/Shutterstock.com

content damages the human infant's immature gastrointestinal tract and puts stress on the kidneys to excrete the excessive amount of protein.

Being a nutrient-dense food (providing a high concentration of nutrients in relation to caloric content), milk supplies significant amounts of protein, calcium, phosphorus, riboflavin, vitamin A, vitamin D, potassium, magnesium, vitamin B_6, vitamin B_{12}, and zinc to the human diet.[18] Additionally, milk/calcium intake has been related to weight control.[19] There appears to be an inverse relationship between intakes of calcium/dairy foods and obesity, but these results remain controversial.[20] Lower dairy intake seems to equal higher amounts of body fat, and higher intakes of milk and dairy foods may have modest benefits in facilitating weight reduction.[21]

Despite all it has going for it (and us!), total per capita milk consumption has declined since 1970. The greatest decline was observed for adolescents age 12 to 19 years, whose average intake of milk decreased by nearly one-half—from about 1¾ cup per day in 1978 to slightly less than 1 cup today.[22] This is attributed to the displacement of milk by carbonated beverages, fruit juices, fruit drinks, flavored teas, and nondairy milks. Innovative advertising campaigns seek to reverse this trend and increase milk consumption, including consumption of flavored milks.[23]

9.4 Caffeinated Beverages: Coffee, Tea, Cocoa, and Soft Drinks

Caffeine is a chemical compound containing four of the most common elements on earth: carbon, hydrogen, nitrogen, and oxygen. At room temperature, caffeine resembles cornstarch in its powdery consistency, is odorless, is slightly bitter to the taste, and is highly soluble in hot water. Caffeine is one of a group of chemicals called *xanthines*.[24] In the United States, most caffeine is consumed in coffee, but significant amounts are also consumed in teas, some carbonated soft drinks, and energy drinks.

In 1657, when merchants first introduced Londoners to a Middle Eastern brew known as *coffee*, they touted it as a "wholesome and physical drink," an elixir of health suitable for treating colds, coughs, gout, and many other ills.[25] Today, at least 8 out of 10 Americans consume caffeine, the most widely used behaviorally active drug in the world. Modern-day coffee drinkers have been subjected to a barrage of reports linking coffee and other caffeine-containing products with both positive and negative health effects.

Scientists have yet to confirm long-standing suspicions that caffeine contributes to any health problems other than jitteriness. One reason for all the controversy is that much of the evidence linking the substance with different diseases has been clouded by a number of methodological issues in the studies. Some studies do not measure caffeine sources except for coffee and tea, excluding soft drinks, chocolate, and certain medications. In addition, most studies fail to account for the fact that the amount of caffeine and other substances in coffee or tea can vary considerably depending on how the beverage is brewed.

For example, consider the widely debated question of whether drinking coffee raises blood cholesterol. Some evidence suggests that the beverage does contribute to high blood cholesterol and therefore to heart disease. The hitch is that most of the evidence comes from Scandinavia, where coffee is boiled rather than brewed in automatic drip coffeemakers or electric percolators. Subsequent research has found that although boiled coffee appears to boost blood cholesterol levels, filtered coffee does not, most likely because substances in boiled coffee other than caffeine may be the cholesterol-raising culprits.[26]

Consuming caffeine day in and day out can be habit forming, as anyone who cannot get going in the morning without a cup of coffee or can of caffeinated soda is well aware. In fact, some researchers have identified a condition called **caffeine dependence syndrome**, characterized by at least three of the four following criteria: withdrawal

caffeine A type of compound, called a methylxanthine, found in coffee beans, cola nuts, cocoa beans, and tea leaves. A central nervous system stimulant, caffeine's effects include increasing the heart rate, boosting urine production, and raising the metabolic rate.

caffeine dependence syndrome Dependence on caffeine characterized by at least three of the four following criteria: withdrawal symptoms such as headache and fatigue; caffeine consumption despite knowledge that it may be causing harm; repeated, unsuccessful attempts to cut back on caffeine; and tolerance to caffeine.

symptoms such as headache and fatigue; caffeine consumption despite knowledge that it may be causing harm; repeated, unsuccessful attempts to cut back on caffeine; and tolerance to caffeine.[27]

Along with people who are dependent on caffeine, people with certain medical conditions would do well to consume caffeine in moderation or avoid it completely. Pregnant women, for example, should limit their caffeine intake.[28] Although it has never been proven to cause birth defects, caffeine does readily cross the placenta and enter the fetus. Some limited research also suggests that the amount of caffeine in three or four cups of coffee could raise the risk of suffering a miscarriage, perhaps by decreasing blood flow through the placenta.[29] Women who drink caffeine during pregnancy are generally advised to limit consumption to less than 200 milligrams per day—the equivalent of about 12 ounces of coffee.[30] In addition, anyone with ulcers should steer clear of both caffeinated *and* decaffeinated coffee, because both stimulate the secretion of acid, which can irritate the stomach lining. Chapter 11 discusses the effect of caffeine on physical performance.

For a healthy person, drinking one to three cups of coffee, tea, or cola a day does not seem to pose any hazard.[31] Only those who are particularly sensitive to caffeine and suffer symptoms such as headaches, nervousness, and insomnia after consuming it really need to consider avoiding it—or at least cutting back (see Table 9-2 to figure out how much caffeine you're taking in each day).

TABLE 9-2 Caffeine Countdown

Drinks and Foods	Average Caffeine Content (milligrams)
Coffee (8-oz cup)	
Brewed, drip method	95–150
Instant	65–75
Decaffeinated, brewed or instant	3
Espresso (2-oz cup)	80
Tea (8-oz cup)	
Brewed, black, steeped for 3 minutes	47
Brewed, green (8 oz cup)	30
Iced tea (8-oz glass)	25
Soft drinks (12-oz can)	
Colas, regular or diet	30–36
Mountain Dew, Mello Yello	45–51
Energy drinks	
Amp; Full Throttle (8 oz)	70
Energy shot (1 oz)	100–350
Jolt; Kick (12 oz)	56–72
Red Bull (8 oz)	80
Chocolate milk or hot cocoa (8 oz)	5–8
Milk chocolate candy (1 oz)	6–15
Drugs*	**Average Caffeine Content (mg)**
Pain relievers (standard extra-strength dose)	
Excedrin, Bayer, Midol	120–130
Stimulants (2 tablets)	
NoDoz, Vivarin	200

*Because products change, contact the manufacturer for an update on products you use regularly.

If you drink coffee or a can or two of cola every day and decide to quit, do it gradually. Even moderate caffeine users who try to stop cold turkey often suffer from withdrawal symptoms, such as splitting headaches, fatigue, moodiness, and nausea. Try instead to cut back gradually by, say, drinking no more than one cup every two or three days. Another way to cut back on caffeine is to mix some decaffeinated grounds in with your regular coffee and gradually use more and more decaf and less regular. Likewise, you can drink a can of decaffeinated soda now and then until you've weaned yourself off the caffeine.

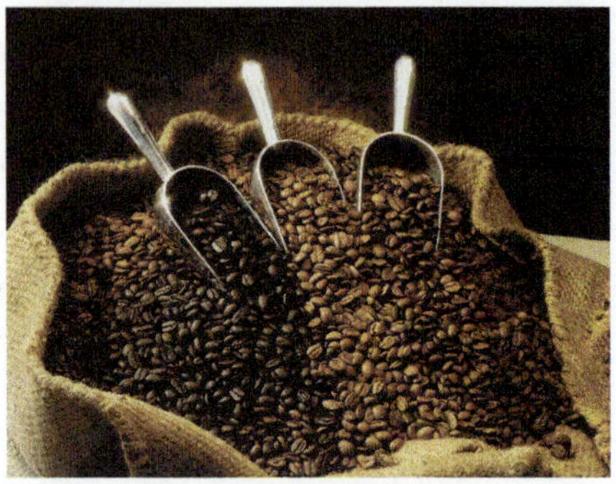
PhotoDisk/Getty Images

Coffee Coffee is one of the most widely consumed beverages in the world. Can it also be a beneficial drink healthwise? According to recent research, the answer may be yes! A growing body of research shows that coffee drinkers, compared to nondrinkers, may be less likely to develop type 2 diabetes, stroke, depression, and other degenerative diseases, including Parkinson's and Alzheimer's.[32] Habitual coffee consumption appears to be associated with a lower risk of type 2 diabetes. It is not known exactly how this apparent protective mechanism works. It may well be that the antioxidant and anti-inflammatory properties of the phytochemicals found in coffee help control cell damage that can be a factor in development of type 2 diabetes. Whatever the mechanism, it is not the caffeine in coffee affording the benefits: Decaffeinated coffee alone offers the same degree of protection.[33]

The antioxidants found in coffee have also been found to inhibit inflammation and thereby reduce risk of cardiovascular and other inflammatory diseases. The most protective effect was found at a dose of 1 to 3 cups of coffee (caffeinated or decaffeinated) per day.[34] Moderate consumption of coffee may also reduce the risk of stroke when compared to non-coffee drinkers.[35] These anti-inflammatory properties of coffee may explain why coffee appears to reduce the risk of alcohol-related cirrhosis and liver cancer.[36] In fact, regular moderate coffee consumption appears to provide a modest protective benefit from all causes of death in both men and women.[37]

To be sure, the antioxidants in coffee may protect us from inflammatory diseases, but it remains prudent to remember that the caffeine in coffee can have negative effects on some people (review the preceding section). For adults consuming 2 to 3 cups of coffee a day, there is little indication of health risks and some suggestion of health benefits. Nevertheless, coffee consumption is linked with increases in cardiovascular disease risk factors such as blood pressure in people with uncontrolled hypertension. This finding implies that individuals with uncontrolled high blood pressure may be more vulnerable to the adverse effects of caffeine.[38]

Tea "Of all the beverages consumed today, tea is undoubtedly one of the oldest, most widely known, and most widely consumed. Consumption was introduced to the world by traders and travelers."[39] The method by which tea is processed determines whether green, black, or oolong is produced. Green tea is made by steaming fresh leaves at high temperatures, followed by a sequence of drying and rolling steps, resulting in tea that is for the most part the same chemical composition as the fresh leaves. Black tea is fermented. The extent of the fermentation period determines the chemical composition of the tea; hence, the chemical composition of most black teas differs.[40] Oolong is produced by "solar withering" of tea leaves followed by partial fermentation.[41]

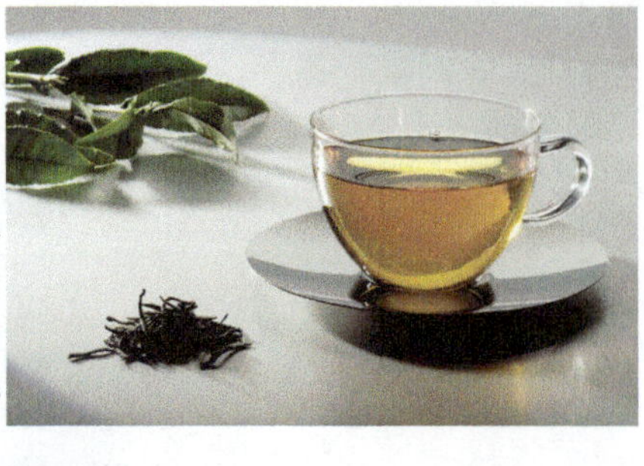
Hugh Threlfall/Alamy Stock Photo

Tea leaves are rich in phytochemicals, antioxidants, and caffeine, among a myriad of other chemicals. The amount of caffeine in a serving of tea is usually less than half the caffeine in a serving of coffee, but actual caffeine content can vary widely depending on the specific blend of tea and the brew strength.[42]

Health benefits most frequently associated with tea include:[43]

- Lowers risk of cardiovascular disease by
    - Reducing inflammation
    - Decreasing total cholesterol
    - Decreasing LDL-cholesterol
    - Protecting against blood clot formation
    - Decreasing blood pressure
- Decreases risk of cancer by
    - Inhibiting carcinogenesis
    - Suppressing formation of carcinogenic substances
    - Increasing the effectiveness of a number of chemotherapeutic agents
- Protects against neurodegenerative diseases by
    - Decreasing plaque formation associated with Alzheimer's disease
    - Raising dopamine levels to ward off Parkinson's disease
    - Protecting against deterioration of brain function

The health benefits of tea appear to be dose dependent, meaning that drinking more tea provides the greatest effect.[44]

Cocoa Cocoa is indigenous to equatorial rain forests of Central and South America, where it was utilized as a beverage, food, and drug by the Olmec, Mayan, and Aztec empires preceding its introduction to Europe in the 1500s. According to Mayan and Aztec religions, cocoa was discovered by the gods and was prepared as a beverage. Perceived as an intoxicating food, the cocoa beverage was reserved for use only by adult males, specifically priests, highest government officials, military officers, distinguished warriors, and occasionally sacrificial victims for ritual purposes.[45]

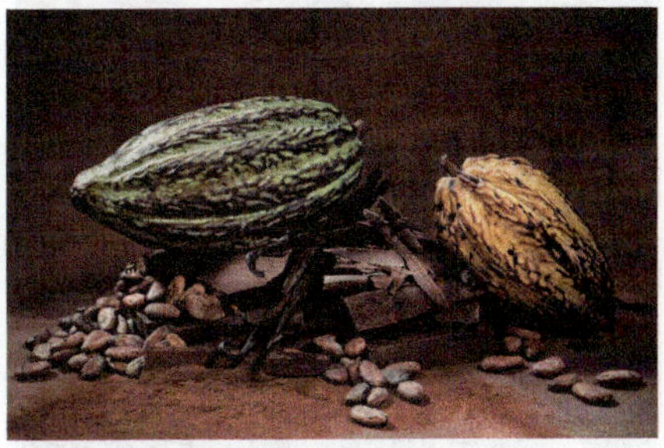

©iStock.com/Maceofoto

Chocolate was introduced to Europe in 1544 by Mayan nobles who were taken to Spain by Dominican friars. Within a century, culinary and medicinal use of chocolate expanded to France, England, and other countries in western Europe.[46] Although the confectionery history of chocolate is familiar to almost everyone, only recently, in the late 20th century, have the health benefits of chocolate returned to the forefront.

Cocoa contains several minerals (potassium, magnesium, phosphorus, and calcium among others), although mineral composition varies among different cocoa varieties and even within the same variety depending on how the cocoa is processed. Other nutrients found in cocoa are fats and proteins, in addition to antioxidants, phytochemicals, and caffeine. As with coffee and tea, cocoa and chocolate (more specifically, dark chocolate) may positively influence cardiovascular health by some of the same mechanisms.[47]

Soft Drinks Whether you call it soda, pop, soda pop, coke, or fizzy drinks (United Kingdom), you are probably talking about a carbonated soft drink. To be precise, a *soft drink* is a beverage that does not contain alcohol; for the purposes of

Miniglossary of Soft-Drink Ingredients

Ever wonder about the ingredients used to make soft drinks? (As with any other food, ingredients used in soft drinks are approved and regulated by the U.S. Food and Drug Administration.) Depending on the product, ingredients may include:

filtered water Regular soft drinks are 90 percent water, and diet soft drinks can contain up to 95 percent water.

carbon dioxide Provides a unique taste (when mixed with water) and the characteristic "pop" you hear and "fizz" you see when you open a bottle or can.

flavors Most soft drinks contain a combination of many individual flavors (some are natural, some are fruit-flavored extracts, others are herbs, spices, or artificial flavors).

colors Obtained from natural and synthetic sources.

acidulants Add tartness and act as a preservative; usually in the form of phosphoric acid and citric acid, although sometimes malic acid or tartaric acid are used.

preservatives The acidity and carbonation of soft drinks usually keep the drinks from spoiling, but some soft drinks contain small amounts of preservatives to improve their shelf life.

potassium Found naturally in the water used to make soft drinks and in some of the flavoring agents and other ingredients used.

sodium Present in small quantities.

regular sweeteners Most soft drinks are sweetened with high-fructose corn syrup (HFCS).

low-calorie sweeteners Aspartame, saccharin, sucralose, stevia, neotame, and acesulfame K are approved for use in soft drinks.

SOURCE: The American Beverage Association. www.ameribev.org.

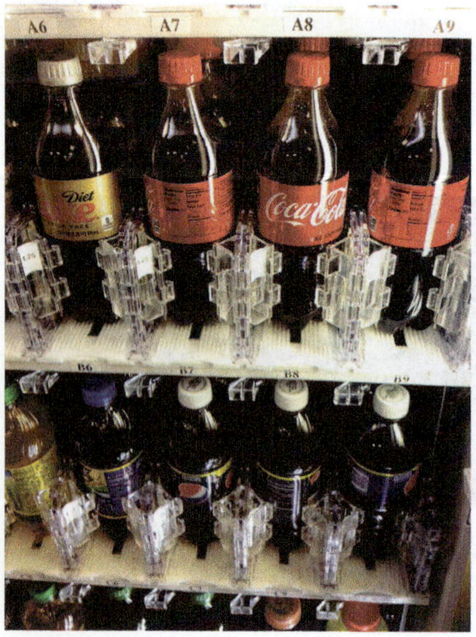
Lissandra Melo/Shutterstock.com

Increase in serving sizes of soft drinks

Standard serving size
- 1950s—6.5 oz
- 1960s—12 oz
- 1990s—20 oz
- 2000+—32 oz & 64 oz

this chapter, though, *soft drink* refers to a cold, carbonated, sweetened (sugar or non-caloric) beverage.

The history of soft drinks dates back to the medieval Middle East. The earliest soft drinks were made of fruit juices or extracts of flowers or herbs combined with sugar and water to form a syrup that was later added to water, ice, or even snow.[48] The first noncarbonated soft drinks appeared in the 17th century, and the process of carbonating water was soon mastered in the 18th century. Carbonated water soon led to flavored carbonated water: American pharmacists began adding herbs and chemicals for flavoring to carbonated water in the 19th century. Root beer, Coca-Cola, Pepsi-Cola, and Dr. Pepper were conceived and sold in pharmacies as health tonics.[49]

Carbonated soft drinks are no longer the unique products of pharmacies—and soft drinks are definitely no longer marketed as health tonics. Until the 1980s, soft drinks were sweetened with refined cane sugar or corn syrup. Today, regular (nondiet) soft drinks get their sweet taste from high-fructose corn syrup (HFCS). The biggest controversy regarding soft drinks in the diet today concerns their contribution to empty-calorie intake in the U.S. population, their replacement of nutrient-dense foods (such as milk), and potential health problems associated with their consumption.

A review of available scientific research regarding the effect of (regular) soft-drink consumption and nutrition and health issues found the following:[50]

- Increased energy consumption
- Increased weight; replacing a sweetened beverage with a zero-calorie beverage can help many people lose weight[51]
- Lower consumption of calcium, protein, riboflavin, fiber
- Lower intake of milk, fruit, fruit juices
- Increased risk of several medical problems
    - Type 2 diabetes (associated with as little as 1 serving per day)
    - Osteoporosis and bone fracture (due to increased calcium excretion in the urine)

  - Dental caries
  - Increased blood pressure
- When regular soft drinks were replaced with diet soft drinks, many of the negative health effects (previously listed) were not seen.

There are more than a few health risks and indications of harm, and *no* indisputable positive health benefits associated with soft-drink consumption. Soft drinks now provide more than one-third of total dietary intake of refined sugar, especially in children. Soft-drink consumption increases caloric intake but decreases total nutrient intake; in particular, soft drinks replace milk in the diet. Increased soft-drink consumption is to a certain extent to blame for the increased rates of obesity, osteoporosis, dental caries, and other health problems.[52]

9.5 Functional Beverages

Beverage choices have exploded! You can find a beverage for just about any need you can ponder. Consumers are asking: "Do I want vitamins or minerals in my water?" "Do I want amino acids in my water?" "Do I want fiber in my water?" "Do I want a beverage to enhance my sports performance?" "Do I want a beverage to help me stay alert and provide energy so I can study?" But are the claims true? What is beneficial? What may be harmful?

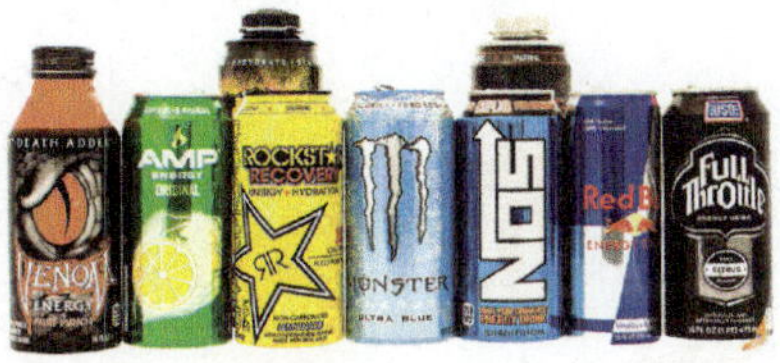

Keith Homan/Shutterstock.com

Energy Drinks

Rip It. Amp. Venom. Full Throttle. Monster Energy. Wired. Red Bull, Rockstar. The names say it all. And they promise even more—unrestrained energy in a can. Need a pick-me-up? Get an energy drink! Want to enhance your workout? Get an energy drink! Need to study all night for that midterm exam? Get an energy drink! Apparently, the ads are working: More than $13 billion a year is spent on energy drinks.[53]

Energy drinks are nonalcoholic beverages containing purportedly energy-enhancing ingredients. The primary ingredients are sugar and caffeine. Other ingredients may include vitamins, amino acids, guarana, carnitine, inositol, ginseng, glutamic acid, ginkgo biloba, royal jelly, and yohimbe, among others.[54]

There are several serious nutrition and health concerns regarding use of energy drinks:

- Energy drinks are not regulated by the Food and Drug Administration. Any amount and any mixture of ingredients can be used without being proven safe or effective.
- The level of caffeine found in most energy drinks is not suitable for children or anyone sensitive to caffeine. Some cans or bottles of energy drinks can exceed 500 milligrams (equivalent to 14 cans of caffeinated soft drinks), and the American Academy of Pediatrics states that children or adolescents should never consume energy drinks.
- Mixing energy drinks with alcohol increases the risk of heart arrhythmias.
- Using energy drinks before or during exercise may cause nervousness, lightheadedness, and nausea.
- Caffeine is a diuretic and may be counterproductive for replacing fluids lost during exercise.
- Mixing several different stimulants (caffeine, guarana, kola nuts, yerba maté) can intensify their effects and cause them to become unsafe.
- Sudden cessation of use of heavily caffeinated energy drinks may cause caffeine withdrawal. Withdrawal symptoms include headaches, mood swings, and trouble concentrating.[55]

Miniglossary of Energy Drink Ingredients

What's in my energy drink?

caffeine Central nervous system stimulant.

carnitine [KAR-nih-teen] Synthesized from the amino acids lysine and methionine in sufficient quantities to meet the needs of most people; it helps the body convert fatty acids into energy.

creatine [KREE-uh-teen] An amino acid synthesized in the body; used as a dietary supplement to increase lean body mass and strength; the amount added to most energy drinks is too small to be of any benefit.

ginkgo biloba [GING-coe bye-LOW-buh] An herb used to treat any number of conditions, including fatigue and failing memory.

ginseng [gin-SING] An herb used to support overall health and boost the immune system; research has not been conclusive enough to prove health claims.

glutamic acid [gloo-TAM-ik] A nonessential amino acid found in plant and animal tissue; used as a flavor-intensifying seasoning.

guarana [gwuh-RAH-nuh] An herb chemically equivalent to caffeine.

inositol [ih-NAH-sih-tall] Once identified in association with the B vitamins; a type of sugar (related to glucose) found synthesized in the body and many foods.

kola nut An herb chemically equivalent to caffeine.

pyruvate [pie-ROO-vate] Fatigue fighter and fat burner.

royal jelly Substance secreted from the saliva glands of honeybees; provides food for all young larvae and is the only food for larvae that will develop into queen bees. It has been incorrectly claimed to impart extra energy and to have restorative properties; can be potentially hazardous for individuals who may suffer allergic reactions.

yerba maté An herb chemically equivalent to caffeine.

yohimbe [yoh-HIM-bee] Touted as an aphrodisiac, a cure-all for sexual dysfunction; also claimed to be able to alter body mass, muscle mass, or exercise performance when combined with resistance training. None of these claims have been proven by research.

SOURCE: L. Bonci, "Energy" drinks: Help, harm, or hype? *Sports Science Exchange* 15 (2002): 1–4.

Energy drinks tend not to live up to most of the claims they make. Don't take the ads at face value. It's also a good idea to question the marketing ethics behind energy drinks. These beverages should be used with caution, and they certainly should not be used by everyone.[56] Want more energy? Want to enhance your workout? Want to be at your best studying for that midterm? Eat a healthful diet, drink plenty of water, and get some sleep!

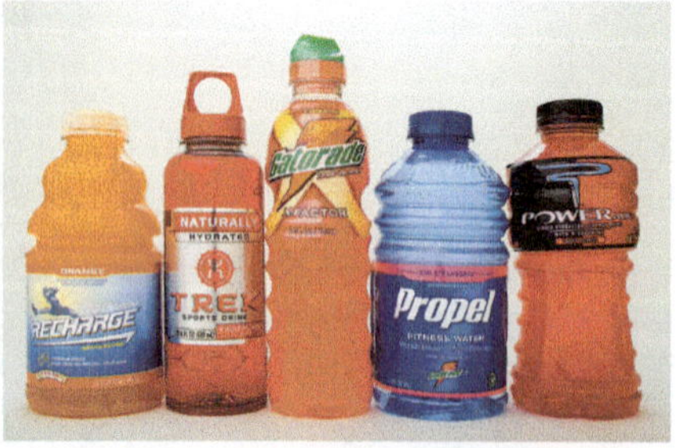

Editorial Image, LLC/Alamy Stock Photo

Sports Drinks

The first sports drink was invented by Dr. Robert Cade and a team of scientists at the University of Florida (UF) in 1965. They were attempting to design a beverage to alleviate dehydration and muscle cramps encountered by their football players. To do this, their beverage had to replace fluids and electrolytes lost due to heat and humidity during practices and games. They named their drink after the UF mascot, and thus Gatorade was born.[57] The sports beverages market exploded in the 1990s, and today it is a $6.8 billion business.[58]

Sports drinks are formulated to replace fluids and electrolytes (minerals) lost through sweat and to provide energy for muscles.[59] They may help delay fatigue and help with postexercise recovery of electrolytes and glycogen synthesis. Flavorings are generally added to enhance fluid intake.

What should you look for in a sports drink?[60]

- Four to seven percent carbohydrate in the form of glucose, sucrose, and fructose
- Low in sodium (55 to 110 milligrams per serving)
- No carbonation
- No caffeine

Sports drinks containing only fructose should be avoided. It slows fluid absorption and causes abdominal cramps. Carbonation can also cause stomach discomfort and therefore should be avoided. Caffeine can cause dehydration and should not be a component of a sports drink.[61] See Chapter 11 for more about water, fluid replacement drinks, and exercise.

"Enhanced" Waters Enhanced water? If you think plain water is boring, you might be tempted to try some of the newest "waters" to hit the market. You might think they taste better, and they certainly are prettier. As you gaze at the display shelf, how do you decide which one to choose? The pink one? The purple one? The peach-colored one? And you just might be convinced that you actually need water with added vitamins, minerals, amino acids, herbs, antioxidants, and fiber.

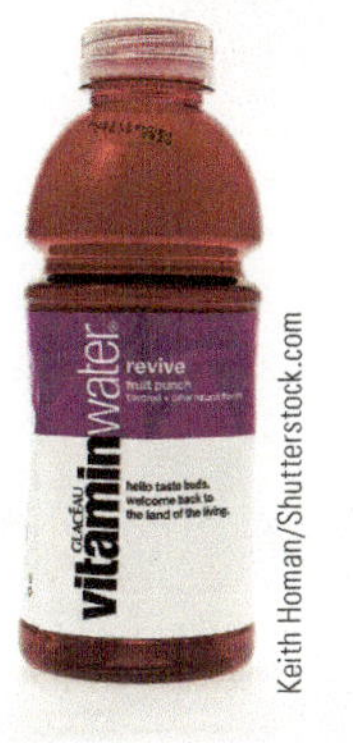

Keith Homan/Shutterstock.com

Let's begin with waters that have added vitamins. Water-soluble vitamins (taken in excess of amounts we need) added to water will flush out of the body along with the water. Fat-soluble vitamins are almost impossible to absorb without the presence of fat (see Chapter 5). The only ingredient in "vitamin waters" that your body just might use is the sugar. If the calories are in excess of what you need for energy, your body will use it to make fat.

How about the water with fiber? Everyone knows Americans don't get the recommended amount of fiber each day. The fiber added to water is maltodextrin. There is no research to demonstrate that maltodextrin works in the same way as fiber from whole grains, vegetables, and beans. Also, because maltodextrin is a soluble fiber (Chapter 4), it won't help with "regularity."[62]

Although no research has ever shown that antioxidant *supplements* help prevent disease, "antioxidant water" is in stores, claiming to "help protect your body." What makes "invigorating" or "energizing" water so invigorating or energizing? It just might be the 50 milligrams of caffeine per bottle (about the same as a small cup of coffee). Herbs added to enhanced water are not added in amounts that might be therapeutic.[63]

Most enhanced waters are no more healthful than other beverages containing added sugar. Adding vitamins and minerals to calorie-dense foods does not make them nutrient dense. Some of the ingredients added to these specialty waters may not have proven health benefits. If you really need enhancement, a vitamin-mineral supplement is a better choice.

9.6 Alcohol

Is alcohol a nutrient? Or is it a drug? **Alcohol** is *not* a nutrient; actually, it is a general term used to describe a group of organic chemicals with common properties. Members of this group include ethanol, methanol, and isopropanol, among others. This chapter discusses the most commonly ingested substance in this group: ethyl alcohol or ethanol (EtOH). Therefore, for the remainder of this chapter, *alcohol* refers to ethanol.

Alcohol is a clear, volatile liquid that burns easily. In fact, it is so flammable that it can easily be used for fuel. It has a slight, characteristic odor and is very soluble in water. Physiologically, alcohol is a sedative and central nervous system depressant. Just as with other drugs, the extent to which central nervous system function is impaired by alcohol consumption is directly related to the amount of alcohol in the blood. Similarly, as with other drugs, any health benefits resulting from alcohol consumption depend on the amount of alcohol consumed.

It's difficult to classify alcohol in terms of nutrition. Like the energy nutrients (carbohydrates, proteins, and fats), alcohol supplies energy (7 calories/gram). Unlike the energy nutrients, alcohol is not an essential nutrient, nor is it stored in the body.

alcohol A clear, colorless, volatile liquid; the most commonly ingested form is ethyl alcohol or ethanol (EtOH).

Absorption and Metabolism of Alcohol

When alcohol is consumed, it passes down the esophagus, through the stomach, and into the small intestine. About 20 percent of the alcohol is absorbed in the stomach, and about 80 percent is absorbed in the small intestine (see Figure 9-4).[64] Alcohol absorbed from the small intestine passes into the portal vein and is transported directly to the liver, where a portion of the alcohol is then metabolized by enzymes. One enzyme in particular, **alcohol dehydrogenase**, facilitates conversion of alcohol into **acetaldehyde** and water. Acetaldehyde is quickly transformed to acetate by other enzymes and then ultimately metabolized to form carbon dioxide and water. Until all the alcohol consumed has been metabolized, it is disseminated throughout the body via the bloodstream and so affects the brain and other tissues.[65]

Nearly all alcohol ingested is metabolized in the liver, but a small amount remains unmetabolized and can be measured in breath (lungs exhale about 5 percent of alcohol, which can be detected by devices such as the Breathalyzer) and urine (kidneys eliminate approximately 5 percent of alcohol in the urine).[66] Alcohol is also eliminated through sweat, feces, breast milk, and saliva.

The liver can metabolize only a limited amount of alcohol per hour, no matter how much is consumed. A healthy average person can eliminate ½ ounce (15 milliliters) of alcohol per hour. The rate of alcohol metabolism depends, in part, on the amount of alcohol dehydrogenase formed in the liver. The amount of alcohol dehydrogenase produced in the liver varies among individuals and appears to depend on a person's genetic makeup.[67] Nonetheless, alcohol is metabolized more slowly than it is absorbed,[68] and

FIGURE 9-4

Alcohol Absorption

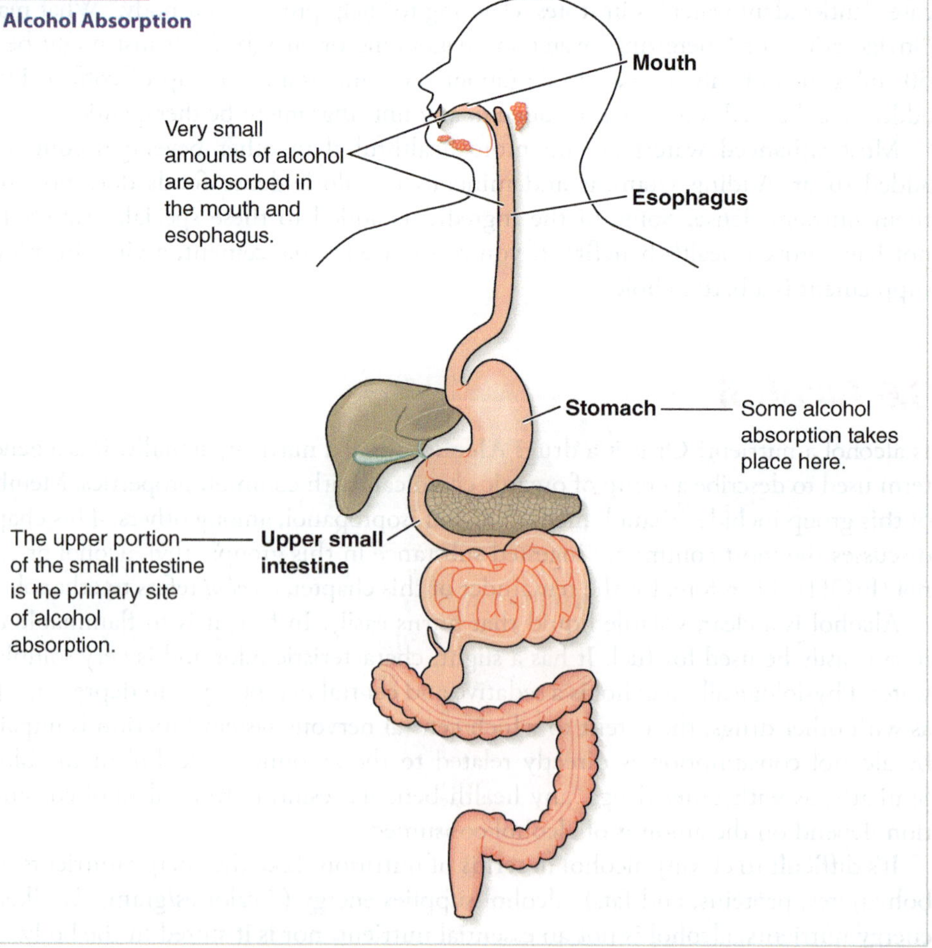

alcohol dehydrogenase A liver enzyme that mediates the metabolism of alcohol.

acetaldehyde (ass-et-AL-duh-hide) A substance into which drinking alcohol (ethanol) is metabolized.

it takes approximately one hour to metabolize one standard drink[69] (see The Savvy Diner feature later in this chapter). Controlled consumption can prevent accumulation of alcohol in the body and, therefore, can prevent intoxication as well.[70]

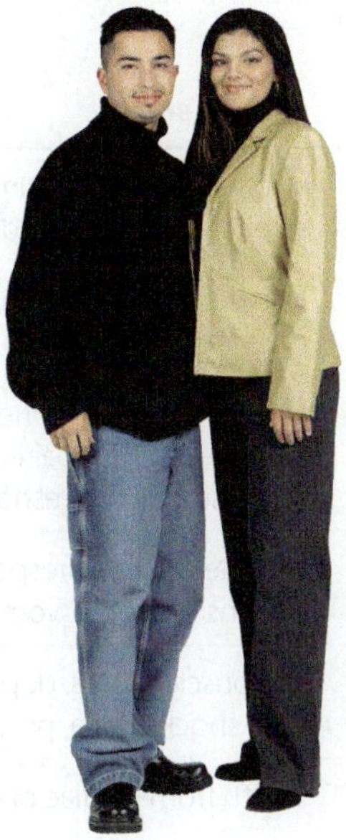

Amos Morgan/Getty Images

Even though this man and woman are the same height and weight, the woman has a lower capacity for metabolizing alcohol.

- Body composition: Because women have less water in their bodies, the concentration of alcohol in their bodies is higher (drink for drink, more alcohol gets into women's bodies).
- Enzymes: Alcohol dehydrogenase is about 40 percent less active in a woman's stomach, allowing more undiluted alcohol to enter the bloodstream.
- Hormones: Alcohol can change estrogen levels during a woman's menstrual cycle, increasing the risk for breast cancer.

Factors Influencing Absorption and Metabolism

Food Presence of food in the stomach slows absorption of alcohol.[71] The rate at which alcohol is absorbed depends on how quickly or slowly the stomach empties its contents into the small intestine. Dietary fat delays emptying time of the stomach and consequently slows absorption of alcohol.

Gender Men and women absorb and metabolize alcohol differently. Women have higher blood alcohol levels after consuming the same amount of alcohol as men. A woman absorbs 30 percent more alcohol into her bloodstream than does a man of the same weight. One drink for a woman could potentially have the same effect as two drinks for a man. Additionally, women are more susceptible to alcoholic liver disease, heart muscle damage,[72] and brain damage.[73] These metabolic differences can be attributed to smaller amounts of body water[74] in women's bodies and a lower activity of alcohol dehydrogenase in the stomach, causing a larger proportion of ingested alcohol to reach the blood.[75]

Ethnicity Native Americans have higher rates of liver damage due to alcohol consumption than do members of other ethnic groups.

Effects of Alcohol

Because it is distributed so quickly and thoroughly in the body, alcohol rapidly affects the central nervous system. Even small amounts of alcohol in the blood can slow reactions (see Figure 9-5). The body responds to alcohol in stages; therefore, higher blood alcohol levels lead to increased loss of mental and physical control (see Table 9-3). If a large amount of alcohol is consumed over a short period of time, a person may lose consciousness or even die.[76]

Alcohol and Medications Use of prescription or over-the-counter medications can increase the effects of alcohol. Chronic, heavy drinking (more than two drinks a day for women or more than four drinks a day for men over a couple of years) appears to activate an enzyme that may be responsible for changing the over-the-counter pain reliever acetaminophen (e.g., Tylenol and many others) into chemicals that can produce liver damage, even when acetaminophen is taken in recommended doses[77] (four to five "extra-strength" pills taken over the course of the day).[78] This interaction is more likely to occur when acetaminophen is taken after, rather than before, the alcohol has been metabolized.

Alcohol and Sex Hormones Alcohol metabolism alters the balance of sex hormones in men and women.[79] In men, alcohol metabolism contributes to testicular injury and impairs testosterone synthesis and sperm production.[80] Prolonged testosterone deficiency may contribute to feminization, such as breast enlargement, in males.[81]

Alcohol and Urine Output Although some people believe it is simply due to the amount of extra liquid they are ingesting, excessive urination when drinking alcohol really has more to do with the alcohol itself. In fact, an ounce of hard liquor will hypothetically cause the same amount of urination as a 12-ounce beer. Alcohol blocks the antidiuretic hormone (ADH), which is secreted from the pituitary gland and is responsible for regulating urine production. ADH works by causing the kidneys to conserve fluids. Thus, when this hormone is blocked, urine output increases

FIGURE 9-5

Alcohol's Effects on the Brain

Alcohol is rightly termed an anesthetic because it puts brain centers to sleep in this order: first the cortex, then the emotion-governing centers, then the centers that govern muscular control, and finally the deep centers that control respiration and heartbeat.

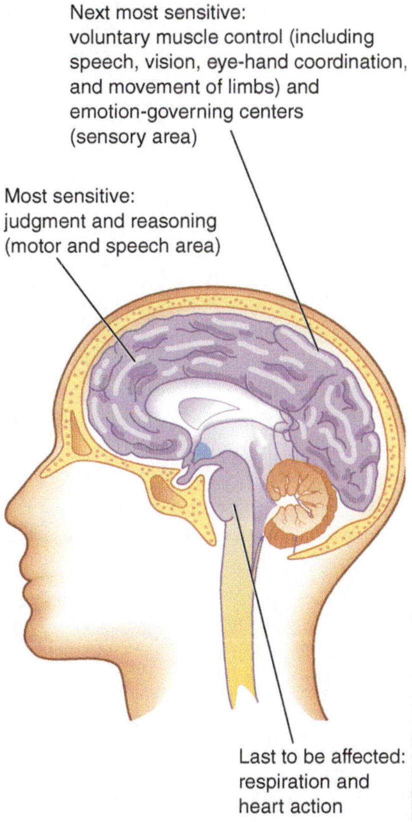

TABLE 9-3 Effects of Drinking Alcohol

Blood Alcohol Level (%)[a]	Stage	Effect on Brain[b]
0.03–0.12[c]	Euphoria	Impaired judgment, impaired fine motor skills, relaxed inhibitions, altered mood, flushed appearance, increased heart rate, shortened attention span
0.09–0.25	Excitement	Impaired coordination, delayed reaction time, blurred vision, sleepiness, impaired ability to operate a vehicle
0.18–0.30	Confusion	Slurred speech, disorientation, impaired vision, exaggerated emotions, dizziness, staggered walk, severely impaired coordination and judgment, inability to comprehend, sleepiness, increased pain threshold
0.25–0.40	Stupor	Double vision, unresponsive to stimuli, inability to walk, uninhibited behavior, lapses in and out of consciousness, vomiting, incontinence
0.35–0.50	Coma	Unconsciousness, depressed reflexes, lowered body temperature, shallow breathing, slow heart rate, shock, coma, possible death
>0.50	Death	Death from cardiac or respiratory failure

[a]Grams per 100 milliliters of blood or grams per 210 liters of breath.
[b]Blood alcohol level (BAL) and effects of drinking alcohol vary from person to person and depend on body weight, amount of food eaten while drinking, and the person's ability to tolerate alcohol.
[c]0.08 = Legal limit defining intoxication in most states.

SOURCE: Adapted from C. C. Freudenrich, *How Alcohol Works*, available online at http://science.howstuffworks.com/alcohol3.htm.

considerably because the kidneys are not properly absorbing fluids. This leads to significant loss of water and eventually to dehydration.

Alcohol and Hangovers A *hangover* actually consists of a group of ailments, usually including but not limited to headache, nausea, vomiting, sensitivity to light and sound, dry mouth, and irritability. As explained earlier, dehydration results from excessive consumption of alcohol, and it is thought to be the main factor contributing to what is referred to as a hangover. In addition, alcohol affects the stomach lining, causing considerable distention. As the depressive effects of alcohol wear off, the person's sensitivity to noise and sound are amplified. Although theories (and myths) abound about how and why hangovers occur and how to subdue their effects, the best way to avoid these unwanted side effects is to drink in moderation.

Alcohol and Blood Alcohol Level Blood alcohol level (BAL) indicates the amount of alcohol in the bloodstream and is measured in milligrams of alcohol per 100 milliliters of blood. This system does not directly relate to how many drinks you consume; instead, it indicates the amount of alcohol actually circulating in the blood at a given time. BAL is affected by the amount of alcohol ingested and how quickly it is consumed. Because the liver can metabolize only one drink per hour, any amount beyond that will hypothetically enter the bloodstream at full strength. As mentioned already, many variables determine the effects of alcohol on a person. Height, weight, and gender all have strong associations with what BAL will be after a given amount of alcohol is consumed. Although a Breathalyzer or urinalysis provides a far more accurate reading, Figure 9-6 provides an estimate of BAL for different people at different levels of alcohol consumption (see Table 9-3 for a reminder of what these levels represent).

Alcohol and Driving The best advice is *never* to drink and drive. Studies have shown that even one drink can considerably impair a driver's response time. Although driving is a very normal task, drivers must remember that behind the wheel of a car, they can do substantial damage to property and can even take people's lives, including their own.

FIGURE 9-6

Estimate of Blood Alcohol Level (BAL) at Different Body Weights and Levels of Alcohol Consumption

[a]A drink is equivalent to ½ ounce of pure ethanol; consumed within about 1 hour.

SOURCE: National Clearinghouse for Alcohol and Drug Information.

Body Weight in Pounds—Men

Drinks[a]	100	120	140	160	180	200	220	240	
	00	00	00	00	00	00	00	00	ONLY SAFE DRIVING LIMIT
1	.04	.03	.03	.02	.02	.02	.02	.02	IMPAIRMENT BEGINS
2	.08	.06	.05	.05	.04	.04	.03	.03	
3	.11	.09	.08	.07	.06	.06	.05	.05	DRIVING SKILLS SIGNIFICANTLY AFFECTED
4	.15	.12	.11	.09	.08	.08	.07	.06	
5	.19	.16	.13	.12	.11	.09	.09	.08	
6	.23	.19	.16	.14	.13	.11	.10	.09	
7	.26	.22	.19	.16	.15	.13	.12	.11	LEGALLY INTOXICATED
8	.30	.25	.21	.19	.17	.15	.14	.13	
9	.34	.28	.24	.21	.19	.17	.15	.14	
10	.38	.31	.27	.23	.21	.19	.17	.16	

Body Weight in Pounds—Women

Drinks[a]	90	100	120	140	160	180	200	220	240	
	00	00	00	00	00	00	00	00	00	ONLY SAFE DRIVING LIMIT
1	.05	.05	.04	.03	.03	.03	.02	.02	.02	IMPAIRMENT BEGINS
2	.10	.09	.08	.07	.06	.05	.05	.04	.04	DRIVING SKILLS SIGNIFICANTLY AFFECTED
3	.15	.14	.11	.10	.09	.08	.07	.06	.06	
4	.20	.18	.15	.13	.11	.10	.09	.08	.08	
5	.25	.23	.19	.16	.14	.13	.11	.10	.09	
6	.30	.27	.23	.19	.17	.15	.14	.12	.11	LEGALLY INTOXICATED
7	.35	.32	.27	.23	.20	.18	.16	.14	.13	
8	.40	.36	.30	.26	.23	.20	.18	.17	.15	
9	.45	.41	.34	.29	.26	.23	.20	.19	.17	
10	.51	.45	.38	.32	.28	.25	.23	.21	.19	

Drinking and driving is simply not worth the risk. In most states, the legal blood alcohol level limit is 0.08; for those under the age of 21, there is zero tolerance for any trace of alcohol. If this limit is exceeded, the driver could receive a citation for DUI (driving under the influence) or DWI (driving while intoxicated), which in some states is a felony.

Alcohol and Tolerance **Tolerance** is the decrease in effectiveness of a drug after a period of prolonged or heavy use. Continued exposure to alcohol causes physiological adaptations that increase tolerance. These adaptations change a person's behavior. Two types of tolerance are at work with alcohol adaptation. **Metabolic tolerance** occurs because, with continued exposure, alcohol is metabolized at a higher rate (up to 72 percent faster). Long-term exposure to alcohol increases levels of alcohol dehydrogenase in the liver, resulting in lower peak blood alcohol concentrations. This means that the body becomes more effective at removing high levels of alcohol from the blood. Even so, it also means the person must drink more alcohol to experience effects comparable to those felt before, which leads to more drinking and can contribute to addiction.[82]

Functional tolerance results from an actual change in sensitivity to a drug. Compared to the average person, chronic alcohol users can have twice the tolerance for alcohol, because the normal chemical and electrical functions of their nerve cells increase to counteract the inhibitory effects of alcohol exposure. The increased nerve activity helps chronic alcohol users function normally when they have a higher blood alcohol level, but it also tends to make them irritable when they are not drinking. Furthermore, the increased nerve activity may make them crave alcohol. Undoubtedly, the increased nerve activity contributes to hallucinations and convulsions (such as delirium tremens) that may occur when alcohol is removed, making it challenging to overcome **alcohol abuse** and **alcohol dependency**.[83]

Impact of Alcohol on Nutrition

If you are a light drinker, in good health, and otherwise well nourished, the occasional consumption of alcohol will probably have little effect on your nutritional status. The biggest risk to you will most likely come from the additional calories provided by alcohol, which may contribute to unwanted weight gain. See Table 9-4 for the calorie content of commonly consumed alcoholic beverages. This is not to say that alcohol has *no effect* on your nutritional status, because it does. Fundamental changes in metabolism occur whenever you

tolerance Decrease in effectiveness of a drug after a period of prolonged or heavy use.

metabolic tolerance Increased efficiency of removing high levels of alcohol from the blood due to long-term exposure; may lead to more drinking and possible addiction.

functional tolerance Actual change in sensitivity to a drug; often results in hallucinations and convulsions when alcohol is withheld.

alcohol abuse Continued use of alcohol despite negative psychological, social, family, employment, or school problems caused by the alcohol use.

alcohol dependency (alcoholism) A condition marked by compulsive, uncontrollable drinking that has negative effects on the affected person's physical health, family relationships, and social health.

TABLE 9-4 Calories in Alcoholic Beverages and Mixers

Beverage	Amount (oz)	Calories
Beer	12	150
Light beer	12	100
Gin, rum, vodka, whiskey (80 proof)	1½	100
Dessert wine	3½	140
Table wine (red, rosé, white)	5	100
Wine cooler	12	170
Liqueurs	1½	155–185
Tonic, ginger ale	8	80
Cola	8	100
Fruit juice	8	110
Club soda, plain seltzer, diet soda	8	0

consume alcohol. The extent to which alcohol affects your nutritional status depends on how much alcohol you consume and your current nutritional and health status.

If you drink excessively on a regular basis, your nutritional status will become compromised. Protein deficiency can develop, both from the depression of protein synthesis in the cells and, in the drinker who substitutes alcohol for food, from poor diet. Alcohol affects every tissue's nutrient metabolism in different ways. Stomach cells become inflamed and vulnerable to ulcer formation. Intestinal cells fail to absorb thiamin, folate, and vitamin B_{12}. Liver cells lose efficiency in activating vitamin D, and they alter their production and excretion of bile. Rod cells in the retina, which normally process vitamin A alcohol (*retinol*) into the form needed for vision (*retinal*), end up processing drinking alcohol (*ethanol*) instead. The kidneys excrete increased quantities of magnesium, calcium, potassium, zinc, and folate. Acetaldehyde interferes with metabolism, too. It dislodges vitamin B_6 from its protective binding protein so that it is destroyed, causing a vitamin B_6 deficiency and thereby lower production of red blood cells.

Health Benefits of Alcohol

Drinking moderate amounts (see The Savvy Diner feature later in this chapter) of alcohol appears to be safe for healthy people who do not have alcohol abuse or dependency problems.[84] People who consume one to two drinks daily have lower mortality rates than nondrinkers.[85] Alcohol, like any other drug, has a beneficial dose and a level (dose) that will cause harm. Whether alcohol consumption will produce beneficial or adverse effects depends on a person's alcohol consumption, age, and background for cardiovascular risk. Rates of death from all causes are lowest among those who report consuming one drink per day.[86] Although most research indicates that wine consumption is the most beneficial, it appears that the benefits are from the alcohol itself, not the other components of each type of alcoholic beverage.[87]

Alcohol and Cardiovascular Health Cardiovascular disease is the leading cause of death worldwide.[88] More than a dozen research studies have demonstrated a consistent, positive correlation between moderate alcohol consumption and decreased incidence of heart disease.[89] The protective effect of alcohol is the result of increased levels of high-density lipoprotein (HDL) cholesterol.[90] HDL-cholesterol removes cholesterol from the lining of artery walls and carries it back to the liver for excretion. Alcohol also inhibits blood from forming clots, reducing risk of death from heart attack.[91] This anticlotting effect of moderate drinking reduces the risk of thrombotic or ischemic stroke (blockage of blood vessel in the brain) but increases the risk of hemorrhagic stroke (rupture of a blood vessel within the brain).

Health Risks of Alcohol

Moderate drinking is not risk-free. Deaths reduced by moderate alcohol consumption are generally found in age groups with high rates of coronary heart disease—in other words, in people 45 years and older. However, most deaths due to alcohol consumption occur in people younger than 45 years.[92] Among young adults, the risks of alcohol consumption (alcohol abuse and dependence, alcohol-related violent behavior and injuries) far outweigh any benefits that may accrue later in life.[93]

Accidents Alcohol affects judgment and slows reflexes, which can lead to falls or accidents with vehicles or other heavy machinery. It can also increase the likelihood of homicide and suicide. Alcohol makes men less able to control impulses toward violence and makes women less capable of recognizing cues to potentially violent behavior.

Drug Interactions Like alcohol, many other **drugs** are metabolized in the liver. The liver has limited processing capacity, and alcohol and drugs may compete with each other for metabolism. Alcohol may hinder the metabolism of another drug, keeping the medication in the system longer than intended and possibly increasing risk of side effects. See Table 9-5 for specific alcohol–drug interactions.

Night Blindness Alcohol blocks formation of retinal, a compound in the eye responsible for vision in low light.

Breast Cancer Even when consumed in moderate amounts (one drink per day for women), alcohol may increase the risk of breast cancer in women.

Other Cancers Heavy alcohol use, especially when combined with smoking, appears to increase risk of cancer of the throat and esophagus. Risk of cancer increases for people who have hepatitis and cirrhosis. Risk of colon cancer also increases with alcohol use.

Liver Damage **Alcoholic hepatitis** (inflammation of the liver) and **cirrhosis** (scarring of liver tissue that interferes with blood flow and liver function) are two common consequences of heavy drinking. Hepatitis can lead to permanent liver damage if alcohol consumption continues.

High Blood Pressure and Stroke Heavy drinking causes high blood pressure (hypertension) as the heart compensates for the initial reduction in blood pressure caused by alcohol consumption. Hypertension is a risk factor for stroke and heart disease.

Pancreatitis Long-term alcohol consumption can result in recurrent attacks of severe pain caused by inflammation of the pancreas. The pancreas is responsible for production of many digestive enzymes. Continued use of alcohol can ultimately cause permanent damage to the pancreas.

Gastrointestinal Symptoms Alcohol irritates the lining of the stomach and impairs intestinal enzymes and transport systems. Thus, alcohol consumption can cause a wide range of common, uncomfortable, but reversible problems, including gastritis (inflammation of the lining of the stomach), stomach and intestinal ulcers, diarrhea, and weight loss.

Brain Damage Brain cells in various parts of the brain die, reducing total brain mass.

Decreased Sex Hormone Production Alcohol causes decreased testosterone secretion from the hypothalamus/pituitary and testes, resulting in decreased sperm production. It can cause infertility in women by disrupting or changing the menstrual cycle.

drugs Substances that can modify one or more of the body's functions.

alcoholic hepatitis Inflammation and injury to the liver due to excess alcohol consumption.

cirrhosis A chronic, degenerative disease of the liver in which the liver cells become infiltrated with fibrous tissues; blood flow through the liver is obstructed, causing back pressure and eventually leading to coma and death unless the cause of the disease is removed; the most common cause of cirrhosis is chronic alcohol abuse.

TABLE 9-5	Specific Alcohol–Drug Interactions
Drug	**Interaction with Alcohol**
Antibiotics	Nausea, vomiting, headache, and possible convulsions
Antidepressants	Increases sedative effect, impairing mental skills used for driving; other interactions can produce a dangerous increase in blood pressure
Oral hypoglycemic drugs (used to treat type 2 diabetes)	Can prolong effects, causing nausea, headache, or a dangerous decrease in blood glucose levels; chronic alcohol consumption can decrease the drug's effect
Over-the-counter antihistamines (such as Benadryl) used to treat symptoms of allergy and insomnia	May intensify the sedation, causing dizziness or drowsiness
Barbiturates	Prolongs sedative effect; chronic alcohol use decreases sedative effect
Cardiovascular medications	Can cause dizziness or fainting upon standing up; chronic alcohol use may decrease therapeutic effect of some cardiovascular drugs
Cocaine/crack	Increases heart rate three to five times as much as when either drug is used alone (cocaine increases metabolism, which in turn increases blood alcohol levels)
Ecstasy/MDMA	Increases dehydration to dangerous levels
GHB	Slows rate of breathing to dangerous levels
Heroin	Can induce heroin overdose, leading to cessation of breathing
Marijuana	Increases suppression of gag reflex (inhibiting vomiting), which can increase risk of alcohol poisoning
Narcotic pain relievers (opiates, morphine, codeine, Darvon, Demerol)	Enhances sedative effect of both substances, increasing risk of death by overdose
Nonnarcotic pain relievers (aspirin and similar nonprescription pain relievers; acetaminophen [Tylenol])	Increases stomach bleeding and inhibition of blood clotting; increases risk of liver damage
Oral contraceptives	May hinder absorption of alcohol into bloodstream, delaying onset of intoxication
PCP/Special K	Compounds central nervous system (CNS) depression
Sedatives and hypnotics (sleeping pills, Valium)	Severe drowsiness, increased risk of household and automotive accidents
Tobacco	Doubles risk of heart attack; increases risk for lung, throat, mouth, and bladder cancers, stroke, high blood pressure, miscarriage, and low birth-weight infants

SOURCE: *Drinking: A Student's Guide*, "Alcohol and Legal Drugs."

Anemia Poor nutrition as a result of excessive alcohol intake decreases levels of iron and B vitamins, leading to anemia.

Emotional and Social Problems Alcohol affects emotional centers in the limbic system, causing anxiety and depression. Emotional and physical effects of alcohol can contribute to marital and family problems, including domestic violence, as well as to work-related problems such as excessive absences and poor work performance.

Weighing the Pros and Cons of Alcohol Consumption

How do you decide if low to moderate alcohol consumption will provide health benefits or health risks for you? One way is to consider the leading causes of death for people of your age group and gender. The leading causes of death for men under the age of 40 and women under the age of 50 (premenopausal) are accidents and breast cancer, respectively. In these cases, the risks of low to moderate alcohol consumption outweigh the benefits. The leading cause of death for men over the age of 40 and women over

THE SAVVY Diner What Is a Drink? (Obj. 9.6)

Ancient Persians ate five almonds to prevent hangovers. For Romans and Greeks, celery was thought to cure a hangover. By the late 1800s, celery still had a medicinal use: Sears, Roebuck & Company advertised a celery tonic to calm the nerves.[94]

According to the *Dietary Guidelines for Americans*, "If alcohol is consumed, it should be consumed in moderation—and only by adults of legal drinking age." But what is drinking in moderation? If you decide to drink alcohol, you should have as much information as possible so that you can drink responsibly.

Moderation is defined as:

- No more than two drinks per day for men
- No more than one drink per day for women

These limits are based on the disparity between men and women in both weight and alcohol metabolism. Whereas drinking in moderation provides little, if any, health benefits for young adults, moderate drinking for men over the age of 40 and women over the age of 50 may lower their risk for coronary heart disease.

More than one drink a day for women or two drinks a day for men can increase risk for motor vehicle accidents, other injuries, high blood pressure, stroke, violence, suicide, and certain types of cancer. Even one drink per day can slightly increase the risk of breast cancer. Alcohol consumption during pregnancy (see the Spotlight feature in this chapter) increases the risk of birth defects.

What Constitutes a Drink?

Alcohol is alcohol is alcohol. It does not matter if the beverage of choice is beer, wine, a wine cooler, a cocktail, or a mixed drink. A standard serving of beer, distilled spirits, and wine each contain the same amount of alcohol (see the photo). A *standard serving* is:

- 12 ounces of regular beer (150 calories)
- 5 ounces of wine (100 calories)
- 1½ ounces of 80-proof distilled spirits (100 calories)
- 10 ounces wine cooler/12 ounces spirit-based cooler (170 to 230 calories)
- 3 ounces of sherry or port (130 calories)
- 9¾ ounces of malt liquor (135 calories)

When it comes to drinking alcohol, the old adage is true: It doesn't matter what you drink, it's really *how much* you drink that counts.

Sometimes responsible drinking means not drinking at all. Some people who should not drink alcoholic beverages include:

- Children and adolescents
- Individuals of any age who cannot restrict their drinking to moderate levels
- Women who *may* become pregnant or who are pregnant. A safe alcohol intake has not been established for women at any time during pregnancy, including the first few weeks (see the Spotlight feature later in this chapter).
- Individuals who plan to drive, operate machinery, or take part in any activities that require attention, skill, or coordination. Most people retain some alcohol in their blood for up to two to three hours after a single drink.
- Individuals who are taking prescription or over-the-counter medications that can interact with alcohol

SOURCES: American Dietetic Association, Alcohol beverages: Making responsible drinking choices; *Dietary Guidelines for Americans* (available online at www.health.gov/dietaryguidelines); National Consumers League, Alcohol: How it all adds up (available online at www.nclnet.org).

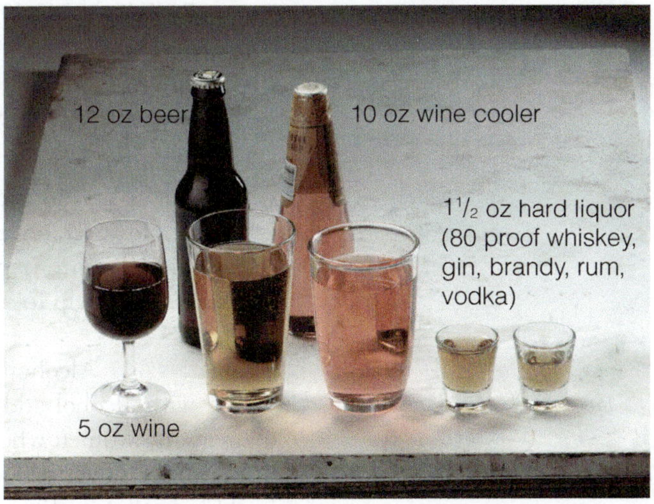

the age of 50 is heart disease. Thus, for these people, the benefits of low to moderate alcohol consumption outweigh the risks.

What Is Alcohol Abuse or Alcoholism? *Alcoholism* is a dependency on alcohol characterized by craving (a strong need to drink), loss of control (being unable to stop drinking despite a desire to do so), physical dependence and withdrawal symptoms, and tolerance (increasing difficulty in becoming drunk).

Although many people stereotype those with alcoholism as people who spend their lives at a bar or as skid-row bums, in fact anyone can suffer from alcoholism. Previous notions of alcoholism as a moral flaw have basically been replaced with the theory that alcoholism is a disease with genetic, psychosocial, and environmental factors and influences. Successful people such as lawyers, doctors, professors, and even college students can suffer from what is commonly known as *alcoholism*.

The following is a scale of alcohol addiction from Narcotics Anonymous (NA) and Alcoholics Anonymous (AA):

> **Use:** Alcohol "use" is considered to be the ingestion of alcohol or other drugs without experiencing any negative consequences. If a college student drinks a beer at a fraternity party, she has used alcohol. (This can also apply to any drug.)
>
> **Misuse:** When a person experiences negative consequences from his or her use of alcohol or other drugs, it is "misuse." A large percentage of the population misuses drugs or alcohol at some point in their lives. However, this does not imply that the negative consequences are minor. For example, the same college student continues to use alcohol on an infrequent basis. Her friends throw her a surprise party and she drinks more than usual. On the way home, she is arrested for DUI. Although she does not really have a problem with alcohol, in this instance the consequences are not minor.
>
> **Abuse:** *Abuse* consists of continued use of alcohol or other drugs in spite of negative consequences. Let's continue to observe the college student who was arrested for DUI. If she does *not* have a substance abuse problem, she will probably cut way back on her alcohol consumption, even if she does not give it up altogether. Getting a DUI should be enough of a deterrent. However, if shortly thereafter she goes to another party, drinks in excess, and then drives her car, it is alcohol abuse.
>
> **Dependency/Addiction:** Compulsive use of alcohol or other drugs, regardless of adverse or negative consequences, represents dependency or addiction. For example, suppose that our college student has received three DUI citations in one year. She is now on probation and will be sentenced to one year in prison if caught using alcohol again. However, she continues to drink at parties and at local establishments. This young woman is clearly addicted to alcohol, because the negative consequences do not affect her decisions or deter her use.[95]

When individuals are clearly in the first or second stage of alcoholism (use or misuse), there are no indications as to whether they will naturally progress to the final stages. However, once individuals reach the abuse stage, it is highly probable that they will progress into dependency on the drugs or alcohol. Such individuals should seek professional help to stop the progression.

What Is AA? Alcoholics Anonymous (AA) is perhaps the best-known method for dealing with alcohol addiction. Alcoholics Anonymous defines itself as "a fellowship of men and women who share their experience, strength, and hope with each other that they may solve their common problem and help others to recover from alcoholism." This not-for-profit organization, established in 1935, has helped millions of people deal with this life-altering disease. Through group meetings, self-proclaimed alcoholics come together for counseling, guidance, and support with the primary purpose of staying sober and helping other people with alcoholism achieve sobriety. Their well-known "12 Step Program" focuses on the physical act of abstaining from alcohol as well as on the psychosocial aspects. To preserve anonymity, membership records do not exist, and people are welcome from all walks of life and at all levels of alcoholism.

SCORE Card Alcohol Assessment Questionnaire (Obj. 9.6)

This screening test is designed to help you determine if you have a problem with alcohol. Read through the following questions about your use of alcoholic beverages during the past year. In the questions, a "drink" is defined as 12 ounces of beer, 5 ounces of wine, or 1 to 1½ ounces of 80-proof liquor. Select the most appropriate answer for each question by checking yes or no.

Early Warning Signs of Alcohol Abuse

	Yes	No
1. Have you missed classes more than once due to a hangover?	☐	☐
2. Have you thought that you should cut down on your drinking?	☐	☐
3. Have you decided to cut down on your drinking and found you could not?	☐	☐
4. Have you been angered by other people's criticism of your drinking?	☐	☐
5. Have you been in fights while drinking?	☐	☐
6. Is excessive alcohol use a significant part of your weekly social and recreational activities?	☐	☐
7. Have you had problems with resident assistants or campus police because of your drinking?	☐	☐
8. Do you routinely "binge" drink? (Binge drinking for women is defined as drinking four or more drinks during an episode of drinking. For men, five or more drinks is considered binge drinking.)	☐	☐
9. Have you ever been unable to account for periods of time during or after drinking occurrences?	☐	☐
10. Have you had sexual experiences after drinking that you felt bad about later?	☐	☐

Give yourself 1 point for each Yes response.

0 Congratulations! Your response on this test suggests that your use of alcohol is not causing you any ongoing negative experiences that indicate early warning signs of alcohol abuse or dependence.

1 Now is the time to evaluate how much you are drinking, how often, and the impact your alcohol consumption is having on you. A score of 1 also indicates that you should probably reduce the quantity of alcohol you consume.

2 or greater More than one yes response indicates the definite need for you to limit your alcohol use by either abstaining or limiting your use to responsible levels of consumption. If you are unable to control your use, then it's time to abstain completely.

What Is Binge Drinking?

What would you think if you were at a party or restaurant and saw someone nearby drink an entire six-pack of a soft drink in one sitting? That's 72 ounces of pop. Strange, right? What will all that sugar do to the person's teeth? What will all of those calories do to his or her waistline? What about all of that caffeine at one time?

Now let's say that same person is drinking a six-pack of beer instead of soft drinks. Sound weird, too? Probably, but many college students do it all the time. It's called *binge drinking*—drinking at least five drinks at one time if you are a man or four drinks at one time if you are a woman, in one sitting. The short-term reactions caused by consuming large amounts of alcohol in a brief period of time are serious: vomiting, dizziness, impaired mental capabilities, and hangover. Other effects can include risky sexual behavior, alcohol-related injuries, or death.

Think it doesn't happen all that often? About 50 percent of college men and 37 percent of college women report drinking more than five drinks at one time in one sitting.

SOURCES: *Drinking: A Student's Guide*, "Binge Drinking," From L. Hickman, Self Tests, Early signs of alcohol abuse.

SPOTLight

9.7 Fetal Alcohol Spectrum Disorders

Scientists first created the term *fetal alcohol syndrome* (FAS) more than 40 years ago to describe a pattern of birth defects found in children of mothers who drank alcohol during pregnancy.[96] Since then, scientists have defined a broad range of birth defects and developmental disabilities caused by prenatal alcohol exposure and now refer to the disorders that fall within that broad range *as fetal alcohol spectrum disorders* (FASD). The following are the disorders under the FASD category:

- FAS—This diagnosis requires a characteristic pattern of facial abnormalities (Figure 9-7), growth deficits, and central nervous system abnormalities.
- Partial FAS—includes some signs and symptoms of FAS but not all three of the characteristics previously noted.
- Alcohol-related birth defects (ARBD)—includes alcohol-related physical abnormalities.
- Alcohol-related neurodevelopmental disorder (ARND)—includes central nervous system abnormalities, as well as cognitive and behavioral problems.[97]

TABLE 9-6 Signs of Fetal Alcohol Spectrum Disorders

Children with FASDs may have the following characteristics and behaviors:

Characteristic Facial Features of Fetal Alcohol Exposure
- Small eyes with drooping upper lids
- Short, upturned nose
- Flattened cheeks
- Small jaw
- Thin upper lip
- Flattened groove in middle of upper lip

Central Nervous System Problems
- Mental retardation
- Hyperactivity
- Delayed development of gross motor skills (rolling over, crawling, walking)
- Delayed development of fine motor skills (grasping objects with the thumb and index finger, transferring objects from one hand to another)
- Impaired language development
- Memory problems, poor judgment, distractibility, impulsiveness
- Learning problems
- Seizures

SOURCE: National Institute on Alcohol Abuse and Alcoholism, *Alcohol Alert: Fetal Alcohol Spectrum Disorders: Understanding the Effects of Prenatal Alcohol Exposure*, No. 82 (Bethesda, MD: National Institute on Alcohol Abuse and Alcoholism, 2011).

FIGURE 9-7

Facial Characteristics Associated with Fetal Alcohol Exposure

These facial traits (low nasal bridge, short eyelid opening, small head circumference, undeveloped groove in center of upper lip) are typical of fetal alcohol syndrome, caused by drinking alcohol during pregnancy. Irreversible abnormalities of the brain and other organs accompany these facial features.

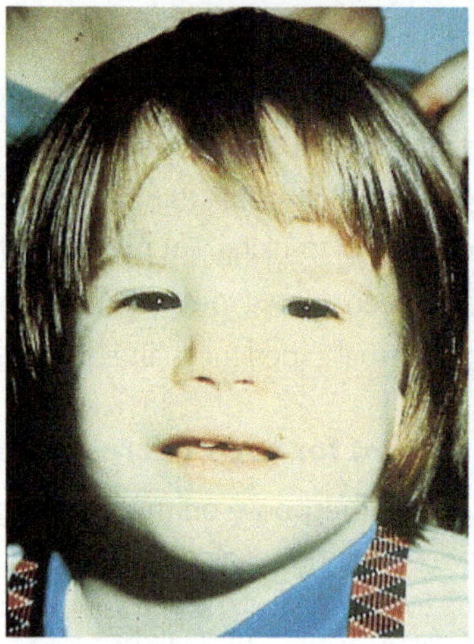

In the United States, FAS is one of the primary causes of birth defects and is considered to be the most common cause of preventable mental retardation. It is defined by four criteria:

- Maternal drinking during pregnancy
- Characteristic pattern of facial abnormalities (see Table 9-6)
- Growth retardation
- Brain damage, often manifested by intellectual difficulties or behavioral problems (see Table 9-6). Studies have demonstrated abnormalities of certain brain regions in babies exposed to alcohol during their mothers' pregnancy (see Figure 9-8).[98]

As you can see, the effects of fetal exposure to alcohol last throughout the child's life.

How does alcohol get into the baby's body?

Alcohol consumed by a pregnant woman travels through her bloodstream and across the placenta to her baby. The unborn baby's body can metabolize the alcohol, but it does so at a much slower rate than the adult body. As a result, the alcohol level in the baby's blood is higher than in the mother's, and the alcohol remains in the baby's blood longer.

FIGURE 9-8

Brain Regions Affected by FAS

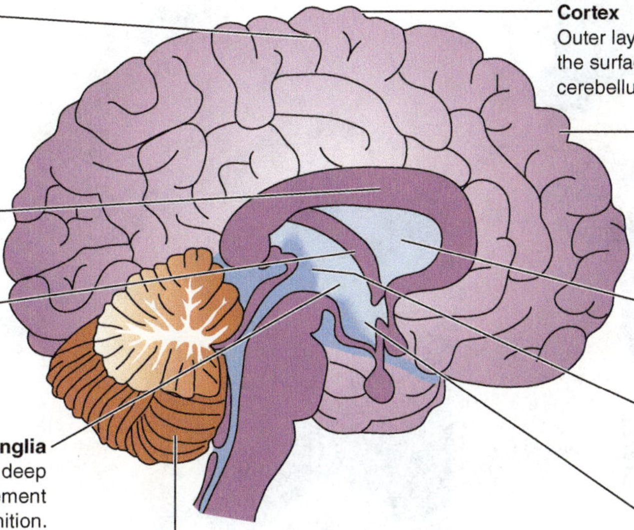

How much alcohol does a woman have to drink to cause FAS?

Women who drink frequently (more than four alcoholic beverages a day) seriously increase the likelihood that their babies will have FAS. Binge drinking (four or more drinks per occasion) is an especially hazardous drinking pattern in terms of FAS risk.[99] However, no quantity of alcohol use during pregnancy has been established to be safe. Effects of FAS have been seen in children whose mothers drank only moderately or lightly during pregnancy. An average of one drink a day increases a baby's risk of FAS. Children with FAS do not outgrow the signs listed in Table 9-6. These problems are lifelong.

How can FAS be prevented?

Unlike most birth defects, FAS is completely preventable, because its direct cause—maternal drinking—is a controllable behavior. Simply put, pregnant women can prevent FAS by *not consuming alcohol.* No amount of alcohol use during pregnancy has been proven to be safe. For that reason, any woman who suspects she might be pregnant should *stop drinking immediately.* Women who are attempting to get pregnant *should not drink* alcohol. Because many women of childbearing age drink regularly, it's likely that their babies will be exposed to alcohol before pregnancy is detected. It is common for a woman to be pregnant for four to six weeks before she knows she is pregnant. Alcohol can hurt a baby even during the first one to two months of pregnancy, and no type of alcoholic beverage—beer, wine, wine coolers, and liquor (whiskey, vodka, tequila, gin, and rum)—is exempt.

The bottom line? Everything a woman eats or drinks affects her baby. Fetal alcohol spectrum disorders could be completely eliminated if pregnant women did not consume alcohol.[100]

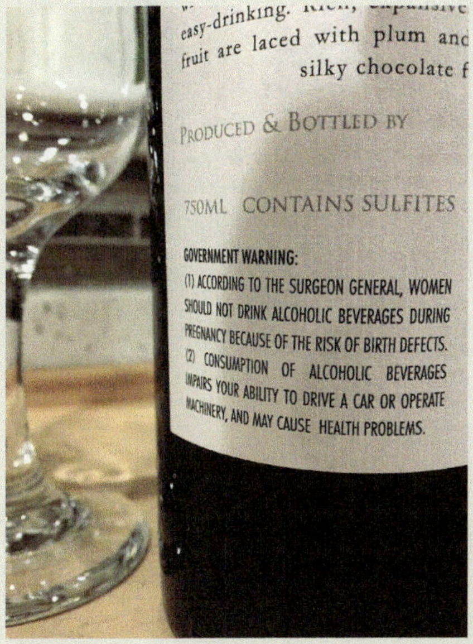

Targeted media campaigns can help increase public awareness of the adverse effects of alcohol use during pregnancy. Because levels of binge and frequent drinking among nonpregnant women have not declined, all women of childbearing age should be warned about the adverse effects of alcohol use to avert early prenatal exposure before women become aware of pregnancy. Additional information about CDC activities to prevent alcohol-exposed pregnancies is available at www.cdc.gov/ncbddd/fasd.

WHAT'S ONLINE

MINDTAP From Cengage

Visit www.cengagebrain.com to access MindTap, a complete digital course that includes Diet & Wellness Plus, interactive quizzes, videos, and more.

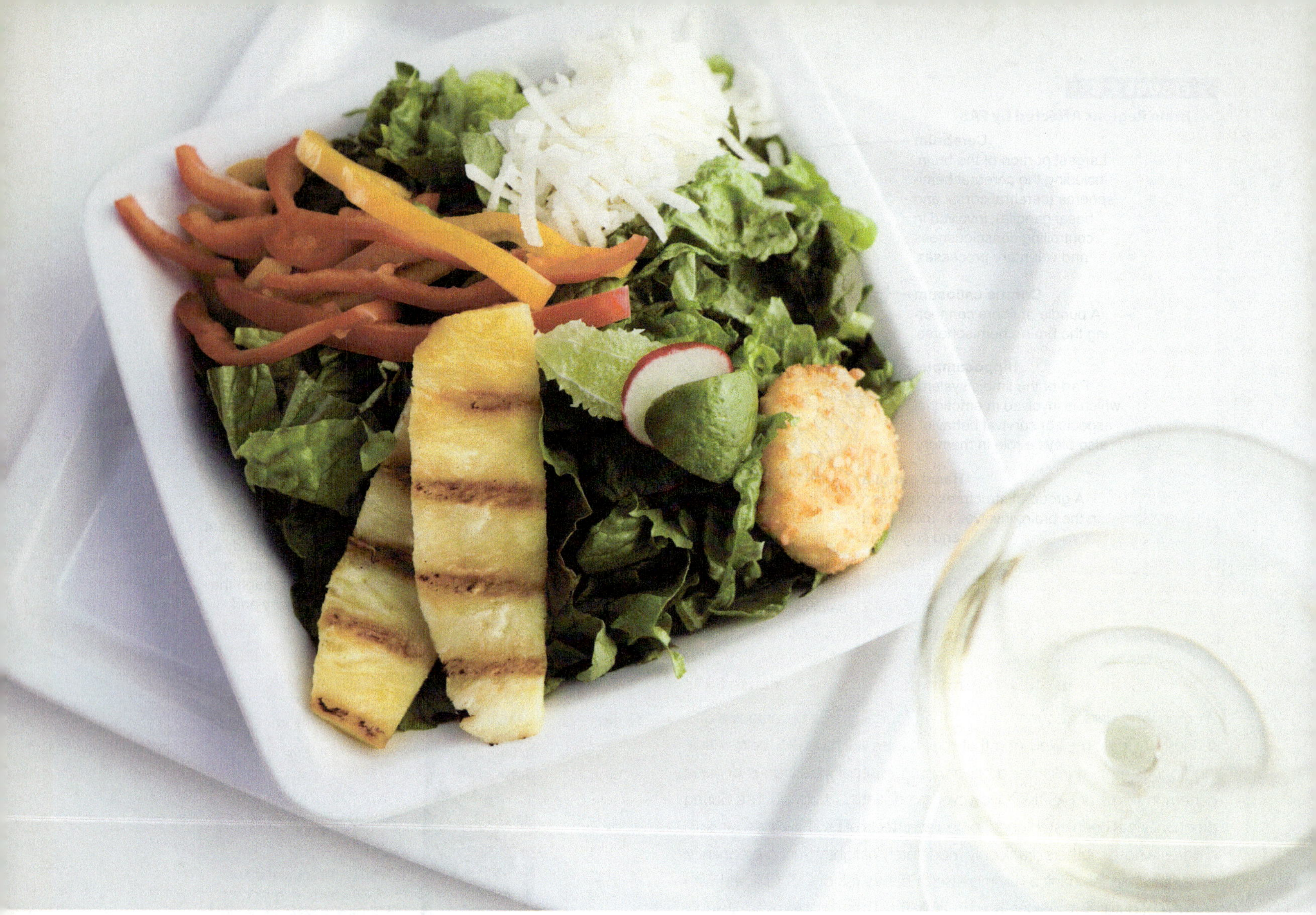

Somos/Jupiter Images

Ask Yourself . . .

Which of the following statements about nutrition are true, and which are false? For each false statement, what would make it true?

1. The less you weigh, the better it is for your health.
2. Basal metabolism contributes only a small percentage of a person's daily energy output.
3. Probably the most important contributor to the obesity problem in our country is underactivity.
4. Fad diets are popular because their followers achieve quick and permanent weight loss.

Answers found on page 286.

Chapter Objectives

10.1 Define overweight and obesity, and discuss their health consequences.

10.2 Discuss the difference between body weight and body fat.

10.3 Define energy balance and its components, and discuss its relationship to weight maintenance.

10.4 Recognize the different factors that interact to cause obesity.

10.5 Compare the physiological processes of weight gain, loss, and maintenance, and describe the medical approaches to weight loss.

10.6 Identify effective weight-loss strategies.

10.7 Identify effective weight-gain strategies.

10.8 Discuss behavior modification and its role in successful weight loss.

10.9 Identify the warning signs of eating disorders.

Weight Management

CHAPTER 10

Say the word *diet*, and most people think "starvation," "deprivation," "hunger," and something to go "on" and "off." As this chapter shows, such thinking is unrealistic and self-defeating. Strict, temporary diets—and the attitudes that go with them—don't work for the great majority of overweight people. In fact, although Americans spend more than $40 billion a year on programs and products aimed at weight loss, obesity rates are higher than ever.[1] More than one-third of all adults and approximately 17 percent of children and adolescents in the United States are obese; that is, exceeding their healthy weight range (see Figure 10-1). The annual costs of overweight and obesity are staggering: more than $190 billion. Overall, medical spending for a person with obesity is approximately 42 percent more than for a person of normal weight.[2]

Before you begin a thing remind yourself that difficulties and delays quite impossible to foresee are ahead. . . . You can see only one thing clearly, and that is your goal. Form a mental vision of that and cling to it through thick and thin.

—K. Norris

10.1 A Closer Look at Obesity

The World Health Organization describes obesity as "an escalating epidemic" and one of the greatest neglected public health problems of our time (see Figure 10-2). Because obesity is a disease with multiple health risks, such as type 2 diabetes, heart disease, and some forms of cancer, the increasing rates of obesity are projected to result in increased rates of disability and preventable deaths.[3] The *Healthy People* national health initiative includes objectives for increasing the proportion of adults who are at a healthy weight and reducing the number of adults and children who are obese by the year 2020.[4]

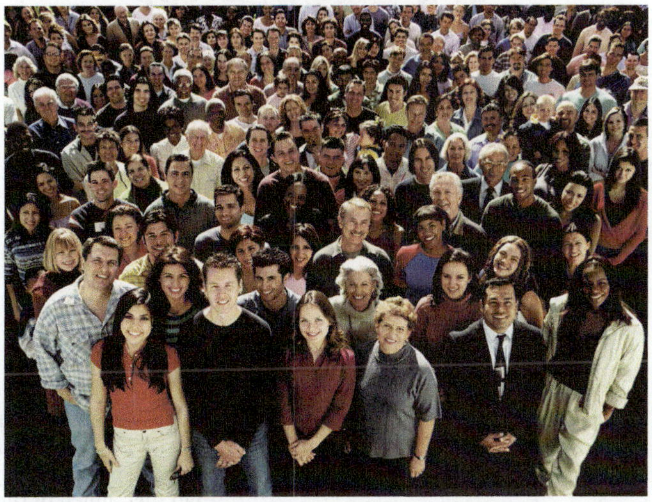
Chabruken/Stone/Getty Images

Bodies come in many shapes and sizes. Which are healthy?

FIGURE 10-1

Trends in Prevalence of Obesity among Children and Adults (1999–2014), United States

A significant increase in obesity was observed in both adults and youth from 1999 through 2014.

SOURCE: C. L. Ogden et al., Prevalence of obesity and youth in the United States, 2011–2014, *NCHS Data Brief*, no. 219, Hyattsville, MD: National Center for Health Statistics, 2015.

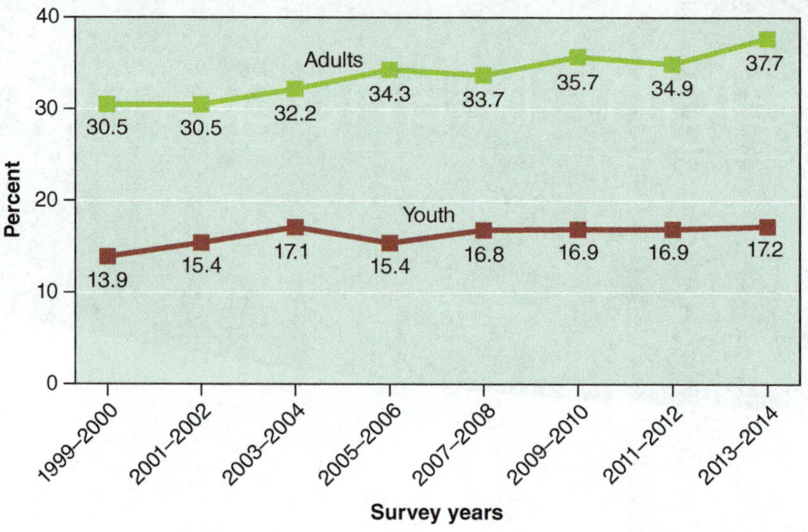

FIGURE 10-2

The Epidemic of Obesity among U.S. Adults

In 1990, 10 states had a prevalence of obesity less than 10%, and no states had prevalence equal to or greater than 15%. By 2011, no state had prevalence of less than 20%, 12 states had a prevalence of obesity between 30 and 34.9%, and no state had prevalence equal to or greater than 35%. By 2015, only 6 states (California, Colorado, Hawaii, Massachusetts, Montana, and Utah) and the District of Columbia, had obesity prevalence ranging from 20% to less than 25%; 19 states had a prevalence of obesity between 25% and less than 30%; obesity prevalence in 21 states was 30% to less than 35%; and four states had an obesity prevalence of 35% or greater. The South had the highest prevalence of obesity (31.2%), followed by the Midwest (30.7%), the Northeast (26.4%), and the West (25.2%).

SOURCE: http://www.cdc.gov/obesity/data/prevalence-maps.html, September 2016.

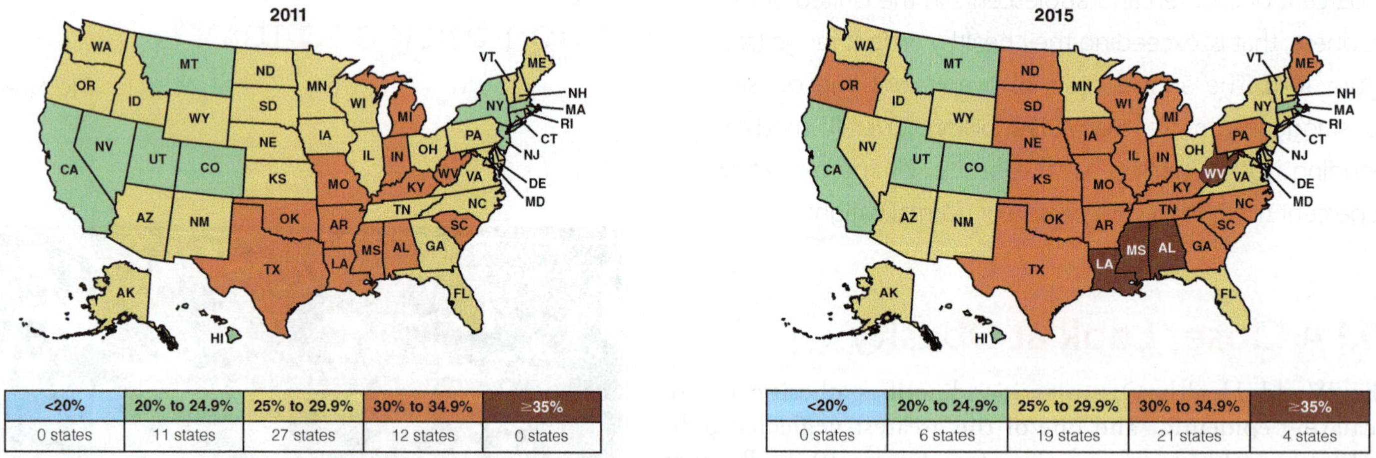

ASK YOURSELF ANSWERS: **1.** False. Being thin is good for health only to a point; being too thin is as risky as being too fat. **2.** False. Basal metabolism contributes about 60 percent or more of the average person's daily energy output. **3.** True. **4.** False. Although you may lose weight quickly on a fad diet, much of the weight you lose may be muscle or water and the weight may soon be regained when the diet ends.

Although many factors (including genetics) influence body weight, excess energy intake and physical inactivity are the leading causes of **overweight** and **obesity**, and they represent the best opportunities for prevention and treatment.[5] Consider how the following trends in our society have increased opportunities for poor nutrition (particularly excess calories) and decreased opportunities for physical activity:

- Food portion sizes and obesity rates have grown at the same rate. In the 1960s, an average fast-food meal of a hamburger, fries, and a 12-ounce cola provided 590 calories; today, large fast-food meals deliver 1,500 calories or more.[6] Although fast-food restaurants have recently made more size options available to customers, portion size still remains an issue. Even an extra 150 calories a day—the calorie cost of a large soft drink—can convert to about 16 extra pounds of body fat every year.
- Vending machines selling soft drinks, high-fat snacks, and highly sugared snacks are common in schools and workplaces. Milk, juices, water, and healthful snacks are far less accessible.
- Adults spend more time in sedentary activities, such as watching television, working on the computer, or commuting to and from work and school.
- Children watch 12 to 14 hours of television a week and spend 7 hours playing video games.[7]
- Schools offer fewer physical education classes for children.
- More families live in communities that are designed for car use but are unsuitable (lack of green space for recreation) and often unsafe (lack of sidewalks, inadequate street lighting) for activities such as walking, biking, and running.

Problems Associated with Weight Clearly, each individual can weigh too much or too little to be healthy. A person who is **underweight** has minimal body fat stores and is at a disadvantage in situations where energy reserves are needed, such as a prolonged period of physiological stress or injury. Other problems for people who are underweight may include menstrual irregularity, infertility, and osteoporosis.

The physical risks of overweight and obesity are greater for some people than for others, depending on inherited predispositions to conditions such as high blood pressure, high blood cholesterol, and diabetes. High blood pressure is made worse by weight gain and can often be normalized by weight loss. Diabetes can be precipitated, in genetically susceptible people, by becoming overweight.

Obesity also increases the risk of heart disease, partly because excess fat tissues crowd the heart muscle and the lungs within the body cavity. This excess fat increases the heart's burden as it beats, requiring it to work harder to deliver oxygen and nutrients to the rest of the body. Also, the lungs cannot expand fully, thus limiting the oxygen intake of each breath and causing the heart to work even harder. Furthermore, because each extra pound of fat tissue must be fed from miles of capillaries, the heart must work extra hard in people with obesity to pump blood through a network of blood vessels that is vastly larger than that of people who are thin. Even a healthy heart is strained by excess fat. When a diseased heart finds itself in this bind, a sudden increase in workload may be more than it can handle.

Gallbladder disease, too, can be brought on in susceptible people merely by excess weight.[8] Similarly, obesity increases a woman's risk of developing breast

overweight Conventionally defined as weight between 10 and 20 percent above the desirable weight for height, or a body mass index (BMI) of 25.0 through 29.9.

obesity Conventionally defined as weight 20 percent or more above the desirable weight for height, or a BMI of 30 or greater.

underweight Weight 10 percent or more below the desirable weight for height, or a BMI of less than 18.5.

TABLE 10-1	Problems Associated with Obesity

- Abdominal hernias
- Accidents
- Certain cancers: colon, rectal, prostate, breast, uterus, cervical, ovarian
- Complications during pregnancy
- Complications with surgical procedures
- Decreased longevity
- Decreased quality of life
- Depression
- Diabetes (type 2)
- Fertility problems
- Gallbladder and liver disease
- Gout
- Heart disease
- High blood cholesterol levels
- Hormonal imbalances
- Hypertension
- Injury to weight-bearing joints
- Kidney abnormalities
- Metabolic syndrome*
- Osteoarthritis (knees, hips, lower spine)
- Poor self-esteem
- Respiratory problems
- Sleep disturbances
- Varicose veins

*Metabolic syndrome is a clustering of risk factors associated with the development of type 2 diabetes and heart disease. These risk factors include excess body weight (especially around the abdomen), insulin resistance, high blood pressure, high levels of triglycerides, low levels of HDL-cholesterol, and increased blood glucose levels.

cancer.[9] Table 10-1 shows additional conditions that can be caused, or worsened, by obesity.

In addition to being at risk for these health hazards, millions of people with obesity incur risks from ill-advised, misguided diet programs. Some fad diets are actually more hazardous to health than obesity! Many claims, treatments, devices, and gadgets for losing weight are, at best, simply ineffective, whereas others are truly dangerous. Over the centuries, "magic" weight-loss plans have been offered time and again, and their success lies in their popularity, not in their results.

Although some people with obesity suffer none of these physical health hazards, no one in our society quite escapes one disadvantage of obesity. In many parts of North America, obesity is a social and economic handicap.[10] Individuals with obesity suffer from discrimination in many areas, including social relationships and the job market. Psychologically, a body size that embarrasses or shames a person can be a private anguish. For people who perceive themselves as fat in a society that prizes thinness, real or imagined obesity can thrust them into withdrawal, shame, humiliation, and isolation.

Then, how thin is too thin—and how fat is too fat? The following section discusses the concept of a healthy weight.

10.2 What Is a Healthy Weight?

The question of what weight is healthy is harder to answer than you might at first think. Although Table 10-2 provides healthy weight ranges, to think merely in terms of weight oversimplifies the issue of body fatness and health. This chapter first asks what range of weights is compatible with wellness and long life and then suggests that personal preferences dictate the choice of a weight within that range.

Body Weight versus Body Fat

Two people of the same sex, age, and height may both weigh the same, yet one may be too fat and the other too thin. The difference lies in their body composition. One may have small, light bones and minimally developed muscles, while the other has big, heavy bones and well-developed muscles. The first person could have too much body fat and the second person too little. For example, football players, bodybuilders, and other athletes may technically be overweight for their height, according to the weight tables. However, they typically have less body fat than would pose a health risk. Likewise, many sedentary people who weigh in as "normal" may actually be too fat. Thus, obesity must be defined by amount of body fat rather than by weight.

The health risks of obesity refer to people who have too much body fat. On the average, men having more than 25 percent body fat and women having more than 33 percent body fat are considered obese.[11] Desirable measures are 12 to 20 percent body fat for most men and 20 to 30 percent body fat for most women.

Measuring Body Fat

Body fatness is hard to measure. One very accurate way is to obtain a measure of the body's density—that is, weight divided by volume. Lean tissue is denser than fat tissue. Weight is easy enough; just step on an accurate scale. To calculate body density, though, you have to immerse the whole body in a tank of water and measure the amount of water displaced. However, not many health professionals have space in their offices for the equipment needed

underwater weighing A measure of density and volume; the less a person weighs underwater compared to the person's out-of-water weight, the greater the proportion of body fat (fat is less dense or more buoyant than lean tissue).

skinfold test A method for measuring body fat in which the thickness of a fold of skin on the back of the arm (the triceps), below the shoulder blade (subscapular), or in other areas is measured with an instrument called a caliper.

bioelectrical impedance Estimation of body fat content made by measuring how quickly electrical current is conducted through the body.

FIGURE 10-3

Hydrostatic (Underwater) Weighing

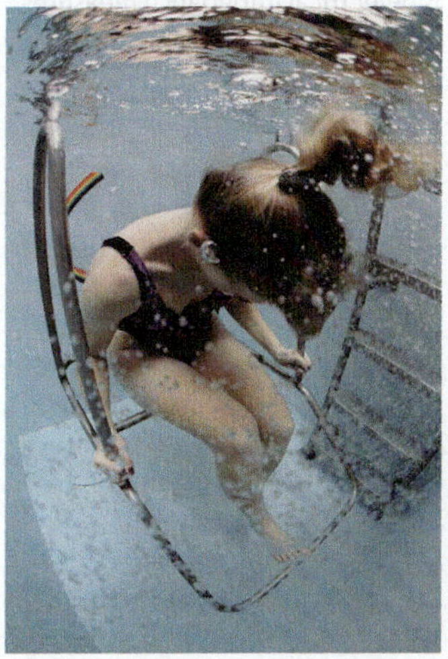

David Madison/Getty Images

FIGURE 10-4

BOD POD

The BOD POD measures body density.

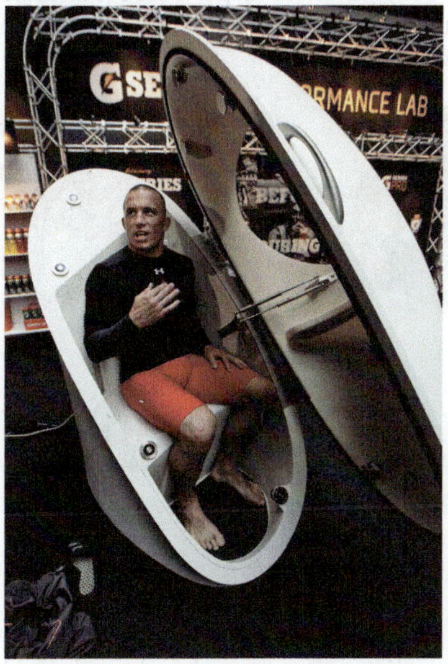

David Cooper/Getty Images

for this procedure, known as *hydrostatic weighing* or **underwater weighing** (see Figure 10-3). Body density can more easily be determined by air-displacement methods* such as the BOD POD, which measures the volume of air displaced by a person seated in a sealed device of known volume (see Figure 10-4).[12] Most professionals employ the **skinfold test**, using a caliper—a pinching device that measures the thickness of a fold of fat in such areas as the back of the arm, below the shoulder blade, and the side of the waist (see Figure 10-5). About 50 percent of the body's fat lies beneath the skin, and its thickness at these locations can be compared with standard tables to give a fair approximation of total body fat, at least for most people.

Although costly, the same technology used to measure bone density—*dual-energy X-ray absorptiometry* (the DEXA test)—can yield an accurate image of the body's fat-free tissue and total fat content. An alternate method for assessing body fatness is **bioelectrical impedance**, in which electrodes are attached to a person's hand and foot. This method measures a person's fat mass by measuring how fast a very low electrical current is conducted through the body (from the ankle to the wrist). Because fat is a poor conductor of electricity, the more fat one has, the more resistance this current encounters in the body.[13] Newer models of machines using this method allow for measurement by stepping on a platform containing the electrodes (see Figure 10-6).

*The air-displacement technique used by the BOD POD relies on the physics of Boyle's law, which states that pressure and volume vary inversely with one another (e.g., as pressure goes up, volume goes down, and vice versa). Measuring air displacement (pressure changes) caused by a person seated in the sealed BOD POD chamber of known volume provides the data needed to calculate the person's body density.

TABLE 10-2 Weight for Height Standards[a]

Healthy Weight Ranges[b]		
Height	**Weight (lb)[c]**	
	Midpoint	**Range**
4′10″	105	91–119
4′11″	109	94–124
5′0″	112	97–128
5′1″	116	101–132
5′2″	120	104–137
5′3″	124	107–141
5′4″	128	111–146
5′5″	132	114–150
5′6″	136	118–155
5′7″	140	121–160
5′8″	144	125–164
5′9″	149	129–169
5′10″	153	132–174
5′11″	157	136–179
6′0″	162	140–184
6′1″	166	144–189
6′2″	171	148–195
6′3″	176	152–200
6′4″	180	156–205

BMI Cutoff Weights for Overweight and Obesity		
Height	**BMI of 25 overweight (lb)**	**BMI of 30 obese (lb)**
4′11″	124	148
5′0″	128	153
5′1″	132	158
5′2″	136	164
5′3″	141	169
5′4″	145	174
5′5″	150	180
5′6″	155	186
5′7″	159	191
5′8″	164	197
5′9″	169	203
5′10″	174	207
5′11″	179	215
6′0″	184	221
6′1″	189	227
6′2″	194	233
6′3″	200	240
6′4″	205	246

[a] See Appendix A for a quick estimation of desirable body weight and a method for determining frame size.
[b] The higher weights in the ranges generally apply to men, who tend to have more muscle and bone; the lower weights more often apply to women, who have less muscle and bone.
[c] Without shoes or clothes.

FIGURE 10-5

Skinfold Test

The skinfold test gives a fair approximation of total body fat. Here, a caliper is used to measure the thickness of a fold of fat at the side of the waist.

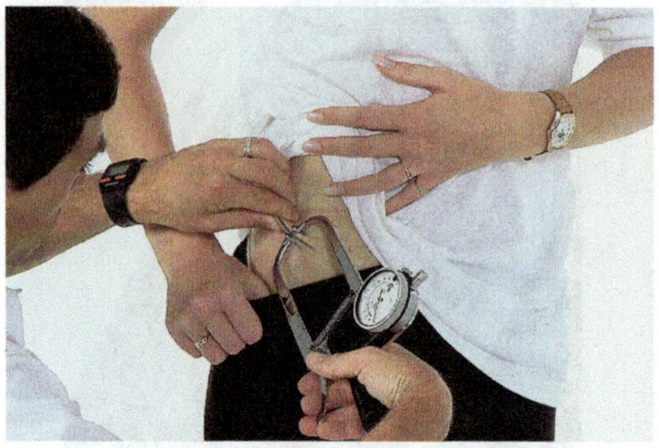

© Fitness & Wellness, Boise, Idaho

FIGURE 10-6

Bioelectrical Impedance

Bioelectrical impedance measures body fat.

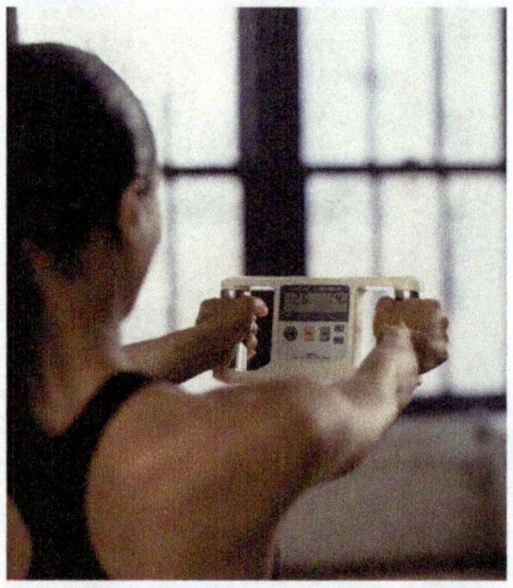

Yoav Levy/Medical Images

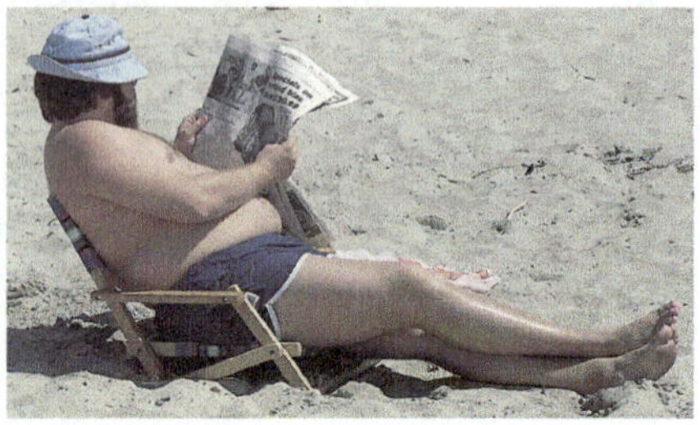

Alan Oddie/PhotoEdit

Central obesity, characterized by an "apple-shaped" body with large abdominal-type fat stores, is a strong risk factor for type 2 diabetes, heart disease, and other problems.

Distribution of Body Fat

Individuals carry body fat in different places. To complicate matters further, how body fat is distributed has health implications. Excess fat around the middle—**central obesity**—is associated with increased health hazards.[14] Body types are described as either apple-shaped or pear-shaped. Apple-shaped people, those who store most of their excess fat around the abdomen (typically men), are at a greater risk for developing diabetes, hypertension, elevated levels of blood cholesterol, and heart disease compared to pear-shaped people, who store excess fat on the hips, thighs, and buttocks (typically women). A simple measurement of a person's waist circumference can be used to assess abdominal fat.

Weighing in for Health

Obesity presents one of the most serious health risks that people face—and one that people should, theoretically, be able to control. In response to the rising epidemic of excessive weight, guidelines for the assessment and treatment of overweight and obesity have been developed.[15] A person's health risk due to weight depends on three factors: body weight, amount and location of body fat, and current health status.

Body weight is assessed using the **body mass index (BMI)**, an index of your weight in relation to your height. *Overweight* is defined as a BMI of 25 to 29.9, and *obesity* is defined as a BMI of 30 or above (refer to Table 10-2 for body weights that equate with these BMI values).[16] Keep in mind that BMI does not account for location of fat in the body; a muscular person with a low percentage of body fat may also have a high BMI (see Figure 10-7). In consideration of this shortcoming of the BMI measurement, the other two factors are taken into account.

The **waist circumference** measurement (see Figure 10-8) provides information about the distribution of fat in the abdomen. Excess abdominal fat poses a greater health risk than excess fat in the hips and thighs. This extra abdominal fat crowds the organs, and its proximity to the liver means that, when metabolized, abdominal fat can raise blood cholesterol levels and lower the body's sensitivity to insulin. Disease risk rises significantly with a waist circumference of more than 35 inches in women and more than 40 inches in men.[17]

central obesity Excess fat on the abdomen and around the trunk. *Peripheral obesity* is excess fat on the arms, thighs, hips, and buttocks.

body mass index (BMI) An index of a person's weight in relation to height that correlates with total body fat content.

waist circumference A measure used to assess abdominal (visceral) fat; excess fat in the abdomen increases a person's risk of health problems.

SCORE Card Healthy Weight (Obj. 10.2)

A wide range of weights is compatible with good health. Within this range, the definition of desirable or healthful weight is up to the individual, depending on such factors as family history, occupation, physical and recreational activities, and personal preferences. To determine if your weight is a healthful weight for you:

1. *Calculate your body mass index (BMI).* Find your height and weight in the following chart.* Your BMI is at the top of the column that contains your weight. Record your BMI here: ____________

BMI:	**19**	**20**	**21**	**22**	**23**	**24**	**25**	**26**	**27**	**28**	**29**	**30**	**35**	**40**
Height							**Weight (pounds)**							
5′0″	97	102	107	112	118	123	128	133	138	143	148	153	179	204
5′1″	100	106	111	116	122	127	132	137	143	148	153	158	185	211
5′2″	104	109	115	120	126	131	136	142	147	153	158	164	191	218
5′3″	107	113	118	124	130	135	141	146	152	158	163	169	197	225
5′4″	110	116	122	128	134	140	145	151	157	163	169	174	204	232
5′5″	114	120	126	132	138	144	150	156	162	168	174	180	210	240
5′6″	118	124	130	136	142	148	155	161	167	173	179	186	216	247
5′7″	121	127	134	140	146	153	159	166	172	178	185	191	223	255
5′8″	125	131	138	144	151	158	164	171	177	184	190	197	230	262
5′9″	128	135	142	149	155	162	169	176	182	189	196	203	236	270
5′10″	132	139	146	153	160	167	174	181	188	195	202	209	243	278
5′11″	136	143	150	157	165	172	179	186	193	200	208	215	250	286
6′0″	140	147	154	162	169	177	184	191	199	206	213	221	258	294
6′1″	144	151	159	166	174	182	189	197	204	212	219	227	265	302
6′2″	148	155	163	171	179	186	194	202	210	218	225	233	272	311
	Healthy Weight						Overweight					Obese		

SOURCE: National Heart, Lung and Blood Institute.

2. Determine if your fat distribution is associated with health risks. Measure your waist circumference by placing a tape measure around your waist just above your belly button. Record your waist in inches here. ____________

3. Is your weight affecting your health? Do you have any of these weight-related health problems or risk factors?

- Heart disease
- Type 2 diabetes
- High blood pressure
- High LDL-cholesterol
- Low HDL-cholesterol
- High triglycerides
- Osteoarthritis
- Recurrent gallstones
- Sleep disturbances
- Cigarette smoking
- Sedentary lifestyle
- Male > 45 years or postmenopausal female

4. How does your current weight measure up to these considerations?

- If your BMI is acceptable for good health and if your waist measurement is not high, you will want to maintain this weight. If you need to lose weight or gain weight, consider the tips offered throughout this chapter for healthfully changing your weight.
- You should consider losing weight if:

  Your BMI is 30 or greater.

  Your BMI is 25 to 29 and you have two or more of the weight-related health problems or risk factors listed previously.

  Your waist circumference exceeds 40 inches (for men) or 35 inches (for women) and you have two or more weight-related health problems or risk factors.
- Weight loss is optional for you if your BMI is 25 to 29 and you do not have two or more weight-related health problems (particularly if your BMI is under 27 or you have large muscles and bones).

*Additional heights and weights are listed at the back of this book, or you can use this formula to calculate your BMI:

$$\frac{\text{weight (in pounds)}}{\text{height}^2\text{ (in inches)}} \times 703$$

EXAMPLE: A 5′8″ person weighing 145 pounds has a BMI of 22.

$$\text{BMI} = \frac{145}{68^2} \times 703$$

$$\text{BMI} = \frac{145}{4624} \times 703$$

BMI = 22 (round)

FIGURE 10-7

Understanding Body Mass Index (BMI)

SOURCE: Adapted from G. Bray, *Contemporary Diagnosis and Management of Obesity* (1998), Handbooks in Healthcare, Co., a division of AAM Co., Inc.

Benefits of Using BMI

BMI correlates strongly with body fatness and risk of disease and death.

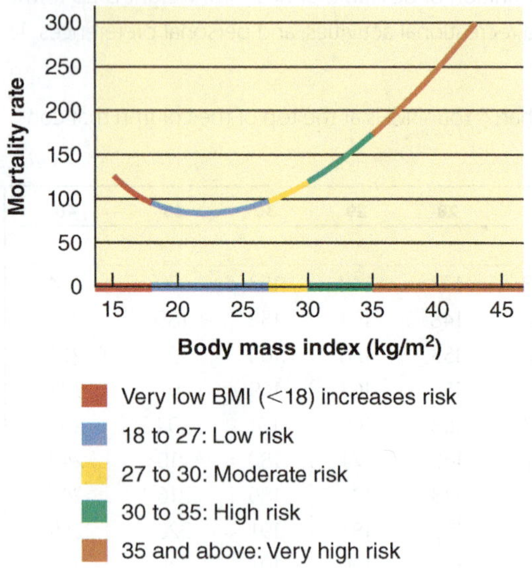

Cautions in Using BMI

May overestimate body fat in athletes and underestimate body fat in adults over 65.

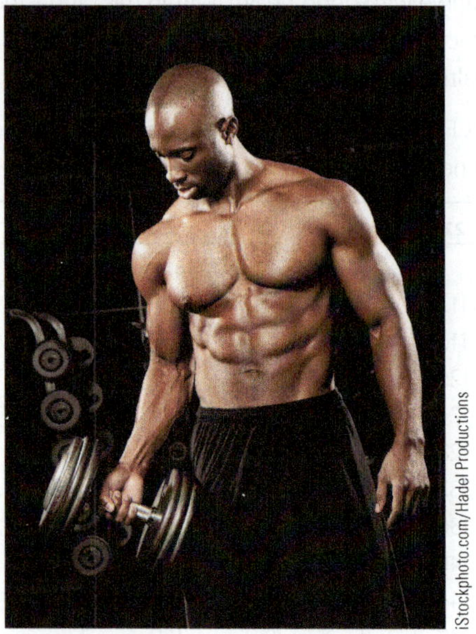

A muscular person, such as this body-builder, often has a low percentage of body fat but a high BMI.

Body Mass Index (BMI) Can Be Calculated As Follows:

BMI = [weight (pounds) ÷ height (inches)^2] × 703

For example, the BMI for a woman who is 5′5″ tall and weighs 145 lb would be:

[145 ÷ (65 × 65)] × 703 = 24

- BMI < 18.5 = underweight
- BMI 18.5 to 24.9 = normal weight
- BMI 25 to 29.9 = overweight
- BMI ≥ 30 = obese
- BMI ≥ 40 = severely obese

FIGURE 10-8

Waist Circumference

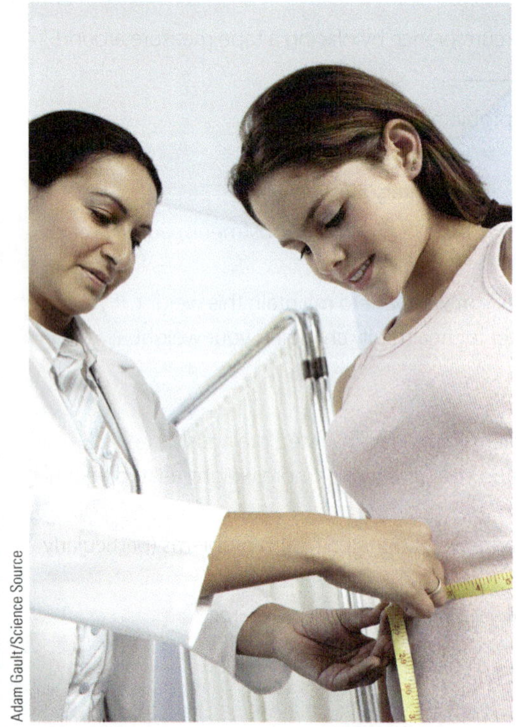

The third factor to consider is current health status: the presence of weight-related health problems and risk factors for diseases. These may include family health history, heart disease, type 2 diabetes, high blood cholesterol, high blood pressure, cigarette smoking, osteoarthritis, gallstones, or sleep apnea (irregular breathing during sleep). According to the treatment guidelines, an initial goal for treatment of people who are overweight and obese with risk factors is to reduce body weight by about 10 percent at a rate of about 1 to 2 pounds per week.[18] For individuals who are overweight, losing as little as 5 to 10 percent of their body weight may improve or even resolve many of the problems linked to overweight, such as diabetes and high blood pressure. The Scorecard feature on page 291 helps you make sense of these guidelines and evaluate your own weight status.

10.3 Energy Balance

Suppose you decide that you are too fat or too thin and that you got that way by having an unbalanced energy budget—that is, by eating either more or less energy from food than you expend. Fatness and thinness are reflections of excess or deficient energy stores. You store extra energy as fat only if you eat *more* food energy in a day than you use to fuel your metabolic and other activities. Similarly, you lose stored fat only if you eat *less* food energy in a day than you use as fuel. A day's energy balance can be stated like this:

Change in energy stores = Energy in − Energy out

You already know about the "energy in" side of this equation. An apple provides you 80 calories; a candy bar, 290 calories. You may also know that for each 3,500 *excess* calories consumed ("excess" meaning more than your body needs), you store 1 pound of body fat.

For the "energy out" side of the equation, the body expends energy in two major ways: to fuel its metabolic activities and to fuel its muscle activities. As shown in Figure 10-9, you also spend a small amount of energy to digest, absorb, transport, process, and store the food you eat, which is known as the *thermic effect of food*. The following three sections discuss the body's needs for energy.

FIGURE 10-9

How the Body Expends Energy

The body expends most of its energy on *basal metabolism*—maintaining basic physiological processes such as breathing, heartbeat, and other involuntary activities. The second largest amount of energy is expended for voluntary *physical activities*—an amount that will vary by activity level. A minor amount of energy is also used for the *thermic effect of food*—the energy needed to digest, absorb, and process the food you eat.

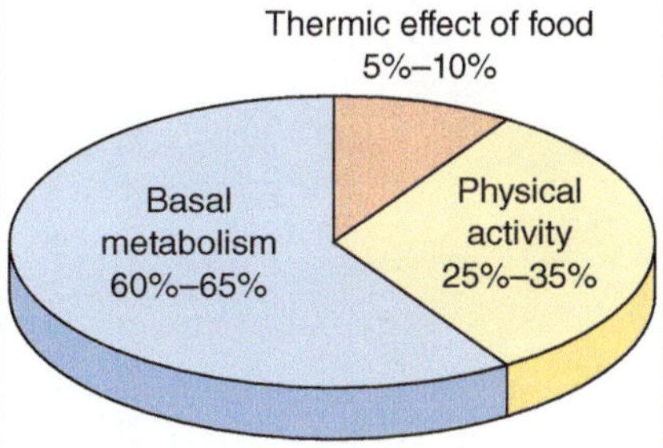

Basal Metabolism

About 60 percent or more of the energy the average person spends goes to support the ongoing metabolic work of the body's cells, the **basal metabolism.**[19] This is the work that goes on all the time, without conscious awareness. The beating of the heart, the inhaling and exhaling of air, the maintenance of body temperature, and the sending of nerve and hormonal messages to direct these activities are the basal processes that maintain life. Basal metabolic needs are surprisingly large. A person whose total energy expenditure amounts to 2,000 calories per day expends as much as 1,200 to 1,400 calories to support basal metabolism.

The **basal metabolic rate** (often abbreviated **BMR**) is influenced by several factors (see Table 10-3). In general, the younger a person is, the higher the basal metabolic rate, partly because of the increased activity of cells undergoing division. The BMR is most pronounced during the growth spurts that take place during infancy, puberty, and pregnancy. Body composition also influences metabolic rate. Muscle tissue is highly active even when it is resting, whereas fat tissue is comparatively inactive. Therefore, when comparing two people of the same body weight, the person with more lean muscle tissue will have a higher BMR, and the person with more fat tissue will have a lower BMR. Lean body mass decreases with age, but consistent physical activity—especially endurance and strength-building activities—may prevent some of the decline.

Gender correlates roughly with body composition. Men generally have a faster metabolic rate than women, and researchers believe that this is because men have a greater percentage of lean tissue. (Also, a female athlete has a greater percentage of lean tissue than a sedentary man of the same weight and so would have a higher metabolic rate.) Fever increases the energy needs of cells, as their increased activities to fight off infection and generate heat speed up the metabolic rate.

Fasting and constant malnutrition lower the metabolic rate because of the loss of lean tissue and the slowdown of activities the body cannot afford to support fully. This slowing of metabolism seems to be a protective mechanism to conserve energy when there is a shortage, and it hampers weight loss in a person who fasts or undertakes a very low-calorie diet.

Some hormones—the stress hormones, for example—influence metabolism. They increase the energy demands of every cell and thus raise the metabolic rate. This raised metabolism partly accounts for the weight loss sometimes seen in people experiencing extreme stress in their life, although other factors, such as upset digestion and loss of appetite, also play a role. The activity of the thyroid gland also influences the basal metabolic rate. The less thyroid hormone secreted, the lower the energy requirement for maintenance of basal functions.

TABLE 10-3 Factors That Influence the Basal Metabolic Rate

Factors That Increase BMR:

- Caffeine
- Fever
- Growth (higher in children and pregnant women)
- Height (higher in tall, thin people)
- High thyroid hormone
- Male gender (more lean tissue)
- Muscle mass (the more lean tissue, the higher the BMR)
- Smoking (nicotine)
- Stress

Factors That Decrease BMR:

- Age (slows down with age)
- Low thyroid hormone
- Reduced energy intake (fasting, starvation, low-calorie diets)
- Sleep (BMR is lowest when sleeping)

© Cengage

basal metabolism The sum total of all the chemical activities of the cells necessary to sustain life, exclusive of voluntary activities; that is, the ongoing activities of the cells when the body is at rest.

basal metabolic rate (BMR) The rate at which the body spends energy to support its basal metabolism. The BMR accounts for the largest component of a person's daily energy (calorie) needs.

Note: For a quick method for calculating your basal energy output:

Men: kg of body weight × 24 = calories/day

Women: kg of body weight × 23 = calories/day

NOTE: To convert pounds to kilograms (kg), divide weight in pounds by 2.2.

Energy Needs

How many calories do you need? This chart helps you calculate the average daily number of calories you need to maintain your current weight. Because energy needs differ among men and women, there are different calculations for each. These calculations are for healthy men and women, ages 19 years and older.

Instructions: Write the answers on the lines below.

Start with these numbers:

Your age in years ________; weight in kilograms* ________; height in meters* ________

FOR MEN:

A. Multiply your age by 9.53 = ________

B. Subtract line A from 662 = ________

C. Multiply your weight by 15.91 = ________

D. Multiply your height by 539.6 = ________

E. Add lines C and D = ________

F. Determine your Physical Activity (PA) Coefficient according to your Physical Activity Level (PAL) (see table below): ________

G. Multiply line E by the PA Coefficient = ________

H. Add lines B and G. This is your total daily caloric maintenance level. ________

FOR WOMEN:

A. Multiply your age by 6.91 = ________

B. Subtract line A from 354 = ________

C. Multiply your weight by 9.36 = ________

D. Multiply your height by 726 = ________

E. Add lines C and D = ________

F. Determine your Physical Activity (PA) Coefficient according to your Physical Activity Level (PAL) (see table below): ________

G. Multiply line E by the PA Coefficient = ________

H. Add lines B and G. This is your total daily caloric maintenance level. ________

	Physical Activity (PA) Coefficient	
Physical Activity Level (PAL)	**Men**	**Women**
Sedentary *No regular activity*	1.00	1.00
Low active *Up to 30 minutes per day*	1.11	1.12
Active *30 to 60 minutes per day*	1.25	1.27
Very active *More than 60 minutes per day*	1.48	1.45

SOURCE: Adapted from the Estimated Energy Requirement calculations established in the *Dietary Reference Intakes for Energy, Carbohydrate, Fiber, Fat, Fatty Acids, Cholesterol, Protein, and Amino Acids* (2005), written by the Panel on Macronutrients; Panel on the Definition of Dietary Fiber; Subcommittee on Upper Reference Levels of Nutrients; Subcommittee on Interpretation and Uses of Dietary Reference Intakes; and the Standing Committee on the Scientific Evaluation of Dietary Reference Intakes, Food and Nutrition Board.

*NOTE: To convert pounds to kilograms, divide weight in pounds by 2.2. For example, 150 lb = 68 kg [150 ÷ 2.2 = 68]; to convert inches to centimeters, multiply height in inches by 2.54, and then to convert centimeters to meters, divide height in centimeters by 100.

Voluntary Activities Muscular activity does not contribute as much to most people's energy outputs as basal metabolism does. On the average, it amounts to only about 30 percent of the total. Unlike basal metabolism, though, which cannot be changed immediately, physical activity can be changed at will. If you want to change your energy balance, this is the component—on the output side—that you can alter significantly in the short term. If you increase physical activity consistently, you will also ultimately increase the energy your body expends on metabolic activity, because you will have an increase in lean body mass.

The energy spent on physical activity is the energy spent moving the body's skeletal muscles—the muscles of the arms, back, abdomen, legs, and so forth—and the extra energy needed to speed up the heartbeat and respiration rate. The number of calories spent depends on three factors: (1) the amount of muscle mass required, (2) the amount of weight being moved, and (3) the amount of time the activity takes. Thus, an activity involving both the arms and the legs requires more calories than an activity of the same intensity involving only the legs; an activity performed by a heavier person requires more energy than the same activity performed by a lighter person; and an activity performed for 40 minutes requires twice as much energy as that same activity performed for 20 minutes.

It may be disheartening for a college student to discover that mental activity requires little energy, even though it may be tiring. Studying for an exam may be hard work, but it doesn't burn body fat. People who are very, very busy—surfing the Internet, making phone calls, riding in their cars—may wonder why they gain weight. Even though they are socially or intellectually active, such activities involve few muscles and therefore little energy expenditure.

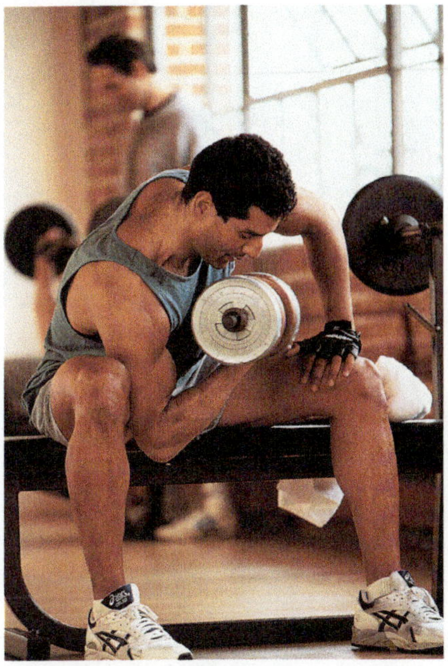
David Madison/Getty Images

Body composition influences metabolic rate. Weight training can help shift your body composition toward more lean tissue, thereby speeding up your metabolism. See Chapter 11 for guidelines on how to get started.

Total Energy Needs A typical breakdown of the total energy spent by a lightly active person (e.g., a student who walks back and forth to classes) might look like this:

Energy for basal metabolism:	1,400 calories
Energy for physical activity:	560 calories
Total:	1,960 calories

The first component (basal metabolism) is larger, and you cannot change it much. You can, however, change the second component—physical activity—and use more calories. To increase your basal metabolic output, make exercise a daily habit. Your body composition will gradually change, and your basal energy output will pick up the pace as well. You can figure out roughly how much energy you need in a day by using the method illustrated in the box—"Energy Needs."

In summary, the amount of fat stored in a person's body depends on the balance between the total food energy the person has taken in and the total energy the person has expended. But why do so many people have excessive fat stores?

10.4 Causes of Obesity

Some people eat more than they need or exercise less than they should to maintain their body weight, and they gain fat. Some eat less or exercise more, and they lose fat. Amazingly, many people eat exactly what they need and stay at the same weight, year after year. Eating a single extra pat of butter each day would make them gain 5 pounds in a year, but if these people overeat by that much on one day, they apparently undereat by the same amount the next day. How do they do this, and (in contrast) why do some people fail to maintain their weight? In general, most experts believe that obesity is associated with both internal causes and environmental factors.[20]

Genetics

The theory that a hereditary, internal factor may promote obesity is supported by the existence of animal strains that are genetically fat. Such animals tend to be fat in any environment; that is, they are fat regardless of the kind or variety of food that is available. In humans, studies have shown that identical twins—whether raised together or apart—tend to have similar weight-gain patterns. Also, twins raised by adoptive parents tend to have body shapes like those of their biological parents. Not all studies confirm this, however.[21] Interestingly, pairs of twins purposefully overfed in clinical experiments tend to respond similarly to the extra calories. Some sets of twins gain considerable weight when fed a certain number of calories, whereas other pairs put on relatively few pounds even on the same diet.[22]

Set-Point Theory One popular internal theory is the so-called **set-point theory**. Noting that many people who lose weight on weight-reducing diets subsequently return to their original weight, some researchers have suggested that the body "wants" to maintain a certain amount of fat and regulates eating behaviors and hormonal actions to defend its "set point." The theory implies that science should search inside people with obesity to find the causes of their excess weight—perhaps in their hunger-regulating mechanisms.

Leptin Researchers have identified a gene—named *ob* (for *obese*)—that produces a hormone called *leptin*, after the Greek word for "slender." When it is released from fat cells, leptin seems to tell the body to stop eating.[23] Researchers report that as body fat stores increase, blood leptin also increases. The brain responds by decreasing appetite and increasing energy expenditure. Likewise, when body fat stores decrease, blood leptin decreases, and the brain responds by stimulating appetite and decreasing energy expenditure. Mice who have a defective form of the gene fail to produce leptin and can weigh as much as three times more than normal mice. People who are overweight, too, may have a defective form of this gene (or may be unresponsive to leptin).[24] More research is needed to clarify this mechanism.

Fat Cell Theory Some infants who are overweight become adults who are overweight, but most outgrow their obesity in childhood. A child who is overweight, however, is more likely to remain overweight into adulthood.[25] Some researchers propose the **fat cell theory**, which holds that childhood obesity is persistent because early overfeeding (during the growing years) may cause fat cells to increase abnormally in *number*. According to this theory, a person's *number* of fat cells is relatively fixed by the time he or she reaches adulthood; after that, a gain or loss of weight either increases or diminishes the size of the fat cells. Unfortunately, people with greater numbers of fat cells are less likely to lose weight successfully. Some researchers suggest that the body triggers hunger signals when the fat stored in these cells begins to decrease. Because fat cells increase in number during childhood, obesity prevention is critical during the growing years.

Additionally, fat cells of people with obesity contain higher levels of the enzyme **lipoprotein lipase (LPL)**, which determines the rate at which adipose cells store fat. The larger the fat cell (and the greater the number of fat cells), the more LPL is available to more easily pull triglycerides into fat cells for storage. Unfortunately, LPL activity rises further with weight loss, enhancing the body's ability to regain the lost weight.[26] A question still to be answered is whether some people develop obesity because their fat cells contain an abnormal amount of LPL from birth.

set-point theory Theory that the body tends to maintain a certain weight by adjusting hunger, appetite, and food energy intake on the one hand and metabolism (energy output) on the other so that a person's conscious efforts to alter weight may be foiled.

fat cell theory Theory that during the growing years, fat cells respond to overfeeding by producing additional fat cells; the number of fat cells eventually becomes relatively fixed, and overfeeding from this point on causes the body to enlarge existing fat cells.

lipoprotein lipase (LPL) An enzyme located on the surfaces of fat cells that enables the cell to convert blood triglycerides into fatty acids and glycerol to be pulled into the cell for reassembly and storage as body fat.

Environment Environmental factors linked with obesity suggest that people overeat or lack exercise because of their surroundings: foremost among them, the ready availability of a multitude of delicious foods and a lack of opportunity for vigorous physical activity.

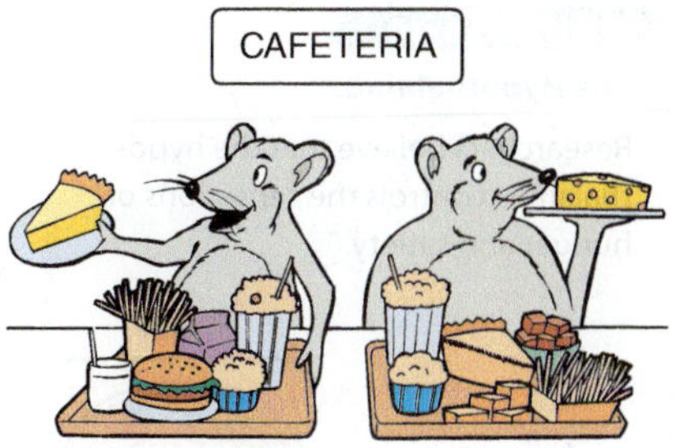

© Cengage

Some people seem to have inherited or learned a way of resisting external stimuli to eat, but others have not. In a classic experiment with "cafeteria rats," ordinary rats who were fed regular rat chow, maintained normal weight (for rats), but when those very same rats were offered free access to a wide variety of rich, highly palatable foods, they greatly overate and became obese. Similarly, one study found a positive correlation between over-fatness and a diet offering a wide variety of snacks and sweets.[27] This is the basis of the **external cue theory**, which suggests that, at least in some people, the internal regulatory systems are easily overridden by environmental influences. Does this mean obesity is hereditary, environmental, or both?

It seems likely that both hereditary and environmental factors influence obesity in human beings. The tendency toward obesity is probably inherited, but the environment is probably influential in the sense that it can prevent or permit the development of obesity when the potential is there.

A Closer Look at Eating Behavior In human beings, learning plays an important role. Although we have genetically inborn instincts, things learned during early childhood experiences, combined with our current environments, may conflict with these instincts. Thus, the **hunger** drive is programmed by heredity, but **appetite** is influenced by learned responses that may cause us to ignore or overrespond to our hunger. In other words, hunger is physiological, whereas appetite is psychological, and the two don't always coincide. We have all experienced appetite without hunger: "I'm not hungry, but I'd love to have some." We also often experience the reverse: "I know I'm hungry, but I don't feel like eating."

The ways people respond to hunger and appetite determine whether they eat too much, too little, or just enough to maintain their weight. A third factor, **satiety**, which signals that it is time to stop eating, also affects our eating patterns and weight issues.

In human physiology, research is beginning to find possible answers to what regulates eating behavior. The stomach's nerves perceive stretching, and you stop eating when your stomach feels stretched full. Blood glucose level is also thought to be involved. You get hungry when your blood glucose level falls—or perhaps when your liver glycogen is beginning to be exhausted. Blood lipids, and possibly amino acids and other molecules, also play a role. When you eat, you secrete hormones to regulate digestive activity; these hormones may also convey the message to the brain that it is time to start or stop eating.*

Where in the brain are these hunger and satiety messages received? One brain area stands out as a regulator for food behavior: the **hypothalamus** (see Figure 10-10). The hypothalamus communicates with the hormone system and the nervous system. It integrates many signals received from the rest of the body, including information about the blood's temperature, sodium content, and glucose content. We know it is important in regulating eating because damage to the hypothalamus produces derangements in eating behavior and body weight. In some cases, it can cause severe weight loss, and in others, it can cause extreme overeating. However, in people with a normal hypothalamus,

external cue theory The theory that some people eat in response to such external factors as the presence of food or the time of day rather than to such internal factors as hunger.

hunger The physiological drive to find and eat food, experienced as an unpleasant sensation.

appetite The psychological desire to find and eat food, experienced as a pleasant sensation, often in the absence of hunger.

satiety The feeling of fullness or satisfaction experienced following a meal.

hypothalamus (high-poh-THALL-ah-mus) A part of the brain that senses a variety of conditions in the blood, such as temperature, salt content, and glucose content, and then signals other parts of the brain or body to change those conditions when necessary.

*Researchers have discovered *ghrelin* (GRELL-in), a protein produced by the stomach cells that acts as a hormone, affecting the hypothalamus and stimulating appetite. Ghrelin levels are high before a meal (reflecting hunger) and fall rapidly after a meal (reflecting satiety). Researchers continue to investigate ghrelin's exact role in food intake regulation.

FIGURE 10-10

The Hypothalamus

Researchers believe that the hypothalamus controls the sensations of hunger and satiety.

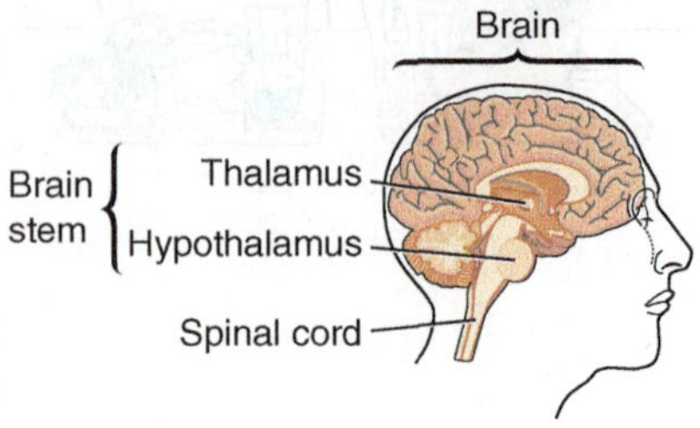

appropriate eating behavior seems to be a response to a whole host of signals rather than a response to a single signal arriving at one location in the hypothalamus. Somehow these many inputs become integrated into a final common path: the act of eating.

A person who eats inappropriately may have established a habitual behavior pattern that inappropriately links certain stimuli to the act of eating. The study of behavior offers insight into the causes of overeating by viewing it as a conditioned response. Sometimes eating behavior is initiated by the wrong triggers. For example, a crying child with a bruised knee who is offered a lollipop may learn to associate food with comfort and inappropriately feel the need for food when experiencing emotional pain later in life.

Eating behavior, then, may be a response not only to hunger or appetite but also to complex human sensations such as yearning, craving, addiction, or compulsion. Often, eating is used to relieve boredom or to ward off depression. Some people respond to anxiety—or, in fact, to any kind of **arousal**—by eating. However, when these people are able to name their aroused condition, they often gain a feeling that they have some control over it and are not as likely to overeat.

Stress may also directly promote the accumulation of body fat. The stress hormones favor the breakdown of energy stores (glycogen and fat) into glucose and fatty acids, which can be used to fuel the human fight-or-flight response. If a person doesn't use the fuel in physical exertion, however, the body cannot turn these pieces of energy back into glycogen. Thus, its only alternative is to convert them to fat. Each time glucose is pulled out of storage, in response to stress and then transformed into fat, the lowered glucose level or exhausted glycogen will signal hunger, and the person will eat again soon after.

Stress eating may appear in different patterns. Some people eat excessively at night, whereas others binge during emotional crises. Some people react oppositely and reject food when stressed. We do not know why these behaviors occur, but research continues.

The many possible causes of obesity mentioned so far all relate to the input side of the energy equation. What about output? Probably the most important contributor to the obesity problem in our country is underactivity.[28] Some people who are obese eat less than people who are lean, but due to extraordinary inactivity, they still manage to store surplus calories. Some people move more efficiently than others, too. Two people of the same age, height, and weight might use different amounts of calories walking five miles because of the different ways in which they move their muscles.

No two people are alike, either physically or psychologically, and the causes of obesity vary as the people themselves. Many causes may contribute to the problem in a single person. Given this complexity, it is obvious that there is no cure-all. The top priority should be prevention, but where prevention has failed, the treatment of obesity must involve a simultaneous attack on many fronts.[29]

10.5 Weight Gain and Loss

When you step on the scale and see that you weigh a pound more or less than you did the last time, you have not necessarily gained or lost body fat. Changes in body weight reflect shifts in many different materials—not only fat but also fluid, bone minerals, and lean tissues such as muscles. The gain of a pound, for example, may reflect gained muscle and bone and an overall shift toward a leaner body type. Because it is so important for people concerned with weight control to realize this, this section discusses the various changes that take place with gains and losses of weight.

A healthy man or woman about 5 feet, 10 inches tall who weighs 150 pounds carries about 90 of those pounds as water and 30 as fat. The other 30 pounds are the so-called *lean tissues*: muscles; organs such as the heart, brain, and liver; and the bones of the skeleton.*

arousal As used in this context, heightened activity of certain brain centers associated with excitement and anxiety.

*For a healthy woman or man 5 feet tall who weighs 100 pounds, the comparable figures would be 60 pounds of water, 20 pounds of fat, and 20 pounds of lean tissue.

Without the water and fat, the person then weighs only 30 pounds. This lean tissue is the body's vital machinery that maintains health and life. When a person who is obese seeks to lose weight, it should be fat, not valuable lean tissue, that is lost. For someone who wants to gain weight, it is desirable to gain lean tissue *and* fat, not just fat.

Weight is gained or lost in different body tissues, depending on how a person goes about it. Most quick-weight-loss diet schemes promote large losses of fluid that create large, temporary changes in a person's scale weight, with little or no real loss of body fat. The rest of this chapter underscores this distinction, and a later section on weight-loss strategy emphasizes exercise as a means of supporting lean tissue during weight loss.

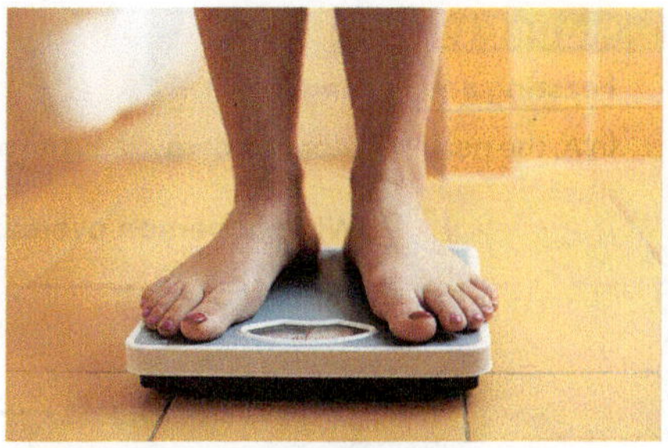
Rostislav_Sedlacek/Shutterstock.com

The loss (or gain) of a pound does not always reflect the loss (or gain) of body fat.

Weight Gain When you eat more calories than you need, where does the excess go? The energy nutrients—carbohydrate, fat, and protein—contribute to body stores as follows:

- Carbohydrate is broken down to glucose for absorption. Inside the body, glucose may be built up to glycogen or converted to and stored as fat.
- Fat is broken down to its component parts (including fatty acids) for absorption. Inside the body, these components are easily converted to storage fat.
- Protein, too, is broken down to its basic units (amino acids) for absorption. Inside the body, these units may be used to replace body proteins. The amino acids that are not used lose their nitrogen and are converted to fat.

Notice in Figure 10-11 that although three kinds of materials enter the body, they are stored for later use in only two forms, glycogen and fat. Also notice that when protein is stored in the form of fat, it cannot be converted back into protein later. The amino acids lose their nitrogen, which is then excreted in the urine. It does not matter whether you are eating hamburgers, brownies, or carrot sticks: If you eat enough of any food, the excess will be turned to fat within hours.

Weight Loss and Fasting When the tables are turned and you stop eating altogether, your body must draw on its stored supplies of nutrients to keep going. Nothing is wrong with this; in fact, it is a great advantage that you can eat periodically, store fuel, and then use up that fuel between meals. The between-meal interval is ideally about 4 to 6 hours (about the length of time it takes to use up most of the available liver glycogen) or 12 to 14 hours at night, when body systems are slowed down and the need for energy is lower. If a person doesn't eat for a longer period of time, like three days or even a week, the body makes one adjustment after another.

The body's first adjustment to fasting is to use the liver's glycogen for needed fuel. (The glycogen in muscles is reserved for the muscles' own use—and they do use it.) The liver's glycogen, remember, is the body's source of blood glucose to fuel brain and nerve activities. Ordinarily, the brain and nerves can use no other fuel, but after about a day without food, the primary supply is gone. Where, then, does the body turn to keep the nervous system going? Whatever it has to do, it will do, for the nervous system runs the body, and when it stops, the body dies.

An obvious alternative source of energy is the abundant fat stores that most people carry. At first, this fat is of no use to the nervous system. The muscles and other organs can use fat as fuel, but the nervous system ordinarily cannot. Nor can the body convert this fat to glucose, because it possesses no enzymes to do so. It does, however, possess enzymes to convert protein to glucose.

When the fast continues, the body turns to its own lean tissues to provide the necessary supply of glucose (see Figure 10-11). One reason people lose weight so

FIGURE 10-11

Feasting and Fasting

In A, the person is storing energy. In B, the person is drawing on stored energy. In C, the person is in ketosis.

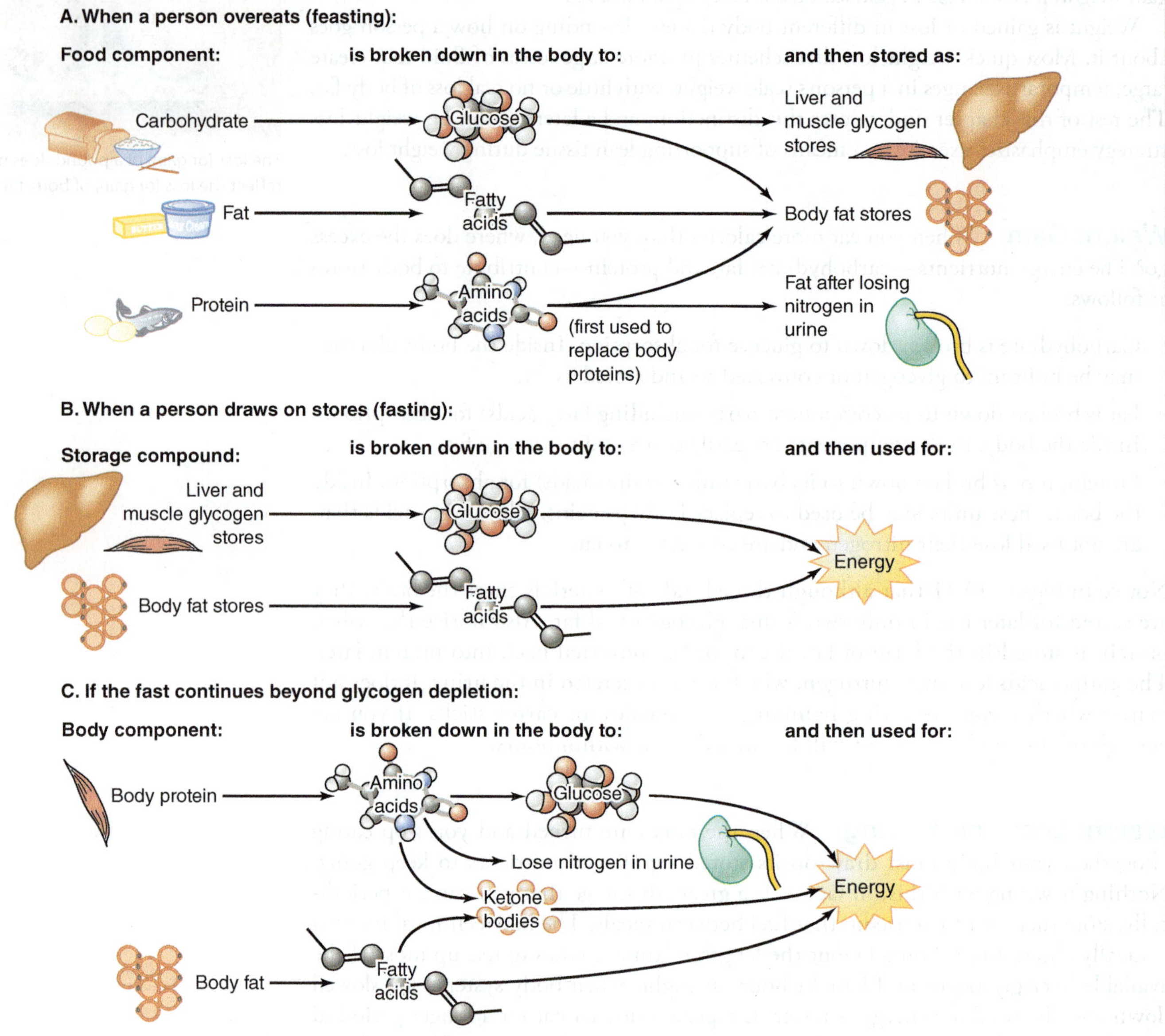

dramatically within the first three days of a fast is that they are using their own protein tissues as fuel. Because protein contains only half as many calories per pound as fat, it disappears twice as fast. Also, with each pound of body protein, three or four pounds of associated water are lost. This same process accounts for the rapid weight loss seen in the early stages of a low-carbohydrate diet.

If the body were to continue to consume itself at this rate, death would occur within about 10 days. After all, the liver, the heart and skeletal muscles, the lung tissue, and the blood—all vital tissues—are being burned as fuel. (In fact, fasting or starving people remain alive only until their body fat is gone or until half their lean tissue is gone, whichever comes first.) But now the body plays its last wild card: It begins converting fat stores into a form it can use to help feed the nervous system and to delay the end. This is known as **ketosis**.

ketosis (key-TOE-siss) An adaptation of the body to prolonged (several days) fasting or carbohydrate restriction; body fat is converted to ketones, which can be used as fuel for some brain cells.

Ketosis is an adaptation to fasting or carbohydrate deprivation. Instead of breaking fat molecules all the way down to carbon dioxide and water as it normally does, the body takes partially broken-down fat fragments, combines them into ketone bodies (compounds that are normally rare in the blood), and lets them circulate in the bloodstream. The advantage for the body is that about half of the brain cells can use these compounds for energy. Thus, indirectly, the nervous system begins to feed on the body's fat stores. This reduces the nervous system's need for glucose, spares the muscle and other lean tissue from being devoured so quickly, and prolongs the starving person's life. Because of ketosis, an initially healthy person who is totally deprived of food can live for as long as six to eight weeks.

Fasting has been practiced as a periodic discipline by respected, wise people in many cultures. However, ketosis may be harmful to the body by upsetting the acid–base balance of the blood. For people who merely want to lose weight, fasting is not the best way. For one thing, even in ketosis, the body's lean tissue continues to be lost at a rapid rate to supply glucose to those nervous system cells that cannot use ketones as fuel. For another, the body becomes conservative during a fast and slows its metabolism so as to lose as little energy as it possibly can. A well-designed, low-calorie diet, accompanied by the appropriate physical activity program, has actually been observed to promote the same rate of *weight* loss as, and a faster rate of *fat* loss than, a total fast. The Nutrition Action feature later in this chapter discusses what to look for in a weight-loss diet, including tips for how *not* to design a diet.

Drugs and Weight Loss

There has been a continuous search to find a safe and effective drug solution to obesity. The ideal drug should be safe, free of undesirable side effects and abuse potential, and effective at reducing body fat. Additionally, as with drug treatments for other chronic disorders (e.g., high blood pressure), the ideal drug should be safe and effective for long-term use. To foster long-term success, any such drug treatment should be combined with lifestyle changes, including physical activity and a healthy diet.[30] Until recently, most of the available drugs were appetite suppressants, which were available as prescriptions or over the counter (see Table 10-4).

TABLE 10-4 Drugs for Weight Loss

	Action in the Body	Potential Side Effects and/or Comments
Prescription Drugs (Trade Name)		
Orlistat (Xenical)[a]	A lipase inhibitor; acts by inhibiting the enzymes—gastric and pancreatic lipase—needed for fat digestion; binds to the enzymes, making them unavailable to digest dietary fat. Because fat absorption is reduced by as much as 30%, people often lose weight.	Bloating, gas, frequent bowel movements, and anal leakage of undigested fats in people who do not adhere to a low-fat diet. Because Xenical may block the absorption of fat-soluble vitamins, users are advised to take a multivitamin supplement. The drug is intended only for people who are obese—with a BMI greater than 30.
Phentermine (Adipex-P or Fastin)	Raises the level of norepinephrine, signals satiety and acts as a stimulant to increase the rate at which calories are burned.	Increased heart rate and blood pressure, dry mouth, insomnia, nausea, agitation, diarrhea, and constipation.
Lorcaserin (Belviq)	Serotonin receptor agonist, which increases serotonin levels and suppresses appetite.	Headache, fatigue, low blood sugar, dry mouth, dizziness, constipation.
Naltrexone and buproprion (Contrave)	Combination reduces appetite (through an opioid antagonist) and curbs food cravings (through an antidepressant)	Nausea, vomiting, insomnia, headache, dry mouth, dizziness, and constipation.
Phentermine and topiramate (Qsymia)	Combination raises the level of norepinephrine (signals satiety) while increasing energy expenditure.	Altered taste, increased heart rate, lack of concentration, insomnia, dry mouth, constipation.

[a]An over-the-counter low-dose form of orlistat is also available (trade name Alli)—to be used only with physician supervision.

Many other diet aids on the market include products with mysterious-sounding ingredients, such as hoodia, chitosan, chromium picolinate, bitter orange extract, "carb blockers," "fat blockers," ginseng, and many others. Manufacturers typically claim or suggest that such products can aid in weight loss, but their ingredients often serve as little more than fillers. To date, none have proven effective in aiding weight loss. For example, manufacturers of products that include chromium picolinate praise its drug-like abilities to reduce fat, build lean tissue, suppress appetite, and increase metabolism, and they imply that our diets lack chromium. However, chromium picolinate has not been approved for weight loss by the FDA, and claims regarding it are not backed by scientific data.[31] The FDA and the Federal Trade Commission have begun taking action against diet aids and products touting false claims for weight loss.[32]

The popularity of herbal supplements for weight loss is on the rise, partly because consumers have the mistaken notion that herbs are a "natural" alternative to prescription drugs. Thus far, herbal preparations in the United States are produced and marketed free of regulation to ensure their safety or effectiveness, and some have been linked to side effects ranging from nausea and headaches to heart attacks and death. For example, the Chinese herb *ma huang*—commonly called ephedra—contains ephedrine, a stimulant that mimics the action of the drug phentermine. Ephedrine can cause tremors, insomnia, severe headaches, high blood pressure, heart attacks, and stroke. Some herbal preparations combine ephedra with other substances (e.g., caffeine-containing guarana), to enhance the ephedrine's effects. More than 800 reports of illness and dozens of deaths are linked to ephedra, and both the FDA and Canada prohibit its use.[33]

Other herbal preparations sold as dieter's tea contain senna, rhubarb root, aloe, cascara, or buckthorn. The "tea" has a laxative effect that can cause dehydration, diarrhea, nausea, fainting, and in some cases, even death.[34] For more about herbs thought to be effective and those that should be avoided, see the Nutrition Action feature in Chapter 7.

Surgery and Weight Loss Sheer desperation prompts some people with obesity to request weight-loss surgery. However, surgery may be an option only for people who cannot lose weight by traditional means and are severely obese (BMI $\geq$ 40) or have a BMI of at least 35 with one or more severe health problems.[35] Three common types of surgery being performed today are gastric bypass, gastric banding, and sleeve gastrectomy (see Figure 10-12). Common side effects include nausea, vomiting, diarrhea, heartburn, abdominal pain, and band slippage or pouch enlargement. Other more severe effects including complications during surgery, infections, and death may occur as well.

Sleeve gastrectomy is currently the most common surgical procedure for obesity in the United States.[36] The surgery involves the removal of a large portion of the stomach so that it becomes shaped like a tube. The second most common procedure would be *gastric bypass.* For this, the surgeon creates a small pouch in the stomach with staples or a plastic band. Next, a Y-shaped section of the small intestine is attached to the pouch to allow food to bypass the lower stomach and the upper portion of the small intestine. These two procedures restrict both food and caloric intake and the amount of nutrients the body absorbs. The third most common operation in the United States for weight loss is called *gastric banding.* The procedure involves placement of an adjustable silicone band around the upper part of the stomach to create a small pouch; this limits food consumption and creates an earlier feeling of fullness.

At first, the small stomach pouch that results from weight-loss surgery holds about 1 ounce of food, though it may later stretch to hold 2 to 3 ounces. Nausea and vomiting occur if the person continues to overeat following surgery. Most people can eat about ½ to 1 cup of food without discomfort or nausea, but the food must be soft, moist, and well chewed. Most people who undergo bariatric surgery lose more than

FIGURE 10-12

Surgical Procedures for Obesity

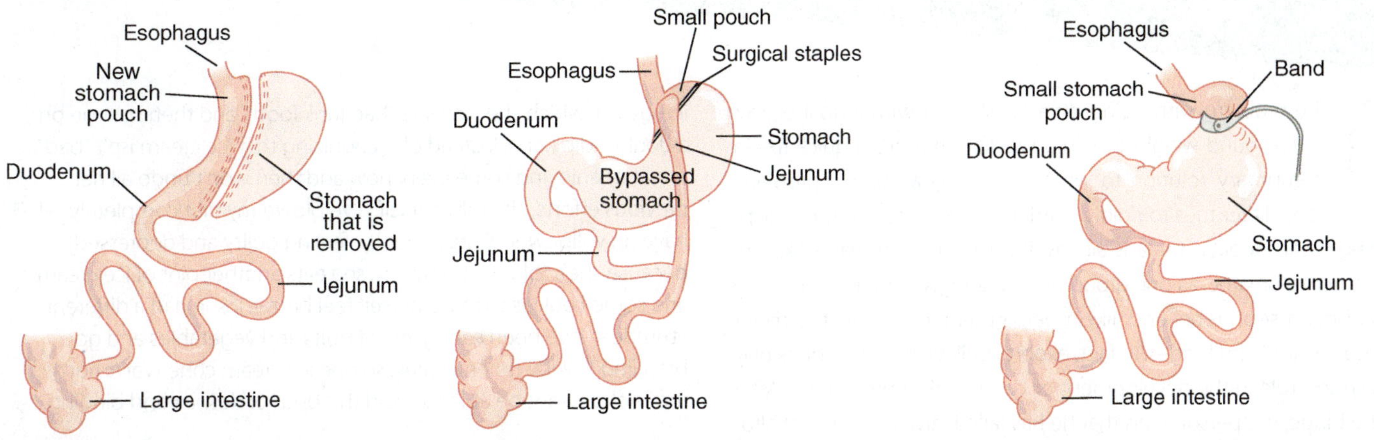

In vertical sleeve gastrectomy, most of the stomach is surgically removed, leaving a narrow banana-shaped stomach pouch.

In gastric bypass (Roux-en-Y) operations, a small pouch near the top of the stomach is created with staples or a plastic band and connected directly to the middle portion of the small intestine (jejunum).

Gastric banding reduces the size of the stomach by using an adjustable silicone band or cuff near the top of the stomach to create a pouch that fills quickly and empties slowly. The inflatable band is connected to an access port placed close to the skin, allowing surgeons to tighten or loosen it to meet an individual's needs.

50 percent of their excess weight and keep that weight off long-term with lifestyle changes toward healthful eating behaviors and regular physical activity.

Another weight-loss approach involves cosmetic surgery. One such procedure is **liposuction**, in which the surgeon uses a small, hollow tube to suction out fatty tissue from beneath the skin. People who wish to remove the fat from a particular area can choose this procedure through consultation with a physician, which sometimes brings pleasing results but can produce a figure in which one part of the body is disproportionately thin relative to the others. However, this fat reduction may be temporary without lifestyle changes and is not an effective strategy over time.

Surgery is appropriate in some instances. Cosmetic surgery can minimize disfigurements, improve self-confidence, and ease the way toward concentration on life issues that are more important than external appearance. However, after surgery, the same person resides within the skin as before. A changed appearance does not guarantee changed eating habits, a better personality, reduced interpersonal conflicts, or any other improvements in the quality of one's life.

10.6 Successful Weight-Loss Strategies

Given that so many approaches are likely to fail, what weight-loss strategies work? How can a person lose weight safely and maintain it? The secret is a sensible (not to say *easy*), three-pronged approach involving healthful eating habits, exercise, and behavior change. Such an approach takes tremendous dedication, especially at first, as a person whose habits promoted weight gain now makes new habits out of the hundred or so behaviors necessary to promote a healthful weight. Even the most effective weight-loss programs reveal a discouraging pattern: Many people complete the program, lose about 10 percent of their body weight, regain two-thirds of it within 1 year, and regain almost all of it within 5 years.[37] Still, many others who resolve to lose weight do so, and they manage to keep it off. Brown Medical School/The Miriam Hospital in Providence, Rhode Island, maintains a National Weight

liposuction A type of surgery (also called lipectomy) that vacuums out fat cells that have accumulated, typically in the buttocks and thighs. If the person continues to eat more calories than are expended, fat will return to the fat cells that remain in those regions.

EAT WELL Be Well Never Say "Diet" (Obj. 10.6)

The problem with going on a "crash" diet with a goal of, say, a 15-pound weight loss in 3 weeks is that it's a quick fix—a temporary solution to what is typically a chronic problem. Often, the dieter tries to rigidly restrict eating by, for example, skipping meals or eating salads all day. But trying not to eat is like trying not to breathe, as one group of psychologists put it.[38] The body and mind soon rebel and, like a person gasping for air, the dieter loses control and binges. In fact, experts believe that rigid diets play a strong role in the development of binge-eating problems.[39] After the binge, the person feels that he has failed, gives up the diet altogether, eats more to make himself feel better, puts on some weight, feels even worse, gains even more weight, decides to try another restrictive diet, and begins the whole cycle all over again. The solution, say many experts, is *not* to focus on losing a certain amount of weight within a set period of time. This feature shows you how.

1 Adopt a Nondiet Approach to Weight Loss.

A more healthful, nondiet approach to weight loss is to gradually develop habits that you can live with permanently and that will help you shed pounds and keep them off over the long run. Instead of measuring your success by the weight on the scale, gauge your progress by the strides you make in adopting good eating and exercise habits as well as healthful attitudes about yourself and your body.

2 Set Achievable Goals.

Most people recognize the importance of the eating and exercise habits discussed in this chapter, but few dieters recognize that the attitude problems that often accompany restrictive dieting can stand in the way of long-term weight loss. One of the most common problems is "all-or-nothing" thinking in which people view the world as black or white, right or wrong, good or bad, and so forth. When it comes to diets, this attitude translates into "good or bad" foods and "on or off" limits to diet food or junk food.[40] Such thinking sets the stage for failure as the dieter tries to live up to extremely rigid, unrealistic goals: "Ice cream is bad, so I must never eat it," "I will jog three miles every day," or "I will never order anything but a salad when I go out to eat." Typically, a person who has an all-or-nothing attitude might go several days without, say, ice cream, which she views as "bad junk food," and then splurge on a double-dip cone. Instead of recognizing that ice cream isn't "bad" and that enjoying some every now and then won't undo all her previous efforts, she tells herself, "I've blown my diet completely—I have no willpower." Consequently, feeling guilty and depressed because she's "blown it" anyway, she eats another pint of ice cream and some cookies to make herself feel better. If she had a different attitude—"I've been eating lots of fruits and vegetables and go bicycling several times a week, so one ice cream cone won't hurt me"—she might be able to avoid this bout of despair and binging.

3 Focus on Health Rather than Appearance.

Many people who are overweight or obese feel that their lives will be more enjoyable once they attain a particular, lower weight. In our society that focuses on thinness or a fit physique, people who are overweight suffer tremendous prejudice and tend to be painfully self-conscious about their bodies. Thus, they may mistakenly believe that all their dreams will come true once they lose weight and that all their problems will be lost along with the pounds. By pinning all their hopes for happiness on losing weight, they put themselves under enormous pressure to shed pounds. In addition, people with this attitude often do not live in the present, because they are so caught up in fantasizing about what they think life will be like once they lose weight.

Using weight and appearance as a measure of self-worth and happiness can be extremely destructive. The person who does so may desperately try to lose weight with restrictive, unrealistic diets or unhealthful, strenuous exercise regimens. Each slipup chips away at the person's self-esteem, which in turn may lead to feelings of rejection, depression, and social isolation, which in turn may prompt a binge, and so forth. Even people who lose a desired number of pounds may find that they still have many of the same life problems as before, and this realization can lead to depression and loss of self-esteem.

Focusing on health, rather than appearance, can help give people a healthier perspective. Although it can be difficult to overcome society's prejudices about weight, striving to achieve a healthy lifestyle, regardless of your weight, can be a major step in helping you take care of your mental and physical health.

Control Registry of more than 10,000 people who have successfully achieved and maintained at least a 30-pound weight loss for at least 1 year. A 2012 survey of registrants found that their average weight loss was 70 pounds upon entering the registry and about 50 pounds after 5 years.[41] Those who succeed typically do so because they have employed many of the techniques described in this chapter, as well as those in the Eat Well Be Well feature—"Never Say Diet."

Weight-Loss Readiness Quiz

Are you ready to lose weight? Your attitude affects your ability to succeed. Take this readiness quiz to see if you're mentally ready before you begin.

Mark each statement as true or false. Be honest with yourself! The answers should reflect the way you really think, not how you'd like to be or think you "should" be!

1. I have thought a lot about my eating habits and physical activities, and I know what I might change.
2. I know that I need to make permanent, not temporary, changes in my eating and activity patterns.
3. I will feel successful only if I lose a lot of weight.
4. I know that it's best if I lose weight slowly.
5. I'm thinking about losing weight now because I really want to, not because someone else thinks I should.
6. I think losing weight would solve other problems in my life.
7. I am willing and able to increase my regular physical activity.
8. I can lose weight successfully if I have no slipups.
9. I am willing to commit time and effort each week to organize and plan my food and activity choices.
10. Once I lose a few pounds but reach a plateau (and can't seem to lose more), I usually lose the motivation to keep going toward my weight goal.
11. I want to start a weight-loss program, even though my life is unusually stressful right now.

Now score yourself:

Look at your answers for items 1, 2, 4, 5, 7, and 9. Score "1" if you answered true and "0" if you answered false. For items 3, 6, 8, 10, and 11, score "0" for each true answer and "1" for each false answer.

No single item indicates if you're ready to start losing weight. But the higher your total score, the more likely you are to be successful.

If you scored 8 or higher, you probably have good reasons to lose weight now, and you know some of the steps that can help you succeed.

If you scored 5 to 7 points, you may need to reevaluate your reasons for losing weight and the strategies you'd follow.

If you scored 4 or less, now may not be the right time for you to lose weight. You may be successful initially, but you may not be able to sustain the effort to reach or maintain your weight goal. Reconsider your reasons and approach.

Interpret Your Score

Your answers can be clues to some stumbling blocks in your weight-management success. Any item you scored as "0" suggests a misconception about weight loss, or a problem area for you. So let's look at each item a bit more closely.

1. You can't change what you don't understand, and that includes your eating habits and activity pattern. Keep records for a week to pinpoint when, what, why, and how much you eat, as well as patterns and obstacles to regular physical activity.
2. You may be able to lose weight in the short run with drastic or highly restrictive changes in your eating habits or activity pattern—but those changes may be hard to live with permanently. Your food and activity plans should be healthful ones that you can enjoy and sustain.
3. Many people fantasize about reaching a weight goal that's unrealistically low. If that sounds like you, rethink your meaning of success. A reasonable goal takes body type into consideration and sets smaller, achievable "mile markers" along the way.
4. If you equate success with fast weight loss, you'll have problems keeping weight off. This "quick-fix" attitude can backfire when you face the challenges of weight maintenance. The best and healthiest approach is to lose weight slowly while learning strategies to keep weight off permanently.
5. To be successful, the desire for and commitment to weight loss must come from you, not your best friend or a family member. People who lose weight and keep it off take responsibility for their weight goals and choose their own approach.
6. Being overweight may contribute to some social problems, but it's rarely the single cause. Although body image and self-esteem are strongly linked, thinking that you can solve all your problems by losing weight isn't realistic. Furthermore, it may set you up for disappointment.
7. A habit of regular, moderate physical activity is a key factor in successfully losing weight and keeping it off. For weight control, physical activity doesn't have to be strenuous to be effective. Any moderate physical activity that you enjoy and will do regularly counts.
8. Most people don't expect perfection in their daily lives, yet they often feel they must stick to a weight-loss program perfectly. Perfection at weight loss isn't realistic. Rather than viewing lapses as catastrophes, see them as opportunities to discover what triggers your problems and to develop strategies for the future.
9. To successfully lose weight, you must take time to assess your problem areas, then develop the approach that's best for you. Success requires planning, commitment, and time.
10. First, a plateau in an ongoing weight loss program is perfectly normal, so don't give up too soon! Before you lose your motivation, think about any past efforts that have failed, then identify strategies that can help you overcome those hurdles.
11. Weight loss itself can be a source of stress, so if you're already under stress, you may find a weight-loss program somewhat difficult to implement right now. Try to resolve other stressors in your life before starting your weight-loss effort.

SOURCE: Chart from the American Dietetic Association's *Complete Food and Nutrition Guide*, 4/E. Copyright © 2012 by the Academy of Nutrition and the Dietetics. Reprinted by permission of Houghton Mifflin Harcourt Publishing Company.

TABLE 10-5 Eating Plan Strategies

1. Get personally involved.
2. Adopt a realistic plan, and then keep track of calories.
3. Make the eating plan adequate.
4. Emphasize high nutrient density.
5. Choose foods that you like.
6. Stress "do's," not "don'ts."
7. Eat regular meals.
8. Take a positive view of yourself.
9. Visualize a healthier future self.
10. Weigh yourself at regular, well-spaced intervals to avoid feeling discouraged.

Personalize Your Weight-Loss Plan The way a person loses weight is highly individualized. Two different weight-loss plans may be equally successful and yet have little or nothing in common. You have to find a plan that's right for you. Because of the personal nature of weight-loss plans, the following sections are written to you as advice, even though you may not need to lose weight at all. To help you understand the issues of weight loss, pretend that you have 10 to 200 pounds to lose and are being competently counseled by someone familiar with the techniques known to be effective. Table 10-5 highlights the principles involved.

No particular diet is magical, and no particular food must be either included or avoided. Because you are the one who has to live with the eating plan, you should be involved in creating it. Don't think of it as going "on" a diet—because then you may be tempted to go "off" it. Lifestyle changes are successful only if the weight does not return. Think of it as an eating plan that you will adopt for life. The diet must consist of foods that you like or can learn to like, that are available to you, and that are within your means.

If you want to lose weight, a deficit of 500 calories a day for 7 days (3,500 calories a week) is enough to lose roughly a pound of body fat each week. If you choose to expend an extra 250 calories a day in some form of exercise, you could increase this energy deficit.

Choose a calorie level you can live with. The "10-calorie rule" will enable you to lose a pound or two a week while still supporting your basal metabolism: Allow 10 calories a day for each pound of your present body weight. As you lose weight, you can gradually adjust calories downward to keep losing at this rate. Thus, a person who weighs 220 pounds should begin with 2,200 calories a day; one who weighs 150 pounds should begin with 1,500 calories a day.

Put nutritional adequacy high on your list of priorities. This is a way of putting yourself first: "I like me, and I'm going to take good care of me." This means including foods that are rich in valuable nutrients, such as vegetables, fruits, whole-grain breads and cereals, and a reasonable amount of protein-rich foods, such as lean meats, skinless poultry, fish, eggs, legumes, low-fat cheeses, and low-fat or fat-free milk. Within these categories, learn what foods you like, and eat them often. If you resolve to include a certain number of servings of food from each of these groups each day, you may be so busy making sure you get what you need that you will have little time or appetite left for high-calorie or empty-calorie foods. Researchers have shown that reducing the intake of fat alone can promote significant weight loss, especially when coupled with a diet high in complex carbohydrates.[42]

A small amount of fat should be included in each meal to make it satisfying and keep you from getting hungry again too soon. You don't have to use pure fat, such as butter, margarine, or oil. Rather, most of the fat should come from protein-rich foods, such as lean meats, eggs, poultry, fish, and low-fat cheeses. Add any pure fat with extra caution. A pat of butter adds more calories than a teaspoon of sugar. Keep concentrated sweets to a minimum, and let your carbohydrate come from fruits, vegetables, and whole-grain foods. Figure 10-13 shows three suitable patterns for weight-loss eating plans.

If you include alcohol or other empty-calorie items in your eating plan, limit them to no more than 150 calories a day. Budget this amount into your chosen calorie level, and remind yourself that successful weight loss may be slow and gradual.

Three meals a day is standard for our society, but no law says you shouldn't have four or five meals—just be sure that they are smaller. What is most important is to eat regularly and, whenever possible, to eat before you become very hungry.

Keep a record of what you have eaten each day for at least a week or two until your new habits are automatic. Try keeping a diet record whenever you need to keep yourself on track.

FIGURE 10-13

Sample Balanced Weight-Loss Diets Using the MyPlate Food Guide[a]

[a]Assumes no alcohol intake.
[b]Not recommended for pregnant or lactating women, children (depending on age), or those who have special dietary needs. At or below this low level of calorie intake, it may not be possible to obtain recommended amounts of all nutrients from foods; therefore, it is important to make careful food choices, and the need for dietary supplements should be evaluated.
[c]The 1,200-calorie and 1,400-calorie plans include a 170 empty-calorie allowance and 4 teaspoons of fats/oils. The 1,800-calorie plan includes 195 empty calories and 5 teaspoons of fats/oils.
[d]For maximum nutritional value, make whole-grain, high-fiber choices.
[e]Choose fat-free or low-fat (1%) dairy products.
[f]Select lean meat and use cooking methods that do not require added fat.

Daily recommendations for a 1,200-calorie diet[b,c]

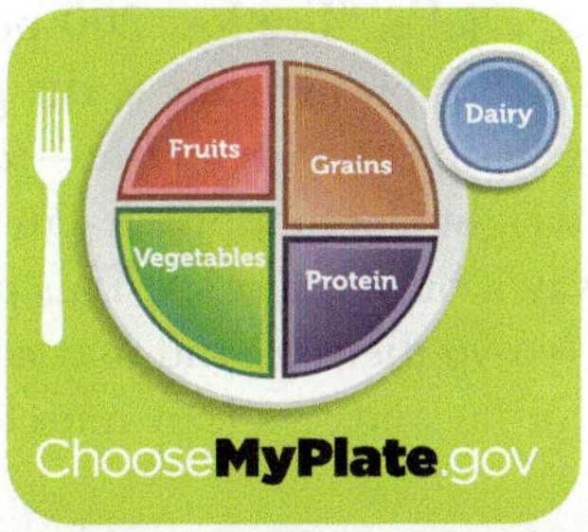

GRAINS	VEGETABLES	FRUITS
4 oz[d]	1.5 cups	1 cup

DAIRY	PROTEIN FOODS
2 cups[e]	3 oz[f]

Daily recommendations for a 1,400-calorie diet[c]

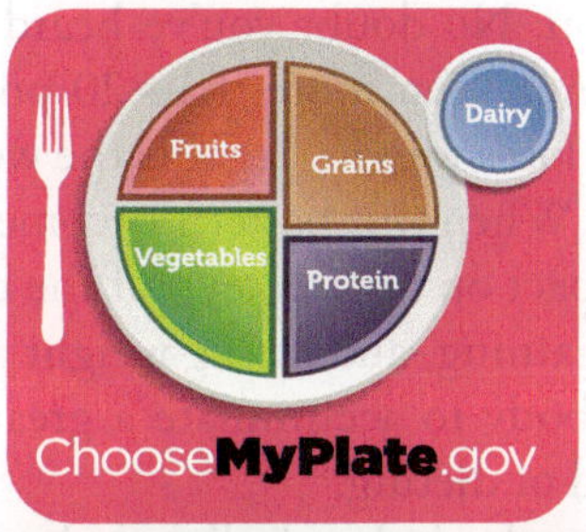

GRAINS	VEGETABLES	FRUITS
5 oz[d]	1.5 cups	1.5 cups

DAIRY	PROTEIN FOODS
2 cups[e]	4 oz[f]

Daily recommendations for a 1,800-calorie diet[c]

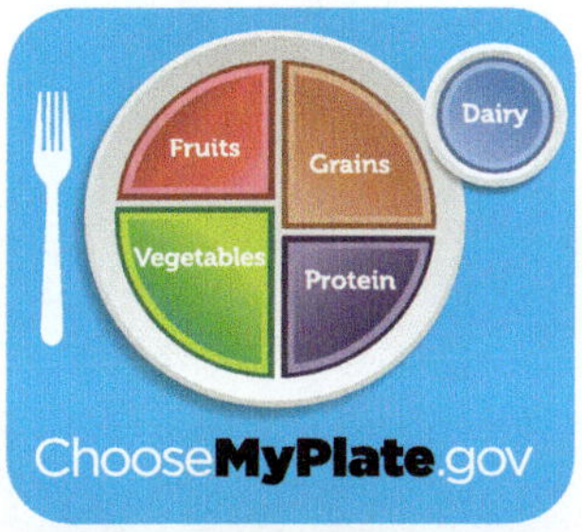

GRAINS	VEGETABLES	FRUITS
6 oz[d]	2.5 cups	1.5 cups

DAIRY	PROTEIN FOODS
3 cups[e]	5 oz[f]

At first, it may seem as if you are spending all your waking hours thinking about and planning your meals. Such a massive effort is always required when you are learning a new skill. After about 3 weeks, however, it will be much easier as your new eating pattern becomes a habit. Some characteristics of successful dieters are listed in Table 10-6.[43] The Savvy Diner feature later in this chapter offers strategies for eating well while dining out.

Aim for Gradual Weight Loss Do not weigh yourself more than once a week. Although approximately 3,500 calories roughly equals a pound of body fat, there is no simple relationship between calorie balance and weight loss over short intervals. A gain or loss of a pound or more in a few days can reverse quickly; the overall average loss is what is real. Don't expect to lose continuously as fast as you did at first. A large water loss is common during the first week, but it will not happen again.

Expect to Reach a Plateau Many dieters experience a temporary plateau after about three weeks—not because they are slipping, but because they have gained water weight temporarily while they are still losing body fat. The fat they are hoping to lose must be used for energy. To use it, the body must combine it with oxygen (oxidize it) to make carbon dioxide and water. These compounds are heavier than the fat they are made from because oxygen has been added to them.* The carbon dioxide

TABLE 10-6 Profile of Successful Dieters

- They know their weight. (They check their scale weight weekly.)
- They are motivated from within.
- They know what they eat. (They keep records.)
- They engage in regular exercise (60 to 90 minutes of moderate exercise on most days).
- They have social support (relationships/groups).
- They control their intake of alcohol, fat, and sugar.
- They follow a personalized diet plan—one that they can enjoy permanently.
- They lose no more than a pound or two a week.
- They set reasonable goals, such as losing just 10 percent of their weight, as a start.
- They accept an occasional lapse rather than aiming for perfection.
- They view weight management as a long-term commitment.

*Water weight accumulates during fat oxidation because one fatty acid weighing 284 units leaves behind water weighing 324 units—14 percent more.

will be exhaled quickly, but the water takes longer to leave the cells. First, it makes its way into the spaces between the cells and finally enters the bloodstream. Only after the water has arrived in the blood do the kidneys remove it and send it to the bladder for excretion. Meanwhile, this excess water creates a temporary weight gain, but one day the plateau will break. The signal that this is happening is frequent urination.

Aim for a Positive Gain in Lean Body Mass If you have been exercising lately, successive weighings may show a slight, occasional gain when you expect a loss. This may reflect a welcome benefit: the gain of lean body mass, just what you want to be healthy. In fact, weight loss without exercise can have a negative effect on body composition. No doubt you've heard someone say as a joke, "I've lost 200 pounds, but I've never been more than 20 pounds overweight." Typically, this is the person who diets, loses weight, regains the weight, and diets again throughout life—*without* exercising. When this pattern becomes a lifetime of weight fluctuations, it can have a lasting impact on the makeup of the body and the way it burns calories. This pattern of losing, gaining, and losing weight again is called "yo-yo dieting" and may actually cause the body to accumulate a greater percentage of fat and less lean muscle with each round of dieting.[44]

If you cut back drastically on the number of calories you consume without exercising for a time, about a month or two, you'll probably lose a great deal of weight each week as fat but also lean muscle. Then, if you later put the weight back on, the regained pounds may be primarily fat, *not* muscle. Thus, you may weigh the same as you did when you began the diet, but your body is now composed of more fat and less muscle. Because muscle burns more calories just to sustain itself than fat does, your body needs fewer calories to maintain its weight than it did before. If you go back to eating the way you used to, chances are you will gain even more weight.

Maintain Bone Health by Increasing Calcium Intake Weight loss—even modest weight loss—can also result in a depletion of bone minerals and hence a loss of bone density.[45] Fat loss may lower the levels of estrogen, a hormone necessary for healthy bone maintenance. Recent research emphasizes the importance of including both adequate calcium intakes and exercise in any weight-loss regimen, particularly weight-bearing exercise such as walking, jogging, stair climbing, and weight lifting. In addition, research suggests that low calcium intakes favor increased deposition of body fat, whereas higher calcium intakes (at levels generally recommended for health) may not only inhibit storage of body fat but also stimulate the use of body fat for energy.[46]

In addition to the risk of changing the body's overall composition during repeated bouts of weight loss, consider that each unsuccessful attempt to keep weight off is often viewed by the dieter as a personal failure, which can erode the person's self-esteem and trigger painful feelings of guilt and depression.[47] A healthier alternative to crash dieting is to gradually develop healthful, permanent lifestyle habits that will help you to lose weight and keep it off.

Adopt a Physically Active Lifestyle Physical activity makes three contributions to a weight-management program. It increases calorie expenditure, improves body composition, and alters metabolism.[48] Physical activity also offers the psychological benefits of looking and feeling healthy, and the increased self-esteem that accompanies these benefits can enhance the motivation to maintain a healthful lifestyle for the long run.

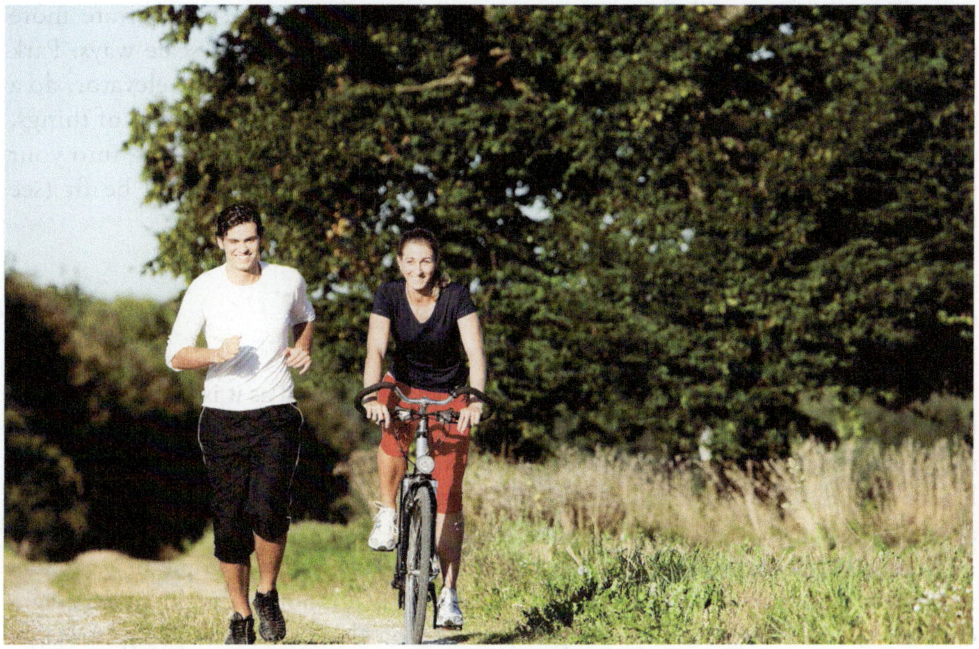

Kzenon/Shutterstock.com

Exercise is essential for weight control.

Compared with lean tissue, fat tissue is relatively inactive metabolically. Metabolic activity burns calories—lots of them. Thus, the more lean tissue you develop, the faster your metabolism becomes, the more calories you spend, and the more you can afford to eat. This brings you both pleasure and nutrients. Physical activity, by shifting body composition toward more lean tissue, speeds up the metabolism *permanently*—that is, for as long as you keep your body conditioned. Furthermore, the more muscle and lean tissue you have, the more fat you will burn—all day long, even when you are resting.

The next chapter offers many pointers about becoming fit, but here are a few pieces of guidance. First, keep in mind that if physical activity is to help with weight loss, it must be *active* exercise of moderate intensity—voluntary moving of muscles. The more muscles you move, the more calories you spend (see Table 10-7). You can tell that the physical activity is moderate if you are breathing a little faster than normal but can still easily carry on a conversation.

People sometimes ask about the possibility of spot reducing: Can you lose fat in specific locations? Unfortunately, muscles cannot control the fat that surrounds them. Because all body fat is shared by all muscles and organs, spot-reducing exercises that work only the flabby parts will not help reduce the fat located there. The good news is, however, that tightening muscles in trouble spots by way of a balanced, all-over exercise program may improve the appearance of the fatty areas.

Another thing to keep in mind is that the number of calories spent in an activity depends more on how much a person weighs than on how fast the person can do the exercise (see Table 10-7). For example, a person who weighs 125 pounds burns off 78 calories by running a 9-minute mile. That same person, walking a mile in 15 minutes, burns almost the same amount: 82 calories. Similarly, a 200-pound person spends 125 calories on the 9-minute mile, and a similar amount—131 calories—on the 15-minute walk. You do not have to work fast to use up calories effectively. If you choose to walk rather than run the distance, you will use up about the same energy; it will just take you longer.

TABLE 10-7 Calories Spent during Various Activities

	Calories Expended per Hour[a]	
Activity	**Man[b]**	**Woman[b]**
Sitting quietly	100	80
Standing quietly	120	95
Light activity:	300	240
Cleaning house		
Office work		
Playing baseball		
Playing golf		
Moderate activity:	460	370
Walking briskly (4 mph)		
Gardening		
Cycling (5.5 mph)		
Dancing		
Playing basketball		
Strenuous activity:	730	580
Jogging (9 min/mile)		
Playing football		
Swimming		
Very strenuous activity:	920	740
Running (7 min/mile)		
Racquetball		
Skiing		

[a]May vary depending on environmental conditions.

[b]Healthy man, 175 lb; healthy woman, 140 lb. (To determine caloric expenditure at a different weight, both men and women should divide their body weight by 175, then multiply by the man's caloric expenditure for the activity.)

SOURCE: U.S. Department of Agriculture, U.S. Department of Health and Human Services, *Dietary Guidelines for Americans*.

A good suggestion that you may have heard already is to incorporate more physical activity into your daily schedule in many simple, small-scale ways. Park the car at the far end of the parking lot; use the stairs instead of the elevator; do a round of sit-ups before you get up in the morning. If you do these types of things, along with incorporating regular aerobic exercise and strength training into your schedule, your heart and lungs as well as your skeletal muscles will be fit (see Chapter 11).

10.7 Weight-Gain Strategies

It is as hard for a person who tends to be thin to gain a pound as it is for a person who tends to be fat to lose one. People who want to gain weight are faced with some of the same challenges as those who want to lose weight: learning new habits, learning to like new foods, and establishing discipline related to meals and mealtimes. But there are major differences.

Knowing that vigorous physical activity costs calories, active people may wonder whether it is advisable to be less active. The answer is no, not unless the underweight condition is so extreme that it endangers your health. The healthful way to gain weight is to build yourself up with patient and consistent training while eating nutritious foods containing enough extra calories to support the weight gain (see Figure 10-14). If you add extra snacks of high-calorie nutritious foods, such as a peanut butter sandwich with a glass of milk before bedtime, and a healthful midafternoon fruit smoothie or milkshake, you can add 700 to 800 extra calories a day and achieve a healthful weight gain of 1 to 1½ pounds per week. Choose calorie-dense snacks, such as fruit yogurt, granola, dried fruits, apple or grape juice, nuts, sunflower seeds, fig bars, and baked potatoes topped with low-fat cheese.

People wanting to gain weight often need to learn to eat different foods. No matter how many helpings of carrots you consume, you will not gain weight very quickly because carrots simply don't offer enough calories. Thus, people who cannot consume much food volume are encouraged to eat calorie-dense foods at meals (the very ones the dieters try to avoid). For example, if you are trying to gain

FIGURE 10-14

Eating Strategies for Weight Gain

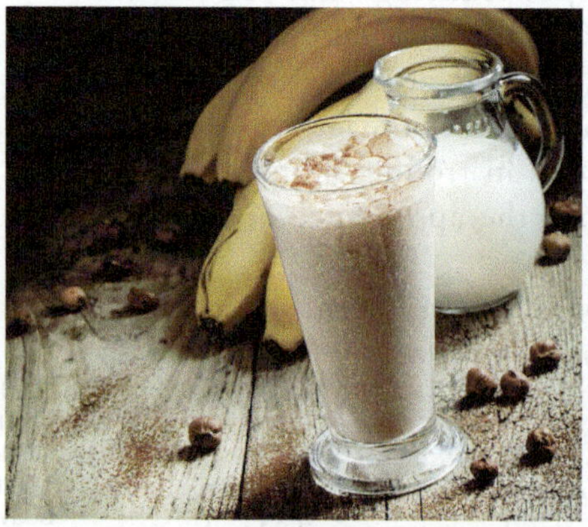

5PH/Shutterstock.com

Add extra calories to the milk or juice you drink by tossing in a frozen banana or other fruit and whipping up a smoothie in the blender.

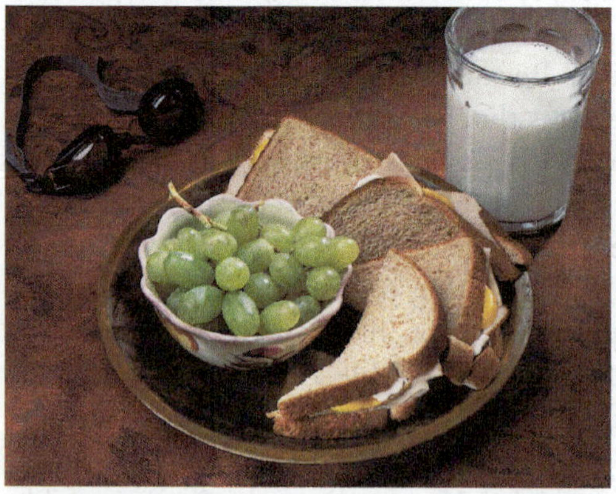

Polara Studios

Try eating more food at each meal. If you normally eat one sandwich for lunch, try eating an extra sandwich between meals.

weight, you should choose a milkshake instead of milk, peanut butter instead of lean meat, an avocado instead of a cucumber, and a blueberry bran muffin instead of whole-wheat bread. When you do eat carrots, dip them in hummus and use creamy dressings on salads, yogurt on fruit, cottage cheese on potatoes, and so forth. Because fat contains twice as many calories per teaspoon as sugar, it adds calories without adding bulk. For heart health, be sure to choose the "good" fats, found in foods such as avocados, olives, peanuts, pistachios, and other nuts and seeds, and limit your intake of saturated fats.

Also, eat more frequently. Make three sandwiches in the morning, and eat them between classes in addition to the day's three regular meals. Spend more time eating each meal. If you fill up fast, eat the highest-calorie items first. Do not start with soup or salad; start with the main course. Finish with dessert. Many underweight people have simply been too busy (for months) to eat enough to gain or maintain weight. These strategies will help you change this behavior pattern.

Whether you need to gain, lose, or maintain weight, paying attention to what you eat will pay off in long-term wellness benefits. This chapter emphasizes the relationship of food and eating to body weight and has the same message as other parts of the book: To support wellness, eat regular, balanced meals composed of a wide variety of foods you enjoy.

10.8 Breaking Old Habits

Starting and maintaining a fitness program is not as simple as putting on your sneakers and running a mile or going to the gym. Sticking to a regular physical activity program for the first time or changing eating habits is not always easy. Most people who successfully quit smoking make three or four attempts before they finally kick the habit; most people make the same New Year's resolution at least five years in a row before they stick to it permanently.[49] Breaking old patterns of behavior and developing new ones involves a number of stages before reaching the point at which you're able to make a permanent change (see Table 10-8).

First, you must accept the belief that you *can* change: "I can lose some weight and try to become more physically fit," you might tell yourself. This might inspire you to *want* to change, which in turn will motivate you to find ways to actually make the change (e.g., talking to a registered dietitian about diet strategies and reading about various forms of physical activity). After you've gone through those steps, you will be ready to take action—that is, to "just do it." Finally, to maintain your behavior change, you can create a game plan to help you handle the inevitable lapses that will occur over time. When you follow these steps and then stick with your plan for a good deal of time, you have successfully made a change.

Behavior Modification

Making lasting, behavioral changes poses ongoing challenges. A process known as **behavior modification** can help. Developed by psychologists to help people change their habits, behavior modification techniques are similar to mapping out a game plan by following the specific steps listed in Table 10-9.

Set a Goal and Get to Know Yourself For *Step 1*, identify your goals. You might decide, for example, that your goal is to lower the fat and calorie content of your diet. Next, in *Step 2*, you record your present behavior pattern and think about the reasons for those behaviors. In this case, for example, you might keep a food diary, writing down everything you eat for five days and describing how you feel each

TABLE 10-8 Elements of Behavior Change

1. *Precontemplation:* You need to change, but you're not yet ready to accept that fact.
2. *Contemplation:* You want to change, but you're not sure how.
3. *Preparation:* You gain knowledge to set up a plan of action for change.
4. *Action:* You jump in and "just do it."
5. *Maintenance:* You work on sticking to your plan of action.
6. *Termination:* You have achieved lasting change and experience few, if any, temptations or relapses.

SOURCE: J. O. Prochaska, *Changing for Good* (New York: William Morrow, 1994), p. 47.

TABLE 10-9 Behavior Modification Steps

Step 1: Identify the goal.

Step 2: Record your present behavior pattern. Identify the reasons you practice these behaviors.

Step 3: Identify the behaviors that will lead to the goal and the rewards of those behaviors.

Step 4: Commit yourself to changing. Face what you'll have to give up or change to make the desired behavior a reality. Envision your changed future self.

Step 5: Plan. Divide the behavior into manageable portions. Set small, achievable goals and plan periodic rewards.

Step 6: Try out the plan. Modify the plan, if necessary, in ways that will help you succeed.

Step 7: Evaluate your progress on a regular basis.

behavior modification A process developed by psychologists that helps people make lasting behavior changes.

TABLE 10-10 Sample Entries in Food Diary				
Food Eaten	**Time and Place**	**With Whom**	**Mood**	**Other Activity**
1 large blueberry muffin	7:30 A.M., doughnut shop	Alone	Stressed—late for class	Skimming notes for upcoming class
1 cup coffee with 1 oz cream & 1 tsp sugar				
1 hot dog with 2 tbsp ketchup	12:45 P.M., cafeteria	2 friends	Relaxed	Talking with friends
1 small bag potato chips				
12-oz can diet soda				
1 candy bar	2:35 P.M., bedroom	Alone	Angry about argument with significant other	Watching TV

time you eat (see Table 10-10 for a sample food diary). This technique will help you understand why you behave the way you do in certain situations. You might find, for instance, that every time you are angry at your significant other or get a bad grade, you eat a candy bar or two to comfort yourself. Or, perhaps without even thinking about it, you nibble on whatever happens to be handy while watching television.

Change Behaviors and Reward Yourself Having identified your goal and current patterns of behavior, you can now move to *Step 3*, which is to determine strategies to help you meet your goal and to choose some rewards for when you follow these strategies. An example of a possible behavior-change strategy might be that you decide to talk to a friend instead of heading to the kitchen cupboard or vending machine when you are angry. You could save hundreds of calories and probably experience emotional relief by getting your feelings off your chest.

This is the time to remind yourself of the progress you are making and the benefits you are gaining: weight loss, increased energy, better health. It is also the time to give yourself a tangible reward, such as a night out at the movies or a new item of clothing. This step is key because behavior research indicates that once you have instituted a change in your life, you will maintain it only by positive reinforcement. Rewards

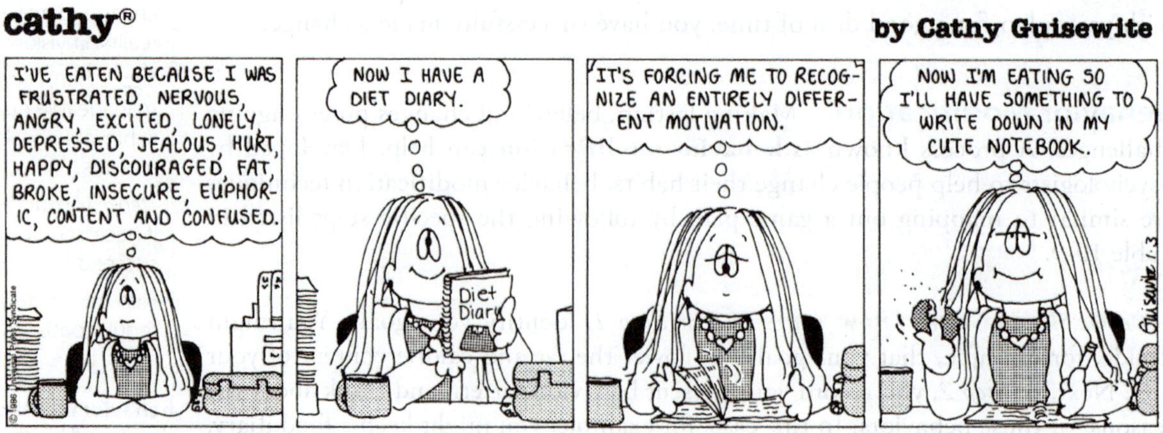

don't have to be expensive. For example, you can take time for a long, relaxing bath, or celebrate with a leisurely Sunday morning curled up with a book you've been wanting to read.

In *Step 4*, after you've pinpointed behaviors you want to alter, you must *commit* yourself to make the changes and take the time to envision the healthier person you'll become as a result.

Plan to Take Small Steps *Step 5* is planning, and the way to do this is to take small steps. Divide your primary goal into smaller goals that can be achieved one at a time. Although you might have identified 10 behaviors that you want to change to meet your overall goal, trying to accomplish all 10 in the first week or two is probably very unrealistic, and it may simply set the stage for disappointment and failure (and cause you to give up completely). To give yourself a more realistic chance for success, choose only one or two of the smaller goals, do your best to stick to them for a time, two weeks for example, and then reward yourself for doing so before going on to work on your next goals (see Table 10-11).

Give It a Try and Adapt Your Plan! In *Step 6* of behavior modification, you put your plan into action. As you meet your goals and reward yourself for doing so, also be aware of when you are not meeting them. If something is not working, do not give up. Instead, go on to *Step 7* and feel free to modify your goals—perhaps those that you initially set were too difficult or too simple to achieve. You may, for example, decide to choose the smaller goal of cutting some of the fat out of your diet for the first two weeks and wait for a later time to work on reducing the calorie count. As you can see, when you evaluate your progress on a regular basis, you offer yourself the flexibility to adapt your plan so that you can continue to move forward to meeting your goal.

Be Prepared for a Relapse While you are working on modifying your behavior, it is critical to keep in mind that you're only human, and there will be days when you slip and revert to an old pattern of behavior. Instead of dwelling on it or being hard on yourself, realize that relapses do happen, forgive yourself, and simply move on. Keep in mind that even though you may have had a setback, you're still moving forward if you learn from your mistakes and get right back on track again. That's why some experts prefer the term *recycle* to the term *relapse*; people who make a mistake and then learn from it can reuse, or recycle, their new knowledge.

Set Priorities Setting priorities helps ensure that you adopt one or two behaviors that you stick to all the time. Also, pay attention to how other areas of your life may be affecting your readiness to make changes and meet your goals. Many people waste a great deal of time and energy trying to make changes at difficult times. Someone who is going through the breakup of a long-term relationship or having difficulties at work or school, for example, may be under too much stress to deal with making a behavior change on top of everything else.

Consider the "Rule of Three" Keep in mind that you might need to try new behaviors more than once before you begin to like them. Dietitians sometimes use a rule of three in counseling. For example, try fat-free milk once, and you may not like it. Try it a second time, and you may be able to tolerate drinking it, even though it

TABLE 10-11 A Recipe for Success

Be Realistic
Make small changes over time in what you eat and your activity level. Aim for losing no more than 1 to 2 pounds per week. Even a small amount of weight loss can bring major health benefits.

Be Adventurous
Expand your tastes to enjoy a wide variety of foods and activities. Get fewer calories by going "large" on flavor and small on portions.

Be Flexible
You don't have to give up your favorite foods to manage your weight. Just balance what you eat and what you do over several days.

Be Sensible
Enjoy all foods; just don't overdo any of them. Slow down when you're eating and listen to your body's signals to know when you're hungry or full.

Be Active
It's not *what* activity you choose, it's whether you enjoy doing it. If you enjoy it, you are likely to do it more often!

SOURCE: Adapted from Weighing In on Health, *Food and Nutrition News* 70 (1998): 6.

does not taste as good as whole milk. Try it a third time, and you may conclude that although it is not as good as whole milk, you don't really mind drinking it. Then you will be able to maintain your new habit more easily.

Stay Motivated Remember, it takes time for change to happen and to last. Hang in there long enough to experience the rewards of making a behavior change, such as an improved self-image and enhanced self-esteem. Always keep in mind where you started, and remember the price of your old behaviors that were not helpful. Look forward, and focus on the benefits of the new behavior.

Strategies for Changing the Way You Eat

The steps in this section are designed specifically to help with weight control. (Chapter 11 includes strategies for modifying exercise behavior.) First, begin by keeping a record of your present eating behavior that you can compare with your future progress. Your eating records will eventually help you see how far you've come in changing your eating habits.

This record will also help you with the second step, which is to identify cues and situations that trigger your behavior of reaching for food. For example, some cues, such as watching television or walking by a vending machine, may prompt you to eat when you are not hungry. Once the cues are identified, you can resolve to stop responding to them and try to eat only in one place in a certain room, such as at the table in the dining room. In addition, try the following tips to eliminate the temptation to eat when you really don't want to:

- Don't buy hard-to-resist foods such as cakes, cookies, and ice cream.
- Don't shop when you're hungry, when you are more likely to buy tempting foods.
- Don't leave large amounts of food within easy reach. Keep serving dishes off the table, for instance, and put the box of cookies out of sight.
- Make small portions of food look large by spreading food out and putting it on smaller plates. Garnish empty space with low-calorie vegetables.
- Try to eat regular meals and snacks instead of skipping them, which reduces the likelihood of your becoming uncomfortably hungry and then overeating later.
- Ask your family and friends to encourage you to eat a healthy diet and not to criticize you if you splurge occasionally.

Third, make it easy for yourself to eat the way you want to eat:

- Keep a variety of nutritious foods, such as fruits and vegetables, readily available.
- If you like to eat between meals, plan snacks that fit easily into your diet, such as low-fat yogurt and fruit.

Fourth, take a look at and then, if necessary, change the way you eat. If you eat quickly, slow down by chewing food thoroughly, pausing between bites, putting down your utensils, and swallowing before reloading your fork or spoon. Eating slowly will give your body a chance to feel full and satisfied.

Finally, reward yourself for positive behaviors. Plan to buy something new to wear or do something you enjoy, such as attending a sporting event or a concert, each time you meet your goals.

THE SAVVY Diner

Aiming for a Healthy Weight While Dining Out (Obj. 10.8)

Pizza Yankee . . . The story goes that a pizza-parlor waitress asked Yogi Berra whether he wanted his pizza cut into six or eight slices. "Six, please," he said. "No way am I hungry enough to eat eight."[50]

Dining out can be a pleasant time to relax, socialize, taste foods of different cultures, and provide a break from your usual schedule—it does not mean that you should overindulge in high-calorie foods. With practice, you can maximize the benefits of eating out by adopting some of the following strategies:

- Examine your options before selecting foods at buffets, cafeterias, or food courts. Otherwise, you may find yourself halfway through the line with a full plate and end up with a mountain of food on your plate when you reach the end of the line.
- Take the edge off hunger by starting with a broth-based soup, small salad, fruit, or light appetizer.
- Make specific requests. Ask for salad dressings, sauces, or gravies *on the side*. This puts you in control of the portions. Ask if reduced-fat or fat-free salad dressings are available.
- Ask for entrées to be broiled, baked, grilled, steamed, or roasted.
- Add fresh or cooked vegetables to your meal, which are flavorful, colorful, filling, and nutritious.
- Request fresh fruit, sorbet, or low-fat frozen yogurt for dessert. It will give you the sweetness you want without excess calories from fat. If you choose to splurge on your favorite chocolate dessert, enjoy it by sharing it with a friend. After the dinner out, go back to your healthful eating habits and exercise program.
- Be a menu sleuth. The following terms typically describe high-fat items: au gratin, Alfredo, batter-dipped, breaded, béarnaise, carbonara, creamy, crispy, croquette, deep-fried, flaky, fritters, parmigiana, tempura, with gravy, or with hollandaise sauce. Order red pasta sauces rather than white.
- Downsize your order. Many restaurants serve portions that are two or more times the recommended serving size. Take half the amount of your order home. Or, consider sharing an entrée with a friend and ordering a salad to go with it. You can also order à la carte: one or two nutritious, low-fat appetizers such as steamed shrimp or raw vegetables and a low-fat dip along with a salad instead of a huge main meal.
- Finally, eat slowly and enjoy your meal, along with the company and conversation. You'll be giving your body time to digest the food, you'll feel satisfied, and you'll have enjoyed yourself at the same time.

Eating Well on the Run

Here are some tips for ordering at quick-service restaurants:

Sandwich shop: Fresh sliced veggies in a pita with low-fat dressing, cup of minestrone soup, turkey breast sandwich with mustard, lettuce, tomato, fresh fruit.

Rotisserie chicken: Chicken breast (remove skin), steamed vegetables, mashed sweet potatoes, tossed salad, fruit salad. Select plain rolls instead of cornbread or biscuits.

Fast food: Grilled chicken breast sandwich (no sauce), single hamburger without cheese, grilled chicken salad, garden salad, low-fat or nonfat yogurt, fat-free muffin, cereal, low-fat milk.

Salad bars: Broth-based soups, fresh bread or bread sticks, fresh greens, chopped veggies, beans, low-fat dressing, fresh fruit salad. Avoid marinated beans and oily pasta salads.

Asian take-out: Wonton soup, pho (Vietnamese noodle soup), hot and sour soup, steamed vegetable dumplings, steamed vegetable mixtures over rice or noodles.

Pizza night: Choose flavorful, low-fat toppings such as peppers, onions, sliced tomatoes, spinach, broccoli, or mushrooms. Ask for your pizza with less cheese.

SOURCE: Adapted from *Healthy Eating Away from Home* (Washington, DC: American Institute for Cancer Research, www.aicr.org).

Nutrition ACTION Diet Confusion—Weighing the Evidence (Obj. 10.5)

Lose weight while you sleep! Lose 30 pounds in just 20 days! Eat the foods you love and lose weight! You will never be hungry! Do these claims sound familiar? With the recent focus on the increased rates of obesity in the United States and the world, diet books, products, and programs are everywhere. The truth is that although most diets enable a short-term weight loss, few people can lose weight and keep it off permanently, and some of these diets may actually be harmful. Nevertheless, dieting is big business in the United States. A November 2013 Gallup poll found that 24 percent of American adults are on a diet, and the weight-loss industry is estimated to be worth more than $60 billion.[51]

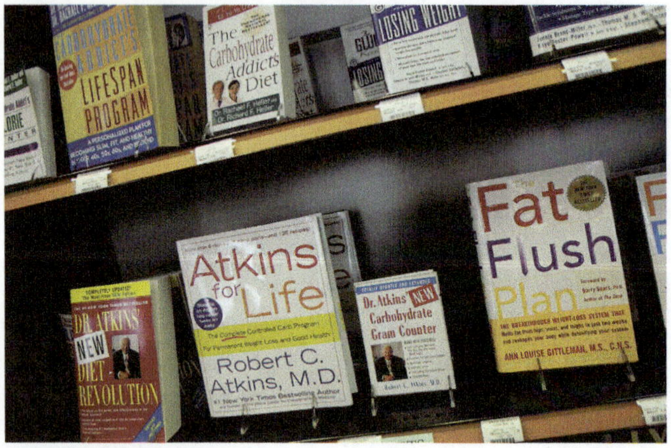

Chris Hondros/Getty Images News/Getty Images

How Do Diets Work?

Diets work because people limit their food consumption. Excess weight is the consequence of an energy imbalance, caused by overconsumption of food or decreased physical activity relative to individual requirements. Limiting dietary intake can take several forms:

- Elimination or restriction of certain food groups, such as carbohydrates
- Portion control through prepackaged meals, snacks, or drinks
- Changes in meal patterns or content
- Control of food intake through monitoring or point systems

A comparison of the approximate caloric content and macronutrient distribution of several types of diets is provided in Table 10-12.

What Are Common Diets?

Although diet fads change quickly, certain types of diets have appeared during the past few years. Here are some of the most common:[52]

- ***The Atkins Diet.*** In this diet, consumption of high-fat meats, cheeses, and fats is encouraged and consumption of carbohydrates (such as fruit, breads, and cereals) is severely limited. The premise of the diet is that elimination of these foods will produce a "benign dietary ketoacidosis," which leads to decreased hunger and slows excessive food consumption. Ketosis can be accompanied by bad breath, nausea, headaches, and fatigue. High protein intakes may exacerbate gout and kidney disease, and high saturated fat intake can increase blood cholesterol levels.
- ***The Zone Diet.*** This rigid eating plan separates foods into "macronutrient blocks."
- ***Volumetrics Diet.*** This diet encourages eating more foods with less calories per gram of food—like fruit, vegetables, cereals, legumes, and low-fat meats—than foods that are high in calories per gram. This allows a person to eat more food volume but with less calories, and gain a feeling of fullness, and more satisfaction overall.
- ***The Flexitarian Diet.*** This diet allows followers to be a flexible vegetarian so that occasional meat consumption will satisfy any cravings. Flexitarians add foods to their diets, rather than take foods away. By focusing on plant proteins in this diet, many feel fuller consuming fewer calories, and dieters follow this plan at their own pace. With fewer calories consumed and increased physical activity, many lose weight or at least maintain their current weight with little difficulty.
- ***Weight Watchers.*** Dieters use a point system to select and eat foods to reduce caloric intake and lose weight. In Weight Watchers, no food is forbidden, but all foods must be balanced with other choices.
- ***Ornish Diet.*** This is a variation of a previous diet designed by Dr. Dean Ornish, which focused on reversing heart disease. The Ornish diet emphasizes an approach that the more dietary changes you make, the more benefits you gain; this makes it flexible. Foods are put into categories ranging from least to most healthful, and the more choices one makes in the most healthful category, the more health benefits will follow. The most strict category still encourages the classic Ornish diet by consuming a very low-fat diet (10 percent of calories from fat), with little meat, oils, nuts, butter, dairy (except nonfat), sweets, or alcohol. This diet plan includes diet together with exercise and stress reduction.

TABLE 10-12	Comparison of Diet Programs/Eating Plans to Typical American Diet		
Type of Diet	**Example**	**General Dietary Characteristics**	**Comments**
Typical American diet		Carb: 50% Protein: 15% Fat: 35% Average of 2,200 cal/day	• Low in fruits and vegetables, dairy, and whole grains • High in saturated fat and refined carbohydrates
Balanced nutrient, moderate-calorie approach	DASH diet or diet based on MyPlate food guide; commercial plans such as Diet Center, Jenny Craig, Nutrisystem, Physicians Weight Loss, Shapedown Pediatric Program, Weight Watchers, Volumetrics	Carb: 55–60% Protein: 15–20% Fat: 20–30% Usually 1,200 to 1,700 cal/day	• Based on set pattern of selections from food lists using regular grocery store foods or prepackaged foods supplemented by fresh food items • Low in saturated fat and ample in fruits, vegetables, and fiber • Recommend reasonable weight-loss goal of 0.5 to 2.0 lb/week • Prepackaged plans may limit food choices • Most recommend exercise plan • Many encourage dietary record-keeping • Some offer weight-maintenance plans/support
Very low-fat, high-carbohydrate approach	Ornish diet (Eat More, Weigh Less), Pritikin diet, Fit or Fat	Carb: 65% Protein: 10–20% Fat: ≤ 10–19% Limited intake of animal protein, nuts, seeds, other fats	• Long-term compliance with some plans may be difficult because of low level of fat • Can be low in calcium • Some plans restrict healthful foods (seafood, low-fat dairy, poultry) • Some encourage exercise and stress-management techniques
Low-carbohydrate, high-protein, high-fat approach	Atkins diet, Protein Power, Stillman diet (The Doctor's Quick Weight Loss diet), Scarsdale diet	Carb: ≤ 20% Protein: 25–40% Fat:≥ 55–65% Strictly limits carbs to less than 100–125 g/day	• Promote quick weight loss (much is water loss rather than fat loss) • Ketosis causes loss of appetite • Can be too high in saturated fat • Low in carbohydrates, vitamins, minerals, and fiber • Not practical for long-term because of rigid diet or restricted food choices
Moderate-carbohydrate, high-protein, moderate-fat approach	The Zone diet, Sugar Busters, South Beach diet, Flat Belly diet	Carb: 40–50% Protein: 25–40% Fat: 30–40%	• Some diets are rigid and difficult to maintain • Enough carbohydrates to avoid ketosis • Can be low in carbohydrates; can be low in vitamins and minerals
Novelty diets	Immune Power diet, rotation diet, cabbage soup diet, paleo diet	Most promote certain foods, or combinations of foods, or nutrients as having unique (magical) qualities	• No scientific basis for recommendations
Very low-calorie diets	Health Management Resources (HMR), Medifast, Optifast	Less than 800 cal/day	• Require medical supervision • For clients with BMI ≥ 30 or BMI ≥ 27 with other risk factors; may be difficult to transition to regular meals
Weight-loss online diets	Nutrio.com, SparkPeople.com, WeightWatchers.com, SouthBeachDiet.com	Meal plans and various online tools available	• Recommend reasonable weight-loss goal of 0.5 to 2.0 lb/week • Most encourage physical activity and weight-maintenance support • Social support can be beneficial

SOURCE: Adapted from Weight-Control Information Network, Choosing a Safe and Successful diet (updated January 2012), NIH Publication No, 8-3007; D. L. Katz and S. Meller, Can we say what diet is best for health? *Ann Rev Pub Health* 35 (2014): 83–103M; Weighing the diet books, *Nutrition Action Newsletter* (January–February 2004): 3–8.

(continued)

- ***The Paleolithic (Paleo) Diet.*** This diet encourages the consumption of foods that were consumed during Paleolithic times, approximately 10,000 years ago, when humans were hunters and gatherers. This plan promotes eating animal proteins and plant foods and shuns dairy and grains, as well as processed and refined products. Excluding food groups can reduce important nutrient intakes.
- ***Dietary Approaches to Stop Hypertension (DASH) Diet.*** This healthy eating pattern was designed to reduce blood pressure but may also promote weight loss. The plan encourages fruits, vegetables, grains, lean proteins, and low-fat dairy while reducing consumption of salt, red meat, and sweets. This diet is considered by experts to be heart-healthy, balanced, and effective.

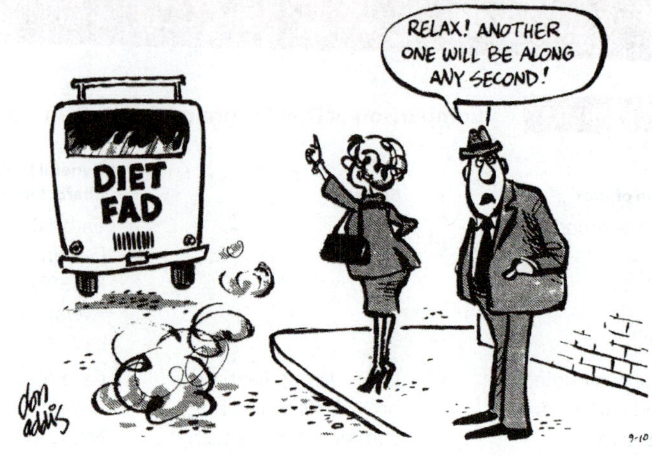

The St. Petersburg Times. Reprinted with Permission.

A study published in the *Journal of the American Medical Association* evaluated four of these diets (the Atkins, Ornish, Weight Watchers, and Zone diets) and found that, after one year on the diet, all four modestly reduced body weight and some cardiac risk factors.[53] Adherence to each diet for the 12-month period varied, ranging from 50 percent for the Ornish diet and 53 percent for the Atkins diet to 65 percent for both the Weight Watchers and Zone diets. The subjects who had the best adherence to the diets had the best results, and cardiac risk factors were more closely associated with weight loss than with diet type. In general, the subjects had more difficulty following the more restrictive diets (the Ornish and Atkins diets). Although this is just one study with small sample sizes, it does suggest that there are many ways to lose weight, that people find it difficult to adhere to very restrictive diets for a long time, and that we need to find methods of keeping people motivated to stay on any new eating plan.

How Can You Determine If a Diet Is Healthful?

What can you do to determine whether a particular diet plan is useful *and* healthful? Use the following checklist:[54]

1. *Does the weight-loss program systematically eliminate one group of foods from a person's eating pattern?* For example, are all carbohydrates systematically eliminated from the diet? Are dairy products eliminated? In general, a diet that eliminates a certain food group is probably lacking in important nutrients and dietary variety, and it will be difficult for a person to adhere to that eating plan.
2. *Does the weight-loss program encourage specific supplements or foods that can be purchased only from selected distributors?* These supplements or foods often contain ingredients that may be harmful or unproven.
3. *Does the weight-loss program tout magic or miracle foods or products that burn fat?* The only way to burn fat is to increase your physical activity levels or decrease the amount of total food that you consume. You cannot "burn" fat with sauna belts, body wraps, thigh-reducing creams, or similar products. If you consume more than you expend, or if you lower your physical activity level and keep your food intake the same, your body will store the extra calories as fat.
4. *Does the weight-loss program promote bizarre quantities of only one food or one type of food?* Some diets require that you eat only one food each day or eat unlimited amounts of certain foods, such as grapefruit or cabbage soup. Such advice runs counter to everything we know about the broad spectrum of human nutritional needs.
5. *Does the weight-loss program have rigid menus?* If a diet has specific meal plans and times to eat, it will be difficult to incorporate individual preferences. People are unique, so no one diet plan will work for everyone. A person who loves Thai food will not succeed on a diet if there is no way to incorporate Thai food into his or her eating plan.
6. *Does the weight-loss program promote specific food combinations?* Some diets include combinations of foods that should or should not be eaten at the same time. These food combinations have no basis in fact and needlessly restrict the dieter's options for reasonable food choices.
7. *Does the weight-loss program promise a weight loss of more than 2 pounds per week for an extended period of time?* If so, the initial weight loss will probably be due to water loss. A more realistic diet plan will aim for a weight loss of 0.5 to 2.0 pounds per week.
8. *Does the weight-loss program provide a warning to people with diabetes, high blood pressure, or other health conditions?* People with preexisting health conditions should consult a physician

TABLE 10-13 Risks Associated with the Very Low-Calorie Diets

- Blood sugar imbalance
- Cold intolerance
- Constipation
- Decreased basal metabolic rate
- Dehydration
- Diarrhea
- Emotional problems
- Fatigue/weakness
- Gallstones and kidney stones
- Headaches
- Heart irregularity
- Ketosis
- Loss of lean body tissue
- Kidney infection
- Menstrual irregularity
- Mineral and electrolyte imbalances
- Sleeplessness
- Sudden death

SOURCE: Adapted from Position of the American Dietetic Association: Very low-calorie weight loss diets, *Journal of the American Dietetic Association* (May 1990), p. 722.

or other health care provider before beginning any diet. Elimination of certain food groups or eating excessive amounts of certain foods can exacerbate these problems and may interfere with the effectiveness of certain medications.

9. *Does the weight-loss program encourage or promote increased physical activity?* Although people can lose weight by limiting food intake alone, research has shown that the most successful weight-loss plans include lifestyle changes, such as increasing exercise.
10. *Does the weight-loss program encourage an intake that is very low in calories (below 800 calories/day) without supervision of medical experts?* Very low-calorie diets should be used only by people with severe obesity or obesity with other health-related problems. Because the calorie intake is so low, the diet must be supplemented with vitamins and minerals. In addition, dieters must be strictly observed by a physician for any of the adverse health effects listed in Table 10-13. Finally, the people need dietary counseling to handle "real" food choices before the end of the diet, or weight gain can quickly ensue.

Don't Give Up!

For some folks, weight loss may seem like a lost cause, but don't give up! Several strategies and diets have been proven successful. The strategies supported by the most evidence are detailed in a recent analysis by the USDA and backed up by data from the National Weight Control Registry, a study that examines people who have lost at least 30 pounds and have maintained that loss for at least a year.[55]

You can take several steps to help you make wise decisions about dieting:

1. Be familiar with the current fad diets, and study any diet that interests you. These food plans often include scientifically based statements mixed with inaccuracies, so you have to know the literature to refute any incorrect claims.
2. Seek out appropriate weight-loss strategies and programs. A recent evidence-based review indicates that most weight loss is associated with diets that include about 1,400 to 1,500 calories per day. It is essential to control energy intake for any weight-loss plan.[56] Weight Watchers has been cited as a good option in many recent studies, because of the variety of foods offered and because its principles are based on scientific evidence. Internet-based programs are available for people who like to keep records and need support but cannot attend group sessions. The DASH diet has been found to significantly reduce high blood pressure and improve other chronic disease outcomes, and it is free on the National Institutes of Health (NIH) website.[57] About half of the people in the National Weight Control Registry (NWCR) lost weight without any formal program, indicating that the more individualized a program, the more likely it is that people will adhere to it for longer periods of time. Finally, most successful attempts to lose weight include some type of regular exercise.
3. The following websites contain good information or handouts that you can use to determine whether or not following a particular diet will be harmful: (1) the Federal Trade Commission (FTC) website, www.consumer.ftc.gov, which includes "Weighing the Claims in Diet Ads"; and (2) the American Heart Association's *Fad Diets*, available at www.heart.org.
4. Report fraudulent or deceptive weight-loss claims. Any weight-loss claims that are distributed via the Internet, television, or print media can be reported at www.ftc.gov.

SOURCE: Adapted from D. M. Hoelscher and C. McCullum-Gomez, Addressing the obesity epidemic: An issue for public health policy, in M. Boyle, *Community Nutrition in Action: An Entrepreneurial Approach*, 7th ed. (Boston, MA: Cengage Learning, 2017).

SPOTLight

10.9 The Eating Disorders

The relentless pursuit of thinness and fear of being fat are a haunting nightmare that drives millions of American teens and adults to starve, vomit, or purge.[58] The illness of **anorexia nervosa**—self-starvation—has been recognized as a psychiatric syndrome since the 1870s. Its companion disease **bulimia nervosa**—gorging on food and then purging—was not recognized as a separate eating disorder until the 1960s and 1970s. Some researchers suspect that a complex interplay between environmental, social, and perhaps genetic factors triggers an eating disorder in victims, who are mostly but not always women. Others question whether the fear of fatness isn't a mask for underlying emotional problems. Experts speculate that focusing on the body diverts these people's attention from and suppresses the painful emotion of anger, feelings of low self-esteem, the inability to express their feelings, or poor family relationships. The acute focus on the body develops into an intense fear of fatness, a characteristic intrinsically linked with food.[59] Thus, for many people, food is seen only as a source of body fat and so becomes carefully controlled. But why food? Why not use some other method of coping with stress?

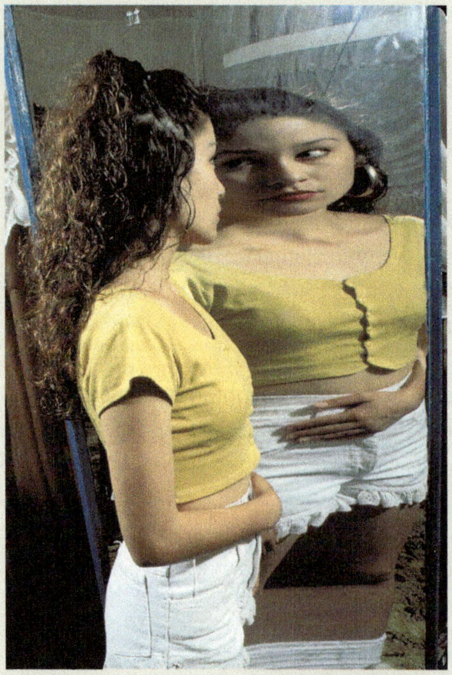
Tony Freeman/PhotoEdit

Looking in the mirror, a woman with anorexia nervosa distorts her body image and overestimates her body fatness.

Enter the societal link. In a society where thinness is equated with material success and even self-worth, especially for women, becoming thin appears to be the path that leads to happiness. Unfortunately, as victims of eating disorders come to learn, practicing self-starvation or gorging and purging leads instead to physical and emotional pain.

What is considered an eating disorder?

The term **eating disorder** comprises a wide spectrum of conditions, including anorexia nervosa, bulimia nervosa, and **binge-eating disorder**.[60] Although the various conditions differ in origin and consequences, they appear to have similarities: All of the conditions involve excessive preoccupation with weight, a fear of fatness, and a distorted body image. Many times, the person with an eating disorder falls short of the diagnostic criteria shown in Table 10-14 for anorexia nervosa or bulimia nervosa. Some of these people, described as having an **other specified feeding** or **eating disorder**, include those who:[61]

- Meet all the criteria for anorexia nervosa except that their weight remains within a normal range.
- Meet all the criteria for bulimia nervosa except that their behaviors are less frequent.
- Meet all the criteria for binge-eating disorder (see Table 10-15)[62] except that their binges are less frequent.

What is the difference between an eating disorder and disordered eating?

Disordered eating occurs when a person eats (or doesn't eat) because of an external stimulus rather than an internal one. For example, an external stimulus might be, "I'm lonely," "I'm angry," or "I'm anxious," and "these chocolate cookies will distract me and help me feel better." An internal stimulus is a physical sensation: a message from your brain about your current state of hunger or satiety, such as "my stomach is growling," or "I feel full." People with eating disorders spend more time in "external eating" than in responding to internal hunger cues.[63] Many people eat for reasons other than hunger from time to time, but if this type of behavior controls someone's thoughts and interferes with their everyday routines, it becomes an eating disorder.

What are the symptoms of anorexia nervosa?

People with anorexia deprive themselves of food except for controlled amounts of very low-calorie foods such as unbuttered toast or popcorn, apples, and green beans. Even intake of these foods is painstakingly

TABLE 10-14 Diagnosis of Eating Disorders

Anorexia Nervosa	Bulimia Nervosa
A person with anorexia nervosa demonstrates the following: 1. Refusal to maintain body weight at or above a minimal normal weight for age and height 2. Intense fear of weight gain or becoming fat, even though underweight 3. Distorted body image, undue influence of body weight or shape on self-evaluation, or denial of the seriousness of the current low body weight **Two types:** *Restricting type*: During the episode of anorexia nervosa, the person does not regularly engage in binge eating or purging behavior (that is, self-induced vomiting or the misuse of laxatives, diuretics, or enemas). *Binge-eating/purging type:* During the episode of anorexia nervosa, the person regularly engages in binge eating or purging behavior (that is, self-induced vomiting or the misuse of laxatives, diuretics, or enemas).	A person with bulimia nervosa demonstrates the following: 1. Recurrent episodes of binge eating characterized by: a. Eating in a discrete period of time an amount of food that is definitely larger than most people would eat during a similar period of time and under similar circumstances b. A sense of lack of control over eating during the episode 2. Recurrent compensatory behavior to prevent weight gain, such as self-induced vomiting; misuse of laxatives, diuretics, enemas, or other medications; fasting; or excessive exercise 3. Binge eating and compensatory behaviors that occur, on an average, at least once a week for three months 4. Self-evaluation unduly influenced by body shape and weight 5. Does not occur exclusively during episodes of anorexia nervosa. **Two types:** *Purging type:* The person regularly engages in self-induced vomiting or the misuse of laxatives, diuretics, or enemas. *Nonpurging type:* The person uses other behaviors, such as fasting or excessive exercise, but does not regularly engage in self-induced vomiting or the misuse of laxatives, diuretics, or enemas.

SOURCE: Adapted from American Psychiatric Association, *Diagnostic and Statistical Manual of Mental Disorders*, 5th ed. (Arlington, VA: American Psychiatric Association, 2013).

TABLE 10-15 Criteria for Diagnosis of Binge-Eating Disorder

A person with a binge-eating disorder demonstrates the following:

1. Recurrent episodes of binge eating. An episode of binge eating is characterized by both of the following:
   a. Eating, in a discrete period of time (for example, within any 2-hour period), an amount of food that is more than most people would eat in a similar period of time under similar circumstances.
   b. A sense of lack of control over eating during the episode (such as a feeling that one cannot stop eating or control what or how much one is eating).
2. Binge-eating episodes are associated with at least three of the following:
   a. Eating much more rapidly than normal.
   b. Eating until feeling uncomfortably full.
   c. Eating large amounts of food when not feeling physically hungry.
   d. Eating alone because of being embarrassed by how much one is eating.
   e. Feeling disgusted with oneself, depressed, or very guilty after overeating.
3. The binge eating causes marked distress.
4. The binge eating occurs, on average, at least once a week for three months.
5. The binge eating is not associated with the regular use of inappropriate compensatory behaviors (purging, fasting, excessive exercise) and does not occur exclusively during the course of anorexia nervosa or bulimia nervosa.

SOURCE: Adapted from American Psychiatric Association, *Diagnostic and Statistical Manual of Mental Disorders*, 5th ed. (Arlington, VA: American Psychiatric Association, 2013).

limited. After three to four days of eating very small amounts of food, hunger pangs subside. Once their appetite is suppressed, people with anorexia report feeling quite energetic, as if on a high, making the strict fast easier to stick to—but the body needs fuel to run. To compensate for the lack of fuel from food, the body turns to itself for fuel and begins to slowly destroy muscle and fat tissue for energy. The following are some of the physical symptoms associated with the starvation seen in people with anorexia:[64]

- Wasting of the whole body, including muscle tissue and bones
- Arrested sexual development and stopping of menstruation due to loss of body fat

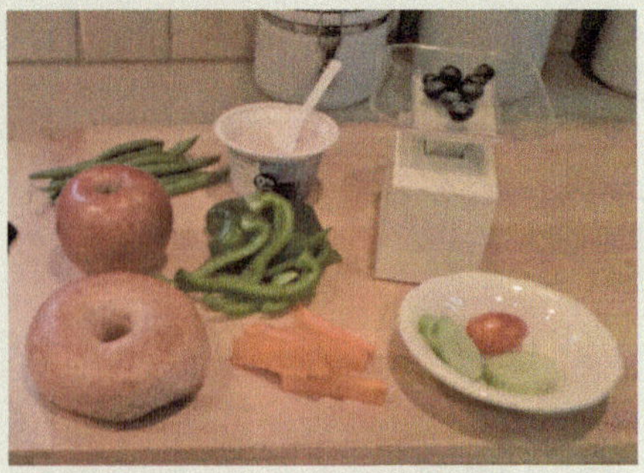

For many people with anorexia nervosa, a full day's diet may consist of no more than three or four items.

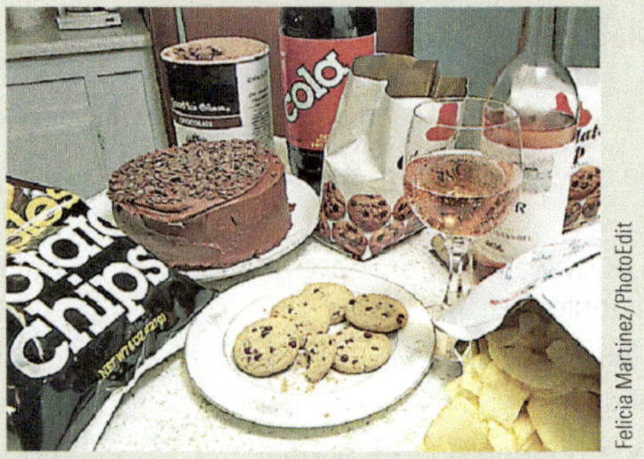

For many people with bulimia, guilt, depression, and self-condemnation follow a binge-eating episode.

- Drying and yellowing of the skin from an accumulation of a stored vitamin A compound released from body fat
- Intolerance to cold weather due to loss of subcutaneous fat
- Growth of hair on the body, perhaps in response to a decrease in body temperature
- Loss of health and texture of hair
- Pain on touch
- Lowered blood pressure and metabolic rate
- Anemia
- Severe sleep disturbance[65]
- Depression, possibly related to changes in neurotransmitter function in the brain[66]

At the same time the physical symptoms appear, distorted psychological symptoms develop. When looking in the mirror, people with anorexia do not see the emaciated body others see, but continue to see themselves as being too fat.[67] A preoccupation with death develops, accompanied by a frantic pursuit of physical fitness by means of stringent exercise routines. People with anorexia deal with parents and family in a manipulative way so they become the center of attention. Diet becomes so totally engrossing that those with anorexia may be quite socially isolated except for friends who stick close by and worry without knowing how to help.

By this time, the person with anorexia may have reached absolute minimum body weight (for example, 65 to 70 pounds for a woman of average height). The person is on the verge of incurring permanent brain damage and chronic debilitation or death. The National Association of Anorexia Nervosa and Associated Disorders (ANAD) estimates that of those with severe eating disorders, 6 percent die, usually because major organs—heart and kidneys—fail.

What are the symptoms of bulimia?

Unlike those with anorexia, people with bulimia usually have a healthy body weight or may even be slightly overweight. People with bulimia also follow rigid rules of dietary restraint, but their routine is not as rigorous as the starvation routine of those with anorexia, and they occasionally break their own rigid rules.

Quickly, and usually privately, people with bulimia gorge on foods that are often sweet, starchy, and high in fat or calories and require little chewing. The binge ends when it would hurt to eat any more, when they are interrupted, or when they go to sleep or induce vomiting to expel the food just eaten.

People with bulimia often feel controlled by the vicious circle that develops: anxiety about being "fat" leads to rigid dietary restraint. Mounting hunger from not eating and an increased preoccupation with food cause them to break their rules, and binging results. After gorging, an intense fear of fatness overtakes the person, who then vomits to get rid of the food and release the fear of becoming "fatter." Feelings of guilt and shame follow the purge, building a new level of anxiety concerning the body, and the cycle begins again. Each binge reinforces the idea that additional rigidity of dietary restraint is required to prevent weight gain. Excessive use of laxatives or diuretics or bouts of vigorous exercise replace vomiting in some cases.

Binge eating is seldom life threatening, but at the extreme, it can be physically damaging, causing lacerations of the stomach, tearing or irritation of the esophagus (in those who vomit frequently), dental caries (from acidic vomit attacking the teeth), electrolyte imbalances, and malnutrition (in those who vomit and those who take laxatives).

People with bulimia also suffer from a distorted body image.[68] They see themselves as fat and needing to restrict food, even though they usually have a healthful body weight. They generally prefer a body size somewhat smaller than normal.

How are anorexia nervosa and bulimia treated?

There are several philosophies regarding the treatment of eating disorders. The four major approaches include individual psychotherapy, hospitalization, family therapy, and behavior modification therapy.[69] Some therapists use more than one approach. Most treatment methods focus on identifying the societal and environmental pressures that triggered the eating disorder and on exposing the emotions masked by it. An interdisciplinary team made up of a psychologist, a social worker, a family therapy counselor, and a dietitian work with the family and the patient to reestablish emotional and nutritional health.[70] Length of treatment varies from two months to two to three years, depending on the patient's readiness for change and the type of treatment. Treatment focuses on the problems of low self-esteem, guilt, anxiety, depression, and a sense of

TABLE 10-16 A Comparison of Eating Disorders

	Anorexia Nervosa	Bulimia Nervosa	Binge-Eating Disorder
Estimated prevalence*			
Males	0.3%	0.5%	2.0%
Females	0.9%	1.5%	3.5%
Usual age of onset	Adolescence	Adolescence into early adulthood	Adulthood
BMI status	Low	Normal to high	High
Family history of eating disorders	Yes	Yes	Yes
Weight loss or maintenance	Inability to maintain a determined body weight	Dramatic shifts in body weight	Difficulty maintaining a determined body weight
Behavioral components	Depression Anxiety Low self-esteem	Depression Anxiety Low self-esteem Substance abuse**	Depression Anxiety Low self-esteem
Body image	Distorted	Poor	Poor

*Note that there is widespread underreporting of all eating disorders, due to their sensitive nature.
**Substance abuse is common among people with bulimia.

SOURCES: Adapted from: S. A. Swanson et al., Prevalence and correlates of eating disorders in adolescents: Results from the National Comorbidity Survey Replication, Adolescent Supplement, *Archives of General Psychiatry* 68 (2011): 714–723; A. D. Ozier et al., Position of the American Dietetic Association: Nutrition intervention in the treatment of eating disorders, *Journal of the American Dietetic Association* 111 (2011): 1236–1241; National Association of Anorexia Nervosa and Associated Disorders, www.anad.org.

helplessness. In addition, family therapy focuses on changing patterns of family interaction.

Normal nutrition must be restored in those with anorexia. After some progress is made in counseling, a dietitian can help the patient gain a new understanding of a healthful eating pattern and clear up misconceptions about food and nutrition.[71]

What are the early warning signs of eating disorders?

Table 10-16 shows the similarities and differences among the eating disorders. Families and friends can be alerted to several possible warning signs of eating disorders (see Table 10-17). Severe dieting often precedes the illness. People with anorexia develop an exaggerated

TABLE 10-17 Warning Signs of an Eating Disorder

- Preoccupation with weight, food, calories, and dieting, to the extent that it consistently intrudes on conversations and interferes with other activities
- Excessive exercise—despite weather, fatigue, illness, and injury
- Dramatic weight loss; arrested growth in children
- Anxiety about being fat that does not diminish with weight loss
- Reluctance to be weighed
- Inability to gain weight
- Difficulty eating in social situations
- Deceptive or secretive behavior
- Alternating periods of severely restrictive dieting and overeating
- Evidence of binge eating or consumption of large quantities of food inconsistent with the person's weight
- Evidence of use of laxatives, diuretics, or agents that cause vomiting (emetics)
- Extreme concern about appearance as a defining feature of self-esteem (for example, I am "thin and good," or "gross and bad")
- Social withdrawal or avoidance of activities because of weight and shape concerns
- Absence from school or work
- Depression
- Disrupted menstruation
- Constipation or diarrhea
- Paleness or lightheadedness not accounted for by other medical conditions
- Susceptibility to fractures

SOURCES: Adapted from Eating Disorders Awareness and Prevention, Inc. materials; and D. Rosen, Dieting disorder, *New England Journal of Medicine* (April 8, 1999).

interest in food but at the same time deny their hunger and stop eating. Their distorted body image makes them feel fat even as weight loss continues. A person with anorexia begins to have sleep problems, shows unusual devotion to schoolwork, and often undertakes a program of unrelenting exercise. People with bulimia may binge and self-induce vomiting or use excessive amounts of laxatives. Reduced food intake usually causes sufficient weight loss to stop menstrual cycles in women.

People with eating disorders were usually good children who did not indulge in rebellion. Not all people with anorexia and bulimia exhibit all symptoms. Early detection is vital. Use the Eating Attitudes Quiz to see if your own eating attitudes and behaviors are within a normal range.

What can be done to prevent eating disorders?

Consider the following suggestions for helping people to remain healthy and for preventing eating disorders altogether:[72]

- Discourage restrictive dieting and meal skipping. Severe dieting may lead to eating disorders, especially in adolescent girls.
- Model a lifestyle of healthful eating and exercise, and never encourage unhealthful "quick-fix" weight loss.
- Promote fitness and a healthy body rather than thinness and numbers on a scale.
- Help teens understand and accept the normal physiological changes in body composition and weight that occur with puberty—changes that may be interpreted as "getting fat."
- Avoid assigning "good" or "bad" labels to food. Don't offer food as a reward. Don't imply that the shape or size of your body, or someone else's, has anything to do with self-worth (e.g., "I'd be happy if I were thin").
- Be sensitive and careful about making weight-related comments or recommendations. Even playful teasing may trigger long-term struggles with disordered eating or eating disorders.
- Encourage normal expression of the basic emotions: joy, anger, fear, sadness, loneliness, guilt, and shame.

What can I do if I am worried that someone I know may have an eating disorder?[73]

If you or others observe behaviors in a friend, roommate, or family member that suggest the possibility of an eating disorder, consider the following:

- Plan to approach the person in a private place when there is no immediate stress and you have time to talk.
- Present in a caring but straightforward way what you have observed and what your concerns are. Tell the person that you are worried and want to help.
- Give the person time to talk, and encourage her or him to verbalize feelings. Listen carefully and accept what is said in a nonjudgmental manner.
- Do not argue about whether there is or is not a problem—power struggles are not helpful. Perhaps you can say, "I hear what you are saying, and I hope you are right that this is not a problem. But I am still very worried about you and your health, and that is not going to go away."
- Provide information about resources for treatment. Offer to go with the person and wait while she or he has a first appointment with a counselor, physician, or dietitian.
- If you are concerned that the eating disorder is severe or life threatening, enlist help from the counseling center, a relative, a friend, or the person's roommate *before* you intervene. Present a united and supportive front together.
- If the person denies the problem, becomes angry, or refuses treatment, understand that this is often part of the illness. You may feel helpless, angry, and frustrated with the person. You might say, "I know you can refuse to go for help, but I am still your friend, and I am worried about you. I may bring this up again later, and maybe we can talk more about it then." Follow through on that—and on any other promise you make.
- Do not try to be a hero or a rescuer; you will probably be resented. Treatment is most effective when the person is truly ready for it. You may have planted a seed that helps the person get ready.

Miniglossary

anorexia nervosa Literally, "nervous lack of appetite," a disorder involving self-starvation to the extreme (*an* = without; *orexis* = appetite).

bulimia nervosa, bulimarexia (byoo-LEE-me-uh, byoo-lee-ma-REX-ee-uh) Binge eating (literally, "eating like an ox"), combined with an intense fear of becoming fat and usually followed by self-induced vomiting or taking laxatives (*buli* = ox).

eating disorder General term for several conditions (anorexia nervosa, bulimia nervosa, binge-eating disorder) that exhibit an excessive preoccupation with body weight, a fear of body fatness, and a poor or distorted body image.

binge-eating disorder An eating disorder characterized by uncontrolled chronic episodes of overeating (compulsive overeating) without other symptoms of eating disorders. Typically, the episodes of binge eating occur at least once a week for a period of three months or more.

other specified feeding or eating disorder Condition in which a person exhibits some but not all of the criteria for specific eating disorders.

disordered eating Eating food as an outlet for emotional stress rather than in response to internal physiological cues.

Eating Attitudes Quiz

Answer the following questions to evaluate your own eating attitudes and behaviors. Do they fall within a normal range? Use these responses:

A = always
U = usually
O = often
S = sometimes
R = rarely
N = never

1. I am terrified about being overweight.
2. I avoid eating when I am hungry.
3. I find myself preoccupied with food.
4. I have gone on eating binges where I feel that I may not be able to stop.
5. I cut my food into very small pieces.
6. I am aware of the calorie content of the foods I eat.
7. I particularly avoid foods with high carbohydrate content.
8. I feel that others would prefer that I eat more.
9. I vomit after I eat.
10. I feel extremely guilty after eating.
11. I am preoccupied with a desire to be thinner.
12. I think about burning up calories when I exercise.
13. Other people think I am too thin.
14. I am preoccupied with the thought of having fat on my body.
15. I take longer than other people to eat my meals.
16. I avoid foods with sugar in them.
17. I eat diet foods.
18. I feel that food controls my life.
19. I display self-control around food.
20. I feel that others pressure me to eat.
21. I give too much time and thought to food.
22. I feel uncomfortable after eating sweets.
23. I engage in dieting behavior.
24. I like my stomach to be empty.
25. I enjoy trying new rich foods.
26. I have the impulse to vomit after meals.

SCORING

Never = 3
Rarely = 2
Sometimes = 1
Always, usually, and often = 0

A total score under 20 points may indicate abnormal eating behavior and the risk of having or developing an eating disorder. Share your results with a health professional for further evaluation.

SOURCE: J. A. McSherry, Progress in the diagnosis of anorexia nervosa, *Journal of the Royal Society of Health* 106 (1986): 8–9; *Eating Attitudes Test* and scoring developed by Dr. P. Garfinkel.

Nutrition on the Web

http://fnic.nal.usda.gov
The Food and Nutrition Information Center (FNIC) provides credible information.

- Under Diet and Health, select Weight and Obesity as well as Disordered Eating.

www.nutrition.gov
Under Browse by Subject, select Weight Management.

www.nhlbi.nih.gov/health/educational/lose_wt
The National Heart, Lung and Blood Institute website provides Aim for a Healthy Weight.

www.cdc.gov/nccdphp/dnpa
The Centers for Disease Control and Prevention (CDC) website contains many topics related to nutrition and weight management.

win.niddk.nih.gov/publications/choosing.htm
The Weight-control Information Network website provides safe and reliable information about successful weight-loss programs.

For more information about anorexia nervosa, bulimia, and associated disorders, go to:

- *Anorexia Nervosa and Related Eating Disorders*: www.anred.com
- *National Eating Disorders Association*: www.nationaleatingdisorders.org
- *National Institute of Mental Health*: www.nimh.nih.gov
- *Canadian National Eating Disorder Information Centre*: www.nedic.ca

WHAT'S ONLINE

MINDTAP From Cengage

Visit www.cengagebrain.com to access MindTap, a complete digital course that includes Diet & Wellness Plus, interactive quizzes, videos, and more.

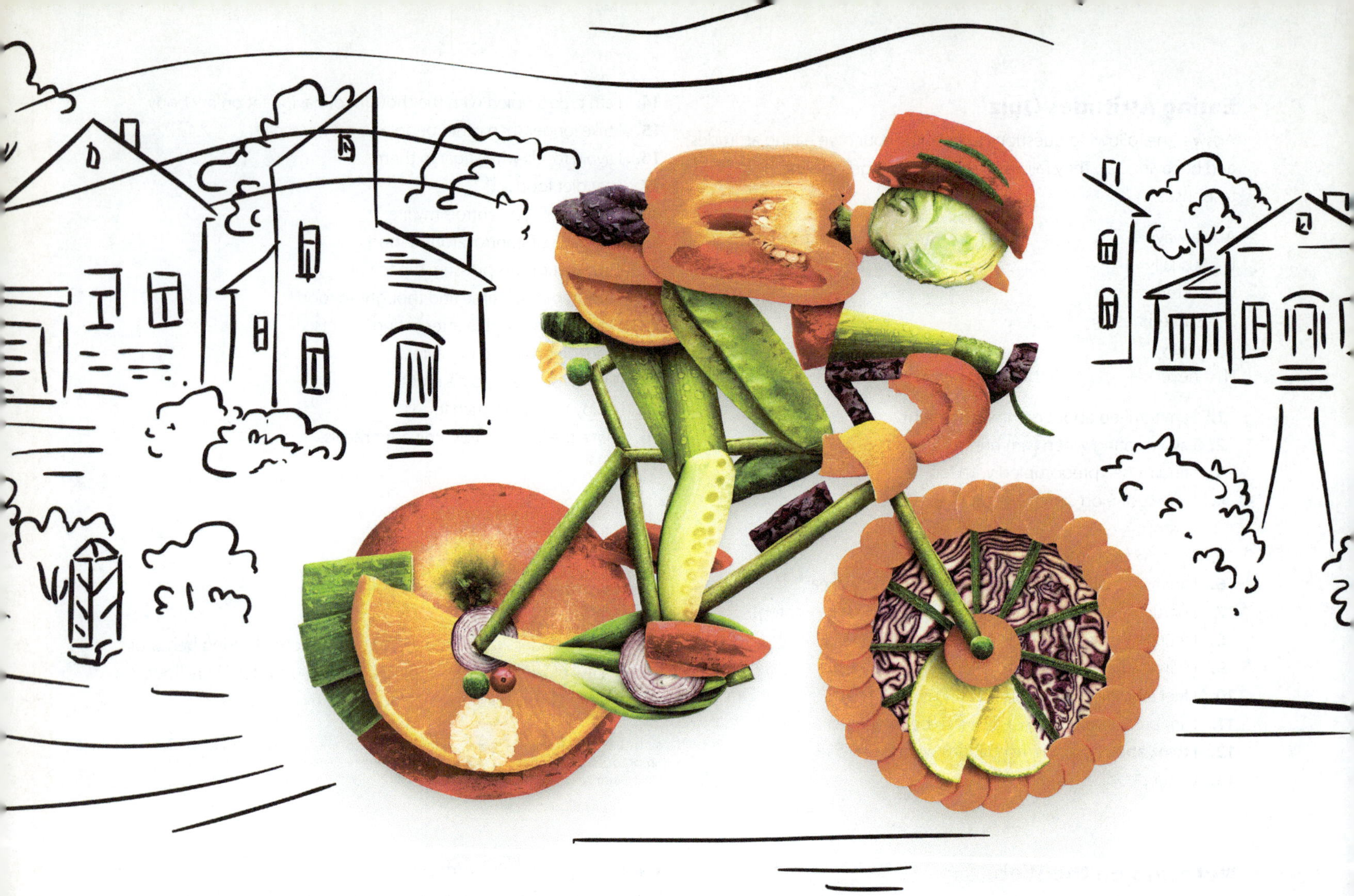

Fisher Photostudio/Shutterstock.com

AskYourself . . .

Which of the following statements about nutrition are true, and which are false? For each false statement, what is true?

1. Less than 25 percent of U.S. adults exercise adequately.
2. People who fail to exercise regularly are more likely to fall prey to degenerative diseases such as heart disease, osteoporosis, and diabetes.
3. Essentially, to be fit means to be at desirable weight and to have strong muscles.
4. If you run out of breath, it is a sign that your heart and lungs are not strong enough to perform the desired tasks.

Answers found on page 328.

ChapterObjectives

11.1 Describe the health benefits of living a physically active lifestyle.

11.2 Identify the five components of fitness and strategies to achieve overall fitness.

11.3 Identify the factors that influence fuel use during physical activity and sport.

11.4 Describe the use of glycogen and body fat for fuel during physical activity and sport.

11.5 Identify the difference in protein needs for active individuals versus competitive athletes.

11.6 Identify the factors that influence fluid needs for the physically active as compared to competitive athletes, and describe the recommended schedule of hydration before, during, and after sport.

11.7 Describe how vitamins and minerals are used by the body during physical activity.

11.8 Discuss the safety and efficacy of popular ergogenic aids.

Nutrition for Fueling Fitness & Sport

CHAPTER 11

How physically active are you? The benefits of regular physical activity make up an impressive list, and the list keeps growing longer as new discoveries are made. People who begin a fitness program to trim fat or add muscle are soon pleasantly surprised to find that they have more energy, feel less tense, sleep better, and feel healthier.[1] And so they keep it up! Most people do not realize the many benefits of regular physical activity. Read the list in Table 11-1 and imagine how being more physically active might change your life for the better.

Get health. No labor, effort, nor exercise that can gain it must be grudged.

— R. W. Emerson (1803–1882, American essayist and poet)

In addition, mounting evidence suggests that our bodies need regular, moderate physical activity that gets our hearts beating and forces our muscles to work harder than they usually do to stay healthy. Physiologically speaking, overall fitness is a balance between different body systems. With respect to the joints, flexibility is important. With respect to muscles, strength and endurance are important. More and more research is proving that sitting, or being sedentary, is the new smoking! Research has linked sitting for long periods of time with several health concerns, including obesity and **metabolic syndrome**—a cluster of conditions that includes increased blood pressure, high blood sugar, excess body fat around the waist, and abnormal cholesterol levels.[2] Too much sitting also seems to increase the risk of death from cardiovascular disease and cancer.

One's overall health can be impacted significantly with even small amounts of increased physical activity and even daily movement.[3] This chapter illustrates the effects of nutrition on one's general fitness and takes a look at the increased nutritional requirements needed for competitive sport. Optimal nutrition contributes to all levels of athletic performance, and, conversely, regular physical activity contributes to a person's ability to use and store nutrients optimally. Together, the two are indispensable for a high quality of life. **Fitness**, like good nutrition, is an essential component of good health.

metabolic syndrome A cluster of conditions that includes increased blood pressure, high blood sugar, excess body fat around the waist, and abnormal cholesterol levels.

fitness The body's ability to meet physical demands; composed of five components: flexibility, muscular strength, muscular endurance, cardiorespiratory endurance, and body composition.

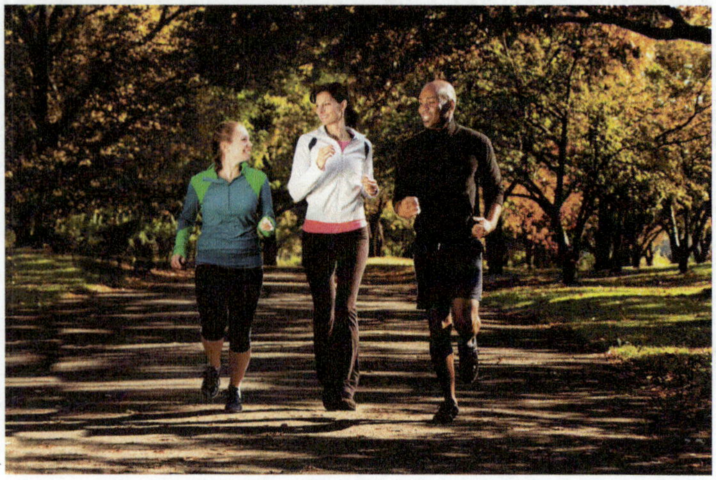

Tyler Olson/Shutterstock.com

Being fit is more than being free of disease; it is feeling full of vitality and enthusiasm for life.

No one can promise that you will receive every potential health benefit from Table 11-1 if you exercise, but almost everyone who exercises reaps at least some of them. Physical activity need not be strenuous to yield health benefits. Moderate amounts of physical activity are recommended for people of all ages. However, at present, only a little more than 20 percent of U.S. adults meet aerobic and muscle strength guidelines, and a little more than 23 percent of adults are not active at all.[4]

11.1 Getting Started on Lifetime Fitness

Although any increase in daily activity is an improvement for our overall health, there is a certain *minimum* daily average amount of activity that is indispensable to health. The *Physical Activity Guidelines for Americans* reports that health benefits occur with at least 2 hours and 30 minutes (150 minutes) per week of moderate-intensity physical activity, which may take any one of numerous forms, including brisk walking (see Figure 11-1).[5] Additional benefits will occur with more physical activity. Just mix and match your preferred activities in periods as short as 10 minutes. Alternatively, adults can choose a minimum of 1 hour and 15 minutes a week of vigorous-intensity aerobic physical activity by doing activities like jogging, aerobic dancing, and jumping rope. These guidelines stress the value of moderate activity and suggest that the total *amount* of activity is more important than the manner in which it is carried out. For total fitness, a physical activity program that incorporates aerobic activity, strength training, and stretching is best. The more active you are, the more fit you are likely to be.

In proceeding with a fitness program, keep in mind that fitness builds slowly, so activity should increase gradually. For beginners, consistency is very important. Establish a regular pattern of physical activity first (e.g., 30 minutes cumulative to start) and plan to increase that amount over time. View your physical activity time as a lifelong commitment.

If you are just starting on a fitness program, a few precautions are important. For most apparently healthy people, moderate physical activity such as walking should not pose any problem. However, medical advice concerning suitable type of activity may be necessary for anyone with any of the risk factors shown in Table 11-2 or for anyone diagnosed with cardiac or other known diseases.[6]

The term *fitness* is not restricted to seasoned athletes. Physical fitness is a general state of health and well-being, and more specifically the ability to perform aspects of sports, occupations, and daily activities.[7] With a basic understanding of the concepts of fitness and a personal commitment to a physically active lifestyle, anyone can become fit. To be fit, you don't have to be able to finish the local marathon, nor do you have to develop the muscles of a Mr. Universe or Miss Olympia. Rather, what you need is a healthy body weight/composition (refer to Chapter 10) and enough flexibility, muscular strength, muscular endurance, and cardiorespiratory endurance to meet the everyday demands that life places on you, plus some to spare. The Scorecard feature later in this chapter helps you evaluate your own level of physical activity.

TABLE 11-1 Benefits of Physical Activity

- Increased self-confidence
- Easier weight control
- More energy
- Less stress and anxiety
- Improved circulation and lung function
- Improved sleep
- Enhanced immunity
- Lowered risk of heart disease
- Lowered risk of certain cancers
- Stronger bones
- Lowered risk of diabetes
- Lowered risk of high blood pressure
- Increased quality of life
- Increased independence in life's later years

© Cengage

TABLE 11-2 Major Risk Factors for Heart Disease

- Sedentary lifestyle
- Family history of heart disease
- Cigarette smoking
- High blood pressure
- High blood cholesterol (>200 mg/dL)
- Obesity (BMI ≥30)
- Diabetes

© Cengage

ASK YOURSELF ANSWERS: **1.** True. **2.** True. **3.** False. To be fit means not only to be at desirable weight and to have strong muscles, but also to be flexible and, most importantly, to have muscular and cardiorespiratory endurance. **4.** False. If you run out of breath, it is not a sign that your heart and lungs are weak but a sign that you are going into oxygen debt.

FIGURE 11-1

Physical Activity Guidelines for Adults

Physical activity helps you feel and perform at your best. The key to sticking with a regular physical activity program is to choose activities that you enjoy. Be flexible. Remember that you don't have to spend 60 consecutive minutes engaged in physical activity—a few minutes here and a few minutes there add to the benefits of moderate activity. Keep in mind that *any* activity is good (for example, "just do something"), but *more* is better. The goal is to have a *physically active* lifestyle.*

SOURCE: Adapted from 2008 Physical Activity Guidelines for Americans, by University of Missouri Cooperative extension, 2009.

*More tips for increasing daily physical activity can be found on the last page of this chapter and at www.ChooseMyPlate.org.

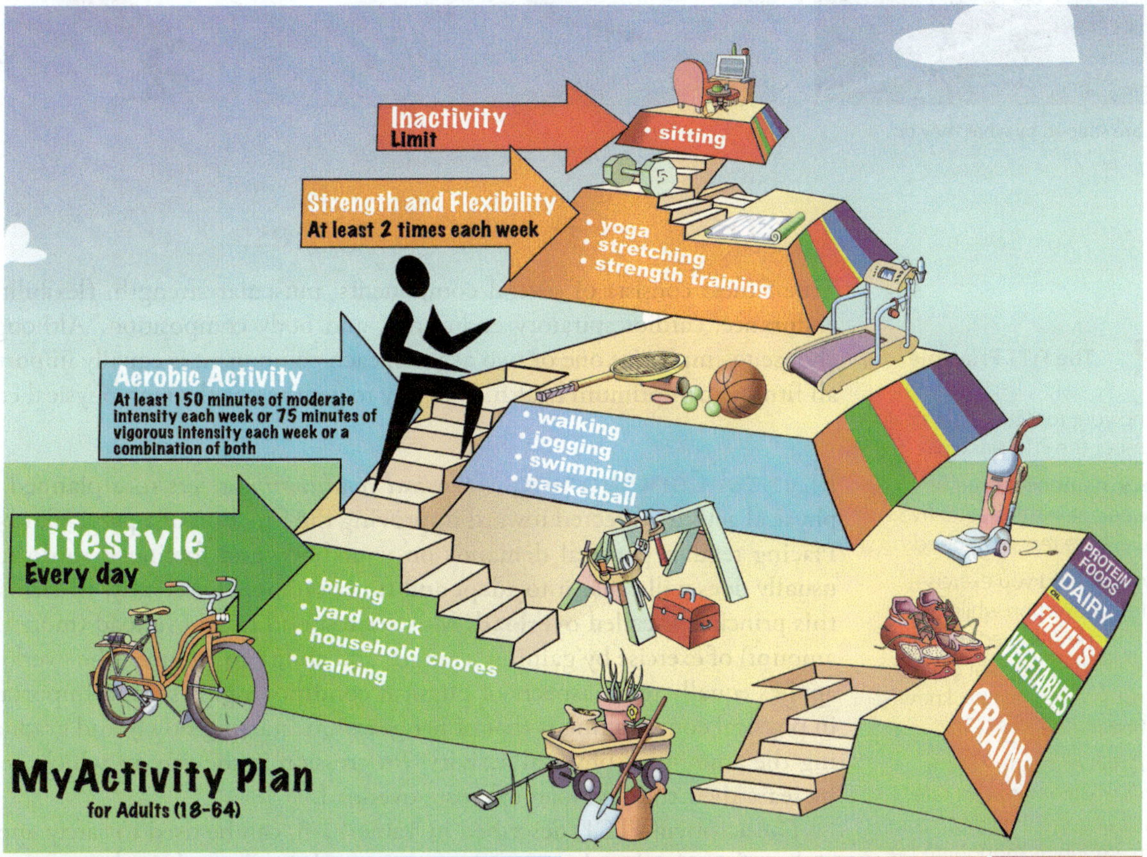

LIFESTYLE ACTIVITIES	AEROBIC ACTIVITY*	STRENGTH & FLEXIBILITY	INACTIVITY
As often as possible.	At least 150 minutes (2 hours and 30 min.) of moderate intensity each week OR At least 75 minutes (1 hour and 15 min.) of vigorous intensity each week	At least 2 times each week	Limit
Pick an activity you like and one that fits your life. Some physical activity is better than none.	What is a moderate-intensity activity? • You can talk while you do it, but you can't sing. What is a vigorous-intensity activity? • You can only say a few words without stopping to catch your breath.	Strength • Include all major muscle groups. • Perform 8–12 repetitions per set (1–3 sets). Flexibility • Perform flexibility activities at least two days each week for at least 10 minutes each day.	Screen time (television, computer, video games). Sitting longer than 60 minutes.

*Most health benefits occur with at least 150 minutes (2 hours and 30 min.) a week of moderate-intensity physical activity.

For additional health benefits, adults should increase their aerobic physical activity to 300 minutes (5 hours) a week of moderate-intensity, or 150 minutes a week of vigorous-intensity aerobic physical activity, or a combination of both. Additional benefits include lower risk of colon and breast cancer and prevention of unhealthy weight gain.

To learn more about these guidelines visit: www.health.gov/paguidelines

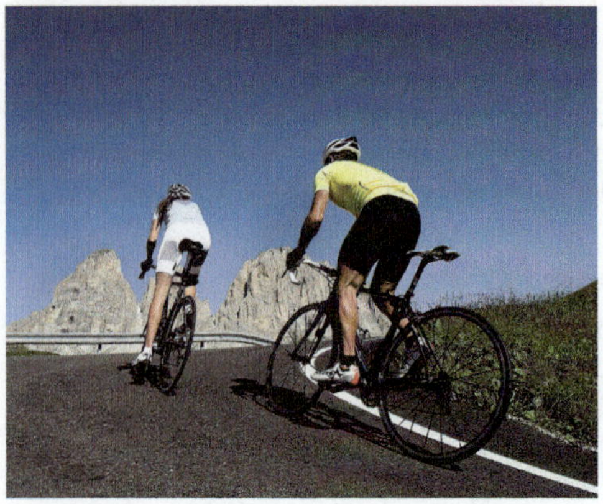

iStock.com/Gorfer

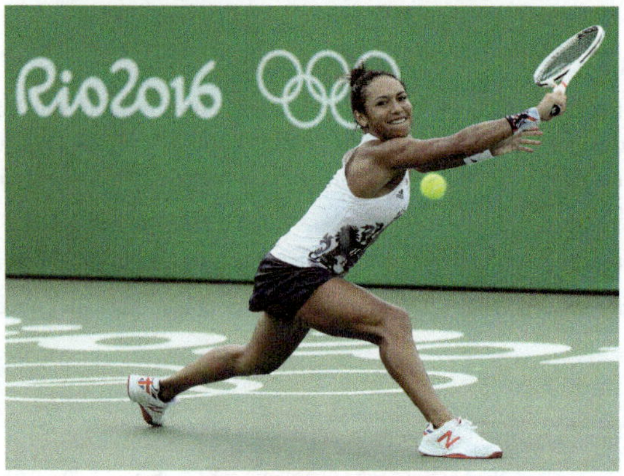

Leonard Zhukovsky/Shutterstock.com

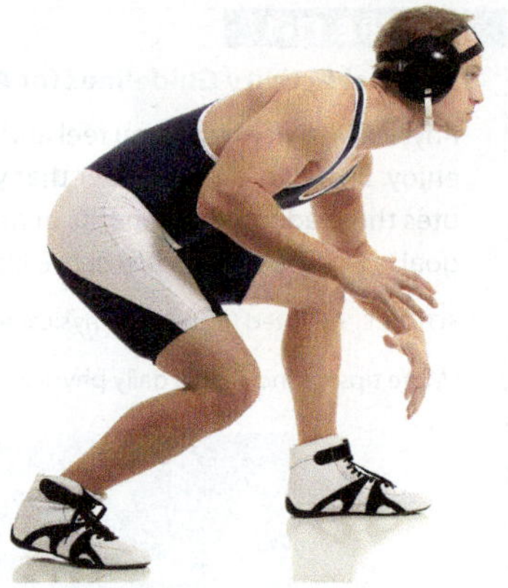

iStock.com/nickp37

People's bodies are shaped by what they do.

11.2 The Components of Fitness

True fitness consists of several components: muscular strength, flexibility, muscular endurance, cardiorespiratory endurance, and body composition.[8] Although you may choose to emphasize one or two aspects, each component is equally important to overall fitness and optimum health. The way to get there is through physical conditioning.

TABLE 11-3 The FITT Principle

For establishing your routine of physical activity remember the FITT principle:

F—Frequency: number of exercise sessions per week; at least three to five sessions per week are recommended.

I—Intensity: how hard you exercise (e.g., the degree of exertion while exercising); it is recommended that you exercise at 50 to 85 percent of your maximum heart rate per minute, known as your target heart rate.

T—Time: duration or length of time that you exercise with your heart rate elevated into your target heart rate zone (the minimum amount is thought to be 20 to 30 minutes per session).

T—Type: specific form of exercise being done such as muscular strength, flexibility, muscular endurance, and/or cardiorespiratory endurance.

Physical Conditioning

Physical conditioning refers to a planned program of physical activity directed toward improving the function of a particular body system. Placing regular physical demands on your body and forcing it to do more than it usually does will cause it to adapt and function more efficiently. In terms of exercise, this principle is called **overload**. Muscles respond to an overload (more than normal amount) of exercise by gaining strength and ability to endure. The overload principle applies equally to all aspects of physical conditioning. A second important principle in physical conditioning is that of **progression**, starting slowly and gradually increasing the amount of physical activity. Progression is the way in which people should increase their training load to create overload.

The acronym FITT, described in Table 11-3, can be used to safely apply the principles of overload and progression to your physical conditioning program.[9] For the type of physical activity preferred, one can apply all three strategies, pick one, or use a combination of the three, depending on your fitness goals. Using any aspects of progression and overload will optimize the results of your conditioning program.

Muscular Strength

Strength is the ability of the muscles to work against resistance, such as pulling yourself out of a swimming pool, carrying a backpack full of books, or opening a jar of pickles. The purpose of resistance training is to build well-toned muscles that let you accomplish daily activities at work and during recreation, as well as to prevent injury. As muscles get stronger, individual fibers thicken and enlarge. This response is called **hypertrophy**. The converse is also true. If muscles are not called on to perform, they decrease in size. This response is called **atrophy**. Our ability to respond to resistance training continues to a very old age.[10] The connective tissues making up muscles, tendons, and ligaments also strengthen and become more efficient at using energy. The benefit is that strong muscles, tendons, and ligaments play a key role in preventing injury. For example, strong quadriceps—the muscles on the front of the thigh—stabilize your knee as you bike. Strong calf muscles and ankle ligaments decrease the risk of an ankle sprain when you walk briskly or jog. Resistance training also helps with weight loss by increasing lean muscle mass and thus increasing your basal metabolic rate.

overload An extra physical demand placed on the body. A principle of training is that for a body system to improve, its workload must be increased by increments over time.

progression To start slowly and gradually increase the amount of exercise performed while also applying the principles of overload.

strength The ability of muscles to work against resistance.

hypertrophy An increase in size in response to use.

atrophy A decrease in size in response to disuse.

Nutrition **ACTION**

Nutrition and Fitness—Forever Young—or You're Not Going to Take Aging Lying Down, Are You? (Obj. 11.1)

No matter how old you are, you have the body of a modern human being—and that body (and how it works) was designed more than 100,000 years ago. One could even conclude that we humans have inherited genes that have been fine-tuned to support a physically active lifestyle. In fact, scientists from the University of Missouri, University of Pennsylvania, and East Carolina University not only hypothesize this to be true, but go on to say "that physical inactivity (defined as the activity equivalent of less than 30 minutes of brisk walking each day) in sedentary societies directly contributes to multiple chronic health disorders."[11] They conclude that physical inactivity is an abnormal state because our bodies have been "programmed" to expect physical activity; this is why inactivity causes the metabolic dysfunctions that lead to a host of chronic health conditions, such as heart disease, cancer, obesity, diabetes, and high blood pressure.

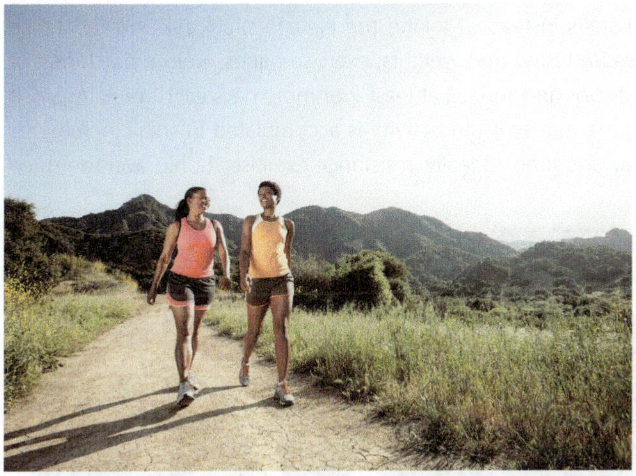

Erik Isakson/Jupiter Images

Finding a type of physical activity you enjoy can make reaching weekly physical activity recommendations fun to do.

Yesterday's Genes, Today's Lifestyle

Nearly all of your biochemistry and physiology (in other words, how you process foods and metabolize energy) was fine-tuned by and for conditions of life that existed more than 10,000 years ago. However, what we eat has changed more in the past 50 years than in the previous 40,000 years. So what's the big problem? Our genes don't know it! We still "process" food the same way our ancestors did—very efficiently (sometimes called the "thrifty gene" hypothesis). To understand this concept, you need only compare "yesterday's" diet and physical activity patterns to "today's" diet and physical activity habits (see Figure 11-2).

FIGURE 11-2

Preagricultural Hunter-Gatherers versus Industrialized Modern Humans

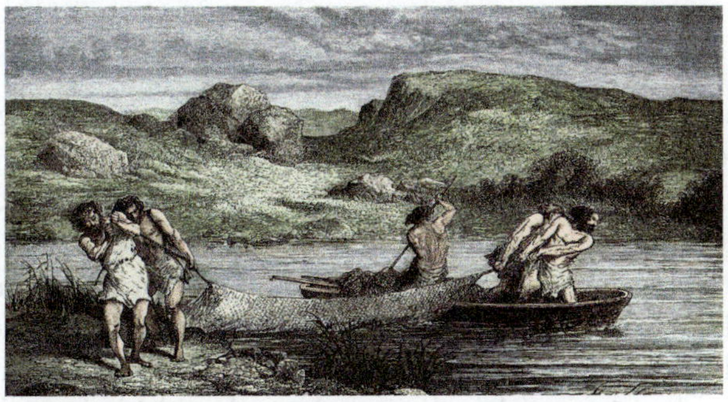

Sheila Terry/Science Source

Preagricultural Hunter-Gatherers

Burned ~3,000 calories per day

Moderate physical activity > 30 minutes per day to provide basic necessities (food, water, shelter, gathering materials for warmth, etc.)

Feast or famine

Lean wild game or fish

Uncultivated fruits and vegetables

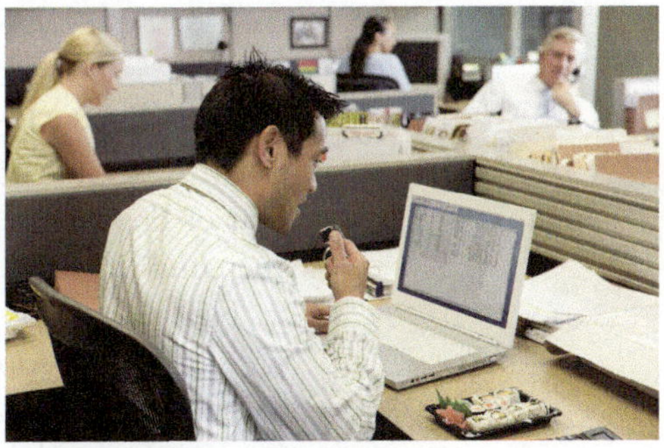

Monkey Business Images/Shutterstock.com

Industrialized Modern Humans

Burn ~1,800 calories per day

Sedentary (desk jobs, computer games, TV, dishwashers, drive-through windows, escalators and elevators, online shopping, remote controls, e-mail/Internet, lawn services, etc.)

Abundance of food (continuous feeding)

Grain-fattened meats

Refined sugar

(Continued)

Choose Your Weapon

You have your choice of weapons against the life-threatening diseases associated with sedentary aging, as listed in Table 11-4. Recommendations for physical activity include 150 minutes or 2 hours and 30 minutes of moderate-intensity activity (brisk walking between classes, bicycling from your dorm to classes, climbing the stairs instead of taking the elevators) a week and resistance exercise (using free weights, exercise bands, weight machines, or push-ups and squats) at least 2 or more days each week. Again, it doesn't matter if the activity is accumulated in small increments or at one time.[12] Ideally, resistance exercise should average three sessions (20 to 45 minutes per session) per week, working one to two muscle groups during each session. The different muscle groups are the chest, shoulders, arms, back, abdominals, and legs. Each session should include one to three sets (8 to 12 repetitions per set), resting 2 to 3 minutes between sets.[13] The photos in Figure 11-3 clearly demonstrate the need for physical activity throughout life.

Get Off Your "Buts"

Perhaps you are thinking, "I can't afford membership to a gym." Or "I don't have any exercise equipment." Or maybe your first thought is,

FIGURE 11-3

Regular Physical Activity Can Prevent Muscle Loss in Aging

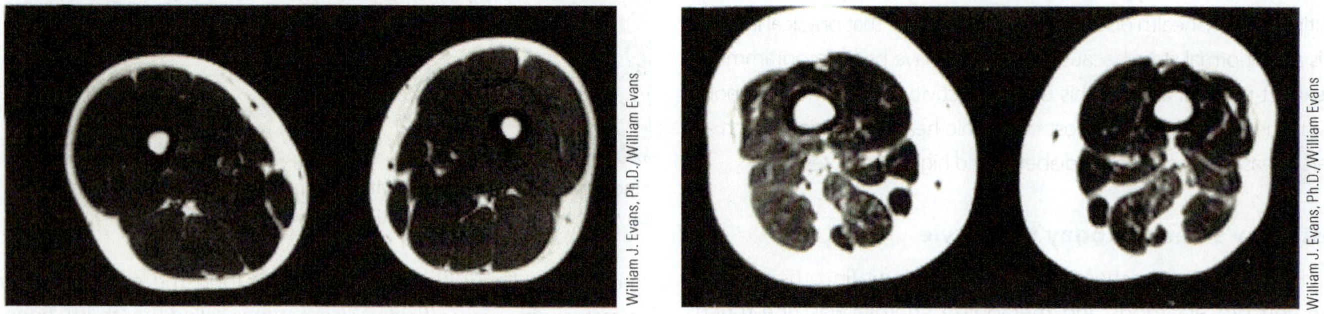

The photo at the left shows cross sections of the thighs of an active 20-year-old woman. The small white circle is the femur or thighbone. The photo at the right shows the thigh muscles of an older, sedentary woman in her late 60s. The older woman's thighs have lost muscle and gained fat. Strength-training activities such as walking, stair climbing, knee extensions, and leg curls can help prevent as well as reverse at least some of the muscle loss that accompanies aging and a sedentary lifestyle.[14] In other words, such a loss of muscle mass and the accompanying decrease in basal metabolism are not inevitable changes that occur with healthy aging. However, as the photos illustrate, these changes will accompany sedentary aging.

Flexibility Keeping your muscles and joints pliable is critical for developing a fit body. A flexible body can move as it was designed to move and will bend rather than tear or break in response to sudden stress. **Flexibility** (range of motion) depends on the condition and interrelationships of bones, ligaments, muscles, and tendons.

Flexibility tends to decrease with age, but improves in response to stretching with progression and overload applied.[15] The degree of flexibility achieved can be maintained in most people when completed with frequency. Stretching activities improve flexibility by increasing muscle and tendon elasticity and length. Stretching should be done slowly. When you feel a slight strain in the muscle, hold the position for 20 to 30 seconds. Bouncy, rapid stretches can cause minute tears in the muscle and often do more damage than good.

Stretching routines are best placed at the beginning and end of physical activity as part of one's warm-up and cooldown routines. Low-intensity preliminary exercise allows your heart—also a muscle—to slowly accelerate and make necessary adjustments in blood flow and oxygen supply, preparing the heart for the work it is about to perform. Using cardiorespiratory or aerobic activities such as walking, marching in place or some other moderate rhythmic activity as a warm-up can prepare your heart muscle for action. After your light warm-up, stretch the muscles that you will

flexibility The ability to bend or extend without injury; depends on the elasticity of the muscles, tendons, and ligaments and on the condition of the joints.

"I just don't have time to exercise." Don't let those thoughts in! You don't need special equipment, special clothes, or membership to a fitness club to stay fit. All you need to do is what we are (physiologically) supposed to be doing: short bouts of activity throughout the day.

For example, walk to your classes instead of driving. When you do have to drive to campus or the mall, park at the far end of the parking lot. Take stairs instead of elevators. Is the weather bad? Go out to the mall and walk. You will be active and will get to window-shop at the same time. Remember, our ancient ancestors didn't have exercise equipment or fitness clubs, either. But the required activities of their lives—hunting food, building shelters, chopping wood—kept them alive, strong, and healthy. The need for physical activity to stay alive hasn't changed today.

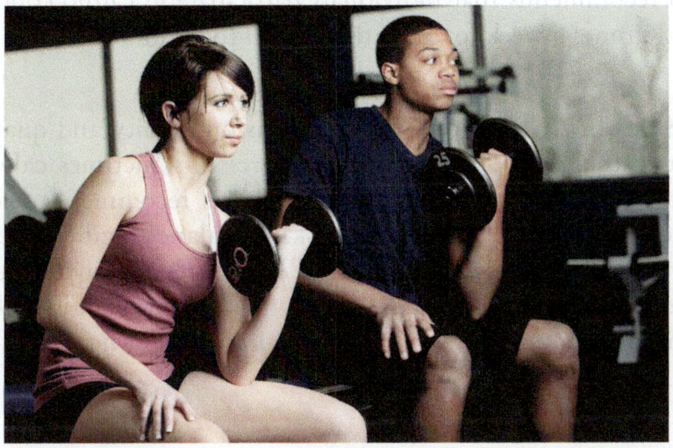

iStockphoto.com/Christopher Futcher

Strength training promotes healthy bones and muscles at any age.

TABLE 11-4 Health Consequences of Physical Inactivity

Cardiovascular Diseases	Coronary artery disease Congestive heart failure Hypertension Stroke Peripheral artery disease
Metabolic Diseases	Type 2 diabetes Obesity Low levels of HDL-cholesterol High levels of triglycerides, LDL-cholesterol, and total cholesterol Gallbladder disease
Cancers	Breast cancer Colon cancer Prostate cancer Pancreatic cancer Melanoma
Pulmonary Diseases	Asthma
Immune Dysfunction	Susceptibility to viral infections
Musculoskeletal Disorders	Osteoporosis Physical frailty
Neurological Disorders	Cognitive dysfunction

be using in your main physical activity. Waiting to stretch until after your warm-up allows blood to move into the muscles, making them easier to stretch. Doing stretches after your activity or in the cooldown phase of physical activity, gives your heart a chance to gradually slow its pace. It also allows you to lengthen any muscles that have become tight and tense from the activity. You can make greater gains in flexibility by stretching after your workout because your muscles are warm and easier to stretch.

Muscular Endurance

Muscular endurance is the ability of a muscle to keep working for long periods. Your muscular endurance influences your performance in the last set of a tennis match, your swing on the 18th hole of a golf game, or your ability to pedal during the last 10 miles of a 100-mile bike tour.

Cardiorespiratory Endurance

Another important aspect of endurance is the length of time that you can keep going with an elevated heart rate—that is, how long your heart can endure a given demand. This kind of endurance is called **cardiorespiratory endurance**. The heart is a muscle, and, like your other muscles, it can respond to applied overload and progressions of repeated demands by becoming larger and stronger.

endurance The ability to sustain an effort for a long time. One type, **muscular endurance**, is the ability of a muscle to contract repeatedly within a given time period without becoming exhausted. Another type, **cardiorespiratory endurance**, is the ability of the cardiovascular system to sustain effort over a period of time.

TABLE 11-5 Activities That Can Develop Cardiorespiratory Fitness

- Aerobic dancing
- Bench stepping
- Bicycling
- Cross-country skiing
- In-line skating
- Rope jumping
- Rowing
- Running
- Speed skating
- Stair climbing
- Swimming
- Walking or jogging

© Cengage

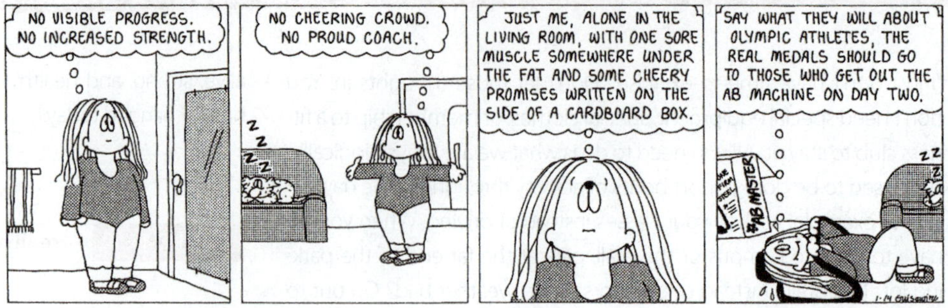

CATHY © 1997 Cathy Guisewite. Reprinted with permission of ANDREWS MCMEELSYNDICATION. All rights reserved

Activities that promote cardiorespiratory endurance are the best for making short-term fitness gains and for long-term health, as well as for weight control. The best activities to develop cardiorespiratory endurance are those that repetitively use large muscle groups—arms and legs—and that last for a continuous 20 to 60 minutes. See Table 11-5 for examples of cardiorespiratory exercise. The American College of Sports Medicine (ACSM) recommends that individuals participate in cardio conditioning activities at least five times a week for a continuous 30 to 60 minutes.[16]

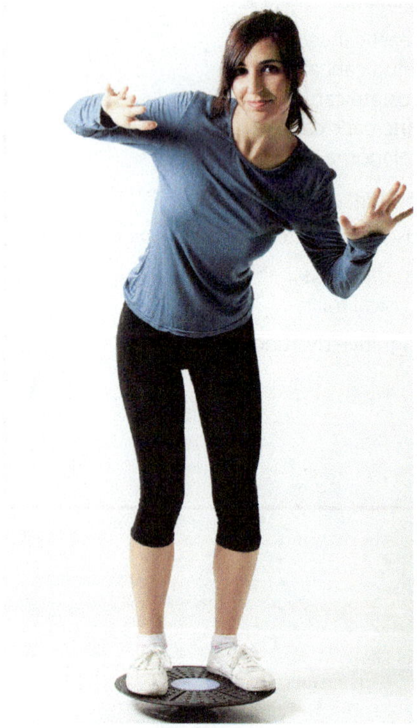

Sebastiano Volponi/Marka/Superstock

Neuromotor Exercise In ACSM's recommendations on quality and quantity of exercise they include the topic of **neuromotor exercise** (sometimes called "functional fitness training"). This form of physical activity is recommended for two or three days per week and should involve motor skills (balance, agility, coordination, and gait), proprioceptive exercise training, and multifaceted activities (tai chi and yoga) to improve physical function and prevent falls in older adults. The ACSM guidelines state that 20 to 30 minutes per day is appropriate for neuromotor exercise.[17]

11.3 Energy for Physical Activity and Sport

Your body runs on water, oxygen, and nutrients from the food you eat—primarily carbohydrates and fats. The chemical process that converts these substances to energy is called *metabolism*. Two interrelated energy-producing systems are at work in your body. One system, which depends on oxygen, is called **aerobic** metabolism. The other system functions without oxygen and is called **anaerobic** metabolism. Understanding how the two systems work is important because it explains why you would choose certain activities over others to strengthen your heart, why you eat what you do, and what factors influence your performance during sporting events.

Aerobic and Anaerobic Metabolism At rest, your muscles burn mostly fats and some carbohydrates for energy. During exercise, though, the amount and type of energy the muscles use depends on the interplay between fuel availability and oxygen availability. To an exercising muscle, oxygen is everything. With ample oxygen, muscles can extract all available energy from carbohydrates and fats by means of the energy processes of aerobic metabolism. During low- and moderately-intense activities, your lungs and circulatory system have no trouble keeping up with the muscles' need for oxygen. You breathe deeply and easily, and your heart beats steadily—the activity is aerobic. Still, the heart and lungs can supply only so much oxygen only so fast.

When the muscles' exertion becomes great enough that their energy demand outstrips the oxygen supply, they must also rely on anaerobic (without oxygen) metabolism for energy. The two types of anaerobic metabolism are the ATP-**PC (phosphocreatine)** system and glycolysis. The ATP-PC system provides immediate

neuromotor exercise Training that incorporates various motor skills, including balance, coordination, gait, agility, and proprioceptive training. The better your neuromotor conditioning, the better you will be at preventing a fall when you slip or lose your balance.

aerobic Requiring oxygen.

anaerobic Not requiring oxygen.

PC or phosphocreatine A high-energy compound stored in muscle cells; its phosphate group can be split and used to replenish ATP for short bursts of anaerobic activity.

energy from **ATP** and PC, which are high-energy compounds stored within muscle cells. This system can provide energy for very short durations, usually up to about 10 seconds. It is the main system behind actions such as a powerful golf swing, a 1-rep powerlifting movement, or a 40-yard dash. **Glycolysis**, the body's primary anaerobic energy metabolism system, is the dominant energy system in exercise lasting under 2 minutes—such as a 400-meter dash. In glycolysis, stored glucose from your cells or glycogen is broken down to produce ATP for energy. Because glycolysis can only burn glycogen for fuel, and one's glycogen stores can be almost fully depleted by an overnight fast, the volume of stored carbohydrate in the body is very important to the ability to perform physical activity. Nevertheless, these systems provide immediate energy without requiring oxygen; this is the defining characteristic of the anaerobic energy pathways. Unfortunately, however, these energy-yielding systems are extremely inefficient. The ATP-PC system only lasts for quick movements, and glycolysis can only harness 5 percent of glucose's energy-producing potential.[18]

Because the anaerobic metabolic pathway only partially burns your carbohydrates, it also litters your muscle with lactic acid—partly broken-down portions of glucose. When lactic acid builds up in the muscles, it causes burning pain and can lead to muscle exhaustion within seconds if it is not drained away. An effective strategy for dealing with lactic acid buildup is to relax the muscles at every opportunity, allowing the circulating blood to carry it away and bring in oxygen to support aerobic metabolism. Fortunately, lactic acid is not a waste product. The blood delivers it to your liver, where it is converted back into glucose.

Neither the aerobic nor the anaerobic metabolic pathway functions exclusively to supply energy to your body. The two work together, complementing and supporting each other. Keep in mind, however, that carbohydrate is absolutely essential for exercise. Without it, your muscles cannot perform. When you exercise aerobically, muscles burn fat and extract energy from carbohydrate sources more efficiently in the presence of oxygen, thereby conserving your body's limited stores of glycogen. Thus, you want to exercise at an intensity that allows your heart and lungs to keep pace aerobically with the oxygen needs of your working muscles.

Aerobic Exercise—Exercise for the Heart

To meet your body's increased oxygen needs during aerobic exercise, your heart must pump oxygen-rich blood to muscles at a faster pace than normal. This increased demand on the heart makes the heart stronger and increases its cardiorespiratory endurance. As Figure 11-4 shows, the oxygen comes from the lungs, which pass it to the blood, which carries it to the muscles. In addition, aerobic exercise improves the endurance of the lungs and the muscles along the arteries and in the walls of the digestive tract and, of course, the muscles directly involved in the activity. These all-over improvements are called **cardiorespiratory conditioning** or the **training effect**. In cardiorespiratory conditioning with progression and overload, the total blood volume increases so that the blood can carry more oxygen. The heart muscle hypertrophies and becomes stronger and larger. Therefore, because each beat of the heart pumps more blood, it needs to pump less often. The muscles that work the lungs gain strength and endurance, and breathing becomes more efficient. Circulation through the body's arteries and veins improves. Blood moves easily, and blood pressure falls. Muscles throughout the body become firmer. Figure 11-4 shows the major relationships among the heart, circulatory system, and lungs.

To make these gains in cardiorespiratory conditioning, you must elevate your heart rate (pulse). There is a range to reach with your heart rate that creates optimal cardiorespiratory conditioning, and this is called your **target heart rate**. The target heart rate range must be considerably faster than the resting rate to push (overload) the heart muscle but not so fast as to strain it. To achieve this goal, it is recommended

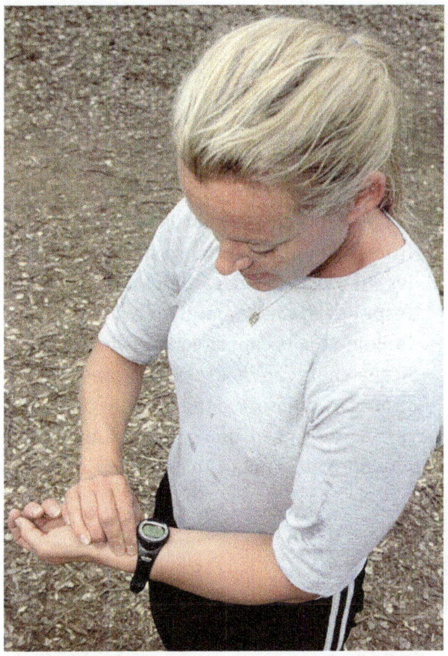
Tom Prettyman/PhotoEdit

To take your pulse and monitor your heart rate during exercise, lightly press your middle and index fingers on the radial artery (on the thumb side of the wrist), as shown here. Count your pulse for 10 seconds, and then multiply by 6 to give beats per minute.

Example: Jennifer, age 25
Maximum heart rate: 220 − age of 25 = 195
Lower limit (50%) of target heart rate range: $0.50 \times 195 = 97$ beats per minute
Upper limit (85%) of target heart rate range: $0.85 \times 195 = 166$ beats per minute
Target heart rate range: 97 to 166 beats per minute. Therefore, when Jennifer exercises aerobically, her heart should beat at least as fast as 97 beats per minute but no faster than 166 beats per minute.

ATP or adenosine triphosphate A high-energy compound present in all body tissues; when the bonds between any of the three phosphate groups in ATP are broken, energy is instantly released to power the activities of cells.

glycolysis An anaerobic energy metabolism pathway for the partial breakdown of glucose for energy. Energy released in glycolysis is used to form the high-energy compound ATP.

cardiorespiratory conditioning or training effect The effect of regular exercise on the cardiovascular system; includes improvements in heart, lung, and muscle function and increased blood volume; also called *cardiorespiratory endurance* or *cardiorespiratory training*.

target heart rate The heartbeat rate that will achieve a cardiorespiratory conditioning effect for a given person: fast enough to push the heart, but not so fast as to strain it.

FIGURE 11-4

Delivery of Oxygen by the Heart and Lungs to the Muscles

The more fit a muscle is, the more oxygen it draws from the blood. That oxygen is drawn from the lungs, so the person with more fit muscles extracts more oxygen from the inhaled air than a person with less fit muscles. The cardiovascular system responds to the demand for oxygen by building up its capacity to deliver oxygen. Researchers can measure cardiorespiratory fitness by measuring the amount of oxygen a person consumes per minute while working out, a measure called VO_2 max.

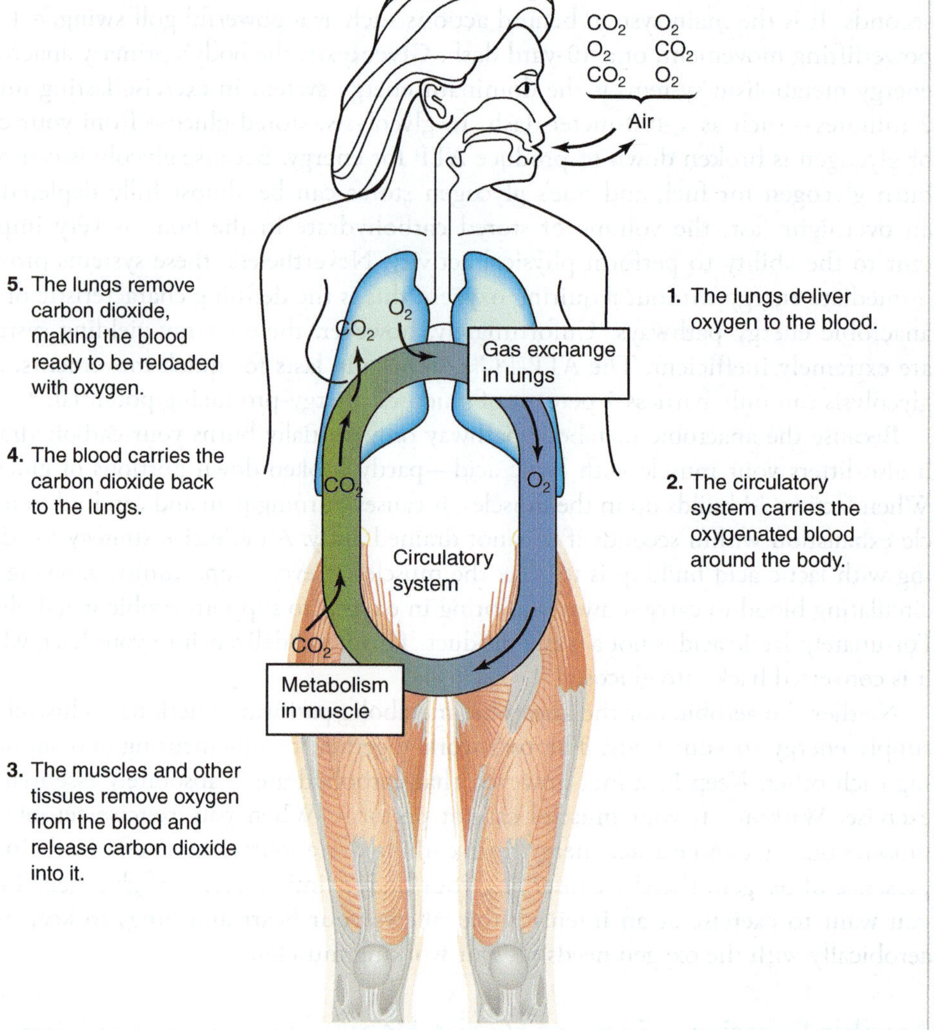

that work is done up to the point at which one can exercise aerobically for at least 20 minutes continuously or even longer. From this point the principles of overload and progression can be applied to continue improving one's cardiorespiratory fitness.

An informal pulse check can give you a starting point regarding your heart's level of conditioning. As a rule of thumb, the average resting heart rate for adults is around 70 beats per minute, but this rate can be higher or lower. Active people who have increased their cardiorespiratory fitness with exercise may have resting pulse rates of 60 or even lower.

For cardiorespiratory conditioning, your starting point for calculating your target heart rate is your age. The older you are, the lower your maximum target heart rate. As your heart becomes stronger and adapts to one load of exercise, more intense exercise will be required to reach the same target rate. For example, at first, walking at a pace of 3 miles per hour may cause you to reach your target heart rate. After 6 to 8 weeks of walking at this pace, you may notice that you no longer reach your target heart rate. That's because your heart is stronger. It now needs more of a challenge to beat faster and reach its target heart rate range. Increasing the intensity of your workout by walking faster can meet this challenge.

To calculate your target heart rate range, take the following steps:

maximum heart rate (MHR) The upper limit of what your cardiorespiratory system can handle during physical activity as represented by your measured heart rate and measured with the following equation: MHR = 220 − current age in years.

1. *Estimate your maximum heart rate (MHR).* Use the following equation: 220 − age in years. This equation provides an estimate of the absolute **maximum heart rate** (MHR) possible for a person your age. Maximum heart rate is the upper

limit of what one's cardiorespiratory system can handle during physical activity. It needs to be stressed that one should NEVER exercise at their maximum heart rate. Exercise goals should be within one's target heart rate range. MHR is determined by the following equation: 220 − current age in years = MHR.

2. *Determine your target heart rate range.* Multiply your MHR by 50 percent and 85 percent to find your lower and upper limits (see example on page 335).

When you can work out at your target heart rate for 20 to 60 minutes, you know that you have arrived at your cardiorespiratory fitness goal.

For endurance training and general aerobic conditioning, the ACSM recommends people calculate 50 to 65 percent of their maximum heart rate if they are a beginner; 60 to 75 percent for intermediate level exercisers; and 70 to 85 percent for established aerobic exercisers.[19]

11.4 Fuels for Physical Activity and Sport

To keep you moving during activity, there are two primary nutrients required to fuel your anaerobic and aerobic pathways—carbohydrates and fatty acids. Your muscles, and to some extent your liver, supply carbohydrate to your muscles from their glycogen stores or stored carbohydrate supply (see Figure 11-5). The fatty acids

FIGURE 11-5

The Use of Glycogen and Body Fat for Energy* during Physical Activity

Training can increase the amount of glycogen a muscle can conserve during exercise. The more fit a muscle is, the more fat it can burn for energy when oxygen is present—sparing the valuable glycogen.

*To perform physical activity, the body generates **ATP (adenosine triphosphate)** from the breakdown of the energy nutrients (primarily carbohydrate and fat). ATP is the "energy molecule" used by all cells of the body. ATP is composed of the compound adenosine plus three phosphate groups attached to each other by high-energy bonds. Energy is released each time a phosphate group is split off from the ATP molecule. For example, ATP converts to ADP (adenosine diphosphate) + PC (phosphocreatine) when a phosphate bond is broken to release energy.

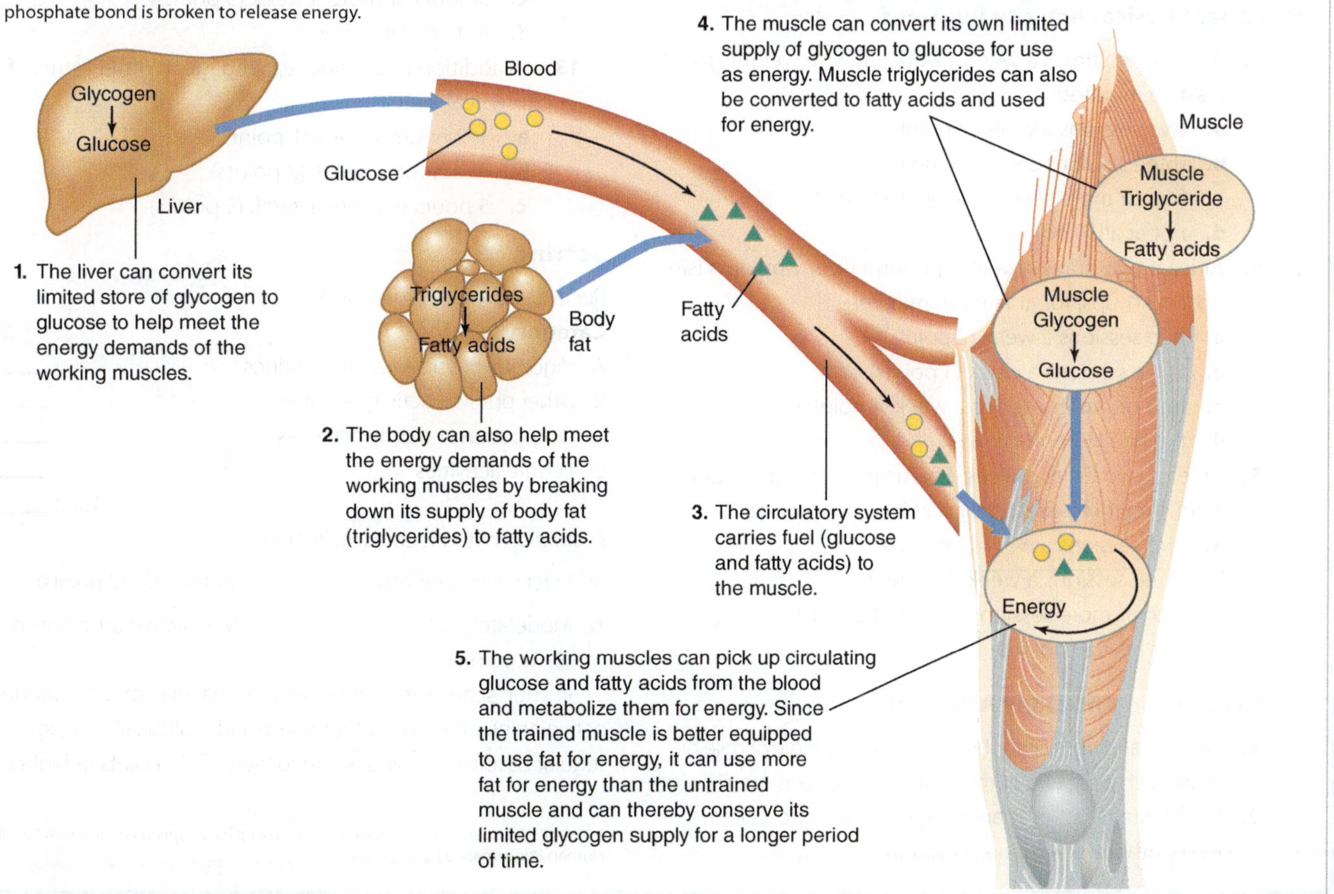

SCORE Card Physical Activity (Obj. 11.2)

How physically active are you? For each answer choice or question answered yes, give yourself the number of points indicated. Then total your points to determine your score.

A. Vigorous Physical Activity Routines

1. I participate in active recreational sports such as tennis or racquetball for an hour or more:

- **a.** about once a week (2 points)
- **b.** about twice a week (4 points)
- **c.** three times a week (6 points)
- **d.** four times a week (8 points)
- **e.** not at all (0 points)

2. I participate in vigorous fitness activities like aerobic dancing, in-line skating, jogging, or swimming (at least 20 minutes each session):

- **a.** about once a week (3 points)
- **b.** about twice a week (6 points)
- **c.** three times a week (9 points)
- **d.** four times a week (12 points)
- **e.** not at all (0 points)

B. Other Physical Activity Routines

3. At least two times a week, I work out with weights for at least 10 minutes:

- **a.** two sessions a week (2 points)
- **b.** three sessions a week (3 points)
- **c.** four or more sessions a week (4 points)
- **d.** not at all (0 points)

4. At least two times a week, I perform floor workouts (sit-ups, push-ups) for at least 10 minutes:

- **a.** two sessions a week (2 points)
- **b.** three sessions a week (3 points)
- **c.** four or more sessions a week (4 points)
- **d.** not at all (0 points)

5. At least two times a week, I participate in yoga or perform stretching exercises for at least 10 minutes:

- **a.** two sessions a week (2 points)
- **b.** three sessions a week (3 points)
- **c.** four or more sessions a week (4 points)
- **d.** not at all (0 points)

C. Occupation And Daily Activities

6. I walk to and from school, work, and shopping (1/2 mile or more each way), two or three times a week or more. (1 point)

7. I climb stairs rather than using elevators or escalators, every other day or more. (1 point)

8. My school, job, or household routine involves physical activity that fits the following description:

- **a.** Most of my day is spent in desk work or light physical activity. (0 points)
- **b.** Most of my day is spent in farm activities, moderate physical activity, brisk walking, or comparable activities. (4 points)
- **c.** My typical day includes several hours of heavy physical activity (shoveling, lifting, etc.). (2 points per day per week)

D. Leisure Activities

9. I do several hours of gardening, lawn work, or similar hobby work each week. (1 point)

10. At least once a week, I dance vigorously (folk or line dancing) for an hour or more. (1 point)

11. In season, I play 9 to 18 holes of golf at least once a week, and I do not use a power cart. (2 points)

12. I walk for physical activity or recreation:

- **a.** 1–2 hours a week (1 point)
- **b.** 3–4 hours a week (2 points)
- **c.** 5 hours or more a week (3 points)
- **d.** not at all (0 points)

13. In addition to the above, I engage in other forms of physical activity:

- **a.** 1–2 hours a week (1 point)
- **b.** 3–4 hours a week (2 points)
- **c.** 5 hours or more a week (3 points)

Scoring

Record your point scores here.

Category	**Score**
A. Vigorous physical activity routines	______
B. Other physical activity routines	______
C. Occupation and daily activities	______
D. Leisure activities	______
Total:	______

Evaluation of total score (circle one):

- Inactive (0–5 points)
- Moderately active (6–11 points)
- Active (12–20 points)
- Very active (21 points or over)

If your score categorizes you as inactive or only moderately active, think of activities that you could realistically engage in on a regular basis to raise your score to "active" (12 points or higher).

SOURCE: Adapted with permission from Russell Pate (University of South Carolina, Human Performance Laboratory).

come mostly from triglycerides stored inside the muscles but partly from triglycerides released from the body's fat stores in adipose tissue. Both glucose and fatty acids are delivered to the muscles by our blood.

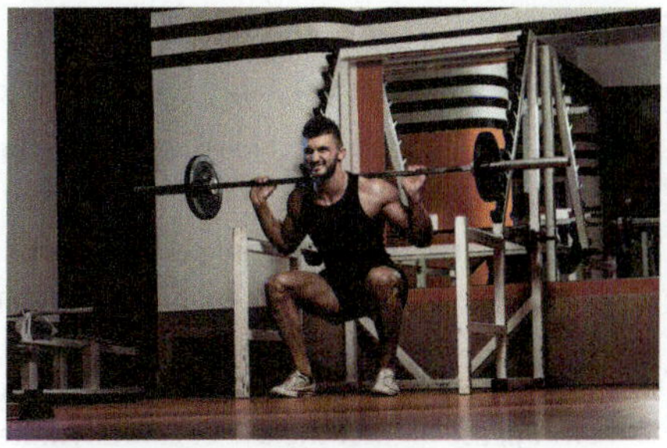

Jasminko Ibrakovic/Shutterstock.com

Anaerobic exercise. Glucose is the principal source of energy for activities of high intensity.

Burning Carbohydrates versus Fats—Intensity Makes the Difference

Glucose found in the body comes from consuming carbohydrate-rich food sources: breads, pasta, rice, legumes, fruits, vegetables, milk, and yogurt. As mentioned previously, your body stores glucose in your liver and muscles in the form of glycogen, a long chain of glucose molecules linked together.

Evaluating the intensity of the activity being completed is crucial to understanding the type of substrate or nutrient that will be preferred to fuel the activity. Low-intensity activity such as walking, which utilizes a higher percentage of aerobic energy pathways, will burn fats (triglycerides) more efficiently. Based upon the conditioning principles mentioned previously in the chapter, intensity of exercise is based upon one's level of conditioning and is very individual to each athlete. The more conditioned people are for an activity, or how "in shape" they are, then the more fats (triglycerides) they will burn as fuel. Fat burning as fuel is heightened at approximately 65 percent of one's maximum heart rate. The higher one's intensity level rises, up to approximately 85 percent maximum heart rate, there will be a significantly larger requirement for carbohydrate use as fuel.[20] So, the longer the activity lasts or the more intense it is, the more glucose people use. Recall that activities done at a higher intensity, which outstrips the ability of the heart and lungs to supply oxygen to working muscles, will rely primarily on glucose for fuel. Thus, activities such as sprinting quickly deplete the body's stores of glycogen. Other activities, such as jogging or brisk walking, in which the body can meet the muscles' oxygen demands, use glycogen more conservatively. Nonetheless, all activities at all intensity levels will require some level of glucose (glycogen) for fuel, and the body can eventually run out of it.

When a person begins exercising, for the first 20 minutes or so, about one-fifth of the body's total glycogen store is rapidly used.[21] If exercise continues beyond 20 minutes, glycogen use slows down (see Figure 11-6). To conserve the remaining glycogen supply, the body begins to rely more on fat (triglycerides) for fuel. At some point, if exercise continues long enough, glycogen will run out almost completely. People who run out of muscle glycogen during an event (e.g., before the finish line in a marathon) "hit the wall." They must slow down their pace because muscle glycogen is no longer available as fuel. Exercise can continue for a short time after that, only because the liver scrambles to produce the minimum amount of glucose needed to briefly forestall body shutdown. When blood sugars dip too low, nervous system function comes almost to a halt, making exercise difficult, if not impossible, even though there would still be plenty of fat left to burn.

Another factor that influences glycogen use during exercise is how well trained the person is. In the beginning stages of building a physical activity program, a person uses more glucose than a trained athlete. This is because their "untrained" muscles can quickly and easily extract energy from glucose. However, for muscles to easily extract energy from fat, the muscle cells must contain abundant fat-burning enzymes. With training, the muscles adapt and pack their cells with more fat-burning enzymes. Thus, trained muscles are able to use more fat and conserve their glucose.

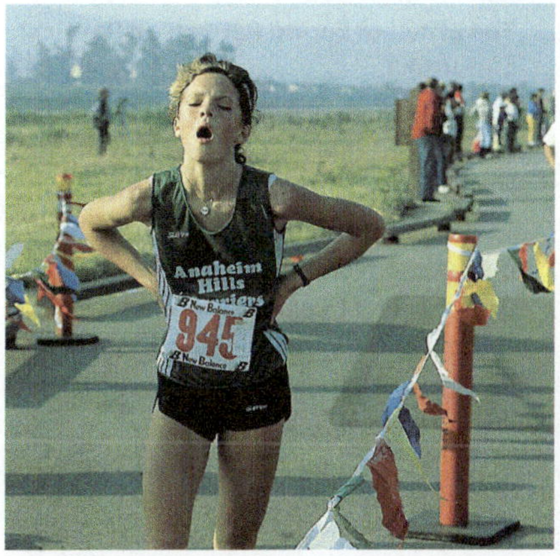

Tony Freeman/PhotoEdit

People who participate in endurance events know to build up their reserves of muscle glycogen before an event, so that they do not run out or "hit the wall" before the finish line.

The amount of glycogen that is present in the muscles before exercise also influences glycogen use. By following the diet prescription in Figure 11-7, athletes can provide their muscles with enough glycogen to support exercise. Casual exercisers engaged in low- to moderate-intensity activities (walking, bicycling, dancing), rarely deplete the glycogen in their stores. Carbohydrate loading—a practice that competitive endurance athletes use to supersaturate their muscles with optimal glycogen levels—may not be beneficial for people who exercise less than 90 minutes per workout

FIGURE 11-6

Fuel Use and Duration/Intensity of Physical Activity

For most people, fat isn't used much as a fuel for exercise until you've been working out aerobically for at least 20 minutes, and it is not used as a primary fuel until after 2 hours.

VO_2 max is the measure of the amount of oxygen a person consumes per minute while engaged in physical activity (see Figure 11-4). Low-intensity and moderate-intensity exercise would be measured up to a reading of 65 percent VO_2 max whereas high-intensity exercise would be above a 65 percent VO_2 max reading. The most optimal VO_2 max for fat burning is 65 percent VO_2 max. The more moderate the intensity of activity (brisk walking, jogging, aerobic dancing), and the longer the duration, the greater the use of fat for fuel. The higher the intensity of activity (sprinting, hurdles, rowing), the greater the use of carbohydrate for fuel. So, if fat burning is your fitness goal, it is definitely more advantageous to exercise at lower to moderate intensity levels for a longer duration. As the saying goes—the slow turtle wins the race!

If you're performing exercise for physical conditioning at high intensity levels, carbohydrates will be essential for optimal fueling as well as optimal use of fat as a fuel source. You cannot maintain optimal energy levels without carbohydrates in your diet if you plan to sustain high-intensity exercise.

SOURCE: Data from J.A. Romijn et al., Regulation of endogenous fat and carbohydrate metabolism in relation to exercise intensity, *American Journal of Physiology*, 265 (1993): E380-E391, Figure 8.

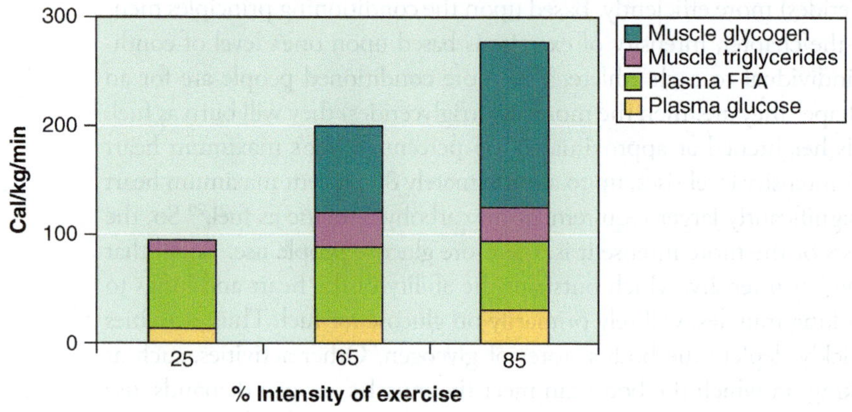

at a low intensity. However, competitive athletes exercising at a high intensity for more than 90 minutes at a time will benefit from carbohydrate loading.[22] The muscles in all athletes typically have enough glycogen to fuel 1½- to 2-hour bouts of activity.

Fat Use during Physical Activity and Sport

When you exercise, the fat your muscles burn comes from the fatty deposits all over the body, especially from those with the

FIGURE 11-7

The Effect of Eating Pattern on Physical Endurance

A high-carbohydrate eating pattern can increase an athlete's endurance. In this study, the fat and protein diet provided 94 percent of calories from fat and 6 percent from protein; the normal mixed diet provided 55 percent of calories from carbohydrate; and the high-carbohydrate diet provided 83 percent of calories from carbohydrate.

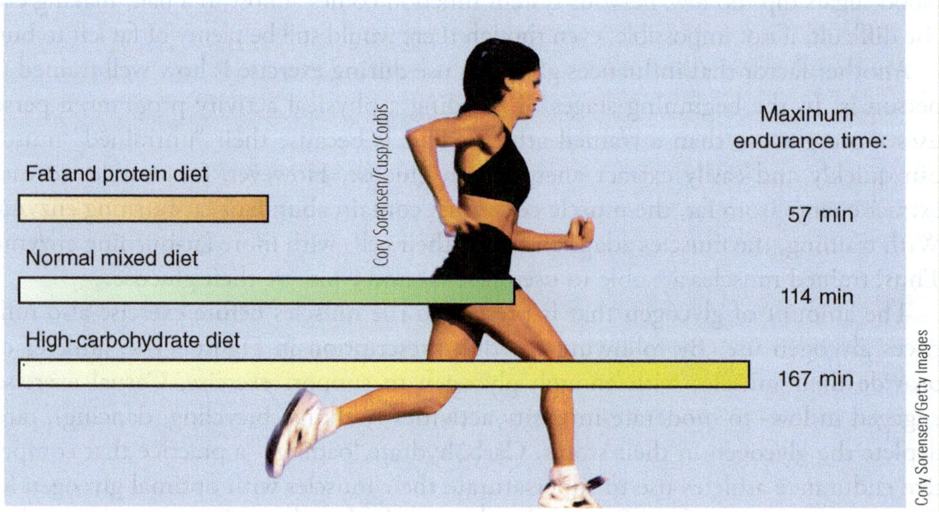

greatest amounts of fat to spare. That is why physically fit people look trim all over: They reduce their fat stores all over the body, not just those overlaying the working muscles.

A person with a desirable body weight may store 25 to 30 pounds of body fat but only about 1 pound of carbohydrate. Although your supply of fat is almost unlimited, the ability of your muscles to use fat for energy is not.

Recall that for a working muscle to burn fat, oxygen and glucose must be present. If you work out at a rate that allows your heart to supply ample oxygen to working muscles, the muscles will draw heavily on fat stores for fuel. When exercise intensity outstrips your oxygen supply, fat still contributes as much energy as ever, but glucose pitches in and is burned by the anaerobic pathway. Thus, the percentage of the total energy supplied by fat declines. Intensity of exercise can be gauged by the percentage of maximum heart rate at which you are performing the activity, but you can also use your breathing rate to signal which fuel is providing most of the energy. A rule of thumb for gauging exercise intensity for aerobic workouts is this: If you cannot talk normally, you are incurring oxygen debt and are burning more glucose than fat; if you can sing, you aren't getting a cardiovascular workout or burning much of anything (so speed up).

Improved physical conditioning also controls the amount of fat used during an exercise period. Exercise training improves the body's ability to deliver fat to working muscles, and trained muscles have an increased ability to use the fat.

Much attention has been focused on the type of fuel used for varying exercise intensities and duration. Research shows that when athletes exercise at a moderate intensity, they initially use more carbohydrate than fat for fuel.[23] Gradually, as exercise continues for more than 20 minutes, the fuel ratio shifts, and the athletes use more fat. For athletes participating in endurance sports, such as marathon runners and long-distance cyclists, who want to conserve their limited supply of carbohydrate, switching to a fat-burning energy system is crucial.

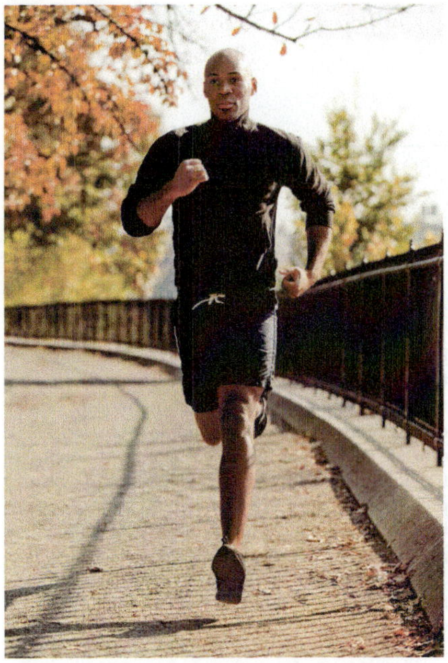

© Tyler Olson/Shutterstock.com

Aerobic activity. Fats are the main source of energy for activities of low to moderate intensity.

11.5 Protein Needs for Fitness and Sport

Fit people can have more muscle than fat; exercise involves muscles; and, muscles are primarily made of protein. It seems logical, then, that to become or stay fit, an athlete might need "more" protein. Although it's true that fat (triglycerides) and glucose are the primary fuels for working muscles, 5 to 10 percent of energy needs for athletes can come from protein sources. But, how much is "more"?

Defining the term "athlete" is very important to the topic of protein consumption for determining who needs "more." Those individuals just starting a physical conditioning regimen as well as high-level competitive and elite athletes will need additional intakes of protein in their daily dietary intakes.

An athlete's body may use slightly more protein, especially during the early stages of training. Initial increases in muscle mass, numbers of red blood cells to carry oxygen, and amounts of aerobic enzymes in muscles to use fuel efficiently may elevate an athlete's protein needs. In addition, hormonal changes during exercise can temporarily slow the amount of protein the muscles make and can encourage muscles to break down their protein stores.[24] How much protein an athlete uses for fuel during hard exercise (endurance exercise and heavy weight lifting) depends on exercise intensity and duration, the athlete's fitness level, and the glycogen stores in the athlete's muscles. Using protein for fuel is inefficient when compared to the use of carbohydrates (glycogen/glucose) or fats (triglycerides). Thus, when glycogen stores are well stocked, protein contributes as little as 5 percent of fuel needs.

During moderate- to high-intensity sport and activity, the need for protein remains mostly as structural repair to muscle tissues. Although muscle protein breakdown

TABLE 11-6 Protein Recommendations for Athletes

	Recommendations
RDA for adults	0.8 g/kg/day
Athletes	1.2–2.0 g/kg /day
Recovery phase (0 to 2 hours after exercise)	0.25–0.3 g/kg (about 15–25 g protein)

Protein intakes should be spread out consistently throughout the day. The higher levels of requirements are necessary for short periods during intensified training (endurance or strength) or when consuming decreased calories. Strenuous training sessions should always be followed with a protein intake of approximately 15 to 25 grams of high biological value (HBV) protein such as whey or other animal sources such as chicken or fish.

NOTE: To convert pounds to kilograms (kg), divide weight in pounds by 2.2.

SOURCE: Adapted from Position of the Academy of Nutrition and Dietetics, Dietitians of Canada, and the American College of Sports Medicine: Nutrition and athletic performance, *Journal of the Academy of Nutrition and Dietetics* 116 (2016): 510–511.

dominates during heavy exercise, muscle *growth* escalates after exercise. The muscles use the available amino acids to repair and build, and the net effect of these changes is muscle protein synthesis. Consistent training enhances muscle protein synthesis after exercise. Optimal nutrient timing before or during and after resistance training can minimize muscle protein breakdown and muscle damage during exercise. It can also optimize muscle growth and repair until the next training session. Current guidance recommends that athletes consume 1.2 to 2.0 grams of protein per kilogram of desirable body weight per day.[25] (see Table 11-6).

There are many misconceptions about protein. Many people believe protein is the main fuel or energy source for our working muscles while others wonder if eating even more protein by itself will help build muscles. Unfortunately, muscles don't respond to excess protein intakes by simply turning it into muscle tissue. Instead, they respond to the hormones that regulate them and to the demands put upon them by physical activity. Muscle building is a supply-and-demand process. Thus, the way to make muscle cells grow is to put a demand on them—that is, to make them work. They will respond by taking up nutrients—amino acids included—so that they can grow or hypertrophy. As mentioned earlier, athletes need a primary fuel source of carbohydrates (glucose/glycogen) to fuel their working muscles.

In summary, it is a combination of macronutrients in our diet that create optimal fueling for physical activity and sport performance. Due to the significant level of variations in duration, intensity, training level, and physical conditioning, a "one diet fits all" approach will not work well. Nutrition goals and requirements for athletes are not static and therefore should be periodized with consideration given to the needs of daily training sessions and overall individual goals. A registered dietitian who has the advanced credentials of a certified specialist in sports dietetics (CSSD) from the Academy of Nutrition and Dietetics can assist you with an individualized plan for success.

11.6 Hydration Practices for Physical Activity and Sport

The water in your blood—known as *plasma volume*, or just *plasma*—serves a function similar to the function of the water in your car's radiator. This particular function of water is critical to humans during physical activity because, as the blood continually circulates throughout your body, it picks up the tremendous amount of heat generated by your working muscles. The plasma then transports this heat to your skin, through which it is expelled from the body primarily by evaporation of sweat. You can think of sweating as your body's air-conditioning system. As sweat evaporates from your skin, it expels large amounts of heat, helping to keep your body cool. However, sweating cools your body only when the sweat evaporates from your skin. If the sweat simply rolls down your face or down your back, body heat is not released. On a humid day, for example, the air is already saturated with water, impairing the evaporation of sweat. Hot, humid days, then, are doubly dangerous because you continue to sweat and lose precious body water, but your body temperature doesn't fall. When exercising on humid days, it is extremely important to pay particular attention to your fluid needs.

Thus, as your body heats up because of the energy released during exercise, it loses water by sweating. How much sweat you lose depends on the intensity and duration of the activity. The more intense the activity, the more heat you generate and the more you sweat. If you don't replace this lost water, your plasma volume will decrease. In its attempt to maintain plasma volume, your body will pull water from your muscles and organs. As water is pulled from muscles, cramps may occur, along with premature fatigue and a noticeable decline in performance.

When plasma levels are low (meaning that blood volume is lower), your heart is forced to beat faster to supply sufficient oxygen to your muscles. Finally, because less plasma is circulating to transport the heat to your skin, the heat builds up, and your body's internal temperature continues to rise. All these changes force your body to work at a higher intensity, leading to early exhaustion. Dehydration of 1 to 2 percent of body weight begins to compromise physiologic function and negatively influence performance. Dehydration of greater than 3 percent of body weight further disturbs physiologic function and increases an athlete's risk of developing an exertional heat illness.[26]

Replenishing fluid lost during exercise is easy, yet many physically active individuals and athletes either don't drink enough or don't drink at all.[27] Ignoring body fluid needs can hinder performance and increase risk of heat-related injury.[28] Table 11-7 shows the various signs and symptoms of dehydration and heat illness.

The amount of fluid needed to prevent dehydration and **heat stroke** can be surprising. Competitive athletes can lose two or more quarts of fluid during every hour of heavy exercise, and they must rehydrate *before*, *during*, and *after* exercise to replace the lost fluid.[29] Even recreational athletes must drink some fluids while exercising. Because the thirst mechanism is strongest after a loss of 1 to 2 percent of one's body weight, it is often a concern that by the time you are thirsty, it is too late. Many athletes are dehydrated to some degree when they begin exercise. During exercise, most drink less than their sweat losses, some drink too much, and a few develop **hyponatremia**.[30] Although there are hydration guidelines for athletes to follow, hydration strategies should be tackled with a very individualized approach. Table 11-8 presents guidelines of proper hydration practices for athletes.

One of the best ways to know how much water you need to replenish fluid losses after a workout is to weigh yourself before and after: The difference in your weight from start to finish is all water. One pound equals roughly 2 cups of fluid. However, it is important to mention that any athlete should not experience weight gain during their activity or sport. Weight loss through water loss up to 2 percent of one's weight is appropriate. If you notice weight gain during physical activity, then you are drinking too much and can cause a serious condition known as hyponatremia.[31] The symptoms of hyponatremia, shown in Table 11-7, resemble dehydration to some extent.

TABLE 11-7 Signs of Dehydration, Heat Stroke, and Hyponatremia

Signs of dehydration and heat stroke include:

- Very high body temperature (104° Fahrenheit or higher)
- Hot, dry, red skin
- Sudden cessation of sweating
- Deep breathing and fast pulse
- Blurred vision
- Confusion, delirium, hallucinations
- Convulsions
- Loss of consciousness

To prevent heat stroke, drink plenty of fluid before, during, and after physical activity; avoid overexercising in hot weather; and stop exercising at any sign of heat exhaustion.

Signs of heat exhaustion include:

- Cool, clammy, pale skin
- Dizziness
- Dry mouth
- Fatigue/weakness
- Headache
- Muscle cramps
- Nausea
- Sweating
- Weak and rapid pulse

Signs of hyponatremia:

- Severe headache
- Nausea, vomiting
- Muscle cramps
- Bloating
- Confusion
- Seizure

TABLE 11-8 Schedule of Hydration for Athletes Before, During, and After Exercise

When to Drink	Amount of Fluid[a]
2–4 hours before exercise	5–10 ml/kg (~2 to 4 ml/lb) Elicits pale yellow or lighter urine color
During exercise	0.4–0.8 L/hour; must be individualized to each athlete Some weight loss is to be expected but weight loss greater than 2% of body weight can impair performance
After exercise	1.25–1.5 L per kg lost (~2 to 2 ½ cups fluid for each pound of body weight lost)
Note: Do not "gain weight" by overhydrating during exercise as this can increase your risk of hyponatremia.	

[a] See Appendix A for conversion factors (e.g., 1 oz = 30 ml; 1L = 1.06 qt; 1 kg = 2.2 lbs).

SOURCE: Adapted from Position of the Academy of Nutrition and Dietetics, Dietitians of Canada, and the American College of Sports Medicine: Nutrition and athletic performance, *Journal of the Academy of Nutrition and Dietetics* 116 (2016): 514–516.

heat stroke An acute and dangerous reaction to heat buildup in the body, requiring emergency medical attention; also called sun stroke.

hyponatremia (HIGH-poe-na-TREE-mee-ah) A decreased concentration of sodium in the blood.

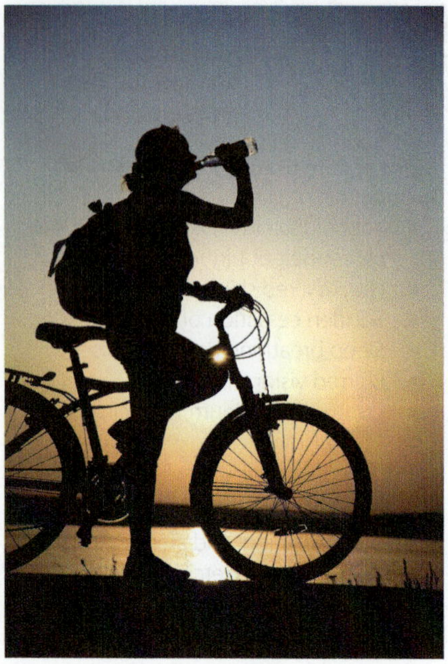

Plan to drink fluids before, during, and after exercise.

Hydration and Electrolyte Replacement Drinks For athletes and active individuals, the choice between water and a sports drink should be based on necessity. Most individuals participating in less than 60 to 90 minutes of continuous activity should only be using water as their primary means of maintaining hydration.[32] When sport or activity does surpass this time frame, sports drinks may become necessary. For those in need of replacing electrolytes as well as additional carbohydrate for muscle fuel, there is solid evidence that consuming a properly balanced sports drink during exercise will enhance energy status and help maintain plasma volume levels better than drinking water does.[33]

How the body manages water and carbohydrate use during exercise determines how well it performs. Sports drinks are designed to enhance the body's use of carbohydrate and water (see Table 11-9). The carbohydrate in a sports beverage serves three purposes during exercise: (1) It becomes an energy source for working muscles, (2) it helps maintain blood glucose at an optimum level, and (3) it helps increase the rate of water absorption from the small intestine, helping better maintain plasma volume. In addition, the drink can supply water and electrolytes lost through sweating.[34]

There are many factors to consider when choosing a sports drink. Sports drinks are very popular in the general population as well as consumed by competitive athletes especially due to their taste. Studies have shown that individuals tend to drink more overall when the beverage tastes good. However, it is more important to consider the functionality of a sports drink than drink excess carbohydrates and electrolytes when they are not needed. Excess calorie intake from caloric beverages is on the list of leading causes of obesity especially in pediatric populations.

The ideal sports drink should leave the digestive tract rapidly and enter circulation, where it is needed. Carbohydrate solutions don't all empty from the stomach at the same rate. The drink should contain at least 4 percent but no more than 8 percent carbohydrate by volume. Drinks containing more than 8 percent carbohydrate, such as sodas, fruit juice, Kool-Aid types of drinks, and some sports drinks, take longer to absorb. Some can cause cramps, nausea, bloating, and diarrhea. Drinks with less than 4 percent carbohydrate may not offer an endurance-enhancing effect. Drinks using a blend of glucose polymers—short chains of carbohydrate—and fructose leave the stomach at the same rate as water, speeding the availability of the carbohydrate and water to working muscles.[35]

Electrolytes (discussed in Chapter 8) are another important factor to consider regarding optimal hydration practices for athletic performance. The main electrolytes required by our body are sodium, potassium, chloride, calcium, magnesium, and phosphate. Sodium plays the largest role with muscle contractions and hydration status in athletes.[36] Water follows the sodium! Although sodium is important, most

TABLE 11-9 Fluid Replacement Drinks

Sports Drink	Calories/Cup	Carbohydrate Percentage	Sodium (mg)
All Sport	60	6.8	55
Gatorade Thirst Quencher	53	6.0	107
Isostar	70	6.9	114
Met-Rx	75	8.0	125
Accelerade	80	6.0	147
Powerade	53	6.2	100

people consume enough salt (sodium chloride) in their regular diet to replace the sodium they lose during exercise. This is yet another area of nutrition where defining an "athlete" is very important in determining the guidelines to follow. Sodium replacement and sports drinks will typically only be required for anyone participating in more than 60 to 90 minutes of continuous activity at a moderate- to high-intensity level.

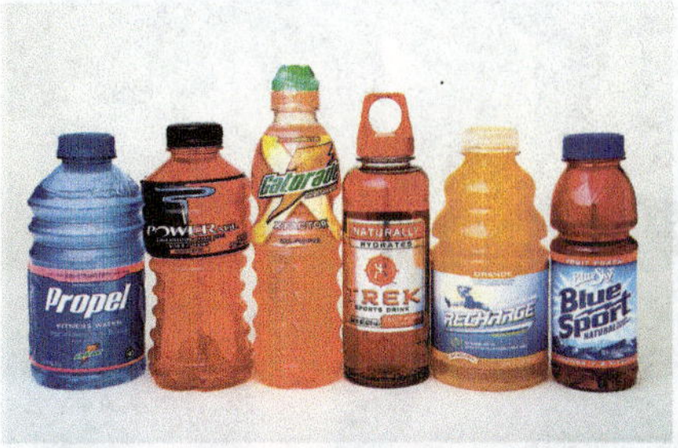

Editorial Image, LLC/Alamy Stock Photo

Sports drinks can enhance fluid and energy status during endurance events.

11.7 Vitamins and Minerals Important for Physical Activity and Sport

Muscles use the macronutrients (carbohydrates, lipids, and protein) from food and oxygen from air to make energy. How well your muscles burn these fuels also depends on your supply of vitamins and minerals. Without small amounts of these potent substances—the micronutrients—your muscles' ability to work is compromised.

Vitamins are the links and regulators of energy-producing and muscle-building pathways. Without them, your muscles' ability to convert food energy to body energy is hindered, and muscle protein formation is slowed. Table 11-10 lists a few vitamins and minerals and their exercise-supporting functions.

The B Vitamins

The B vitamins are of special interest to athletes and exercisers because they govern the energy-producing reactions of metabolism. There can be confusion due to marketing that makes it seem these vitamins have calories to "give you more energy." The B vitamin complex will only support the energy-producing pathways in our body and will not supply direct energy on their own. Needs for these vitamins increase proportionally with energy expenditure. A person who expends 4,000 calories per day needs twice as much of the B vitamins as someone who expends 2,000 calories. A well-balanced diet that meets athletes' energy needs

TABLE 11-10 Exercise-Related Functions of Vitamins and Minerals

Vitamin or Mineral	Function
Thiamin, riboflavin, pantothenic acid, niacin, magnesium	Energy-releasing reactions
Vitamin B_6, zinc	Building of muscle protein
Folate, vitamin B_{12}, copper	Building of red blood cells to carry oxygen
Biotin	Fat and glycogen synthesis
Vitamin C	Collagen formation for joint and other tissue integrity; antioxidant ability may reduce oxidative tissue damage
Vitamin E	Protect cell membranes from oxidative damage
Iron	Transport of oxygen in blood and in muscle tissue
Calcium, vitamin D, vitamin A, phosphorus	Building of bone structure; muscle contractions; nerve transmissions
Sodium, potassium, chloride	Maintenance of fluid balance; transmission of nerve impulses for muscle contraction
Chromium	Assistance in insulin's glucose-storage function
Magnesium	Cardiac and other muscle contraction

NOTE: This is just a sampling. All vitamins and minerals play indispensable roles in exercise.

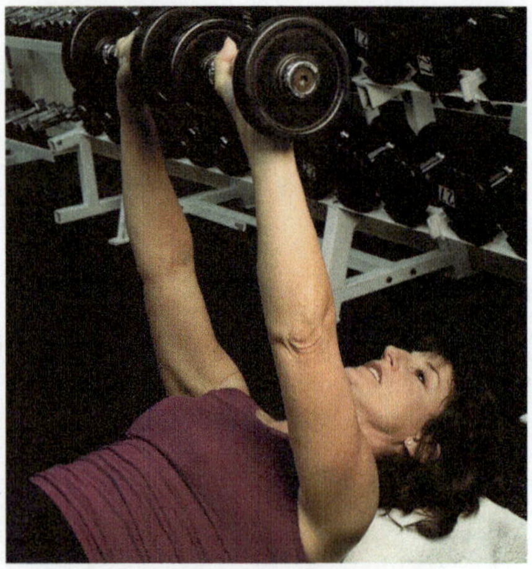

Muscles grow in response to work, not to eating protein. Several vitamins regulate the muscle-building pathways.

and that features complex carbohydrate-rich foods will ensure B vitamin intakes proportional to energy intake. If you are falling short on eating your carbohydrates from whole-grain foods and low-fat dairy products, then you are likely falling short on obtaining adequate B vitamins in your daily diet.

The Antioxidants Researchers continue to study the protective effects of antioxidants on recovery from exercise and performance. Because the body uses oxygen at a higher rate during exercise, the generation of free radicals and the potential for exercise-induced tissue damage increase in the body. Although more research is needed, preliminary studies support a role for the antioxidant nutrients, which may enhance recovery from exercise by reducing exercise-induced oxidative injury.[37] Consuming the recommended intake of fruits and vegetables each day will help athletes meet recommended intakes for the antioxidant nutrients. Some of the highest antioxidant foods and substances include citrus fruits, berries, and green tea.

An Important Mineral: Iron Iron is a core component of the body's oxygen taxi service: hemoglobin and myoglobin. A lack of oxygen compromises the muscles' ability to perform. Iron deficiency has not been reported as a problem for active individuals who exercise moderately.[38] Male and female endurance athletes, though, may be prone to developing mild iron deficiency, diagnosed by low blood ferritin levels (a measure of the body's store of iron). Menstruating female athletes are at particular risk. Growth and menstruation combined with strenuous training can take a toll on a woman's iron stores.[39]

A combination of factors increases athletes' chances of depleting their iron stores. Inadequate dietary intakes of iron-rich foods combined with iron losses due to physical activity can compromise iron status. Physical activity may cause increased iron losses in sweat, feces, and urine, plus increased destruction of red blood cells that occurs during exercise. (Chapter 8 contains numerous suggestions for obtaining sufficient iron from foods.)

Sometimes iron deficiencies can be corrected only with iron supplements. If you are concerned about your iron level, see a physician. Iron supplements should not be taken without medical supervision. High iron intakes can induce deficiencies of trace minerals, such as copper and zinc, and can produce an iron overload in some people.

Calcium and Your Bones Bones absorb great stresses during physical activity and sport, and like the muscles, they respond by growing thicker and stronger. Weight-bearing activities—running, walking, dancing, rope skipping, or activities such as strength training in which significant muscular force can be generated against the long bones of the body—encourage bone development. A bone that is not strong enough to withstand the strain of an athletic exertion can suffer from an overuse injury known as a **stress fracture**. When a person suffers from a stress fracture, there can be various causes: unbalanced muscle development, bone weakness caused by inadequate calcium intake, and reduced estrogen concentration that leads to bone mineral loss in postmenopausal women.[40]

stress fracture Bone damage or breakage caused by stress on bone surfaces during exercise.

Balanced muscle development can protect the bones from undue stresses. Each set of muscles pulling against bone should be kept in check by an equally strong set of opposing muscles. Thus, when you work one set of muscles in training, you should also work the opposing muscles. For example, if you work your back and leg muscles (by jogging or walking, for example), also work your abdominal muscles, too (do sit-ups). Bones, like muscles, take time to develop strength. To avoid the likelihood of stress fractures, give your bones and muscles plenty of time to build up to one level of performance before moving up to the next level. Maintaining adequate calcium and vitamin D intakes throughout life may be one of the primary defenses against developing weak bones. For achieving adequate calcium intakes, focus on consuming low-fat dairy products such as milk and yogurt as well as other fortified foods such as breakfast cereal. Certain vegetables also contain some calcium such as collard greens, kale, and broccoli.

Individuals who exercise strenuously yet consume inadequate calories can develop low energy availability.[41] For women, this may cause menstruation to cease, a condition called **amenorrhea**. Such women have lower than normal amounts of estrogen, a hormone essential for maintaining the integrity of the bones. With low estrogen levels, the mineral structures of the bones are rapidly dismantled, weakening the skeleton. Female athletes who have amenorrhea are at risk for stress fractures now and adult bone loss later in life.[42] The conditions of energy insufficiency, menstrual dysfunction, and decreased bone mineralization are causative to the condition known as the Female Athlete Triad.[43] Any athlete or active individual whose menstrual cycle is absent for more than 3 months should seek evaluation from a health care provider who specializes in sports medicine and receive appropriate treatment. Resumption of menses and improved bone mineral density are usually achieved through adequate caloric intakes.

Eating disorders are sometimes related to the occurrence of an energy deficit.[44] A logical part of diagnosis is to look carefully but fully at the athlete's diet. Additional medical attention and working with a registered dietitian with specific experience assisting recovery from an eating disorder would be necessary. However, overall treatment remains the same with goals of adequate caloric intakes, appropriate exercise participation, maintaining adequate body fat stores, and having an appropriate daily intake of calcium between 1,000 and 1,300 milligrams per day.[45]

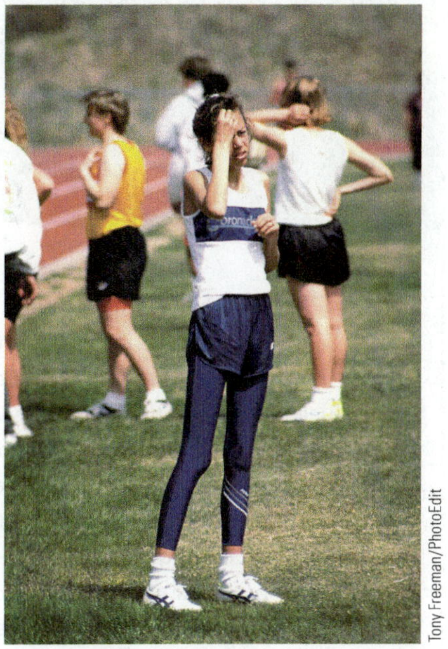

The condition characterized by the potentially fatal combination of disordered eating, amenorrhea, and low bone density is referred to as the female athlete triad.

amenorrhea Cessation of menstruation that can be associated with the occurrence of a relative energy deficit in sport.

Nutrition on the Web

http://fnic.nal.usda.gov
The Food and Nutrition Information Center (FNIC) provides credible information. Select Diet and Health, scroll down, and click on Fitness and Sports Nutrition.

www.fitness.gov
The President's Council on Fitness, Sports, and Nutrition website contains information about healthy eating, fitness, physical activity, and sports.

www.acefitness.org/acefit/nutrition
The American Council on Exercise provides fact sheets, a newsletter, recipes, and an information resource center.

www.acsm.org
Click on the tab for Public Information to access research and publications from the American College of Sports Medicine.

www.kidshealth.org
This website provides information about nutrition and fitness for parents, children, and educators. Choose the Parents Site and click on the Nutrition and Fitness link.

www.cdc.gov/nccdphp/dnpao/index.html
The Centers for Disease Control and Prevention houses the Division of Nutrition, Physical Activity, and Obesity, which provides information on various health and wellness topics.

www.scandpg.org
SCAN is the Sports, Cardiovascular and Wellness Nutrition practice group of the Academy of Nutrition and Dietetics. Click on the Nutrition Info tab for resources and help in finding an expert in your area.

EAT WELL Be Well

Defining Sports Nutrition: Active Individuals versus Competitive Athletes (Obj. 11.4)

When looking at sports nutrition principles, it is crucial to look at when they should be applied. Just because one is completing exercise does not mean that additional fueling or nutrient requirements will be necessary. As a rule of thumb, sports nutrition guidelines are applied when activity of a moderate to high intensity is completed for more than 60-90 *continuous* minutes. Thus, an individual walking for 30 minutes, 3 days per week is not going to require additional fueling or need to adhere to precise timing protocols to have enough energy for the activity. However, a basketball player practicing for 2.5 hours, 5 days each week will need to consider fueling strategies for optimal performance.

For discerning between individuals and their need for sports nutrition education, we will use the following definitions: physically active individual, recreational athlete, competitive athlete, and elite athlete (see Figure 11-8). A *physically active individual* participates in planned, consistent, and repeated movements that are done to improve and maintain a healthful level of physical fitness. Physically active individuals will not often require additional nutrients to cover the physical cost of their activity. A *recreational athlete* is physically active, however, and trains at a higher level of consistency and intensity than a physically active individual. These individuals may not compete in their chosen activity or sport, but train for fitness as well as being socially involved on a team. Many recreational athletes of all ages are individuals who no longer play on a structured, competitive team or league. Recreational athletes may have additional nutritional requirements based on activity. Typically if activity is not done for at least 60 to 90 continuous minutes, then sports nutrition principles may not apply. A *competitive athlete* participates in structured sport with a structured training and conditioning schedule for improved performance typically longer than 60 to 90 minutes per activity or sport session.

FIGURE 11-8

Everyday Athlete versus Elite Athlete

Stay fit and engage in a physical activity you love! Nutritional requirements will vary depending upon your status as an "athlete":

- Swimming in your backyard pool for up to 60 minutes each day = **physically active individual**
- Swimming on a structured club team 2 to 3 days per week for 60 minutes each practice = **recreational athlete**
- Swimming for a collegiate team 6 days per week for 120 minutes or more each practice with additional dry land conditioning 2 days each week = **competitive athlete**
- Swimming on schedule with Michael Phelps up to 8 hours each day when training for the Olympics = **elite athlete**

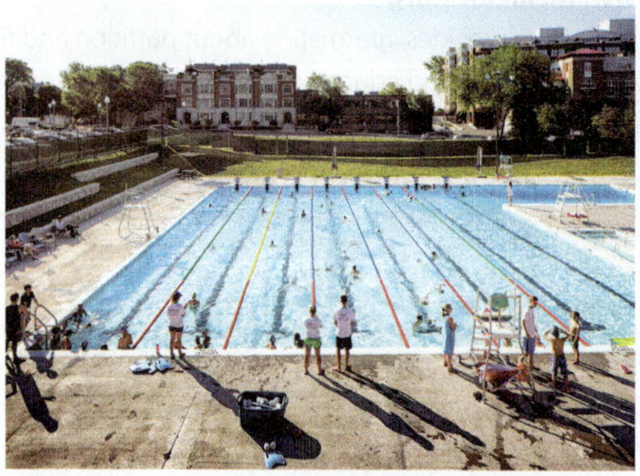

iStock.com/NicolasMcComber

Physically active individuals or recreational athletes will not typically need additional nutritional requirements.

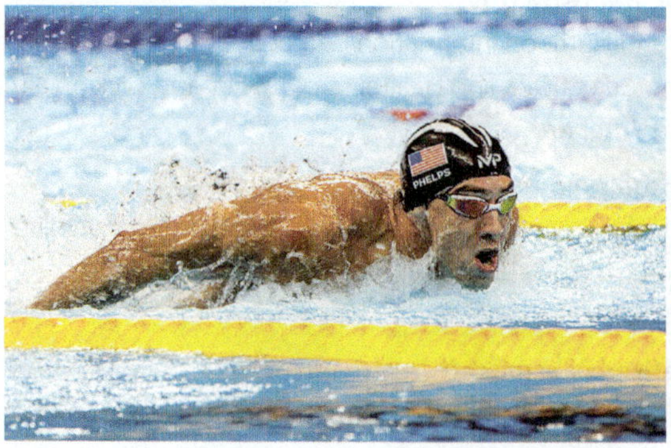

Petr Toman/Shutterstock.com

However, competitive or elite athletes will need to focus on meeting the increased nutritional demands from their activity in order to achieve optimal performance (see The Savvy Diner feature that follows).

Although fitness level is important to these athletes, the ultimate goal is improving physical strength, agility, and/or stamina for optimal sport performance. Lastly, *elite athletes* take training to the "next level." The majority of hours in their day will be dedicated to aspects of training and conditioning for competition in their sport. Both competitive and elite athletes will need to apply sports nutrition practices to their daily nutrient intakes for optimal health and performance.[46] Let's use an example of swimming (see Figure 11-8) to decipher an "athlete."

By looking at the examples in Figure 11-8, it is easy to see how one's level of fueling will need to adjust with each level of sport participation. For application of sports nutrition principles, start by deciphering your status as an "athlete." Unless you're completing more than 60 to 90 minutes of moderate- to high-intensity activity, then sports nutrition guidelines may not apply.

When looking to become a more physically active individual, it is important to make sure that your body is prepared for additional levels of physical activity. See the tips that follow for individuals just getting started.

1. Check with your physician before starting any physical activity program. Your doctor can assess your ability for a given level of activity and refer you to qualified professionals such as physical therapists, exercise physiologists, registered dietitians, and/or certified personal trainers to assist you in reaching your fitness goals.
2. Find an exercise buddy and be SMART. Although a buddy can help with some motivation and accountability, it is important to remember that no one can reach your goals for you. Use a gradual approach and set SMART goals. Small but achievable goals can be built upon for continued success! **SMART** goals are specific, measurable, action oriented, realistic, and set within a time frame as shown in Figure 11-9.[47]
3. Don't overdo it, especially in the beginning! Listen to your body and let it set the pace while still challenging yourself. "No pain, no gain" is a myth that can be dangerous.
4. Don't focus only on weight loss. Focus on your new energy level and how much better you feel!

FIGURE 11-9
SMART Goals

SMART Goal = **S**pecific + **M**easurable + **A**ction-oriented + **R**ealistic + **T**ime frame

Specific
- What exactly are you going to do?
- Describe your activity plan.

Measurable
- Define success; how will you measure progress (e.g., minutes completed)?

Action-oriented
- Define the activity you will be completing (e.g., walking, biking, or swimming).

Realistic
- Will the activity plan lead to the desired results?
- Do you have the resources needed to achieve the goal?

Time frame
- When do you begin?
- When do you re-evaluate your progress?

Example of a SMART goal:

I will walk four days per week beginning on Monday in my neighborhood from 6:30 A.M. to 7:00 A.M. The loop I will walk is 1.0 mile (be specific with location) and I will walk two loops on every Monday, Wednesday, Friday, and Saturday. I will time myself and record the time of completion in my activity log.

(Continued)

Don't jump out of bed tomorrow morning and expect to be able to run 10 miles. Set a realistic initial goal and use it as motivation to set your next goal. Experiment a little to find the time that is right for you to exercise. Many people like to exercise in the morning before their day begins. If you try that and it doesn't work, don't give up. You might have more luck with a lunchtime routine or an after-work exercise schedule.

Regardless of whether you are a physically active individual or an elite athlete, the benefits of a fitness routine can be exponential. The word *routine* almost always accompanies *exercise plan* when the goal is to enhance health through physical activity. It should be no surprise that positive health effects cannot be realized with inconsistent physical activity. Sporadic binges of activity are of little or no benefit and often do more harm than good. But how do you find time and motivation to get fit and stay fit in today's hectic lifestyle? Many people are dying to tell you how, and they claim to have just the plan for you! Look at any late-night infomercial or shopping channel to see the many exercise gurus with videos, equipment, and supplements to allegedly keep you motivated and provide great results in a short amount of time. But just as fad diets come and go, the promised success with these gizmos and gadgets is usually unsustainable, and the equipment that works for one person may not work for another.

What's usually missing from these infomercials is the whole story. Although many products and programs promise to burn loads of fat in minimal time, they typically fail to mention that success with their product *must* be combined with a total fitness routine—which would mean that their product wasn't necessary in the first place! Don't be swayed by commercials that liberally use the phrase "scientific research." If their "scientific research" is not peer reviewed and published in a respected scientific journal, the results are most likely invalid or, at the very least, biased. Those who market these programs and products are skilled with their presentations, and their real goal is to separate you from your hard-earned money. If their product sounds too good to be true, it probably is!

Instead, pay attention to the guidelines in this text, do additional reading, consult experts, talk to your physician, and let education and common sense guide your fitness routine. Even though physical activity is not always easy, it is worthwhile and can change your life! In your physical activity program, consistency is the key, and no amount of gizmos or gadgets can replace that. Get moving and stay moving throughout your life to maximize your long-term health!

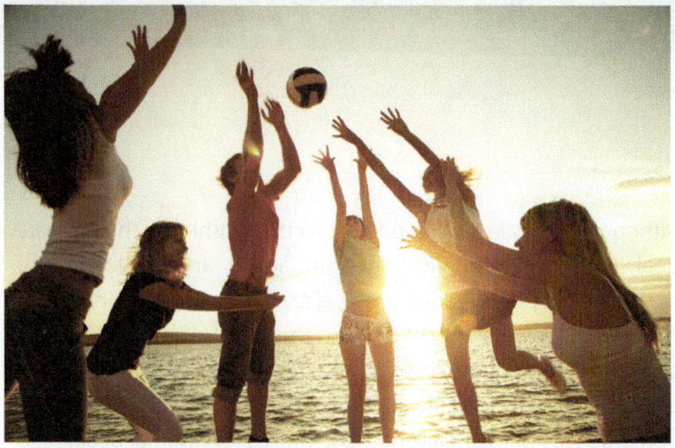

YanLev/Shutterstock.com

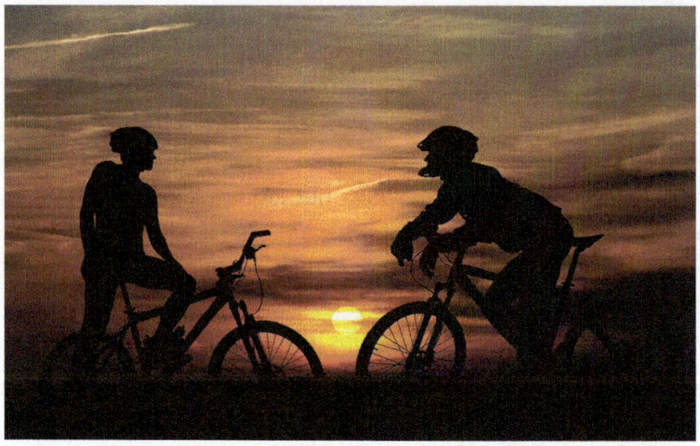

Vaclav Volrab/Shutterstock.com

Make physical activity a habit; finding an exercise buddy may help.

THE **SAVVY** Diner

Sports Nutrition Basics for Athletes (Obj. 11.7)

The best nutrition prescription for peak performance is a well-balanced diet. Although no eating plan meets every athlete's needs, certain components are common to all well-balanced diets (see Figure 11-10). An athlete's diet should account for increased energy needs, vitamin and mineral needs, the relative efficiency of various foods as fuels, and current knowledge about long-term health. However, nutritional needs can vary greatly for competitive and elite athletes depending on their training season.

One area of sports nutrition focus for athletes is periodization.[48] *Periodization* is the strategic use of specific nutritional intakes for the ultimate purpose of obtaining training adaptations that optimize sport performance. A cycle of heavy lifting will require different fueling strategies as compared to optimal fueling for high-intensity competition. Whereas individuals may require one eating plan to optimize health and performance at recreational levels, high-level athletes may need to address multiple meal plans to meet the shifting needs of their training and competition schedules.

The Athlete's Plate

Similar to the MyPlate food guide discussed in Chapter 2, athletes can visualize an Athlete's Plate to meet their sports nutrition goals. The plates in Figure 11-10 show the differences between light training, weight management, standard training, heavy training, and event day fueling strategies. Eating a balanced plate at each meal and utilizing the fueling guidelines that follow will help to optimize an athlete's performance.

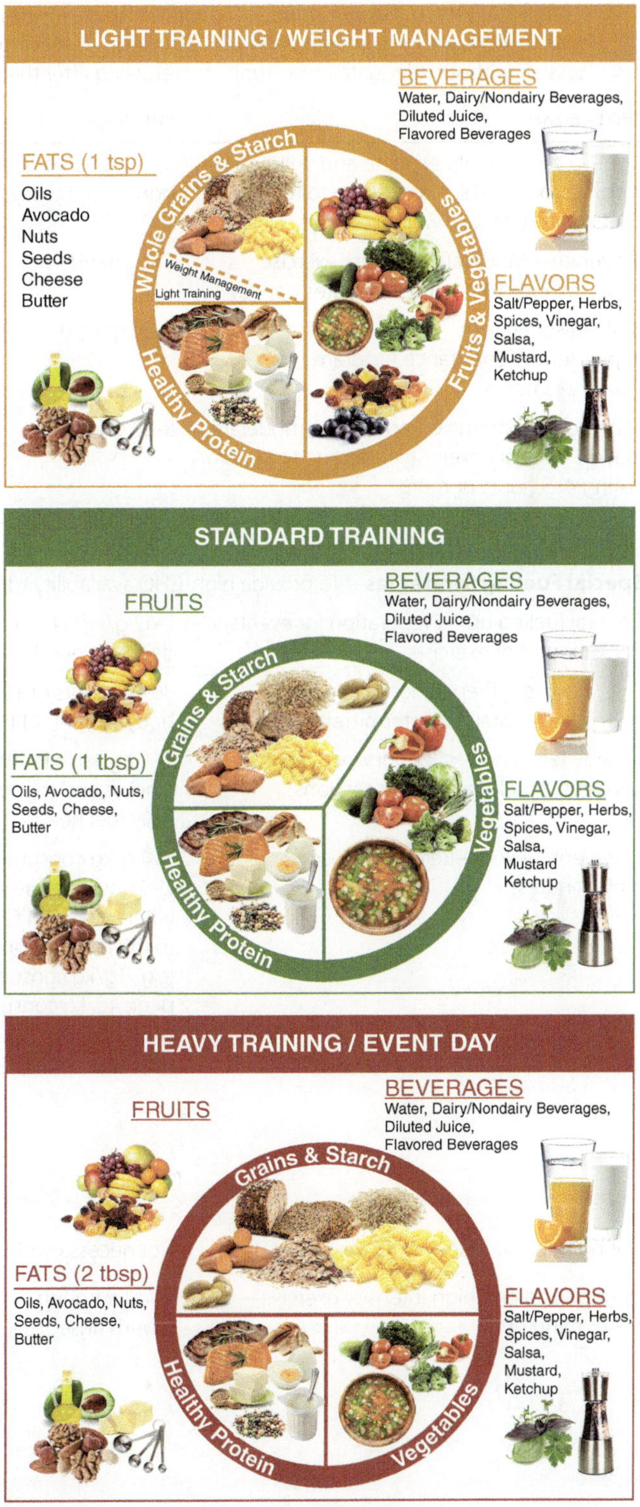

FIGURE 11-10

MyPlate for Athletes

Visually, it is easy to notice that as training intensity increases so does an athlete's carbohydrate intakes, especially from grains and starches. At levels of heavy training, grains and starches become half of an athlete's plate to meet the elevated energy demands for working muscles. Whereas for weight management or light training, fruits and vegetables comprise half of the plate. Notice that an athlete's protein intake remains consistent throughout their plates.

SOURCE: Adapted from The Athlete's Plates, a collaboration between the United States Olympic Committee Sport Dietitians and the University of Colorado Sport Nutrition Graduate Program.

Tetiana Shpuryk/Shutterstock.com; panuwat panyacharoen/Shutterstock.com; mylisa/Shutterstock.com; Somchai Som/Shutterstock.com; Olyina/Shutterstock.com; ArtCookStudio/Shutterstock.com; Nattika /Shutterstock.com; Slawomir Zelasko/Shutterstock.com; Robyn Mackenzie/Shutterstock.com; Madlen /Shutterstock.com; Elena Elisseeva/Shutterstock.com; Ewais/Shutterstock.com; Sergey Chayko/Shutterstock.com; Tiger Images/Shutterstock.com; ifong/Shutterstock.com; Fotyma/Shutterstock.com; Jag_cz /Shutterstock.com; Viktor1/Shutterstock.com; Nattika/Shutterstock.com; amenic181/Shutterstock.com; Room's Studio/Shutterstock.com; JIANG HONGYAN/Shutterstock.com; johnfoto18/Shutterstock.com; TrotzOlga/Shutterstock.com; Chamille White/Shutterstock.com; AlinaMD/Shutterstock.com; Rtstudio /Shutterstock.com; kaiskynet/Shutterstock.com; bergamont/Shutterstock.com; matkub2499/Shutterstock.com

TABLE 11-11 **Summary Guidelines for Carbohydrate Intake by Athletes[a]**

Daily needs for fuel and exercise recovery

1. The carbohydrate (CHO) recommendations presented here are intended to meet the CHO needs of the muscle and central nervous system (CNS) for different exercise situations when high-quality or high-intensity exercise is vital.
2. When exercise quality or intensity is less important, CHO choices should be based on energy goals, food preferences, or food availability.
3. If enhancing the training stimulus or adaptive response is desired, low CHO availability may be deliberately achieved by reducing total CHO intake, or by manipulating CHO intake in relation to training sessions (such as fasted state training or a second training session without adequate opportunity for refueling after the first).

CHO Demand	CHO Target	Comments on Type and Timing of CHO
Light—Low intensity exercise and skill-based activities; or for athletes needing to reduce energy intake to lose weight.	3–5 grams/kg of athlete's body weight/day	• The pattern of intake should be adjusted to meet the athlete's total energy needs, specific training needs, as well as for convenience and personal preference. • Athletes should make nutrient-dense CHO choices spread out over the course of the day to meet nutrient needs and promote fuel availability for before, during, and after exercise. • The timing and glycemic index of CHO foods and meals may be manipulated to promote high-CHO availability for a specific session. • Energy and CHO needs are often greater during training than during competition to meet heavier training demands.
Moderate—Moderate-intensity exercise program approximately 60 minutes per day	5–7 g/kg/d	
High—Moderate to high-intensity endurance program lasting 1–3 hours	6–10 g/kg/d	
Very High—Extreme commitment; moderate to high-intensity exercise endurance program lasting 4–5 hours or more	8–12 g/kg/d	
Special Fueling Strategies—To provide high-CHO availability to support optimal performance during competition or training sessions		
General fueling up—Preparation for events <90 minutes of exercise	7–12 g/kg/24 hours as for daily fuel needs	• Choose CHO-rich foods and drinks low in fiber and easily consumed to meet fuel targets and goals for gut comfort, or to achieve a lighter "racing weight."
CHO loading—Preparation for events >90 min of sustained/intermittent exercise	36–48 hours of 10–12 g/kg body weight/24 h	
Speedy refueling—<8 hours recovery between 2 fuel-demanding sessions	1–1.2 g/kg/h for first 4 hours and then resume daily fuel needs	• Eating small, regular snacks may be beneficial.
Pre-event fueling—Before exercise >60 minutes	1–4 g/kg consumed 1–4 hours before exercise, where grams of CHO are equal to the hours prior to exercise (e.g., 1g/kg consumed 1 hour prior; 4g/kg consumed 4 hours prior)	• Timing, amount, and type of CHO foods and drinks should meet personal preferences and the practical needs of event. • May need to avoid CHO items high in fat/protein/fiber to reduce gastrointestinal concerns during the event. • Choose low glycemic index foods and drinks for a more sustained source of fuel for times when CHO cannot be consumed during exercise. • If unable to eat breakfast prior to early morning exercise, consuming ~30g of easily digested CHO 5 minutes prior may improve performance.
During brief exercise—< 45 min	Not necessary or practical	
During sustained high intensity exercise—45–75 minutes	Small amounts, including mouth rinse	• Various drinks and sports products can provide easily consumed CHO options. • Frequent contact of CHO with mouth and oral cavity can stimulate brain and CNS to enhance perceptions of well-being and increase performance.

(Continued)

CHO Demand	CHO Target	Comments on Type and Timing of CHO
During endurance exercise, including "stop and start" sports—1–2.5 hours	30–60 g/hour	• CHO intake supplements the body's glycogen stores. • Access to foods and drinks vary with each sport. • Personal dietary CHO choices and liquid and solid sports products may be useful. • Athletes should develop a refueling plan that suits their goals, hydration needs, and gut comfort.
During ultra-endurance exercise—>2.5–3 hours	Up to 90 g/hour	• As above • Higher-CHO intake is associated with improved performance. • Products providing glucose:fructose mixtures achieve high rates of CHO oxidation during exercise.

[a]These general recommendations should be adapted for an individual's total energy needs, specific training needs, and personal experience with training performance.

SOURCE: Adapted from Position of the Academy of Nutrition and Dietetics, Dietitians of Canada, and the American College of Sports Medicine: Nutrition and athletic performance, *Journal of the Academy of Nutrition and Dietetics* 116 (2016): 508–509.

Optimal Fueling Pointers

- A diet rich in complex carbohydrates and low in fat provides the best balance of nutrients for health and also the best support for sport. Olympic training tables are laden with foods such as breads, whole-grain cereals, pasta, rice, potatoes, low-fat dairy options and fresh fruit. Table 11-11 outlines carbohydrate intake guidelines for athletes.
- Choose foods to provide nutrients as well as calories—extra milk for calcium and riboflavin, whole grains for B vitamins, meat or alternates for iron and other vitamins and minerals, and a wide variety of vegetables for magnesium and chromium. Maximize your nutrition by spacing your food throughout your day.
- Any meal of mixed composition, but predominantly carbohydrates, should be consumed at least 4 hours before sport participation because digestion requires routing the blood supply to the digestive tract to pick up nutrients. During training, it is optimal to have blood circulating freely to carry oxygen and fuel to the muscles. This meal should also be lower in fiber because fiber will slow digestion.
- Include plenty of fluids—two or more 8-ounce glasses of water per meal—to ensure adequate hydration. If you are adequately hydrated, urine color should be pale yellow. Check your first void in the morning to evaluate your hydration status. You can use many visual charts to assess urine color (see Figure 11-11).
- Space your protein intake throughout your entire day. Consume at least 20 grams of protein at each meal to satisfy the need for 1.0 to 2.0 g/kg/day of protein (see Table 11-6).

FIGURE 11-11

Hydration Status

SOURCE: Adapted from L. E. Armstrong, *Performing in Extreme Environments*. Champaign: Human Kinetics, 2000.

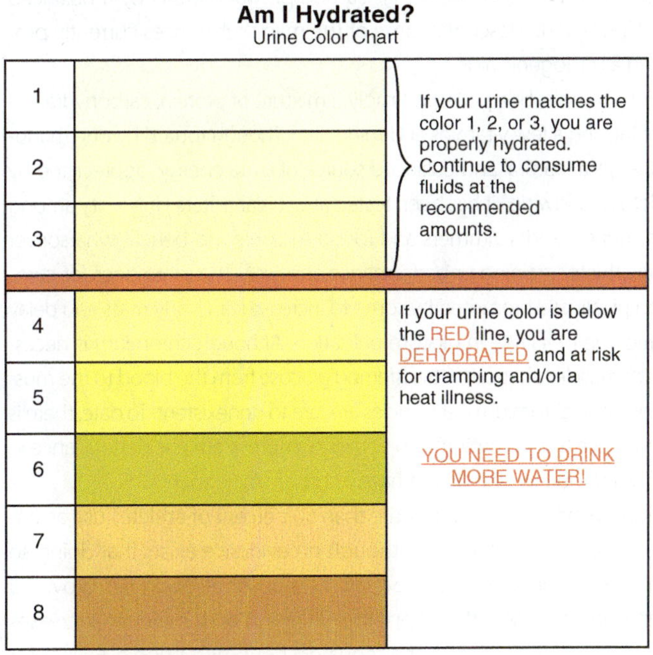

SPOTLight

11.8 Athletes and Nutritional Supplements—Help or Hype?

Competitors in the ancient Greek Olympiad reportedly used mushrooms and herbs.[49] Since then, virtually every food has at one time or another been touted as the "magic bullet" that will enhance athletic performance. Athletes have been known to swallow everything from bee pollen to brewer's yeast to kelp to wheat germ in their quest to gain the competitive edge. Although the idea of using pills and potions to achieve peak performance (to run faster or jump higher) may be seductive, scientific evidence supporting such claims is sorely lacking.[50]

Can nutritional supplements enhance the benefits I achieve from my everyday workouts?

Most so-called **ergogenic aids**—that is, any substances that increase the ability to exercise harder—are costly versions of vitamins, minerals, sugar, and other substances that can be provided easily by a balanced diet.[51] Table 11-12 describes some of the many substances currently promoted as ergogenic aids.

For example, bee pollen is simply a mixture of protein, carbohydrate, a bit of fat, and a few vitamins and minerals.[52] Though touted by one manufacturer as a "natural and balanced source of extra energy" appreciated by "athletes worldwide," it has been tested at Louisiana State University among both runners and swimmers and found to confer no benefit whatsoever on an athlete's training or performance abilities.[53] The same goes for chromium picolinate, promoted by some to increase lean body mass and delay fatigue due to its role in glucose utilization. Although chromium is necessary for muscle function by transferring glucose from the blood to the muscle cells, true chromium deficiencies are rare to nonexistent. To date, there is no evidence that chromium supplements improve athletic performance in healthy individuals who do not have a chromium deficiency.[54]

Surveys have found that more than 50 percent of athletes use a vitamin or mineral supplement, although no evidence exists that doing so improves performance.[55] More than 40 years of research has provided no strong evidence that popping vitamins and minerals increases energy or athletic prowess of adequately nourished people. Except for iron, clinical vitamin and mineral deficiencies are rare among athletes and active individuals. Because most athletes eat more food than nonathletes eat to meet their increased energy demands, the extra food intake usually provides the additional vitamins, minerals, and other beneficial substances required. That is, if they choose a well-balanced diet.

Of course, when athletes firmly hold that one or another ergogenic aid does indeed improve performance, convincing them otherwise can be extremely difficult. One reason for this is that their profound belief that a particular substance is effective can actually produce a psychological benefit. This phenomenon is known as the **placebo effect**.

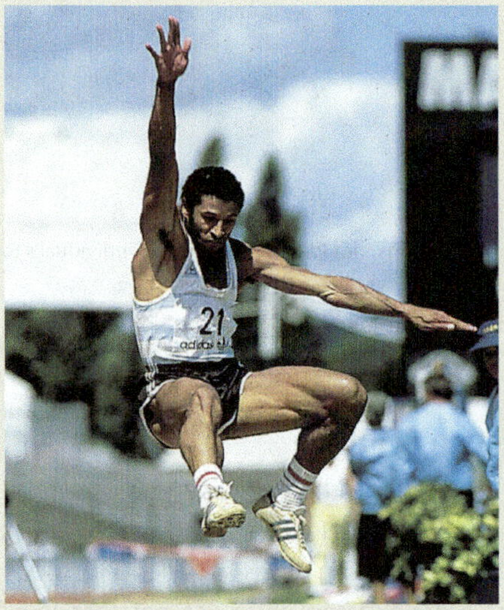

Felicia Martinez/PhotoEdit

Athletes rank as prime targets of supplement manufacturers, whose products typically promote false hopes.

I see many claims about amino acids and athletic ability. Can I improve my performance by using amino acid supplements?

Athletes rank as prime targets for amino acid supplement manufacturers. Pick up any copy of one of the bodybuilding magazines, and you'll probably see ads for supplements packed with "free-form," "predigested," and "peptide-bond" amino acids touted as optimum sources of protein for athletes. Scientific-sounding names notwithstanding, such products have never been proven to increase muscle size or enhance athletic prowess. Consider that one comparison of U.S. Marine officer candidates given protein supplements with another set of trainees who received a placebo indicated that the groups performed equally well before, during, and after the program.[56] (Refer to the Spotlight feature in Chapter 1 for some tips on how to spot fraudulent nutritional products.)

An additional important fact is that your body cannot store extra amino acids, whether they come from food you eat or from supplements. Your body converts the excess into stored calories or fat mass. Another negative impact from excess amino acid intakes is that the breakdown of amino acids generates urea, which is a waste product that must be excreted, thus increasing your body's need for water. Increased use of

TABLE 11-12 A Sampling of Popular Sports Foods, Supplements, and Ergogenic Aids[a,b,c,d]

Category	Examples	Use	Concerns
Sports food	• Sports drinks • Sports bars • Sports confectionery • Sports gels • Electrolyte supplements • Protein supplements • Liquid meal supplements	Useful when access to food or gastrointestinal (GI) concerns make consumption of regular foods and beverages difficult; may help in rapid delivery of fluid or CHO for rehydration or recovery	Cost is more than whole foods; may not be necessary; supplements are not strictly regulated and may contain banned substances
Nutritional supplement	Supplements of • Iron • Calcium • Vitamin D • Multivitamin-mineral • Omega-3 fatty acids	Prevention or treatment of nutrient deficiency	Often self-prescribed but not necessary; potential risk increased if used without supervision of physician or registered dietitian
Performance Supplement	**Ergogenic Effects**	**Physiological Effects**	**Concerns**
β-alanine[1] (a nonessential amino acid)	Improves anaerobic performance that would otherwise be limited by the effects of lactic acid buildup during high-intensity events (exercise lasting 1 to 4 minutes); may enhance training capacity by delaying neuromuscular fatigue	May increase muscle carnosine—a buffer synthesized in skeletal muscle from the amino acids histidine and ß-alanine that helps buffer acid in muscles—thereby increasing the muscle's ability to buffer the acidity produced during anaerobic high-intensity events	Some products with rapid absorption may cause a tingling or "pins and needles" sensation for ≤ 60 minutes
Branched-chain amino acids (BCAA)—a group of three essential amino acids (leucine, isoleucine, and valine)[2]	May delay fatigue and improve muscle recovery time by reducing exercise-induced muscle fatigue and delayed-onset muscle soreness by reducing protein breakdown and stimulating muscle protein synthesis in the exercised muscle	Skeletal muscle metabolizes the BCAAs for energy during prolonged endurance exercise when glycogen stores are low; BCAAs compete with tryptophan, an amino acid associated with mental fatigue	A diet adequate in protein will provide plenty of BCAAs; side effects of excessive doses (>20g/d) are not yet known
Caffeine[3] (a central nervous system stimulant)	Reduces perception of fatigue and increases the threshold for pain; may improve endurance performance, especially in those engaged in high-intensity activities lasting 1 to 20 minutes	Stimulant that increases blood levels of epinephrine with effects on many body targets, including central nervous system, resulting in a heightened sense of awareness and a decreased perception of effort; may have glycogen sparing responses with larger doses	High doses may cause dehydration, headache, muscle tremors, anxiety, increased heart rate, increased blood pressure, insomnia, gastrointestinal distress; some products do not disclose caffeine dose or may contain other stimulants

(continued)

TABLE 11-12 A Sampling of Popular Sports Foods, Supplements, and Ergogenic Aids *(continued)*

Performance Supplement	Ergogenic Effects	Physiological Effects	Concerns
Creatine[4] (The nitrogen containing substance made by the body that combines with phosphate to form the high energy compound phosphocreatine [PC])	Improves performance of repeated bouts of short-term (< 30 seconds) high-intensity exercise with short recovery periods (e.g., sprinting, weight lifting); may help to maintain force output for a longer period of time, resulting in a greater ability to complete more repetitions	May increase PC production in muscles; may enhance glycogen storage; may directly affect muscle protein synthesis	Long-term effects are unknown; may cause acute weight gain (undesirable in weight-sensitive sports); may cause GI discomfort and muscle cramping; may not contain appropriate amounts or forms of creatine; may cause kidney impairment in individuals with pre-existing kidney disease
Nitrate[5] (an ion composed of one nitrogen and three oxygen atoms)	Improves exercise tolerance; may improve performance in endurance exercise in nonelite athletes, resulting in an increased time to exhaustion	Reduces oxygen demand during moderate-intensity exercise by increasing plasma nitrite levels to increase production of nitric oxide with various vascular and metabolic effects	Concentrated sources (e.g., beetroot juice) may cause GI distress; efficacy in elite athletes is unclear; not known whether long-term intake of high-nitrate products may pose harm due to formation of potentially carcinogenic nitrosamines in the body
Sodium bicarbonate (a salt composed of sodium and bicarbonate ions)	Improves anaerobic performance that would otherwise be limited by lactic acid buildup—a major cause of muscle fatigue—during high-intensity events of 1 to 10 minutes (brief) and 30 to 60 minutes (prolonged)	May increase extracellular buffering capacity by increasing the muscle's ability to dispose of excess hydrogen ions when taken before high-intensity events	High sodium load may cause GI side effects (e.g., diarrhea); effects of repeated ingestion are unknown

[a] Although items may perform as claimed and may have evidence-based uses in sports nutrition, their inclusion in this table does not imply endorsement.
[b] Note: If you are a competing NCAA athlete, consult your certified athletic trainer or campus sports dietitian before using any dietary supplement or ergogenic aid. Over-the-counter dietary supplements may contain NCAA-banned ingredients and disqualify you from competition. For example, NCAA rules prohibit the intake of large doses of caffeine that produce urinary caffeine levels exceeding 15 μg/mL.
[c] Athletes should perform a cost-to-benefit analysis before using any sports food and/or supplement. Consider any potential benefits versus the potential risks, including the risk of contamination with unsafe or illegal chemicals.
[d] Consult with a registered dietitian who is also a Certified Specialist in Sports Dietetics (CSSD) to create a protocol for optimal sport performance.

Table Notes: 1. G. Artioli et al., The role of beta-alanine supplementation on muscle carnosine and exercise performance, *Medicine and Science in Sports and Exercise* 42 (2010): 1162–1173; 2. S. Jackman et al., Branched-chain amino acid ingestion can ameliorate soreness from eccentric exercise, *Medicine and Science in Sports and Exercise* 42 (2010): 962–970; 3. M. Tarnopolsky, Effect of caffeine on the neuromuscular system—Potential as an ergogenic aid, *Applied Physiology, Nutrition, and Metabolism* 33 (2008): 1284–1289; M. Ganio et al., Effect of caffeine on sport-specific endurance performance: A systematic review, *Journal of Strength and Conditioning Research* 23 (2009): 315–324; 4. J. Volek and E. Rawson, Scientific basis and practical aspects of creatine supplementation for athletes, *Nutrition* 20 (2004): 609–614; 5. K. Lansley et al., Acute dietary nitrate supplementation reduces the O_2 cost of walking and running: A placebo-controlled study, *Journal of Applied Physiology* 110 (2011): 591–600; K. Lansley et al., Acute dietary nitrate supplementation improves cycling time trial performance, *Medicine and Science in Sports and Exercise* 43 (2011): 1125–1131.

SOURCES: Adapted from Position of the Academy of Nutrition and Dietetics, Dietitians of Canada, and the American College of Sports Medicine: Nutrition and athletic performance, *Journal of the Academy of Nutrition and Dietetics* 116 (2016): 518–519; M. Dunford and E.Coleman, Ergogenic Aids, Dietary Supplements, and Exercise, in *Sports Nutrition A Practice Manual for Professionals*, 5th ed., edited by C. Rosenbloom and E. Coleman (Chicago: The Academy of Nutrition and Dietetics, 2012), 128–161; L. Burke and V. Deakin. Supplements and Sports Foods, in *Clinical Sports Nutrition*, 5th ed. (Australia: McGraw-Hill, 2015), 419–500.

body water for the excretion process will leave your organs and muscles vulnerable to dehydration, which impedes training and performance.

What risks are associated with protein and/or amino acid supplements?

Based on available research, the American College of Sports Medicine, the Academy of Nutrition and Dietetics, and the Dietitians of Canada, in their recent joint position stand on nutrition and athletic performance, concluded that protein requirements are higher in very active individuals.[57] Despite this need for "more," it is often found that the recommended amounts are compatible with the current recommendations (10 to 35 percent of energy from protein) and may be easily obtained from foods in the diet.[58]

However, dietary protein is composed of 20 different amino acids that, if ingested individually, have been theorized to possess ergogenic potential and have been marketed as sports supplements to physically active individuals. Indeed, amino acids are among the top five most popular sports supplements. Amino acids are theorized to enhance performance in a variety of ways, such as increasing the secretion of anabolic hormones, modifying fuel use during exercise, preventing adverse effects of overtraining, and preventing mental fatigue.[59] The use of a high-protein diet (defined as 2.8 grams protein/kg or less) by well-trained athletes does not appear to impair renal function, as indicated by various measures of renal function. Outside of predisposing conditions such as renal disease and diabetes mellitus, most amino acid supplements are safe in recommended dosages, but may interfere with protein metabolism if consumed in excess.[60] Because risks have not been proven, the use of amino acid supplements is not prohibited by the World Anti-Doping Agency (WADA).[61]

Health risks aside, it can be noted that most protein and/or amino acid supplements are very expensive. Conversely, foods are relatively much less expensive and offer more than adequate amounts of protein. For example, 6 ounces of yogurt, 4 ounces of tofu, or a 3-ounce portion of fish, all provide a generous helping of all nine essential amino acids for less than half the price of an amino acid supplement. So, are protein and amino acid supplements harmful—not likely if consumed in moderation. However, they are definitely not necessary.

What about arginine and other amino acid products advertised for weight control? Do these products work?

Arginine is an amino acid that has been promoted as "causing weight loss overnight" by stimulating secretion of a substance called *human growth hormone*, which in turn supposedly promotes weight loss. Although it's true that arginine can prompt the release of the hormone, it does so only when people take whopping doses that are unlikely to be found in supplements. Furthermore, even if a person were to take enough arginine to prompt a surge of the hormone in the body, he or she wouldn't automatically shed pounds. Human growth hormone has not been found to cause weight loss. Thus, claims that arginine "burns fat" are spurious at best. An FDA advisory panel on over-the-counter weight-loss products investigated arginine along with 11 other amino acids touted as diet aids—cysteine, histidine, isoleucine, leucine, L-lysine, methionine, phenylalanine, threonine, tryptophan, tyrosine, and valine—and found no basis for the claims about the effectiveness of any of these products in controlling weight.

What about energy drinks or pre-workout energy powders? They seem perfect for athletic performance!

Carbohydrates, vitamins, minerals, and hydration all in one bottle or in a scoop of powder . . . sounds too good to be true! Well, for athletes who use "energy drinks" or "pre-workouts" for an extra edge, it probably is.[62] For more than a decade, energy drinks have increased in variety and market share of beverage sales across the United States (see discussion in Chapter 9). More recently, pre-workout energy powders have become popular. Their formulations of high amounts of caffeine, simple carbohydrates, and mixtures of vitamins and minerals have caused many people to use them as a "pick-me-up" to get through their day. In particular, manufacturers target athletes because of their desire to gain an advantage over the competition. Unfortunately, however, energy drinks or "pre-workouts" are not properly formulated to increase athletic performance, and the "energy boost" felt from any of the many stimulants in the various drinks are not actually fueling your muscles. For energy drinks, the minimal potential benefit does not outweigh the risks.

Caffeine Thought of as the central ingredient in almost all "energy drinks," caffeine is a central nervous system stimulant that has been shown to increase athletic ability slightly when consumed in moderate amounts within 1 hour prior to activity. However, higher doses are considered "doping" in most athletic organizations, and they cause unwanted side effects such as light-headedness and twitchiness, along with laxative and diuretic effects. Even though energy drinks do not all have exactly the same ingredients, nearly all contain higher than desirable levels of caffeine.[63] When looking for real energy for activity or sport, you will need to focus on your intake of complex carbohydrates to actually fuel your muscles.

Simple Sugars Although complex carbohydrates are the preferred source of fuel for athletes, high levels of simple sugars in an energy drink pose undesirable side effects. One problem is that absorption of water is slowed considerably, putting the athlete's hydration status at risk. Furthermore, like caffeine, simple carbohydrate ingestion greater than the threshold of 8 percent carbohydrate immediately before physical exertion might cause gastrointestinal distress and create a laxative effect.

Vitamins and minerals There is little chance that an athlete who consumes a normal diet will be at risk for a vitamin or mineral deficiency. A daily multivitamin/mineral supplement and a balanced diet are far less costly than relying on fortified energy drinks as a source of nutrition.

Other ingredients It is important to realize that these drinks sometimes include additional ingredients such as amino acids and herbal supplements. Even though they may be catchy items to list on the label, few, if any, have been proven to increase athletic performance. In fact, herbal ingredients may increase the risk of serious drug–nutrient interactions if the athlete is also taking medication.[64] Additionally, because of these "other ingredients," energy drinks may contain banned substances for various sports organizations and cause an athlete to lose eligibility due to a positive drug test.

What questions should I ask if I'm considering consuming energy drinks or "pre-workouts"?[65]

- Does the drink contain herbal ingredients that will affect a medication I am currently taking?
- Does any research back up the claimed or proposed benefits of this beverage?
- Does the beverage label include a Nutrition Facts panel? If not, avoid this product!
- Can I do anything else to positively affect my energy level when training? (e.g., am I eating a balanced diet, getting enough rest and hydration, and training for the proper length of time?)
- Is the cost of the product really worth what I am getting?
- How high is the caffeine level? Will it cause me to fail a doping test?
- Are there any other ingredients that may be on a banned substance list for competitive sport?

Some athletes use caffeine or alcohol instead of popping pills to promote athletic prowess. Can these substances improve my athletic performance?

Many exercisers drink caffeine-containing beverages such as coffee, tea, or cola to enhance performance and endurance. Despite this widely held belief, there is conflicting information to call this an undisputed fact. By some accounts, caffeine apparently stimulates the release into the blood of fats that the body can then use instead of glycogen as a source of energy.[66] Thus, the glycogen is "spared," or saved, for later use, and the amount of time an exerciser can endure physical activity before running out of fuel is prolonged. However, some studies show that caffeine does not have a significant impact on fat oxidation.[67]

Information supporting the ergogenic effects of caffeine suggests that the glycogen-sparing effect is beneficial only for athletes who exercise for more than 1½ to 2 hours at a time. As noted earlier, the muscles generally store enough glycogen to fuel as much as 90 minutes of activity. Moreover, even endurance athletes consuming caffeine can experience certain downsides, such as tachycardia or rapid heart rate, increased anxiety, or "jitters" that can interfere with performance. Athletes would also do well to remember that caffeine is a drug that neither the American College of Sports Medicine nor the International Olympic Committee condones for use among athletes.

Along with caffeinated beverages, alcoholic drinks are often touted as choice fluids for athletes. Beer, for example, is sometimes portrayed as the perfect carbohydrate-containing complement to both before- and after-competition meals. Despite such images, alcoholic drinks rank as poor sources of fluid and energy, for several reasons. For one, alcohol is a diuretic that can bring about fluid loss and dehydration. More importantly, the amount of alcohol in just one beer or glass of wine depresses the nervous system, thereby slowing an athlete's reaction time and interfering with reflexes and coordination. Also, one can of beer provides only 50 carbohydrate calories. The rest of the calories come from alcohol, which must be metabolized by your liver, not your muscles. The American College of Sports Medicine and the Academy of Nutrition and Dietetics both conclude that use of alcohol hinders performance. (Chapter 9 presents a detailed explanation of how alcohol affects the body.)

The special supplements discussed here are just a sampling of the many "magic" pills and potions promoted to athletes. A nutritious diet and regular physical activity enhance performance far better than these products that are supposed to help you gain the competitive edge. If you're in doubt about a particular product you see touted as an ergogenic aid, ask yourself some of the following questions:

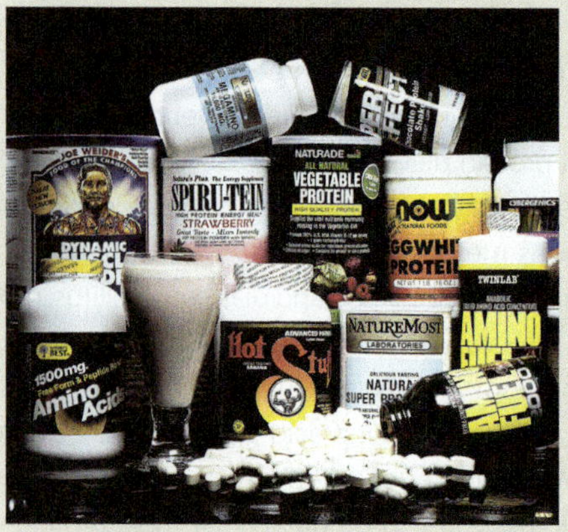

Charles D. Winters/Science Source

An endless array of ergogenic aids are marketed to athletes and other sports enthusiasts. Although big on claims, few are based on scientific evidence.

1. Is the promised action of the product based on magical thinking? ("Develop a trim body with no exercise.")
2. Does the promotion claim that "doctors agree" or "research has determined," without clarification? (Which doctors? What research?)
3. Does the promoter use scare tactics to pressure you into buying the product? ("It's the only one available without poisons.")
4. Is the product advertised as having a multitude of different beneficial effects? ("Makes bigger muscles; gives that pumped-up feeling; improves digestion, coordination, and breathing.")
5. Is the product available only from the sponsor by mail order and with payment in advance?
6. Does the promoter use many case histories or testimonials from grateful users?

Every yes answer is a point against the claimant—a warning signal that you are dealing with misinformation or **nutritional quackery**. Three or more points is a sure sign that it's too good to be true!

Miniglossary

ergogenic aids Anything that helps increase the capacity to work or exercise (*ergo* = work; *genic* = give rise to).

placebo effect An improvment in a person's sense of well-being or physical health in response to the use of a placebo (a substance having no medicinal properties or medicinal effects).

nutritional quackery A type of health fraud that promotes products and services that have questionable and unproven scientific bases.

WHAT'S ONLINE

MINDTAP From Cengage

Visit www.cengagebrain.com to access MindTap, a complete digital course that includes Diet & Wellness Plus, interactive quizzes, videos, and more.

USDA
United States Department of Agriculture

10 tips
Nutrition Education Series

physical activity at home, work, and play

10 tips to make physical activity a regular part of the day

Adding activity into your day is possible. Choose activities that you enjoy. Adults should aim for at least 2½ hours or 150 minutes of physical activity each week. Every little bit adds up, and doing something is better than doing nothing. Most important—have fun while being active!

1 take 10
Do at least 10 minutes of activity at a time to reach your weekly goal. Walk the dog for 10 minutes before and after work and add a 10-minute walk at lunchtime.

2 mix it up
Start the week with a swim at the pool, take a yoga class during a weekday lunch, lift weights in the evening, and end the week by working in the garden.

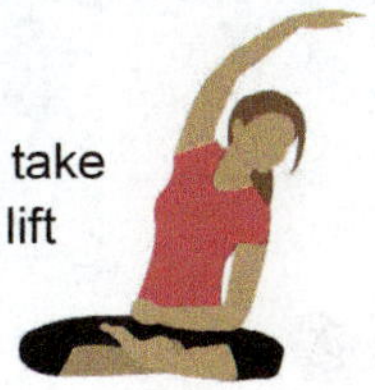

3 be ready anytime
Keep comfortable clothes and walking or running shoes in the car and at the office.

4 find ways to move
Take a brisk walk around the parking lot, jog to the bus stop, or ride your bike to the subway station. If you have an infant or toddler, take a long walk using the stroller and everyone gets some fresh air.

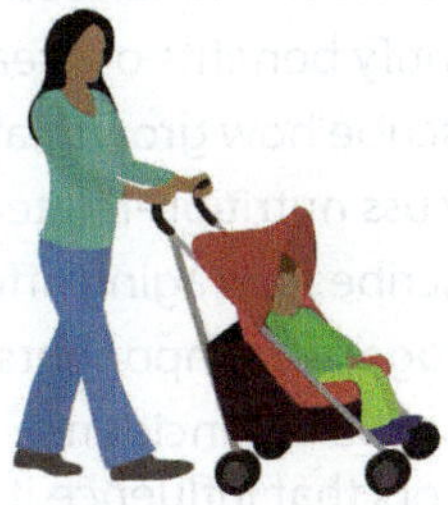

5 work out during TV time
Watch a movie while you jog on a treadmill or download a video on your phone and watch while you ride a stationary bike.

6 be an active parent
Instead of standing on the sidelines, walk up and down the soccer, football, or softball field while the kids play their game.

7 find support
Join a walking group, play wheelchair sports, practice martial arts, or sign up for an exercise class in your community. Recruit family or friends for support.

8 enjoy the great outdoors
Tumble in the leaves, build a snowman with your kids, or ski cross-country. Visit a county or national park and spend time hiking, canoeing, or boating.

9 look for wellness at work
Find a softball, basketball, or volleyball team at your job. You can also take the lead by starting a wellness or exercise group in your office.

10 the chores count, too!
Clean the house, wash the car, or mow the lawn with a push mower. Know that these activities count toward your goal of at least 150 minutes each week.

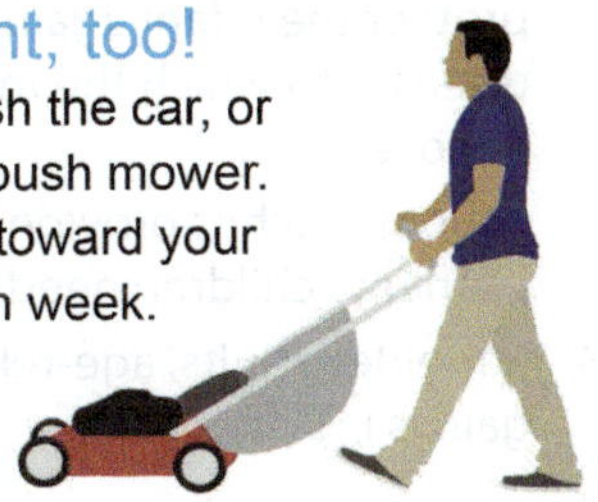

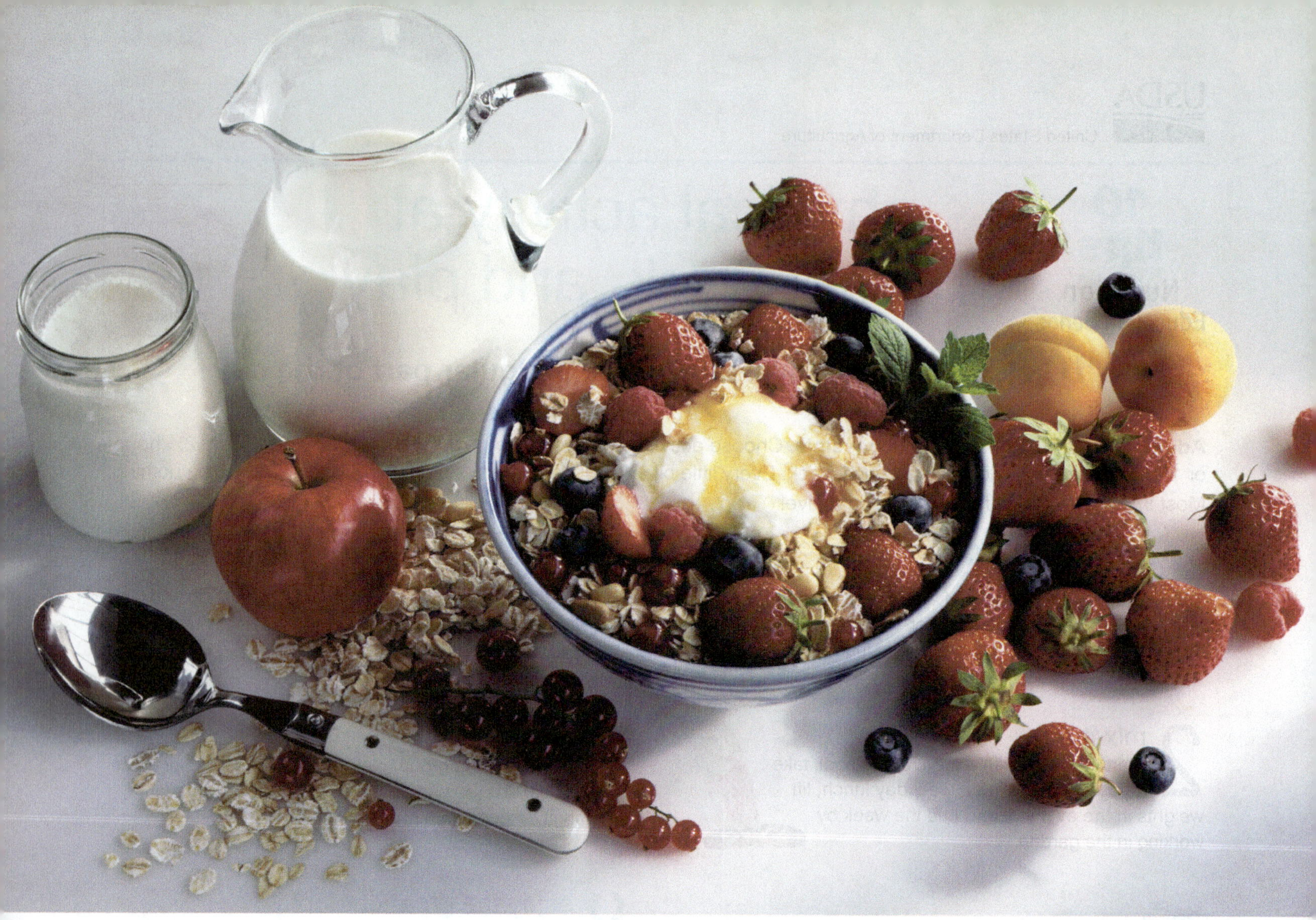
Maximilian Stock Ltd./Getty Images

AskYourself . . .

Which of the following statements about nutrition are true, and which are false? For each false statement, what is true?

1. A woman needs twice as many calories per day in late pregnancy as she did before she was pregnant.
2. Substances in a mother's milk can protect the infant against certain diseases to which the mother has been exposed.
3. School lunches provide all of the nutrients children need in a day.
4. For older adults, age-related weight gain is inevitable.

Answers found on page 362.

ChapterObjectives

12.1 Describe nutrient needs during pregnancy and lactation.
12.2 Identify benefits of breastfeeding.
12.3 Describe how growth affects the nutrient needs of children.
12.4 Discuss nutrition-related problems of adolescents.
12.5 Describe how aging affects nutrient needs.
12.6 Recognize components of successful aging.
12.7 Describe the incidence of childhood obesity and environmental factors that influence its development.

The Life Cycle: Conception through the Later Years

CHAPTER 12

Nutrition shares the responsibility for maintaining good health with other lifestyle factors. The complete prescription for good health presented in Chapter 1 reads as follows: Avoid excess alcohol, don't smoke, maintain a healthy weight, exercise regularly, get regular sleep, and eat nutritious, regular meals. A person who practices good health habits can expect to delay the onset of even minimal disability by several years, compared with a person who practices few or none of them.[1] If you believe in accepting the things you cannot control and controlling the things you can, you are in luck. Your nutritional health can be controlled, and it deserves your conscientious attention. This chapter follows people through the life cycle, considering their special nutritional needs at each stage.

How far you go in life depends on your being tender with the young, compassionate with the aged, sympathetic with the striving, and tolerant of the weak and the strong. Because someday in life you will have been all of these.

—George Washington Carver (1864–1943, American botanist)

12.1 Pregnancy: Nutrition for the Future

The only way nutrients can reach the developing fetus in the uterus is through the **placenta**, the special organ that grows inside the uterus to support the new life. If a mother's nutrient stores are inadequate early in pregnancy when the placenta is developing, the fetus will develop poorly, no matter how well the mother eats later.

Infants born to malnourished mothers are more likely to become ill, to have birth defects, and to suffer delayed mental or physical development than infants who are born to healthy women. Malnutrition in the **prenatal** and early **postnatal** periods also affects learning ability and behavior. According to the fetal origins hypothesis, if a woman's nutrient intake is undersupplied or oversupplied—particularly at critical phases of fetal development—long-term alterations in tissue function may occur. For example, if a woman's energy intake is low during the third trimester of pregnancy, pancreatic cell development may be hindered, resulting in impaired glucose tolerance

placenta (pluh-SEN-tuh) The organ inside the uterus in which the mother's and fetus's circulatory systems intertwine and in which exchange of materials between maternal and fetal blood takes place. The fetus receives nutrients and oxygen across the placenta; the mother's blood picks up carbon dioxide and other waste materials to be excreted via her lungs and kidneys.

prenatal Prior to birth.

postnatal After birth.

TABLE 12-1 Nutrition-related Risk Factors in Pregnancy

- Pregnancy at age 15 years or under
- Preconception nutrition and lifestyle behaviors (folate intake, smoking, alcohol intake)
- Diet quality
- Underweight or overweight prepregnancy
- Insufficient or excessive weight gain in pregnancy
- Physical activity practices
- Pregnant with more than one fetus
- Iron-deficiency anemia during pregnancy
- Health conditions during pregnancy (gestational diabetes, preeclampsia)
- Cigarette smoking
- Alcohol or drug dependency
- History of or current eating disorder
- Poverty (increased risk for food insecurity)
- Lack of access to health care

SOURCE: Adapted from Position Paper of the Academy of Nutrition and Dietetics: Nutrition and lifestyle for a healthy pregnancy outcome, *Journal of the Academy of Nutrition and Dietetics,* 114 (2014): 1099–1103; Practice Paper of the Academy of Nutrition and Dietetics: Nutrition and lifestyle for a healthy pregnancy outcome, Published July 1, 2014.

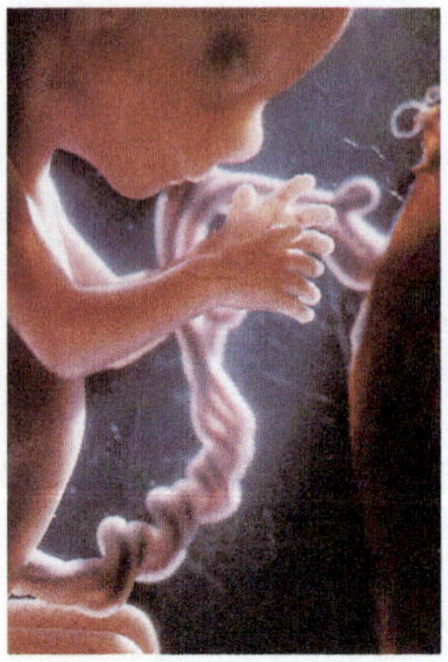

Notice the umbilical cord connecting this 16-week-old fetus with the placenta. The placenta is the organ inside the uterus in which maternal blood vessels lie side by side with fetal blood vessels entering it through the umbilical cord. This close association between the two circulatory systems permits the mother's bloodstream to deliver nutrients and oxygen to the fetus and to carry away fetal waste products.

for the baby and increased risk of developing diabetes later in life.[2] Clearly, it is critical to provide the best nutrition at the early stages of life. Ideally, a woman will start pregnancy at a healthful weight, with optimal nutrient stores, and with the established habit of eating a balanced and varied diet. The Scorecard feature in this chapter helps women evaluate their nutritional readiness for pregnancy and identify which of their eating habits might need improvement. Table 12-1 lists nutrition-related risk factors in pregnancy.

Nutritional Needs of Pregnant Women

For pregnant and lactating women, nutrient needs are higher than at any other time in their adult life, and they have greater need for certain nutrients than for others (see Figure 12-1). Notice that although their nutrient needs are much higher than usual, their energy needs are not. To support the metabolic demands of pregnancy and fetal development, the recommended average increase is only about 17 percent higher than recommended maintenance calories. An additional 340 calories during the second **trimester** and an additional 450 calories per day during the third trimester are recommended.[3]

Nearly all nutrients are recommended in increased amounts during pregnancy and lactation. The nutrient needs of pregnancy are best met by the routine intake of a variety of foods (see Figure 12-2). The nutrients deserving special attention in the diets of pregnant women include protein, folate, iron, zinc, and calcium as well as vitamins known to be toxic in excess amounts.[4]

The recommended protein intake is about an additional 25 grams per day more than nonpregnant requirements. Many women already eat enough protein to cover the increased demand of pregnancy.

A pregnant woman's recommended folate intake is 50 percent greater than the normal requirement due to her large increase in blood volume and the rapid growth of the fetus. Adequate intake of folate is important both before and during pregnancy to lower the risk of **neural tube defects**, such as spina bifida.

trimester One-third of the normal duration of pregnancy; the first trimester is 0 to 13 weeks, the second is 13 to 26 weeks, and the third trimester is 26 to 40 weeks.

neural tube defects Any of a number of birth defects in the orderly formation of the neural tube during early gestation. Both the brain and the spinal cord develop from the neural tube, and defects cause various central nervous system disorders.

ASK YOURSELF ANSWERS: **1**. False. A woman needs only 17 percent more calories per day during pregnancy than she did before. **2**. True. **3**. False. School lunch is designed to provide one-third of the nutrients schoolchildren need in a day. **4**. False. Although age-related weight gain is a fact of life for many people, it is not inevitable. Consuming nutritionally balanced meals within your calorie allowance and making physical activity part of your daily routine can help.

FIGURE 12-1

Comparison of Nutrient Needs of Nonpregnant, Pregnant, and Lactating Women*

*For actual values, turn to the DRI tables at the back of this book.

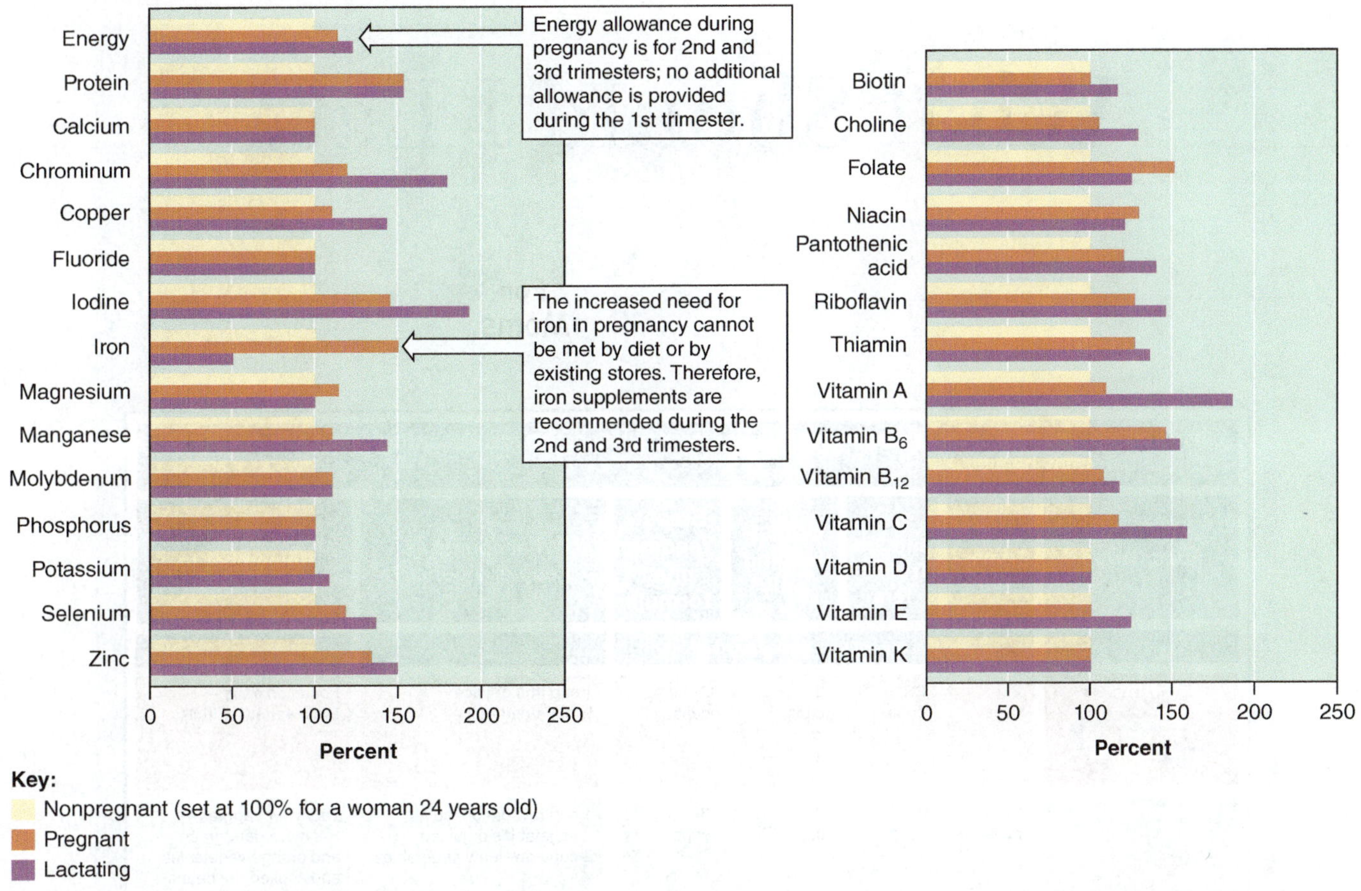

Folate is found naturally in green leafy vegetables, citrus fruits, legumes, and in refined grain products (bread, cereal, cornmeal, farina, flour, grits, pasta, and rice) fortified with folic acid. The folic acid contained in fortified foods and supplements is almost twice as well absorbed as the folate that is naturally available in foods. It is recommended that women of reproductive age get 400 to 800 micrograms of folic acid daily from fortified foods or a daily supplement in addition to consuming a diet rich in vegetables, fruits and grains.[5] Because high folate intake can mask a vitamin B_{12} deficiency, folate intake should not exceed 1 milligram per day.

The body conserves iron even more than usual during pregnancy. Menstruation ceases, and absorption of iron increases up to threefold. However, the developing fetus draws on its mother's iron stores to create stores of its own to carry it through the first 3 to 6 months of life. This drain on the mother's iron supply can precipitate a deficiency. Furthermore, she will lose blood when she gives birth.

The recommended iron intake during pregnancy is 27 milligrams per day—an increase of 50 percent above standard recommendations—to meet maternal and fetal needs. Consuming a well-balanced diet that includes good sources of iron (red meat, fish, dried fruits, legumes, whole-grain and fortified breads and cereals, and dark-green leafy vegetables) can contribute to the body's iron stores. Because iron deficiency is a common problem among nonpregnant women, many women begin pregnancy with diminished iron stores. For this reason, an iron supplement of

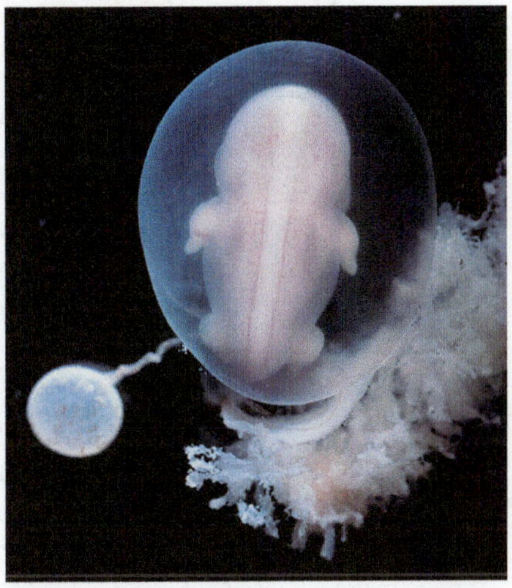

The neural tube (outlined by the delicate red arteries) has successfully closed after only 6 weeks of pregnancy.

FIGURE 12-2

A Food Guide for Pregnant and Lactating Women[a]

[a] Refer to Figure 2-9 and Figure 2-12 in Chapter 2 for a summary of foods in each group and serving sizes.
[b] Most pregnant and lactating women need a total of 2,200 to 2,900 calories per day; see "MyPlate for Moms" at www.ChooseMyPlate.gov.

What Should I Eat?

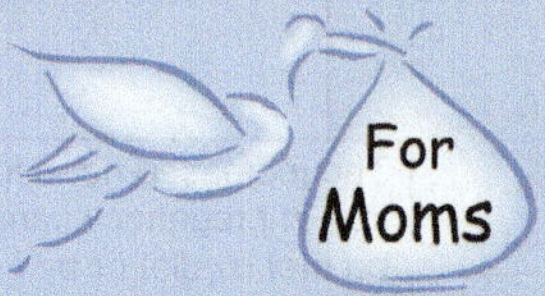

When you are pregnant or breastfeeding, you have special nutritional needs. Follow the plan below to help you and your baby stay healthy.

Food Group	1st Trimester	2nd and 3rd Trimesters	Breastfeeding only	Breastfeeding plus formula	What counts as 1 cup or 1 ounce?	Remember to...
	Eat this amount from each group daily.*					
Fruits	2 cups	2 cups	2 cups	2 cups	1 cup fruit or juice ½ cup dried fruit	*Focus on fruits*—Eat a variety of fruits.
Vegetables	2½ cups	3 cups	3 cups	3 cups	1 cup raw or cooked vegetables or juice 2 cups raw leafy vegetables	*Vary your veggies*—Eat more dark-green and orange vegetables and cooked dry beans.
Grains	6 ounces	8 ounces	8 ounces	7 ounces	1 slice bread 1 ounce ready-to-eat cereal ½ cup cooked pasta, rice, or cereal	*Make half your grains whole*—Choose whole instead of refined grains.
Protein Foods	5½ ounces	6½ ounces	6½ ounces	6 ounces	1 ounce lean meat, poultry, or fish ¼ cup cooked dry beans ½ ounce nuts or 1 egg 1 tablespoon peanut butter	*Go lean with protein*—Choose low-fat or lean meats and poultry.
Dairy	3 cups	3 cups	3 cups	3 cups	1 cup milk 8 ounces yogurt 1½ ounces cheese 2 ounces processed cheese	*Get your calcium-rich foods*—Go low-fat or fat-free when you choose milk, yogurt, and cheese.

*These amounts are for an average pregnant woman.[b] You may need more or less than the average. Check with your doctor to make sure you are gaining weight as you should.

In each food group, choose foods that are low in "extras"—solid fats and added sugars.

Pregnant women and women who may become pregnant should not drink alcohol. Any amount of alcohol during pregnancy could cause problems for your baby.

Most doctors recommend that pregnant women take a prenatal vitamin and mineral supplement every day **in addition to** eating a healthy diet. This is so you and your baby get enough folic acid, iron, and other nutrients. But don't overdo it. Taking too much can be harmful.

Get a Food Guide Plan for Moms designed just for you.
Go to www.ChooseMyPlate.gov for your Plan and more.
Click on "Pregnancy and Breastfeeding."

U.S. Department of Agriculture
Center for Nutrition Policy and Promotion
May 2008
CNPP-21
USDA

USDA is an equal opportunity provider and employer.

SCORE Card Pregnancy Readiness (Obj. 12.1)

Are you nutritionally ready for pregnancy? Score each question. A score of 21 is perfect; scores below 3 per question identify areas for improvement.

1. My body weight is desirable for my height:
   - **a.** Right on target (3 points)
   - **b.** Within 10 percent (2 points)
   - **c.** 10 to 20 percent above (1 point)
   - **d.** More than 20 percent above or 20 percent below (0 points)
2. I drink milk or use milk alternatives every day:
   - **a.** Equivalent of 3 cups or more a day (3 points)
   - **b.** About 2 cups a day (2 points)
   - **c.** About 1 cup a day (1 point)
   - **d.** No milk or milk substitutes (0 points)
3. I eat vegetables daily:
   - **a.** Five servings a day (3 points)
   - **b.** Four servings a day (2 points)
   - **c.** Three servings a day (1 point)
   - **d.** Two or fewer servings a day (0 points)
4. I eat fruits daily:
   - **a.** Four servings a day (3 points)
   - **b.** Three servings a day (2 points)
   - **c.** Two servings a day (1 point)
   - **d.** One or fewer servings a day (0 points)
5. I eat folate-rich foods, such as green leafy vegetables, orange juice, cantaloupe, legumes, and fortified grain products, daily:
   - **a.** Three to four servings, or enough to provide 400 µg daily (3 points)
   - **b.** Two to three servings, or enough to meet half the recommended intake (1 point)
   - **c.** One or fewer servings, or less than half the current recommended intake (0 points)
6. I eat iron-rich foods, such as meats, legumes, or fortified cereals, daily:
   - **a.** Two servings, or enough to meet the recommended intake (3 points)
   - **b.** One serving, or enough to meet about half the recommended intake (1 point)
   - **c.** Less than one serving, or less than half the recommended intake (0 points)
7. I am physically fit because I have a well-established habit of exercising daily, and I will be able to continue exercising during pregnancy:
   - **a.** I am as fit as I can be (3 points)
   - **b.** I am fairly fit (2 points)
   - **c.** I am not fit (0 points)

30 milligrams ferrous iron daily during the second and third trimesters is recommended. To facilitate absorption from the supplement, iron should be taken between meals with vitamin C-rich fruit juices or at bedtime.

The Dietary Reference Intakes (DRI) for calcium during pregnancy are 1,300 milligrams for teens and 1,000 milligrams for adults over 18 years of age. Intestinal absorption of calcium doubles early in pregnancy, and the mineral is stored in the mother's bones. Later, during the last trimester of pregnancy, when fetal skeletal growth is at maximum and teeth are being formed, the fetus draws approximately 300 milligrams of calcium per day from the maternal blood supply.[6] Dairy products are a recommended calcium source because they include valuable vitamin D and riboflavin as well. Other food sources include legumes, fortified juice or soy milk, and certain brands of tofu. This increased calcium intake is particularly important for women under 25 years of age because their bone mineral density is still increasing. For women who normally consume less than 600 milligrams of calcium a day, a 600-milligram supplement of calcium per day during pregnancy is recommended.

Routine use of vitamin supplements during pregnancy is not advised, and excess intakes of certain vitamins, especially in early pregnancy, can cause fetal complications.[7] Supplements should not contain more than one to two times the recommended levels. For example, taking more than three times the recommended intake of vitamin A per day early in pregnancy may cause malformations of the newborn.[8]

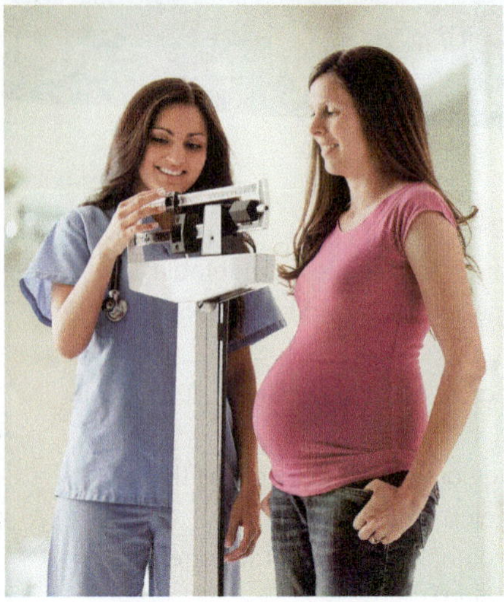
Mike Kemp/Glow Images

In some situations nutrient supplements may be recommended. For example, a multivitamin-mineral supplement (providing 100 percent of the DRI) beginning in the second trimester may be recommended for women who do not ordinarily consume an adequate diet or who are in high-risk categories (such as women carrying more than one fetus, or those who are heavy cigarette smokers or have alcohol or other drug dependencies).[9]

Because energy needs increase less than nutrient needs, pregnant women must select foods of high nutrient density. A woman who already eats well can simply increase her servings of nutritious foods to meet her increasing nutrient needs (refer to Figure 12-2).

Maternal Weight Gain

Normal weight gain and adequate nutrition support the health of the mother and the development of the fetus. The recommendations for weight gain take into account a mother's pre-pregnancy weight for height or body mass index (BMI), as shown in Table 12-2. A woman who begins pregnancy at a healthful weight should gain between 25 and 35 pounds. A woman pregnant with twins needs to gain 35 to 45 pounds. An underweight woman needs to gain between 28 and 40 pounds; an obese woman, between 11 and 20 pounds. Weight gains at the upper end of the range are recommended for pregnant teenagers because of their increased risk of low weight gains and delivery of low-birthweight infants.

Low weight gain in pregnancy is associated with increased risk of delivering an infant of **low birthweight (LBW)**. Not all small babies are unhealthy, but birthweight and length of gestation are the primary indicators of an infant's future health status. A low-birthweight baby is more likely than a normal-weight baby to experience complications during delivery and has a statistically greater chance of having physical and mental birth defects, developing diseases, and dying early in life.

Excessive weight gain during pregnancy increases the risk of complications during labor and delivery as well as of postpartum obesity.[10] Women who are obese also have an increased risk for complications during pregnancy, including hypertension and gestational diabetes.

An infant at birth weighs only about 6½ to 8 pounds, but the mother's built-up body tissues (blood, blood vessels, muscle, fat stores, and others) that provided a healthful environment for the developing fetus weigh more than 20 pounds (see Table 12-3). Weight gain should be lowest during the first trimester—1 to 4.5 pounds for the entire trimester—followed by a steady gain of about 1 pound per week (for BMI = normal) thereafter. A *sudden* large weight gain may indicate the onset of pregnancy-induced

low birthweight (LBW) A birthweight of 5½ lb (2,500 g) or less; used as a predictor of poor health in a newborn and as a probable indicator of poor nutrition status of the mother during and/or before pregnancy. Normal birthweight for a full-term baby is 6½ to 8¾ lb (about 3,000 to 4,000 g). LBW infants are either born premature or have suffered growth failure in the uterus; they may or may not be born early, but they are small.

TABLE 12-2 Recommended Weight Gain for Pregnant Women

Weight Category[a]	Recommended Gain (lb)	Weight Gain Rates 2nd & 3rd Trimester[b] lb per week (range)
Underweight	28–40	1 (1–1.3)
Normal weight	25–35	1 (0.8–1)
Overweight	15–25	0.6 (0.5–0.7)
Obese	11–20	0.5 (0.4–0.6)

[a]Underweight is defined as BMI <18.5; normal weight as BMI 18.5 to 24.9; overweight as BMI 25.0 to 29.9; and obesity as BMI ≥30.0.

[b]Assume a 1.1- to 4.4-lb weight gain in the first trimester.

SOURCE: Adapted from Weight gain during pregnancy, Committee Opinion No. 548, American College of Obstetricians and Gynecologists, *Obstetrics and Gynecology*, 121 (2013): 210–212.

hypertension (discussed later). A woman who experiences this type of weight gain should see her health care provider. It is recommended that women receive education on their individual weight gain goals and the benefits of diet and physical activity to support a healthy pregnancy outcome.[11]

Some of the weight a woman gains in pregnancy is lost at delivery. For the woman who has gained only the recommended 25 to 35 pounds, the remainder is generally lost within a few months as her blood volume returns to normal and she loses the fluids she has accumulated.

TABLE 12-3 An Example of the Pregnant Woman's Weight Gain

Development	Weight Gain (lb)
Infant at birth	7–8
Placenta	1
Increase in mother's blood volume to supply placenta	4
Increase in mother's fluid volume	4
Increase in size of mother's uterus and the muscles to support it	2
Increase in size of mother's breasts	2
Fluid to surround infant in amniotic sac	2
Mother's fat stores (varies)	3–12
Total	25–35

NOTE: The pattern of gain should be about 1 pound a month for the first 3 months and 1 pound a week thereafter. Different patterns of weight gain are suggested for women who are underweight, normal weight, or overweight.

Practices to Avoid

Optimal pregnancy outcome is influenced by maternal nutrient intake, but it can also be affected by maternal use of nonfood substances, excess caffeine, low-calorie diets, megadoses of certain vitamins, tobacco, alcohol, and illicit drugs. See Chapter 9 for recommendations regarding caffeine and pregnancy.

The term **pica** refers to the craving for and ingestion of nonfood items that have little or no nutritional value. When pica occurs during pregnancy, it typically involves the consumption of dirt, clay, laundry, or other starches, but episodes of pica have included compulsive ingestion of such things as ice, paper, and coffee grounds.[12] The medical consequences of pica can include malnutrition (as nonfood items replace nutritious foods in the diet), obesity (from overconsumption of items such as starch), poisoning (from ingestion of toxic compounds), or intestinal obstruction (due to consuming large amounts of clay or starch).

Additional practices may also have a potential impact on pregnancy outcome. For example, low-carbohydrate or low-calorie diets that cause ketosis can deprive the fetus's brain of needed glucose and cause congenital deformity. Protein deprivation can cause children's height and head circumference to diminish markedly and irreversibly.

Another harmful maternal practice is smoking, which restricts the blood supply to the growing fetus, thereby limiting the delivery of nutrients and removal of wastes. Smoking stunts fetal growth, thus increasing the risk of premature delivery, low birthweight, delayed development, and spontaneous abortions.[13] Sudden infant death syndrome (SIDS) has been linked to smoking during pregnancy and to postnatal exposure to secondhand smoke.[14]

As discussed in Chapter 9, research confirms that alcohol consumption adversely affects fetal development. Even as few as one or two drinks daily can cause **fetal alcohol syndrome (FAS)**—a range of physical and mental disabilities in the fetus. The most severe impact of maternal drinking is likely to occur in the first month, before the woman is even sure she is pregnant. Data from the Behavioral Risk Factor Surveillance System (BRFSS) shows that 10.2 percent of pregnant women reported consuming alcohol.[15] Birth defects, low birthweight, and spontaneous abortions occur more often in pregnancies of women who drink even as little as 2 ounces of alcohol daily during pregnancy. Accumulating evidence that even one drink during any trimester of pregnancy may be too much has led the American Academy of Pediatrics to take the position that women should stop drinking as soon as they *plan* to become pregnant.[16]

Drugs other than alcohol taken during pregnancy can also cause birth defects. A particularly dramatic example is the acne medication Accutane (isotretinoin), which causes major deformities during fetal development. Pregnant women should avoid taking all drugs except on the advice of their physician.

Although some pregnant women may view herbal products as safe and natural alternatives to over-the-counter medications, few studies have been done to evaluate

pica The craving of nonfood items such as clay, ice, and laundry starch; does not appear to be limited to any particular geographic area, race, sex, culture, or social status.

fetal alcohol syndrome (FAS) The cluster of symptoms seen in an infant or child whose mother consumed alcohol during pregnancy; includes retarded growth, impaired development of the central nervous system, and facial malformations. A lesser condition—called *fetal alcohol effect (FAE)*—causes learning impairment and other more subtle abnormalities in infants exposed to alcohol during pregnancy.

how they might affect pregnancy. As with prescription and nonprescription medications, pregnant women should talk to their health care provider before taking any herbal products.[17] See the Nutrition Action feature in Chapter 7 for more information on the use of herbal remedies, including safety and regulatory issues.

Pregnant women and young children are particularly vulnerable to the effects of environmental contaminants, notably lead and mercury. Increased levels of lead in pregnant women may lead to spontaneous abortion, premature delivery, or a low-birthweight infant. To reduce exposure to lead during pregnancy, the Food and Drug Administration (FDA) advises pregnant women to avoid the use of imported lead-glazed ceramic pottery, lead crystal glassware, and pewter or brass containers and exposure to lead-based paint from renovations or repairs to older homes.

High levels of mercury can impair an unborn child's developing nervous system. To reduce exposure to mercury, the FDA advises that children under 12 years of age, pregnant or lactating women, and women planning pregnancy within a year should do the following:

- Avoid eating tilefish, shark, swordfish, and king mackerel due to their high mercury content.
- Consume up to 8 to 12 ounces per week from a variety of fish and shellfish. Commonly eaten fish that are low in mercury are cod, flounder, shrimp, canned light tuna, salmon, pollock, and catfish.[18]

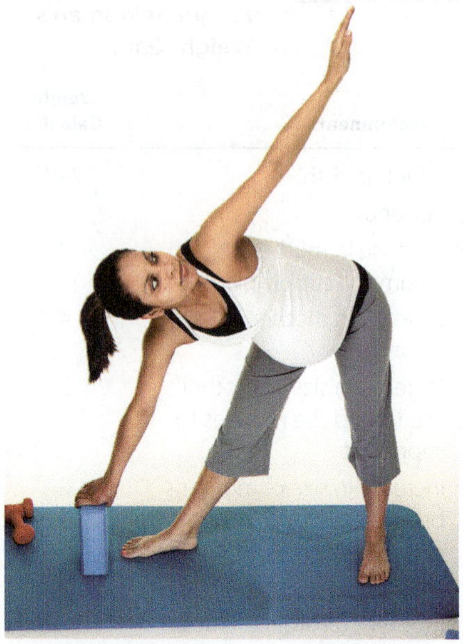

Ken Hurst/Shutterstock.com

For most women, the surest way to have a healthy baby is to follow a healthy lifestyle: Get early prenatal care, eat a well-balanced diet, exercise regularly with your doctor's permission, and avoid cigarettes, alcohol, and other drugs.

Common Nutrition-Related Problems of Pregnancy

Common physical problems in pregnancy include morning sickness and, later, constipation. The nausea of morning sickness seems unavoidable because it arises from the hormonal changes taking place early in pregnancy, but it can sometimes be alleviated. Suggested strategies to alleviate the nausea and vomiting of morning sickness include eating small, frequent meals, consuming low-fat, low-fiber foods, and avoiding any specific foods (especially highly seasoned foods or foods with strong odors) that trigger nausea or vomiting.[19] Severe vomiting, especially in early pregnancy, may be an indication of a condition known as **hyperemesis gravidarum**, which requires medical treatment and possibly hospitalization.

Later, as the hormones of pregnancy alter her muscle tone and the growing fetus crowds her intestinal organs, an expectant mother may complain of constipation. A high-fiber diet, plentiful fluid intake, and regular exercise will help relieve this condition.

Alterations in taste and smell sensitivities may result in changes of food preferences during pregnancy. Some women may experience food aversions, a sudden dislike for foods that were ordinarily consumed prior to pregnancy. Commonly reported food aversions are for meats, eggs, and bitter foods. Others may experience cravings for certain tastes, especially sweet or salty foods.[20] More serious problems requiring control during pregnancy include hypertension and diabetes.

hyperemesis gravidarum Nausea and vomiting during pregnancy that is severe enough to cause effects such as acidosis, dehydration, and weight loss.

pregnancy-induced hypertension (PIH) High blood pressure that develops during the second half of pregnancy.

preeclampsia A condition characterized by hypertension, fluid retention, and protein in the urine.

eclampsia A severe extension of preeclampsia characterized by convulsions; may lead to coma.

Hypertension in Pregnancy

Ideally, a woman with preexisting hypertension has her blood pressure under control before becoming pregnant. Otherwise, she may have an increased risk of delivering a low-birthweight baby. Some women develop a *transient hypertension of pregnancy* during the second half of their pregnancy. Usually, this is a mild form of hypertension with no adverse effects on pregnancy outcome, and the mother's blood pressure returns to normal shortly after the baby is born. Sometimes, however, high blood pressure in a pregnant woman signals the onset of **pregnancy-induced hypertension (PIH)**. **Preeclampsia** and **eclampsia** are hypertensive conditions induced by pregnancy. Preeclampsia is characterized by high blood pressure, protein in the urine, and generalized edema that may cause sudden, large weight gain from retained water. Fluid retention alone, which is quite common in pregnant women, is not sufficient for a diagnosis of preeclampsia.[21] Warning signs of preeclampsia include severe and constant headaches; sudden weight gain (1 lb/day); swelling of face, hands, and feet; dizziness; and blurred vision. Eclampsia, the most severe form of pregnancy-induced hypertension, is characterized by convulsions that may lead to coma. PIH can retard fetal growth and cause the placenta to separate from the uterus, resulting in stillbirth. Both conditions present serious health risks to mother and fetus and demand careful medical treatment.

Diabetes Infants born to women with diabetes are at greater risk for premature birth, excessively high birthweight, low blood glucose at birth, and birth injury.[22] Metabolic control of diabetes before and throughout pregnancy is critical. In some women, pregnancy can alter carbohydrate metabolism and precipitate a condition known as **gestational diabetes**. The abnormal blood glucose levels usually occur during the second half of pregnancy and return to normal after pregnancy for most women with the condition. However, some women with gestational diabetes are at increased risk of developing type 2 diabetes after pregnancy, especially if too much weight is gained. Risk factors include a previous history of gestational diabetes, obesity, and a strong family history of diabetes (see Table 12-4). Some women with gestational diabetes have the classic symptoms of diabetes—increased thirst, hunger, urination, weakness—but other women have no warning signs. For this reason, the American Diabetes Association recommends that screening for diabetes using standard diagnostic criteria be conducted in women with risk factors for diabetes at the first prenatal examination. If they are not diagnosed with diabetes at their initial prenatal visit, they should follow the recommendations for pregnant women not previously known to have diabetes and be tested at 24 to 28 weeks' gestation.[23]

Adolescent Pregnancy

The encouraging news is that the birthrate in the United States for teens aged 15 to 19 declined 9 percent between 2013 and 2014, the lowest rate ever reported. Despite these statistics, the teen birthrate in the United States is higher than that of many other industrialized countries.[24] This is a concern as the complexity of social, emotional, and physical factors makes teen pregnancy a very challenging situation for meeting nutritional needs. Medical and nutritional risks are particularly high when the teenager is within 2 years of menarche (usually 15 years of age or younger). Risks for pregnant teens include higher rates of pregnancy-induced hypertension, iron-deficiency anemia, premature birth, stillbirths, low-birthweight infants, and prolonged labor.

Pregnancy places adolescent girls, who are already at risk for nutrition problems, at even greater risk because of the increased energy and nutrient demands of pregnancy.

TABLE 12-4 Maternal Risk Factors for Gestational Diabetes

Obesity
Increased maternal age
First-degree relative with diabetes
Member of an ethnic or racial group with high prevalence of diabetes (Hispanic, Native American, South or East Asian, African American, or Pacific Islander)
Previously delivered a baby weighing >9 pounds
Personal history of gestational diabetes

SOURCE: V. A. Moyer, Screening for gestational diabetes: U.S. Preventive Services Task Force Recommendation Statement, *Annals of Internal Medicine* 160 (2014): 414–420.

gestational diabetes The appearance of abnormal glucose tolerance during pregnancy.

To support the needs of both mother and infant, adolescents are encouraged to strive for pregnancy weight gains at the upper end of the ranges recommended for pregnant women (refer to Table 12-2). Those who gain between 30 and 35 pounds during pregnancy have lower risks of delivering low-birthweight infants.[25] Nutrition education and access to healthy foods can substantially improve the course and outcome of adolescent pregnancy.[26] A model program for providing nutritional help to teenage mothers is the Women, Infants, and Children (WIC) program, a federally funded program that provides nutrition education and low-cost, nutritious foods to low-income pregnant women, mothers, and their children.

Nutrition of the Breastfeeding Mother Adequate nutrition for the mother makes a highly significant contribution to successful lactation. A nursing mother produces 30 ounces of milk a day, on the average, with wide variations possible. Current recommendations suggest that 400 of the calories needed to support this milk production come from added food and that the rest come from the stores of fat the mother's body has accumulated during pregnancy for this purpose. (Figure 12-2 shows a food pattern that will meet the lactating woman's nutrient needs.)

The period of lactation is the natural time for a woman to lose the extra body fat she has accumulated during pregnancy. Once lactation is established, if her food choices are judicious, a nursing mother can tolerate a calorie deficit and a gradual loss of weight (1 pound per week) without any effect on her milk output. Fat is mobilized slowly, however, and an energy deficit that is too large will inhibit lactation.

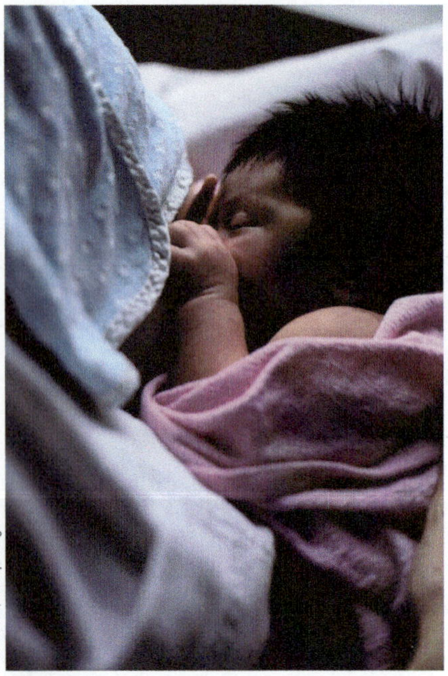
PhotoDisk/Getty Images

Breast milk supports infants' immune and digestive systems.

12.2 Healthy Infants

The growth of infants directly reflects their nutritional well-being and is the major indicator of their nutrition status. A baby grows faster during the first year of life than it ever will again, doubling its birthweight during the first 4 to 6 months and tripling its birthweight by the end of the first year. Adequate nutrition during infancy is critical to support this rapid rate of growth and development. This section provides an overview of nutrient requirements, current recommendations for feeding healthy infants, and the relationship between infant feeding and selected pediatric nutrition issues.

Milk for the Infant: Breastfeeding Breastfeeding has both emotional and physical health advantages. Emotional bonding is facilitated by many events and behaviors of mother and infant during the early months and years; one of the first can be breastfeeding.

During the first 2 or 3 days of lactation, the breasts produce **colostrum**, a premilk substance containing antibodies and white cells from the mother's blood. Because it contains immunity factors, colostrum helps protect a newborn infant from those infections against which the mother has developed an immunity—precisely those in the environment against which the infant needs protection. Upon entering the infant's body with the milk, these antibodies inactivate bacteria within the digestive tract, where they could otherwise cause intestinal infections. Breast milk also contains antibodies, although not as much as colostrum contains.

Colostrum and breast milk both contain the **bifidus factor** that favors growth of "friendly" probiotic bacteria, such as *Lactobacillus bifidus*, in the infant's digestive tract so that other, harmful bacteria cannot grow there. (Probiotics are discussed in Chapter 7.) Breast milk also contains **lactoferrin**, a protein that enhances iron

colostrum (kuh-LAHS-trum) A milk-like secretion from the breast, rich in protective factors, present during the first day or so after delivery and before milk appears.

bifidus factor (BIFF-id-us) A factor in colostrum and breast milk that favors growth in the infant's intestinal tract of the "friendly" bacteria *Lactobacillus bifidus*; colonization with friendly bacteria means that other, less desirable intestinal inhabitants will not flourish.

lactoferrin (lak-toe-FERR-in) A protein in breast milk that binds and helps absorb iron and keeps it from supporting the growth of the infant's intestinal bacteria.

absorption and functions as an antibacterial agent by binding to iron and making it unavailable to bacterial pathogens. Other factors found in breast milk include several enzymes, hormones, and lipids that help protect infants against infection. Breast-fed infants have lower rates of hospital admissions, ear infections, diarrhea, rashes, allergies, asthmatic disease, and other health problems than bottle-fed infants.[27]

Breast milk is superior to other feeding preparations in meeting the nutrient needs of the young infant. It offers carbohydrate in the easy-to-assimilate form of lactose; the fat contains a generous proportion of the essential omega-6 fatty acid linoleic acid; and the protein, alpha-lactalbumin, is one that infants can easily digest. Depending on the mother's diet, breast milk can also deliver beneficial omega-3 fatty acids to an infant. Except for vitamin D, its vitamin contents are ample. As for minerals, calcium, phosphorus, and magnesium are present in amounts appropriate for the rate of growth expected in human infants, and breast milk is low in sodium. Its iron is highly absorbable, and the presence of a zinc-binding protein facilitates absorption of the zinc it contains.

The American Academy of Pediatrics recommends that infants receive exclusive breastfeeding for the first 6 months of life, and breastfeeding with complementary foods for at least 12 months.[28] The national health objective plan, *Healthy People 2020,* has identified several objectives for breastfeeding. Data show that breastfeeding rates for children born in 2013 have risen from prior years. Four out of five infants had initiated breastfeeding, slightly over half were breastfeeding at 6 months and nearly one third were breastfeeding at 12 months.[29] Although the overall rate of breastfeeding is improving, that rate differs by race/ethnicity and region. Breastfeeding rates continue to be the highest among women who are older, well educated, relatively affluent, and/or live in the western United States. Among those least likely to breastfeed are women who are in low-income groups, black, under age 20, and/or live in the southeastern United States.[30]

A number of barriers to achieving the nation's health objective for increasing the incidence of breastfeeding have been identified. They include lack of knowledge, an absence of work policies and facilities that support lactating women (e.g., extended maternity leave, part-time employment, facilities for pumping breast milk or breastfeeding, and on-site child care), and the portrayal of bottle-feeding rather than breastfeeding as the norm in the American society. Additional support is needed for mothers to initiate and continue to breastfeed. La Leche League offers trained volunteer mothers to provide support for breastfeeding. Child care settings and workplaces can make provisions to accommodate lactating mothers. The Baby Friendly Hospital Initiative (BFHI) encourages hospitals and birthing centers to offer mothers the information and skills to initiate and continue breastfeeding based on the Ten Steps to Successful Breastfeeding (see Table 12-5).

Contraindications to Breastfeeding Breastfeeding is not recommended in certain circumstances. A woman should not breastfeed if she has a communicable disease such as active untreated tuberculosis, if she takes a medication that is secreted in breast milk and is known to affect the infant, or if she is using drugs of abuse. Mothers who are undergoing radiation treatments or chemotherapy also should not breastfeed.

Because the human immunodeficiency virus (HIV), which is responsible for AIDS, can be passed to an infant through breast milk, HIV-infected mothers should not breastfeed. Unfortunately, sometimes the nutritional and immunologic benefits of breast milk outweigh the risks of HIV transmission through breastfeeding. Such is the case in many developing countries, where lack of safe drinking water to make formula increases the risk of diarrhea and disease for infants. However, the World Health Organization encourages HIV-positive mothers in developing countries to

TABLE 12-5	Baby-Friendly Hospitals: 10 Steps to Successful Breastfeeding

To promote breastfeeding, every maternity facility should:

- Develop a written breastfeeding policy that is routinely communicated to all health care staff.
- Train all health care staff in the skills necessary to implement the breastfeeding policy.
- Inform all pregnant women about the benefits and management of breastfeeding.
- Help mothers initiate breastfeeding within ½ hour of birth.
- Show mothers how to breastfeed and how to maintain lactation, even if they need to be separated from their infants.
- Give newborn infants no food or drink other than breast milk, unless medically indicated.
- Practice rooming-in, allowing mothers and infants to remain together 24 hours a day.
- Encourage breastfeeding on demand.
- Give no artificial nipples or pacifiers to breastfeeding infants.*
- Foster the establishment of breastfeeding support groups and refer mothers to them at discharge from the facility.

*Compared with nonusers, infants who use pacifiers breastfeed less frequently and stop breastfeeding at a younger age.

SOURCE: United Nations Children's Fund and World Health Organization.

feed formula whenever their circumstances ensure a regular supply of infant formula and safe drinking water.[31]

Most prescription drugs taken by mothers do not reach nursing infants in sufficiently large quantities to affect them adversely. As a precaution, however, a nursing mother should consult with her physician before taking any drug. Occasional use of a small, single serving of alcohol is compatible with breastfeeding, but both alcohol and nicotine can enter breast milk. These substances also adversely affect maternal production and composition of breast milk. It is important not to expose the infant to secondhand smoke, due to the risk of health problems such as impaired growth, respiratory problems, and sudden infant death. Coffee drinking is fine in moderation (two to three cups a day), as is eating foods such as garlic and spices. Sometimes, a particular food may affect the baby's liking for the mother's milk, but this matter requires individual detective work. (Examples are chocolate for some babies, excess caffeine for others, and foods that cause gas in the mother for still others.)

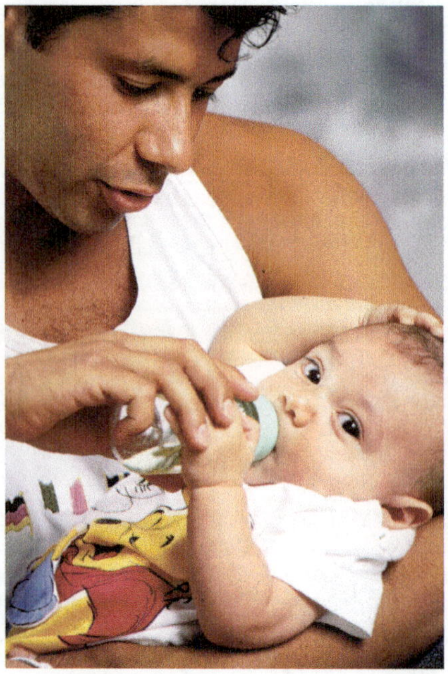

Vic Bider/PhotoEdit

Pumping breast milk into a bottle or using formula feeding allows other family members to enjoy feeding the infant.

Feeding Formula

Like the breastfeeding mother, a mother who offers formula to her baby has reasons for making that choice, and her feelings should be honored. Infant formulas are manufactured to approximate the nutrient composition of breast milk. National and international standards have been set for the nutrient content of infant formulas. The immunologic protection of breast milk, however, cannot be duplicated. One major advantage of formula feeding is the relief it provides to mothers whose attempts at breastfeeding have been met with frustration. Formula provides adequate nourishment for infants, and mothers can choose this alternative with confidence.

Many mothers breastfeed at first and then wean the baby within the first 1 to 6 months. When a woman chooses to wean her infant during the first 12 months of life, it is imperative that she shift to *infant formula*. Cow's milk, whether whole or reduced-fat, is not recommended during the first year of life, according to the American Academy of Pediatrics (AAP).[32] Cow's milk is an inappropriate replacement for breast milk or infant formula because it provides insufficient vitamin C and iron and excessive sodium and protein. Feeding cow's milk to infants may increase the risk of iron-deficiency anemia and cow's milk protein allergy.

For infants with special problems, many variations of infant formulas are available. Special formulas based on soy protein are available for infants allergic to milk protein, and formulas with the lactose replaced can be used for infants with lactose intolerance.

Supplements for the Infant Breast milk or formula and the infant's own internal stores will meet most nutrient needs for the first 6 months. Thereafter, the introduction of properly chosen foods will normally keep up with the infant's changing requirements. At 6 months, infants require additional iron, preferably in the form of iron-fortified cereal.

Breast milk does not provide enough vitamin D for infants, and vitamin D deficiency causes impaired bone mineralization in children. Manufacturers fortify infant formulas with vitamin D, but due to the low concentration of vitamin D in breast milk, pediatricians routinely prescribe a vitamin D supplement for breast-fed infants whose mothers are vitamin D deficient.

Supplementary fluoride should not be given during the first 6 months. From 6 months to 3 years of age, the pediatrician may prescribe fluoride if the water supply is severely deficient.

Food for the Infant The infant's rapid growth and metabolism demand an adequate supply of all essential nutrients.[33] Because of their small size, infants need smaller total amounts of the nutrients than adults do, but when comparisons are made based on body weight, infants need more than twice as much of many of the nutrients. Figure 12-3 compares a 5-month-old baby's needs with those of an adult man.

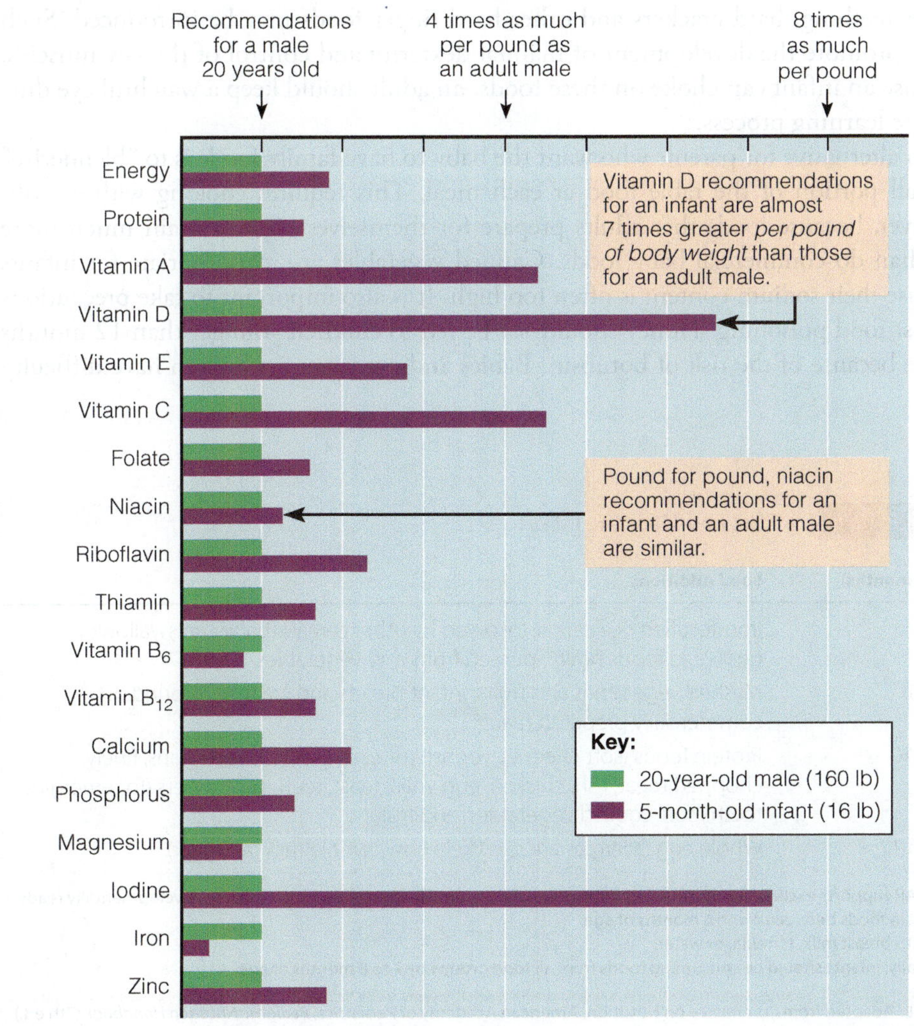

FIGURE 12-3

Recommended Intakes of Nutrients for an Infant and an Adult Compared on the Basis of Body Weight

SOURCE: Adapted with permission from E. Whitney and S. Rolfes, *Understanding Nutrition*, 14th ed.

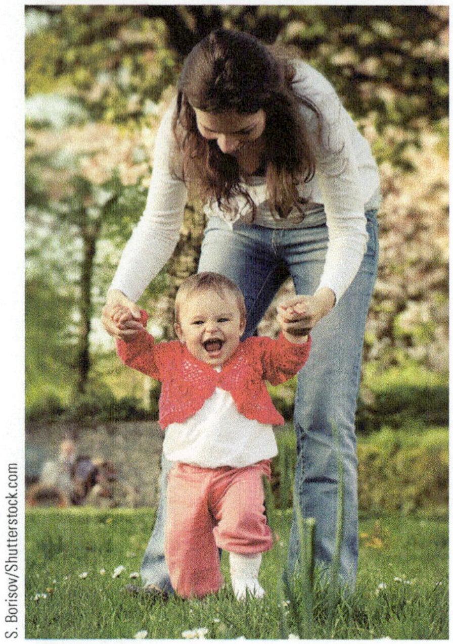

Energy saved by slower growth is spent in increased activity.

As you can see, some of the differences are extraordinary. After 6 months, calorie needs increase less rapidly as the growth rate begins to slow down, but some of the energy saved by slower growth is spent on increased activity.

Solid foods may normally be added to a baby's diet when the baby is about 6 months old, depending on readiness. The addition of foods to a baby's diet should be governed by three considerations: the baby's nutrient needs, the baby's physical readiness to handle different forms of foods, and the need to detect and control allergic reactions. All babies are different, and the program of food additions should depend on the individual baby, not on any rigid schedule. Table 12-6 presents a suggested sequence for feeding infants.

Solid foods are a source of important nutrients such as iron, zinc, and vitamin C. Because a baby's stored iron supply from before birth runs out after the birthweight doubles, breast milk or iron-fortified formula, followed by iron-fortified cereals—and, later, meat or meat alternates such as legumes—are recommended. Fruits and fruit juices are a good source of vitamin C, which helps with absorption of iron. However, the AAP recommends avoiding the use of fruit juice before 1 year of age and limiting intake to 4 ounces per day for toddlers 1 to 3 years of age and 4 to 6 ounces per day for children ages 4 through 6 to avoid the displacement of other important nutrients from their diets.[34]

A baby's physical readiness to handle foods develops in many small steps. For example, the ability to swallow solid food develops at around 4 to 6 months, and experience with solid food at 6 months helps develop swallowing ability by desensitizing the gag reflex. Later still, when a baby can sit up, can handle finger foods, and is teething, hard crackers and other hard finger foods may be introduced. Such foods promote the development of manual dexterity and control of the jaw muscles. Because an infant can choke on these foods, an adult should keep a watchful eye during the learning process.

An alternative for parents who want the baby to have family foods is to "blenderize" a small portion of the table food at each meal. This requires cooking without salt, however, because foods that adults prepare for themselves often contain much more salt than do commercial baby foods. Canned vegetables are inappropriate for infants because their sodium content is often too high. It is also important to take precautions against food poisoning. Honey should *not* be fed to children younger than 12 months of age because of the risk of botulism. Babies and even young children have difficulty

TABLE 12-6 First Foods for the Infant

Age (months)	Food Additions
4 to 6[a]	Iron-fortified rice cereal, followed by other cereals (baby can swallow nonliquid foods now);[b] pureed fruits and vegetables
6 to 8	Mashed vegetables and fruits; infant breads and crackers; ground or commercially prepared meat[c]
8 to 10	Protein foods (soft cheeses, yogurt, tofu, mashed cooked beans, finely chopped meat, fish, chicken, egg yolk); toast, teething crackers (for emerging teeth); soft-cooked vegetables, and fruit
10 to 12	Whole egg (allergies are less likely now), whole milk (at 1 year)

[a] The AAP supports exclusive breastfeeding for 6 months but acknowledges that infants may be developmentally ready for certain foods between 4 and 6 months of age.
[b] Mix with breast milk, formula, or water.
[c] Generally, infants should be consuming foods from all food groups by 7 to 8 months of age.

SOURCE: Adapted from Committee on Nutrition, American Academy of Pediatrics, *Pediatric Nutrition Handbook* (7th ed.), eds. R. E. Kleinman, F.R. Greer (Elk Grove Village, IL: American Academy of Pediatrics, 2014).

swallowing certain foods: popcorn, whole grapes, hard candies, bite-size hot dogs, nuts, and spoonfuls of peanut butter may be a choking hazard and are best avoided.

At 1 year of age, milk can be a source of most of the nutrients the baby needs; 2 to 3 cups a day are now sufficient. Infants less than 2 years old should drink whole milk rather than low-fat or fat-free milk. They need the fat and vitamins A and D of fortified whole milk until 2 years of age. The other foods—meat, iron-fortified cereal, enriched or whole-grain bread, fruits, and vegetables—should be supplied in variety and in sufficient amounts to round out total calorie needs. Ideally, a 1-year-old is sitting at the table and eating many of the same foods everyone else eats. Table 12-7 shows a meal plan that meets the requirements for 1-year-olds.

The wise parent of a 1-year-old offers nutrition and love together. Both promote growth. It is literally true that "feeding with love" produces better growth in both weight and height of children than feeding the same food in an emotionally negative climate. It also promotes better brain development. The formation of nerve-to-nerve connections in the brain depends both on nutrients and on environmental stimulation.

A person feeding a 1-year-old should keep in mind that the baby is also developing eating habits that will persist throughout life.[35] Mealtimes should be relaxed and leisurely. Children should learn to eat slowly, pause and enjoy their table companions, and stop eating when they are full. Physical activity should be encouraged on a daily basis to promote strong skeletal and muscular development and to establish habits that will promote good health throughout life.

TABLE 12-7 Meal Plan for a 1-Year-Old

Breakfast
¼ c whole milk
½ c iron-fortified cereal
1–2 tbsp fruit
Snack
½ c yogurt
Teething crackers
½ c fruit
Lunch
½ c whole milk
½ c vegetables
1 egg or 1 oz chopped meat or well-cooked mashed legumes
½ c noodles
Snack
½ c whole milk
½ slice toast
1 tbsp apple butter
Supper
½ c whole milk
1 oz chopped meat or well-cooked mashed legumes
¼ c potato or rice
½ c vegetables
2 to 3 tbsp fruit

Nutrition-Related Problems of Infancy

Iron deficiency and food allergies are two significant nutrition-related problems of infants.

Iron Deficiency Iron deficiency remains a prevalent nutritional problem for infants, although it has declined in recent years largely due to the increasing use of iron-fortified formulas. Feeding cow's milk earlier than recommended in infancy can cause iron deficiency because of its poor iron content and the potential to cause gastrointestinal blood loss in susceptible infants.[36] Other factors contributing to iron deficiency in infancy include breastfeeding for more than 6 months without providing supplemental iron, feeding infant formula that is not fortified with iron, the infant's rapid rate of growth, low birthweight, and low socioeconomic status. To prevent iron deficiency, the American Academy of Pediatrics recommends that infants be fed breast milk or iron-fortified formula for the first year of life, with appropriate foods added as shown in Table 12-6.

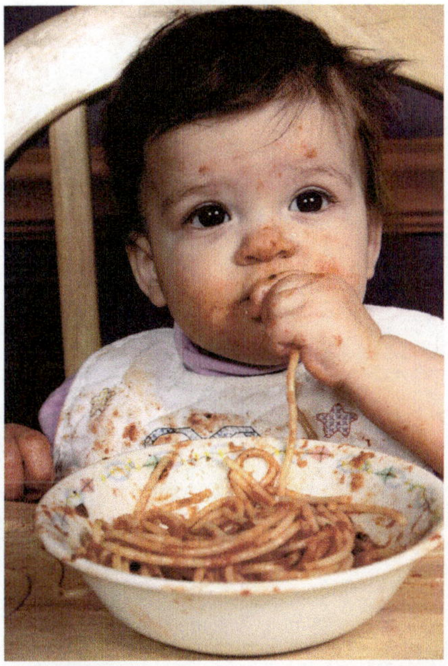

Let infants handle food as they become ready.

Food Allergies Genetics and environmental factors are believed to be the main causes of food allergies. A diagnosis of food allergy is confirmed based on history of possible allergic response and clinical diagnostic testing. As described earlier, recommendations for early infant feeding include exclusive breastfeeding for the first 6 months. At-risk infants (have eczema or a first-degree relative with allergy) can be fed partially hydrolyzed formula rather than cow's milk if breastfeeding is not an option.[37] New foods should be introduced one at a time to facilitate prompt detection of allergies or sensitivities to foods. For example, when cereals are introduced, rice cereal may be tried first for 3 to 5 days as it causes allergy least often. Wheat cereal is a common offender and so may be introduced last. If a cereal causes irritability from skin rash, digestive upset, or respiratory discomfort, its use should be discontinued before going on to the next food. It is possible that the allergic response may not be evident immediately but will manifest itself in vague symptoms occurring up to 5 days after the offending food is eaten. Allowing several days to lapse between the introduction of each new food will provide time for the clinical symptoms to appear so that the offending food may be identified. The Nutrition Action feature in Chapter 6 provides more information about food allergies and intolerances in children and adults.

12.3 Early and Middle Childhood

Childhood is a critical time in human development. Children typically grow taller by 2 to 3 inches and heavier by 5 or more pounds each year between the age of 1 and adolescence. They master fine motor skills (including those related to eating and drinking), become increasingly independent, and learn to express themselves appropriately. This section describes the nutrient requirements of children and the primary nutritional problems of this population.

Growth and Nutrient Needs of Children

After age 1, a child's growth rate slows, but the body continues to change dramatically. At age 1, most babies have just learned to stand and toddle; by age 2, they can take long strides with solid confidence and are learning to run, jump, and climb. The internal change that makes these new accomplishments possible is the accumulation of a larger body mass and greater density of bone and muscle tissue. These changes are obvious in the photos of the two young boys.

Children generally become leaner between the ages of 6 months and 6 years, after which time there is a gradual increase in fat thickness in both males and females until puberty. Females have a greater body fat content than males at all stages of development. The energy requirements of children are determined by their individual basal metabolic rates, activity patterns, and rates of growth. Toddlers (ages 1 to 3 years) need about 1,000 calories per day. By the age of 10, children need about 2,000 calories per day. Appetite decreases markedly around the age of 1 year, in line with the great reduction in growth rate. Thereafter, the appetite fluctuates; a child will need and demand much more food during periods of rapid growth than during slow periods.

To provide the gradually increasing needs for all nutrients during the growing years, the MyPlate food guide recommends a balance among dairy products, meats and meat alternates, fruits, vegetables, and grains. "Sometimes foods" have empty calories from ingredients like solid fats or added sugars; they provide calories with low nutritional value and should be consumed in moderation. The importance of daily physical activity is also emphasized (see Figure 12-4). In addition, the

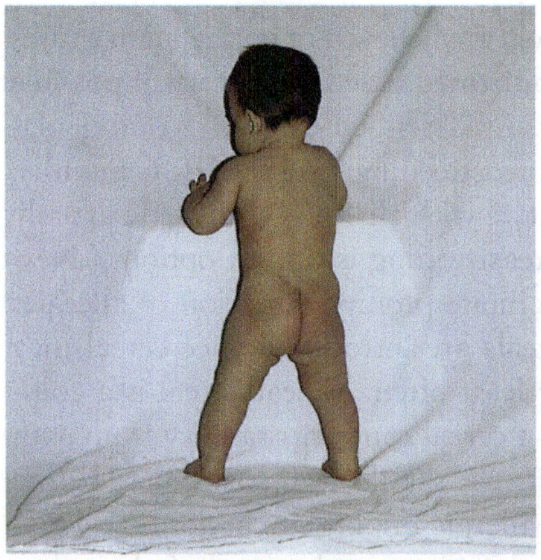

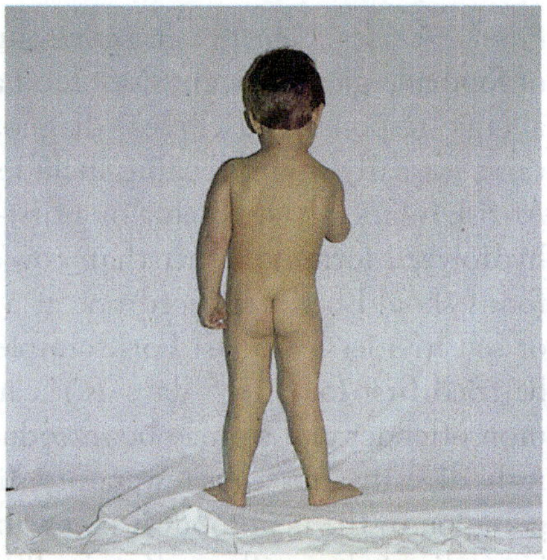

1-Year-Old and 2-Year-Old

The 2-year-old has lost much of the baby fat; the muscles (especially in the back, buttocks, and legs) have firmed and strengthened, and the leg bones have lengthened and increased in density.

FIGURE 12-4

A Food Guide for Young Children

SOURCE: United States Department of Agriculture, Food and Nutrition Service, available at www.fns.usda.gov/multimedia/tn/sump_level1.pdf.

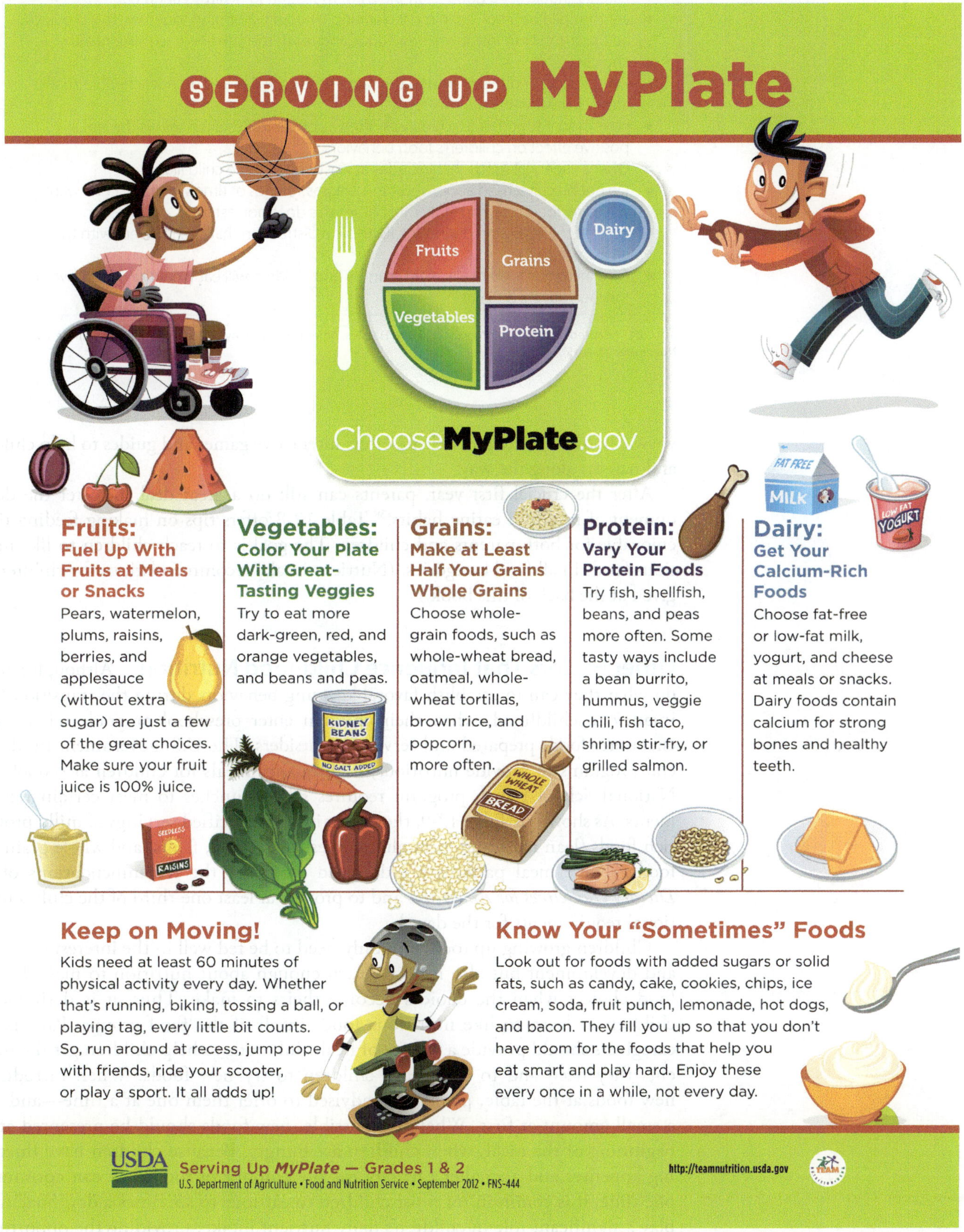

TABLE 12-8 **Strategies to Foster Healthful Eating Habits and Happy Mealtimes**

These tips may make feeding time easier and more relaxing for both parent and child:

- Parents should set a good example by demonstrating healthy eating habits.
- Let the child be involved in meal planning by going shopping together. This provides an opportunity to introduce new foods and teach the child how to make healthy choices.
- Serve snacks and meals around the same time each day and do not schedule snacks close to mealtime.
- Have dinner together as a family as often as possible. Research shows this has a positive effect on children's food behaviors.
- Offer a variety of foods that includes at least one that the child likes.
- Do not be concerned about short food jags, stretches of time when the child wants the same food over and over; most times this does not last long.
- Turn off the television during meals; this is a distraction that can interfere with the child's eating.
- Offer healthful food in a relaxed manner and children will eat what they need, avoid forcing your child to eat.

SOURCE: Adapted from Tips for Preventing Food Hassles, American Academy of Pediatrics, HealthyChildren.org (updated November 21, 2015).

www.ChooseMyPlate.gov website offers interactive games and guides to help children and parents along the way.

After the crucial first year, parents can still do a great deal to foster the development of healthful eating habits.[38] Table 12-8 offers tips on making feeding times enjoyable for both parents and children. The goal is to teach children to like nutritious foods in all food categories. (Nutrient intake recommendations for children are given at the back of this book.)

Other Factors That Influence Childhood Nutrition Although parents do what they can to establish favorable eating behaviors during the transition from infancy to childhood, when their children enter preschool or grade school, they encounter foods prepared and served by outsiders. The U.S. government funds several programs to provide nutritious, high-quality meals for children at school. The National School Lunch program requires school lunches to meet certain requirements. As shown in Table 12-9, they must include specified servings of milk, protein-rich foods (lean meat and meat alternatives), vegetables, fruits, and whole grain-rich foods. These meal patterns are designed to follow the recommendations of the *Dietary Guidelines for Americans* and to provide at least one-third of the child's nutritional requirements for the day.[39]

Children growing up today not only need to be fed well in the interest of growth and development but also need to learn enough about nutrition to make healthy food choices when the choices become theirs to make. Thus, it is desirable for children to learn to like nutritious foods in all of the food groups. Parents and caregivers should provide a variety of healthful foods to help children get the nutrients they need and to encourage children to try new foods. When introducing new foods at the table, parents are advised to offer them one at a time—and only a small amount at first. Whenever possible, new foods should be presented at the beginning of the meal, when children are hungry. Because children have fluctuating appetites and a smaller capacity for the amount of food they can consume at one time, it is common for most children to eat four to six times a day. Snacks can play a significant role in children's daily nutrient intake; providing the opportunity

TABLE 12-9 School Meal Patterns for Different Ages

	Breakfast Meal Pattern			Lunch Meal Pattern		
	Amount of Food per Week (Minimum per Day)					
	Grades K–5	Grades 6–8	Grades 9–12	Grades K–5	Grades 6–8	Grades 9–12
Fruits (cups)[a,b]	5 (1)	5 (1)	5 (1)	2½ (½)	2½ (½)	5 (1)
Vegetables (cups)[a,b]	0	0	0	3¾ (¾)	3¾ (¾)	5 (1)
Dark green[c]	0	0	0	½	½	½
Red/orange[c]	0	0	0	¾	¾	1¼
Beans/peas/legumes[c]	0	0	0	½	½	½
Starchy[c]	0	0	0	½	½	½
Other[c,d]	0	0	0	½	½	¾
Additional vegetable to reach total[e]	0	0	0	1	1	1½
Grains (oz equivalent)[f]	7–10 (1)	8–10 (1)	9–10 (1)	8–9 (1)	8–10 (1)	10–12 (2)
Meats/meat alternatives (oz equivalent)	0	0	0	8–10 (1)	9–10 (1)	10–12 (2)
Fluid milk (cups)[g]	5 (1)	5 (1)	5 (1)	5 (1)	5 (1)	5 (1)
Minimum-maximum calories (cal)[h]	350–500	400–550	450–600	550–650	600–700	750–850
Saturated fat (% of total calories)	<10	<10	<10	<10	<10	<10
Sodium (mg)	≤430	≤470	≤500	≤640	≤710	≤740
Trans fat	0	0	0	0	0	0

[a] One quarter-cup of dried fruit counts as ½ cup of fruit; 1 cup leafy greens counts as ½ cup vegetables. No more than half the fruit and vegetable offers may be in the form of juice. All juice must be 100% full strength.
[b] For breakfast, vegetables may be substituted for fruits, but the first two cups per week of any substitution must be from the dark-green, red/orange, beans and peas (legumes), or "other vegetables."
[c] Larger amounts of these vegetables may be served.
[d] This category consists of other vegetables as defined in the standards. For the purposes of the lunch "other vegetables," requirements may be met with any additional dark-green, red/orange, and beans/peas (legumes).
[e] Any vegetable subgroup may be offered to meet the total weekly vegetable requirement.
[f] At least half of the grains offered must be whole-grain rich.
[g] Fluid milk must be low-fat (1% fat or less, unflavored) or fat-free (unflavored or flavored).
[h] Discretionary sources of calories (solid fats and added sugars) may be added to the meal pattern if within the specifications for calories, saturated fat, *trans* fat, and sodium. Foods of minimal nutritional value and fluid milk with fat content greater than 1% milk fat are not allowed.

SOURCE: U.S. Department of Agriculture, Food and Nutrition Service, Nutrition Standards in the National School Lunch and School Breakfast Programs, 7 CFR Parts 210 and 220, *Federal Register* Vol. 77, No. 17, January 26, 2012.

for children to choose their snacks from two or three options can also promote greater acceptance of a variety of foods.

Nutrition-Related Problems of Childhood Nutrition plays a critical role in the development and growth of children. The Healthy Eating Index (HEI) is a tool used to measure how well people's diets meet the *Dietary Guidelines* for consumption of fruits, vegetables, whole grains, dairy, and other foods or nutrients. The HEI also considers intake of foods that are high in sodium or are of low nutritional quality, which should be consumed in moderation. Recent results show the diet quality of most children and adolescents aged 2 to 17 is less than optimal. The average scores for all of the categories were below recommendations. Consumption of dairy products and protein foods were closest to the standards; intake of green vegetables and beans were farthest from recommendations. It is recommended that children and adolescents increase their consumption of vegetables, replace refined grains with whole grains, and decrease the amount of sodium and empty calories from solid fats and sugar.[40]

National surveys show that overall calorie intake has increased significantly for children and adolescents over the past few decades, and much of that comes from

FIGURE 12-5

Percent of Total Daily Calories Consumed from Sugar-Sweetened Beverages by Age in Children and Adolescents age 2 to 19, United States, 2011–2014

The percentage of total daily calories consumed from sugar-sweetened beverages increased with age for both boys and girls. Children and adolescents consumed an average 7% of their total daily calories from sugar-sweetened beverages. Boys and girls consumed a similar percentage of total calories from sugar-sweetened beverages: 4% of total daily calories consumed for boys and girls aged 2–5; 6.6% for boys and 5.8% for girls aged 6–11; and 9.3% for boys and 9.7% for girls aged 12–19.

SOURCE: A. Rosinger et al., Sugar-sweetened beverage consumption among U.S. youth, 2011–2014. *NCHS data brief,* no. 271, Hyattsville, MD: National Center for Health Statistics, 2017.

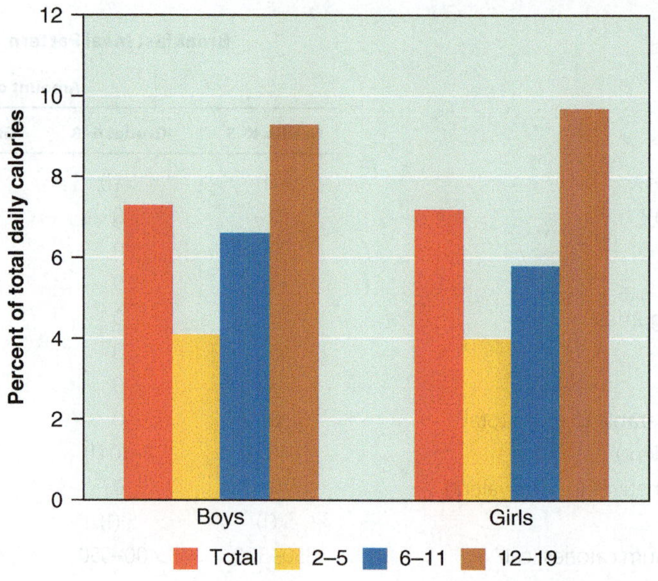

the consumption of high-calorie, low-nutrient-density foods.[41] On any given day, approximately 64 percent of boys and 61 percent of girls aged 2 to 19 consume soft drinks, which can account for more than 7 percent of their total calorie intake. The amount of beverages consumed increased significantly with age in both boys and girls (see Figure 12-5).[42] Consumption of sugar-sweetened beverages is associated with dental caries, weight gain, type 2 diabetes, and fatty liver in children. In 2011–2012 over one-third of children and adolescents consumed fast food in a given day.[43] Foods that are high in solid fats, such as grain-based desserts, pizza, full-fat cheese, and fried white potatoes are an additional source of empty calories for this age group. The *Dietary Guidelines for Americans* 2015–2020 recommends reducing the intake of calories from added sugars and solid fats.

The most common nutrition-related problems among U.S. children include overweight and obesity, iron-deficiency anemia, and high blood cholesterol levels. The high rate of obesity among U.S. children requires a multifaceted strategy to address the health, social, physical, and environmental issues that may prevent and treat this escalating public health problem.[44] See the Spotlight feature later in this chapter for more about the problem of obesity in children and adolescents.

Iron-Deficiency Anemia The majority of iron is found in hemoglobin, the protein in red blood cells that carries oxygen to the body's tissues. Low iron stores can affect cognitive development in infants and adolescents and can lead to iron-deficiency anemia. It is estimated that approximately 7 percent of children aged 1 to 5 years have iron deficiency.[45] The prevalence is higher in Mexican American children compared to non-Hispanic black and non-Hispanic white children. Iron in the diet is present in the form of heme iron found in foods from animal sources, nonheme iron found in some plant foods, and in foods that have been iron-enriched or fortified. To ensure adequate iron intake, parents should offer their children an abundance of iron-rich foods such as lean meats, fish, poultry, eggs, legumes, and whole-grain or enriched-grain products.

High Blood Cholesterol Considerable evidence exists that certain risk factors identified in children and adolescents, such as high cholesterol, obesity, hypertension, tobacco use, and diabetes, are linked to the development of atherosclerosis and heart disease in adulthood.[46] A panel of experts from major U.S. health and professional organizations has identified the importance of addressing these risk factors early on. Good nutrition starting at birth and continuing through childhood and early adulthood has many health benefits, including reducing the likelihood for heart disease. Exclusive breastfeeding from birth to 6 months of age and continued breastfeeding to 1 year of age with the gradual addition of solid foods at approximately 6 months is recommended. It is also recommended that children aged 1 and older eat diets containing no more than 30 percent of total calories from fat and less than 10 percent of total calories from saturated fat daily. However, from birth to 1 year of age, a child's fat consumption should *not* be restricted, because fat is a concentrated source of the calories needed to ensure proper physical development.

The panel also advises that children with certain risk factors have their blood cholesterol measured between the ages of 2 and 8. All other children should have their initial cholesterol screening done between the ages of 9 and 11.[47] For children and adolescents, a total of 200 milligrams per deciliter of blood or more is considered high; 170 to 199 is borderline high; and less than 170 is acceptable.

12.4 The Importance of Teen Nutrition

Adolescence is a time of change. Between the ages of about 10 and 18 years in girls and 12 and 20 years in boys, marked changes take place in physical, intellectual, and emotional growth and development. The maturation process is initiated and controlled by a variety of hormones such as growth hormone, prolactin, estrogen, testosterone, and the thyroid hormones. Many aspects of the maturation process are influenced by dietary intake and nutritional status. This section reviews the nutrient requirements and special nutrition-related problems of teenagers.

Nutrient Needs of Adolescents

The dramatic changes in body composition and the rate of growth that occur during early adolescence give rise to the familiar phrase "the adolescent growth spurt." The magnitude of these changes is such that the linear growth increments during adolescence can contribute about 15 to 25 percent of adult stature. The rate of weight gain can contribute anywhere from 40 to 50 percent of the adult body mass. This remarkable growth rate requires adequate intakes of energy and nutrients.[48] The individual energy needs for teenagers are influenced by body size, activity levels, and biological factors affecting growth. Consult the DRI table shown at the back of this book for the energy and nutrient intake recommendations for adolescents.

The rates and patterns of growth for individual teenagers vary widely. The only way to be sure teenagers are growing normally is to compare their heights and weights with previous measures taken at intervals and note whether reasonable progress is being made. Physical growth charts for children and adolescents and information on assessing children's growth status can be accessed at www.cdc.gov/growthcharts.

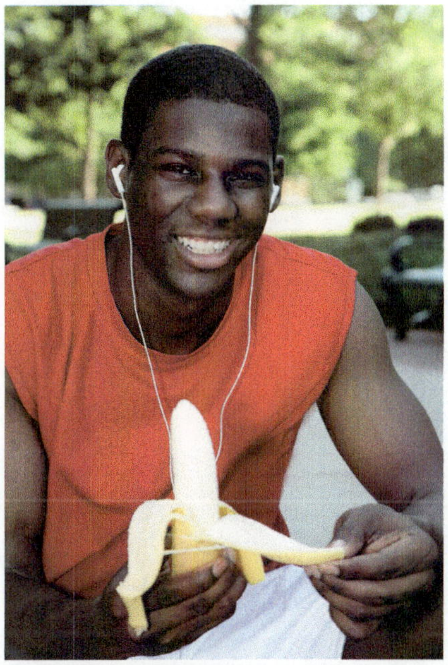
iStockphoto.com/Steve Debenport

Nutritious snacks can supply added nutrients to the active teenager's diet.

Nutrition-Related Problems of Adolescents

Most adolescents in the United States are perceived as "healthy." However, many U.S. adolescents experience a variety of health and nutrition problems, some related to their risk-seeking behaviors and an inability to deal with abstract notions such as "good health" and the link between current behaviors and long-term health. Nutrition-related problems among U.S. adolescents include overweight and obesity (discussed later in this chapter's Spotlight feature), undernutrition, iron-deficiency anemia, low dietary calcium intakes, high blood cholesterol levels, dental caries, and eating disorders.

Undernutrition Some groups of adolescents, such as those who are from low-income families, have run away from home, or abuse alcohol or other drugs, are at risk for reduced energy and food intakes. Households with incomes at or below the poverty line are much more likely to have less access to adequate food due to lack of money or other resources.[49] Approximately 23 percent of youth aged 18 or younger are estimated to be living below the poverty line. African American and Hispanic teenagers are more than twice as likely to live in poverty as are white youth. This is a population that is highly susceptible to inadequate or poor nutrition. Adolescents who practice unhealthy weight control behaviors such as dieting or restricting their intake are also at risk for undernutrition. Data from the Youth Risk Behavior Surveillance System show that between 2014 and 2015, 60 percent of female and 31 percent of male students in 9th through 12th grades reported some form of unhealthy weight control behavior.[50] This is especially concerning as it has been suggested that these behaviors tend to increase into young adulthood.[51]

Iron-Deficiency Anemia Iron needs increase during adolescence, especially for females as they start to menstruate. In boys, the requirements for absorbed iron increase because of an expanding blood volume and rise in hemoglobin concentration that accompanies the development of larger muscles and sexual maturation. (After the adolescent growth spurt, a male's need for iron falls off.) Whereas most males have an adequate iron intake during adolescence, many females between 12 and 22 years of age have iron intakes below the current recommended intake. Girls typically consume fewer total calories and less meat than boys do.

Low Calcium Intakes Another problem nutrient during the teen years is calcium. Low intakes of calcium-rich foods during adolescence compromise peak bone mass development and increase the risk of osteoporosis later in life. Adolescents need a minimum of 1,300 milligrams of calcium each day to achieve an optimal peak bone mass and healthy bones. However, the actual calcium intake by many teenagers, especially girls, is below the recommended amount.[52] Adolescent girls on low-calorie diets who drink diet soft drinks instead of milk are at particular risk for age-related bone loss and subsequent fractures. See the Spotlight feature in Chapter 8 for more about calcium and osteoporosis.

High Blood Cholesterol Teenagers have many of the same risk factors for high blood cholesterol as adults: family history of coronary heart disease; diets high in *trans* fat, saturated fat, and cholesterol; hypertension; low activity levels; and smoking. Although the process of atherosclerosis is not completely understood, it is believed that the fatty streaks in blood vessels that develop in young people progress to the fibrous plaques of adulthood.[53] For more information about diet and heart disease, see the Spotlight feature in Chapter 5.

Dental Caries Although dental caries are largely preventable, this remains the most common chronic disease of children aged 5 to 17 years.[54] By age 5, 60 percent of all children have had tooth decay, and more than 90 percent of 18-year-olds have experienced decay.[55] Children in low-income households, and especially those who are American Indian, African American, or Hispanic, have three times the risk of tooth decay because they lack access to or encounter barriers to accessing dental services. Fortunately, the incidence of dental caries has decreased, partly because of fluoridation of public drinking water, improved dental hygiene, and the use of fluoride in toothpastes and mouthwashes.

Eating Disorders Eating disorders have become a serious health problem in recent years. The most common eating disorders are anorexia nervosa and bulimia nervosa. A constellation of individual, familial, sociocultural, and biological factors contribute to these disorders, which threaten physical health and psychological well-being. See the Spotlight feature in Chapter 10 for more information about eating disorders.

Some individuals are more predisposed to developing an eating disorder than others. For example, about 90 percent of people with eating disorders are female. Most are Caucasian, with few cases seen among blacks and other minority groups. Most individuals who develop eating disorders are adolescents or young adults who typically began experiencing food-related and self-image problems between the ages of 14 and 30 years. Because these syndromes are often surrounded by secrecy, their prevalence is not known with certainty, although it has increased dramatically within the past three decades.[56] Estimates in the general population range from 0.9 percent of women and 0.3 percent of men for anorexia nervosa to 1.5 percent of women and 0.5 percent of men for bulimia nervosa.[57] These two eating disorders are also sometimes seen in adolescent athletes, many of whom compete in sports such as gymnastics, wrestling, distance running, diving, and swimming, which demand a rigid control of body weight.

12.5 Nutrition in Later Life

The life expectancy in the United States is 78 years (76 years for men and 81 years for women).[58] To what extent is aging inevitable? Apparently, aging is an inevitable, natural process programmed into our genes at conception. Nevertheless, we can adopt lifestyle habits, such as consuming a healthful diet, exercising, and paying attention to our work and recreational environments, that will promote healthy aging.[59] Clearly, good nutrition can support healthy aging in many significant ways.

One approach to understanding healthy aging has been to study other cultures in the hope of finding an extremely long-lived race of people and then learning their secrets. (See The Savvy Diner feature in Chapter 1 for more insights regarding nutrition and longevity.) The views of the experts are summed up best by simply saying that disease can *shorten* people's lives, and poor nutrition practices make diseases more likely to occur. Thus, by postponing and slowing disease processes, optimal nutrition can help prolong life and can promote health to make later years more enjoyable.[60] This section focuses on the nutrient requirements of older adults, the diseases associated with aging, their risk factors, and the relevance of nutrition to these diseases.

Demographic Trends and Aging

In 2000, people aged 65 and over accounted for 12.4 percent of the population, and this proportion is expected to grow to 21.7 percent by 2040. The number of people aged 85 and older is expected to triple from 6 million in 2013 to 14.6 million in 2040. The increased growth in the older adult population in the United States is illustrated in Figure 12-6.[61]

Improved life expectancy and the baby boom that took place between 1946 and 1964 are important contributors to the growing older adult population in the United States. Baby boomers increased the numbers of the older middle-aged

FIGURE 12-6

The Aging of the Population

In 1900, 4 percent of the U.S. population (3.1 million people) were more than 65 years of age; in 2015, 14.9 percent (47.8 million people) were more than 65; by 2040, 21.7 percent (about 82.3 million people) will have reached age 65.

SOURCE: Data from *A Profile of Older Americans, 2016;* available at https//aoa.acl.gov/aging_statistics/profile/index.aspx.

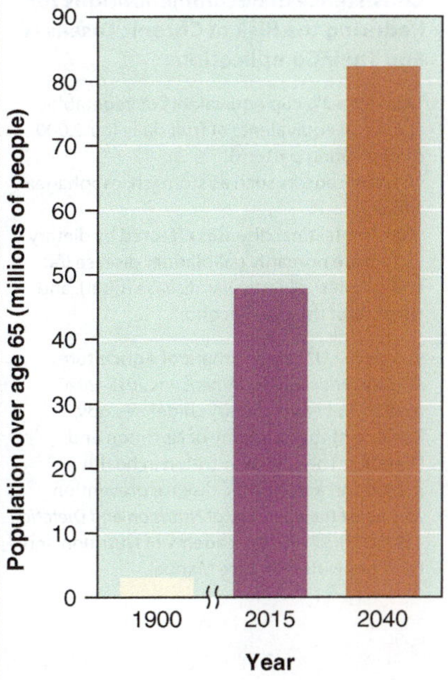

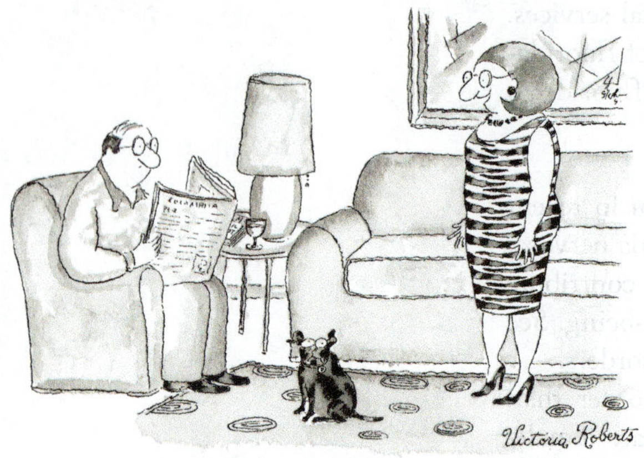

"Good news, honey—seventy is the new fifty."

(ages 46 through 63) until 2010; now they swell the ranks of the retired population. Improved life expectancy has resulted from better prenatal and postnatal care and more effective means of combating disease in older adults. For example, the death rate from heart disease began to decline in the 1960s and continues to fall today. More than half of the drop is attributed to a decline in smoking and fewer people with high blood pressure or high blood cholesterol.

Healthy Adults

Many of the health problems associated with the later years can be affected by diet and lifestyle choices made throughout the life span. Of the leading causes of death for adults aged 65 and older, one-half are directly influenced by nutrition-related factors.[62] For example, incorporating physical activity and a healthful diet into one's lifestyle can contribute to controlling three important risk factors for heart disease: high saturated fat intake, overweight, and a sedentary lifestyle. Figure 12-7 illustrates how the same set of dietary recommendations can promote general health and help prevent a broad spectrum of chronic diseases.[63]

Aging and Nutrition Status

Aging is often associated with frailty, sickness, and a loss of vitality. Although the aging members of our society do experience chronic illness and the associated disabilities, there is great heterogeneity among this population. That is, older people vary greatly in their social, economic, and lifestyle situations as well as their capacity to function and their physical condition.[64] Each person ages at a different rate, sometimes making chronological age different from biological age. Most older people live at home, are fully independent, and believe their health is excellent or very good.[65] Older people sometimes have problems with the **activities of daily living (ADL)**. Because they depend on others to perform these essential activities, they are more likely to be at risk for malnutrition.

activities of daily living (ADL) Self-care activities including bathing, dressing, grooming, transferring from bed to chair, going to the bathroom, and feeding oneself.

FIGURE 12-7

Consistency of Recommendations for Reducing the Risk of Chronic Diseases and Their Complications

Diet Recommendations → / Reduce risk ↓	Adequate fruits/ vegetables[a]	Reduce saturated & *trans* fats	Control calories	Reduce sodium	Control alcohol
Heart disease	🍎	🍎	🍎	🍎	🍎
Cancer[b]	🍎	🍎	🍎	🍎	🍎
Stroke	🍎	🍎	🍎	🍎	🍎
Diabetes	🍎	🍎	🍎		
Gastrointestinal diseases[c]	🍎	🍎	🍎		🍎

[a] Aim for a 2½ cup equivalents of vegetables and 2 cup equivalents of fruit daily (for 2,000 calorie eating pattern).

[b] Certain cancers such as stomach, esophageal, and colon.

[c] Gastrointestinal diseases affected by dietary factors are primarily gallbladder disease (fat and calories), diverticular disease (fiber), and cirrhosis of the liver (alcohol).

SOURCES: U.S. Department of Agriculture, *Dietary Guidelines for Americans 2015–2020*, available at www.dietaryguidelines.gov; Position of the Academy of Nutrition and Dietetics: The role of nutrition in health promotion and chronic disease prevention, *Journal of the Academy of Nutrition and Dietetics*, 113 (2013): 972–979; Academy of Nutrition and Dietetics Nutrition Care Manual.

Nutritional Needs and Intakes Many of the nutrient needs of older adults are the same as for younger people, but some special considerations deserve emphasis. Calorie needs decline with age because of a decrease in basal metabolism related to loss of lean tissue and a decrease in physical activity. According to the Dietary Reference Intake recommendations, energy intake should decrease by 10 calories per day for males and 7 calories per day for females for each year of age above 19.[66] Given their lower energy allowances, older adults are advised to select mostly nutrient-dense foods to be sure their nutritional needs are met. General nutrition guidelines for older adults are shown in Figure 12-8.[67] The recommended eating pattern reflects

FIGURE 12-8

MyPlate for Older Adults[a]

MyPlate for Older Adults provides examples of foods that are recommended by the *2015–2020 Dietary Guidelines for Americans* for a well-balanced diet that meets the unique needs of older adults. This food guide highlights the nutritional requirements for older adults. Half of the plate has icons for a variety of fruits and vegetables in a range of colors that include representations of frozen, pre-peeled fresh, dried, and low-sodium, low-sugar canned options as they are affordable and convenient. The other half provides examples of whole, enriched, and fortified grains that are good sources of fiber and lean protein sources such as beans, fish, lean meat, and low-fat and fat-free dairy products. Water, tea, coffee, and soup are represented to emphasize the importance of adequate fluid intake because decline in thirst is a common issue with the older population. Because overall calorie requirements decline with age due to a slowing of metabolism and physical activity, it is important to consume a variety of foods that are good sources of vitamins and minerals but low in *trans* and saturated fats and added sugars to meet nutrition and calorie needs.

[a] MyPlate for Older Adults was developed in collaboration with the AARP Foundation to target the demographic and food access issues associated with individuals 50+ years.

SOURCE: Tufts University Jean Mayer USDA Human Nutrition Research Center on Aging, available at http://hnrca.tufts.edu/myplate/#.

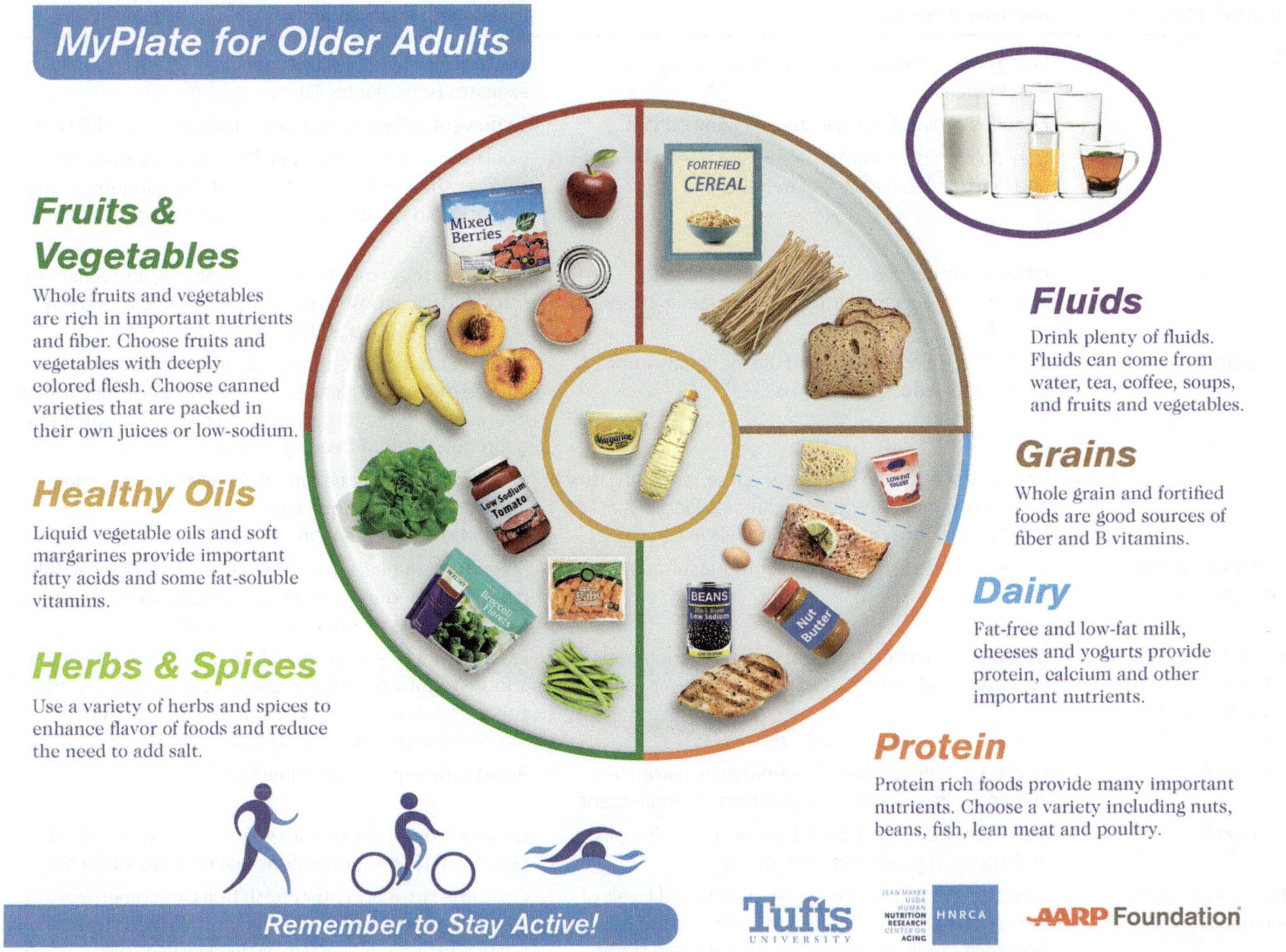

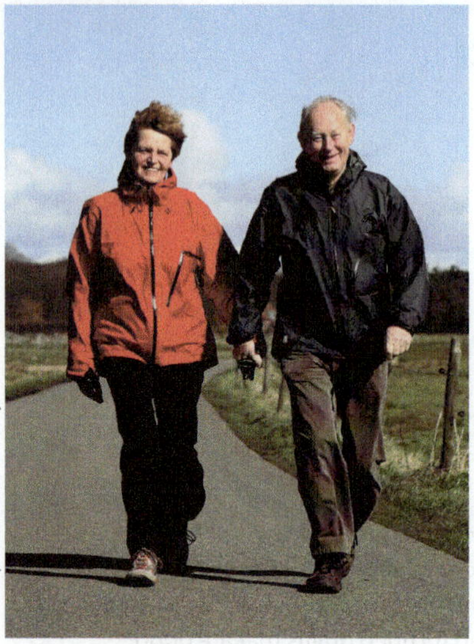

Any form of physical activity—even a 10-minute walk—is beneficial.

the lower caloric needs of most healthy older adults and emphasizes the need for regular physical activity and adequate fluid intake.

On one side of the energy budget, energy is taken in; and on the other side, it is spent. Regular physical activity is important for healthy aging. Studies have shown that up to 2½ hours a week of moderate-intensity physical activity can result in substantial health benefits for older adults, including improvement in conditions such as high blood pressure, arthritis, heart disease, and diabetes.[68]

Although caloric needs may decrease with age, the need for certain nutrients—such as calcium, vitamin D, vitamin C, vitamin B_{12}, and vitamin B_6—may actually increase with the effects of aging (see Table 12-10).[69] For example, as many as 30 percent of people older than 50 years may experience reduced stomach acidity, which can interfere with their ability to absorb vitamin B_{12}, calcium, and iron from foods. In addition, older adults who have low intakes of fortified dairy products may have increased needs for vitamin D because their skin has become less efficient at making vitamin D when exposed to sunlight.[70]

Assessing the diet quality of older adults is important for identifying issues relevant to their health and nutrition status. According to the Healthy Eating Index,

TABLE 12-10 The Impact of Aging on Nutrient Needs

Nutritional Concern	Age-Related Finding	Implications for Healthy Aging
Energy	Energy needs decrease due to decline in amount of lean tissue.	Get regular physical activity, including strength-training exercises (see Chapter 11).
Water	Reduced sense of thirst; increased urine output.	To prevent dehydration, drink 6 to 8 glasses of fluid a day.
Fiber	Constipation is a common complaint due to low fiber and fluid intakes and lack of exercise.	Consume 21 to 38 grams of fiber from a variety of sources such as fresh fruits, vegetables, legumes, and whole-grain products; get adequate amounts of fluid and exercise.
Vitamin D	Intakes may be low; skin becomes less able to synthesize the vitamin from sunlight; less exposure to sunlight.	Choose fortified milk and cereals, salmon, and other fatty fish; get daily exposure to sunlight if possible; or use a supplement [600 to 800 IU (15-20 μg) per day].
Calcium	Intakes typically low; reduced gastric acidity impairs absorption; reduced bone mass.	To offset bone loss, choose calcium-rich foods (low-fat or fat-free milk, yogurt, cheese), fortified sources of calcium (orange and other juices), or take a calcium supplement; get regular weight-bearing exercise.
Iron	Anemia less common after menopause; reduced gastric acidity may impair absorption; chronic blood loss or low energy intakes may increase risk of deficiency.	Consume adequate calories from a variety of nutrient-dense foods with a source of vitamin C to enhance absorption of dietary iron.
Protein, vitamin E, vitamin B_6, zinc	Intakes may be low; decline in immune function.	Meet nutrient needs from low-fat servings of meat, fish, poultry, and legumes; use nuts in moderation; choose at least 6 servings of whole-grain products.
Antioxidants: vitamin C, vitamin E, carotenoids (beta-carotene, lutein)	Decline in vision (cataracts, macular degeneration); increased oxidative stress to body tissues.	Eat at least 5 to 9 servings of fruits and vegetables a day; choose regular servings of green leafy vegetables, brightly colored fruits and vegetables, and citrus fruits; choose whole-grain products; use nuts in moderation.
Vitamin A	Decline in liver's uptake of vitamin A; increased absorption may lower the aging body's requirement.	Avoid supplements of vitamin A.
Vitamin B_{12}	Intakes may be low; reduced gastric acidity impairs absorption of food-bound vitamin B_{12}.	Choose foods fortified with vitamin B_{12} (e.g., breakfast cereals), or take a supplement that contains vitamin B_{12}.
Folate, vitamin B_6, vitamin B_{12}	Intakes may be low, causing elevated blood levels of homocysteine and increased risk of heart disease; use of certain medications may impair B-vitamin status.	Consume citrus and other fresh fruits and green leafy vegetables, legumes, whole grains, and foods fortified with folate and vitamin B_{12} (such as breakfast cereals).

THE SAVVY Diner

Make MyPlate Your Plate (Obj. 12.5)

Proper nutrition is vital for maintaining good health and quality of life in the later years. The MyPlate for Older Adults illustrates the components of a balanced meal pattern based on the *2015–2020 Dietary Guidelines for Americans* that meets the unique needs of older adults. The following tips can help people of any age incorporate healthy choices from each category of MyPlate into their daily meal pattern.[71]

Fruits and Vegetables

- Shop for deeply colored fruits and vegetables, for example:

asparagus	kale
beets	peaches
blackberries	spinach
butternut squash	strawberries
carrots	sweet potatoes
cranberries	tomatoes

- Frozen and canned vegetables are less likely to spoil if not used quickly—be sure to watch for added salt and sugar.
- Sprinkle frozen berries on top of your cereal—they thaw quickly.
- Keep ready-to-eat raw vegetables in a clear container in the front of your refrigerator for snacks.
- Have bags of frozen broccoli, spinach, peppers, or other vegetables available to add to tomato sauce, soups, or stews.
- Keep fruit readily available on the table or counter.
- Try unfamiliar seasonal fruits and vegetables that appear in the market; you may find out there is something you really enjoy!
- Choose a variety of vegetables when dining out.

Grains

- Look for whole grains like:

barley	popcorn
brown rice	quinoa
cornmeal	rye
oats, oatmeal	whole-wheat bread

- When purchasing a grain-based product, read the ingredient list on the label to ensure that "whole grain" is the first ingredient listed.

Dairy Products

- These products are good sources of protein, calcium, and other important nutrients.
- Eat a variety of fat-free and low-fat (1%) dairy products daily, including milk, yogurt, and cheese.
- Substitute nonfat yogurt for cream cheese or sour cream.
- Sweeten nonfat yogurt with fruits.
- Make a smoothie with fresh or frozen fruit and nonfat or low-fat plain yogurt.

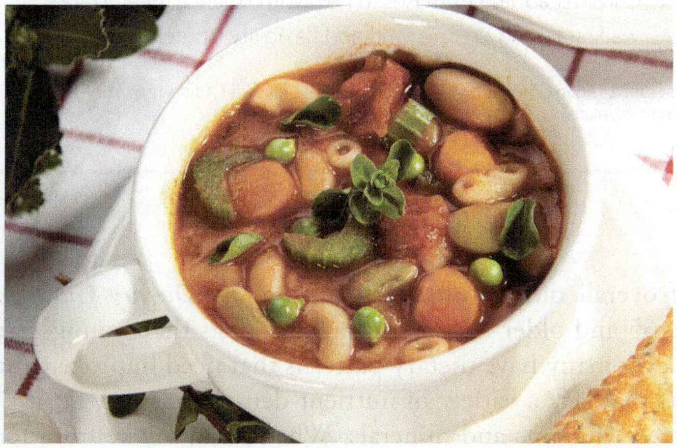

Bochkarev Photography/Shutterstock.com

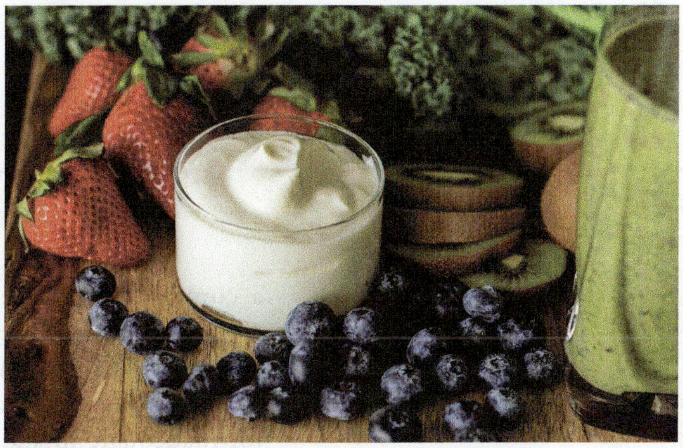

dashkin14/Shutterstock.com

(Continued)

Protein

- Choose a variety of protein-rich foods throughout the week including seafood, lean meats and poultry, eggs, legumes (beans and peas), nuts, seeds, and soy products.
- Prepare protein foods with the least amount of added salt and saturated fat (butter, cheese).
- Try new herbs and spices for added flavor.
- Good sources of lean protein:

fish and shellfish	nut butters
beans (black, kidney, pinto, etc.)	lean meat
eggs	skinless poultry

Healthy Oils

- Substitute liquid oils and soft margarines for solid fats.
- Use oils to dress salads, brown meats, and to sauté vegetables.
- Common liquid oils are:

canola	sesame
olive	soybean
peanut	walnut

Fluids

- Fluids can come from water, tea, coffee, soups, fruits, and vegetables.
- Add lemon, lime, or orange wedges to your container or glass of water to add flavor.
- Think about adding a small bowl of low-sodium soup to dinner or have soup for lunch.
- Increase your intake of fresh fruits and vegetables, especially those that are fluid-filled:

apricots	nectarines
bell peppers	spinach
cherries	strawberries
grapes	tomatoes
lettuce	watermelon

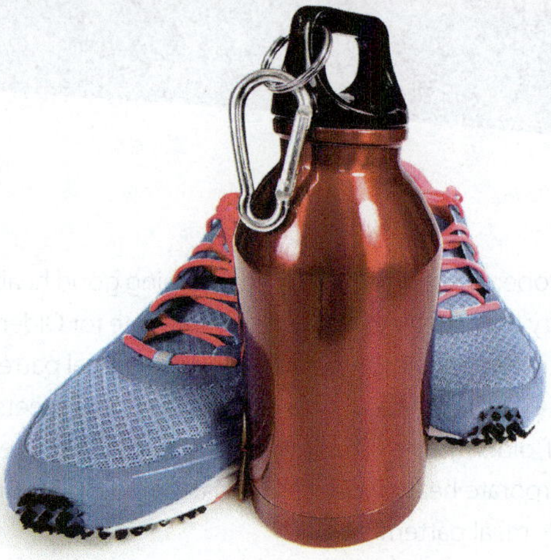

Leena Robinson/Shutterstock.com

- Purchase a refillable water bottle to use throughout the day.
- Drink unsweetened water-based beverages such as coffee or tea.

Physical Activity

- Anyone with a health condition should talk to their doctor to see if this limits their ability to be physically active.
- Aim for at least 150 minutes a week of moderate-intensity aerobic activity like brisk walking, dancing, jogging, swimming, biking, playing tennis.
- Include muscle-strengthening activities at least 2 days a week. Examples include lifting weights, using a resistance band, yoga.
- Find an activity that you enjoy and consider doing it with a partner or a friend.
- Even 10 minutes at a time of moderate-intensity aerobic activity can be beneficial.
- Consider adding exercises to help with balance (heel-to-toe walk, standing on one foot) and flexibility (stretches, yoga).

SOURCE: Adapted from Tufts University, MyPlate for Older Adults http://hnrca.tufts.edu/myplate/

a composite measure of overall dietary quality based on the *Dietary Guidelines for Americans*, adults age 65 and older have better-quality diets than younger and middle-aged adults; however many have dietary patterns that need improvement.

Older adults with diets that lack a variety of nutrient-dense foods may be at risk for inadequate intake of key vitamins and minerals. When usual intake from food and beverages does not meet a person's needs, health care providers may recommend the use of supplements. It is important to assess the intake of all the sources of nutrients such as regular and fortified foods and dietary supplements to be sure that overall consumption is adequate and does not exceed the Tolerable Upper Intake Levels (ULs) of the Dietary Reference Intakes.

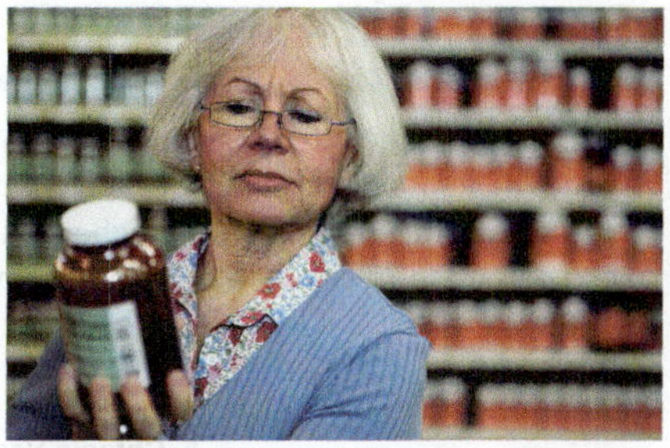
Keith Brofsky/Getty Images

The evidence for using dietary supplements to slow the aging process is not as strong as the evidence supporting a diet rich in fruits, vegetables, and other nutrient-dense foods along with a physically active lifestyle.

Nutrition-Related Problems of Older Adults Although aging is not completely understood, we know that it involves progressive changes in every body tissue and organ: the brain, heart, lungs, digestive tract, and bones. After age 35, functional capacity declines in almost every organ system. Some changes, such as loss of appetite and oral problems, interfere with nutrient intake; others affect absorption, storage, and utilization of nutrients; still others increase the excretion of and need for specific nutrients. Examples of various changes associated with aging that can affect nutritional status include sensory impairments and altered endocrine, gastrointestinal, and cardiovascular functions, as well as changes in the renal and musculoskeletal systems. Both genetic and environmental factors contribute to these declines. Many of the changes are inevitable, but a healthful lifestyle that combines regular physical activity with adequate intakes of all essential nutrients can forestall degeneration and improve the quality of life into the later years.

As a person gets older, the chances of suffering a chronic illness or functional impairment become greater. In the United States, 22 percent of older people in 2014 reported some type of disability (e.g., difficulty in hearing, vision, cognition, communication, mobility, or self-care).[72] A majority of older people have at least one chronic condition, and many have multiple conditions. Among the most frequently occurring conditions in older people are hypertension, diagnosed arthritis, all types of heart disease, any cancer, and diagnosed diabetes (see Figure 12-9).[73] Other chronic conditions contributing to disability include strokes and disorders of vision and hearing. Dementia (especially Alzheimer's disease) is a major contributor to disability and nursing home placement for those over the age of 75. As noted in Table 12-11, malnutrition can occur secondary to these conditions, many of which require special diets that can further compromise nutrition status in the older adult.

Socioeconomic, psychological, and environmental factors can also influence the nutritional status of older adults. Financial resources, living arrangements, and a social support network, including availability of caregivers, can directly affect a person's nutrition status. Poverty and social isolation in particular impair the nutrition status of many older adults. About 9 percent of the population 65 years and older lives in poverty, and the same percentage of seniors living alone experienced food insecurity.[74] Older women are more likely than older men to live in poverty. In addition, older women are almost twice as likely as older men to live alone (36 percent and 20 percent, respectively).[75] In addition, older adults can have difficulties with basic activities (e.g., preparing meals and taking medications). All of these factors place older people at risk for malnutrition (see Table 12-12).

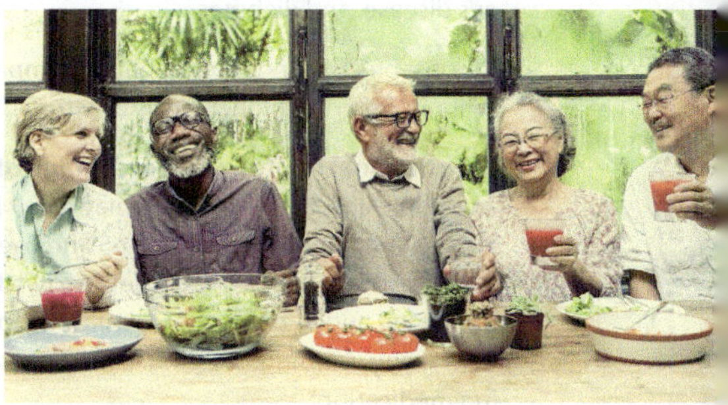
Rawpixel.com/Shutterstock.com

As noted perceptively by a professor of psychiatry:[76]
It is not what the older person eats but with whom that will be the deciding factor in proper care for him. The oft-repeated complaint of the older patient that he has little incentive to prepare food for only himself is not merely a statement of fact but also a rebuke to the questioner for failing to perceive his isolation and aloneness and to realize that food . . . for one's self lacks the condiment of another's presence which can transform the simplest fare to the ceremonial act with all its shared meaning.

Sources of Nutritional Assistance Socioeconomic problems—low income, inadequate facilities for preparing food, lack of transportation, and inability to afford dental care, among others—trouble many older adults and may lead to malnutrition. In response, federal, state, and local agencies have mandated nutrition programs for older adults.

The Supplemental Nutrition Assistance Program (SNAP)—formerly the Food Stamp program—enables people who qualify to obtain electronic benefits in the form of a "credit" card they can use to buy food. In many areas, food banks allow older people on limited incomes to buy good food for less money. A food bank buys industry "irregulars"—products that have been mislabeled, underweighted, redesigned, or mispackaged and would otherwise be thrown away. Nothing is wrong

FIGURE 12-9

Chronic Health Conditions and Functional Limitations in U.S. Older Adults

Aging adults are at increased risk for chronic conditions. The number of people reporting a disability increases with age. Given the size of the baby boom generation, the number of adults with a disability is likely to increase along with the need for appropriate medical and public health services, as the baby boomers enter into higher-risk age groups (≥65 years) over the next decade. Increasing physical activity and reducing or preventing obesity and tobacco use can eliminate some of the underlying causes of disability for some people and prevent secondary conditions in those already affected.

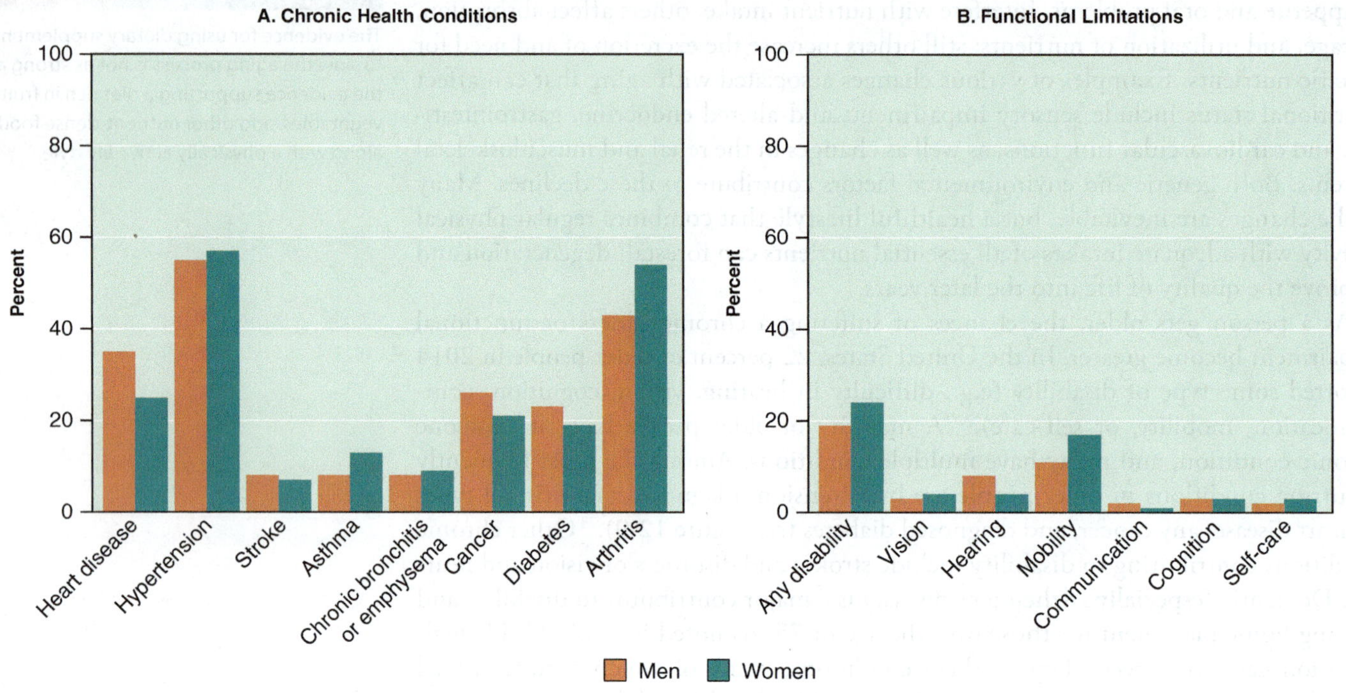

A. Percentage of people age 65 and over who reported having selected chronic health conditions, 2014

The six leading causes of death among people age 65 and over were chronic conditions: heart disease, cancer, chronic lung diseases, stroke, Alzheimer's disease, and diabetes.

Chronic health conditions negatively impact quality of life, contributing to declines in functional status and the inability to live independently. Women reported higher levels of asthma, arthritis, and hypertension than men. Men reported higher levels of heart disease, cancer, and diabetes.

B. Functional limitations: Percentage of people age 65 and over with a disability, 2014[a]

As people age, illness or injury may result in disability, defined by limitations in vision, hearing, mobility, communication, cognition, or self-care. In 2014, 22 percent of people age 65 and over reported having a disability. Women were more likely to report any disability than men (24 percent versus 19 percent). Difficulties with mobility (walking or climbing stairs) were the most commonly reported disability for those age 65 and over (17 percent of women and 11 percent of men). Some of these disabilities may be minor but others cause people to require assistance to perform basic activities of daily living (bathing, dressing, eating, getting around the house) and other related activities (preparing meals, shopping, managing money, and taking medication).

[a] Disability is defined as "a lot" or "cannot do/unable to do" when asked about difficulty with seeing, even if wearing glasses (vision); hearing, even if wearing hearing aids (hearing); walking or climbing steps (mobility); communicating, for example, understanding or being understood by others (communication); remembering or concentrating (cognition); and self-care, such as washing all over or dressing (self-care). Any disability is defined as having difficulty with at least one of these activities.

DATA SOURCE: These data refer to the civilian noninstitutionalized population. Centers for Disease Control and Prevention, National Center for Health Statistics, National Health Interview Survey.

SOURCE: Adapted from Federal Interagency Forum on Aging-Related Statistics, *Older Americans 2016: Key Indicators of Well-Being*, Washington, DC: U.S. Government Printing Office, August 2016.

TABLE 12-11 Malnutrition That Is Secondary to Disease or Physiological State

Disease or Condition	Effects on Nutrition Status
Congestive heart failure	Fluid may accumulate in lungs or abdominal cavity causing shortness of breath, fatigue, chest pain, or nausea leading to loss of appetite.
Cancer	Weight loss, lack of appetite, and secondary malnutrition are common.
Dental and oral disease	May alter the ability to chew and thus reduce dietary intake. Increased likelihood of choking and aspiration.
Depression and dementia	Increased or decreased food intakes are common. A person with dementia may have decreased ability to obtain or prepare food, or the appetite may be very small or very great. Judgment and balance in meal planning may be absent.
Diabetes mellitus	Increased risk of other diet-related diseases.
Emphysema	May be difficult to eat because of breathing problems.
End-stage kidney disease	Alters fluid and electrolyte needs. Infections and low-grade fever may increase energy output and weight loss.
Gastrointestinal disorders	Increased risk of malabsorption of nutrients and consequent undernutrition.
Osteoarthritis	Makes motion difficult, including those activities related to purchasing, serving, eating, and cleaning up after meals. Predisposes people to a sedentary lifestyle and may give rise to obesity.
Osteoporosis	Limits the ability to purchase and prepare food if mobility is affected. If severe scoliosis is present, the appetite may be altered.
Stroke	May alter abilities in the cognitive and motor realms related to food and eating.

SOURCE: B. Shatenstein, Impact of health conditions on food intakes among older adults, *Journal of the Elderly* 27 (2008): 333–61; Position of the Academy of Nutrition and Dietetics: Food and nutrition for older adults: Promoting health and wellness, *Journal of the Academy of Nutrition and Dietetics* 112 (2012): 1255–77; G.B. Huffman, Evaluating and treating unintentional weight loss in the elderly, *American Family Physician* 65 (2002): 640–50.

TABLE 12-12 Factors Influencing Nutritional Status of Older Adults

Physiological	Socioeconomic	Psychological	Environmental
Dietary intake	Cultural beliefs	Cognitive impairment	Inadequate housing
Loss of appetite	Poverty	Dementia	Inadequate cooking facilities
Involuntary weight loss or gain	Limited education	Depression	Lack of transportation
Inactivity/immobility	Limited access to health care	Loss of spouse	Lack of access to health services/programs
Poor taste and smell acuity	Institutionalization	Social isolation	
Alcohol or drug abuse			
Presence of chronic disease			
Polypharmacy (multiple medications)			
Disability			
Oral health problems			
Need of assistance for self-care			

with this food; the industry can credit it as a donation, and the buyer (often a food-preparing site) can obtain the food for a small handling fee and make it available at a greatly reduced price.

The Older Americans Act (OAA) Nutrition Services are intended to improve older people's nutrition status, help them avoid medical problems, and enable them to continue living independently in communities of their own choice. Its specific goals are to provide:

- Low-cost, nutritious meals
- Opportunities for social interaction

- Nutrition education and shopping assistance
- Counseling and referral to other social and rehabilitation services
- Transportation services

The OAA provides funding to the Administration on Aging to support various nutrition programs. Congregate Nutrition Services provides meals and other nutrition services for adults age 60 and over in congregate settings. The congregate meal sites are often community centers, senior centers, religious facilities, schools, extended care facilities, or retirement housing complexes. Additional nutrition-related services such as screenings, assessments, education, and counseling are also provided. Volunteers may also deliver meals to those who are homebound either permanently or temporarily; these efforts are known as the Home-Delivered Nutrition Services. Home-delivered meals are often the first in-home service that an older adult receives and may lead to participation in other types of home- and community-based services. In 2013, 2.4 million older adults received 219 meals—62 percent of meals were home-delivered and 38 percent were served at congregate settings.[77] Evaluations of the congregate and home-delivered meals programs generally show that they improve the dietary intake and nutrition status of their clients.[78] Participants generally have greater diversity in their diets and higher intakes of essential nutrients and are less likely to report food insecurity than nonparticipants. Additional benefits come as a result of screening and the referrals generated by such programs, as well as from the activities associated with the congregate meals: diet counseling, physical activity, adult education, and activities. Participants also benefit from the opportunity for improved socialization.

12.6 Looking Ahead and Aging Wisely

Between 2014 and 2060, the U.S. older population age 65 and older is projected to double. The number of people 85 years and older is anticipated to nearly triple from 6.2 million in 2014 to 14.6 million in 2040.[79] Aging is associated with declines in functional and health status, which can affect one's quality of life; however, studies have shown that a number of older adults feel they are aging successfully.[80] Having a healthy and engaged lifestyle early on in life can support individuals as they approach older age. The goal is to arrive at maturity with as healthy a mind and body as possible; this means cultivating good nutrition status and maintaining a program of daily physical activity. Refer to Figure 12-10 for lifelong habits that can support aging well.

In general, the ability of older adults to function well varies from person to person and depends on several factors. The following "life advantages" seem to contribute to good physical and mental health in later years:

- Genetic potential for extended longevity. Some people seem to have inherited a reduced susceptibility to degenerative diseases.
- A continued desire for new knowledge and new experiences. Some studies suggest that active minds, ever involved in learning new things, may be more resistant to decline.
- Socialization, intimacy, and family integrity. Older people thrive in situations that nurture love, understanding, shared responsibility, and mutual respect.
- Adhering to a healthy eating pattern while avoiding excess food energy, saturated fat, *trans* fat, cholesterol, and sodium. A diet with adequate intakes of all essential nutrients has a positive impact on health and weight management.
- Avoiding substance abuse.

FIGURE 12-10

Successful Aging

The time to prepare for old age is early in life. Practice the "lifelong habits" at the top of the circle to achieve an optimal sense of well-being. Use the other compartments to create a balance among all aspects of your life: nutrition, physical activity, cognitive health, social health, and emotional and spiritual well-being.

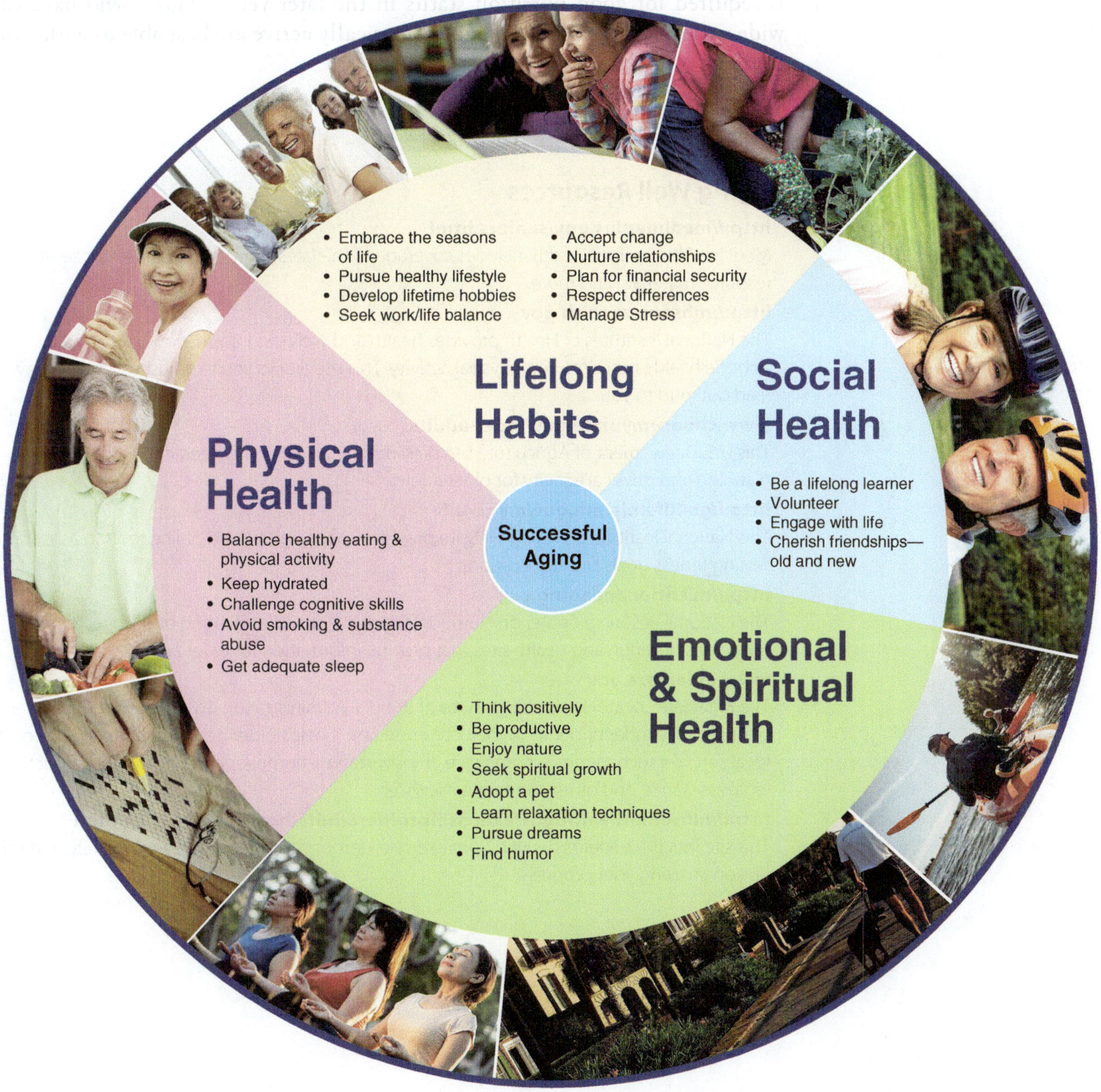

- Acceptable living arrangements.
- Financial independence.
- Access to health care, including a family physician, health clinic, public health nursing service providing home health care, dentist, podiatrist, physical therapist, pharmacist, and registered dietitian.[81]

Everyone knows older people who have maintained many contacts—through relatives, friends, religious institutions, or fraternal orders—and have not allowed themselves to drift into isolation. This favorable environment most likely came from a lifetime of effort. These people spent time reaching out to others and practicing the art of weaving others into their own lives. Likewise, a lifetime of effort is required for good nutrition status in the later years. Those who have eaten a wide variety of foods and remained physically active are best able to withstand the challenges of change.

Aging Well Resources

http://medlineplus.gov/seniors.html
MedLine Plus Seniors' Health includes coverage of the latest news topics on senior health issues, resource materials, and more.

http://nihseniorhealth.gov
The National Institutes of Health provides health and wellness information on many topics, such as bone health, nutrition, and physical activity. This site allows you to adjust text size or have it read out loud to you.

www.choosemyplate.gov/older-adults
This U.S. Department of Agriculture site provides information and interactive tools for meal planning and physical activity for older adults.

http://go4life.nia.nih.gov/mygo4life
This National Institute on Aging website provides coaching tips and online tools to assist in setting fitness goals and track progress.

http://nutritionandaging.org
The National Resource Center on Nutrition, Physical Activity, and Aging offers direct links to numerous nutrition and health sites that provide information for older adults.

www.eldercare.gov
The Eldercare Locator is a public service of the U.S. Administration on Aging to enable older people to live independently in their communities. It helps older people and caregivers locate local services such as meals, home care, transportation, home repair, recreation, social activities, legal assistance, and other community services.

http://nihseniorhealth.gov/exerciseforolderadults/healthbenefits/01.html
This site lists the benefits derived from exercise, demonstrates how to exercise safely, and offers tips on charting your progress.

SPOTLight

12.7 Addressing Weight Problems in Children and Adolescents

"With every healthy meal and snack you provide for kids in your community, you're not just nourishing them today; you are shaping their habits and their tastes for the rest of their lives."

—Former First Lady Michelle Obama at the Let's Move! Cities, Towns and Counties Event, November 16, 2015

For the past three decades, the health status of U.S. children and adolescents has generally improved, as seen in reduced infant mortality rates and a decline in the nutrient deficiency diseases of the past. However, despite the significant decline in obesity rates in preschool-aged children, approximately 17 percent of children and adolescents aged 2 to 19 are obese.[82] The increasing prevalence of overweight is now among the most important public health challenges in the United States.

Exactly how many children are overweight?

Two terms are used to refer to children and adolescents whose excess body weight could pose medical risks:

- *Overweight* is defined as a BMI at or above the 85th percentile and lower than the 95th percentile.
- *Obesity* is defined as a BMI at or above the 95th percentile for children of the same age and sex.

Results from the National Health and Nutrition Examination Survey show that the rate of obesity among children aged 2 to 5 years actually decreased from 13.9 percent in 2003–2004 to 9.4 percent in 2013–2014. Unfortunately, the prevalence in children in the older age groups did not change significantly and remains high.[83] The rate of obesity is greater in certain ethnic and racial groups (particularly Hispanics and non-Hispanic blacks) as well as in certain regions of the country (notably the South). Figure 10-1 in Chapter 10 illustrates the increasing trend toward overweight in U.S. children.

So why should we be concerned?

Overweight in childhood involves significant risks to physical and emotional health. It has been estimated that one in three children born in the United States is at risk for being diagnosed with type 2 diabetes at some point in life. This risk increases for minority children. One out of two children born in 2000 will develop diabetes sometime in life.[84] The same conditions associated with overweight adults, such as type 2 diabetes, high blood lipids, high blood pressure, and gallbladder disease, are now appearing with greater frequency in young children and teens. Overweight children are also at risk for injury to weight-bearing joints, decreased quality of life, depression, poor self-esteem, respiratory problems and sleep disturbances, and other serious health problems. Because overweight children and adolescents are more likely to become overweight and obese adults, experts project that the rate of chronic diseases will skyrocket even higher in the United States if the current rate of overweight and obesity remain unchanged.[85]

What has caused this problem?

The rapid increases in overweight and obesity over the past three decades are due primarily to societal and environmental factors.[86] Factors in the environment that may contribute to overweight include increased calorie intake due to increased portion sizes; increased consumption of foods and meals away from home; excessive consumption of soft drinks; lack of positive role models; and physical inactivity. The way a community is built can affect the availability of a safe place for children to be physically active. Nearly half of the children in the United States do not have parks or playground areas, community centers, sidewalks, or walking paths in their neighborhoods to provide a space for physical activity.[87] Some communities, especially in rural or low-income areas, have limited access to grocery stores and other large food retailers, making it difficult for them to purchase healthy, affordable foods like fresh fruits and vegetables.

What are children and adolescents eating, and how is it affecting their health?

Eating practices influence a child's physical growth, cognitive development, and overall health. Reports from a number of organizations have shown that children are failing to meet the recommended nutrition guidelines by not consuming enough fruits and vegetables and by eating too many foods high in solid fat and added sugars. Children's eating habits have changed over the past three decades. Dietary data, collected in large nationwide surveys to determine trends in nutrient intakes, have shown most children and adolescents have either poor diets or diets that need improvement. Children's consumption of solid fats, added sugars and sodium exceed recommendations. Many children and adolescents consume inadequate amounts of dietary fiber, calcium, vitamin D, and potassium.[88]

Over the past 25 years, the portion sizes of commonly consumed foods, such as soft drinks and hamburgers, have increased. Large food portions that provide more calories than smaller portions may be contributing to the increasing prevalence of overweight in children and teens. For example, children 3 to 5 years of age consumed 25 percent more of an entrée when they were presented with portions that were double an age-appropriate standard size.[89]

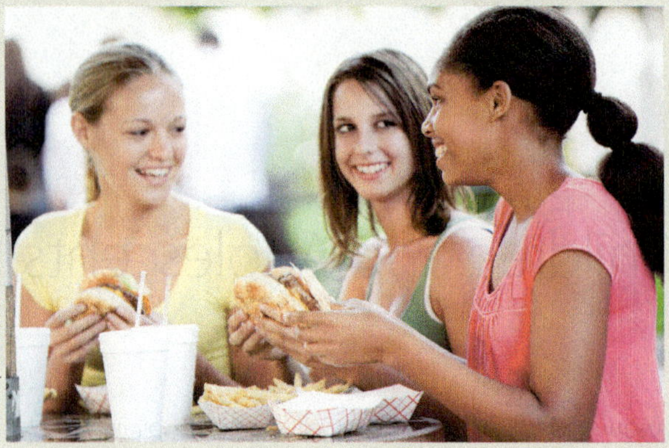

The popularity of fast-food meals poses a challenge to the nutritional quality of diets, because these meals are typically high in saturated fat, sodium, added sugar, and calories and lacking in fruits and vegetables.

Today, many busy parents rely on fast-food meals to nourish their children. Research shows that children who ate fast food consumed more total energy and had poorer diet quality (e.g., more added sugars, more sugar-sweetened beverages, less milk, and fewer fruits and nonstarchy vegetables) on days when they ate fast food, compared to days without fast food.[90]

How does the media factor into this?

Children, especially adolescents, spend a large amount of their leisure time using various media, including television, video games, computers (for social media, gaming), and cell phones. Billions of advertising dollars targeting children and adolescents are spent each year in an effort to influence their food and beverage choices. Food and beverage companies draw from a variety of advanced digital marketing strategies intended to expose young people to advertisements. The majority of the advertisements promote foods and beverages such as candy, fast food, snack foods, soft drinks, and sweetened breakfast cereals that are high in sugar, saturated fat, and sodium and low in essential nutrients. Studies have shown that marketing of foods and beverages influences the nutrition preferences and choices of children, that obese children may be more susceptible to advertising than normal-weight children, and that child-directed advertising could be used to promote healthy foods.[91] In response to the growing concern regarding the impact of the advertising industry on childhood obesity, several major food companies have chosen to join the industry-based Children's Food and Beverage Advertising Initiative (CFBAI). The CFBAI has developed voluntary nutrition guidelines for food and beverage products that are advertised on children's programs. The member companies agree to comply with nutrition criteria that identify healthy nutrition components to promote and to limit calories, saturated fat, sugar, and sodium.[92] This is a positive step for the industry; however, there is more work to be done.

The more time children spend in sedentary behaviors like watching television or using screen-based media, the less time they have for physical activity. Research shows that children who watch television more often had lower activity levels, were less likely to participate in organized sports or community activities, and were more likely to gain excess weight. Parents can encourage physical activity in children, and thereby help prevent overweight, by participating in activities with their children, such as cycling, swimming, rollerblading, skating, and hiking, and helping them find physical activities they enjoy.

What are some simple tips for helping children learn good eating habits?

- Parents can set good examples with their own eating habits.
- Discourage children from eating while watching TV, working/playing on the computer, or doing homework.
- Eat meals together as a family when possible; keep fast-food meals to a minimum.
- Encourage children to "listen to their bodies (stomachs)" and eat only when hungry.
- Limit consumption of high-fat or high-sugar foods, including soft drinks.
- Include children in food purchasing and preparation of meals as a way of helping them become more interested in and aware of what they eat.

Can school food play a role?

The school nutrition environment can have an influence on children's food choices and preferences and the development of healthy dietary habits. Studies have shown that children typically consume more than one-third of their daily calorie intake at school; for the children eating both breakfast and lunch at school, that amount can be close to one-half.[93] The Institute of Medicine's Committee on Accelerating Progress in Obesity Prevention recommends making schools a national focal point for obesity by requiring quality physical education and opportunities for physical activity, ensuring nutritional standards for all foods and beverages in the schools, and ensuring food literacy and skill development.[94]

Since its establishment in 1946, the National School Lunch program has become the second largest food and nutrition assistance program in the United States, feeding millions of children every day. The main goal of the program is to promote the health and well-being of the nation's children by providing nutritious and appealing lunches. Over 72 percent of the 30.5 million lunches served each day are free or reduced price to low-income students.[95] Since 1966 the School Breakfast program has also provided meals to students at participating schools. Like the National School Lunch program, participation in the breakfast program has grown over the years, especially for low-income students. Recent data show that 85 percent of the 14.5 million breakfasts served each day were free or at reduced cost.[96]

Even though school meal programs appeared to have a positive effect on children's consumption of milk, fruit, vegetables, and some vitamins and minerals, early on, there was evidence that school meals contributed excess fat in menu items such as pizza, chicken sandwiches, French fries, and baked goods. The 2010 Healthy, Hunger-Free Kids Act established new standards for school meals based on recommendations from a panel of experts convened by the Institute of Medicine and the *Dietary Guidelines for Americans*. To meet the new nutrition standards, menus now offer both fruits and vegetables each day, offer increased choices of foods rich in whole grains, include only fat-free or low-fat milk varieties, limit calories based on the age of the children, and contain reduced amounts of saturated fat, *trans* fat, and sodium.[97] In 2013 amendments to the Healthy, Hunger-Free Kids Act extended these standards to include foods that are in competition with the school lunch program, such as foods sold à la carte in the cafeteria, from vending machines, or in school stores. Through this regulation, all foods sold on the school campus at any time during the school day are required to meet the competitive food nutrient standards.

Schools participating in the National School Lunch and/or School Breakfast programs are required to develop a school wellness policy to promote a healthy lifestyle in their students. Effective policies provide an integrated program that focuses on nutrition education and promotion, physical activity, and school and community partnerships that promote student wellness.[98] The Yale Rudd Center for Food Policy and Obesity provides a sample model wellness policy that recommends:

- Teachers should integrate nutrition education into core curricula.
- Nutrition promotion should be provided that includes participatory activities such as contests, farm visits, and experience working in school gardens.
- Students should have the opportunity to taste foods that are low in saturated and *trans* fats, sodium, and added sugar.
- Skills such as label reading and meal planning should be developed.
- All K–12 students should receive daily physical education for the entire school year.
- Classroom health education should be provided that reinforces the knowledge and skills needed to maintain a physically active lifestyle.[99]

How can child obesity be prevented?

Prevention of overweight and obesity involves a focus on *energy balance*—calories consumed versus calories expended—so taking action against overweight in childhood must address the factors that influence both eating and physical activity.[100] In general, most interventions for prevention of overweight in children have been conducted through the schools.[101] Effective interventions among children tend to include a component on decreasing the amount of "screen time"—hours spent in front of the television or computer or using other forms of media. School-based programs that increase physical activity also appear effective in reducing body size, especially when physical activity is for an hour or more. Most interventions involve a family component. For small children, the parents are often "gatekeepers" for diet and physical activity because they control the types of foods in the house, the access and availability of those foods, opportunities for activity or inactivity, and meal patterns. In addition, parents often serve as role models for their children. Although family is important for preschool and elementary-aged children, adolescents are often more interested in peer relationships and influences, so interventions for adolescents should include a peer component as well.[102] See the accompanying box for additional recommendations from the Institute of Medicine regarding the prevention of childhood obesity. For additional information, visit the listed websites.

Key Recommendations for the Prevention of Childhood Obesity

- The business community should reduce foods and beverages that are calorie dense and low in nutrients and increase the availability of healthier options at affordable prices.
- Nutrition labeling should be clear and useful so that parents and youth can make informed product comparisons to achieve and maintain energy balance at a healthful weight.
- Marketing by the food, beverage, restaurant, and media industries aimed at children should support a diet that corresponds with the *Dietary Guidelines for Americans* to prevent obesity and risk factors for chronic disease.
- Schools should be a national focal point for obesity prevention by requiring quality physical education, ensuring strong nutritional standards for all foods and beverages sold, and ensuring food literacy and skill development by providing nutrition science education from grades K–12.
- Local governments, schools, and community organizations should collaboratively develop programs that encourage healthful eating behaviors and regular physical activity.
- Local governments, private developers, and community groups should expand opportunities for physical activity, including recreational facilities, parks, playgrounds, sidewalks, and bike paths.[103]

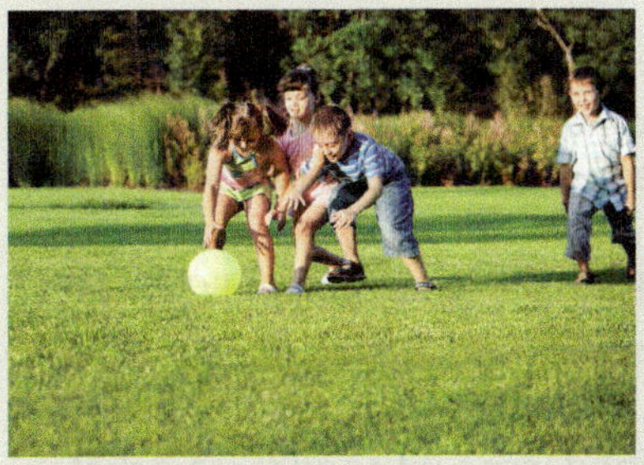

2xSamara.com/Shutterstock.com

Physical activity builds lean muscle and strong bones and decreases the risk of obesity. Children need 60 minutes of play with moderate to vigorous activity every day to grow up to a healthy weight.

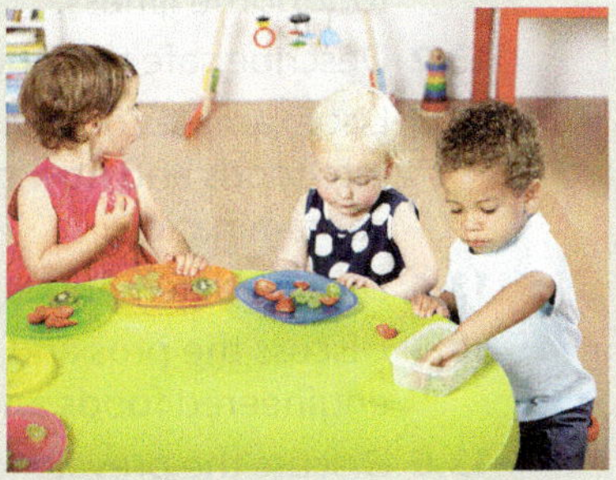

istockphoto.com/Jonas Unruh

Parents and caregivers play a key role in teaching children to make healthy food choices for themselves—for example, choosing colorful fruit slices as an easy snack option.

Websites

- *2015–2020 Dietary Guidelines for Americans:* health.gov/dietaryguidelines/2015
- *USDA General Information and Resources for Weight and Obesity:* www.nal.usda.gov/fnic/general-information-and-resources-weight-and-obesity
- *Center for Disease Control and Prevention Strategies to Prevent Obesity:* www.cdc.gov/obesity/strategies/index.html
- *Center for Disease Control and Prevention Healthy Weight:* www.cdc.gov/healthyweight/index.html
- *Coordinated Approach to Child Health:* www.catchinfo.org
- *Team Nutrition:* www.fns.usda.gov/team-nutrition

WHAT'S ONLINE

MINDTAP From Cengage

Visit www.cengagebrain.com to access MindTap, a complete digital course that includes Diet & Wellness Plus, interactive quizzes, videos, and more.

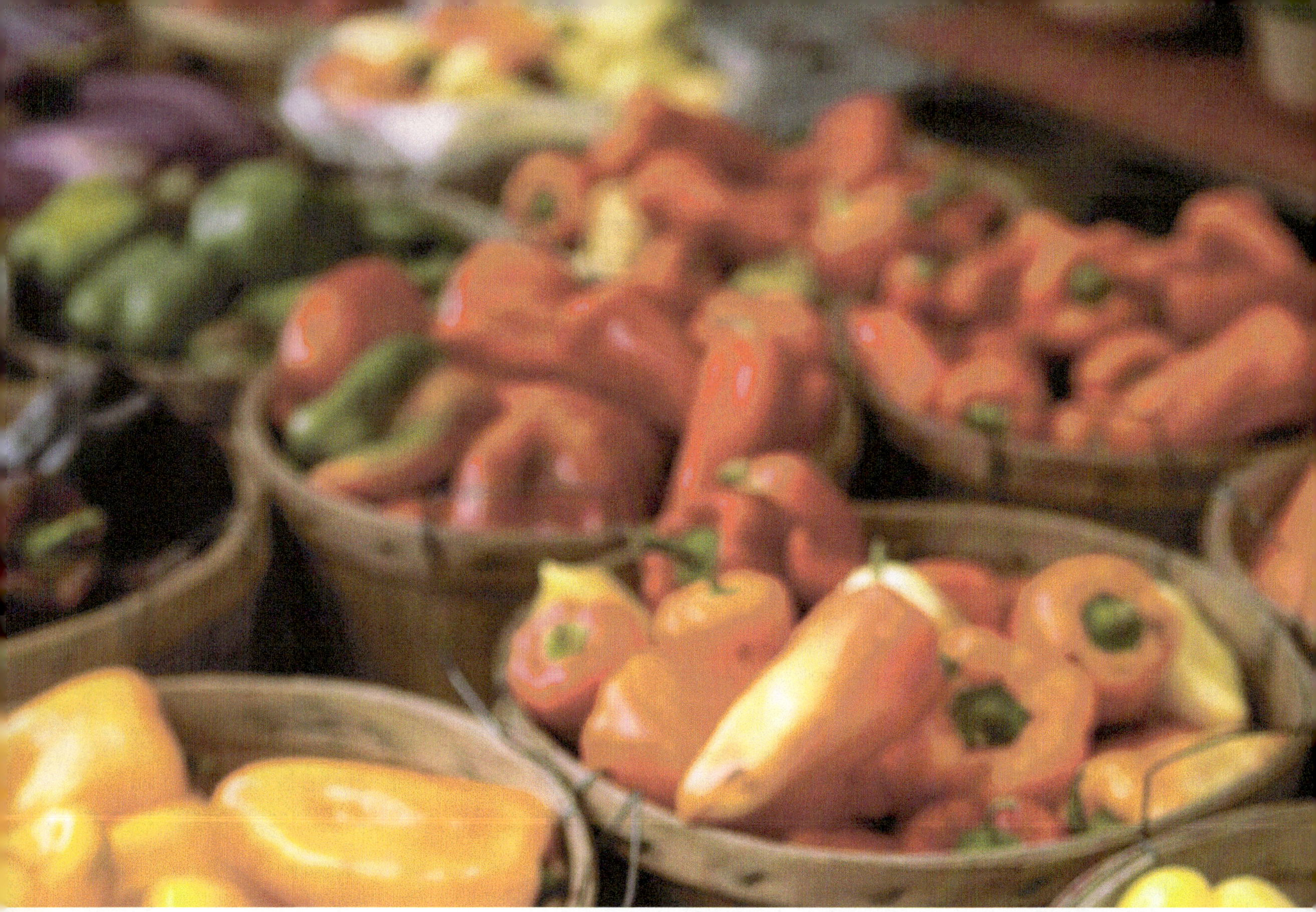

Roderick Chen/Getty Images

AskYourself . . .

Which of the following statements about nutrition are true, and which are false? For each false statement, what is true?

1. Two frequent causes of foodborne illness in homes and restaurants are inadequate cooking and improper cooling of foods.
2. Imported foods may contain residues of pesticides that are illegal in the United States.
3. Lead poisoning ranks as one of the most common childhood environmental health problems.
4. Food insecurity in the United States almost exclusively afflicts unemployed homeless people.

Answers found on page 400.

ChapterObjectives

13.1 Identify common pathogens that cause foodborne infections and intoxications, and list the foods that cause the most cases of foodborne illness.

13.2 Describe safe methods of storage and preparation of food.

13.3 List examples of environmental contaminants that may get into foods and how people can reduce their exposure to contamination.

13.4 Differentiate between intentional and indirect food additives.

13.5 Discuss the pros and cons surrounding irradiation and genetically engineered foods and crops.

13.6 Discuss the prevalence of global food insecurity and factors that contribute to food insecurity.

Food Safety and the Global Food Supply

CHAPTER 13

So far this book has dealt primarily with nutrients and how your body handles them. This chapter takes the study of nutrition one step further and examines some nonnutrient components of food—bacteria, additives, and pesticides, to name a few—and how they affect the food supply. In addition, the chapter takes a global view of the science of nutrition, looking at how foodways in different countries influence each other and how some of our food habits affect the environment.

What additives do foods contain, and what are the effects of those additives? Are foods ever contaminated? How can you reduce your risk of food poisoning? What potential do food technologies, such as irradiation and genetic engineering, hold for our lives and for the health of the environment? This chapter addresses these and other questions.

The role of the infinitely small is infinitely large.

— Louis Pasteur (1822–1895, French chemist and microbiologist who developed the pasteurization process)

13.1 Foodborne Illnesses and the Agents That Cause Them

North America has one of the safest, most plentiful food supplies in the world, thanks to the concerted efforts of food suppliers, food processors, and federal, state, and local governments, all of which are concerned with food safety. North Americans also enjoy the most diverse food supply in the world, consisting of an incredible array of fresh and processed foods. Most American supermarkets stock a variety of foods from other countries: cookies and crackers from Denmark and the United Kingdom, Belgian chocolates, Italian cheeses, beef and veal products from New Zealand and Australia, goose liver paté from France, and specialty foods from Japan, Mexico, and China. Our international food interests can be seen in the produce section as well, where exotic star fruit, papaya, and mango from overseas markets are widely available. Still, the diverse mix of fresh and processed foods coming from local, national, and international markets underscores the need to understand where the culprits behind foodborne illnesses originate.

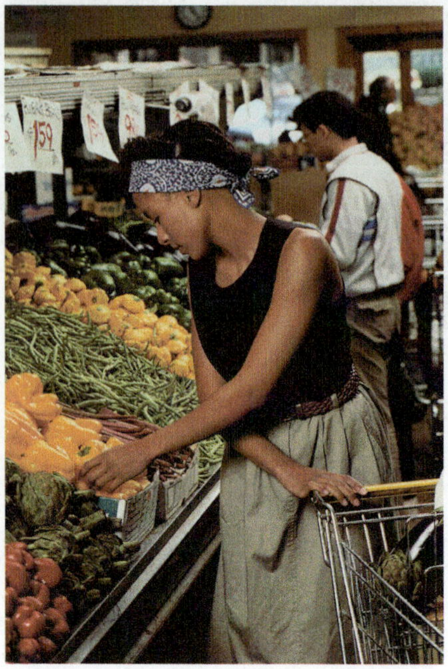
Doug Menuez/Forrester Images/Getty Images

Americans enjoy one of the safest, most diverse food supplies in the world.

Within hours of the September 11, 2001, attacks on the Pentagon and New York City, the nation's food and water supplies were identified as likely targets of terrorists. *Food safety* today refers to a food supply that is free of foodborne pathogens as well as one that is safe from bioterrorism.[1] As part of a heightened awareness of bioterrorism threats, the Food and Drug Administration (FDA) has created a special website that links to information about bioterrorism as well as other information sources. See www.fda.gov/Food/default.htm.

Foodborne illness is one of the greatest concerns of public health experts and the food industry.* According to the Centers for Disease Control and Prevention, as many as 48 million Americans experience foodborne illness each year, 128,000 are hospitalized, and an estimated 3,000 deaths are linked to tainted foods.[2] Incredible as these figures are, they probably represent only a fraction of the whole picture. For a number of reasons, many mild cases of foodborne illness are never reported: Those affected pass off the symptoms as flu and do not seek medical attention, the illness is misdiagnosed as another problem with similar symptoms, the victim fails to recognize food as the source of the illness, or the physician doesn't report the illness to local health agencies. Diarrhea, nausea, abdominal pain, or vomiting without fever or upper respiratory distress is often taken to be flu, but people who experience such symptoms are highly likely to be suffering from foodborne illness.

The fact that more people aren't afflicted with foodborne illness is surprising because disease-producing microorganisms proliferate in our environment. Consider that all raw foods contain microbes, and foods often pick up more microbes during production, processing, packaging, transport, storage, and preparation. For this reason, the food industry uses various control measures to limit the risk of foodborne illness. Bacteria or their spores are destroyed or inactivated by heat treatments such as **pasteurization** and canning. Freezing, dehydrating, and refrigerating food also halt or slow down bacterial growth. In addition, special packaging techniques and antimicrobial preservatives help control food-related pathogens.

What causes most cases of foodborne illness? Many people believe that chemical additives and pesticide residues added during the growing and processing of food pose the greatest risk. However, most foodborne disease is actually caused by mishandling of food, either in food service establishments such as restaurants or in homes. In fact, food from restaurants, cafeterias, and other food service establishments accounts for at least half of all reported outbreaks of foodborne illness, whereas food eaten at home accounts for about one-fourth.[3] Most cases of foodborne disease are caused by faulty handling, cooking, and storing of food long after it has left the manufacturer or processor. Table 13-1 ranks the most common food hazards.

Experts classify foodborne diseases into two types: intoxications and infections. **Food intoxications** occur when a chemical or toxin transmitted by way of food causes the body to malfunction. An example of food intoxication is the vomiting, nausea, abdominal cramping, sweating, and chills that result from eating food contaminated with a strain of bacteria called *Staphylococcus aureus*. This bacterium produces what is known as an **enterotoxin**, a toxin that causes severe gastrointestinal distress. Other types of bacteria can produce **neurotoxins**, or toxins that afflict the nervous system. Food intoxication can also be caused by eating food that has been contaminated with a chemical, such as lead or some other heavy metal.

foodborne illness Illness occurring as a result of ingesting food or water contaminated with a poisonous substance, such as a toxin or chemical (*food intoxication*) or an infectious agent, such as bacteria, viruses, or parasites (*foodborne infection*); commonly called *food poisoning*.

pasteurization The process of sterilizing food via heat treatment.

food intoxications Illnesses caused by eating food that contains a harmful toxin or chemical.

enterotoxin A toxic compound, produced by microorganisms, that harms mucous membranes, as in the gastrointestinal tract (*entero* = intestine).

neurotoxin A poisonous compound that disrupts the nervous system (*neuro* = nerve).

*The FDA Food Safety Modernization Act was signed into law on January 4, 2011. It aims to ensure the U.S. food supply is safe by shifting the focus of federal regulators from responding to contamination to preventing it.

ASK YOURSELF ANSWERS: 1. True. **2.** True. **3.** True. **4.** False. Food insecurity in the United States affects not only the unemployed homeless but also homeowners and the working poor.

TABLE 13-1 **FDA's Rank of Areas of Concern in the Food Supply**

Although most people think that chemicals such as pesticides and additives rank as the most dangerous, illness-producing substances in our food supply, the real hazard comes from naturally occurring bacteria and other microbes.

Most dangerous:

1. Microbial foodborne illness
2. Naturally occurring toxins in foods
3. Residues in foods, including:
   - Environmental contaminants, such as industrial chemicals
   - Pesticide residues
   - Animal drugs, such as hormones or antibiotics
4. Food processing and nutrients in foods

Least dangerous:

5. Intentional food additives approved for use
6. Genetically engineered foods

© Cengage

Foodborne infections, in contrast, occur as a result of eating a food that contains living microorganisms, such as bacteria, viruses, or parasites that are capable of multiplying and thriving in the body. When ingested in large amounts, such microorganisms can wreak havoc in the digestive tract or other areas of the body. An example of this type of foodborne illness is infection with *Vibrio* bacteria, which often reside in raw seafood such as oysters and clams. Inside the body, the bacteria settle in quickly and cause abrupt onset of chills, fever, or vomiting. The following section provides an overview of the various agents that can cause a foodborne illness, be it intoxication or an infection.

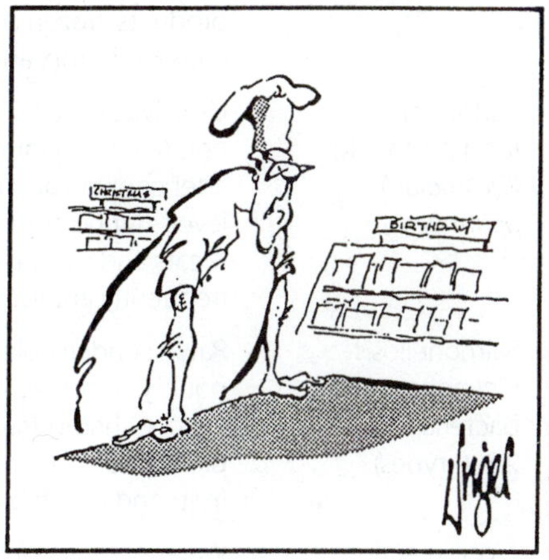

"I need 148 get-well cards."

LaughingStock Licensing Inc.

Microbial Agents

When we order a meal at a restaurant or reach for an egg or glass of milk from the refrigerator at home, we don't usually think about the microorganisms that might be lurking in the foods or their potential to cause illness. We tend to assume that the foods and beverages we consume are safe to eat or drink. Granted, most of the time we don't need to worry. Typically, a food must harbor thousands of microorganisms before it causes nausea, diarrhea, cramps, or other symptoms of foodborne illness. What's more, a healthy body can usually defend itself against small amounts of the "bad bugs."

However, when proper food-handling procedures are not followed carefully, the risk of food poisoning from bacteria or other microbial agents soars. When food items are not cooked or stored properly, they provide the perfect medium in which microorganisms can flourish. For children, older adults, people with compromised immune systems, and other vulnerable people, it might take only small amounts of the offending microorganisms to cause trouble. Table 13-2 summarizes the common food sources of the microbial agents responsible for most outbreaks of foodborne illness.

Among the 31 known foodborne pathogens:

- *Salmonella*, *Toxoplasma*, *Listeria*, norovirus, and *Campylobacter* contribute to the most deaths.
- *Salmonella,* norovirus, *Campylobacter, Toxoplasma,* and *E. coli* contribute to the most hospitalizations.
- Norovirus, *Salmonella*, *Clostridium*, *Campylobacter,* and *Staphylococcus* contribute to the most illnesses.[4]

foodborne infections Illnesses caused by eating a food containing bacteria or other microorganisms capable of growing and thriving in a person's tissues.

TABLE 13-2 Microbial Food Agents: Organisms that Can Bug You

Disease and Organism that Causes It	Source of Illness	Onset and Symptoms	Prevention
Bacteria			
Botulism (*Botulinum* toxin produced by *Clostridium botulinum* bacteria)	Improperly canned foods, especially vegetables (corn, beets, asparagus, mushrooms, peppers), tuna, and liver paté; also found in luncheon meats, ham, sausage, stuffed eggplant, lobster, smoked fish, bottled garlic, and herb-flavored oils.	Onset: 4–72 hours. Vomiting, diarrhea, double vision, muscle weakness, speech and swallowing difficulties, progressive paralysis of the respiratory system. Often fatal.	Do not use damaged canned foods or canned foods showing signs of swelling, leakage, punctures, holes, denting, or extensive deep rusting. Do not feed honey to infants. Follow guidelines for canning low-acid foods.
Campylobacteriosis (*Campylobacter jejuni*)	Raw or undercooked poultry, meat, eggs, and unpasteurized milk, contaminated water.	Onset: 2–5 days. Diarrhea, abdominal cramps, fever, vomiting, sometimes bloody stools. Lasts 2–10 days.	Cook meat and poultry to a safe temperature; use pasteurized milk/milk products; wash hands and use safe food handling practices.
Listeriosis (*Listeria monocytogenes*)	Fresh soft cheeses, raw meat and seafood, unpasteurized milk, deli meats, hot dogs, imported seafood products, frozen cooked crabmeat, cooked shrimp, and cooked surimi.	Onset: 9–48 hours (though symptoms can strike 2–6 weeks after eating). Fever, muscle aches, headache, nausea, diarrhea, and vomiting.	Cook raw meat, poultry, and seafood to a safe temperature; prevent cross-contamination; wash hands before and after handling raw meat, poultry, seafood, and egg products. Use pasteurized milk/milk products.
Perfringens food poisoning (*Clostridium perfringens*)	Usually caused by failure to keep food hot. A few organisms are often present after cooking and multiply to toxic levels during cooldown and storage. Meats and meat products are most frequently implicated.	Onset: 8–12 hours. Abdominal pain and diarrhea and sometimes nausea and vomiting.	Keep hot food hot and cold food cold! Once food is cooked, it should be held hot, at an internal temperature of 140°F or above. Discard all perishable foods left at room temperature longer than 2 hours; 1 hour in temperatures above 90°F.
Salmonellosis (*Salmonella* bacteria—over 2,300 types)	Raw or undercooked eggs, meats, poultry, unpasteurized milk or juice, cheese, shrimp, frog legs, yeast, coconut, pasta, chocolate, contaminated raw fruits and vegetables.	Onset: 6–48 hours. Nausea, abdominal cramps, diarrhea, fever, and headache.	Cook raw meat, poultry, and egg products to a safe temperature. Do not eat raw or undercooked eggs. Use pasteurized milk. Wash produce thoroughly.
E. coli infection (shiga toxin-producing *E. coli* [STEC] released by *Escherichia coli* O157:H7 and others)	Water or food contaminated with human feces. Undercooked ground beef, unpasteurized milk and juice, raw apple cider, mayonnaise, raw fruits and vegetables.	Onset: 1–8 days. Abdominal cramps, vomiting, nausea, bloody diarrhea, fever, and, in severe cases, kidney failure, strokes, and seizures.	Cook hamburgers and ground beef to a safe temperature of 160°F. Drink only pasteurized milk, juice, or cider. Rinse fruits and vegetables under running tap water. Wash your hands with soap and warm water after changing diapers or using the bathroom.
Shigellosis (*Shigella* bacteria)	Raw produce, contaminated drinking water, uncooked foods and cooked foods that are not reheated after contact with an infected food handler.	Onset: 4–7 days. Abdominal cramps, diarrhea, fever, sometimes vomiting, and blood and mucus in stools.	Always wash your hands with soap and warm water for 20 seconds before handling food and after using the bathroom, changing diapers, or having contact with an infected person.
Staphylococcal food poisoning (staphylococcal toxin produced by *Staphylococcus aureus* bacteria)	Toxin produced when food contaminated with the bacteria is left too long at room temperature. Meats, poultry, egg products, tuna, potato and macaroni salads, puddings, and cream-filled pastries are good environments for these bacteria to produce toxin.	Onset: 1–6 hours. Sudden onset of severe nausea, diarrhea, vomiting, abdominal cramps. Fever may be present.	Because the toxins produced by this bacterium are resistant to heat, preventing the contamination of food before the toxin can be produced is important. Keep hot food hot (over 140°F) and cold food cold (40°F or below). Wash hands with warm water and soap, and follow safe food handling practices.
Vibrio infection (*Vibrio vulnificus*)	The bacteria live in coastal waters and can infect humans either through open wounds or through consumption of contaminated undercooked or raw seafood (especially oysters).	Onset: 1–7 days. Chills, fever, abdominal cramps, vomiting, diarrhea. Can be fatal to people with liver disease or impaired immunity.	Do not eat raw oysters or other raw shellfish; cook shellfish (oysters, clams, mussels) thoroughly. Prevent cross-contamination by separating cooked seafood and other foods from raw seafood. Refrigerate food within 2 hours after cooking.

TABLE 13-2	Microbial Food Agents: Organisms that Can Bug You *(continued)*		
Disease and Organism that Causes It	**Source of Illness**	**Onset and Symptoms**	**Prevention**
Parasite			
Cryptosporidiosis (*Cryptosporidium parvum*)	Swimming in or drinking contaminated water; contaminated raw fruits and vegetables, unpasteurized milk, juices, and ciders.	Onset: 2–10 days. Diarrhea, nausea, fever; can be symptomless.	Wash hands and follow safe food handling practices. Do not drink untreated water from shallow wells, lakes, rivers, and streams.
Toxoplasmosis (*Toxoplasma gondii*)	Raw or undercooked contaminated meat (especially pork, lamb, and venison) or oysters, mussels, or clams; contaminated water or unwashed produce; unpasteurized goat's milk.	Onset: 7–21 days. Fever, headache, swollen glands, muscle pain, stiff neck.	Cook foods thoroughly; use safe food handling practices. Wash hands with soap and warm water after gardening or contact with soil.
Giardiasis or "traveler's diarrhea" (*Giardia intestinalis*)	Contaminated water, or may be transmitted by uncooked foods that become contaminated while growing or after cooking by infected food handlers.	Onset: 12 hours to several days. Sudden onset of explosive watery stools, abdominal cramps, anorexia, nausea, and vomiting.	Wash your hands before, during, and after preparing food and after changing diapers or going to the bathroom. Avoid water that might be contaminated.
Virus			
Hepatitis (hepatitis A virus)	Raw produce, contaminated drinking water, shellfish from contaminated waters, uncooked foods and cooked foods that are not reheated after contact with an infected food handler.	Onset: 15–50 days. Malaise, appetite loss, nausea, vomiting, and fever. After 3–10 days, person develops jaundice. Severe cases can cause liver damage and death.	Wash hands thoroughly after using the bathroom, changing diapers, and before preparing or eating food.
Norovirus or "stomach flu"*	Raw produce, contaminated drinking water, salads, sandwiches, or other foods contaminated by infected food handlers; raw oysters and other shellfish from contaminated waters.	Onset: 12–48 hours. Headache, fever, nausea, vomiting, diarrhea, abdominal pain.	Use safe food handling practices.

*A misnomer; unrelated to influenza.

SOURCES: Adapted from A. Hecht, *The Unwelcome Dinner Guest: Preventing Foodborne Illness* (Washington, DC: U.S. Government Printing Office, DHHS Publication No. (FDA) 91-2244); and USDA, FSIS, *Foodborne Illness: What Consumers Need to Know*.

Symptoms of the illness caused by *Campylobacter jejuni*, called campylobacteriosis, usually begin 2 to 5 days after the contaminated food is eaten and last for 2 to 10 days. Many cases of campylobacteriosis probably go unreported because the illness's characteristic diarrhea, abdominal pain, and fever mimic flulike gastrointestinal ills.

In the past, egg products were a major source of salmonellosis—an illness caused by *Salmonella* bacteria. However, this is no longer the case, because of the mandatory pasteurization of eggs used in the commercial preparation of ice cream, baked goods, and other egg-containing food products. Eggs sold commercially are washed and sanitized before packing, however, some raw eggs have been implicated in outbreaks of salmonellosis, as has raw, unpasteurized milk. (Because of this concern, the sale of raw milk is banned in most states.) Today, most outbreaks of salmonellosis are caused by faulty handling of raw meat and poultry, unpasteurized juice, and contaminated fresh, raw produce.

Staphylococcus aureus is another strain of bacteria responsible for many of the reported cases of foodborne illnesses that occur in the United States. The bacterium, found in the nose and throat and on the skin of most people, can be transmitted to

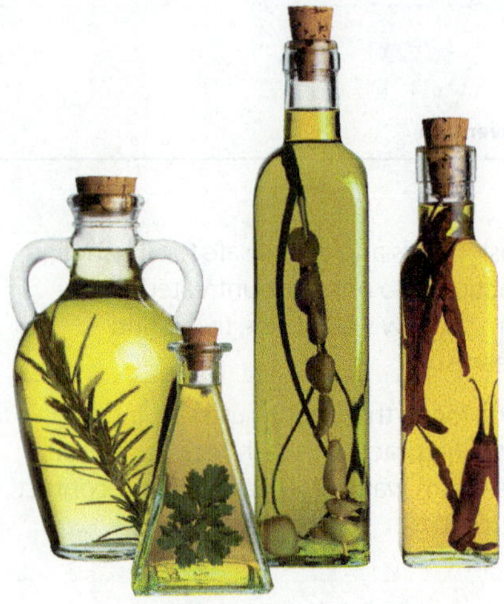
C Squared Studios/Getty Images

Covered, bottled garlic in oil left at room temperature provides the perfect warm, oxygen-free, low-acid environment for the toxin-releasing spores of *Clostridium botulinum*.

food when an individual with an infected wound or boil or a respiratory infection handles food improperly. The bacterium itself isn't directly responsible for the illness, however. Rather, it produces staphylococcal enterotoxin, which causes food poisoning within 1 to 6 hours of eating a contaminated food. The foods typically implicated in *S. aureus* intoxication include meat and poultry products, egg products, tuna, potato and macaroni salads, and cream-filled pastries.

Another particularly deadly foodborne pathogen is *Clostridium botulinum*, the agent that causes the nausea, vomiting, dizziness, and muscle paralysis known as *botulism*. This severe illness results from eating food in which the bacterium has flourished and produced a neurotoxin. The toxin binds irreversibly to nerve endings and causes progressive paralysis, which makes swallowing and breathing difficult. Botulism typically develops within 4 to 36 hours of eating the contaminated food. Because it can be fatal, botulism requires immediate medical attention.

Spores of *C. botulinum* are ubiquitous, having been detected in everything from shellfish to fruits and vegetables to honey to corn syrup.* However, the *botulinum* bacteria produce the deadly neurotoxin only if they are in a warm, oxygen-free, low-acid environment. That's why improperly sterilized, low-acid canned goods are the most common culprits in cases of botulism. Note also that trendy oils flavored with garlic or herbs can harbor *C. botulinum*. Manufacturers of such mixtures must add antibacterial agents to their preparations, but people who make their own flavored oils should be sure to store them in the refrigerator.

Another especially virulent pathogen that is a major public health concern is *Escherichia coli* O157:H7.** First recognized as a cause of foodborne illness in 1982, *E. coli* garnered national attention about a decade later when it caused a major outbreak of foodborne illness in the northwest part of the United States. Undercooked, contaminated hamburgers sold at a major fast-food chain prompted the scare, which ultimately led to more than 500 reported cases of illness, some 150 hospitalizations, and 3 deaths. The outbreak sparked a national debate about the safety of the U.S. meat and poultry supply.[5]

Found in the intestinal tracts of mammals, *E. coli* is usually transmitted via animal feces. It poses special concern because it is so dangerous. Unlike most other illness-producing microorganisms, *E. coli* need not be present in large numbers to make a person sick; just a few bacteria seem to do the trick. Once ingested, the bacterium clings to the intestinal wall, where it releases an enterotoxin that causes abdominal pain and watery diarrhea that often turns bloody. In vulnerable people, such as children and older adults, *E. coli* may cause serious complications, including kidney failure and death.

Most *E. coli* outbreaks have been linked to undercooked beef, particularly hamburger. Some contaminated fresh produce (Alfalfa sprouts, spinach) raw milk, and fresh apple cider, presumably made from apples exposed to tainted animal manure, have also been implicated in more recent outbreaks.[6] As with all illness-causing microorganisms, the best defense against *E. coli* is careful food handling.

Mold is another potential microbial food contaminant. Certain molds produce poisonous compounds called **aflatoxins**. These compounds are powerful liver toxins in animals, are known to be carcinogenic in some species, and can be lethal if consumed in large doses. Aflatoxins have been found on peanuts, wheat, corn, meat pies, dry beans, and even refrigerated and frozen pastries. Molds that produce the

aflatoxins Poisonous toxins produced by molds.

*Honey has been found to contain dormant bacterial spores, which can awaken in the human body to produce botulism. In adults, this is not a hazard, but infants under 1 year of age should never be fed honey. Honey has been implicated in several cases of sudden infant death.

***Escherichia coli* O157:H7 is a particular strain of *E. coli* bacteria. When *E. coli* is mentioned throughout the rest of this chapter, it refers to the O157:H7 strain.

aflatoxins typically flourish when foods such as corn and peanuts get wet and are then stored in a warm place, such as a grain silo or railroad boxcar. Control of aflatoxins in food is difficult, but it is given high priority by the food industry and regulatory agencies.

To be sure, not all microorganisms are bad. A mold called *Penicillium roquefortii* imparts the special, pungent flavor of Roquefort cheese. Another mold strain, *P. camembertii*, lends flavor to Camembert cheese. Likewise, a strain of mold called *Acetobacter* causes the alcohol in wine and hard cider to turn to vinegar.[7] What's more, yogurt owes its existence to active cultures of bacteria added during processing, and a new area of research—called probiotics—suggests that the "good bugs" in the yogurt may help fight "bad bugs" that cause yeast infections and other ills.[8]

Natural Toxins

Most people assume that products derived from plants are safe because they are "natural." Nevertheless, natural food **toxicants** in plants—especially herbs—are sometimes to blame for poisonings. Even familiar foods that are generally safe sometimes harbor potential toxicants. For example, potatoes contain a substance called *solanine*, a powerful inhibitor of nerve impulses. The green substance accumulates just beneath the vegetable's skin, usually in harmless amounts. When potatoes are exposed to light, however, they sometimes develop excess solanine. When this happens, the green area and about one-half inch of potato around it should be removed before cooking.

When plants are transformed into powders and potions, their components become more concentrated, as do their potentially harmful effects. Nevertheless, people often assume that because they come from plants, these substances must be safe. Unlike the chemical composition of standard pharmaceutical drugs, however, the composition of herbal products is not regulated—by the government or anyone else. This lack of safety standards for herbal pills, powders, teas, and other potions, which have become increasingly popular in recent years, ranks as a major concern among public health officials. The potential risks are amplified when an herb is mislabeled, misidentified, or mixed with another potentially toxic substance.

For example, several children and adults suffered life-threatening respiratory problems and liver malfunctions as a result of taking a Chinese herb called Jin Bu Huan. Investigators found, among other problems, that the plant from which the product was derived had been misidentified and that the product carried false and misleading medical claims.[9] Along the same lines, the FDA has banned the use of a plant derivative called ma huang, which contains ephedrine (an amphetamine-like substance often used in weight-loss products) because it has been linked to rapid heart rate, stroke, nerve damage, and several deaths.[10]

These are just a few of the herb-related problems that continue to surface. They highlight the need to be cautious about using herbs of any sort. Adults should not take large amounts of a particular herbal product or take more than one product at a time without consulting a competent professional regarding the various effects of that product. Pregnant and breastfeeding women should avoid using herbs because they can expose a fetus or an infant to a toxic dose.[12] In addition, people with any type of liver disease or condition should be wary of herbal products; liver failure is one of the hallmarks of an herbal overdose, because toxins accumulate in that organ.

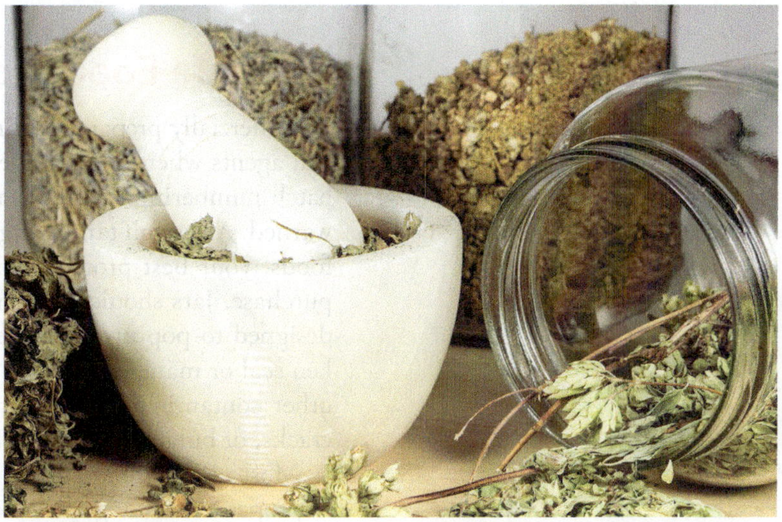

Alonso Aguilar/Shutterstock.com

Numerous herbs have been implicated in liver failure and other health problems. Here are just a few:

- Chaparral
- Kava
- Jin Bu Huan
- Ma huang
- Germander
- Comfrey
- Mistletoe
- Skullcap
- Margosa oil
- Maté tea
- Gordolobo yerba tea
- Pennyroyal (squawmint) oil[11]

See Chapter 7 for more information about herbal remedies.

toxicants Poisons; that is, agents that cause physical harm or death when present in large amounts.

In addition to plant foods, other types of food, notably seafood, often harbor natural toxicants. For example, a type of fish called puffers, long considered a delicacy in Japan, contains a potent poison—tetrodotoxin—which doesn't harm the fish but can be lethal to people and other animals. Tetrodotoxin, which is 275 times deadlier than cyanide, works by blocking nerve impulses. Over a period of several hours, it eventually closes down a person's entire nervous system. The toxin is so deadly that sale of puffers is illegal in the United States.[13]

Puffer poisoning is just one example of a foodborne disease traced to eating a toxic sea creature; there are others as well. For instance, paralytic shellfish poisoning can occur after eating mollusks (clams, mussels, oysters, and scallops) contaminated with marine algae that produce a neurotoxin. The mollusks themselves don't become ill; but people who eat them do, experiencing such symptoms as nausea, vomiting, cramps, and muscle weakness. In each of these cases, the toxin is not destroyed by the heat of cooking. Fish can also harbor viruses, including hepatitis viruses, worms, and other parasites. For these reasons, it is especially important to buy seafood from reputable vendors and to handle it with care.

13.2 Safe Food Storage and Preparation

Commercially prepared, canned, or packaged food is usually free of harmful microbial agents when it leaves the manufacturer. When a batch of food is contaminated, batch numbering ensures that it can be recalled quickly, and the public can be forewarned. Although tampering with food products is unlikely to occur in grocery store foods, your best protection is to carefully inspect the seals and wrappers of every purchase. Jars should be firmly sealed (many have safety buttons—areas of the lid designed to pop up once opened). Packages should be free of holes or tears. A broken seal or mangled package does not provide protection against microorganisms or other contaminants. Likewise, do not purchase any canned goods that have dents, cracks, or bulges, which can indicate possible contamination with *C. botulinum*.

Most cases of food poisoning occur in the home or the restaurant and are caused by improper food storage or handling (see Table 13-3). Food poisoning caused by kitchen mistakes can be avoided by doing three simple things: keep cold food cold; keep your hands, the utensils, and the kitchen clean; and keep hot food hot. Most bacteria flourish in warm environments, but heat kills them and cold temperatures halt their growth.

Keep Cold Foods Cold The first step, keeping cold food cold, starts when you leave the grocery store. If you are running errands in a car, do the grocery shopping last so that the food does not stay in the car too long, especially in hot weather. As soon as

TABLE 13-3 Common Food Safety Mistakes

- Excessive store-to-refrigerator lag time
- Not washing hands before food handling
- Unclean equipment or utensils
- Countertop thawing
- Room-temperature marinating
- Using same spoon to stir and taste
- Cross-contamination:
  - Using the same board or knife to cut raw meat and vegetables or fruits
  - Using the same plate for raw and cooked foods
- Inadequate cooking or reheating
- Failure to keep hot foods at high temperature
- Improper cooling: leftovers and "doggie bags" left out

you get home, put foods in a refrigerator set at 40 degrees Fahrenheit or a freezer kept at 0 degrees Fahrenheit, and be sure not to leave food in the refrigerator too long before eating it (see Figure 13-1). Place packages of raw meat, poultry, or fish on a plate before refrigerating, or store them in plastic storage bags to prevent bacteria-containing juices from dripping onto other foods. Thaw frozen food in the refrigerator or microwave oven—not on the kitchen counter. Because bacteria can multiply at room temperature, they can thrive in the relatively warm exterior of a food before the interior has thawed.

Wash Hands and Surfaces Often Along with keeping foods properly chilled, keeping the kitchen clean prevents contamination of otherwise wholesome foods. Before you handle food, wash your hands in warm, soapy water. In addition, be sure to wash your hands after touching meat, poultry, or fish to prevent the spread of any bacteria that your hands have picked up. Likewise, keep countertops and all kitchen equipment clean with soap and hot water. Because bacteria love to nestle down in the fibers of kitchen cloths, sponges, and wooden cutting boards, take particular care to keep such items clean.

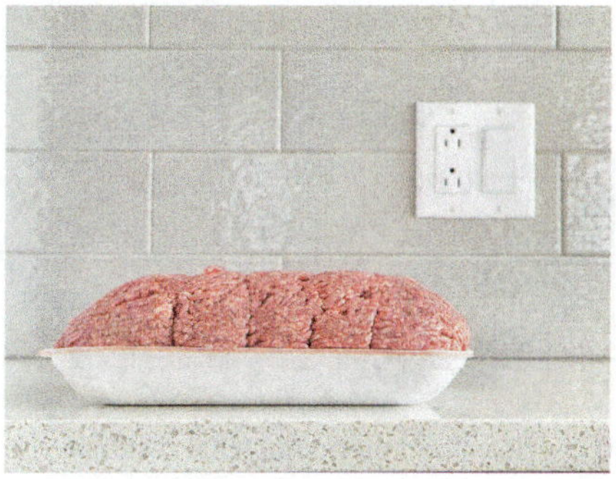

DD Images/Shutterstock.com

Follow food safety recommendations when preparing and eating foods to reduce the risk of foodborne illnesses. Never thaw food on a kitchen counter. Bacteria can flourish at room temperature.

FIGURE 13-1

Take Control of Home Food Safety

Was it a 24-hour bug? Or something you ate? Very often what seems like the flu may be foodborne illness. The following four simple actions will help you take control of food safety in your kitchen.

SOURCE: Adapted from the Academy of Nutrition and Dietetics and the ConAgra Foundation's *Home Food Safety . . . It's In Your Hands* program. For more information, visit www.homefoodsafety.org and www.fightbac.org.

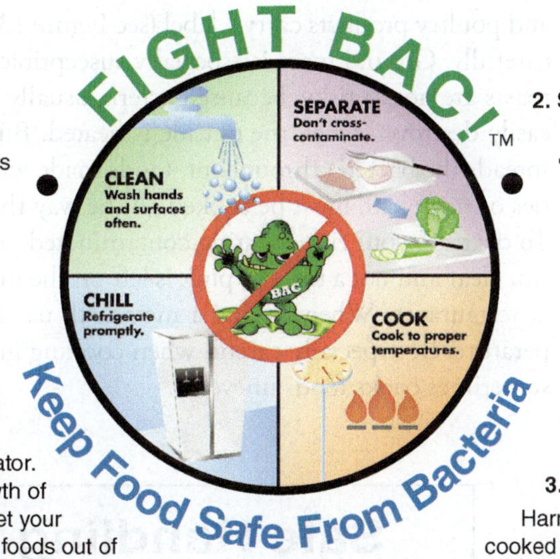

1. CLEAN: Wash Hands and Surfaces Often Using Hot Soapy Water.

Hand washing may eliminate half of all cases of foodborne illness and reduce the spread of the common cold and flu.

- Wash hands in warm, soapy water for a minimum of 20 seconds before preparing foods and after handling raw meat, poultry, and seafood.

2. SEPARATE: Keep Raw Meats and Ready-to-Eat Foods Separate.

- Never work with raw meat, poultry, or seafood on the same surface that you use for other foods without cleaning the surface after you've finished.
- Use different cutting boards: one to cut raw meat, poultry, and seafood and another for ready-to-eat foods, such as breads and vegetables. Discard old cutting boards that have cracks, crevices, and excessive knife scars.

3. COOK: Cook to Proper Temperatures.

Harmful bacteria are destroyed when food is cooked to proper temperatures. Buy a meat thermometer and use it!

4. CHILL: Refrigerate Promptly Below 40°F.

- Defrost foods in the refrigerator or in the microwave. Marinate foods in the refrigerator. Refrigerate foods quickly to slow the growth of bacteria and prevent foodborne illness. Set your refrigerator below 40°F to keep perishable foods out of the "danger zone"—40° to 140°F.

General Guidelines for Leftovers

Perishable food	Keeps up to
Cooked fresh vegetables	3–4 days
Cooked pasta	3–5 days
Cooked rice	1 week
Deli counter meats	5 days
Greens	1–2 days
Meat	
Ham, cooked and sliced	3–4 days
Hot dogs, opened	1 week
Lunch meats, prepackaged, opened	3–5 days
Cooked beef, pork, poultry, fish, meat casseroles	3–4 days
Cooked patties and nuggets, gravy and broth	1–2 days
Seafood, cooked	2 days
Soups and stews	3–4 days
Stuffing	1–2 days

When in doubt, throw it out!

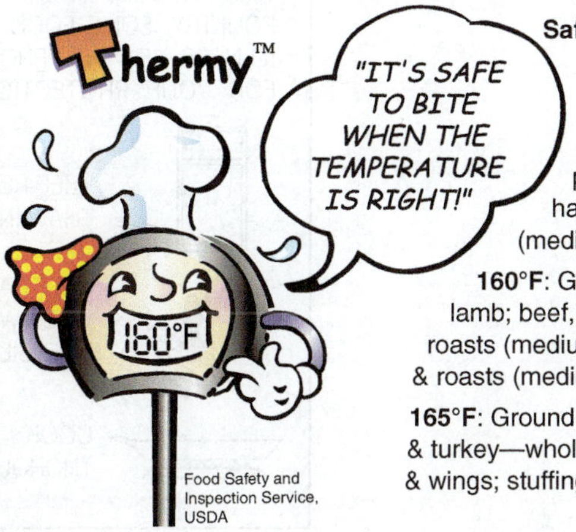

Safe Cooking Temperatures

140°F: Ham, fully-cooked (to reheat)

145°F: Beef, lamb, veal & pork (includes raw cured ham) steaks, chops, roasts (medium rare), fish

160°F: Ground beef, pork, veal & lamb; beef, lamb & veal steaks & roasts (medium-done); pork chops, ribs & roasts (medium-done); egg dishes

165°F: Ground chicken & turkey; chicken & turkey—whole bird, breasts, legs, thighs & wings; stuffing & casseroles; leftovers

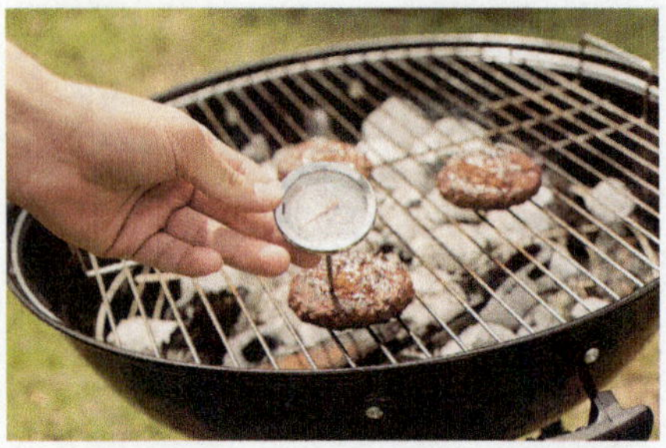

ESB Professional/Shutterstock.com

Use a clean food thermometer to test that the internal temperature has reached 160°F when cooking hamburgers or 165°F when baking a meat loaf or casserole or warming up leftovers. Allow meat to rest for at least 3 minutes before carving or consuming because its temperature can continue to rise and destroy pathogens during that time frame.

Keep Hot Foods Hot Keeping hot food hot means first cooking food thoroughly to ensure that the heat destroys any bacteria that might have been present in the uncooked food. See Figure 13-1 for proper cooking temperatures. After cooking, foods must be kept hot at 140 degrees Fahrenheit or above until serving to prevent bacterial growth. Never leave perishable food at room temperature for more than 2 hours. Before refrigerating a large quantity of hot food, such as a pot of chili or a large casserole, divide it up and place it in shallow containers to allow easy cooling. Otherwise the food inside the pot may stay warm for a dangerously long time, even in the refrigerator.

Prevent Cross-Contamination Meat, poultry, and fish require special handling because they often harbor high levels of bacteria. In addition, they provide a moist, nutritious environment—just right for microbial growth. Wash anything that has come into contact with such foods to prevent **cross-contamination**. For instance, after marinating raw meat in a dish, don't put the meat back in the same dish after cooking it, and don't use the marinade unless it has been cooked thoroughly. Wash the dish in hot, soapy water before reusing it; otherwise, the bacteria inevitably left in the dish from the raw meat can contaminate and grow in the cooked product or other food—a classic example of cross-contamination. Similarly, wash a cutting board (and your hands) after, say, skinning chicken on it. If you don't, and you use the contaminated board to chop raw vegetables for a salad, the vegetables can pick up the bacteria from the poultry. Because the salad won't be heated, the bacteria won't be killed.

cross-contamination The inadvertent transfer of bacteria from one food to another that occurs, for instance, by chopping vegetables on the same cutting board that was used to skin poultry.

Food Safety for Meats The U.S. Department of Agriculture requires that all fresh meat and poultry products carry a label (see Figure 13-2) as a reminder to handle the products carefully. Ground meat is especially susceptible to bacterial contamination. Steaks and roasts are not as risky, because bacteria usually settle on the outside of the cuts and are easily destroyed when the outside is heated. But, because the process of grinding meat spreads the bacteria throughout, foods made with ground meat, such as hamburger patties or meat loaf, must be cooked all the way through to kill the bacteria in the middle. To decrease your risk of eating contaminated ground beef, cook burgers until the juices run clear and not a trace of pink is left on the inside, and always order burgers well done at restaurants. When baking a meat loaf, use a thermometer to test the internal temperature. Be especially careful when cooking ground meat in a microwave oven, which sometimes cooks foods unevenly.

FIGURE 13-2
Safe Handling Instructions for Raw Meat and Poultry

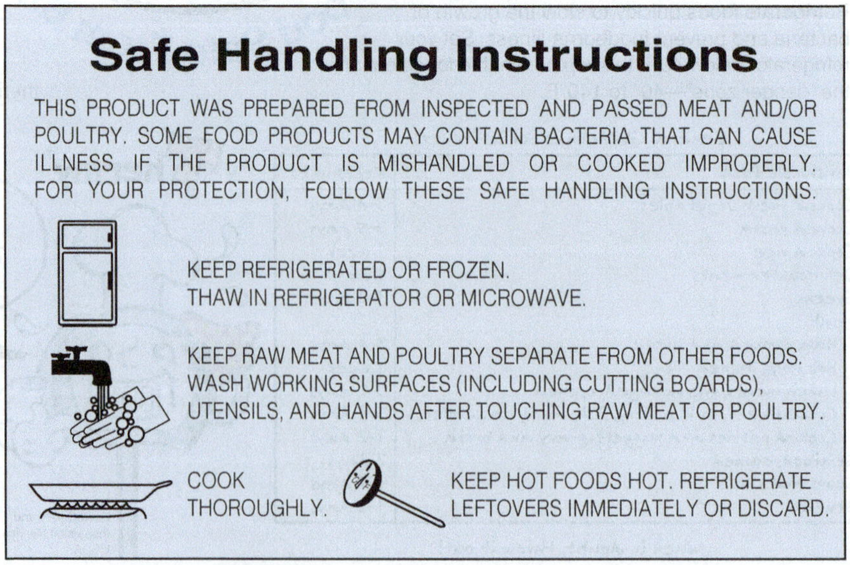

© Cengage

Reports of outbreaks of **mad cow disease**, primarily in the United Kingdom but in other countries as well, raise concerns among American consumers regarding the safety of consuming meat from infected animals. Agricultural officials in the United Kingdom now prohibit the addition of mammalian meat and bone meal to the feed of any food-producing animals, because these tissues are suspected to be the source of the disease. As a result, the rate of newly reported cases of the disease is decreasing. The USDA also bans the use of most mammalian protein tissues in the manufacture of animal feed given to ruminant animals (e.g., cows, sheep, and goats).[14]

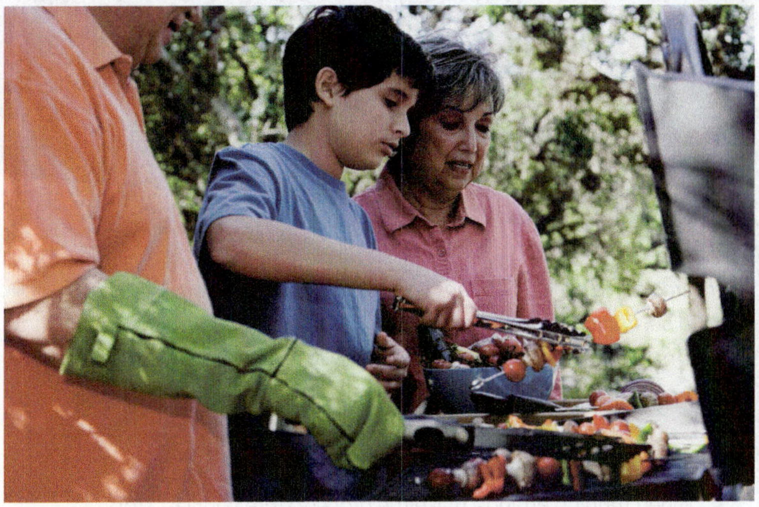
Blend Images/Alamy

Handle raw meat and poultry with care, and cook it thoroughly to destroy any bacteria present. Place it on a clean plate when it is cooked.

Food Safety for Seafood Seafood also should be handled with care, especially fish intended to be eaten raw or only lightly steamed. The dangerous foodborne diseases that may lurk in normal-appearing seafood—worms, parasites, severe viral intestinal disorders, and hepatitis—can be much worse than those resulting from normal bacterial spoilage. Raw fish dishes such as sushi and sashimi are safe for most healthy people to eat if they are prepared with fresh fish that has been commercially frozen at temperatures lower than most home freezers can attain. This type of freezing kills any parasites that might be present. However, eating raw or undercooked oysters, clams, mussels, and whole scallops is especially risky because these types of seafood sometimes carry a strain of bacteria known as *Vibrio*, which can multiply even during refrigeration. Although *Vibrio* bacteria are destroyed by thorough cooking, they can thrive in raw shellfish and cause serious illness, sometimes even causing a deadly blood poisoning that can kill a person within a day or two.[15] Thus, the hazards of eating raw or undercooked seafood are especially serious for vulnerable people, such as those with liver disease, diabetes, gastrointestinal disorders, and HIV infection. People with these and other diseases that may compromise the body's immune system, and hence its ability to defend itself against food poisoning (see Table 13-4), need to be especially cautious when preparing and consuming seafood.

TABLE 13-4 Individuals at High Risk for Foodborne Illness and Foods They Should Avoid

High-Risk Patient Categories	Foods to Avoid
Young children	Raw fish or shellfish
Pregnant women	Raw or unpasteurized milk or cheeses
Older adults	Soft, French-style cheeses and patés
Immunocompromised individuals	Raw or undercooked eggs or foods containing raw or lightly cooked eggs (e.g., certain salad dressings, cookie and cake batters, sauces, and beverages such as unpasteurized eggnog) Raw or undercooked meat or poultry Precooked processed meats that have not been reheated (e.g., deli meats, hot dogs) Raw sprouts (alfalfa, clover, and radish) Unpasteurized fruit or vegetable juices

SOURCE: Data from *Diagnosis and Management of Foodborne Illnesses: A Primer for Physicians and Other Health Care Professionals*, available at www.cdc.gov/mmwr/pdf/rr/rr5304.pdf; Nutrition and the MD (Hagerstown, MD: Lippincott & Wilkins, 2003), p. 8.

mad cow disease Also called *bovine spongiform encephalopathy* (BSE); a rare and fatal degenerative disease first diagnosed in 1986 in cattle in the United Kingdom. The bovine disease may be passed to humans who eat the meat of infected animals and may lead to death due to brain and nerve damage.

THE SAVVY Diner Keep Food Safe to Eat (Obj. 13.2)

The tradition of tea drinking has been popular for more than 2,000 years in China. Contaminated water may have been one of the reasons. A hot drink made with boiled water was less likely to cause digestive problems than plain water.[16]

To Prevent Foodborne Illness

- When running errands, make the grocery store your last stop. When you get home, refrigerate perishables immediately.
- Refrigerate leftovers promptly, and heat them thoroughly to at least 165°F before serving. Refrigerate leftovers within 2 hours of serving (or 1 hour if it is warmer than 90°F).
- Use clean eggs with intact shells, and cook eggs before eating them (soft-boiled for 7 minutes, poached for 5, or fried for 3 minutes on each side).
- Keep hot foods hot (140°F or above). Keep cold foods cold (40°F or below).
- Do not prepare food if you have a skin infection or infectious disease. Anyone, though, may be a carrier of bacteria and should avoid coughing or sneezing over food.
- When in doubt, throw it out. Do not even taste food that is suspect. (An "off" odor, however, is not necessarily detectable in a food containing toxins.)
- Discard food from cans that leak or bulge. Dispose of the food in a manner that will protect other people and animals from accidental use.
- Cook all meat and poultry to 160°F or higher, until the flesh is no longer pink and all the juices run clear. Order hamburgers and other beef items well done when eating out.
- Wash fruits and vegetables thoroughly before eating.

To Ensure a Safe Catch: Seafood Safety Tips

- Choose fresh fish steaks and fillets that are moist, with no drying or browning around the edges.
- Buy seafood only from reputable dealers, and cook fish within 2 days of purchase. Use packaged, frozen seafood before the expiration date.
- Make sure the fish odor is fresh and mild. Fresh fish and shellfish should not have an overly "fishy" odor. Refrigerate seafood below 40°F immediately after buying.
- Cook fish to 145°F or until the flesh is opaque and separates easily with a fork.
- Refrigerate smoked, pickled, vacuum-packed, and modified-atmosphere-packed fish products.

Food Safety for Picnics When planning picnics, choose foods that last without refrigeration, such as fresh fruits and vegetables, breads and crackers, and canned spreads and cheeses that can be opened and used on the spot. Aged cheeses, such as cheddar and Swiss, do well for an hour or so, but they should be kept in an ice chest for longer periods. Chill dishes containing mayonnaise or other types of dressing before, during, and after the picnic. Burgers, chicken breasts, and other foods intended for grilling should not be partially cooked ahead of time. Partial cooking may not kill all the bacteria, and if these half-cooked items are not heated thoroughly later, chances of bacterial contamination run high. Partial cooking is a safe method only when, for example, you take a burger or other food *directly* from the microwave oven to the grill.[17]

In general, remember that fresh food smells fresh. Do not eat any food that carries an "off" odor, because the smell is probably the result of bacterial wastes and indicates a dangerous number of bacteria in the food. To be sure, not all types of food poisoning are detectable by odor; but if a food smells bad, chances are high that it is spoiled. Refer to The Savvy Diner feature for recommendations about preventing foodborne illness. See also the Scorecard feature in this chapter to help you rate your food-safety knowledge.

13.3 Pesticides and Other Environmental Contaminants

Food producers and food processors exert major efforts to maintain a safe food supply. Some risk of consuming undesirable substances, or **contaminants**, however, is unavoidable. Our industrial society's reliance on chemical processes means that foods may become contaminated by a variety of chemicals introduced into the environment. In addition, pesticides used in agricultural techniques affect the food supply. The following section examines some of the major chemical players in the food supply and looks at some ways that scientists hope to reduce them.

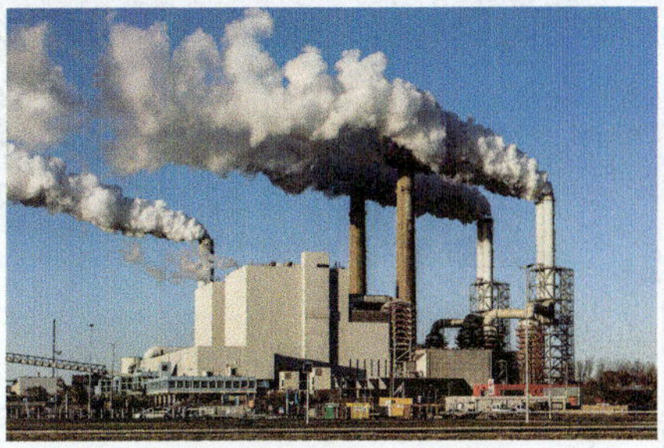
Corine van Kapel/Shutterstock.com

Many of the chemicals that contaminate foods are the waste products of industry.

Chemical Agents Some of the problem industrial chemicals prevalent in the environment and food supply are **organic halogens**, such as polychlorinated biphenyl (PCB) and polybrominated biphenyl (PBB); and **heavy metals**, such as lead and mercury. Fortunately, episodes of direct, excessive chemical contamination such as chemical spills are rare. However, when contamination *does* occur, the effects can be far-reaching. Table 13-5 presents a list of several chemical contaminants of particular concern in foods.

Under normal circumstances, even though a chemical substance is toxic, it tends to pose only a small hazard because it is usually carefully controlled. However, when

contaminants Potentially dangerous substances, such as lead, that can accidentally get into foods.

organic halogens Compounds that contain one or more of a class of atoms called *halogens*, including fluorine, chlorine, iodine, or bromine.

heavy metals Any of a number of mineral ions, such as mercury and lead, so named because of their relatively high atomic weight. Many heavy metals are poisonous.

TABLE 13-5 Examples of Contaminants in Foods

Name and Description	Sources	Toxic Effects	Typical Route to Food Chain
Cadmium (heavy metal)	Used in industrial processes, including electroplating, plastics, batteries, alloys, pigments, smelters, and burning fuels; present in cigarette smoke	No immediately detectable symptoms; slowly and irreversibly damages kidneys and liver	Enters air in smokestack emissions, settles on ground and is absorbed into plants, consumed by farm animals, and eaten in meat and produce by people. Sewage sludge and fertilizers leave large amounts in the soil; runoff contaminates shellfish.
Lead (heavy metal)	Lead crystal, improperly manufactured and old ceramic ware, paint, old plumbing, and leaded gasoline	Displaces calcium, iron, zinc, and other minerals from their sites of action in the nervous system, bone marrow, kidneys, and liver, causing failure to function; causes breakage of red blood cells (anemia) and interferes with the immune response	Air and soil pollution from industrial plants and the former use of leaded gasoline, water pipes, improperly manufactured and old ceramic ware, and lead crystal.
Mercury (heavy metal)	Widely dispersed in gases from the Earth's crust; local high concentrations from industry, electrical equipment, paints, and agriculture	Poisons the nervous system, especially in fetuses	Inorganic mercury released into waterways by industry and acid rain is converted to methylmercury by bacteria and ingested by fish.*
Polychlorinated biphenyl (PCB) (organic compound)	No natural source; produced for use in electrical equipment	Causes long-lasting skin eruptions, eye irritation, growth retardation in children of exposed mothers, anorexia, fatigue, and other effects	Discarded electrical equipment, accidental industrial leakage, or reuse of PCB containers for food.

*The FDA recommends that women of childbearing age, especially pregnant women and lactating women eliminate from their diets certain species of large, predatory fish, because these fish may contain high levels of mercury that can cause neurological damage during sensitive stages of fetal brain development. These include shark, swordfish, king mackerel, orange roughy, tilefish, marlin, and tuna (bigeye). Visit www.fda.gov/food/default.htm for more information and updates. Some fish caught by family and friends, such as larger carp, catfish, trout, and perch, are more likely to have fish advisories due to mercury or other contaminants. State advisories will tell you how often you can safely eat those fish.

SCORE Card Food Safety (Obj. 13.2)

Improper storage of food not only increases the risk of food poisoning but also almost always results in a loss of nutrients and good taste. The following quiz is designed to measure your food-safety savvy.

1. If you're packing a picnic, it's okay for the cold foods to be at room temperature before packing as long as they are placed in a cooler with ice or ice packs. *True or False?*
2. Foods prepared with mayonnaise—macaroni salad, potato salad, and coleslaw—are common sources of food poisoning. *True or False?*
3. Raw ground meat or poultry can be stored in the refrigerator, but these items should be used within:
   - **a.** 1–2 days.
   - **b.** 2–3 days.
   - **c.** 3–4 days.
   - **d.** 1 week.
4. What sign indicates that canned foods may be contaminated?
   - **a.** Bulging
   - **b.** Leaking
   - **c.** Spurting of liquid when opened
   - **d.** All of the above
5. Which of the following foods has been linked to food poisoning?
   - **a.** Cooked rice
   - **b.** Apple cider
   - **c.** Shellfish
   - **d.** All of the above
6. The best place in the refrigerator to store milk is in the door. *True or False?*
7. When bringing home groceries from the market, it's a good idea to rewrap meat and poultry before placing them in the refrigerator or freezer. *True or False?*
8. Fresh fish should smell "fishy." *True or False?*
9. The best way to handle green-skinned potatoes is to
   - **a.** throw them away.
   - **b.** soak them in cold water.
   - **c.** peel the skin and remove some of the flesh before cooking.
   - **d.** remove the green section after cooking.
10. Canned foods can be stored in the pantry indefinitely. *True or False?*
11. You can tell if a food is contaminated by the way it looks, smells, or tastes. *True or False?*
12. What is the maximum time perishable foods can be kept at room temperature?
    - **a.** ½ hour
    - **b.** 1 hour
    - **c.** 2 hours
    - **d.** 24 hours
13. It's okay to thaw frozen ham on the kitchen counter because salted, and smoked meats are free of bacteria. *True or False?*
14. You can reduce your exposure to chemical contaminants in whole fish by proper cleaning. *True or False?*

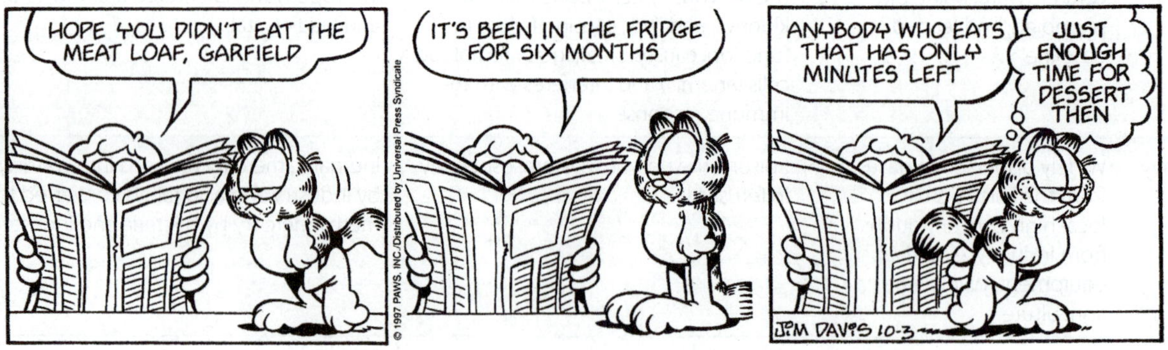

toxicity The ability of a substance to harm living organisms. All substances are toxic if present in high enough concentrations.

hazard State of danger; used to refer to any circumstance in which harm is possible.

a chemical spill or other accident occurs, the risk can suddenly soar. That's why scientists differentiate between **toxicity** (a property of all substances) and **hazard** (the likelihood of a substance's actually causing harm). All substances are potentially toxic, but they are hazardous only if consumed in large enough quantities. In other words, the dose makes the poison. Thus, a chemical that is present in foods in minuscule

15. Cloudy liquid around packaged hot dogs indicates that bacteria have started growing. *True or False?*

Answers

1. False. Be sure food is cold or frozen before placing it in a cooler. This minimizes the chance of microbial growth. Use ice packs between food items. Frozen juice boxes can also be packed and enjoyed later in the day after they have thawed.
2. False. Adding mayonnaise to food does not increase the chance of food poisoning. Most store-bought mayonnaise contains ingredients (vinegar, lemon juice, and salt) that actually slow bacterial growth.
3. (a) Ground meat and ground poultry are more perishable than other meats. They should be refrigerated and cooked (or frozen) within 1 to 2 days of purchase.
4. (d) Never buy or use products with bulging lids, leaking cans, or cracked jars. All are warning signs that a product may be contaminated with the bacteria that cause deadly botulism.
5. (d) Although the most common offenders are poultry, meat, and shellfish, any food can cause food poisoning, including cooked rice, if mishandled.
6. False. The refrigerator door does not stay as cold as the rest of the refrigerator. Highly perishable foods like milk and eggs should be stored on an inside shelf. Use the door for condiments.
7. False. Leave meat and poultry in store wrapping. The less you handle it, the better. This is especially true for ground meat and ground poultry.
8. False. Fresh fish should smell like a fresh sea breeze. If it smells "fishy," don't buy it.
9. (c) Green-skinned potatoes contain a natural toxin called solanine, which develops when potatoes are exposed to sunlight. It imparts a bitter taste and may cause stomach upset if eaten in large quantities. Before cooking, simply remove the green area and about ½ inch of flesh around it.
10. False. Canned foods have an extended but not infinite shelf life. Remember to place newly purchased cans behind older ones. To be safe, throw out beans and high-acid foods (for example, pineapple, tomatoes) after 1 year and other canned foods after 2 years. Use canned fish within 6 months.
11. False. Food spoilage may leave telltale signs such as changes in looks, smell, or taste, but contaminated food does not. Remember this rule of thumb: "When in doubt, throw it out."
12. (c) The longer a perishable food is kept at room temperature, the greater the likelihood that bacteria will multiply to dangerous levels. Food kept unrefrigerated for more than 2 hours is a prime target for bacterial growth.
13. False. Many people think that salted or smoked meats are immune to bacterial contamination. That's not so, especially because many manufacturers have gradually lowered the salt content of cured meats. With any meat or poultry, the safest way to thaw it is in the refrigerator overnight.
14. True. By removing the skin and trimming the fatty tissue along the back and belly, where chemicals tend to concentrate, you can reduce your exposure to contaminants.
15. True. Although hot dogs are processed to last longer than other meat products, *Listeria monocytogenes* can grow even under refrigeration. If you notice cloudy liquid, discard the franks. Freeze hot dogs if you don't plan to use them within 2 weeks. If opened, use within a week.

How Did You Score?

Count up the number of questions you answered correctly.

12–15	Congratulations! You're quite the food-safety scholar.
8–11	You're fairly savvy when it comes to food safety, but don't push your luck. Brush up on the questions you had trouble with.
7 or below	You're a likely target for food poisoning. Mend your ways; it's never too late.

SOURCE: Adapted with permission from A. Schepers, "What's your food safety I.Q.?" *Environmental Nutrition* 22 (1999): 1, 6. © Copyright 1999 by Environmental Nutrition, Inc., 52 Riverside Drive, New York, NY 10024, www.environmentalnutrition.com

amounts does not pose a significant hazard until for some reason it becomes concentrated in the food, that is, in toxic amounts.

Most experts agree that although chemicals in foods pose a small hazard, the chief concern is accidental gross contamination. In some instances, however, chemical contamination can be subtle and insidious. The problem of chronic low-level lead

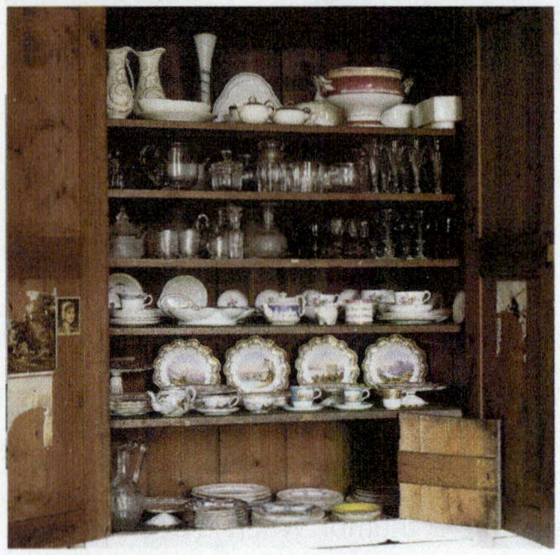

Andreas von Einsiedel/Corbis Documentary/Getty Images

Some antique ceramic and crystal items are best left on the shelf. The older the piece, the higher the chances that it leaches lead.

TABLE 13-6 Getting the Lead Out

To protect against overexposure to lead:

- Do not store fruit juices or other acidic foods in ceramic containers.
- Do not store beverages in lead crystal containers.
- Do not eat or drink from items that show a dusty or chalky gray residue on the glaze after they are washed.
- Do not feed babies from crystal bottles.
- Run cold water for a minute before using it for drinking or cooking.

For more information, call the National Lead Information Center at 1-800-424-LEAD or go to www.epa.gov/lead.

poisoning is a prime example. In the United States, lead poisoning ranks as one of the most common childhood environmental health problems. More than 535,000 children under the age of 6 have lead levels in their blood high enough to increase risk for behavioral, mental, and other health problems.[18]

Lead contamination usually does not poison a person all at once; rather, low levels build up gradually in the soft tissues of the kidneys, bone marrow, liver, and brain. Over time, the accumulated lead can cause such health problems as diminished intelligence and impaired development.

Historically, lead has entered the food and water supply largely through leaded gasoline exhaust, which contaminates rainfall, which in turn pervades crop soil and water supplies. Lead contamination of the water supply continues to be a source of concern (refer to the discussion on water in Chapter 9). In addition, lead solder used to seal the seams of cans was a source of the contaminant for many years. Fortunately, a 25-year process to phase out lead in gasoline reached its goal in 1995, and lead-soldered cans have been eliminated. Today the levels of lead in foods and beverages are the lowest in history.

Nevertheless, lead paint abounds in older housing, and new sources of lead contamination have surfaced during recent years. When it comes to lead exposure via food and beverages, scientists have identified ceramic holloware, lead crystal, and foil capsules on wine bottles as potential sources. Lead can leach from the glaze of ceramic bowls, mugs, and pitchers that have not been properly formulated or fired—especially when the food or beverage inside is hot and acidic, such as coffee, tea, or tomato soup. Wine and other alcoholic beverages also promote the leaching of lead, so experts advise against storing alcohol in pitchers and other containers made with lead crystal. In addition, it's a good idea to use a damp cloth to wipe the rims of wine bottles capped with foil, which has been shown to leach lead. For help on lowering your own risk, see the tips in Table 13-6.

Although chemical contamination is not the greatest hazard posed by the food supply, there are still many unknowns. For example, what are the effects of prolonged exposure? Despite the uncertainties, keep in mind that more often than not, healthful eating habits and overall good health protect against the toxicity of food contaminants and other environmental pollutants. Eating a wide variety of food ensures an adequate supply of essential nutrients and minimizes exposure to potential environmental contaminants.

Pesticide Residues

Pesticides are substances used to prevent, destroy, or repel harmful pests, including insects, spiders, bacteria, weeds, molds and mildews, rodents, and other living things. Unlike many other chemicals present in the food supply, pesticides are intended specifically to poison living things. The trouble with pesticides, of course, is that they can inadvertently harm wildlife, people, and other species.

When farmers first began using pesticides, they chose potent ones: chemicals designed to keep on killing for as long as they remained in the soil. Unfortunately, after years of widespread pesticide use, some unsettling side effects of the chemicals surfaced. They washed from the soil into lakes, rivers, and oceans, contaminating water supplies; they poisoned farmworkers, who breathed the chemicals day in and day out; they endangered many species of wildlife, disrupting the animals' abilities to reproduce and wiping out entire populations; and, most disturbing, they would not go away.

For example, in the 1960s, scientists observed that a popular pesticide called DDT had begun accumulating in the body fat of animals. DDT threatened the survival of the American eagle by weakening eggshells to the point of collapse, killing the developing chicks inside. DDT also appeared in big fish, carnivorous animals, people, and human breast milk. Finally, after years of widespread agricultural use, the United States banned DDT. However, the pesticide still lingers in the environment. Many

pesticides Chemicals intentionally applied to plants, including foods, to prevent or eliminate pest damage. *Pests* include all living organisms that destroy or spoil foods: bacteria, molds and fungi, insects, and rats and other rodents, to name a few.

foreign countries continue to use DDT, including countries from which the United States buys produce. Regrettably, despite the U.S. ban on DDT, U.S. companies are still allowed to sell it (as well as other banned pesticides) to countries where DDT use remains legal. This practice may come back to haunt us, however, when we buy imported produce that has been exposed to DDT. In addition, the DDT situation illustrates the need to consider environmental issues from a global perspective; residues of chemicals banned in one country can travel the entire world not only through the imported and exported foods but also through wind, rain, and waterways.

DDT taught us another lesson about pesticides: A contaminant that builds up in the body carries the greatest potential risk. In the body, a contaminant that is quickly broken down to some harmless compound poses the least risk to health. Likewise, if the body can easily and rapidly excrete a pesticide residue, the body may not be harmed by it. But if the residue enters the body and stays there, all the while interacting with the body's cells and systems, it may wreak havoc. Additional doses piled on top of the first ones compound the damaging effects. Moreover, when a substance resists breakdown either inside the body (by the body's own enzymes) or outside (by microorganisms) and furthermore accumulates from one species to the next, it builds up in the food chain (see Figure 13-3). DDT causes all these problems, which is why it is so deadly.

Careful use of pesticides often boosts crop yields, which in turn helps keep the price of fruits and vegetables down and the availability of a wide variety of produce high. Still, as the DDT experience illustrates, pesticides must be evaluated scrupulously and used judiciously. The ideal pesticide destroys the target pest and then breaks down quickly into other products that pose minimal hazard to people and other animals. Scientists have made many strides in developing relatively innocuous pesticides over the years, and the search for better, safer pesticides continues. What's more, since the introduction of pesticides decades ago, many national and international agencies have adopted strict **regulations** on pesticide use.

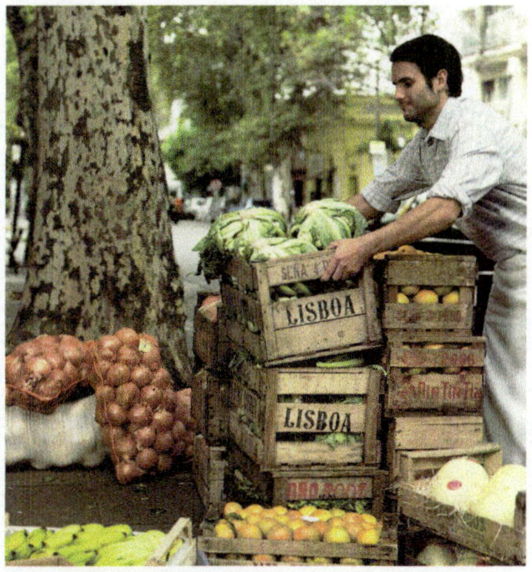

Michael Blann/Getty Images

Foods imported from other countries may harbor residues of pesticides that have been banned for use in the United States.

regulations Legal mandates that must be obeyed. Failure to follow a regulation brings about legal consequences.

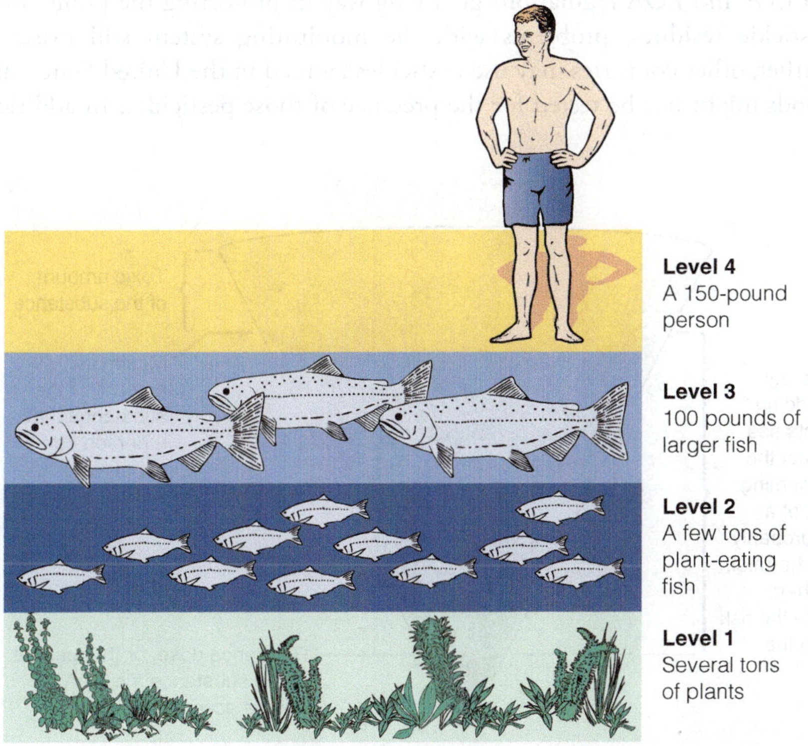

FIGURE 13-3

How a Food Chain Works

A person who eats fish regularly may consume about 100 pounds of it in a year. These fish will, in turn, have eaten a few tons of small plant-eating fish during their lifetime. The little plant eaters will have ingested several tons of plants. If the plants have been contaminated with toxic chemicals, the bodies of the small fish that eat them will contain high concentrations of the chemicals; the larger fish that eat the little fish will harbor even higher amounts of the chemicals; and so on through the food chain. If none of the chemicals are lost along the way, the person at the top of the food chain ultimately eats the same amount of chemical contaminants that was contained in the original *several tons* of plants at the bottom of the food chain.

In the United States, the Environmental Protection Agency (EPA) determines whether a particular chemical may be used on U.S. crops. In deciding whether to approve a pesticide, the EPA scrutinizes dozens of studies that assess the possible effects of the substance on people, wildlife, fish, or plants, as well as its potential to cause such problems as cancer and birth defects. To do so, the EPA examines the estimated amount of a pesticide residue that a person might be exposed to during the course of a 70-year lifetime and the **risk** of harm that amount of exposure might pose. If the risk is unacceptably high, the pesticide is ruled out. This extensive research process often requires years of research and costs millions of dollars.[19]

Once the EPA approves a pesticide for use, it sets forth safety standards. For those pesticides it allows, the EPA determines which crops may be treated with it and how much may be applied. It also establishes a **tolerance**—that is, the maximum amount of a pesticide residue allowed in or on a food. The EPA identifies what is called a **reference dose** for the pesticide: the amount that could be consumed daily without posing any health risk. First, scientists use animal studies to estimate the maximum amount of the chemical that a person could take in daily without suffering harm. Next, to ensure an extra **margin of safety**, they calculate a small fraction of this amount, usually $\frac{1}{100}$, which becomes the reference dose. In other words, the reference dose is $\frac{1}{100}$ of the maximum amount of the substance that appears to be safe. Scientists factor in this large margin of safety as a precaution to help ensure that even highly vulnerable people won't be harmed by the substance in question (see Figure 13-4).[20]

After the EPA approves a pesticide, the FDA, in its ongoing monitoring program, begins to check for residues. Inspectors collect samples from packers, shippers, and other food handlers and test them for pesticide residues. If a food contains residues that exceed the EPA's tolerance limits, the FDA can seize the entire shipment and press criminal charges. Meanwhile, how can you protect yourself against unacceptably high levels of pesticides? The Nutrition Action feature later in this chapter offers a perspective.

Although EPA and FDA regulations go a long way in protecting the public from harmful pesticide residues, problems with the monitoring system still exist. As explained earlier, other countries may use pesticides banned in the United States, and imported foods might not be tested for the presence of those pesticides. In addition,

risk For pesticide residues, the harm a substance may cause. Scientists estimate risk by assessing the amount of a chemical that each person in a population might consume over time (also called *exposure*) and by considering how toxic the substance might be (*toxicity*).

risk = exposure × toxicity

exposure = amount of substance in food × amount of food eaten

tolerance The maximum amount of a particular substance allowed in food.

reference dose The estimated amount of a chemical that could be consumed daily without causing harmful effects.

margin of safety From a food-safety standpoint, the *margin* is a zone between the maximum amount of a substance that appears to be safe and the amount allowed in the food supply.

FIGURE 13-4

Margin of Safety

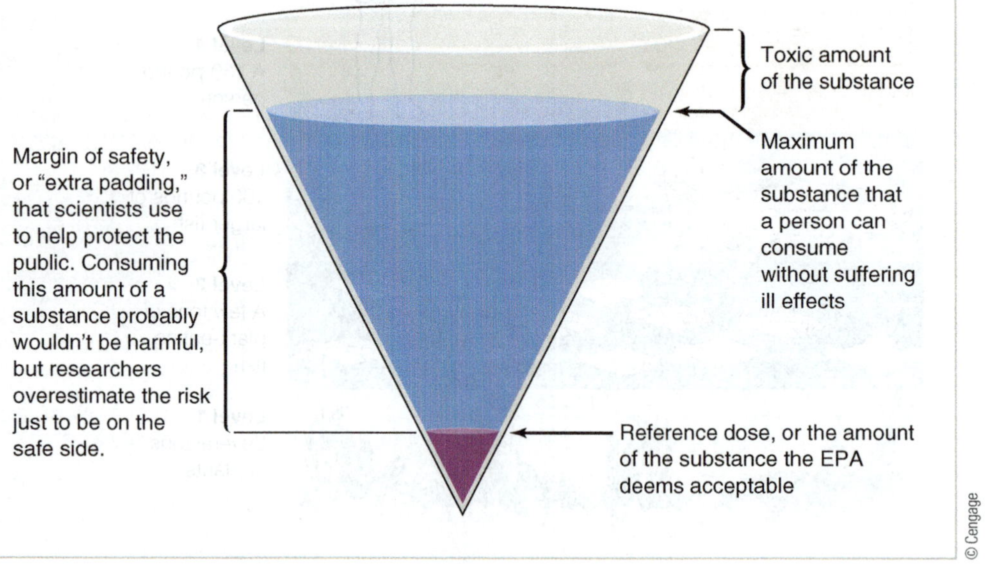

TABLE 13-7 Handling Produce Safely*

Wash produce to remove dirt, dislodge bacteria, and keep pesticide residues to a minimum. Use the following tips:

- Rinse produce thoroughly with running water just before eating, cutting, or cooking. Scrub the skin or rind of firm produce, such as melons or cucumbers, with a clean vegetable brush while you wash it. Peel produce to which wax has been applied.
- Dry produce with a clean cloth towel or paper towel; wet produce can allow any remaining microbes to multiply faster.
- Discard the outer leaves of lettuce, cabbage, and other leafy vegetables. Rinse the interior leaves thoroughly to remove dirt and debris.
- Use a knife to peel an orange or grapefruit; do not bite into the peel.
- Eat a variety of fruits and vegetables. Farmers use different chemicals for different crops, so eating a wide variety of produce helps decrease exposure to any particular pesticide residue.
- Consider purchasing certified organic foods, especially for items most likely to contain pesticide residues (such as peaches, apples, spinach, cucumbers, cherry tomatoes, snap peas [imported], celery, nectarines [imported], strawberries, and grapes).

*Raw seafood, meat, and poultry should not be rinsed before cooking, to avoid spreading bacteria to other foods, utensils, and surfaces. To reduce pesticide residue intake from meats, trim fat from meat and remove the skin from poultry and fish (pesticide residues concentrate in the animals' fat tissues). Discard fats and oils in broths and pan drippings.

SOURCE: Adapted from *Daily Tip: Protection from Pesticides* (Chicago: American Dietetic Association, July 13, 2007); U.S. Department of Health and Human Services and U.S. Department of Agriculture, *2015–2020 Dietary Guidelines for Americans*, 8th ed. December, 2015.

consider that the National Academy of Sciences issued the results of a large-scale, 5-year study on the risk of pesticide residues in the diets of infants and children who may be more susceptible than adults to adverse effects from pesticides. Although it concluded that the U.S. food supply is safe for children, it called for changes in the methods used to assess health risks from pesticides to better account for differences between adults and children.[21] To keep pesticide residues from all types of produce to a minimum, use the produce-handling tips in Table 13-7.

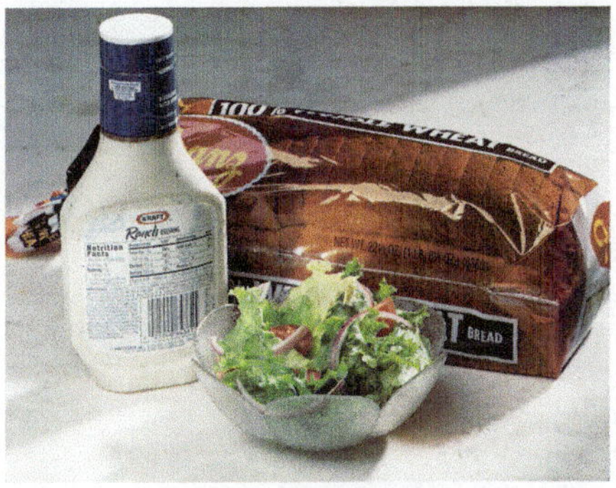

Polara Studios

Food additives extend the shelf life of many commonly eaten foods.

13.4 Food Additives

From a safety standpoint, **food additives** rank among the least hazardous substances in food, although consumers tend to rank them high on their list of food-related concerns. The great majority of food additives enhance the color, flavor, texture, or stability of foods or even improve the nutritional value of certain items, as shown in Table 13-8. Many additives are common substances such as vitamins, herbs, and spices, deliberately added to foods and called *direct* or **intentional food additives**.

In contrast, **incidental food additives**, such as packaging materials or processing chemicals, often accidentally get into foods during processing. The federal government regulates all food additives and requires that food processors perform tests to determine whether additives are present in safe levels.

Manufacturers must go through a lengthy, costly process to get FDA approval for a new food additive. The manufacturer must conduct extensive research to show that the additive in question does what it is supposed to do, that it can be detected and measured in foods to which it has been added, and that it is safe in the amounts in which it will be used.

As with pesticide residues, many food additives are allowed only in amounts that ensure a wide margin of safety. Most additives that pose any potential risk

food additives Any substances added to food, including substances used in production, processing, treatment, packaging, transportation, or storage.

intentional food additives Substances intentionally added to food; examples include nutrients, colors, spices, and herbs.

incidental food additives (indirect additives) Substances that accidentally get into food as a result of contact with it during growing, processing, packaging, storing, or some other stage before the food is consumed.

TABLE 13-8 **Major Uses of Food Additives**

Function of Additive	Examples	Foods in Which Often Used
Impart or maintain consistency	Stabilizers, thickeners, anticaking agents, and emulsifiers including alginates, lecithin, mono- and diglycerides, glycerine, pectin, guar gum	Baked goods, cake mixes, salad dressings, ice cream, processed cheese, table salt, chocolate
Improve or maintain nutritional value	Vitamins A and D, thiamin, niacin, folic acid, ascorbic acid (vitamin C), calcium citrate, zinc oxide, iron, iodine	Flour, bread, biscuits, breakfast cereals, pasta, margarine, milk, iodized salt, juices
Maintain palatability and wholesomeness	Ascorbic acid, butylated hydroxyanisole (BHA), butylated hydroxytoluene (BHT), benzoates, sulfites	Bread, crackers, frozen and dried fruit, margarine, lard, potato chips, cake mixes, meat
Produce light texture; control acidity or alkalinity	Yeast, sodium bicarbonate, citric acid, lactic acid, phosphoric acid	Cakes, cookies, quick breads, crackers, butter, soft drinks
Enhance flavor or impart desired color	Cloves, ginger, fructose, aspartame, MSG, FD&C Red No. 40, caramel, turmeric, vegetable dyes	Spice cake, gingerbread, soft drinks, yogurt, soup, candy, cheese, jams, gum

SOURCE: Adapted from *Food Additives* (Rockville, MD/Washington, DC: Food and Drug Administration in cooperation with International Food Information Council, www.ific.org).

are allowed in foods only at levels $\frac{1}{100}$ of those at which the risk is still known to be zero. Even nutrient food additives are subject to the margin-of-safety concept. For example, even though iodine has long been added to salt to prevent iodine deficiency, the amounts added have been controlled because excess iodine can be deadly.

Substances Generally Recognized As Safe (GRAS) Attention to certain aspects of food law will help you to better understand the issues surrounding the use of additives in foods. For the first half of the 20th century, scientists evaluated the safety of food additives using a simple approach: an added substance was either "safe" and therefore permitted for use in foods or "poisonous and deleterious" and therefore banned. As the study of toxic agents advanced, scientists realized that eventually they would be able to show that virtually every substance poses a health hazard if the dose is large enough. Consequently, they recognized that simply classifying an additive as "safe" or "poisonous" was not an effective means of evaluation.

To get around the problem, Congress proposed the bill that later became the Food Additives Amendment of 1958. As the members of Congress debated the bill, a question arose as to how to deal with the additives already in use. Congress decided that a "safe" substance in use before 1958 would be deemed a "Substance Generally Recognized as Safe" (a GRAS substance) and be put on the **GRAS list**. Substances not in use before that time would be classified as food additives and subject to regulation under the Food Additives Amendment.

With the establishment of the amendment, the FDA put hundreds of substances on the GRAS list. Everything from vegetable oils, salt, pepper, sugar, caffeine, vinegar, and baking powder to meat, poultry, eggs, milk, seafood, cereals, vegetables, and fruit was—and still is—classified as GRAS substances.

The GRAS list came under scrutiny in 1969, however, when safety questions arose about the GRAS substance cyclamate, an artificial sweetener. After reviewing hundreds of studies, the FDA decided to ban cyclamate from use in foods and beverages. As a result of this incident, President Richard Nixon ordered a reevaluation of the

GRAS (Generally Recognized As Safe) list A list of ingredients, established by the FDA, that had long been in use and were believed safe. The list is subject to revision as new facts become known.

safety of all substances on the GRAS list. The FDA conducted a sweeping review and removed about 300 substances from the list. Today, the more than 400 substances classified as GRAS are continually subject to reexamination as new facts and concerns arise.

The FDA requires that the labels of irradiated foods carry this internationally known radura symbol for radiation. The circle in the middle represents an energy source, the five breaks in the outer circle symbolize rays generated by the energy source, and the two petals signify food. For unpackaged irradiated meat, the statement and logo must be displayed at the point of sale for consumers. The labeling requirements do not pertain to food service establishments such as restaurants. The FDA approves irradiation of beef, lamb, pork, poultry, citrus fruits, eggs, flour, fresh or frozen red meats, iceberg lettuce, mushrooms, onions, potatoes, seafood (clams, oysters, mussels, scallops), spices, spinach, strawberries, tea, tomatoes, tropical fruits, and wheat.

13.5 Food Technologies

Back in the 1860s, a French scientist named Louis Pasteur came up with a radical, "newfangled" process by which the disease-producing microorganisms in a food could be destroyed by exposing the food to heat. Dubbed *pasteurization*, after Dr. Pasteur, the process marked a major breakthrough in the science of food safety. At the time, however, Dr. Pasteur's discovery met with widespread fear and opposition. In fact, it wasn't accepted as a vital public health measure until 1909, when the city of Chicago set forth the first U.S. law requiring pasteurization of milk.

Today, of course, few consumers question the wisdom of drinking pasteurized milk. Still, according to many experts, technologies such as irradiation have prompted a public outcry similar to the turn-of-the-century resistance to pasteurization.[22] As public health organizations strive to feed a fast-growing world population while ensuring a safe food supply, debate about new ways of doing so is sure to heat up. The following sections explore some of the food technologies that may help improve the safety of our food supply and maintain the nutritional value of the foods available in the marketplace.

Irradiation

Irradiation is one of the foremost technologies earmarked by food-safety experts for increased use in the United States. The process involves exposing food to low doses of radiation, which destroys insects and several types of bacteria, including *Salmonella*. Contrary to popular belief, irradiation does not make a food radioactive. Rather, the radiation rays pass through food, leaving behind no radioactive residues.

A common concern about irradiation is that it might alter the nutritional value of a food. The World Health Organization (WHO), along with numerous other public health agencies, points out that nutrient losses, if any, are insignificant.[23]

That's not to say, however, that irradiation poses no risks. One of the most troublesome is that the radioactive materials used in the irradiation process may put workers and communities at undue risk. However, as with any technology, the risk of irradiation must be weighed carefully against the benefits and risks of alternate technologies. Consider spices, which typically harbor high levels of pathogens. Often, manufacturers douse them with a toxic, explosive chemical called *ethylene oxide* to rid them of bacteria. Yet because of its toxic, explosive nature, ethylene oxide puts workers at risk, may pollute the air, and may leave residue on the spices. In fact, the gas, which was once used to sterilize medical supplies, has been deemed so dangerous that most manufacturers now use irradiation instead. (Cotton swabs, tampons, teething rings, and a number of other consumer goods are also sterilized via irradiation.)[24] The USDA authorizes irradiation of meat already inspected by the agency and approved as safe for consumption. As a result, food companies have the option of using irradiation on raw meat and meat products (e.g., ground beef, frozen hamburger patties, or frozen poultry).

The WHO, the Food and Agriculture Organization (FAO) of the United Nations, the FDA, and numerous other agencies encourage the use of irradiation in the fight

irradiation The process of exposing a substance to low doses of radiation, using gamma rays, X-rays, or electricity (electron beams) to kill insects, bacteria, and other potentially harmful microorganisms.

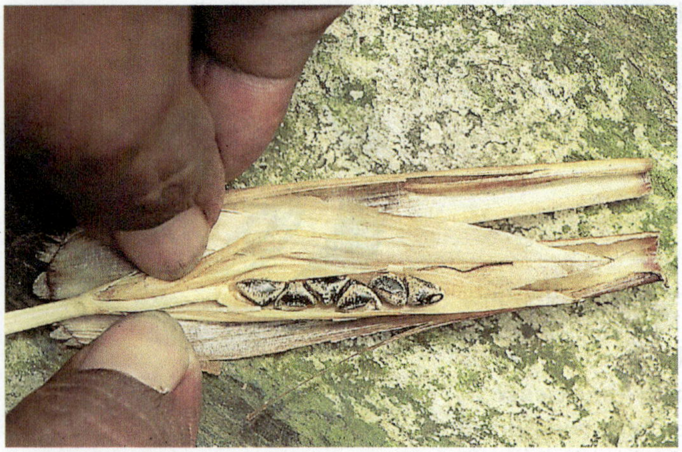

Antonio Mortaner/Smithsonian Tropical Research Institute

Farmers bred corn as we know it today from this wild corn.

against foodborne disease and food loss, and some 40 countries have approved it for use. According to WHO, each year spoilage, insect infestation, and the like lead to losses of as much as 50 percent of the world's food supply—losses that could be eliminated with irradiation. What's more, the process may help prevent deaths resulting from foodborne illness. Clearly, as the pressures to feed the world safely continue to mount, the public and scientific community will continue to examine the pros and cons of irradiation.

Biotechnology and Genetic Engineering In May 1994, a new breed of tomato made headlines. Called the Flavr Savr, the product garnered national repute as the first food created via **genetic engineering** to hit the market. It wasn't so much the product itself, which is simply a slow-ripening tomato, that caused such a stir; but rather the opening of the regulatory door that could pave the way to a whole new crop of genetically engineered products. What are these high-tech foods, and will we see more of them in the future?

Just as a person's genes determine hair color, eye color, and other characteristics, a plant's genes dictate the plant's structure, resistance to spoilage, and other qualities. With genetic engineering, scientists can alter a plant's genes to make a particular trait more desirable. To create the Flavr Savr tomato, scientists first identified the gene that causes ripe tomatoes to soften and rot. Then they isolated the gene, reversed it (or turned it backward, so to speak), and inserted the reversed gene back into tomato plants. The backward gene in the new tomatoes suppresses, or "turns off," the rotting gene. As a result, the Flavr Savr tomato stayed ripe longer than regular tomatoes (see Figure 13-5). This allowed growers more time to ship it to consumers without refrigeration.[25]

genetic engineering The use of biotechnology to alter the genes of a plant in an effort to create a new plant with different traits; also called *genetic modification*. In some cases, a plant's genes may be deleted or altered, or genes may be introduced from different organisms or species. The foods or crops produced are called genetically engineered (GE) or genetically modified (GM) foods or crops.

FIGURE 13-5

Creating the Flavr Savr Tomato

SOURCE: Adapted from Calgene's recipe for genetically engineered tomatoes, *FDA Consumer* (April 1995): 9.

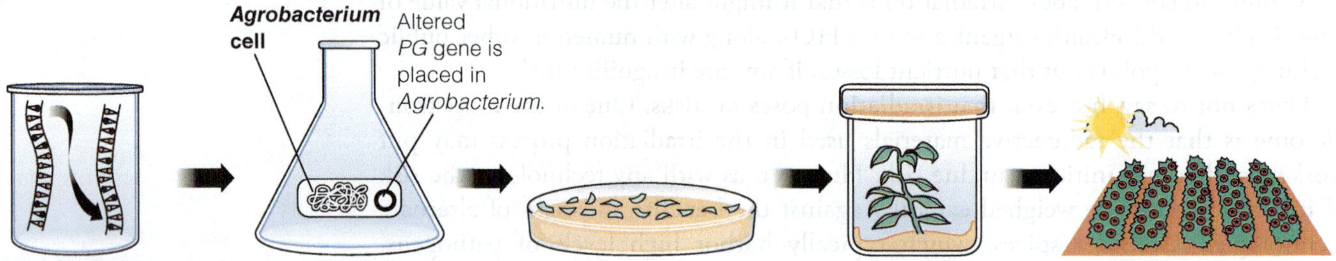

1. The *PG* (polygalacturonase) gene, which causes ripe tomatoes to soften and rot, is isolated and cloned. The sequence of *PG* gene is reversed so that the gene is backward (in what scientists call the "antisense" orientation).

2. The reversed *PG* gene is put into *Agrobacterium*, which is a bacterium that infects plants and is commonly used by genetic engineers to insert modified or foreign genes into other target cells.

3. The *Agrobacteria* are then placed in a petri dish with pieces of leaf from a tomato plant. The cut edges of the leaves absorb the *Agrobacteria* and antisense *PG* gene. Antisense gene thus becomes part of the genetic material of the tomato plant cells.

4. The leaf cuttings regenerate into tomato plants that contain the reversed *PG* gene. The new plants sprout roots, are transplanted to soil, and grow to mature tomato plants. The seeds collected from these greenhouse tomatoes are planted outdoors for field trials and more seed production.

5. In the genetically engineered tomato, the natural *PG* gene's production of the fruit-rotting *PG* enzyme is repressed by the reversed gene. This gives the commercial tomato extended shelf life, allowing it to ripen more fully on the vine and still have time to get to market before it spoils.

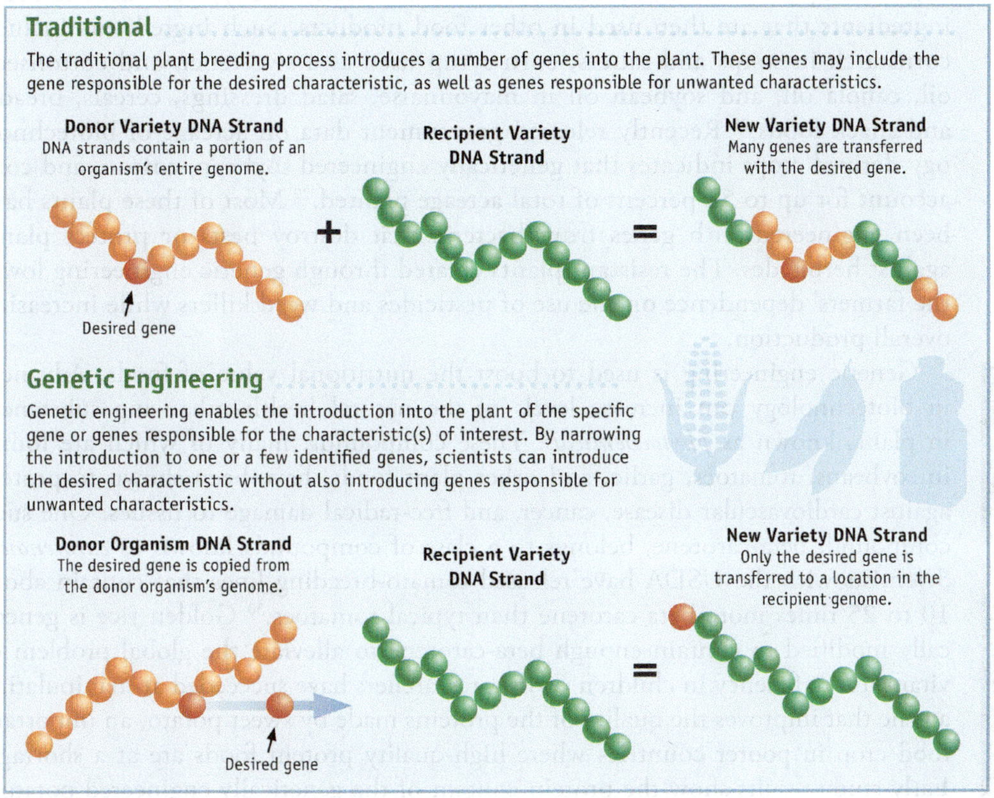

FIGURE 13-6

Methods of Plant Breeding

SOURCE: U.S. Food and Drug Administration, FDA's role in regulating safety of GE foods, May 2013.

Although the idea of altering a plant's genes to create a different version sounds new, scientists have used a crude version of the concept for centuries. In the 1500s, farmers crossed, say, a good food crop with another plant, which was resistant to disease, to form a hybrid that contained traits of both plants. Many of the fruits and vegetables we enjoy today were produced by this sort of cross-breeding. For example, corn as we know it today came from cross-breeding it with a type of corn that has a much harder outer shell on the kernel; kiwi was originally a small, hard berry; and nectarines are modified peaches.[26] Genetic engineering is different, however, because of its speed and the precision it affords scientists (see Figure 13-6). Whereas cross-breeding typically takes more than a decade, genetic engineering can yield new products in about 5 years.

In addition, genetic engineering allows scientists to "mix and match" genes from different species—say, mixing a gene from a fish with the genes of a vegetable. This type of research, called **transgenetics**, raises many ethical questions, especially among vegetarians and other people who fear that inserting an animal gene into a fruit or vegetable makes a food that is on some level both vegetable and animal. The possibilities created by this technology are seemingly endless. It has been suggested that ultimately, the world will obtain most of its food, fuel, fiber, and some of its pharmaceuticals from genetically altered vegetation and trees.[27] Major companies spend billions of dollars annually on **biotechnology** as researchers continue to develop new applications for genetically engineered products.

The U.S. Department of Agriculture reports that more than 40 new genetically engineered agricultural products have completed all the federal regulatory requirements and are now sold commercially. The majority of genetically

transgenetics The process of transferring genes from one species to another unrelated species.

biotechnology The use of biological systems or living organisms to make or modify products. Includes traditional methods used in making products such as wine, beer, yogurt, and cheese; cross-breeding to enhance crop production; and modification of living plants, animals, and fish through the manipulation of genes (genetic engineering).

engineered plants—corn, canola, soybean, and cotton—are typically used to make ingredients that are then used in other food products. Such ingredients include cornstarch in soups and sauces, corn syrup used as a sweetener, and cottonseed oil, canola oil, and soybean oil in mayonnaise, salad dressings, cereals, breads, and snack foods.[28] Recently released government data on acreage of biotechnology-derived crops indicates that genetically engineered soybean, cotton, and corn account for up to 52 percent of total acreage planted.[29] Most of these plants have been engineered with genes from bacteria that destroy pests or protect plants against herbicides. The resistant plants created through genetic engineering lower the farmers' dependence on the use of pesticides and weed killers while increasing overall production.

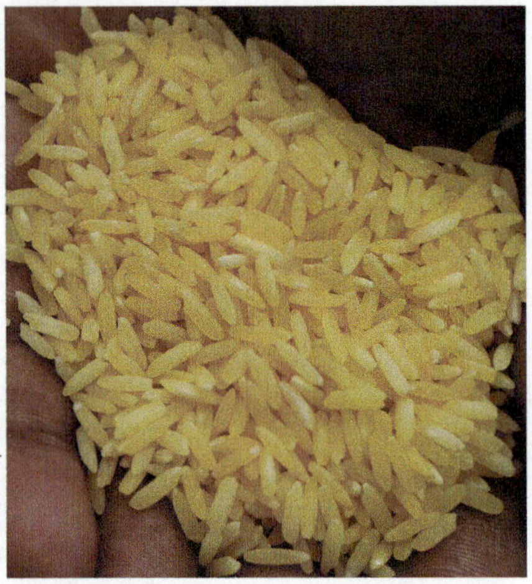

REUTERS/Alamy Stock Photo

Transgenic "golden rice" has the potential to reduce vitamin A deficiency.

Genetic engineering is used to boost the nutritional value of foods. Advances in biotechnology can increase levels of the natural health-enhancing substances in plants known as *phytochemicals*. These compounds, many of which are found in soybeans, tomatoes, garlic, and other plant foods, have been shown to protect against cardiovascular disease, cancer, and free-radical damage to tissues. One such compound, beta-carotene, belongs to a class of compounds known as *carotenoids*. Scientists with the USDA have released tomato-breeding lines that contain about 10 to 25 times more beta-carotene than typical tomatoes.[30] Golden rice is genetically modified to contain enough beta-carotene to alleviate the global problem of vitamin A deficiency in children.[31] Also, researchers have succeeded at manipulating a gene that improves the quality of the proteins made by sweet potato, an important food crop in poorer countries where high-quality protein foods are at a shortage. Early study results show the protein content of the genetically engineered potatoes increased as much as fivefold.[32]

Scientists are now developing plants that will produce edible vaccines. Such plants could be extremely valuable in developing countries where some environmental conditions can make conventional vaccine administration impractical. Also, an edible vaccine is being investigated that will, it is hoped, protect against diarrhea, a major cause of infant mortality in developing countries.[33]

The introduction of genetically engineered food has encountered several problems. Some people are concerned about the potential impact of an organism that would not have evolved under normal conditions. We cannot know the long-term environmental consequences as these genetically engineered plants multiply and mutate. Some people fear that naturally occurring cross-pollination between genetically engineered plants with nearby weeds may spread traits from plants to weeds. Potentially, this so-called superweed would be resistant to insects and herbicides.

People with food allergies express concern that new varieties of food produced by transgenetics may introduce allergens not found in the food before it was altered. Indeed, researchers have shown that allergens can be transferred through bioengineering, as in one case where an allergic protein showed up in soybeans that had been genetically altered with proteins from Brazil nuts.[34]

Another widely debated issue surrounding genetic engineering involves labeling. Many consumer groups have called for across-the-board labels on genetically engineered foods. But according to the FDA, with some exceptions, the food must carry distinct consequences to consumers who eat it before it requires special labeling. When genes from peanuts and other foods known to be common causes of allergies are put into a food, the label must indicate that the food contains an allergen, unless the manufacturer can prove that the item's potential to cause allergies has not been transferred via the gene. In addition, a food that

Risks versus Benefits: The Debate over Genetically Engineered (GE) Foods and Crops

Some Currently Available GE Crops*

- **Corn:** Insect resistance (reduced insect damage)
- **Soybean, Cotton, Corn:** Herbicide tolerance (greater weed control)
- **Cotton:** Insect resistance (reduced insect damage)
- **Rice:** Pro-vitamin A (increase vitamin A supply)

Potential Benefits of GE Foods and Crops

- **Increased nutritional value of staple foods:** Genes are being inserted into rice to make it produce beta-carotene, which the body converts into vitamin A. This experimental transgenic "golden rice" has the potential to reduce vitamin A deficiency, a leading cause of blindness and a significant factor in many child deaths.
- **Reduced environmental impact:** Scientists are developing trees with modified cell lignin content. When used to make pulp and paper, the modified wood requires less processing with harsh chemicals.
- **Increased fish yield:** Researchers have modified the gene that governs growth hormones in tilapia, a farmed fish, offering the prospect of increased yield and greater availability of fish protein in local diets.
- **Increased nutrient absorption by livestock:** Animal feed under development will improve animals' absorption of phosphorus. This reduces the phosphorus in animal waste, which pollutes groundwater.
- **Tolerance of poor environmental conditions:** Scientists are working to produce drought-resistant or salt-tolerant transgenic crops, which can then be grown on marginal land.

Potential Risks of GE Foods and Crops

- **Inadequate controls:** Although safety regimes are being improved, control over GE crop releases is not completely effective. In 2000, for example, a maize variety cleared only for animal consumption was found in food products.
- **Transfer of allergens:** Allergens can be transferred inadvertently from an existing to a target organism, and new allergens can be created. For example, when a Brazil nut gene was transferred to soybean, tests found that a known allergen had also been transferred. However, the danger was detected during testing, and the soybean was not released.
- **Unpredictability:** GE crops may have unforeseen effects on farming systems, for example, by taking more resources from the soil or using more water than normal crops use.
- **Undesired gene movement:** Genes brought into a species artificially may cross accidentally to an unintended species. For example, resistance to herbicide could spread from a GE crop into weeds, which could then become herbicide resistant themselves.
- **Environmental hazards:** GE fish might alter the composition of natural fish populations if they escape into the wild. For example, fish that have been genetically modified to eat more in order to grow faster might invade new territories and displace native fish populations.

*A full biotechnology glossary is available at www.fao.org/biotech/biotech-glossary/en/

SOURCE: Adapted from *World Food Summit Fact Sheet: Biotechnology and Food Security* (Rome, Italy: The Food and Agriculture Organization of the United Nations, WFS FS 01-E).

has been genetically engineered to significantly change—say, its fiber content or nutrient composition—must bear a label that states the nature of the change.[35] Currently, food manufacturers may indicate through voluntary labeling whether foods have or have not been developed through genetic engineering, provided that such labeling is truthful and not misleading.[36] A number of petitions currently calling for required labeling of foods with genetically engineered ingredients may lead to FDA approval of required labeling for these foods in the future.[37] The "Risks versus Benefits" box lists some examples of currently available genetically engineered crops and highlights some of the potential benefits and risks associated with them.

Despite the concerns, many scientists are hopeful that careful use of genetic engineering will confer long-term benefits. For instance, the development of insect- and disease-resistant plants may allow farmers to grow crops with fewer chemicals. The possibilities are enormous, and each new product considered for entry into the marketplace will require careful scrutiny.

Nutrition ACTION

Eat Fresh Eat Local (Obj. 13.3)

It's Saturday morning in Any-town, USA, and in the center of the old "downtown," a large gathering of community members bustle around, chat, and enjoy their morning out. No, it's not a flashback to the 1950s. These people are buying locally grown produce and goods from farmers in their community.

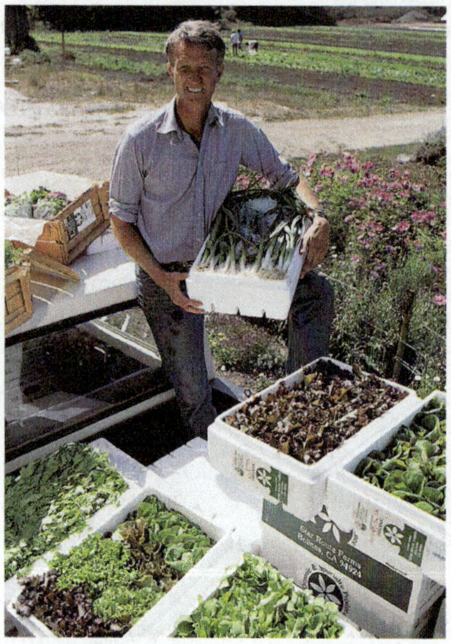

Nancy Richmond/The Image Works

Farmers' markets have existed in different forms for many years and have enjoyed remarkable growth in recent years. Through these markets, farmers are able to build a local clientele and reap profits without a middleman. Buyers also benefit from consuming produce that is ultra-fresh and in season. In addition, programs like the USDA's Senior Farmers' Market and WIC Farmers' Market provide vouchers for low-income participants to buy fresh, nutritious produce from farmers' markets. Communities as a whole benefit from farmers' markets because of the small investment and potential boost to their economies.

Farmers' markets are much more than a place to buy produce, however. In an age when mega-supermarkets have overtaken the landscape, these markets provide a great locale for a community gathering place. Farmers' markets give customers the unique experience of being able to converse with the actual growers of the produce. In doing so, these consumers can make suggestions about produce they would like to buy in the future and learn how different food items are grown.

Why Choose a Farmers' Market?*

1. They help develop a food culture—a variety of foods that are commonly grown in the local area can be displayed and purchased seasonally.
2. Foods are less processed, and less packaging is used. This creates less waste, which is good for the environment. Moreover, energy resources used to transport foods produced in more distant areas can be saved, thus helping to diminish the size of the region's ecological footprint. According to the United Nations, the ecological footprint is a measure of the resources needed to support a region's consumption of food, materials, and energy—in other words, its impact on the environment. The box on page 426 offers tips for reducing your own ecological footprint. Take the *Ecological Footprint Quiz* at www.footprintnetwork.org/resources/footprint-calculator to estimate how much productive land and water you need to support what you use and what you discard.
3. Foods are usually fresher. Most of the foods have been picked within 24 hours of purchase and have not been frozen or treated with preservatives.
4. Farmers' markets encourage healthier food choices by promoting fresh-picked seasonal fruit and vegetables.
5. Farmers' markets boost local economies because the food distributor (middleman) is eliminated. Thus, the farmers' income is more likely to be reinvested within the community.

Should You Buy Organically Grown Produce or Meats?

Once sold only in health food stores, organic fruits, vegetables, meats, and other **certified organic foods** can now be found in most mainstream markets nationwide. Sales of organic food products have grown from $78 million in 1980 to more than $30 billion today. Fresh produce is the best-selling organically grown food worldwide, but organic dairy products, soy foods, eggs, meat, and poultry are also popular.

Organically grown foods have been available for more than 40 years, but they have only recently been regulated. The United States Department of Agriculture (USDA) has created a national reference standard to define what is and what is not organic. Organic crops must be raised without the use of pesticides, petroleum-based fertilizers, or sewage sludge-based fertilizers. Animals raised on organic farms must be fed organic feed and given access to the outdoors. Additionally, they may not be given antibiotics or growth hormones.[38]

These regulations were put into place in October 2002 to regulate foods labeled "organic," whether grown in the United States or imported from other countries. The regulations mandate certification of organic products by USDA-approved state or private regulating authorities and set strict labeling standards for processed organic food. For manufacturers to use the USDA organic seal on labels, raw products must be 100 percent organic, and processed

*To locate your local farmers' market, visit www.ams.usda.gov/farmersmarkets.

FIGURE 13-7

Consumer Information about Organic Foods and Product Labels

The USDA organic seal is intended to provide information to consumers. It will help organic farmers and ranchers further expand their already growing markets.

These sample cereal boxes show the four labeling categories. Look for the name and address of the government-approved certifier on all packaged products that contain at least 70 percent organic ingredients.

SOURCE: Adapted from the National Organic Program: Labeling Packed Products, January 9, 2003; available at www.ams.usda.gov/nop/ProdHandlers/LabelTable.htm.

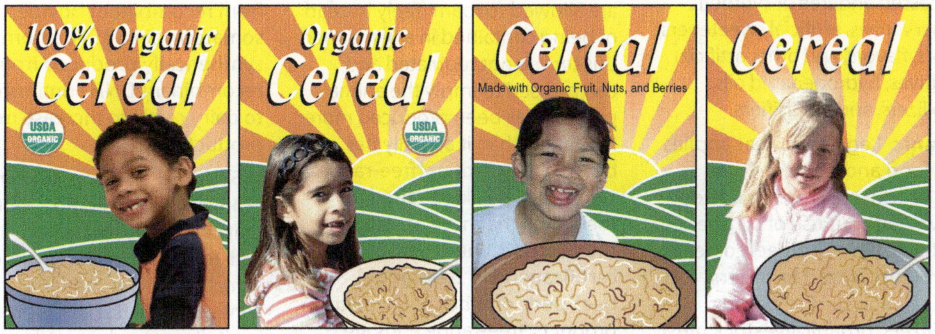

Foods made with 100 percent organic ingredients may claim "100% organic" and use the USDA seal.

Foods made with at least 95 percent organic ingredients may claim "organic" and use the USDA seal.

Foods made with at least 70 percent organic ingredients may list up to three of those ingredients on the front panel.

Foods made with less than 70 percent organic ingredients may list them on the side panel but may not make any claims on the front.

foods must contain 95 percent organic ingredients. If a food contains between 70 and 95 percent organic contents, the label can read "product made with organic ingredients." Additionally, irradiated or genetically engineered products cannot be labeled as organic.[39] See Figure 13-7 for more about consumer information on food labels. The USDA makes no claims that organically grown food is safer or more nutritious than conventionally produced foods.

However, buying organically grown food casts a vote in favor of agricultural techniques that promote the well-being of the environment and farming communities over the long run. Reputable organic farmers typically use more "eco-friendly" techniques, such as crop rotation, to help keep pests under control than do conventional farmers. These practices help protect the soil, the groundwater, and the farmworkers themselves against chemical contamination. The following box lists some of the pros and cons of buying organic foods.

Still, many farmers who don't meet "organic" standards per se use other techniques to keep pesticide use to a minimum. For example, more and more farmers have adopted a system called **integrated pest management**, a technique by which farmers cut back on chemical use by combining strategies such as crop rotation, genetic engineering, and biological controls such as the release of a predator insect on a crop to get rid of a pest.

certified organic foods Crops or livestock grown and processed according to USDA regulations concerning use of pesticides, herbicides, fungicides, fertilizers, preservatives, other synthetic chemicals, growth hormones, and antibiotics or other drugs.

integrated pest management The use of biological controls, crop rotation, genetic engineering, and other tactics to reduce chemical use in the growing and production of crops.

Advantages of Certified Organic Foods

- Less synthetic pesticide, hormone, and other chemical fertilizer residues in foods and waterways
- Beneficial to the environment: Improved soil fertility and crop diversity; increased water and energy conservation
- Farmers may follow more humane animal welfare standards
- May be higher in certain phytochemicals

Disadvantages of Certified Organic Foods

- More expensive
- Tend to spoil faster, because they contain no preservatives
- May be fertilized with improperly composted animal manure containing potentially harmful organisms, such as *E. coli*
- May be cross-contaminated with pesticides from nearby conventionally sprayed fields

(Continued)

Miniglossary of Organic Buzz Words

natural Most foods labeled "natural," except for meat and poultry, are not subject to government regulations; this term applies broadly to foods minimally processed and free of synthetic preservatives, artificial sweeteners, colors, flavors, and other artificial additives, hydrogenated oils, stabilizers, and emulsifiers.

organic Legal term that applies to a food and how the food was produced; crops must be grown without use of synthetic pesticides, bioengineered genes, petroleum-based fertilizers, and sewage sludge-based fertilizers; organic livestock must have access to outdoors and be given no antibiotics or growth hormones; organic foods may not be irradiated.

free range A method of producing livestock where animals are allowed to roam freely instead of being contained in any manner; this term is not regulated and can be used to imply the animal product has been produced more humanely than it actually has been. USDA certifies "free-range" chickens as chickens raised for their meat that have access to the outdoors; there is no USDA certification for "free-range" beef, pork, or other non-poultry products; free-range eggs also have no legal definition.

grass-fed Refers to livestock allowed to forage on pasture grass; not legally defined.

hormone-free Generally refers to products free from recombinant bovine somatotropin (rBST), a hormone synthetically produced from recombinant DNA administered to dairy cattle to increase milk production.

rBST-free Refers to milk (dairy products) produced from cattle that have not been treated with recombinant BST (bovine somatotropin hormone); all milk contains some BST as it is produced in pituitary glands of cattle.

genetically modified organisms (GMOs)/genetically engineered organisms (GEOs) Organisms from bacteria, plants, or animals that have been genetically changed in a laboratory through DNA technology. Genetically engineered plants have been developed to increase nutritional value, be resistant to pests, herbicides, or harsh environmental conditions like drought, and for other purposes.

non-GMO Term used to imply a food contains no ingredients made from GMO/GEO products; not legally defined and therefore cannot be enforced.

How to Reduce Your Ecological Footprint

Electricity

1. Turn all lighting, appliances, and electronics off when not in use.
2. Unplug things when not in use and when traveling.
3. Keep the heat at or below 68°F in the winter and keep the air conditioner at or above 75°F in the summer. Don't open windows when the heat or A/C is on!
4. Use the clothes dryer as seldom as possible and wash clothes in cold water.
5. Use compact fluorescent lightbulbs.

Food and Water

1. Eat local. Type in your zip code at Local Harvest (www.localharvest.org) to see a list of all the sustainably farmed foods in your area.
2. Eat in season. It reduces the amount of energy (and associated CO_2 emissions) needed to grow and transport the food we eat. To find out which foods, go to www.eattheseasons.com.
3. Grow it yourself, shop farmers' markets, and/or join a farm share program.
4. Make it yourself. Enjoy cooking and baking.
5. Eat lower on the food chain. The single greatest thing you can do to help stop climate change is to eat less meat or none at all.
6. Take shorter showers. Limit yourself to five minutes.
7. Turn off the water while brushing your teeth and while washing dishes. Use it only for rinsing.

Transportation

1. Keep your car clean and tuned up. Check your tire pressure and air filter regularly.
2. Drive efficiently (don't speed; avoid idling).
3. Carpool or use public transportation; fly less often.
4. Walk, jog, bike, skateboard, Rollerblade…
5. Plan ahead. Try to consolidate all your weekly errands into one outing to reduce the number of trips you take.

Goods [Reduce, Reuse, Recycle]

1. **REDUCE.** There's a reason it comes first. The less we use in the first place, the fewer resources are required and the less space we take up in landfills.
   a. Cancel any catalog and magazine subscriptions you can live without.
   b. Use both sides of sheets of paper.
   c. When shopping, take a list to avoid impulse purchases.
   d. Forgo convenience-oriented products such as individually packaged snack foods and single-use cleaning wipes.
2. **REUSE.** There's a reason it comes second.
   a. Take cloth bags to the store; carry a reusable coffee mug and water bottle, set of utensils, and food container.
   b. Opt for real dishes and utensils and cloth towels and napkins that you can launder instead of paper and plastic goods.
3. **RECYCLE.** There's a reason it comes last. Recycling should only happen once a product is absolutely not usable by anyone any longer.

Always

1. Think hard about whether or not you really need it, what went into it, and where it came from.
2. Read labels! Check out http://greenerchoices.org/labels.

SOURCE: *How to Reduce Your Ecological Footprint On (and Off) Campus*; www.smcm.edu/sustainability.

SPOTLight

13.6 Global Food Insecurity

This book emphasizes the problems of *overnutrition*: obesity, heart disease, cancer, and others—diseases of economically developed nations. However, many people in developing nations, as well as people in the less privileged parts of developed nations, suffer from problems of **undernutrition**, which is characterized by chronic debilitating hunger and malnutrition. These conditions are most visible in times of **famine**, but they are widespread and persistent even when famine does not occur.

All people need food. Regardless of our race, religion, gender, or nationality, our bodies react similarly to the effects of hunger and its companion, **malnutrition**: listlessness, weakness, failure to thrive, stunted growth, mental retardation, muscle wastage, scurvy, pellagra, beriberi, anemia, rickets, osteoporosis, goiter, tooth decay, blindness, and a host of other effects, including death.

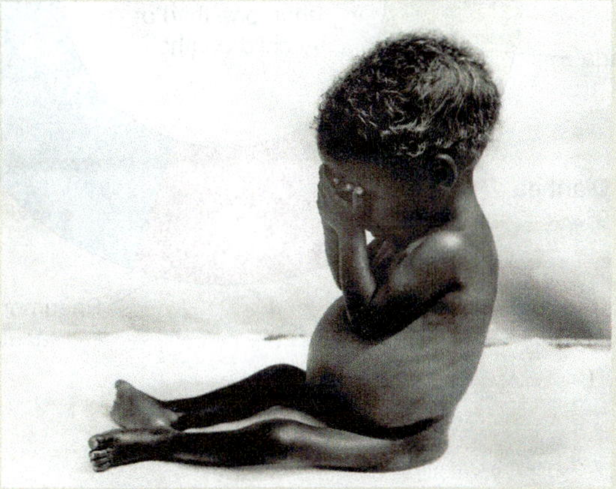

Louise Gubb/The Image Works

Children can be the first to show the signs of undernutrition due to their high nutrient needs. No famine, no flood, no earthquake, no war has ever claimed the lives of 200,000 children in a single week. Yet UNICEF estimates that malnutrition and disease claim more than that number of child victims under the age of 5 years every week at the rate of one every three seconds.

How are hunger and poverty related?

The phenomenon of hunger today is being discussed in terms of **food security** or **food insecurity**. *Food security* is defined as access by all people at all times to enough food for an active, healthy life and at a minimum includes (1) the ready availability of nutritionally adequate and safe foods, and (2) the ability to acquire personally acceptable foods in a socially acceptable way.[40] Food insecurity was once viewed as a problem of overpopulation and inadequate food production, but now many people recognize it as a problem of **poverty**. Food is *available* but is not *accessible* to the poor, who have neither land nor money. **Nutrition security** requires that all people have access to a variety of nutritious foods and potable drinking water; knowledge, resources, and skills for healthy living; prevention, treatment, and care for diseases affecting nutrition status; and safety-net systems during crisis situations, such as natural disasters or deleterious social and political systems.[41] Poverty is much more than an economic condition; it exists for many reasons, including overpopulation, greed, unemployment, and the lack of productive resources such as land, tools, and credit. Consequently, if we are to provide adequate nutrition for all the Earth's hungry people, we must transform the economic, political, and social structures that limit food production, distribution, and consumption and create a gap between rich and poor.

Approximately how many people worldwide are affected by food insecurity?

The Food and Agriculture Organization (FAO) estimates that of the more than 7.5 billion people in the world, at least 795 million people suffer from chronic, severe malnutrition, consuming too little food each day to meet even minimum energy requirements (see Figure 13-8). Three micronutrient deficiencies are of particular concern worldwide: vitamin A deficiency, the world's most common cause of preventable child blindness and vision impairment; iron-deficiency

FIGURE 13-8

Undernourishment in 2014–2016, by region (millions)

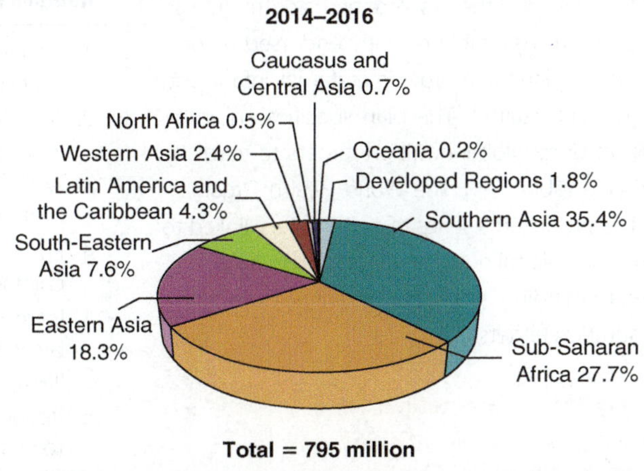

SOURCE: Food and Agriculture Organization (FAO), 2016.

FIGURE 13-9
Causes of Child Mortality

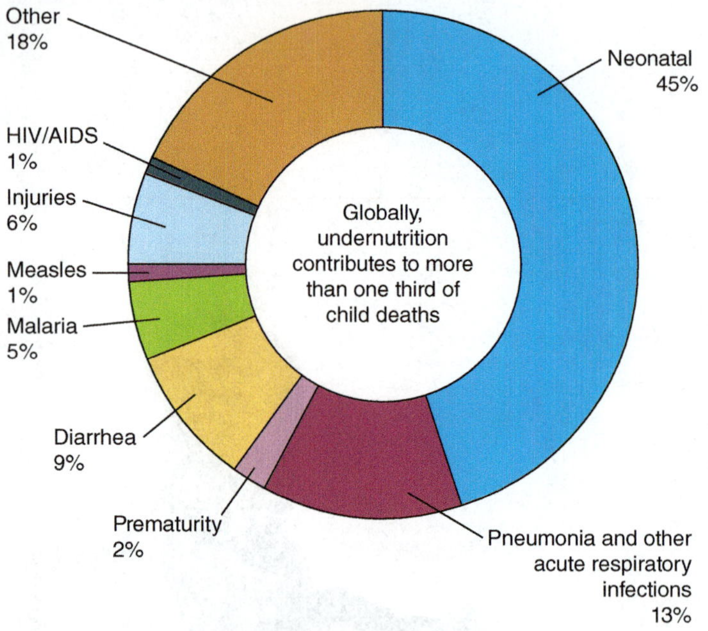

SOURCE: World Health Organization, 2015.

anemia; and iodine deficiency, which causes high levels of goiter and child retardation.[42]

Worldwide, 10 million people die every year of hunger and hunger-related diseases. Millions of children die each year from the diseases of poverty: parasitic and infectious diseases such as dysentery, whooping cough, measles, tuberculosis, cholera, and malaria (see Figure 13-9). These diseases interact with poor nutrition to form a vicious cycle in which the outcome for many is death.

Undernutrition reduces a nation's economic development by at least 8 percent because of direct losses in work productivity, as well as indirect losses from poorer cognition and missed schooling.[43] Accelerated action is needed to resolve the problem of malnutrition. The World Health Assembly recently endorsed a comprehensive plan for improving maternal, infant, and young child health.[44] The plan specifies an ambitious set of six global nutrition targets to reach by 2025 (see Table 13-9). The World Health Organization has produced a series of policy briefs, linked to each of the global nutrition targets to guide policy-makers regarding strategies necessary to achieve the nutrition targets.

What are the characteristics of protein-energy malnutrition?

Protein deficiency and energy deficiency very often go hand in hand and are called **protein-energy malnutrition (PEM)**—the world's main form of malnutrition. The condition involves a depletion of both the body's energy stores and tissue proteins and is usually accompanied by multiple vitamin and mineral deficiencies as well. Historically, severe child malnutrition was characterized as either protein deficiency called **kwashiorkor**, the disease of the weaned child, or **marasmus**, the emaciation caused by energy deficiency. Today, child malnutrition is described in terms of **chronic malnutrition**, evidenced by stunting and long-term undernutrition, and **severe acute malnutrition (SAM)**, characterized by rapid weight loss, wasting, and **edema** from recent or sudden food deprivation.[45]

Apathy is one of the earliest signs of protein-energy malnutrition. As PEM progresses, all growth ceases, and the child is no larger at age 4 than at age 2. As the protein and energy deficits worsen, new hair grows without the protein pigment that gives hair its color. The skin also loses its color, and open sores fail to heal. Digestive enzymes are in short supply, the digestive tract lining deteriorates, and absorption fails. The child cannot assimilate what little food is eaten. Proteins and hormones that previously kept the fluids correctly distributed among the compartments of the body now are diminished so that fluid leaks out of the blood (edema) and accumulates in the belly and legs. Blood proteins, including hemoglobin, are not synthesized, so the child becomes anemic, which increases the child's weakness and apathy. Antibodies to fight off invading bacteria are degraded to provide amino acids for other uses; hence, the child becomes an easy target for any infection. The child is often sick because his or her resistance to disease is low. Measles, which might make a healthy child sick for a week or two, can kill a malnourished child within 2 or 3 days. If PEM is caught in time, the starving child's life may be saved by careful nutrition therapy.

TABLE 13-9 Global Nutrition Targets, 2025

Nutrition Target	Baseline (2012)	Target for 2025
1. Achieve a 40% reduction in the number of children under five who are stunted.	162 million	~100 million
2. Achieve a 50% reduction of anemia in women of reproductive age.	29%	15%
3. Achieve a 30% reduction in low birthweight.	15%	10%
4. Ensure that there is no increase in childhood overweight.	7%	≤ 7%
5. Increase the rate of exclusive breastfeeding in the first six months of life up to at least 50%.	38%	≥ 50%
6. Reduce and maintain childhood wasting to less than 5%.	8%	< 5%

SOURCE: WHO, Global Nutrition Targets 2025: Policy Brief Series (WHO/NMH/NHD/14.2) (Geneva: World Health Organization, 2014).

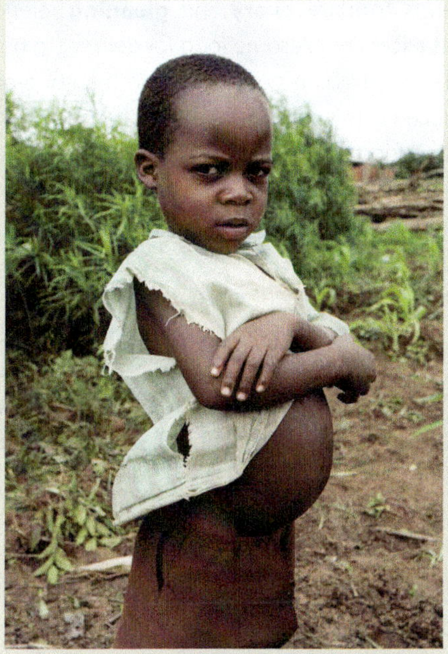
Stephen Dorey ABIPP/Alamy Stock Photo

This child has the characteristic edema and swollen belly often seen with kwashiorkor.

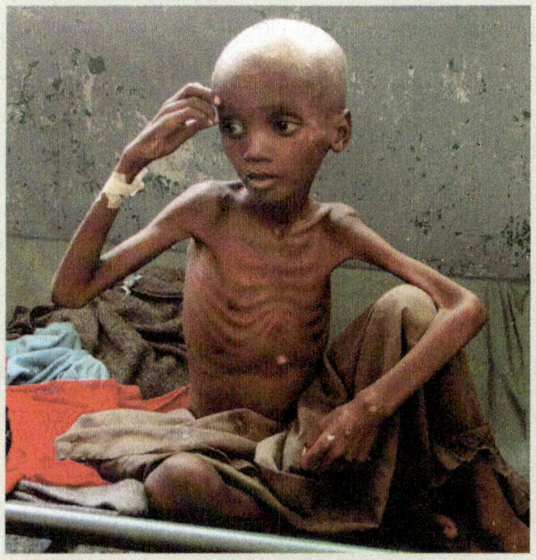
Farah Abdi Warsameh/AP Images

This child is suffering from the extreme emaciation of marasmus.

When is the risk for undernutrition highest?

Undernutrition runs high when the body's nutrient needs are high, as in times of rapid growth. If family food is limited, pregnant and lactating women, infants, and children are the first to show the signs of undernutrition. Undernutrition (low birthweight, insufficient breastfeeding, **stunting**, **wasting**, and deficiencies of vitamin A and zinc) contributes to 45 percent of the deaths worldwide of children less than 5 years of age.[46] **UNICEF** refers to the **under-5 mortality rate (U5MR)** as the best indicator of children's overall health and well-being. UNICEF argues that the U5MR reflects a country's overall resources directed at children:

> The U5MR reflects the nutritional health and the health knowledge of mothers; the level of immunization and use of **oral rehydration therapy**; the availability of maternal and health services (including prenatal care); income and food availability in the family; the availability of clean water and safe sanitation; and the overall safety of the child's environment.[47]

Until the middle of the 20th century in most of the developing countries, babies were breastfed for their first year of life, and supplements of other milk and cereal gruel were added to their diets after the first several months. Today, only about half of all infants are exclusively breastfed to the age of 4 months.[48] A number of factors contributed to this unfortunate decline, including the aggressive promotion and sale of infant formula to new mothers; the encouragement by health care practitioners for mothers to bottle-feed (hospitals sent home free samples after delivery of the newborn); and the global pattern of urbanization and the accompanying loss of cultural ties supporting breastfeeding combined with more women working outside the home. Overall, WHO estimates that more than 1.5 million children's lives could be saved each year if all mothers gave their babies nothing but breast milk for the first 6 months of life.[49]

Breastfeeding permits infants in many developing countries to achieve weight and height gains equal to those of children in developed countries until about 6 months of age. Even if infants are protected by breastfeeding at first, they must eventually be weaned. The weaning period is one of the most dangerous periods for children in developing countries. Newly weaned infants often receive nutrient-poor diluted cereals or starchy root crops, and the infants' foods are often prepared with contaminated water, making infection almost inevitable.

What is the status of food insecurity in the United States?

In 2015, more than one in six households experienced food insecurity. This represents 42.2 million people, including more than 13 million children (see Figure 13-10). Food insecurity rates are higher than average in female-headed households, households with children (especially African American and Hispanic households), and households in inner-city areas.[50] A recent analysis of state hunger surveys found consistent results across all surveys and evidence for several broad conclusions:

- Food insecurity is a chronic problem in the United States.
- Food insecurity is not due to food shortages. Hunger results from unequal distribution of economic resources, that is, poverty.
- People who lack access to a variety of resources—not just food—are most at risk of hunger. When income is inadequate to meet the costs of housing, utilities, health care, and other fixed expenses, these items compete with and may take precedence over food.
- Private charity cannot solve the food insecurity problem. Voluntary activities are limited in expertise, time, and resources and are likely to require government support to continue.[51]

What are the causes of food insecurity in the United States?

The most compelling single reason is poverty. Poverty and food insecurity are interdependent. Nutrition surveys investigating people's nutritional health in the United States have demonstrated consistently that the lower a family's income, the less adequate the family's nutrition status.

Although poverty is the major cause of food insecurity in the United States, other problems contribute as well, including, among others, homelessness; the reluctance of people to accept what they perceive as "welfare" or "charity"; delays in receiving public assistance benefits; health problems of older adults; lack of access to assistance programs; insufficient community

FIGURE 13-10

Prevalence of Food Security and Food Insecurity in U.S. Households, 2015.

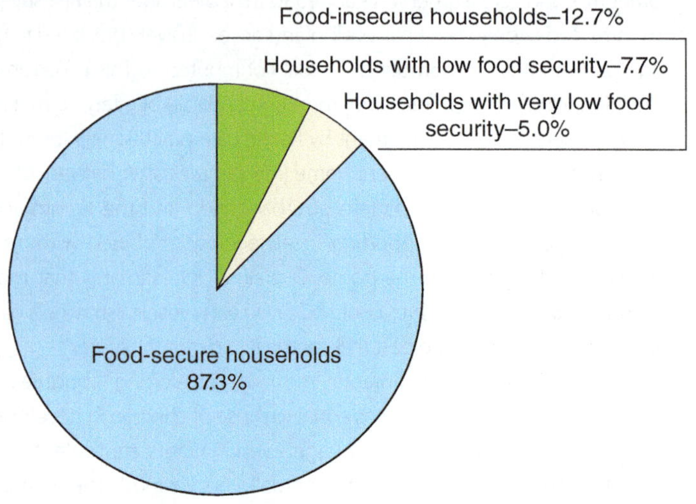

SOURCE: A. Coleman-Jensen, M. Rabbitt, C. Gregory, and A. Singh, Household Food Security in the United States in 2015, ERR-215, U.S. Department of Agriculture, Economic Research Service, September 2016.

food resources for the hungry; and insufficient community transportation systems to deliver food to people who have no transportation.

What is being done to help reduce problems of food insecurity?

The U.S. Department of Agriculture's (USDA) Food and Nutrition Service (FNS) implements an array of programs as a "food safety net," to provide children and low-income people with food or the means to purchase food.[52] Five programs—the Supplemental Nutrition Assistance Program (SNAP), previously called the food stamp program; National School Lunch Program; Special Supplemental Nutrition Program for Women, Infants, and Children (WIC); Child and Adult Care Food Program; and School Breakfast Program—account for 94 percent of all federal expenditures for food assistance. Other food assistance programs for older adults (Congregate and Home-Delivered Meal Programs) are administered by the Department of Health and Human Services.

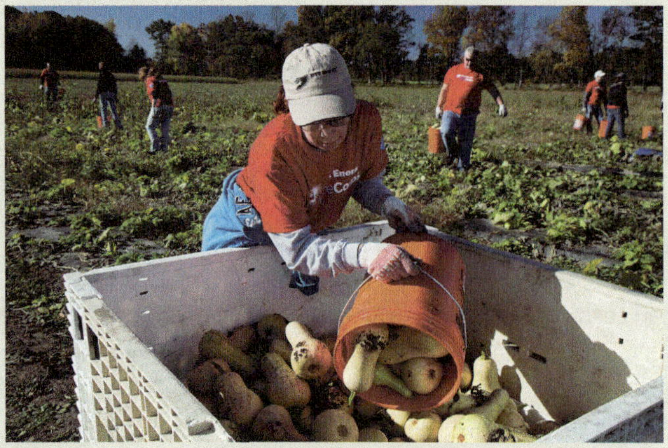

Jim West/Alamy Stock Photo

Volunteers harvest excess squash from a farmer's field for a charity that provides fresh food to soup kitchens, food banks, and other social service agencies.

The terms **food recovery** and **gleaning** refer to programs that collect excess wholesome food for delivery to hungry people. Approximately 70 billion pounds—more than one-quarter of the food produced in this country for human consumption—are lost at the retail and food service levels. In an effort to reduce food waste, the National Summit on Food Recovery and Gleaning set a goal of providing an additional 500 million pounds of food a year to feeding organizations.

Additionally, concerned citizens work through community programs and churches to provide meals to the hungry. **Feeding America**, the nation's largest supplier of surplus food, distributed more than 2 billion pounds of food to nearly 200 **food banks** and some 60,000 feeding programs for direct distribution around the nation in 2015 (see Figure 13-11).[53]

How does food insecurity in developing countries differ from food insecurity in the United States?

Global food insecurity is more extreme than domestic food insecurity. In fact, most people would find it hard to imagine the severity of poverty in the developing world:

> Many hundreds of millions of people in the poorest countries are preoccupied solely with survival and elementary needs. For them, work is frequently not available, or pay is low, and conditions barely tolerable. Homes are constructed of impermanent materials and have neither piped water nor sanitation. Electricity is a luxury. Health services are thinly spread, and in rural areas only rarely within walking distance. Permanent insecurity is the condition of the poor . . . in the wealthy countries, ordinary men and women face genuine economic problems. . . . But they rarely face anything resembling the total deprivation found in the poor countries.[54]

Food insecurity in developing nations is a problem of supply and demand, of inappropriate technology, of environmental abuse, of demographic distribution, of unequal access to resources, of extremes in dietary patterns, and of unjust economic systems. People who are poor are often powerless to change their situation because they have less access to vital resources such as education, training, food, and health services.

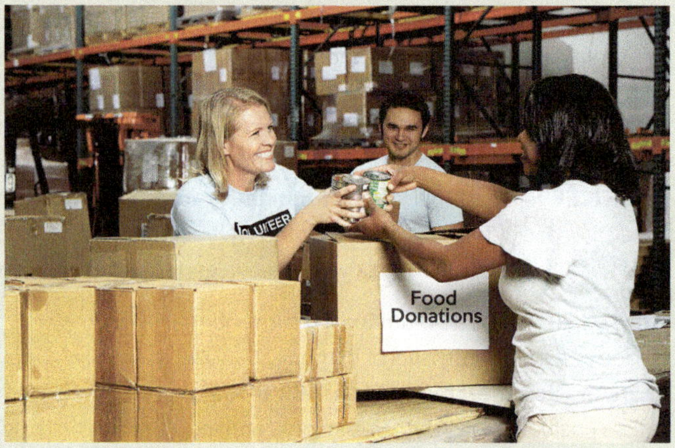

Monkey Business Images/Shutterstock.com

Volunteers accept donations and sort foods and beverages into boxes available for clients at a local food pantry.

FIGURE 13-11

What Is a Community Food Bank?

With extra groceries, hot meals, or day care snacks, hundreds of thousands of individuals benefit from a food bank's partnerships with industry and the community.

How We Work

THE DONORS AND PARTNERS

- Growers
- Processors
- Restaurants
- Manufacturers
- Distributors
- Retailers
- Convenience Stores
- Wholesalers
- Food Industry Associations
- Foodservice Operators
- Food Drives
- U.S. Department of Agriculture

→

FEEDING AMERICA

Using the latest technology, the Feeding America network distributes and tracks donated food to more than 200 certified member food banks nationwide.

→

THE AGENCIES

- Food Pantries
- Youth Programs
- Community Kitchens
- Senior Centers
- Daycare Centers
- Rehabilitation Centers
- Homeless Shelters
- Kids Cafés
- Residential Shelters
- Other Charitable Organizations

→

46.5 MILLION AMERICANS IN NEED

- Victims of Disaster
- Children
- Working Poor
- Single-Parent Families
- Unemployed
- Homeless
- Persons with Disabilities
- Older Persons

Program Types

	GROCERY	MEAL	FOOD-RELATED BENEFITS	NON-FOOD
MIXED AGE GROUP	• Community Garden • Food Bank-Operated Pantry Program • Food Pantry • Home-Delivered Grocery Program • Mobile Market/Mobile Pantry • Other Pantry Program • School Pantry Program	• Community Kitchen • Food Bank-Operated Meal Program • Group Home • Rehabilitation Program • Residential Program • Shelter • Soup Kitchen • Transitional Housing	• Nutrition Education • Special Supplemental Nutrition Program for Women, Infants, and Children (WIC) Outreach • Supplemental Nutrition Assistance Program (SNAP) Assistance and Outreach	• Clothing/Furniture Assistance • Financial Assistance • General Educational Development (GED) Programs • General Information and Referrals • Health Clinics • Housing Assistance • Job Training • Legal Assistance • Medicaid/Children's Health Insurance Program (CHIP) • Transportation Assistance • Utility/Heat Assistance
CHILDREN	• Backpack Program	• After-School Snack • Child Congregate Feeding Program (Non-Kids Café) • Daycare • Kids Café • Summer Food Service Program (SFSP)	• National School Lunch Program (NSLP) Outreach • School Breakfast Program (SBP) Outreach	
SENIORS	• Commodity Supplemental Food Program (CSFP) • Senior Brown Bag • Senior Grocery Program • Senior Mobile Pantry	• Home-Delivered Meal (or Meals on Wheels) • Senior Congregate Meal		

SOURCE: Adapted from *Hunger in America*, 2014 (Chicago: Feeding America, 2014); www.feedingamerica.org.

How are international trade and debt connected to food insecurity?

Over the years, developing countries have seen the prices of imported fuels and manufactured items rise much faster than the prices they receive for their export goods (such as bananas, coffee, and various raw materials) on the international market. The combination of high import costs with low export profits often pushes a developing country into accelerating international debt that sometimes leads to bankruptcy.

Debt and trade are closely related to the progress a country can make toward achieving an adequate diet for its people. As import prices increase relative to export prices, more of a country's total money base moves abroad to pay for the imports. With more and more of its money abroad, the country is forced to borrow money, usually at high interest rates, to continue functioning at home. As more and more of its financial resources are used to pay off interest on the country's trade debts, less and less money is available to deal with food insecurity at home. Each year, the debt crisis worsens and leads to further problems with hunger.

What about the role of multinational corporations in this issue?

Typically, large landowners and **multinational corporations** hire indigenous people for below-subsistence wages to work in the fertile farmlands growing crops to be exported for profit—leaving little fertile land for the local farmers to use to grow their own food. The local people work hard cultivating cash crops for others, not food crops for themselves. The money they earn is not even enough to buy the products they help to produce. They do not adequately share in the profits realized from the marketing of products grown with their labor. The end results of this process are that imported foods—bananas, beef, cocoa, coconuts, coffee, pineapples, sugar, tea, winter tomatoes, and others—fill the grocery stores of developed countries, while the people who labored to grow and produce these foods have less food and fewer resources than when they farmed the land for their own use. Additional cropland is diverted for nonfood, cash crops such as tobacco, rubber, cotton, and other agricultural products. These practices have also adversely affected the financial status of many U.S. farmers. The foreign cash crops often undersell the same U.S.-grown produce. The U.S. farmer cannot compete against these lower-priced imported foods and may be forced out of business.

How does overpopulation fit into the picture?

The current world population is approximately 7.5 billion, and the United Nations projects this figure to be approximately 9 billion by the year 2050. The Earth may not be able to adequately support this many people. The world's present population is certainly a concern, as is the projected population increase. As serious as the population problem is, it is only one cause of the world food problem. Poverty seems to be at the root of both hunger and overpopulation.

Three major factors affect population growth: birthrates, death rates, and standards of living. Low-income countries have high birthrates, high death rates, and low standards of living.

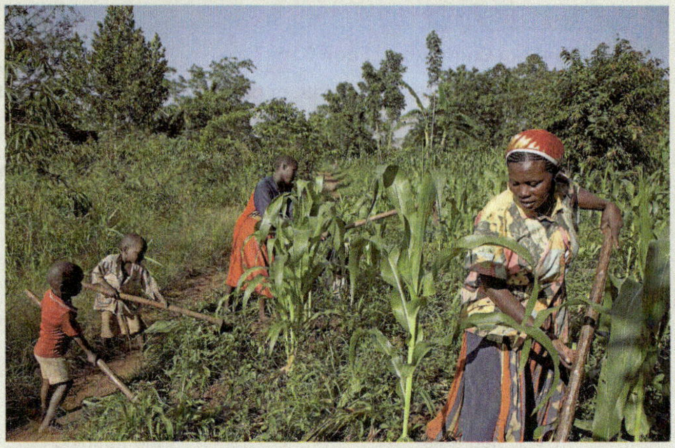

Sean Sprague/Alamy Stock Photo

A family depends on its children to cultivate the land, secure food and water, and provide for the adults in their old age.

When a people's standard of living rises, giving them better access to health care, family planning, and education, the death rate falls. In time, the birthrate also falls. As the standard of living continues to improve, the family earns sufficient income to risk having smaller numbers of children. A family depends on its children to cultivate the land, secure food and water, and provide for the adults in their old age. Under conditions of ongoing poverty, parents choose to have many children to ensure that some will survive to adulthood. Children represent the "social security" of the poor. Improvements in economic status help relieve the need for this "insurance" and thus help reduce the birthrate.

Is there a better way to distribute world resources?

Land reform—for example, giving people a meaningful opportunity to produce food for local consumption—can combine with population control to increase everyone's assets. Poor nations must be allowed to increase their agricultural productivity. Much is involved, but to put it simply, poor nations must gain greater access to five things simultaneously: land, capital, water, technology, and knowledge.[55] Equally important, each nation must adopt the political priority of improving the conditions of all its people. International food aid may be required during the development period, but eventually this aid will become less and less necessary.

Governments can learn from history the importance of developing local agricultural technology. A major effort made in the 1960s and 1970s—the green revolution—demonstrated the potential for increased grain production in Asia. It was an effort to bring the agricultural technology of the industrial world to the developing countries, but the high-yielding strains of wheat and rice that were selected required irrigation, chemical fertilizers, and pesticides—all costly and beyond the economic means of too many of the farmers in the developing world.

Instead of transplanting industrial technology into the developing countries, small, efficient farms and local structures for marketing, credit, transportation, food storage, and agricultural education should be developed. International research centers need to examine the conditions of tropical countries and orient their research toward **appropriate technology**: labor-intensive rather than energy-intensive agricultural methods. For example, labor-intensive technology, such as the use of manual grinders for grains, is appropriate in some places because it makes the best use of human, financial, and natural resources. A manual grinder can process 20 pounds of grain per hour, replacing the mortar and pestle, which in the same time can pound a maximum of only 3 pounds.[56] The specific technology that is appropriate varies from situation to situation.

Environmental concerns must be taken more seriously as well. As important as the amount of land available for crop production is the condition of the soil and the availability of water. Soil erosion is now accelerating on every continent at a rate that threatens the world's ability to continue feeding itself.[57] Erosion of soil has always occurred; it is a natural process. In the past, however, processes that build up the soil, such as the growth of trees, have compensated for erosion.

Is there hope for a world without hunger for women and children?

Women make up 50 percent of the world's population. Any solution to the problems of poverty and food insecurity is incomplete and even hopeless if it fails to address the role of women in developing countries, because women and their children represent the majority of those living in poverty.

Women play a vital role in the nutrition of their nation's people. Their nutrition during pregnancy and lactation determines the future health of their children. If women are weakened by malnutrition, the consequences ripple outward to affect many other individuals. The importance of the role women play in these countries is increasingly appreciated, and many countries now offer development programs with women in mind.

Seven basic strategies are at the heart of women's programs:

- Removing barriers to financial credit
- Providing access to time-saving technologies
- Providing appropriate education and training to promote self-reliance
- Teaching management and marketing skills
- Making health and day care services available
- Forming women's support groups[58]
- Providing information and technology to promote planned pregnancies

The recognition of women's needs by some development organizations is an encouraging trend in the efforts to fight the global malnutrition crisis.

There is hopeful news for children in developing countries—the group that is most strongly affected by poverty, malnutrition, and food insecurity and its relationship to the environment.[59] **GOBI**, a child survival plan set forth by UNICEF, has made outstanding progress in cutting the number of hunger-related child deaths. GOBI is an acronym formed from four simple, but profoundly important, elements of UNICEF's Child Survival campaign: **g**rowth charts, **o**ral rehydration therapy, **b**reast milk, and **i**mmunization.

In this program, a mother learns to weigh her child every month and chart the child's growth on a specially designed paper chart. She can learn to detect the early stages of hidden malnutrition.

Oral rehydration therapy (ORT) is important because most children who die of malnutrition do not starve to death; rather, they die because their health has been compromised by dehydration due to infections that cause diarrhea. The spread of ORT is preventing an estimated 1 million dehydration deaths each year.[60] Oral rehydration therapy is the administration of a simple solution that mothers can make up themselves, using locally available ingredients, that increases a body's ability to absorb fluids 25-fold.[61] International development groups also provide mothers with packets of premeasured salt and sugar to be mixed with water in rural and urban areas. A safe and sanitary supply of drinking water is a prerequisite for the success of the ORT program.

The promotion of breastfeeding among mothers in developing countries has many benefits. Breast milk is hygienic, is readily available, is nutritionally sound, and provides infants with immunologic protection specific for their environment. In the developing world, the advantages of breastfeeding over formula feeding can mean the difference between life and death.

Immunizations (the *I* of GOBI) could prevent most of the 5 million deaths each year from measles, diphtheria, tetanus, whooping cough, poliomyelitis, and tuberculosis. The immunization achievements of the last two decades are credited with the prevention of approximately 3 million deaths a year, as well as the protection of many millions more from disease, malnutrition, blindness, deafness, and polio.[62]

Organizations have come together to ensure children and families get a healthy start at life through the *Scaling-Up Nutrition* network of maternal and child health programs from conception to 2 years (see Table 13-10).[63] Many governments have actively adopted the child survival strategies of UNICEF: universal immunization; oral rehydration therapy; a massive effort to promote breastfeeding as the ideal food for at least the first 6 months of an infant's life; an attack on malnutrition involving nutrition surveillance focusing on growth monitoring and weighing of infants at least once every month for the first 18 months of the child's life; and nutrition and literacy education that will empower women in developing countries and lead to a reduction in nutrition-related diseases among vulnerable children.[64]

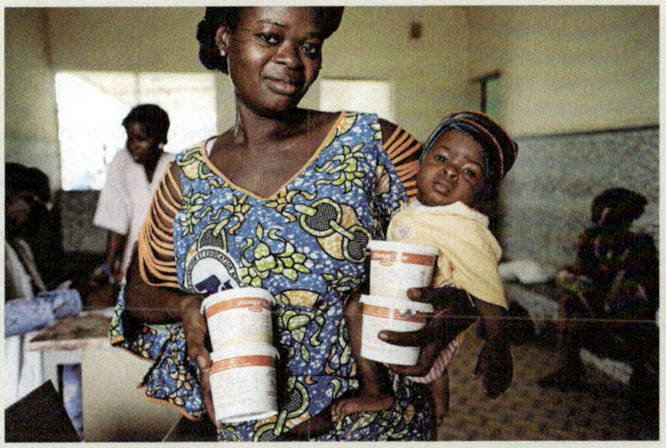

© Michaël Zumstein/Agence Vu

Ready-to-use supplementary feedings such as Plumpy'Doz® are intended to be used as a nutritional supplement to the regular diet.

TABLE 13-10 **Examples of 13 Cost-Effective Interventions to Reduce Malnutrition**

Type of Intervention	Example of Intervention or Practice	Target Population
Behavior Change Interventions		
1. Breastfeeding promotion and support	• Early initiation of breastfeeding • Exclusive breastfeeding for 6 months and continued breastfeeding until 2 years of age	Pregnant women and parents of infants under 6 months of age
2. Promotion of complementary feeding	Delivery of educational messages	Pregnant women and parents of infants and young children under 2 years of age
3. Safe hygiene behaviors, including hand washing with soap	Delivery of educational messages	Entire population
Micronutrient Supplementation and Deworming Interventions		
4. Vitamin A supplementation	Semi-annual doses for children	Children 6 months to 5 years of age
5. Therapeutic zinc supplements	As part of diarrhea management	Children 6 months to 5 years of age
6. Supplements for pregnant women	• Iron-folic acid supplements • Calcium supplements	Pregnant women
7. Deworming (to reduce loss of micronutrients)	Treat with deworming drugs (1 or 2 rounds per year)	Children 6 months to 5 years of age
Home and Community Food Fortification Interventions		
8. Home and community food fortification	• Multiple micronutrient powders (sachets or "Sprinkles")[a] for in-home fortification of complementary foods • Ready-to-use supplementary feeding (RUSF) (e.g., Plumpy'Doz®); intended to be an adjunct to the diet; provides energy with the full daily requirement of micronutrients[b]	Children aged 6–24 months and pregnant women; or may provide the complete recommended nutrient intake for children aged 6 months to 5 years of age
Mass or Universal Fortification[c] Interventions		
9. Iron fortification of staples	Iron fortification of staples (e.g., flour, rice, oil, condiments)	Entire population
10. Salt iodization	Salt iodization	Entire population
11. Iodine supplements	Iodized oil capsules	Pregnant women in highly endemic areas if iodized salt is not available
Complementary and Therapeutic Feeding Interventions		
12. Prevention or treatment of moderate malnutrition (underweight)	• Screening to determine circumstances in which food supplementation is needed • Provision of complementary foods	Populations with high prevalence of children 6–24 months with low weight-for-age measures
13. Treatment of severe acute malnutrition (severe wasting)	• Screening to identify cases of severe acute malnutrition • Therapeutic feeding with high-energy, fortified, ready-to-use therapeutic foods (RUTF)[d]—e.g., Plumpy'Nut®	Children 6 months to 5 years of age with very low weight-for-height measures

[a] Large-scale distribution has been limited to a small number of countries thus far, but the number of sachets bought and supplied by UNICEF and the World Food Programme (WFP) increased from just over 50 million in 2008 to around 810 million in 2016.

[b] Home fortification is recommended where children have low dietary diversity or when a child has infectious diseases or worm infestation. Supplementary feedings are energy and nutrient dense with essential fats and recommended micronutrients. Also known as lipid-based nutrient supplements (LNS), they are usually pastes made from oil seed or peanuts that are enriched with nutrients. One example is Plumpy'Doz®, which has about 245 calories per recommended dose and comes in tubs containing a weekly ration. It contains peanut paste, vegetable fat, skimmed milk powder, whey, maltodextrins, and sugar, and is designed to be eaten in small quantities, as a supplement to the regular diet.

[c] Biofortification is the development of staple crops that are rich in micronutrients through traditional or conventional agricultural breeding practices or through modern biotechnology. Biofortification is an area in need of further research, including whether farmers would accept the new technology and whether consumers would buy and eat biofortified foods. An example is the large-scale introduction in Mozambique of the orange-flesh sweet potato, which is rich in vitamin A. Other commercial or market-driven fortification involves food companies voluntarily fortifying products, such as cereals or porridge for infants and young children, within regulatory limits set by the national government.

[d] Plumpy'Nut® is a ready-to-use therapeutic spread packaged in individual sachets of 500 calories each. It is a paste of groundnut composed of vegetable fat, peanut butter, skimmed milk powder, sugar, minerals, and vitamins.

SOURCES: Adapted from UN Standing Committee on Nutrition, *Scaling Up Nutrition: A Framework for Action* (Geneva: United Nations Standing Committee on Nutrition, 2010); *The Lancet Maternal and Child Nutrition Series,* June 2013; S. Horton, M. Shekar, C. McDonald, A. Mahal, and J. K. Brooks, *Scaling Up Nutrition: What Will It Cost?* (Washington, DC: The International Bank for Reconstruction and Development, 2010); Save the Children, *A Life Free from Hunger: Tackling Child Malnutrition* (Westport, CT: The Save the Children Fund, 2012).

What can I do to help alleviate hunger problems?

"Our lives begin to end the day we become silent about things that matter."

—*Dr. Martin Luther King*

The problems of hunger can appear so great that they sometimes seem approachable only by way of worldwide political decisions. To this end, many individuals and groups are working to improve the chances of the future well-being of the world and its people through a number of national and international organizations. Check out the resources available from the organizations listed in the Nutrition on the Web section at the end of this chapter.

Regardless of the type and level of involvement a person chooses, each person can make a difference. Consider working with others who have similar interests, raising awareness of world food security issues, following current hunger-related legislation, and calling for change by writing and telephoning local and national political representatives and expressing concern about foreign aid, trade, and other domestic policy issues relevant to world food security. Encourage your church, synagogue, or mosque to support both overseas work and domestic outreach efforts to address food insecurity; support these efforts with monetary contributions.[65]

Individuals can also help change the world through the personal choices they make each day. Our choices affect the way the rest of the world's people live and die. People in affluent nations have the freedom and means to choose their lifestyles. We can find ways to reduce our consumption of the world's nonrenewable resources and use only what is absolutely required. As one person put it, "The widespread simplification of life is vital to the well-being of the entire human family."[66] Personal lifestyles do matter, for a society is nothing more than the sum of its individuals. As we go, so goes our world.

The late George McGovern, former U.S. senator and former U.S. ambassador to the UN Agencies on Food and Agriculture in Rome, called us all to action with the following words—excerpted from his book, *The Third Freedom: Ending Hunger in Our Time*:[67]

> Hunger is a political condition. The Earth has enough knowledge and resources to eradicate this ancient scourge. Hunger has plagued the world for thousands of years. But ending it is a greater moral imperative now than ever before, because for the first time humanity has the instruments in hand to defeat this cruel enemy at a very reasonable cost.
>
> What will it cost if we don't end the hunger that now afflicts so many of our fellow humans? The World Bank has concluded that each year malnutrition causes the loss of 46 million years of productive life, at a cost of $16 billion annually, several times the cost of ending hunger and turning this loss into productive gain.
>
> Of course it is impossible to evaluate with dollars the real cost of hunger. What is the value of a human life? The twentieth century was the most violent in human history. With nearly 150 million people killed by war. But in just the last half of that century nearly three times as many died of malnutrition or related causes. How does one put a dollar figure on this terrible toll silently collected by the Grim Reaper? What is the cost of 850 million hungry people dragging through shortened and miserable lives, unable to study, work, play, or otherwise function normally because of the ever-present drain of hunger and malnutrition on body, mind, and spirit? What is the cost of millions of young mothers breaking under the despair of watching their children waste away and die from malnutrition? This is a problem we can resolve at a fraction of the cost of ignoring it. We need to be about that task now. I give you my word that anyone who looks honestly at world hunger and measures the cost of ending it for all time will conclude that this is a bargain well worth seizing. More often than not, those who look at the problem and the cost of its solution will wonder why humanity didn't resolve it long ago.

Miniglossary

appropriate technology A technology that utilizes locally abundant resources in preference to locally scarce resources. For developing countries, which usually have a large labor force and little capital, the appropriate technology would therefore be labor intensive.

chronic malnutrition A condition characterized by chronic growth retardation or stunting as reflected in low weight or low height for age.

edema (eh-DEEM-uh) Swelling of body tissue caused by leakage of fluid from the blood vessels, seen in (among other conditions) protein deficiency.

famine Widespread lack of access to food caused by natural disasters, political factors, or war; characterized by a large number of deaths due to starvation and malnutrition.

Feeding America A national food-banking network to which most food banks belong.

food banks Nonprofit community organizations that collect surplus commodities from the government as well as edible but often unmarketable foods from private industry for use by nonprofit charities, institutions, and feeding programs at nominal cost.

food insecurity The inability to acquire or consume an adequate quality or sufficient quantity of food in socially acceptable ways, or the uncertainty that one will be able to do so.

food recovery Such activities as salvaging perishable produce from grocery stores and wholesale food markets; rescuing surplus prepared food from restaurants, corporate cafeterias, and caterers; and collecting nonperishable, canned, or boxed processed food from manufacturers, supermarkets, or people's homes. The items recovered are donated to hungry people.

food security Access by all people at all times to enough food for an active and healthy life. Food security has two aspects: ensuring that adequate food supplies are available and ensuring that households have the ability to acquire food, either by producing it themselves or by being able to purchase it.

gleaning The harvesting of excess food from farms, orchards, and packing houses to feed the hungry.

GOBI An acronym formed from the elements of UNICEF's Child Survival campaign: **g**rowth charts, **o**ral rehydration therapy, **b**reast milk, and **i**mmunization.

kwashiorkor (kwash-ee-OR-core) Severe malnutrition caused by inadequate protein and calories leading to apathy, anemia, loss of body proteins, and poor growth.

malnutrition The impairment of health resulting from a relative deficiency or excess of food energy and specific nutrients necessary for health.

marasmus (muh-RAZ-mus) Severe emaciation from energy deficiency with chronic wasting of fat, muscle, and other tissues; starvation.

multinational corporations International companies with direct investments and/or operative facilities in more than one country. U.S. oil and food companies are examples.

nutrition security Condition in which all people have access to a variety of nutritious foods and potable drinking water; knowledge, resources, and skills for healthy living; prevention, treatment, and care for diseases affecting nutrition status; and safety-net systems during crisis situations, such as natural disasters or deleterious social and political systems.

oral rehydration therapy (ORT) The treatment of dehydration (usually due to diarrhea caused by infectious disease) with an oral solution; ORT as developed by UNICEF is intended to enable a mother to mix a simple solution for her child from substances that she has at home.

poverty The state of having too little money to meet minimum needs for food, clothing, and shelter. The U.S. Department of Agriculture defined the poverty level in the United States as an annual income of $24,600 for a family of four in 2017.

protein-energy malnutrition (PEM) The world's most widespread malnutrition problem; characterized by a depletion of both energy stores and tissue proteins; usually accompanied by micronutrient deficiencies.

severe acute malnutrition (SAM) A condition characterized by very low weight for height, severe wasting, and/or edema associated with recent severe food deprivation.

under-5 mortality rate (U5MR) The number of children who die before the age of 5 for every 1,000 live births.

undernutrition (also called hunger) As used in this discussion, a term that describes the domestic and world food problem of a continuous lack of the food energy and nutrients necessary to achieve and maintain health and protection from disease.

stunting (short for age) Children aged 0 to 59 months with a low height for age measure; a measure of chronic malnutrition (long-term food deprivation).

wasting (thin for height) Children aged 0 to 59 months with a low weight for length/height measure; a measure of severe acute malnutrition—indicating recent rapid weight loss or a failure to gain weight.

UNICEF The United Nations International Children's Emergency Fund, now referred to as the United Nations Children's Fund.

WHAT'S ONLINE

MINDTAP From Cengage

Visit www.cengagebrain.com to access MindTap, a complete digital course that includes Diet & Wellness Plus, interactive quizzes, videos, and more.

Nutrition on the Web: Food Safety

http://fnic.nal.usda.gov

The Food and Nutrition Information Center: Click on Food Safety.

www.foodsafety.gov

This website is the gateway to government food-safety information.

www.cdc.gov/foodsafety

Food-safety information and tips for international travelers.

www.fda.gov/Food/default.htm

Information on food safety from the Center for Food Safety and Applied Nutrition.

www.fsis.usda.gov

Information about ensuring the safety of the U.S. food supply.

http://publications.usa.gov

Food-safety resources.

www.fightbac.org

The Partnership for Food Safety Education provides consumer information about food safety.

Nutrition on the Web: Food Insecurity

www.who.int/en

The World Health Organization website provides resources on food insecurity, poverty, and overpopulation.

http://feedingamerica.org

This website addresses food distribution, community food banks, and food security topics.

http://frac.org

The Food Research and Action Center website provides information on U.S. food security issues and food assistance programs.

www.fns.usda.gov/fns

This website provides information about U.S. food assistance and food recovery programs.

www.unicef.org

Visit this website for information on child survival programs worldwide.

www.bread.org

This website addresses domestic and world food insecurity issues.

www.fao.org/home/en

At this website, FAO provides information about global food issues.

www.wfp.org

The United Nations World Food Programme website provides resources about food insecurity.

www.oxfamamerica.org

This website provides information about global food insecurity and poverty.

Appendix A

Aids to Calculations, the Food Lists for Diabetes and Weight Management, and the USDA Healthy Eating Patterns

This appendix aims to help with the use of the metric system and with calculation problems not fully explained elsewhere. Chapter 2 introduced several diet-planning tools. This appendix also provides more detail about the *Choose Your Foods: Food Lists for Diabetes and Weight Management* (formerly, The Exchange System), and presents several eating patterns that meet the *Dietary Guidelines for Americans.*

Conversion Factors*

Conversion factors are useful mathematical tools in everyday calculations, like the ones encountered in the study of nutrition. A conversion factor is a fraction in which the numerator (top) and the denominator (bottom) express the same quantity in different units. For example, 2.2 pounds and 1 kilogram are *equivalent;* they express the same weight. The conversion factor used to change pounds to kilograms or vice versa is:

$$\frac{2.2 \text{ lb}}{1 \text{ kg}} \text{ or } \frac{1 \text{ kg}}{2.2 \text{ lb}}$$

Because either of these factors equals 1, a measurement can be multiplied by the factor without changing the value of the measurement. Thus its units can be changed.

The correct factor to use in a problem is the one with the unit you are seeking in the numerator (top) of the fraction. Following are three examples of problems commonly encountered in nutrition study; they illustrate the usefulness of conversion factors.

Example 1

Convert ¼ cup to an approximate number of milliliters for use in a recipe.

1. The conversion factor is:

$$\frac{1 \text{ c}}{250 \text{ mL}} \text{ or } \frac{250 \text{ mL}}{1 \text{ c}}$$

2. Multiply ¼ cup by the factor:

$$\tfrac{1}{4} \text{ c} \times \frac{250 \text{ mL}}{1 \text{ c}} = 62.5 \text{ mL, or about } 60 \text{ mL}$$

Example 2

Convert the weight of 130 pounds to kilograms.

1. Choose the conversion factor in which the unit you are seeking is on top:

$$\frac{1 \text{ kg}}{2.2 \text{ lb}}$$

*For a listing of specific conversion factors, see Table A-1 on page A-4.

2. Multiply 130 pounds by the factor:

$$130 \text{ lb} \times \frac{1 \text{ kg}}{2.2 \text{ lb}} = \frac{130 \text{ kg}}{2.2} = 59 \text{ kg (rounded off to nearest whole number)}$$

Example 3

How many grams of saturated fat are contained in a 3-ounce hamburger? A 4-ounce hamburger contains 7 grams of saturated fat.

1. You are seeking grams of saturated fat; therefore, the conversion factor is:

$$\frac{7 \text{ g saturated fat}}{4 \text{ oz hamburger}}$$

2. Multiply 3 ounces of hamburger by the conversion factor:

$$3 \text{ oz hamburger} \times \frac{7 \text{ g saturated fat}}{4 \text{ oz hamburger}} = \frac{3 \times 7 \text{ g}}{4} = \frac{21}{4}$$
$$= 5 \text{ g saturated fat (rounded off to nearest whole number)}$$

Percentages

A *percentage* is a comparison between a number of items (perhaps your intake of calories) and a standard number (perhaps the number of calories recommended for your age and gender). The standard number is the number you divide by. The answer you get after the division must be multiplied by 100 to be stated as a percentage (*percent* means "per 100").

Example 4

What percentage of the DRI for energy (EER) is your calorie intake?

1. We'll use 2,400 calories to demonstrate. (The EER are lised at the back of the book.)
2. Total your calorie intake for a day—for example, 1,200 calories.
3. Divide your calorie intake by the EER calories:

$$1{,}200 \text{ cal (your intake)} \div 2{,}400 \text{ cal (EER)} = 0.50$$

4. Multiply your answer by 100 to state it as a percentage:

$$0.50 \times 100 = 50.0 = 50\%$$

In some problems in nutrition, the percentage may be more than 100. For example, suppose your daily intake of vitamin C is 500 mg and your RDA (male) is 90 mg. Your intake as a percentage of the RDA is more than 100 percent (that is, you consume more than 100 percent of your vitamin C RDA). The following calculations show your vitamin C intake as a percentage of the RDA:

$$500 \div 90 = 5.55$$
$$5.55 \times 100 = 555\% \text{ of RDA}$$

Sometimes the comparison is between a part of a whole (e.g., your calories from protein) and the total amount (your total calories). In this case, the total number is the one you divide by as shown in Example 5.

Example 5

What percentages of your total calories for the day come from protein, fat, and carbohydrate?

1. Using the Table of Food Composition in MindTap and your diet record, find the total grams of protein, fat, and carbohydrate you consumed—for example, 60 grams protein, 80 grams fat, and 285 grams carbohydrate.
2. Multiply the number of grams by the number of calories from 1 gram of each energy nutrient (conversion factors):

$$60 \text{ g protein} \times \frac{4 \text{ cal}}{1 \text{ g protein}} = 240 \text{ cal}$$

$$80 \text{ g fat} \times \frac{9 \text{ cal}}{1 \text{ g fat}} = 720 \text{ cal}$$

$$285 \text{ g carbohydrate} \times \frac{4 \text{ cal}}{1 \text{ g carbohydrate}} = 1{,}140 \text{ cal}$$

$$240 + 720 + 1{,}140 = 2{,}100 \text{ cal}$$

3. Find the percentage of total calories from each energy nutrient (see Example 4):

$$\text{Protein: } 240 \div 2{,}100 = 0.114$$
$$0.114 \times 100 = 11.4 = 11\% \text{ of calories}$$

$$\text{Fat: } 720 \div 2{,}100 = 0.343$$
$$0.343 \times 100 = 34.3 = 34\% \text{ of calories}$$

$$\text{Carbohydrate: } 1{,}140 \div 2{,}100 = 0.543$$
$$0.543 \times 100 = 54.3 = 54\% \text{ of calories}$$

$$11\% + 34\% + 54\% = 99\% \text{ of calories (total)}$$

The percentages total 99 percent rather than 100 percent because a little was lost from each number in rounding off. Either 99 or 101 is a reasonable total.

Daily Values (DV) for Food Labels[a]

The Daily Values are standards developed by the Food and Drug Administration (FDA) for use on food labels. The values are based on 2,000 calories a day for adults and children over 4 years old.

DV for Food Components			DV for Vitamins			DV for Minerals		
Component	**Old DV[b]**	**New DV**	**Nutrient**	**Old DV**	**New DV**	**Nutrient**	**Old DV**	**New DV**
Protein[c]	50 g	50 g	Thiamin	1.5 mg	1.2 mg	Calcium	1,000 mg	1,300 mg
Fat	65 g	78 g	Riboflavin	1.7 mg	1.3 mg	Iron	18 mg	18 mg
Saturated fat	20 g	20 g	Niacin	20 mg	16 mg NE	Zinc	15 mg	11 mg
Cholesterol	300 mg	300 mg	Biotin	300 µg	30 µg	Iodine	150 µg	150 µg
Total carbohydrate	300 g	275 g	Choline	550 mg	550 mg	Copper	2 mg	0.9 mg
Added sugars	—	50 g	Pantothenic acid	10 mg	5 mg	Chromium	120 µg	35 µg
Fiber	25 g	28 g	Vitamin B_6	2 mg	1.7 mg	Selenium	70 µg	55 µg
Sodium	2,400 mg	2,300 mg	Folate	400 µg	400 µg DFE	Molybdenum	75 µg	45 µg
Potassium	3,500 mg	4,700 mg	Vitamin B_{12}	6.0 µg	2.4 µg	Manganese	2.0 mg	2.3 mg
Calculation factors:			Vitamin C	60 mg	90 mg	Chloride	3,400 mg	2,300 mg
Fat	78 g	35% of calories	Vitamin A	5,000 IU[d]	900 µg RAE	Magnesium	400 mg	420 mg
Saturated fat	20 g	10% of calories	Vitamin D	400 IU[d]	20 µg	Phosphorus	1,000 mg	1,250 mg
Total Carbohydrate	275 g	55% of calories	Vitamin E	30 IU[d]	15 mg			
Added sugars	50 g	10% of calories	Vitamin K	80 µg	120 µg			
Protein	50 g	10% of calories						

[a]Abbreviations used: g = grams, mg = milligrams, mg NE = milligrams niacin equivalents, µg = micrograms, µg DFE = micrograms dietary folate equivalents, IU = International Units, µg RAE = micrograms retinol activity equivalents
[b]Formerly the U.S. RDA, based on National Academy of Sciences' 1968 Recommended Dietary Allowances.
[c]The Daily Values for protein vary for different groups of people: children 1 to 4 years: 16 g; infants under 1 year: 14 g; pregnant women: 60 g; nursing mothers: 65 g.
[d]Equivalent values for the nutrients expressed as IU are: vitamin A, 1,500 RAE (assumes a mixture of 40% retinol and 60% beta-carotene); vitamin D, 10 µg; vitamin E, 20 mg.

SOURCE: Food and Drug Administration, Food Labeling: Revision of the Nutrition and Supplement Facts Labels, *Federal Register* Vol. 81, No. 103, May 27, 2016.

Nutrient Units and Unit Conversions

International Units (IU)	Folate
To convert IU to: µg vitamin D: divide by 40 or multiply by 0.025. mg αTE:[a] divide by 1.5 or multiply by 0.67	To convert micrograms of synthetic folate in supplements and enriched foods to Dietary Folate Equivalents (µg DFE): µg synthetic folate × 1.7 = µg DFE For naturally occurring folate, assign each microgram folate a value of 1 µg DFE: µg folate = µg DFE Total DFE = µg food folate + (1.7 × µg synthetic folate)
Sodium	**Niacin**
To convert milligrams of sodium to grams of salt mg sodium ÷ 400 = g of salt The reverse is also true g salt × 400 = mg sodium	1 mg NE (niacin equivalent) = 1 mg niacin = 60 mg dietary tryptophan (an amino acid)
Vitamin A	
1 µg RAE[b] = 1 µg retinol = 12 µg beta-carotene = 24 µg other vitamin A carotenoids	1 IU = 0.3 µg retinol = 3.6 µg beta-carotene = 7.2 µg other vitamin A carotenoids

[a]Alpha-tocopherol equivalents (vitamin E).
[b]Retinol activity equivalents (vitamin A).

TABLE A-1 **Conversion Factors**

Length	Volume	Temperature
1 inch = 2.54 centimeters (cm) 1 ft = 30.48 cm 1 meter (m) = 39.37 inches	1 tbsp = 3 tsp or 15 milliliters (mL) 1 oz = 2 tbsp or 30 mL ½ c = about 125 mL 1 c = 16 tbsp or about 250 mL 1 qt = 4 c or 0.95 liter (L) 1 qt = 32 oz (fluid) 1 L = 1.06 qt or 1000 mL 1 gal = 16 c or 4 qt or 3.79 liter	Celsius (Centigrade) / Fahrenheit Steam: 100°C / 212°F Body temperature: 37°C / 98.6°F Ice: 0°C / 32°F $t_F = \frac{9}{5} t_c + 32$ $t_c = \frac{5}{9}(t_F - 32)$
Weight		**Energy**
1 oz = about 30 grams (g) (28.35 g) 1 lb = about 454 g 1 kilogram (kg) = 1000 g 1 kg = 2.2 lb 1 g = 1000 mg 1 milligram (mg) = 1000 µg 1 microgram (µg or mcg) = $\frac{1}{1000}$ mg	1 tsp any powder or liquid = about 5 g or 5 mL 1 tbsp any powder or liquid = about 15 g or 15 mL ½ c any vegetable, fruit, or fluid weighs about 100 g	1 calorie (cal) = 4.2 kilojoule (kJ) = 0.004 megajoule (mJ) 1 mJ = 240 cal 1 kJ = 0.24 cal 1 g carbohydrate = 4 cal = 17 kJ 1 g fat = 9 cal = 37 kJ 1 g protein = 4 cal = 17 kJ 1 g alcohol = 7 cal = 29 kJ

Body Weights: Quick Estimation of Desirable Body Weight

Men	Women
For 5 ft, consider 106 lb a reasonable weight. For each inch over 5 ft, add 6 lb. Subtract 6 lb for each inch under 5 ft. Add 10% for a large-framed individual; subtract 10% for a small-framed individual. *Example:* A man 5 ft 8 inches tall (medium frame) would start at 106 lb, add 48, and arrive at a reasonable weight of 154 lb.	For 5 ft, consider 100 lb a reasonable weight. For each inch over 5 ft, add 5 lb. Subtract 5 lb for each inch under 5 ft. Add 10% for a large-framed individual; subtract 10% for a small-framed individual. For each year under 25 (down to 18), subtract 1 lb. *Example:* A woman 21 years old, 5 ft 4 inches tall (medium-frame), would start at 100 lb, add 20, and subtract 4, arriving at a reasonable weight of 116 lb.

Table A-2 shows how to determine frame size.

TABLE A-2 Frame Size

To make a simple approximation of your frame size:

Extend your arm and bend the forearm upward at a 90-degree angle. Keep the fingers straight and turn the inside of your wrist away from your body. Place the thumb and index finger of your other hand on the two prominent bones on either side of your elbow. Measure the space between your fingers against a ruler or a tape measure.[a] Compare the measurements with the following standards. (These standards represent the elbow measurements for medium-framed men and women of various heights. Measurements smaller than those listed indicate you have a small frame, and larger measurements indicate a large frame.[b])

Men		Women	
Height in 1-in. Heels	**Elbow Breadth**	**Height in 1-in. Heels**	**Elbow Breadth**
5 ft 2 in. to 5 ft 3 in.	$2\frac{1}{2}$ to $2\frac{7}{8}$ in.	4 ft 10 in. to 4 ft 11 in.	$2\frac{1}{4}$ to $2\frac{1}{2}$ in.
5 ft 4 in. to 5 ft 7 in.	$2\frac{5}{8}$ to $2\frac{7}{8}$ in.	5 ft 0 in. to 5 ft 3 in.	$2\frac{1}{4}$ to $2\frac{1}{2}$ in.
5 ft 8 in. to 5 ft 11 in.	$2\frac{3}{4}$ to 3 in.	5 ft 4 in. to 5 ft 7 in.	$2\frac{3}{8}$ to $2\frac{5}{8}$ in.
6 ft 0 in. to 6 ft 3 in.	$2\frac{3}{4}$ to $3\frac{1}{8}$ in.	5 ft 8 in. to 5 ft 11 in.	$2\frac{3}{8}$ to $3\frac{5}{8}$ in.
6 ft 4 in. and over	$2\frac{7}{8}$ to $3\frac{1}{4}$ in.	6 ft 0 in. and over	$2\frac{1}{2}$ to $3\frac{3}{4}$ in.

[a]For the most accurate measurement, have your health care provider measure your elbow breadth with a caliper.

[b]A simple estimate of frame size can be derived by circling your wrist with the thumb and middle finger of your other hand. If the thumb and finger do not meet, you most likely have a large frame. If the thumb and finger just meet, you most likely have a medium frame, and if the fingers overlap greatly, you may have a small frame.

Choose Your Foods: Food Lists for Diabetes and Weight Management

The food lists (formerly food exchange system) divide the foods suitable for use in planning a healthy diet into several lists—the starch; fruit; milk; sweets, desserts, and other carbohydrates; nonstarchy vegetables; protein; and fat lists.* The food lists are shown in Table A-3. Figure A-1 provides examples of foods, portion sizes, and energy-nutrient contributions for each of the food lists.

TABLE A-3 The Food Lists

List	Portion Size	Carbohydrate (CHO) (g)	Protein (g)	Fat (g)	Energy (cal)
Carbohydrate Group					
Starch	1 slice; ½ c	15	3	1	80
Fruit	varies	15	—	—	60
Milk and Milk Substitutes	1 c				
Fat-free, low-fat, 1%		12	8	0–3	100
Reduced-fat, 2%		12	8	5	120
Whole		12	8	8	160
Nonstarchy Vegetables	½ c	5	2	—	25
Sweets, Desserts, and Other Carbohydrates	varies	15	varies	varies	varies
Protein Group	1 oz				
Lean		0	7	2	45
Medium-fat		0	7	5	75
High-fat		0	7	8	100
Plant-based Proteins	varies	varies	7	varies	varies
Fat Group	1 tsp pure fat	—	—	5	45
Alcohol	varies	varies	—	—	100

*The food lists presented here are based on material in *Choose Your Foods: Food Lists for Diabetes*, 2014, and *Choose Your Foods: Food Lists for Weight Management*, 2014, prepared by committees of the American Diabetes Association and the Academy of Nutrition and Dietetics.

FIGURE A-1

The Food Lists: Example Foods, Portion Sizes, and Energy-Nutrient Contributions

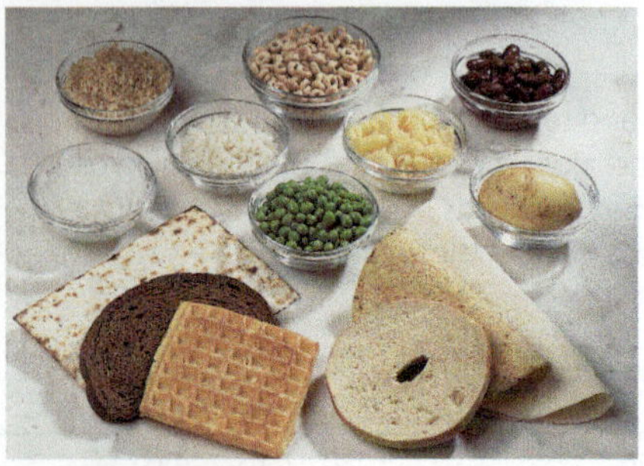

Starch

1 starch choice is like:

1 slice bread

3/4 c ready-to-eat cereal

½ c cooked grits, rice noodles, or bulgur

½ c cooked rice or pasta

½ c cooked beans[a]

½ c corn, peas, or yams

1 small (3 oz) potato

½ bagel, English muffin, or bun

1 tortilla, waffle, roll, taco, or matzoh

(1 starch = 15 g carbohydrate, 3 g protein, 1 g fat, and 80 cal.)

[A] ½ c cooked beans = 1 lean protein choice *plus* 1 starch choice.

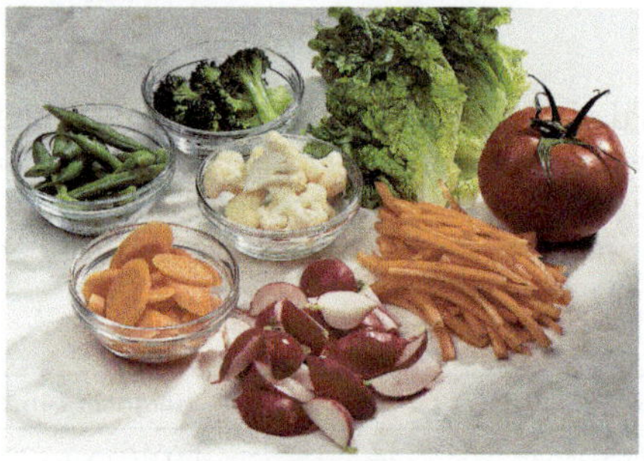

Nonstarchy Vegetables[b]

1 vegetable choice is like:

½ c cooked carrots, greens, green beans, brussels sprouts, beets, broccoli, cauliflower, or spinach

1 c raw carrots, radishes, or spinach

1 lg tomato

(1 vegetable = 5 g carbohydrate, 2 g protein, and 25 cal.)

[B] Salad greens are on the Free Foods list.

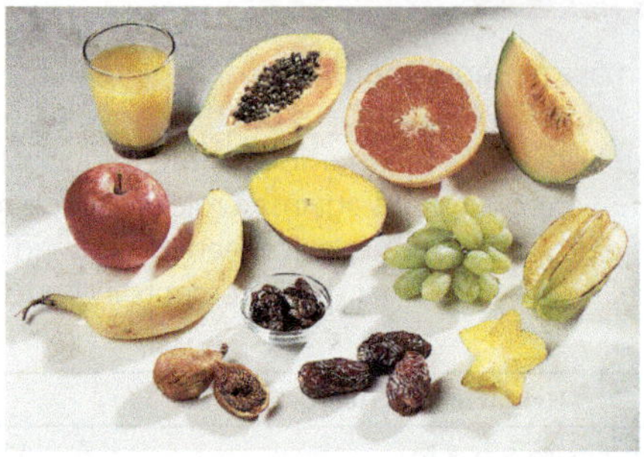

Fruits

1 fruit choice is like:

1 small banana, nectarine, apple, or orange

½ large grapefruit, pear, or papaya

½ c orange, apple, or grapefruit juice

17 small grapes

1/3 cantaloupe (or 1 c cubes)

2 tbs raisins

1½ dried figs

3 dates

1½ carambola (star fruit)

(1 fruit = 15 g carbohydrate and 60 cal.)

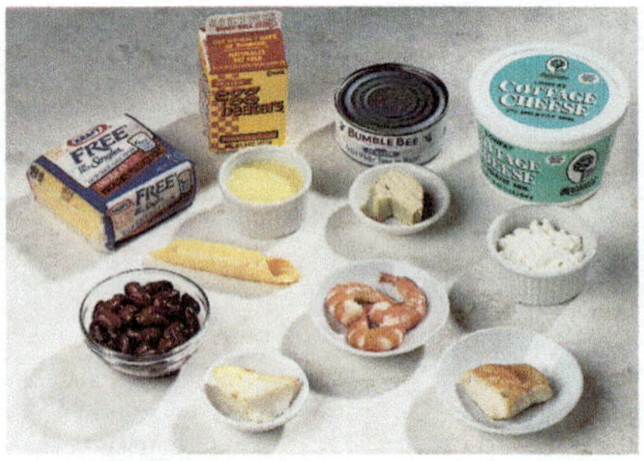

Lean Proteins

1 lean protein choice is like:

1 oz cod, flounder, or trout

1 oz clams, crab, lobster, scallops, shrimp, or imitation seafood

1 oz cheese with 3 g fat or less

2 egg whites (or ¼ c egg substitute)

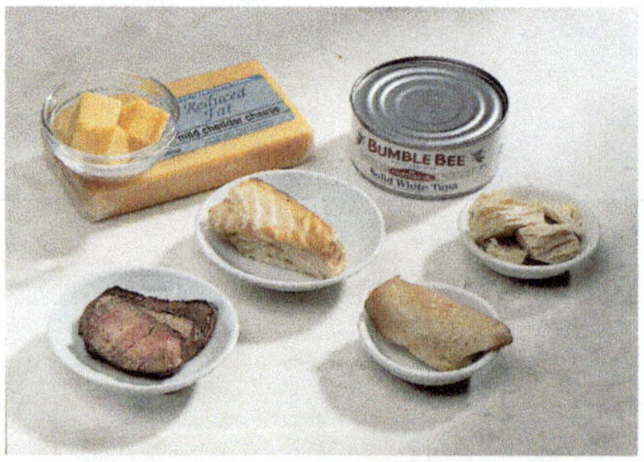

1 oz beef or pork tenderloin trimmed of fat

¼ c cottage cheese

1 oz game meat

1 oz chicken without skin

1 oz tuna (canned in water or oil, drained)

(1 lean protein = 7 g protein, 2 g fat, and 45 cal.)

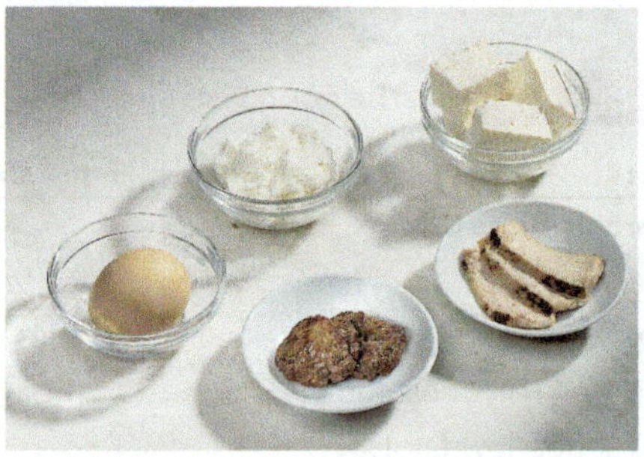

Medium-fat Proteins

1 medium-fat protein choice is like:

1 oz ground beef

1 oz pork cutlet

1 egg

¼ c ricotta cheese

(1 medium-fat protein = 7 g protein, 5 g fat, and 75 cal.)

FIGURE A-1

The Food Lists: Example Foods, Portion Sizes, and Energy-Nutrient Contributions—*Continued*

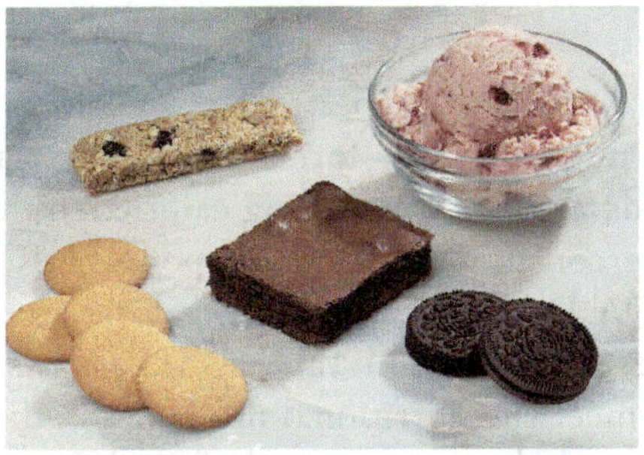

Sweets, Desserts, and Other Carbohydrates

1 other carbohydrates choice is like:
2 small cookies
1 small brownie or cake
5 vanilla wafers
1 granola bar
½ c ice cream
(1 other carbohydrate = 15 g carbohydrate and may be exchanged for 1 starch, 1 fruit, or 1 milk. Because many items on this list contain added sugar and fat, their fat and calorie values vary, and their portion sizes are small.)

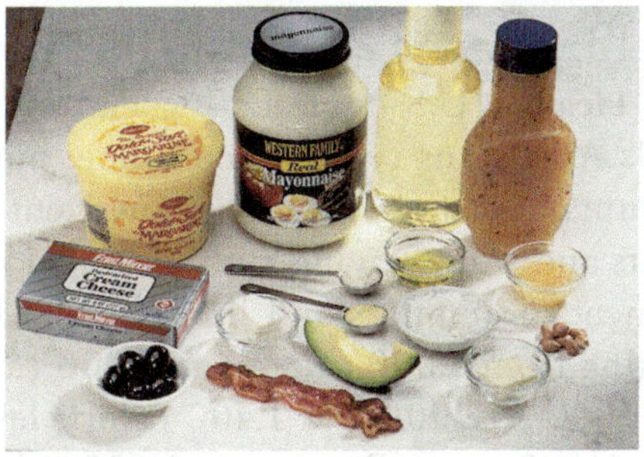

THE FAT GROUP

Fats

1 fat choice is like:
1 tsp butter
1 tsp margarine or mayonnaise (1 tbs reduced fat)
1 tsp any oil
1 tbs salad dressing (2 tbs reduced fat)
8 large black olives
10 large peanuts
⅛ medium avocado
1 slice bacon
2 tbs shredded coconut
1 tbs cream cheese (1½ tbs reduced fat)
(1 fat = 5 g fat and 45 cal.)

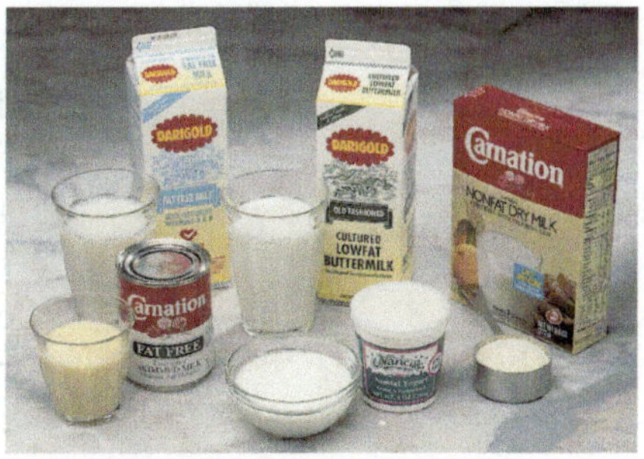

Milks (fat-free and low-fat, 1%)

1 fat-free milk choice is like:
1 c fat-free or 1% milk
¾ c fat-free yogurt, plain
1 c fat-free or low-fat buttermilk
½ c evaporated fat-free milk
⅓ c dry fat-free milk
(1 fat-free milk = 12 g carbohydrate, 8 g protein, 0–3 g fat, and 100 cal.)

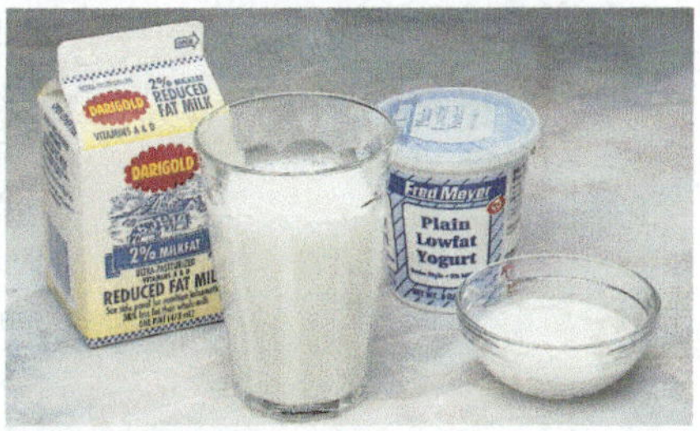

Milks (reduced-fat, 2%)

1 reduced-fat milk choice is like:
1 c 2% milk
6 oz reduced-fat yogurt, plain
(1 reduced-fat milk = 12 g carbohydrate, 8 g protein, 5 g fat, and 120 cal.)

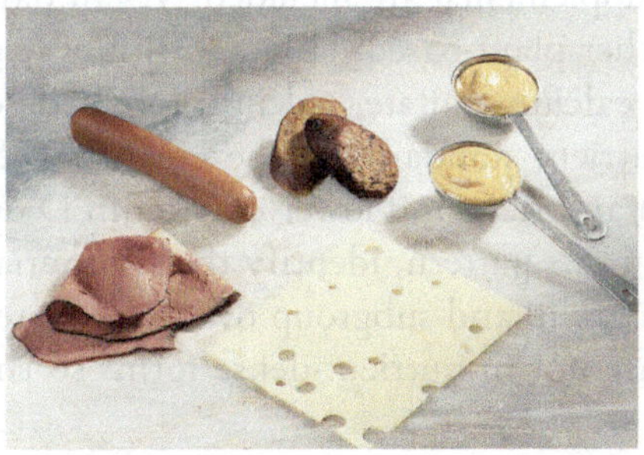

High-fat Proteins

1 high-fat protein choice is like:
2 slices pork bacon
3 slices turkey bacon
1 oz American cheese
1 hot dog (turkey or chicken) [c]
1 oz pork sausage
(1 high-fat protein = 7 g protein, 8 g fat, and 100 cal.)

[c]A beef or pork hot dog counts as 1 high-fat protein choice *plus* 1 fat choice.

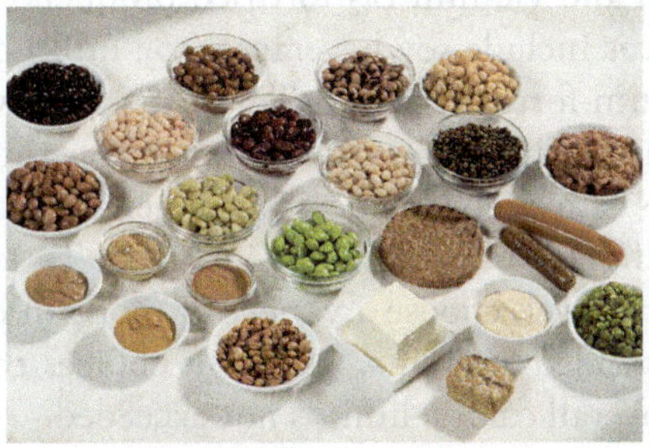

Plant-based Proteins

1 plant-based protein choice is like:
½ c baked beans (1 starch + 1 lean protein)
½ c edamame (½ CHO + 1 lean protein)
⅓ c hummus (1 CHO + 1 high-fat protein)
3 oz meatless burger, soy based (½ CHO + 2 lean proteins)
1 tbs peanut butter (1 high-fat protein)
½ c refried beans, canned (1 CHO + 1 lean protein)
4 oz (½ c) tofu (1 medium-fat protein)

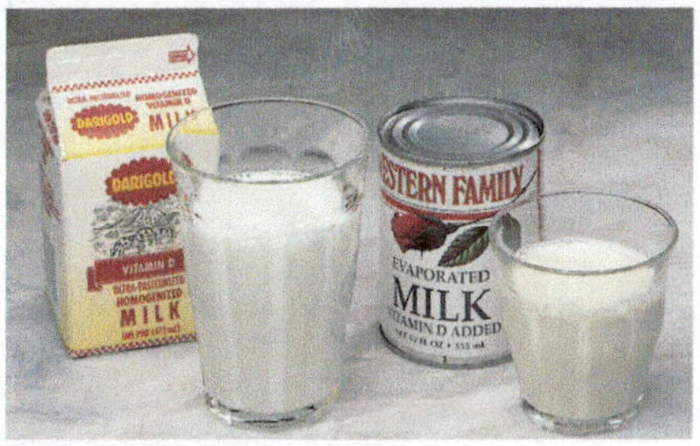

Milks (whole)

1 whole milk choice is like:
1 c whole milk
½ c evaporated whole milk
(1 whole milk = 12 g carbohydrate, 8 g protein, 8 g fat, and 160 cal.)

The USDA Food Patterns to Meet the Dietary *Guidelines for Americans*

Healthy U.S.-Style Eating Pattern

The Healthy U.S.-Style Eating Pattern is based on the types and proportions of foods Americans typically consume, but in nutrient-dense forms and appropriate amounts. It is designed to meet nutrient needs while not exceeding calorie requirements and while staying within limits for overconsumed dietary components. Recommended amounts and limits in the USDA Food Patterns at 12 calorie levels, ranging from 1,000 calories to 3,000 calories, are shown in Table A-4. Patterns at the 1,000-, 1,200-, and 1,400-calorie levels meet the nutritional needs of children ages 2 to 8 years. Patterns at 1,600 calories and above meet needs for adults and children ages 9 years and older. Individuals should follow a pattern that meets their estimated calorie needs.

USDA Food Patterns: Healthy Vegetarian Eating Pattern

A healthy vegetarian eating pattern is shown in Table A-5. The vegetarian pattern relies on fortified foods for some nutrients. The Healthy Vegetarian Eating Pattern is adapted from the Healthy U.S.-Style Eating Pattern, modifying amounts recommended from some food groups to more closely reflect eating patterns reported by self-identified vegetarians in the National Health and Nutrition Examination Survey (NHANES). This analysis allowed development of a pattern that is based on evidence of the foods and amounts vegetarians consume, in addition to meeting the same nutrient and *Dietary Guidelines* standards as the Healthy U.S.-Style Pattern. Based on a comparison of the food choices of these vegetarians to nonvegetarians in NHANES, amounts of soy products (particularly tofu and other processed soy products), legumes, nuts and seeds, and whole grains were increased, and meat, poultry, and seafood were eliminated. Dairy and eggs were included because they were consumed by the majority of these vegetarians. This pattern can be vegan if calcium-fortified and vitamin B_{12}-fortified products (or supplements) are included. Vegan dairy choices include soy beverages (soy milk) or other plant-based dairy substitutes (e.g., calcium-fortified rice milk, tofu made with calcium-sulfate, calcium-fortified soy yogurt). The pattern is similar in meeting nutrient standards to the Healthy U.S.-Style Pattern, but somewhat higher in calcium and fiber and lower in vitamin D due to differences in the foods included. To follow this pattern, identify the appropriate calorie level, choose a variety of foods in each group and subgroup over time in recommended amounts, and limit choices that are not in nutrient-dense forms so that the overall calorie limit is not exceeded.

TABLE A-4 Healthy U.S.-Style Eating Pattern

For each food group or subgroup,[a] recommended average daily intake amounts[b] are provided at all calorie levels. Recommended intakes from vegetable and protein foods subgroups are per week. For more information and tools for application, go to ChooseMyPlate.gov.

Calorie level of pattern[c]	**1,000**	**1,200**	**1,400**	**1,600**	**1,800**	**2,000**	**2,200**	**2,400**	**2,600**	**2,800**	**3,000**	**3,200**
Fruits	1 c	1 c	1½ c	1½ c	1½ c	2 c	2 c	2 c	2 c	2½ c	2½ c	2½ c
Vegetables[d]	1 c	1½ c	1½ c	2 c	2½ c	2½ c	3 c	3 c	3½ c	3½ c	4 c	4 c
Dark-green vegetables	½ c/wk	1 c/wk	1 c/wk	1½ c/wk	1½ c/wk	1½ c/wk	2 c/wk	2 c/wk	2½ c/wk	2½ c/wk	2½ c/wk	2½ c/wk
Red and orange vegetables	2½ c/wk	3 c/wk	3 c/wk	4 c/wk	5½ c/wk	5½ c/wk	6 c/wk	6 c/wk	7 c/wk	7 c/wk	7½ c/wk	7½ c/wk
Legumes (beans and peas)	½ c/wk	½ c/wk	½ c/wk	1 c/wk	1½ c/wk	1½ c/wk	2 c/wk	2 c/wk	2½ c/wk	2½ c/wk	3 c/wk	3 c/wk
Starchy vegetables	2 c/wk	3½ c/wk	3½ c/wk	4 c/wk	5 c/wk	5 c/wk	6 c/wk	6 c/wk	7 c/wk	7 c/wk	8 c/wk	8 c/wk
Other vegetables	1½ c/wk	2½ c/wk	2½ c/wk	3½ c/wk	4 c/wk	4 c/wk	5 c/wk	5 c/wk	5½ c/wk	5½ c/wk	7 c/wk	7 c/wk
Grains[e]	3 oz-eq	4 oz-eq	5 oz-eq	5 oz-eq	6 oz-eq	6 oz-eq	7 oz-eq	8 oz-eq	9 oz-eq	10 oz-eq	10 oz-eq	10 oz-eq
Whole grains	1½ oz-eq	2 oz-eq	2½ oz-eq	3 oz-eq	3 oz-eq	3 oz-eq	3½ oz-eq	4 oz-eq	4½ oz-eq	5 oz-eq	5 oz-eq	5 oz-eq
Refined grains	1½ oz-eq	2 oz-eq	2½ oz-eq	2 oz-eq	3 oz-eq	3 oz-eq	3½ oz-eq	4 oz-eq	4½ oz-eq	5 oz-eq	5 oz-eq	5 oz-eq
Protein foods[d]	2 oz-eq	3 oz-eq	4 oz-eq	5 oz-eq	5 oz-eq	5½ oz-eq	6 oz-eq	6½ oz-eq	6½ oz-eq	7 oz-eq	7 oz-eq	7 oz-eq
Seafood	3 oz/wk	4 oz/wk	6 oz/wk	8 oz/wk	8 oz/wk	8 oz/wk	9 oz/wk	10 oz/wk	10 oz/wk	10 oz/wk	10 oz/wk	10 oz/wk
Meats, poultry, eggs	10 oz/wk	14 oz/wk	19 oz/wk	23 oz/wk	23 oz/wk	26 oz/wk	28 oz/wk	31 oz/wk	31 oz/wk	33 oz/wk	33 oz/wk	33 oz/wk
Nuts, seeds, soy products	2 oz/wk	2 oz/wk	3 oz/wk	4 oz/wk	4 oz/wk	5 oz/wk	5 oz/wk	5 oz/wk	5 oz/wk	6 oz/wk	6 oz/wk	6 oz/wk
Dairy	2 c	2½ c	2½ c	3 c	3 c	3 c	3 c	3 c	3 c	3 c	3 c	3 c
Oils[f]	15 g	17 g	17 g	22 g	24 g	27 g	29 g	31 g	34 g	36 g	44 g	51 g
Limit on calories for other uses[g] **calories (% of calories)**	150 (15%)	100 (8%)	110 (8%)	130 (8%)	170 (9%)	270 (14%)	280 (13%)	350 (15%)	380 (15%)	400 (14%)	470 (16%)	610 (19%)

Notes:

[a]All foods are assumed to be in nutrient-dense forms, lean or low-fat and prepared without added fats, sugars, or salt. Solid fats and added sugars may be included up to the daily maximum limit on calories for other uses identified in the table. See Figure 2-12 on p. 46 for food items in each group and subgroup.

[b] Food group amounts are shown in cup (c) or ounce-equivalents (oz-eq). Oils are shown in grams (g); 1 tsp = about 4.5 grams. Quantity equivalents for each food group are listed in Figure 2-12 on p. 46.

[c] See Table 2-3 on p. 44 for estimated calorie needs per day by age, gender, and physical activity level. Food intake patterns at 1,000, 1,200, and 1,400 calories meet the nutritional needs of children ages 2 to 8 years. Patterns from 1,600 to 3,200 calories meet the nutritional needs of children ages 9 years and older and adults. If a child ages 4 to 8 years needs more calories and, therefore, is following a pattern at 1,600 calories or more, the recommended amount from the dairy group can be 2½ cups per day. Children ages 9 years and older and adults should not use the 1,000-, 1,200-, or 1,400-calorie patterns.

[d] Vegetable and protein foods subgroup amounts are shown in this table as weekly amounts because it would be difficult for consumers to select foods from all subgroups daily.

[e] Whole-grain subgroup amounts shown in this table are minimums. More whole grains up to all of the grains recommended may be selected, with offsetting decreases in the amounts of enriched refined grains.

[f] Oils and soft margarines include vegetable, nut, and fish oils and soft vegetable oil table spreads that have no *trans* fats.

[g] The limit on calories for other uses is the remaining amount of calories in each food pattern after selecting the specified amounts in each food group in nutrient-dense forms (forms that are fat-free or low-fat and with no added sugars). The number of calories is lower in the 1,200-, 1,400-, and 1,600-calorie patterns than in the 1,000-calorie pattern. The nutrient goals for the 1,200- to 1,600-calorie patterns are higher and require that more calories be used for nutrient-dense foods from the food groups.

SOURCE: Reprinted from U.S. Department of Agriculture and U.S. Department of Health and Human Services, 2015–2020 *Dietary Guidelines for Americans, 8th ed.* (Washington, DC: U.S. Government Printing Office, 2015). Appendix 3, pp. 80–82.

TABLE A-5 **USDA Food Patterns: Healthy Vegetarian Eating Pattern**

For each food group or subgroup,[a] recommended average daily intake amounts[b] are provided at all calorie levels. Recommended intakes from vegetable and protein foods subgroups are per week. For more information and tools for application, go to ChooseMyPlate.gov.

Calorie level of pattern	**1,000**	**1,200**	**1,400**	**1,600**	**1,800**	**2,000**	**2,200**	**2,400**	**2,600**	**2,800**	**3,000**	**3,200**
Fruits	1 c	1 c	1½ c	1½ c	1½ c	2 c	2 c	2 c	2 c	2½ c	2½ c	2½ c
Vegetables	1 c	1½ c	1½ c	2 c	2½ c	2½ c	3 c	3 c	3½ c	3½ c	4 c	4 c
Dark-green vegetables	½ c/wk	1 c/wk	1 c/wk	1½ c/wk	1½ c/wk	1½ c/wk	2 c/wk	2 c/wk	2½ c/wk	2½ c/wk	2½ c/wk	2½ c/wk
Red and orange vegetables	2½ c/wk	3 c/wk	3 c/wk	4 c/wk	5½ c/wk	5½ c/wk	6 c/wk	6 c/wk	7 c/wk	7 c/wk	7½ c/wk	7½ c/wk
Legumes (beans and peas)	½ c/wk	½ c/wk	½ c/wk	1 c/wk	1½ c/wk	1½ c/wk	2 c/wk	2 c/wk	2½ c/wk	2½ c/wk	3 c/wk	3 c/wk
Starchy vegetables	2 c/wk	3½ c/wk	3½ c/wk	4 c/wk	5 c/wk	5 c/wk	6 c/wk	6 c/wk	7 c/wk	7 c/wk	8 c/wk	8 c/wk
Other vegetables	1½ c/wk	2½ c/wk	2½ c/wk	3½ c/wk	4 c/wk	4 c/wk	5 c/wk	5 c/wk	5½ c/wk	5½ c/wk	7 c/wk	7 c/wk
Grains	3 oz-eq	4 oz-eq	5 oz-eq	5½ oz-eq	6½ oz-eq	6½ oz-eq	7½ oz-eq	8½ oz-eq	9½ oz-eq	10½ oz-eq	10½ oz-eq	10½ oz-eq
Whole grains	1½ oz-eq	2 oz-eq	2½ oz-eq	3 oz-eq	3½ oz-eq	3½ oz-eq	4 oz-eq	4½ oz-eq	5 oz-eq	5½ oz-eq	5½ oz-eq	5½ oz-eq
Refined grains	1½ oz-eq	2 oz-eq	2½ oz-eq	2½ oz-eq	3 oz-eq	3 oz-eq	3½ oz-eq	4 oz-eq	4½ oz-eq	5 oz-eq	5 oz-eq	5 oz-eq
Protein foods	1 oz-eq	1½ oz-eq	2 oz-eq	2½ oz-eq	3 oz-eq	3½ oz-eq	3½ oz-eq	4 oz-eq	4½ oz-eq	5 oz-eq	5½ oz-eq	6 oz-eq
Eggs	2 oz-eq/wk	3 oz-eq/wk	3 oz-eq/wk	3 oz-eq/wk	3 oz-eq/wk	3 oz-eq/wk	3 oz-eq/wk	3 oz-eq/wk	3 oz-eq/wk	4 oz-eq/wk	4 oz-eq/wk	4 oz-eq/wk
Legumes (beans and peas)[c]	1 oz-eq/wk	2 oz-eq/wk	4 oz-eq/wk	4 oz-eq/wk	6 oz-eq/wk	6 oz-eq/wk	6 oz-eq/wk	8 oz-eq/wk	9 oz-eq/wk	10 oz-eq/wk	11 oz-eq/wk	12 oz-eq/wk
Soy products	2 oz-eq/wk	3 oz-eq/wk	4 oz-eq/wk	6 oz-eq/wk	6 oz-eq/wk	8 oz-eq/wk	8 oz-eq/wk	9 oz-eq/wk	10 oz-eq/wk	11 oz-eq/wk	12 oz-eq/wk	13 oz-eq/wk
Nuts and seeds	2 oz-eq/wk	2 oz-eq/wk	3 oz-eq/wk	5 oz-eq/wk	6 oz-eq/wk	7 oz-eq/wk	7 oz-eq/wk	8 oz-eq/wk	9 oz-eq/wk	10 oz-eq/wk	12 oz-eq/wk	13 oz-eq/wk
Dairy	2 c	2½ c	2½ c	3 c	3 c	3 c	3 c	3 c	3 c	3 c	3 c	3 c
Oils	15 g	17 g	17 g	22 g	24 g	27 g	29 g	31 g	34 g	36 g	44 g	51 g
Limit on calories for other uses, calories (% total calories)	190 (19%)	170 (14%)	190 (14%)	180 (11%)	190 (11%)	290 (15%)	330 (15%)	390 (16%)	390 (15%)	400 (14%)	440 (15%)	550 (17%)

Notes:

[a] All foods are assumed to be in nutrient-dense forms, lean or low-fat and prepared without added fats, sugars, or salt. Solid fats and added sugars may be included up to the daily maximum limit identified in the table. See Figure 2-12 on p. 46 for food items in each group and subgroup.

[b] Food group amounts are shown in cup (c) or ounce-equivalents (oz-eq). Oils are shown in grams (g); 1 tsp = about 4.5 grams. Quantity equivalents for each food group are listed in Figure 2-12 on p. 46.

[c] Total recommended legumes (beans and peas) amounts would be the sum of amounts recommended in the vegetable and the protein foods groups. An ounce-equivalent of beans and peas in the protein foods group is ¼ cup, cooked. For example, in the 2,000-calorie pattern, total weekly beans and peas recommendation is (6 oz-eq/4) + 1½ cups = about 3 cups, cooked.

SOURCE: Reprinted from U.S. Department of Agriculture and U.S. Department of Health and Human Services, 2015–2020 *Dietary Guidelines for Americans, 8th* ed. (Washington, DC: U.S. Government Printing Office, 2015). Appendix 3, pp. 87–88.

Appendix B

Canadian Nutrition and Physical Activity Guidelines

Canada's Guidelines for Healthy Eating

Canada's Guidelines for Healthy Eating encourage healthy Canadians over 2 years of age to

- Enjoy a variety of foods.
- Emphasize cereals, breads, other grain products, vegetables, and fruits.
- Choose lower-fat dairy products, leaner meats, and foods prepared with little or no fat.
- Achieve and maintain a healthy body weight by enjoying regular physical activity and healthy eating.
- Limit salt, alcohol, and caffeine.

Canada's Recommended Nutrient Intakes

The Dietary Reference Intakes (DRI) are presented at the back of this book.

Eating Well with Canada's Food Guide

Figure B-1 presents the 2011 *Eating Well with Canada's Food Guide*, which gives detailed information for selecting foods to meet *Canada's Guidelines for Healthy Eating*. The *Food Guide* was designed to meet the nutritional needs of all Canadians 2 years of age and older and takes a total diet approach. The *Food Guide* shows the four food groups with pictorial examples of foods in each group and shows the number of servings recommended for each food group.

For more detailed information and interactive tools using the *Food Guide*, go to www.healthcanada.gc.ca/foodguide. Additional publications are available from Health Canada's Office of Nutrition Policy and Promotion at www.hc-sc.gc.ca.

FIGURE B-1

Eating Well with Canada's Food Guide

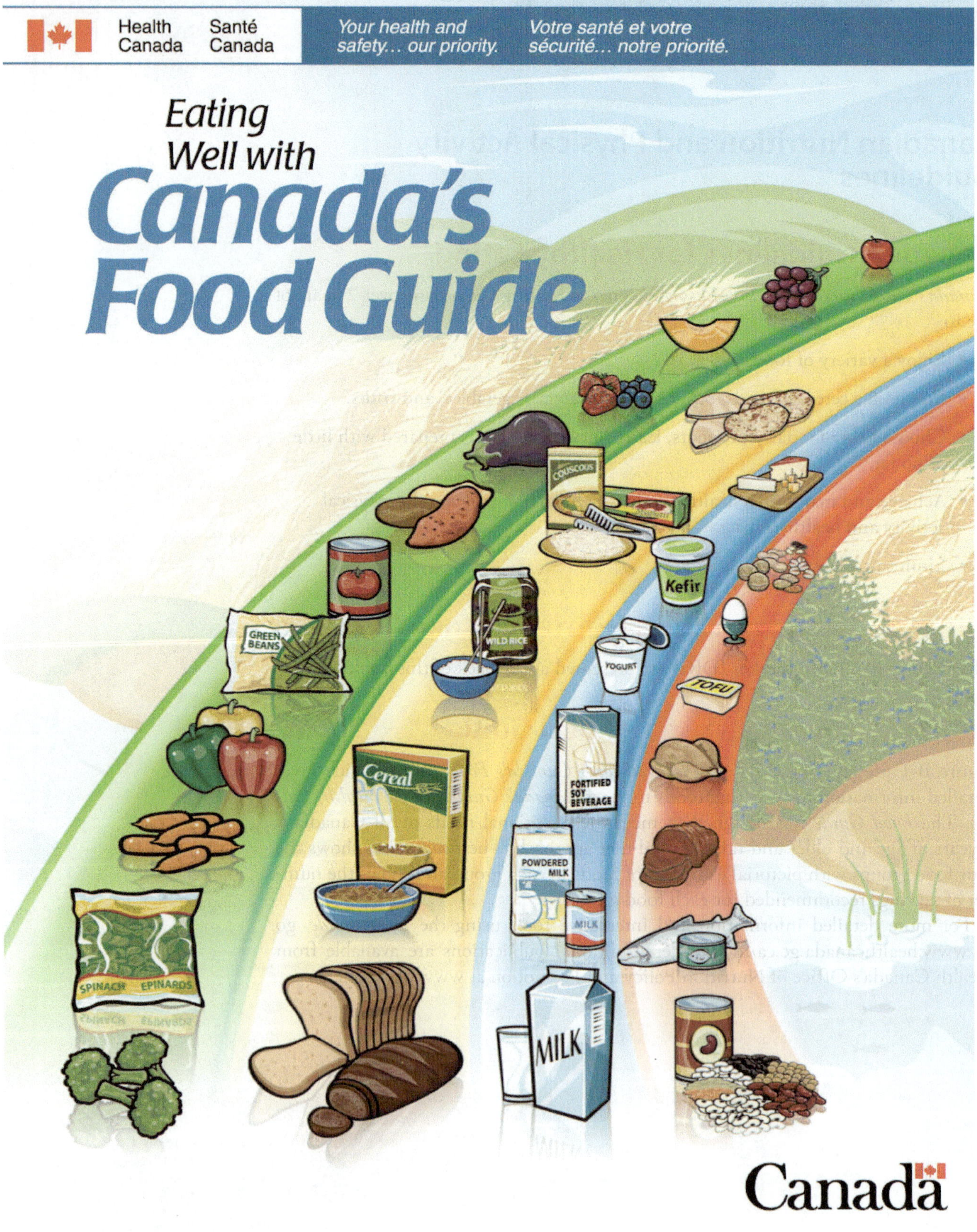

APPENDIX B

FIGURE B-1

Eating Well with Canada's Food Guide—*Continued*

Recommended Number of **Food Guide Servings** *per Day*

	Children			Teens		Adults			
Age in Years	2-3	4-8	9-13	14-18		19-50		51+	
Sex	Girls and Boys			Females	Males	Females	Males	Females	Males
Vegetables and Fruit	4	5	6	7	8	7-8	8-10	7	7
Grain Products	3	4	6	6	7	6-7	8	6	7
Milk and Alternatives	2	2	3-4	3-4	3-4	2	2	3	3
Meat and Alternatives	1	1	1-2	2	3	2	3	2	3

The chart above shows how many Food Guide Servings you need from each of the four food groups every day.

Having the amount and type of food recommended and following the tips in *Canada's Food Guide* will help:

- Meet your needs for vitamins, minerals and other nutrients.
- Reduce your risk of obesity, type 2 diabetes, heart disease, certain types of cancer and osteoporosis.
- Contribute to your overall health and vitality.

APPENDIX B

FIGURE B-1

Eating Well with Canada's Food Guide—*Continued*

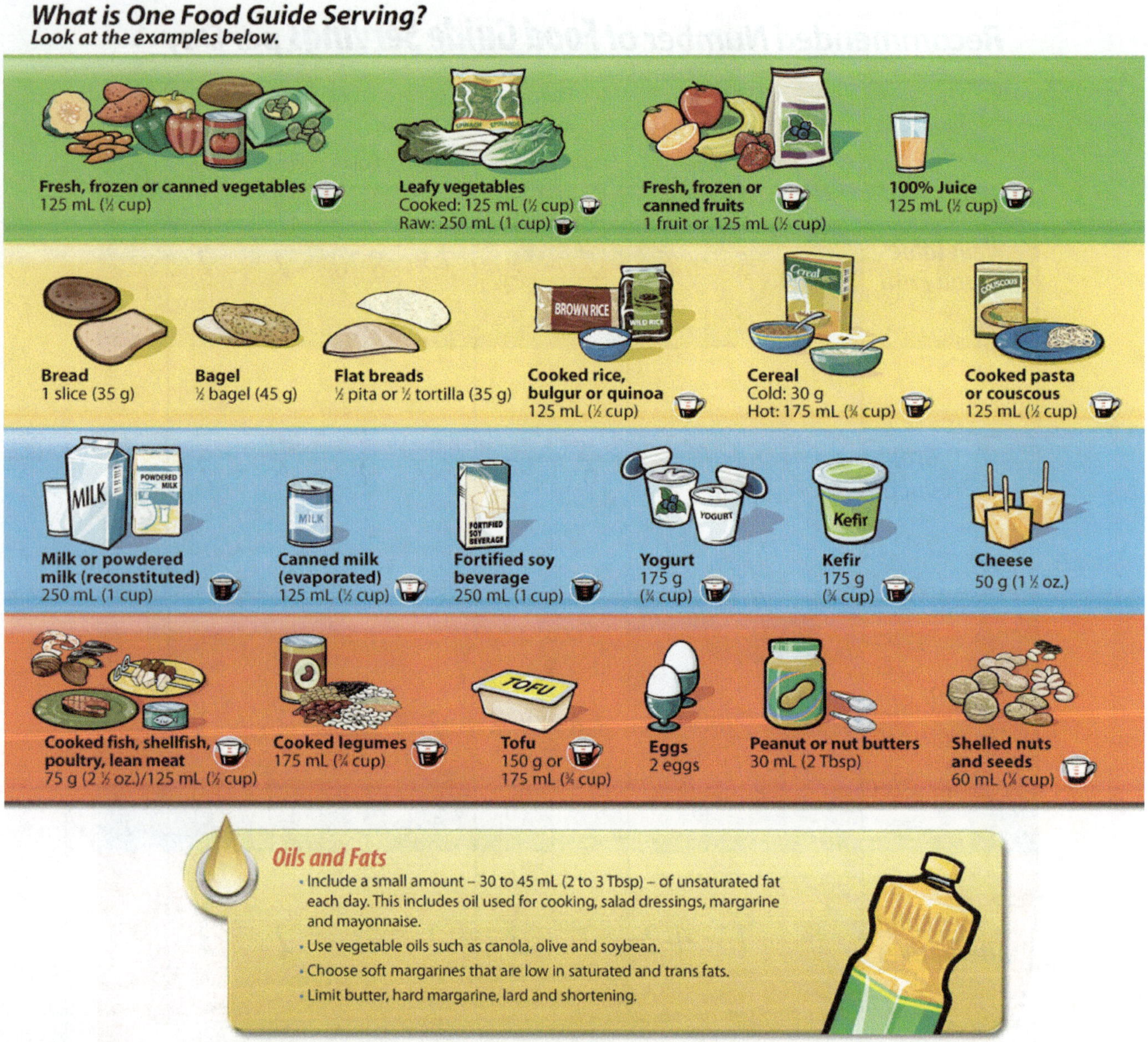

FIGURE B-1
Eating Well with Canada's Food Guide—*Continued*

Make each Food Guide Serving count…
wherever you are – at home, at school, at work or when eating out!

- **Eat at least one dark green and one orange vegetable each day.**
  - Go for dark green vegetables such as broccoli, romaine lettuce and spinach.
  - Go for orange vegetables such as carrots, sweet potatoes and winter squash.
- **Choose vegetables and fruit prepared with little or no added fat, sugar or salt.**
  - Enjoy vegetables steamed, baked or stir-fried instead of deep-fried.
- **Have vegetables and fruit more often than juice.**

- **Make at least half of your grain products whole grain each day.**
  - Eat a variety of whole grains such as barley, brown rice, oats, quinoa and wild rice.
  - Enjoy whole grain breads, oatmeal or whole wheat pasta.
- **Choose grain products that are lower in fat, sugar or salt.**
  - Compare the Nutrition Facts table on labels to make wise choices.
  - Enjoy the true taste of grain products. When adding sauces or spreads, use small amounts.

- **Drink skim, 1%, or 2% milk each day.**
  - Have 500 mL (2 cups) of milk every day for adequate vitamin D.
  - Drink fortified soy beverages if you do not drink milk.
- **Select lower fat milk alternatives.**
  - Compare the Nutrition Facts table on yogurts or cheeses to make wise choices.

- **Have meat alternatives such as beans, lentils and tofu often.**
- **Eat at least two Food Guide Servings of fish each week.***
  - Choose fish such as char, herring, mackerel, salmon, sardines and trout.
- **Select lean meat and alternatives prepared with little or no added fat or salt.**
  - Trim the visible fat from meats. Remove the skin on poultry.
  - Use cooking methods such as roasting, baking or poaching that require little or no added fat.
  - If you eat luncheon meats, sausages or prepackaged meats, choose those lower in salt (sodium) and fat.

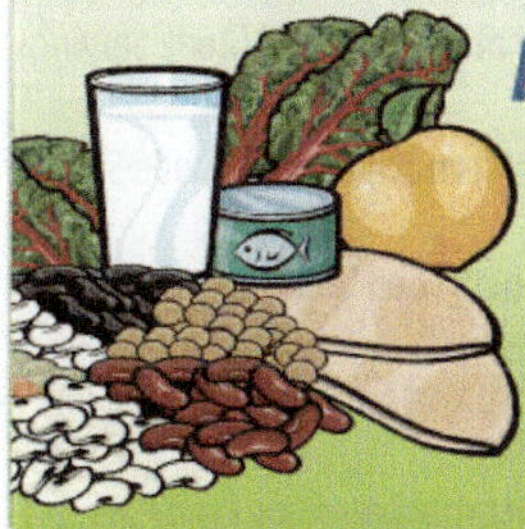

Enjoy a variety of foods from the four food groups.

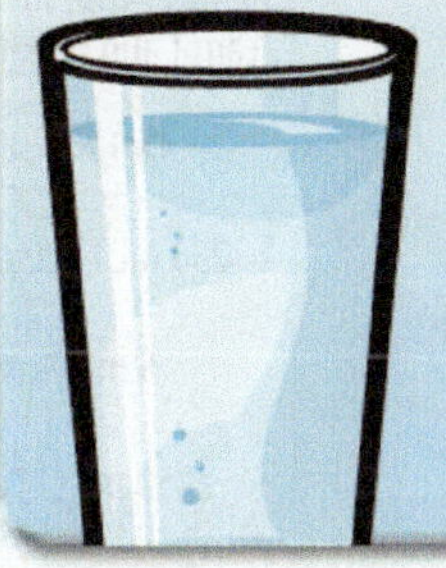

Satisfy your thirst with water!

Drink water regularly. It's a calorie-free way to quench your thirst. Drink more water in hot weather or when you are very active.

* Health Canada provides advice for limiting exposure to mercury from certain types of fish. Refer to www.healthcanada.gc.ca for the latest information.

APPENDIX B

FIGURE B-1

Eating Well with Canada's Food Guide—*Continued*

Advice for different ages and stages...

Children

Following *Canada's Food Guide* helps children grow and thrive.

Young children have small appetites and need calories for growth and development.

- Serve small nutritious meals and snacks each day.
- Do not restrict nutritious foods because of their fat content. Offer a variety of foods from the four food groups.
- Most of all... be a good role model.

Women of childbearing age

All women who could become pregnant and those who are pregnant or breastfeeding need a multivitamin containing **folic acid** every day. Pregnant women need to ensure that their multivitamin also contains **iron**. A health care professional can help you find the multivitamin that's right for you.

Pregnant and breastfeeding women need more calories. Include an extra 2 to 3 Food Guide Servings each day.

Here are two examples:

- Have fruit and yogurt for a snack, or
- Have an extra slice of toast at breakfast and an extra glass of milk at supper.

Men and women over 50

The need for **vitamin D** increases after the age of 50.

In addition to following *Canada's Food Guide*, everyone over the age of 50 should take a daily vitamin D supplement of 10 µg (400 IU).

How do I count Food Guide Servings in a meal?

Here is an example:

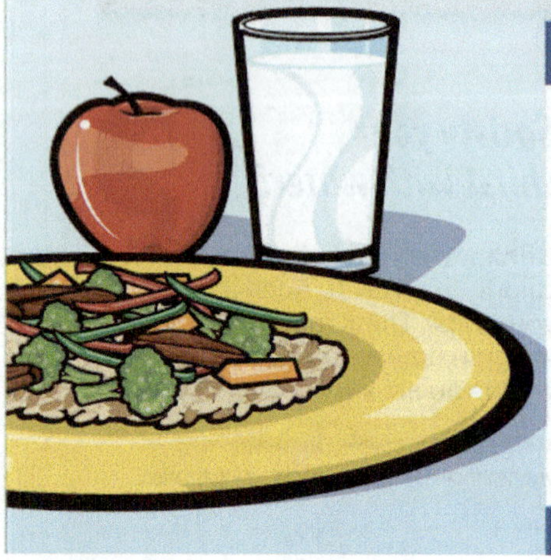

Vegetable and beef stir-fry with rice, a glass of milk and an apple for dessert		
250 mL (1 cup) mixed broccoli, carrot and sweet red pepper	=	2 **Vegetables and Fruit** Food Guide Servings
75 g (2 ½ oz.) lean beef	=	1 **Meat and Alternatives** Food Guide Serving
250 mL (1 cup) brown rice	=	2 **Grain Products** Food Guide Servings
5 mL (1 tsp) canola oil	=	part of your **Oils and Fats** intake for the day
250 mL (1 cup) 1% milk	=	1 **Milk and Alternatives** Food Guide Serving
1 apple	=	1 **Vegetables and Fruit** Food Guide Serving

FIGURE B-1

Eating Well with Canada's Food Guide—*Continued*

Eat well and be active today and every day!

The benefits of eating well and being active include:

- Better overall health.
- Lower risk of disease.
- A healthy body weight.
- Feeling and looking better.
- More energy.
- Stronger muscles and bones.

Be active

To be active every day is a step towards better health and a healthy body weight.

Canada's Physical Activity Guide recommends building 30 to 60 minutes of moderate physical activity into daily life for adults and at least 90 minutes a day for children and youth. You don't have to do it all at once. Add it up in periods of at least 10 minutes at a time for adults and five minutes at a time for children and youth.

Start slowly and build up.

Eat well

Another important step towards better health and a healthy body weight is to follow *Canada's Food Guide* by:

- Eating the recommended amount and type of food each day.
- Limiting foods and beverages high in calories, fat, sugar or salt (sodium) such as cakes and pastries, chocolate and candies, cookies and granola bars, doughnuts and muffins, ice cream and frozen desserts, french fries, potato chips, nachos and other salty snacks, alcohol, fruit flavoured drinks, soft drinks, sports and energy drinks, and sweetened hot or cold drinks.

Read the label

- Compare the Nutrition Facts table on food labels to choose products that contain less fat, saturated fat, trans fat, sugar and sodium.
- Keep in mind that the calories and nutrients listed are for the amount of food found at the top of the Nutrition Facts table.

Nutrition Facts

Per 0 mL (0 g)

Amount	% Daily Value
Calories 0	
Fat 0 g	0 %
Saturates 0 g + Trans 0 g	0 %
Cholesterol 0 mg	
Sodium 0 mg	0 %
Carbohydrate 0 g	0 %
Fibre 0 g	0 %
Sugars 0 g	
Protein 0 g	

Vitamin A	0 %	Vitamin C	0 %
Calcium	0 %	Iron	0 %

Limit trans fat

When a Nutrition Facts table is not available, ask for nutrition information to choose foods lower in trans and saturated fats.

Take a step today…

✓ Have breakfast every day. It may help control your hunger later in the day.

✓ Walk wherever you can – get off the bus early, use the stairs.

✓ Benefit from eating vegetables and fruit at all meals and as snacks.

✓ Spend less time being inactive such as watching TV or playing computer games.

✓ Request nutrition information about menu items when eating out to help you make healthier choices.

✓ Enjoy eating with family and friends!

✓ Take time to eat and savour every bite!

For more information, interactive tools, or additional copies visit Canada's Food Guide on-line at:
www.healthcanada.gc.ca/foodguide

or contact:

Publications
Health Canada
Ottawa, Ontario K1A 0K9
E-Mail: publications@hc-sc.gc.ca
Tel.: 1-866-225-0709
Fax: (613) 941-5366
TTY: 1-800-267-1245

Également disponible en français sous le titre : Bien manger avec le Guide alimentaire canadien

This publication can be made available on request on diskette, large print, audio-cassette and braille.

 HC Pub.: 4651 Cat.: H164-38/1-2007E ISBN: 0-662-44467-1

APPENDIX B

Glossary

absorption The passage of nutrients or substances into cells or tissues; nutrients pass into intestinal cells after digestion and then into the circulatory system (e.g., into the bloodstream).

acceptable daily intake (ADI) The estimated amount of a sweetener that can be consumed daily over a person's lifetime without any adverse effects.

Acceptable Macronutrient Distribution Range (AMDR) A range of intakes for a particular energy source (carbohydrates, fat, protein) that is associated with a reduced risk of chronic disease while providing adequate intakes of essential nutrients.

accreditation Approval; in the case of hospitals or university departments, approval by a professional organization of the educational program offered. There are phony accrediting agencies; the genuine ones are listed in a directory called *Accredited Institutions of Postsecondary Education.*

acetaldehyde (ass-et-AL-duh-hide) A substance into which drinking alcohol (ethanol) is metabolized.

acid–base balance Equilibrium between acid and base concentrations in the body fluids.

acidosis (a-sih-DOSE-is) Blood acidity above normal, indicating excess acid.

acids Compounds that release hydrogens in a watery solution; acids have a low pH.

activities of daily living (ADL) Self-care activities including bathing, dressing, grooming, transferring from bed to chair, going to the bathroom, and feeding oneself.

added sugars Sugars and other caloric sweeteners that are added to foods during processing or preparation. Added sugars do not include naturally occurring sugars such as those found in milk and fruits.

adequacy The characteristic of a diet that provides all of the essential nutrients, fiber, and energy (calories) in amounts sufficient to maintain health.

Adequate Intake (AI) The average amount of a nutrient that appears to be adequate for individuals when there is not sufficient scientific research to calculate an RDA. The AI exceeds the EAR and possibly the RDA.

ADL *See* activities of daily living.

adverse reaction An unusual response to food, including food allergies and food intolerances.

aerobic Requiring oxygen.

aflatoxins Poisonous toxins produced by molds.

agave (uh-GAH-vee) A plant with spiny-margined leaves and flower.

age-related macular degeneration Oxidative damage to the central portion of the eye (the *macula*) that allows you to focus and see details clearly (peripheral vision remains unimpaired). The carotenoids lutein and zeaxanthin (found in broccoli, Brussels sprouts, kale, spinach, corn, lettuce, and peas) may protect normal macular function.

AI *See* Adequate Intake.

alcohol A clear, colorless, volatile liquid; the most commonly ingested form is ethyl alcohol or ethanol (EtOH).

alcohol abuse Continued use of alcohol despite negative psychological, social, family, employment, or school problems caused by the alcohol use.

alcohol dehydrogenase A liver enzyme that mediates the metabolism of alcohol.

alcohol dependency (alcoholism) A condition marked by compulsive, uncontrollable drinking that has negative effects on the affected person's physical health, family relationships, and social health.

alcoholic hepatitis Inflammation and injury to the liver due to excess alcohol consumption.

alkalosis (al-kuh-LOW-sis) Blood alkalinity above normal.

alpha-lactalbumin The chief protein in human breast milk.

alternative sweeteners Nutritive (calorie-containing) sweeteners such as fructose and the sugar alcohols (e.g., sorbitol, mannitol, and xylitol) that are absorbed more slowly and metabolized differently than other sugars in the body.

amaranth A golden-colored grain.

AMDR *See* Acceptable Macronutrient Distribution Range.

amenorrhea Cessation of menstruation that can be associated with the occurrence of a relative energy deficit in sport.

amine (a-MEEN) **group** The nitrogen-containing portion of an amino acid.

amino (uh-MEEN-oh) **acids** Building blocks of protein; each is a compound with an amine group at one end, an acid group at the other, and a distinctive side chain.

anabolic steroids Synthetic male hormones (related to testosterone) that stimulate growth of body tissues, with many adverse effects.

anaerobic Not requiring oxygen.

anaphylaxis (an-uh-feh-LACKS-is) A potentially fatal reaction to a food allergen that causes reduced oxygen supply to the heart and other body tissues. Symptoms include difficulty breathing; low blood pressure; pale skin; a weak, rapid pulse; and loss of consciousness.

anemia Any condition in which the blood is unable to deliver oxygen to the cells of the body. Examples include a shortage or abnormality of the red blood cells. Many nutrient deficiencies and diseases can cause anemia.

anorexia nervosa Literally, "nervous lack of appetite," a disorder involving self-starvation to the extreme (*an* = without; *orexis* = appetite).

antibodies Large proteins of the blood and body fluids that are produced by one type of immune cell in response to invasion of the body by unfamiliar molecules (mostly foreign proteins). Antibodies inactivate the foreign substances and so protect the body. The foreign substances are called *antigens.*

antioxidant A compound that protects other compounds from oxygen by itself reacting with oxygen; that is, antioxidants help prevent damage done to the body as a result of chemical reactions involving oxygen.

antioxidant nutrients Vitamins and minerals that protect other compounds from damaging reactions involving oxygen by themselves reacting with oxygen. The antioxidant nutrients are vitamin C, vitamin E, and beta-carotene. The mineral selenium also has a role in antioxidant reactions in the body.

appendicitis Inflammation and/or infection of the appendix, a sac protruding from the large intestine.

appetite The psychological desire to find and eat food, experienced as a pleasant sensation, often in the absence of hunger

appropriate technology A technology that utilizes locally abundant resources in preference to locally scarce resources. For developing countries, which usually have a large labor force and little capital, the appropriate technology would therefore be labor intensive.

arousal As used in this context, heightened activity of certain brain centers associated with excitement and anxiety.

artesian water or **artesian well water** Water drawn from a well that taps a confined water-bearing rock or rock formation.

atherosclerosis (ATH-er-oh-skler-OH-sis) A type of cardiovascular disease characterized by the formation of fatty deposits, or plaques, in the inner walls of the arteries.

ATP or adenosine triphosphate A high-energy compound present in all body tissues; when the bonds between any of the three phosphate groups in ATP are broken, energy is instantly released to power the activities of cells.

atrophic gastritis An age-related condition characterized by the stomach's inability to produce enough acid, which in turn leads to vitamin B_{12} deficiencies.

atrophy A decrease in size in response to disuse.

β-alanine A nonessential amino acid that may improve anaerobic performance that would otherwise be limited by the effects of lactic acid buildup during high-intensity events (exercise lasting 1 to 4 minutes).

balance A feature of a diet that provides a number of types of foods in harmony with one another, such that foods rich in one nutrient do not crowd out the diet foods that are rich in another nutrient.

basal metabolic rate (BMR) The rate at which the body spends energy to support its basal metabolism. The BMR accounts for the largest component of a person's daily energy (calorie) needs.

basal metabolism The sum total of all the chemical activities of the cells necessary to sustain life, exclusive of voluntary activities; that is, the ongoing activities of the cells when the body is at rest.

bases Compounds that accept hydrogens from a watery solution; bases have a high pH.

behavior modification A process developed by psychologists that helps people make lasting behavior changes.

beriberi The thiamin deficiency disease, characterized by irregular heartbeat, paralysis, and extreme wasting of muscle tissue.

beta-carotene An orange pigment found in plants that is converted into vitamin A inside the body. Beta-carotene is also an antioxidant.

bialy A flat breakfast roll that is softer than a bagel.

bicarbonate A chemical that neutralizes acid; a secretion of the pancreas.

bifidus factor (BIFF-id-us) A factor in colostrum and breast milk that favors growth in the infant's intestinal tract of the "friendly" bacteria *Lactobacillus bifidus*; colonization with friendly bacteria means that other, less desirable intestinal inhabitants will not flourish.

bile A compound made from cholesterol by the liver, stored in the gallbladder, and secreted into the small intestine. Bile emulsifies lipids to ready them for enzymatic digestion and helps transport them into the intestinal wall cells.

binders In foods, compounds that can combine with nutrients to form complexes the body cannot absorb. For example, *phytates* (FYE-tates) in whole grains and *oxalates* (in vegetables) may bind iron and calcium and interfere with their absorption to a minor extent.

bing Thin pancakes.

binge-eating disorder An eating disorder characterized by uncontrolled chronic episodes of overeating (compulsive overeating) without other symptoms of eating disorders. Typically, the episodes of binge eating occur at least once a week for a period of three months or more.

bioelectrical impedance Estimation of body fat content made by measuring how quickly electrical current is conducted through the body.

biotechnology The use of biological systems or living organisms to make or modify products. Includes traditional methods used in making products such as wine, beer, yogurt, and cheese; cross-breeding to enhance crop production; and modification of living plants, animals, and fish through the manipulation of genes (genetic engineering).

bisphosphonates Drugs that decrease the risk of fractures by acting on the bone-dismantling cells (osteoclasts) and inhibiting their resorption of bone tissue; examples are Fosamax, Actonel, Boniva, and Reclast.

black-eyed peas Small, oval-shaped, creamy-white peas with a black spot. They have a vegetable flavor with mealy texture. Use in salads with rice and greens.

black, Cuban, or turtle beans Medium-size, black-skinned oval beans that have a rich, sweet taste. They are best served in Mexican and Latin American dishes or thick soups and stews.

BMI *See* body mass index.

BMR *See* basal metabolic rate.

body mass index (BMI) An index of a person's weight in relation to height that correlates with total body fat content.

bok choy A vegetable with broad, white or greenish-white stalks and dark-green leaves; also called *Chinese chard.*

bolillo (buh-LEE-oh) A roll-like bread often used instead of tortillas or to make sandwiches.

bone density A measure of bone strength that reflects the degree of bone mineralization. The DEXA (dual-energy X-ray absorptiometry) bone-density test compares your bone density to that of a healthy young adult. Bone-density tests—using a dual beam of low-level X-rays—take a snapshot of bone density in the spine, wrist, and hip.

branched-chain amino acids (BCAAs) A group of 3 essential amino acids (isoleucine, leucine, and valine). Skeletal muscle metabolizes the BCAAs for energy during prolonged endurance exercise when glycogen stores are low. It is touted as an ergogenic aid that may delay fatigue and improve muscle recovery time by reducing exercise-induced muscle fatigue and delayed-onset muscle soreness by reducing protein breakdown and stimulating muscle protein synthesis in the exercised muscle.

buffers Compounds that help keep the acidity (amount of acid) or alkalinity (amount of base) of a solution constant.

bulimia nervosa, bulimarexia (byoo-LEE-me-uh, byoo-lee-ma-REX-ee-uh) Binge eating (literally, "eating like an ox"), combined with an intense fear of becoming fat and usually followed by self-induced vomiting or taking laxatives (*buli* = ox).

burritos Warm flour tortillas stuffed with a mixture of egg, meat, beans, and/or avocado.

caffeine A type of compound, called a methylxanthine, found in coffee beans, cola nuts, cocoa beans, and tea leaves. A central nervous system stimulant, caffeine's effects include increasing the heart rate, boosting urine production, and raising the metabolic rate.

caffeine dependence syndrome Dependence on caffeine characterized by at least three of the four following criteria: withdrawal symptoms such as headache and fatigue; caffeine consumption despite knowledge that it may be causing harm; repeated, unsuccessful attempts to cut back on caffeine; and tolerance to caffeine.

calcitonin A hormone used as a drug to decrease the rate of bone loss in osteoporosis. Administered as a nasal spray (Miacalcin) or by injection, calcitonin works by inhibiting the bone resorption activity of osteoclasts.

calorie The unit used to measure the energy in foods.

calorie control A feature of a diet that achieves balance between calories consumed in foods and beverages and calories expended through physical activity.

capillaries Minute, weblike blood vessels that connect arteries to veins and permit transfer of materials between blood and tissues.

carbohydrates Compounds made of single sugars or multiple sugars and composed of carbon, hydrogen, and oxygen atoms (*carbo* = carbon [C]; *hydrate* = water [H_2O]).

cardiorespiratory conditioning or **training effect** The effect of regular exercise on the cardiovascular system; includes improvements in heart, lung, and muscle function and increased blood volume; also called *cardiovascular endurance.*

carnitine (KAR-nih-teen) A compound synthesized in the body from two amino acids (lysine and methionine) and required in fat metabolism. Falsely claimed to increase the use of fatty acids and spare glycogen during exercise, delay fatigue, and decrease body fat.

carotenoids (kah-ROW-teh-noyds) A group of pigments (yellow, orange, and red) found in foods.

cassava A starchy root that is never eaten raw because it must be cooked to eliminate its bitter smell.

cellophane noodles Thin, translucent noodles made from mung beans.

cells The smallest units in which independent life can exist. All living things are single cells or organisms made of cells.

central obesity Excess fat on the abdomen and around the trunk. *Peripheral obesity* is excess fat on the arms, thighs, hips, and buttocks.

certified organic foods Crops or livestock grown and processed according to USDA regulations concerning use of pesticides, herbicides, fungicides, fertilizers, preservatives, other synthetic chemicals, growth hormones, and antibiotics or other drugs.

challah (KAH-luh) An egg-containing yeast bread, often braided, typically served on the Sabbath and holidays.

chapatti A flat, unleavened bread made with finely milled whole-meal flour.

cherimoya A fruit with a rough green outer skin and sherbet-like flesh.

chickpeas *See* garbanzo beans.

chilaquiles (chee-lah-KEE-lehs) Tortilla casserole often made with eggs or meat.

chiles relleños (CHEE-lehs Ray-EN-yose) Roasted mild green chili peppers stuffed with cheese, dipped in egg batter, and fried.

Chinese broccoli A green leafy vegetable often stir-fried; also called *Chinese kale.*

chitterlings (chitlins) Pig intestine.

chlorophyll The green pigment of plants that traps energy from sunlight and uses this energy in photosynthesis (the synthesis of carbohydrate by green plants).

cholesterol (koh-LESS-ter-all) One of the sterols, manufactured in the body for a variety of purposes.

choline A nonessential nutrient used by the body to synthesize various compounds, including the phospholipid lecithin; the body can make choline from the amino acid methionine.

chorizo (chuh-REE-zoh) Spicy beef or pork sausage.

choy sum A bright green vegetable commonly stir fried; also called *field mustard* or *Chinese flowering cabbage.*

chronic malnutrition A condition characterized by chronic growth retardation or stunting as reflected in low weight or low height for age.

chylomicron (KIGH-loh-MY-cron) A type of lipoprotein that transports newly digested fat—mostly triglyceride—from the intestine through lymph and blood.

chyme The semi-liquid mixture of food and gastric secretions resulting from the actions of the stomach after consuming food.

cirrhosis A chronic, degenerative disease of the liver in which the liver cells become infiltrated with fibrous tissues; blood flow through the liver is obstructed, causing back pressure and eventually leading to coma and death unless the cause of the disease is removed; the most common cause of cirrhosis is chronic alcohol abuse.

club soda Artificially carbonated water containing added salts and minerals.

coenzyme Q10 A lipid made by the body and used by cells in energy metabolism; falsely touted to increase exercise performance and stamina in athletes; potential antioxidant role. May increase oxygen use and stamina in patients with heart disease, but no significant effect is seen in healthy athletes.

coenzymes Enzyme helpers; small molecules that interact with enzymes and enable them to do their work. Many coenzymes are made from water-soluble vitamins.

cofactor A mineral element that, like a coenzyme, works with an enzyme to facilitate a chemical reaction.

collagen (KAHL-uh-jen) The characteristic protein of connective tissue (*kolla* = glue; *gennan* = to produce).

colon cancer Cancer of the large intestine (colon), the terminal portion of the digestive tract.

colostrum (kuh-LAHS-trum) A milk-like secretion from the breast, rich in protective factors, present during the first day or so after delivery and before milk appears.

complementary proteins Two or more food proteins whose amino acid assortments complement each other in such a way that the essential amino acids limited in or missing from each are supplied by the others.

complex carbohydrates Long chains of sugars (glucose) arranged as starch or fiber; also called *polysaccharides* (*poly* = many; *saccharide* = sugar unit).

conjugated linoleic acid (CLA) An altered form of the omega-6 fatty acid linoleic acid, CLA is falsely promoted to support lean muscle retention, weight loss, and increased exercise recovery. Research does not scientifically support these notions even in long-term use.

constipation Hardness and dryness of bowel movements associated with discomfort in passing them.

contaminants Potentially dangerous substances, such as lead, that can accidentally get into foods.

contamination iron Iron found in foods as the result of contamination by inorganic iron salts from iron cookware, iron-containing soils, and the like.

control group A group of individuals with characteristics that match those of the group being treated in an intervention study but who receive a placebo or no treatment at all.

correlation A simultaneous change in two factors, such as a decrease in blood pressure with regular aerobic activity (a direct or positive correlation) or the decrease in incidence of bone fractures with increasing calcium intakes (an inverse or negative correlation).

correspondence school A school from which courses can be taken and degrees granted by mail (or online). Schools that are accredited offer respectable courses and degrees.

cortex An outer covering; in the brain, that part in which conscious thought takes place.

cortical bone The dense outer ivory-like layer of bone that provides an exterior shell over trabecular bone.

CP or creatine phosphate *See* PC or phosphocreatine.

creatine A nitrogen-containing substance made by the body that combines with phosphate to form the high-energy compound phosphocreatine (PC). PC is stored and used by muscle for ATP production. Touted as ergogenic aid that may increase PC production in muscles and improve performance of repeated bouts of short-term (< 30 seconds) high-intensity exercise with short recovery periods (e.g., sprinting, weight lifting).

cretinism (CREE-tin-izm) Severe mental and physical retardation of an infant caused by iodine deficiency during pregnancy.

cross-contamination The inadvertent transfer of bacteria from one food to another that occurs, for instance, by chopping vegetables on the same cutting board that was used to skin poultry.

cross-reaction The reaction of one antigen with antibodies developed against another antigen.

culture Knowledge, beliefs, customs, laws, morals, art, and literature acquired by members of a society and passed along to succeeding generations.

daily limit for discretionary calories The balance of calories remaining in a person's energy allowance, after accounting for the number of calories needed to meet recommended nutrient intakes through consumption of nutrient-dense foods.

Daily Value The amount of fat, sodium, fiber, and other nutrients health experts say should make up a healthy diet. The "% Daily Values" that appear on food labels tell you the percentage of a nutrient that a serving of the food contributes to a healthy diet.

degenerative disease Chronic disease characterized by deterioration of body organs as a result of misuse and neglect. Poor eating habits, smoking, lack of exercise, and other lifestyle habits often contribute to degenerative diseases including heart disease, cancer, osteoporosis, and diabetes.

denaturation A change in the shape of a protein brought about by heat, alcohol, acids, bases, salts of heavy metals, or other agents.

denosumab A drug (brand name Prolia) in a class of medications called RANK ligand (RANKL) inhibitors. Administered by injection every six months, denosumab works by stopping the development of osteoclasts and thereby inhibiting their ability to damage bone.

dental caries Decay of the teeth; tooth cavities (*caries* = rottenness).

dental plaque A colorless film, consisting of bacteria and their by-products, that is constantly forming on the teeth.

designer estrogens Drugs that act like estrogen on *estrogen receptors* in osteoblasts to promote an increase in bone mass; an example is raloxifene (Evista). *Estrogen receptors* are cellular molecules that bind to estrogen, estrogen agonists/antagonists, or phytoestrogens and deliver these compounds to the nucleus of the cell.

DHEA (dehydroepiandrosterone) A precursor of the hormones testosterone and estrogen; falsely promoted to increase production of testosterone, build muscle, burn fat, and delay the effects of aging. Long-term effects unknown; self-supplementation not recommended.

diabetes (dye-uh-BEET-eez) A disorder characterized by insufficiency or relative ineffectiveness of insulin, which renders a person unable to regulate the blood glucose level normally.

Dietary Reference Intakes (DRI) A set of reference values for energy and nutrients that can be used for planning and assessing diets for healthy people.

dietetic technician, registered (DTR) Nutrition professionals who work as part of health care and food service management teams. DTRs have completed at least a two-year associate's degree at a U.S. regionally accredited college or university and an accredited dietetic technician program, and passed a national examination.

digestion The process by which foods are broken down into smaller, absorbable products.

digestive system The body system composed of organs and glands associated with the ingestion and processing of food for absorption of nutrients into the body.

dim sum Dumplings stuffed with pork, shrimp, beef, sweet paste, or preserves and steamed or fried.

dipeptides (dye-PEP-tides) Protein fragments two amino acids long. A peptide is a strand of amino acids.

diploma mill A correspondence school that grinds out degrees (sometimes worth no more than the paper they are printed on) the way a grain mill grinds out flour.

disaccharide A double sugar (sucrose, maltose, and lactose); *di* = two.

disordered eating Eating food as an outlet for emotional stress rather than in response to internal physiological cues.

diuretics (dye-you-RET-iks) Medications and other substances causing increased water excretion (*dia* = through; *ouron* = urine).

diverticulosis (dye-ver-tik-you-LOH-siss) Outpocketings of weakened areas of the intestinal wall that can rupture, like blowouts in a tire, causing dangerous infections.

DRI *See* Dietary Reference Intakes.

drugs Substances that can modify one or more of the body's functions.

EAR *See* Estimated Average Requirement.

eating disorder General term for several conditions (anorexia nervosa, bulimia nervosa, binge-eating disorder) that exhibit an excessive preoccupation with body weight, a fear of body fatness, and a poor or distorted body image.

eating pattern The combination of foods and beverages that constitute an individual's complete dietary intake over time; may describe a usual way of eating or a combination of foods recommended for consumption.

eclampsia A severe extension of preeclampsia characterized by convulsions; may lead to coma.

edema (eh-DEEM-uh) Swelling of body tissue caused by leakage of fluid from the blood vessels, seen in (among other conditions) protein deficiency.

EER *See* Estimated Energy Requirement.

electrolytes Compounds that partially dissociate in water to form ions; examples are sodium, potassium, and chloride.

empty-calorie foods Foods that supply calories but negligible nutrients.

emulsifier A compound with both water-soluble and fat-soluble portions that can attract lipids into water to form an emulsion.

endocrine (EN-doh-krin) A term to describe a gland secreting or a hormone being secreted into the blood.

endurance The ability to sustain an effort for a long time. One type, **muscle endurance**, is the ability of a muscle to contract repeatedly within a given time period without becoming exhausted. Another type, **cardiovascular endurance**, is the ability of the cardiovascular system to sustain effort over a period of time.

energy The capacity to do work, such as moving or heating something.

energy metabolism All reactions by which the body obtains and expends the energy from food or body stores.

enriched Refers to the process by which the B vitamins thiamin, riboflavin, niacin, folic acid, and the mineral iron are added to refined grains and grain products at levels specified by law.

enterotoxin A toxic compound, produced by microorganisms, that harms mucous membranes, as in the gastrointestinal tract (*entero* = intestine).

enzyme A protein catalyst. A *catalyst* is a compound that facilitates (speeds up the rate of) a chemical reaction without itself being altered in the process.

epidemiological study A study of a population that searches for possible correlations between nutrition factors and health patterns over time.

epithelial (ep-ih-THEE-lee-ul) **tissue** The cells that form the outer surface of the body and line the body cavities and the principal passageways leading to the exterior. Examples include the cornea, digestive tract lining, respiratory tract lining, and skin. The epithelial cells produce mucus to protect these tissues from bacteria and other potentially harmful substances. Without this mucus, infections become more likely.

ergogenic aids Anything that helps increase the capacity to work or exercise (*ergo* = work; *genic* = give rise to).

essential amino acids Amino acids that cannot be synthesized by the body or that cannot be synthesized in amounts sufficient to meet physiological need.

essential fatty acid A fatty acid that cannot be synthesized in the body in amounts sufficient to meet physiological need.

essential nutrient A compound that must be obtained from food because it cannot be synthesized by the body in amounts sufficient to meet physiological needs.

Estimated Average Requirement (EAR) The amount of a nutrient that is estimated to meet the requirement for the nutrient in half of the people of a specific age and gender. The EAR is used in setting the RDA.

Estimated Energy Requirement (EER) The average calorie intake that is predicted to maintain energy balance in a healthy adult of a defined age, gender, weight, height, and level of physical activity, consistent with good health.

estrogen A hormone; important in connection with nutrition because it maintains calcium balance and because its secretion abruptly declines at menopause.

estrogen/hormone therapy (ET/HT) Administration of estrogen to replace the natural hormone that declines with menopause. Because ET may increase the risk of uterine and breast cancer, *hormone replacement therapy* (the administration of a combination of estrogen with the hormone progesterone) is often used. However, the FDA recommends that HT and ET be considered only for women with significant risk of osteoporosis that outweighs the risk of the drugs.

ethnic cuisine The traditional foods eaten by the people of a particular culture.

exchange lists Now known as Food Lists. Lists of foods with serving sizes specified. The foods on a single list are similar with respect to nutrient and calorie content and thus can be mixed and matched in the diet.

exocrine (EX-oh-krin) Describes glands that secrete chemical messengers through a duct into a body cavity or onto the surface of the skin; *exo* means "out."

experimental group The participants in a study who receive the real treatment or intervention under investigation.

external cue theory The theory that some people eat in response to such external factors as the presence of food or the time of day rather than to such internal factors as hunger.

famine Widespread lack of access to food caused by natural disasters, political factors, or war; characterized by a large number of deaths due to starvation and malnutrition.

fat cell theory Theory that during the growing years, fat cells respond to overfeeding by producing additional fat cells; the number of fat cells eventually becomes relatively fixed, and overfeeding from this point on causes the body to enlarge existing fat cells.

fats Lipids that are solid at normal room temperature.

fatty acids Basic units of fat composed of chains of carbon atoms with an acid group at one end and hydrogen atoms attached all along their length.

Feeding America A national food-banking network to which most food banks belong.

fetal alcohol spectrum disorder (FASD) A spectrum of behavioral, cognitive, and physical disabilities caused by prenatal exposure to alcohol.

fetal alcohol syndrome (FAS) The cluster of symptoms seen in an infant or child whose mother consumed excess alcohol during pregnancy; includes retarded growth, impaired development of the central nervous system, and facial malformations. A lesser condition—called *fetal alcohol effect (FAE)*—causes learning impairment and other more subtle abnormalities in infants exposed to alcohol during pregnancy.

fibers The indigestible residues of food, composed mostly of polysaccharides. The best known of the fibers are cellulose, hemicellulose, pectin, and gums.

First Amendment The amendment to the U.S. Constitution that guarantees freedom of the press.

fitness The body's ability to meet physical demands; composed of four components: flexibility, muscular strength, muscle endurance, and cardiorespiratory endurance.

flexibility The ability to bend or extend without injury; depends on the elasticity of the muscles, tendons, and ligaments and on the condition of the joints.

fluid balance Distribution of fluid among body compartments.

fluorosis (floor-OH-sis) Discoloration of the teeth from ingestion of too much fluoride during tooth development.

foam cells Cells from the immune system containing scavenged oxidized LDL-cholesterol; thought to initiate arterial plaque formation.

food additives Any substances added to food, including substances used in production, processing, treatment, packaging, transportation, or storage.

food allergen A substance in food (usually a protein) that is seen by the body as harmful and causes the immune system to mount an allergic reaction.

food allergy An adverse reaction to an otherwise harmless substance that involves the body's immune system.

food banks Nonprofit community organizations that collect surplus commodities from the government as well as edible but often unmarketable foods from private industry for use by nonprofit charities, institutions, and feeding programs at nominal cost.

food group plan A diet-planning tool, such as MyPlate, that groups foods according to similar origin and nutrient content and then specifies the amount of food a person should eat from each group.

food insecurity The inability to acquire or consume an adequate quality or sufficient quantity of food in socially acceptable ways, or the uncertainty that one will be able to do so.

food intolerance A general term for any adverse reaction to a food or food component that does not involve the body's immune system.

food intoxications Illnesses caused by eating food that contains a harmful toxin or chemical.

food recovery Such activities as salvaging perishable produce from grocery stores and wholesale food markets; rescuing surplus prepared food from restaurants, corporate cafeterias, and caterers; and collecting nonperishable, canned, or boxed processed food from manufacturers, supermarkets, or people's homes. The items recovered are donated to hungry people.

food security Access by all people at all times to enough food for an active and healthy life. Food security has two aspects: ensuring that adequate food supplies are available and ensuring that households have the ability to acquire food, either by producing it themselves or by being able to purchase it.

foodborne illness Illness occurring as a result of ingesting food or water contaminated with a poisonous substance, such as a toxin or chemical *(food intoxication)* or an infectious agent, such as bacteria, viruses, or parasites *(foodborne infection)*; commonly called *food poisoning*.

foodborne infections Illnesses caused by eating a food containing bacteria or other microorganisms capable of growing and thriving in a person's tissues.

fortified Term for foods to which nutrients have been added. Typically, commonly eaten foods are chosen for fortification with added nutrients to help prevent a deficiency (iodized salt, milk with vitamin D) or to reduce the risk of chronic disease (juices with added calcium).

fortified foods Foods to which nutrients have been added, either because they were not already present or because they were present in insignificant amounts; foods to which manufacturers have added 10 percent or more of the Daily Value for a particular nutrient. Examples: margarine with added vitamin A, milk with added vitamin D, certain brands of orange juice with added calcium, and breakfast cereals with added nutrients and nonnutrients.

free radicals Highly toxic compounds created in the body as a result of chemical reactions that involve oxygen. Environmental pollutants such as cigarette smoke and ozone also prompt the formation of free radicals.

free range A method of producing livestock where animals are allowed to roam freely instead of being contained in any manner; this term is not regulated and can be used to imply the animal product has been produced more humanely than it actually has been. USDA certifies "free-range" chickens as chickens raised for their meat that have access to the outdoors; there is no USDA certification for "free-range" beef, pork, or other nonpoultry products; free-range eggs also have no legal definition.

from a community water system or **from a municipal source** Statement that must appear on bottles containing water derived from a municipal water supply. The phrase must conspicuously precede or follow the name of the brand.

fructose (FROOK-toce) Fruit sugar; the sweetest of the monosaccharides.

functional tolerance Actual change in sensitivity to a drug; often results in hallucinations and convulsions when alcohol is withheld.

fusion cuisine A term used to describe food that combines the elements of two or more cuisines—say, European and Oriental—to create a new one.

galactose (guh-LACK-toce) A monosaccharide that occurs bonded to glucose in the sugar of milk.

garbanzo beans or chickpeas Large, round, tan-colored legumes that have a nutty flavor and crunchy texture. Use in soups and stews and puréed for dips.

gefilte fish (guh-FIL-tuh) A chopped fish mixture often made with pike and whitefish as well as matzoh crumbs, eggs, and seasonings.

gene A unit of a cell's inheritance; made of a chemical, DNA, that is copied faithfully so that every time the cell divides, both its offspring get identical copies. Genes direct the cells' machinery to make the proteins that form each cell's structures and enable the cell to do its work.

genetic engineering The use of biotechnology to alter the genes of a plant in an effort to create a new plant with different traits; also called *genetic modification*. In some cases, a plant's genes may be deleted or altered, or genes may be introduced from different organisms or species. The foods or crops produced are called genetically engineered (GE) or genetically modified (GM) foods or crops.

genetically modified organisms (GMOs)/ genetically engineered organisms (GEOs) Organisms from bacteria, plants, or animals that have been genetically changed in a laboratory through DNA technology. Genetically engineered plants have been developed to increase nutritional value, be resistant to pests, herbicides, or harsh environmental conditions like drought, and for other purposes.

gestational diabetes The appearance of abnormal glucose tolerance during pregnancy.

ghee A clarified butter without any milk solids or water.

GI *See* glycemic index.

ginkgo biloba (GING-coe bye-LOW-buh) An herb used to treat any number of conditions, including fatigue and failing memory.

gleaning The harvesting of excess food from farms, orchards, and packing houses to feed the hungry.

glucagon (GLOO-kuh-gahn) A hormone released by the pancreas that signals the liver to release glucose into the bloodstream.

glucose (GLOO-koce) The building block of carbohydrate; a monosaccharide used in both plant and animal tissues as quick energy.

glutamic acid (gloo-TAM-ik) A nonessential amino acid found in plant and animal tissue; used as a flavor-intensifying seasoning.

glutinous rice Short-grained, opaque white rice that turns sticky when cooked.

glycemic effect (also called *glycemic response)* The effect of food on a person's blood glucose and insulin response; how fast and how high the blood glucose rises and how quickly the body responds by bringing it back to normal.

glycemic index (GI) A ranking of foods based on their potential to raise blood glucose levels.

glycerol (GLISS-er-all) An organic compound that serves as the backbone for triglycerides.

glycogen (GLEYE-ko-jen) A polysaccharide composed of chains of glucose, manufactured in the body and stored in liver and muscle. As a storage form of glucose, liver glycogen can be broken down by the liver to maintain a constant blood glucose level when carbohydrate intake is inadequate.

glycolysis An anaerobic energy metabolism pathway for the partial breakdown of glucose for energy. Energy released in glycolysis is used to form the high-energy compound ATP.

GOBI An acronym formed from the elements of UNICEF's Child Survival campaign: **g**rowth charts, **o**ral rehydration therapy, **b**reast milk, and **i**mmunization.

goiter (GOY-tur) Enlargement of the thyroid gland caused by iodine deficiency.

GRAS (Generally Recognized As Safe) list A list of ingredients, established by the FDA, that had long been in use and were believed safe. The list is subject to revision as new facts become known.

grass-fed Refers to livestock allowed to forage on pasture grass; not legally defined.

grazing Eating small amounts of food at intervals throughout the day rather than or in addition to eating regular meals.

Great Northern beans A medium-white, kidney-shaped bean. Enjoy the delicate flavor and firm texture in salads, soups, and main dishes.

green soybeans (edamame) These large soybeans are harvested when the beans are still green and sweet and can be served as a snack or a main vegetable dish, after boiling in water for 15 to 20 minutes. They are high in protein and fiber and contain no cholesterol.

grits Coarsely ground cornmeal.

ground water Water that comes from an underground body of water that does not come into contact with any surface water.

guarana (gwuh-RAH-nuh) An herb chemically equivalent to caffeine.

guava A sweet, juicy fruit with green or yellow skin and red or yellow flesh.

hard water Water that has a high mineral (calcium and magnesium) content.

hazard State of danger; used to refer to any circumstance in which harm is possible.

HDL (high-density lipoprotein) Lipoprotein that carries cholesterol in the blood back to the liver for recycling or disposal.

health claim A statement on the food label linking the nutritional profile of a food to a reduced risk of a particular disease, such as osteoporosis or cancer. Manufacturers must adhere to strict government guidelines when making such claims.

health fraud Conscious deceit practiced for profit, such as the promotion of a false or an unproven product or therapy.

health promotion Helping people achieve their maximum potential for good health.

heat stroke An acute and dangerous reaction to heat buildup in the body, requiring emergency medical attention; also called *sun stroke*.

heavy metals Any of a number of mineral ions, such as mercury and lead, so named because of their relatively high atomic weight. Many heavy metals are poisonous.

heme (HEEM) **iron** The iron-holding part of the hemoglobin protein, found in meat, fish, and poultry. About 40 percent of the iron in meat, fish, and poultry is bound into heme. Meat, fish, and poultry also contain a factor (MFP factor) other than heme that promotes the absorption of iron, even of the iron from other foods eaten at the same time as the meat.

hemoglobin (HEEM-uh-glow-bin) The oxygen-carrying protein of the blood; found in the red blood cells.

hemorrhoids (HEM-or-oyds) Swollen, hardened (varicose) veins in the rectum, usually caused by the pressure resulting from constipation.

high-density lipoprotein *See* HDL.

high-quality proteins Proteins containing all the essential amino acids in the right proportion relative to need. The *quality* of a food protein is judged by the proportions of essential amino acids that it contains relative to our needs. Animal and soy proteins are the highest in quality.

histamine A substance released by cells of the immune system during an allergic reaction to an antigen; causes inflammation, itching, hives, dilation of blood vessels, and a drop in blood pressure.

hominy Hulled, dried corn kernels.

homocysteine (hoe-moe-SIS-teen) A chemical that appears to be toxic to the blood vessels of the heart. High blood levels of homocysteine have been associated with low blood levels of vitamin B_{12}, vitamin B_6, and folate.

hormones Chemical messengers, secreted by one organ (a gland) in response to a condition in the body, that acts on another organ or organs to change that condition. Each affects one or more target tissues or organs and elicits specific responses to restore normal conditions.

hormone-free Generally refers to products free from recombinant bovine somatotropin (rBST), a hormone synthetically produced from recombinant DNA administered to dairy cattle to increase milk production.

hunger The physiological drive to find and eat food, experienced as an unpleasant sensation.

hydrogenation (high-drah-jen-AY-shun) The process of adding hydrogen to unsaturated fat to make it more solid and more resistant to chemical change.

hydrolyzed vegetable protein (HVP) A protein obtained from any vegetable, including soybeans. The protein is broken down into amino acids by a chemical process called *acid hydrolysis*. HVP is a flavor enhancer that can be used in soups, broths, sauces, gravies, flavoring and spice blends, canned and frozen vegetables, and meats and poultry.

hyperemesis gravidarum Nausea and vomiting during pregnancy that is severe enough to cause effects such as acidosis, dehydration, and weight loss.

hyperglycemia An abnormally high blood glucose concentration, often a symptom of diabetes.

hypertension Sustained high blood pressure (*hyper* = too much; *tension* = pressure).

hypertrophy An increase in size in response to use.

hypoglycemia (HIGH-po-gligh-SEEM-ee-uh) An abnormally low blood glucose concentration, below 60 to 70 mg/100 mL.

hyponatremia (HIGH-poe-na-TREE-mee-ah) A decreased concentration of sodium in the blood.

hypothalamus (high-poh-THALL-ah-mus) A part of the brain that senses a variety of conditions in the blood, such as temperature, salt content, glucose content, and others, and signals other parts of the brain or body to change those conditions when necessary.

immunity Specific disease resistance derived from the immune system's memory of prior exposure to specific disease agents and its ability to mount a swift response against them.

incidental food additives (indirect additives) Substances that accidentally get into food as a result of contact with it during growing, processing, packaging, storing, or some other stage before the food is consumed.

ingredients list A listing of the ingredients in a food, with items listed in descending order of predominance by weight. All food labels are required to bear an ingredients list.

innate immunity Type of immunity that is naturally existing and does not require prior sensitization to an antigen.

inorganic Being or composed of matter other than plant or animal.

inositol (ih-NAH-sih-tall) Once identified in association with the B vitamins; a type of sugar (related to glucose) found synthesized in the body and many foods.

insoluble fiber Fiber category that includes the fiber types called cellulose, hemicellulose, and lignin. Insoluble fibers do not dissolve in water.

insulin A hormone secreted by the pancreas in response to high blood glucose levels; it assists cells in drawing glucose from the blood.

integrated pest management The use of biological controls, crop rotation, genetic engineering, and other tactics to reduce chemical use in the growing and production of crops.

intentional food additives Substances intentionally added to food; examples include nutrients, colors, spices, and herbs.

intervention study A population study examining the effects of a treatment on experimental subjects compared to a control group.

intestinal flora The normal bacterial inhabitants of the digestive tract (*flora* = plant inhabitants).

intrinsic factor A compound made in the stomach that is necessary for the body's absorption of vitamin B_{12}.

ions (EYE-onz) Electrically charged particles, such as sodium (positively charged) and chloride (negatively charged).

iron overload A condition in which the body contains more iron than it needs or can handle; excess iron is toxic and can damage the liver. The most common cause of iron overload is the genetic disorder hemochromatosis.

iron-deficiency anemia A reduction of the number and size of red blood cells and a loss of their color because of iron deficiency.

irradiation The process of exposing a substance to low doses of radiation, using gamma rays, X-rays, or electricity (electron beams) to kill insects, bacteria, and other potentially harmful microorganisms.

jicama (HE-cah-mah) A crisp root vegetable of the bean family that is tan outside and white inside and is always eaten raw; as popular in Mexico as the potato is in the United States.

jujube (JOO-joob) Chinese date.

kasha Cracked buckwheat, barley, millet, or wheat that is served as a cooked cereal or potato substitute.

kefir A fermented milk made by adding *Lactobacillus acidophilus* and other bacteria that break down lactose.

ketosis (key-TOE-siss) An adaptation of the body to prolonged (several days) fasting or carbohydrate restriction; body fat is converted to ketones, which can be used as fuel for some brain cells. Caused by abnormal amounts of ketone bodies in the blood and urine; ketone bodies are produced from the incomplete breakdown of fat when glucose is unavailable for the brain and nerve cells.

kidney beans These familiar beans are large, red, and kidney shaped (the white variety is called cannellini). They have a bland taste and soft texture but tough skins. Use in chili, bean stews, and Mexican dishes (for red) or Italian dishes (for white).

knish A potato pastry filled with ground meat, potato, or kasha.

kola nut An herb chemically equivalent to caffeine.

kosher Fit, proper, or in accordance with religious law.

kwashiorkor (kwash-ee-OR-core) Severe malnutrition caused by inadequate protein and calories leading to apathy, anemia, loss of body proteins, and poor growth.

lacto-ovovegetarian A person who includes milk and milk products and eggs in their diet, but excludes meat, poultry, fish, and seafood.

lacto-vegetarian A person who includes milk and milk products in their diet, but excludes meat, poultry, fish, seafood, and egg.

lactoferrin (lak-toe-FERR-in) A factor in breast milk that binds and helps absorb iron and keeps it from supporting the growth of the infant's intestinal bacteria.

lactose A disaccharide composed of glucose and galactose; commonly known as *milk sugar.*

lactose intolerance Inability to digest lactose as a result of a lack of the necessary enzyme lactase.

lassi A milkshake-like drink made from yogurt.

LBW *See* low birthweight.

LDL (low-density lipoprotein) Lipoprotein that carries cholesterol (much of it synthesized in the liver) to body cells. A high blood cholesterol level usually reflects high LDL.

lecithin (LESS-ih-thin) A phospholipid, a major constituent of cell membranes; manufactured by the liver and also found in many foods.

legumes (LEG-yoomz or leh-GYOOMZ) Plants of the bean and pea family having roots with nodules containing bacteria that can trap nitrogen from the air in the soil and make it into compounds that become part of the seed. The seeds are rich in high-quality protein compared with those of most other plant foods.

lentils Small, flat, and round legumes. Usually brown, lentils can also be green, pink, or red. They have a mild taste with firm texture. Best used when combined with grains or vegetables in salads, soups, or stews.

leptin An appetite-suppressing hormone produced in the fat cells that communicates information about the body's fat content to the brain (*leptos* means slender).

lifestyle diseases Conditions that may be aggravated by modern lifestyles that include too little exercise, poor diets, excessive drinking, and smoking. Lifestyle diseases are also referred to as *diseases of affluence.*

lima or butter beans Limas are soft and mealy in texture. They are flat, oval shaped, and white tinged with green. The smaller variety has a milder taste. Use in soups and stews.

limiting amino acid A term given to the essential amino acid in shortest supply (relative to the body's need) in a food protein; it therefore *limits* the body's ability to make its own proteins.

linoleic (lin-oh-LAY-ik) **acid, linolenic** (lin-oh-LEN-ik) **acid** Polyunsaturated fatty acids, essential for human beings.

lipids A family of compounds that includes triglycerides (fats and oils), phospholipids (lecithin), and sterols (cholesterol).

lipoprotein lipase (LPL) An enzyme located on the surfaces of fat cells that enables the cell to convert blood triglycerides into fatty acids and glycerol to be pulled into the cell for reassembly and storage as body fat.

lipoproteins (LYE-poh-PRO-teenz) Clusters of lipids associated with protein that serve as transport vehicles for lipids in blood and lymph. The four main types of lipoproteins are chylomicrons, VLDL, LDL, and HDL.

liposuction A type of surgery (also called lipectomy) that vacuums out fat cells that have accumulated, typically in the buttocks and thighs. If the person continues to eat more calories than are expended, fat will return to the fat cells that remain in those regions.

litchi (LEE-chee) Small, round fruits with orange-red skin and opaque white flesh; also called *litchee* or *lychee.*

liver The large, lobed organ that lies under the ribs and filters the blood, in the process removing, processing, and readying for redistribution many of its materials.

longan A small round fruit with smooth brown skin and clear pulp.

low birthweight (LBW) A birthweight of 5½ lb (2,500 g) or less; used as a predictor of poor health in a newborn and as a probable indicator of poor nutrition status of the mother during and/or before pregnancy. Normal birthweight for a full-term baby is 6½ to 8¾ lb (about 3,000 to 4,000 g). LBW infants are either born premature or have suffered growth failure in the uterus; they may or may not be born early, but they are small.

low-density lipoprotein *See* LDL.

lox Smoked salmon.

LPL *See* lipoprotein lipase.

lymph (LIMF) The fluid outside the circulatory system that bathes the cells; derived from the blood by being pressed through the capillary walls; similar to the blood in composition but without red blood cells; this body fluid transports the products of fat digestion toward the heart and eventually drains back into the bloodstream.

macrobiotic diet Extremely restrictive diet based on metaphysical beliefs and consisting mostly of legumes, whole grains, and certain vegetables.

mad cow disease Also called *bovine spongiform encephalopathy* (BSE); a rare and fatal degenerative disease first diagnosed in 1986 in cattle in the United Kingdom. The bovine disease may be passed to humans who eat the meat of infected animals and may lead to death due to brain and nerve damage.

major mineral An essential mineral nutrient found in the human body in amounts greater than 5 grams.

malnutrition Any condition caused by an excess, deficiency, or imbalance of calories or nutrients; the impairment of health resulting from a relative deficiency or excess of food energy and specific nutrients necessary for health.

maltose A disaccharide composed of two glucose units.

mantou Steamed bread.

marasmus (muh-RAZ-mus) Severe emaciation from energy deficiency with chronic wasting of fat, muscle, and other tissues; starvation.

margin of safety From a food-safety standpoint, the *margin* is a zone between the maximum amount of a substance that appears to be safe and the amount allowed in the food supply.

matzoh A cracker-like bread eaten most often at Passover.

maximum heart rate The upper limit of what your cardiorespiratory system can handle during physical activity as represented by your measured heart rate and measured with the following equation: MHR = 220 – current age in years.

meat alternatives/analogs Meat alternatives made from soybeans contain soy protein or tofu and other ingredients mixed together to simulate various kinds of meat. These meat alternatives are sold as frozen, canned, dried or refrigerated foods.

meat analogs Textured vegetable protein products formulated to look and taste like meat, fish, or poultry. Many of these are designed to match the known nutrient contents of animal protein foods.

menopause The time of life at which a woman's menstrual cycle ceases, usually at about 45 to 50 years of age.

metabolic syndrome A cluster of conditions that includes increased blood pressure, high blood sugar, excess body fat around the waist, and abnormal cholesterol levels.

metabolic tolerance Increased efficiency of removing high levels of alcohol from the blood due to long-term exposure; may lead to more drinking and possible addiction.

metabolism Collective term for all the chemical and physical reactions occurring in living cells, including the reactions by which the body obtains and uses energy from foods.

microvilli (MY-croh-VILL-ee, MY-croh-VILL-eye) Tiny hairlike projections on each cell of the intestinal tract lining that can trap nutrient particles and translocate them into the cells (singular: *microvillus*).

mineral water Water that is drawn from an underground source and contains at least 250 parts per million of dissolved solids. If the water contains between 250 and 500 parts per million total dissolved solids, the statement "low mineral content" must appear. If it contains more than 1,500 parts per million, the statement "high mineral content" must appear. If a cup of the water contains at least 20 milligrams of calcium, 0.36 milligram of iron, or 5 milligrams of sodium, the product must carry nutrition labeling.

minerals Naturally occurring, inorganic, chemical elements; serve as structural components of the body and are used in many vital body processes.

miso A rich, salty condiment that characterizes the essence of Japanese cooking. A smooth paste, miso is made from soybeans and a grain such as rice, plus salt and a mold culture, and then aged in cedar vats for 1 to 3 years. Miso should be refrigerated. Use miso to flavor soups, sauces, dressings, marinades, and pâtés.

moderation The attribute of a diet that provides no unwanted constituent in excess.

monoglyceride (mahn-oh-GLISS-er-ide) A glycerol molecule with one fatty acid attached to it. A *diglyceride* is a glycerol molecule with two fatty acids attached to it.

monosaccharides The single sugars (glucose, fructose, and galactose); *mono* = one.

monounsaturated fatty acid A fatty acid containing one point of unsaturation; found mostly in vegetable oils such as olive, canola, and peanut.

mucus (MYOO-kuss) A thick, slippery coating of the intestinal tract lining (and other body linings) that protects the cells from exposure to digestive juices. The adjective form is *mucous,* and the coating is often called the *mucous membrane.*

multinational corporations International companies with direct investments and/or operative facilities in more than one country. U.S. oil and food companies are examples.

natural Most foods labeled "natural," except for meat and poultry, are not subject to government regulations; this term applies broadly to foods minimally processed and free of synthetic preservatives, artificial sweeteners, colors, flavors, and other artificial additives, hydrogenated oils, stabilizers, and emulsifiers.

neural tube defects Any of a number of birth defects in the orderly formation of the neural tube during early gestation. Both the brain and the spinal cord develop from the neural tube, and defects cause various central nervous system disorders.

neuromotor exercise Training that incorporates various motor skills, including balance, coordination, gait, agility, and proprioceptive training. The better your neuromotor conditioning, the better you will be at preventing a fall when you slip or lose your balance.

neurotoxin A poisonous compound that disrupts the nervous system (*neuro* = nerve).

night blindness Slow recovery of vision following flashes of bright light at night; an early symptom of vitamin A deficiency.

nitrate An ion composed of one nitrogen and three oxygen atoms; touted as ergogenic aid that may improve exercise tolerance and improve performance in endurance exercise in nonelite athletes. Reduces oxygen demand during moderate-intensity exercise by increasing plasma nitrite levels to increase production of nitric oxide with various vascular and metabolic effects.

non-GMO Term used to imply a food contains no ingredients made from GMO/GEO products; not legally defined and therefore cannot be enforced.

nondairy soy frozen dessert Nondairy frozen desserts are made from soy milk or soy yogurt. Soy ice cream is one of the most popular desserts made from soybeans and can be found in many grocery stores.

nonheme iron The iron found in plant foods.

nonnutritive sweeteners Synthetic or natural ingredients added to foods and beverages to provide sweetness with negligible, if any, calories (sometimes referred to as artificial sweeteners or sugar substitutes), such as aspartame, saccharin, stevia, and sucralose.

nursing bottle syndrome (also called *baby bottle tooth decay*) Decay of all the upper and sometimes the back lower teeth that occurs in infants given carbohydrate-containing liquids when they sleep. The syndrome can also develop in toddlers given bottles of liquid to carry around and sip all day.

nutrient content claims Claims such as "low-fat" and "low-calorie" used on food labels to help consumers who don't want to scrutinize the Nutrition Facts panel get an idea of a food's nutritional profile. These claims must adhere to specific definitions set forth by the Food and Drug Administration.

nutrient density A measure of the nutrients a food supplies relative to the number of calories it provides. The higher the level of nutrients and the fewer the number of calories, the higher the nutrient density.

nutrients Substances obtained from food and used in the body to promote growth, maintenance, and repair. The nutrients include carbohydrates, fats, proteins, vitamins, minerals, and water.

nutrition The study of foods, their nutrients and other chemical components, their actions and interactions in the body, and their influence on health and disease.

Nutrition Facts panel A detailed breakdown of the nutritional content of a serving of a food that must appear on virtually all packaged foods sold in the United States.

nutrition security Condition in which all people have access to a variety of nutritious foods and potable drinking water; knowledge, resources, and skills for healthy living; prevention, treatment, and care for diseases affecting nutrition status; and safety-net systems during crisis situations, such as natural disasters or deleterious social and political systems.

nutritional quackery A type of health fraud that promotes products and services that have questionable and unproven scientific bases.

nutritional yeast A fortified food supplement containing B vitamins, iron, and protein; can be used to improve the quality of a vegetarian diet.

nutritionist A person who claims to be capable of advising people about their diets. Some nutritionists are registered dietitians, whereas others are self-described experts whose training is questionable.

o-LDL *See* oxidized LDL-cholesterol.

obesity Conventionally defined as weight 20 percent or more above the desirable weight for height, or a BMI of 30 or greater.

oils Lipids that are liquid at normal room temperature.

olestra An artificial fat derived from sucrose and fatty acids combined in such a way that the body cannot break them down. Sold under the brand name Olean, olestra does not contribute calories to food.

omega-3 fatty acids Polyunsaturated fatty acids that have their endmost double bonds after the third carbon in the chain.

omega-6 fatty acids Polyunsaturated fatty acids that have their endmost double bonds after the sixth carbon in the chain.

oral rehydration therapy (ORT) The treatment of dehydration (usually due to diarrhea caused by infectious disease) with an oral solution; ORT as developed by UNICEF is intended to enable a mother to mix a simple solution for her child from substances that she has at home.

organic Legal term that applies to a food and how the food was produced; crops must be grown without use of synthetic pesticides, bioengineered genes, petroleum-based fertilizers, and sewage sludge-based fertilizers; organic livestock must have access to outdoors and be given no antibiotics or growth hormones; organic foods may not be irradiated.

organic halogens Compounds that contain one or more of a class of atoms called *halogens*, including fluorine, chlorine, iodine, or bromine.

Oriental radish A large, cylindrically shaped vegetable with smooth skin; also called *daikon.*

osteoblast A bone-building cell; responsible for formation of bone.

osteoclast A bone-destroying cell; responsible for resorption and removal of bone.

osteomalacia (os-tee-oh-muh-LAY-shuh) The disease resulting from vitamin D deficiency in adults and characterized by softening of the bones. (Its counterpart in children is called rickets.) Symptoms include bowed legs and a curved spine.

osteoporosis (OSS-tee-oh-pore-OH-sis) Also known as *adult bone loss;* a disease in which the bones become porous and fragile (*osteo* = bones; *poros* = porous).

other specified feeding or eating disorder Condition in which a person exhibits some but not all of the criteria for specific eating disorders.

overload An extra physical demand placed on the body. A principle of training is that for a body system to improve, its workload must be increased by increments over time.

overnutrition Calorie or nutrient overconsumption severe enough to cause disease or increased risk of disease; a form of malnutrition.

overweight Conventionally defined as weight between 10 and 20 percent above the desirable weight for height, or a body mass index (BMI) of 25.0 through 29.9.

ovovegetarian A person on this diet includes eggs, but excludes milk and milk products, meat, poultry, fish, and seafood.

oxidized LDL-cholesterol (o-LDL) The cholesterol in LDLs that is attacked by reactive oxygen molecules inside the walls of the arteries; o-LDL is taken up by scavenger cells and deposited in plaque.

pancreas A gland that secretes the endocrine hormone insulin and also produces the exocrine secretions that aid digestion in the small intestine. (See also *endocrine; exocrine.*)

parathyroid hormone A hormone used as a drug to stimulate new bone formation; administered by injection once a day. Daily injections of teriparatide (brand name Forteo) lead to increased bone mineral density.

pasteurization The process of sterilizing food via heat treatment.

PC or phosphocreatine A high-energy compound stored in muscle cells; its phosphate group can be split and used to replenish ATP for short bursts of anaerobic activity.

peak bone mass The highest bone density achieved for an individual; accumulated over the first three decades of life; typically occurs by 30 years of age. After age 30, bone resorption slowly begins to exceed bone formation.

pellagra (pell-AY-gruh) Niacin deficiency characterized by diarrhea, inflammation of the skin, and, in severe cases, mental disorders and death.

PEM *See* protein-energy malnutrition.

peptide bond A bond that connects one amino acid with another.

periodization The strategic use of specific nutritional intakes for the ultimate purpose of obtaining adaptations that optimize sport performance.

periodontal disease Inflammation or degeneration of the tissues that surround and support the teeth.

peristalsis (pair-ih-STALL-sis) The wavelike squeezing motions of the stomach and intestines that push their contents along the digestive tract.

pesticides Chemicals intentionally applied to plants, including foods, to prevent or eliminate pest damage. *Pests* include all living organisms that destroy or spoil foods: bacteria, molds and fungi, insects, and rats and other rodents, to name a few.

pH The concentration of hydrogen ions. The lower the pH, the stronger the acid: pH 2 is a strong acid, pH 7 is neutral, and a pH above 7 is alkaline (a base).

phenylketonuria (FEN-il-KEY-toe-NYOO-ree-ah) or **PKU** An inborn error of metabolism, detectable at birth, in which the body lacks the enzyme needed to convert the amino acid phenylalanine to the amino acid tyrosine. If it is not detected and treated, derivatives of phenylalanine accumulate in the blood and tissues, where they can cause severe damage, including mental retardation.

phospholipid (FOSS-foe-LIP-id) A lipid similar to a triglyceride but containing phosphorus; one of the three main classes of lipids.

phytochemicals (FIGHT-oh-KEM-ih-kulz) Nonnutritive compounds in plants that confer color and other characteristics. Some phytochemicals provide health-protecting benefits in the body; also called *phytonutrients (phyto* = plant).

pica The craving of nonfood items such as clay, ice, and laundry starch; does not appear to be limited to any particular geographic area, race, sex, culture, or social status.

pigment A molecule capable of absorbing certain wavelengths of light. Pigments in the eye permit us to perceive different colors.

PIH *See* pregnancy-induced hypertension.

pinto beans These medium-size, oval beans are mottled beige and brown and have an earthy flavor. They are most often used in Mexican dishes, such as refried beans, stews, or dips.

PKU *See* phenylketonuria.

placebo (plah-SEE-bo) An inert, harmless "treatment" given to a control group in a research study that the group's members cannot recognize as different from the actual treatment or intervention given to the experimental group.

placebo effect An improvement in a person's sense of well-being or physical health in response to the use of a placebo (a substance having no medicinal properties or medicinal effects).

placenta (pluh-SEN-tuh) The organ inside the uterus in which the mother's and fetus's circulatory systems intertwine and in which exchange of materials between maternal and fetal blood takes place. The fetus receives nutrients and oxygen across the placenta; the mother's blood picks up carbon dioxide and other waste materials to be excreted via her lungs and kidneys.

plantain A greenish, starchy banana; because it is starchy even when ripe, it is never eaten raw and is usually pan-fried.

polysaccharide A long chain of 10 or more glucose molecules linked together in straight or branched chains; another term for *complex carbohydrates.*

polyunsaturated fatty acid (sometimes abbreviated PUFA) A fatty acid in which two or more points of unsaturation occur; found in nuts and vegetable oils such as safflower, sunflower, and soybean as well as in fatty fish.

postnatal After birth.

poverty The state of having too little money to meet minimum needs for food, clothing, and shelter. The U.S. Department of Agriculture defined the poverty level in the United States as an annual income of $23,550 for a family of four in 2013.

precursor A compound that can be converted into another compound. For example, beta-carotene is a precursor of vitamin A (*pre* = before; *cursor* = runner, forerunner).

preeclampsia A condition characterized by hypertension, fluid retention, and protein in the urine.

preformed vitamin A Vitamin A in its active form.

pregnancy-induced hypertension (PIH) High blood pressure that develops during the second half of pregnancy.

prenatal Prior to birth.

progression The process of starting slowly and gradually increasing the amount of physical activity.

protein quality A measure of the essential amino acid content of a protein relative to the essential amino acid needs of the body.

protein synthesis The process by which cells assemble amino acids into proteins. All individuals are unique because of minute differences in the ways their body proteins are made. The instructions for making all the proteins in our bodies are transmitted in the genetic information we receive at conception.

protein-energy malnutrition (PEM) The world's most widespread malnutrition problem; characterized by a depletion of both energy stores and tissue proteins; usually accompanied by micronutrient deficiencies.

protein-sparing A description of the effect of carbohydrate and fat, which, by being available to yield energy, allow amino acids to be used to build body proteins.

proteins Compounds composed of atoms of carbon, hydrogen, oxygen, and nitrogen and arranged as strands of amino acids. Some amino acids also contain atoms of sulfur.

purified water Water from which all minerals have been removed, thereby eliminating the possibility that the minerals might corrode pipes or appliances (such as a steam iron). Also known as *demineralized water, distilled water, deionized water, or reverse osmosis water.*

purslane A leafy vegetable that can be used in salads or cooked like spinach.

pylorus (pie-LORE-us) Muscle that regulates the opening of the bottom of the stomach.

quackery Health fraud; a quack is a person who practices health fraud (quack = to boast loudly).

queso blanco, fresco, or Mexicano Soft white cheese made of part-skim milk.

RAE *See* retinol activity equivalents.

rBST-free Refers to milk (dairy products) produced from cattle that have not been treated with recombinant BST (bovine somatotropin hormone); all milk contains some BST as it is produced in pituitary glands of cattle.

RD *See* registered dietitian.

Recommended Dietary Allowance (RDA) The average daily amount of a nutrient that is sufficient to meet the nutrient needs of nearly all (97 to 98 percent) healthy individuals of a specific age and gender.

red beans These versatile beans are medium-size, dark-red oval. The taste and texture are similar to kidney beans. Use in soups and stews, and serve with rice.

reference dose The estimated amount of a chemical that could be consumed daily without causing harmful effects.

refined grains Grains that have been milled to remove the husk, bran, and germ from the grain—leaving only the endosperm—to yield a finer texture and improved shelf life. The process also removes dietary fiber, iron and other minerals, and many B vitamins. The recommended amount of refined grains is no more than 3 ounce-equivalents per day.

registered dietitian/nutritionist (RD/RDN) A professional who has graduated from a program of dietetics accredited by the Accreditation Council for Education in Nutrition and Dietetics (ACEND) of the Academy of Nutrition and Dietetics, has completed an internship program or the equivalent to gain practical skills, has passed a registration examination, and maintains competencies through continuing education. Some states require licensing for dietitians, thereby requiring anyone who wants to use the title "dietitian" to receive permission to do so by passing a state examination.

regulations Legal mandates that must be obeyed. Failure to follow a regulation brings about legal consequences.

requirement The minimum amount of a nutrient that will prevent the development of deficiency symptoms. Requirements differ from the RDA and AI, which include a substantial margin of safety to cover the requirements of different individuals.

retina (RET-in-uh) The paper-thin layer of light-sensitive cells lining the back of the inside of the eye.

retinal (RET-in-al) One of the active forms of vitamin A that functions in the pigments of the eye. Other active forms of vitamin A include retinol and retinoic acid.

retinol One of the active forms of vitamin A.

retinol activity equivalents (RAE) A measure of the amount of retinol the body will derive from a food containing preformed vitamin A or beta-carotene and other vitamin A precursors. Note that some tables list vitamin A in terms of *International Units (IU)*. (See Appendix A for methods of converting from one measure to another.)

rice sticks Flat, opaque, wide noodles made from rice flour.

rice vermicelli (vur-mi-SEL-ee) Thin white noodles made from rice flour.

rickets A disease that occurs in children as a result of vitamin D deficiency; characterized by abnormal growth of bone, which in turn leads to bowed legs and an outward-bowed chest.

risk For pesticide residues, the harm a substance may cause. Scientists estimate risk by assessing the amount of a chemical that each person in a population might consume over time (also called *exposure*) and by considering how toxic the substance might be (*toxicity*).

roti An unleavened flatbread, resembling a tortilla, usually made from whole-wheat flour.

royal jelly Substance secreted from the saliva glands of honeybees; provides food for all young larvae and is the only food for larvae that will develop into queen bees. It has been incorrectly claimed to impart extra energy and to have restorative properties; can be potentially hazardous for individuals who may suffer allergic reactions.

salt A pair of charged mineral particles, such as sodium (Na^+) and chloride (Cl^-), that associate together. In water, they dissociate and help carry electric current; that is, they become *electrolytes*.

satiety (sah-TIE-eh-tee) The feeling of fullness and satisfaction that occurs after a meal.

saturated fatty acid A fatty acid carrying the maximum possible number of hydrogen atoms (having no points of unsaturation). Saturated fats are found in animal foods such as meat, poultry, and full-fat dairy products as well as in tropical oils such as palm and coconut.

schmaltz Chicken fat.

scurvy The vitamin C-deficiency disease characterized by bleeding gums, tooth loss, and, in severe cases, death.

selective estrogen receptor modulators (SERMs) *See* designer estrogens.

seltzer Tap water injected with carbon dioxide and containing no added salts.

semivegetarian A person on this diet includes some but not all groups of animal-derived products, such as meat, poultry, fish, seafood, eggs, milk, and milk products.

serving The standard amount of food used as a reference to give advice regarding how much to eat (such as a 1-cup serving of milk); serving sizes also allow comparisons to be made when reading food labels.

set-point theory Theory that the body tends to maintain a certain weight by adjusting hunger, appetite, and food energy intake on the one hand and metabolism (energy output) on the other so that a person's conscious efforts to alter weight may be foiled.

severe acute malnutrition (SAM) A condition characterized by very low weight for height, severe wasting, and/or edema associated with recent severe food deprivation.

simple carbohydrates (sugars) The single sugars (*monosaccharides*) and the pairs of sugars (*disaccharides*) linked together.

skinfold test A method for measuring body fat in which the thickness of a fold of skin on the back of the arm (the triceps), below the shoulder blade (subscapular), or in other areas is measured with an instrument called a caliper.

small intestine A long, tubular organ of digestion that is the site of nutrient absorption.

social group A group of people, such as a family, who depend on one another and share a set of norms, beliefs, values, and behaviors.

sodium bicarbonate A salt composed of sodium and bicarbonate ions; touted as ergogenic aid that may increase extracellular buffering capacity by increasing the muscle's ability to dispose of excess hydrogen ions when taken before high-intensity events. High sodium load may cause GI side effects (e.g., diarrhea); effects of repeated ingestion are unknown.

soft water Water containing a high sodium concentration and little or no calcium or magnesium.

solid fats Fats that are usually solid at room temperature, such as butter, lard, and shortening. These fats may be visible or may be a constituent of foods such as milk, cheese, meats, or baked products. Common solid fats include butter, beef fat, chicken fat, pork fat (lard), stick margarine, and shortening. The fat in whole milk is also considered to be solid fat because it is solid at room temperature, but suspended in milk by the process of homogenization.

soluble fiber Fiber category that includes the fiber types called pectin, gums, mucilages, some hemicelluloses, and algal substances (e.g., carrageenan). Soluble fibers either dissolve or swell when placed in water.

sopa Rice or pasta that is fried and cooked in consommé.

soy cheese Cheese made from soy milk. The standard soy cheese products (sandwich slices, shreds, blocks) have a firm texture and are substitutes for firm dairy cheese. Soy cream cheese and soy sour cream products are available as well.

soy flour Flour made from roasted soybeans ground into a fine powder. Soy flour gives a protein boost to recipes. Soy flour is gluten-free, so yeast-raised breads made with soy flour are denser in texture.

soy milk, soy beverages Soybeans that are soaked, ground fine, and strained produce a fluid called *soybean milk*. Soy milk is an excellent source of high-quality protein and B vitamins. Look for calcium-fortified varieties.

soy-nut butter Made from roasted, whole soy nuts, which are then crushed and blended with soy oil and other ingredients. Soy-nut butter has a slightly nutty taste, contains significantly less fat than peanut butter, and provides many other nutritional benefits.

soy nuts Whole soybeans that have been soaked in water and then baked until browned. High in protein and isoflavones, soy nuts are similar in texture and flavor to peanuts.

soy protein, texturized *Texturized soy protein* usually refers to products made from texturized soy flour. Texturized soy flour is made by running defatted soy flour through an extrusion cooker, which allows the creation of many different forms and sizes. When hydrated, it has a chewy texture. It is widely used as a meat extender.

soy yogurt Yogurt made from soy milk. Its creamy texture makes it an easy substitute for sour cream or cream cheese. Soy yogurt can be found in a variety of flavors in many food stores.

soybeans As soybeans mature in the pod, they ripen into a hard, dry bean. Most soybeans are yellow. However, brown and black varieties are also available. Whole soybeans can be cooked and used in sauces, stews, and soups. They have a firm texture and bland flavor; found in numerous food products, such as tofu, soy flour, soy grits, and soy milk.

sparkling bottled water Water in which carbon dioxide (the ingredient that makes soda pop bubbly) is naturally present; that is, carbonation is not added from an outside source.

split peas Green or yellow, these small, halved peas supply an earthy flavor with a mealy texture. They are best used in soups and with rice or grains.

sports anemia A temporary condition of low blood hemoglobin level, associated with the early stage of athletic training.

spring water Water derived from an underground formation from which water flows naturally to the surface of the earth and to which minerals have not been added or taken away. It may be collected either at the spring itself or through a hole tapping the underground formation feeding the spring.

staple grain A grain used frequently in the diet; for example, corn (in Mexico), rice (in Asia), or wheat (in the United States).

starch A plant polysaccharide composed of hundreds of glucose molecules, digestible by human beings.

sterols (STEER-alls) Lipids with a structure similar to that of cholesterol; one of the three main classes of lipids.

strength The ability of muscles to work against resistance.

stress fracture Bone damage or breakage caused by stress on bone surfaces during exercise.

strict vegetarian *See* vegan.

structure function claim A statement allowed on food and dietary supplement labels that describes the effect that a nutrient or dietary ingredient has on the structure or function of the body, but cannot mention a disease or symptom. Example: "probiotics help regulate your digestive system." These claims are not pre-approved by FDA,

stunting (short for age) Children aged 0 to 59 months with a low height for age measure; a measure of chronic malnutrition (long-term food deprivation).

sucrose (SOO-krose) A disaccharide composed of glucose and fructose.

Sugar alcohols Alternative sweeteners including mannitol, sorbitol, isomalt, xylitol; can be derived from fruits or commercially produced from dextrose and are absorbed more slowly and metabolized differently than other sugars in the human body. The sugar alcohols are not readily used by bacteria ordinarily found in the mouth and therefore are associated with less cavity formation. Although the sugar alcohols are used as sugar substitutes, they do add calories (about 1.5 to 3 calories per gram) to a food product.

target heart rate The heartbeat rate that will achieve a cardiorespiratory conditioning effect for a given person: fast enough to push the heart, but not so fast as to strain it.

taro A starchy vegetable with brown, hairy skin and a pink-purple interior.

tempeh A chunky, tender soybean cake; a traditional Indonesian food. Whole soybeans, sometimes mixed with another grain such as rice or millet, are fermented into a rich cake of soybeans with a smoky, nutty flavor. Tempeh can be marinated and grilled and added to soups, casseroles, or chili.

tofu and tofu products *Tofu*, also known as *soybean curd*, is a soft, cheese-like food made by curdling fresh, hot soy milk with a coagulant. Tofu is a bland product that easily absorbs the flavors of other ingredients with which it is cooked. Tofu is rich in high-quality protein and B vitamins and is low in sodium.

Tolerable Upper Intake Level (UL) The maximum amount of a nutrient that is unlikely to pose any risk of adverse health effects to most healthy people. The UL is not intended to be a recommended level of intake.

tolerance (1) Decrease in effectiveness of a drug after a period of prolonged or heavy use. Increased efficiency of removing high levels of alcohol from the blood due to long-term exposure; may lead to more drinking and possible addiction. (2) the maximum amount of a particular substance allowed in food.

tonic water Artificially carbonated water with added sugar and/or high-fructose corn syrup, sodium, and quinine.

toxicants Poisons; that is, agents that cause physical harm or death when present in large amounts.

toxicity The ability of a substance to harm living organisms. All substances are toxic if present in high enough concentrations.

trabecular (tra-BECK-you-lar) **Bone** The lacy inner network of calcium-containing crystals; spongelike in appearance, it supports the bone's structure.

trace mineral An essential mineral nutrient found in the human body in amounts less than 5 grams.

trans fat A type of fatty acid created when an unsaturated fat is hydrogenated. Found primarily in margarines, shortenings, commercial frying fats, and baked goods, *trans* fatty acids have been implicated by research as culprits in heart disease.

transgenetics The process of transferring genes from one species to another unrelated species.

transport proteins Proteins that either carry nutrients and other molecules in body fluids or reside in cell membranes and act as "pumps" by picking up compounds on one side of the membrane and releasing them on the other side as needed.

triglycerides (try-GLISS-er-ides) The major class of dietary lipids, including fats and oils. A triglyceride is made up of three units known as *fatty acids* and one unit called *glycerol.*

trimester One-third of the normal duration of pregnancy; the first trimester is 0 to 13 weeks, the second is 13 to 26 weeks, and the third trimester is 26 to 40 weeks.

tripeptides (try-PEP-tides) Protein fragments three amino acids long.

UL *See* Tolerable Upper Intake Level.

under-5 mortality rate (U5MR) The number of children who die before the age of 5 for every 1,000 live births.

undernutrition Severe underconsumption of calories or nutrients, leading to disease or increased susceptibility to disease; a form of malnutrition.

underwater weighing A measure of density and volume; the less a person weighs underwater compared to the person's out-of-water weight, the greater the proportion of body fat (fat is less dense or more buoyant than lean tissue).

underweight Weight 10 percent or more below the desirable weight for height, or a BMI of less than 18.5.

UNICEF The United Nations International Children's Emergency Fund, now referred to as the United Nations Children's Fund.

unsaturated fatty acid A fatty acid with one or more points of unsaturation. Unsaturated fats are found in foods from both plant and animal sources. Unsaturated fatty acids are further divided into monounsaturated fatty acids and polyunsaturated fatty acids.

unspecified eating disorders Condition in which a person exhibits some but not all of the criteria for specific eating disorders.

urea (yoo-REE-uh) The principal nitrogen excretion product of metabolism, generated mostly by the removal of amine groups from unneeded amino acids or from those amino acids being sacrificed to a need for energy.

variety A feature of a diet in which a wide selection of foods from within and among the different food groups are consumed; the opposite of *monotony.*

vegan A person who excludes all animal-derived foods, including meat, poultry, fish, seafood, eggs, milk, and milk products from their diet.

veins Blood vessels that carry used blood from the tissues back to the heart.

very-low-density lipoprotein *See* VLDL.

villi (VILL-ee, VILL-eye) Fingerlike projections of the sheet of cells that line the GI tract; the villi make the surface area much greater than it would otherwise be (singular: *villus*).

vitamins Organic, or carbon-containing, essential nutrients that are vital to life but needed only in relatively minute amounts. Vitamins perform various body functions that promote growth and reproduction and maintain health. (*vita* = life; *amine* = containing nitrogen).

VLDL (very-low-density lipoprotein) Lipoprotein that carries fats packaged or made by the liver to various tissues in the body.

waist circumference A measure used to assess abdominal (visceral) fat; excess fat in the abdomen increases a person's risk of health problems.

wasting (thin for height) Children aged 0 to 59 months with a low weight for length/height measure; a measure of severe acute malnutrition—indicating recent rapid weight loss or a failure to gain weight.

water Fluid that provides the medium for life processes.

well water Ground water derived from a rock formation by way of a hole bored, drilled, or otherwise constructed in the ground.

white navy beans These small, white, oval beans are best used in soups and stews and as baked beans.

whole food A food that is altered as little as possible from the plant or animal tissue from which it was taken; examples are milk, oats, potatoes, and apples.

whole grain A grain that is milled in its entirety (all but the husk), not refined. Whole grains include whole wheat, bulgur, corn, brown rice, whole rye, oats, amaranth, barley, buckwheat, quinoa, sorghum, and millet.

yard-long beans Thin, tender string beans that grow to as long as 18 inches.

yerba maté An herb chemically equivalent to caffeine.

yohimbe (yoh-HIM-bee) Touted as an aphrodisiac, a cure-all for sexual dysfunction; also claimed to be able to alter body mass, muscle mass, or exercise performance when combined with resistance training. None of these claims have been proven by research.

zapote (sah-POH-tay) An apple-sized fruit with green skin and black flesh.

Index

Analyze Your Diet

Diet & Wellness Plus shows you how your current diet relates to recommended health goals. Use *Diet & Wellness Plus* to track your diet, generate reports, and analyze the nutritional value of the food you eat.

Assignment Objectives:

1. Gain experience in keeping a food record and utilizing a computer database
2. Collect and analyze food intake data and determine solutions for any dietary shortcomings identified

Instructions

Part I: Create a 3-Day Food Intake Record

1. Record all foods, snacks, and beverages that you consume on 3 consecutive days (include 2 weekdays and 1 weekend day). Do not include any vitamin, mineral, or protein supplements that you are taking so that you can accurately evaluate your dietary intake. Write down the information as soon as you finish eating.
2. Estimate amounts, as closely as possible, of each food item. Weigh or use household measuring cups and spoons to estimate amounts and, where needed, refer to food labels to determine ingredients. For casseroles, soups, or hot dishes, estimate the amount of each ingredient that you consumed.
3. Remember to list any salt added to foods; sugar added to cereal and beverages; milk or cream in coffee or tea; and any margarine, butter, oils, or gravies that you add to foods.

Tips: When recording your intake, be sure to include **everything** you eat, including serving sizes (cups, ounces, etc.). Also remember to include your snacks and beverages. Describe the type of food you have eaten, giving as many details as possible. For example, if you drank milk, indicate whether you had whole, skim, 2%, or 1% milk. Here is an example format for recording intake:

Time	Food	Amount (cups, oz, tsp, etc.)	Notes

Part II: Perform Computerized Diet Analysis

1. Sign in to *Diet & Wellness Plus* from www.cengagebrain.com and create a profile following the directions given in the program.
2. Click on the "Track Diet" tab and enter the foods you ate for each meal on each day.
3. Click on **Reports,** then select and print or save the following **Reports:**
   a. **Intake Spreadsheets** (one for each day)
   b. **Intake vs. Goals** (reporting your 3-day average intake compared to recommendations)
   c. **MyPlate Analysis**, which compares your intake with your recommendations
   d. **Energy Balance**
   e. **Fat Breakdown**
   f. **Macronutrient Ranges**
   g. **Daily Food Log**

Part III: Complete an Analysis of Your Diet Based on Your Reports

Using your analysis reports, respond to the questions in each section.

A. Energy (calories)

1. What was your energy (calorie) intake?
2. What is your DRI recommendation for energy (calorie) intake on your Intake vs. Goals report?
3. Is this a realistic caloric recommendation for you? Why or why not?

B. Carbohydrates

1. Did your carbohydrate intake meet the minimum of 130 grams per day?
2. How many grams of fiber did you consume? How does your intake compare to the DRI?
3. List two good sources of fiber in your diet. See each day's intake spreadsheet.
4. What changes could you make to improve your fiber intake?
5. Take a look at your daily food logs and list three foods that contain naturally occurring sugars (e.g., milk) and those that contain added sugars (e.g., soda).
6. What changes, if any, could you make in your sugar intake?

C. Fats

1. Fill in Table 1 using the data in your reports.

TABLE 1 Fat Intake

Type of Fat	Recommended Amount	% Recommended
Total fat (g)		
Saturated (g)		
Polyunsaturated (g)		
Monounsaturated (g)		
Trans (g)		

2. Which types of fat in your diet need to be decreased and/or increased and why?
3. If your overall intake of fat exceeded the recommended amount (20 to 35 percent of total calories), what changes could you make to improve your fat intake?

D. Protein

1. Calculate your DRI for protein. ________ grams per day.
2. How many grams of protein did you consume on average per day? ________ grams per day.
3. Does your protein intake need to be altered? If so, how?
4. How well did you balance your protein intake from animal sources vs. plant sources?

E. Vitamin and Mineral Intake

1. List ALL vitamins and minerals that were under 75% or were over 200% of your recommended intake, or above your Tolerable Upper Intake Level in Table 2.

TABLE 2

Vitamins	
Under 75%	**>200% or >UL**
Minerals	
Under 75%	**>200% or >UL**

2. Why do you think that you did not achieve the recommended intakes for the vitamins or minerals listed above? What foods could you add to your diet to increase your intake of these vitamins and minerals?
3. For the nutrients listed above that are in excess (over 200%), what foods contributed to this excess? Can you adjust your diet to create a better balance of vitamins and minerals?

F. Your Overall Diet

1. Use the MyPlate Analysis report for your 3-day average to complete Table 3.

TABLE 3 **MyPlate Analysis**

	Recommended Amount	My Intake	% Recommended Amount
Grains, ounce equivalents			
Vegetables, cup equivalents			
Fruits, cup equivalents			
Dairy, cup equivalents			
Protein foods, oz. equivalents			

2. How well does your MyPlate analysis reflect the five characteristics of a healthy diet (adequacy, balance, calorie control, moderation, and variety) discussed in your textbook? Briefly discuss **each** one as it applies to your diet.

G. Design a Healthy Diet

Take a look at your food records and analysis reports and think about the changes that you could make to address any concerns and improve your overall diet.

1. Using Table 4, evaluate your deficiencies and excesses. Add new rows if needed. You do not need to run any new printouts. Use your intake spreadsheets to help you.

TABLE 4 **Diet Evaluation**

Nutrients under 75%	What will you change?	Nutrients over 200%	What will you change?
Ex: Calcium is 350 mg short	Add 8 oz. milk = 300 mg	Sodium 1000 mg over	Subtract 1 c. canned soup = 950 mg

2. In one or two paragraphs, summarize what changes you would make to your diet to improve it.

H. Assignment Completion. Assemble the following items to complete this assignment:

1. LOGS and REPORTS:
   - Daily Food Logs (one for each day)
   - Intake Spreadsheets (one for each day)
   - Intake vs. Goals
   - MyPlate Analysis (3-day average)
2. DIET ANALYSIS QUESTIONS (SECTIONS A to G): Your responses to the questions in sections A through G.

Body Mass Index (BMI)

Height	18	19	20	21	22	23	24	25	26	27	28	29	30	31	32	33	34	35	36	37	38	39	40
	Body Weight (pounds)																						
4′10″	86	91	96	100	105	110	115	119	124	129	134	138	143	148	153	158	162	167	172	177	181	186	191
4′11″	89	94	99	104	109	114	119	124	128	133	138	143	148	153	158	163	168	173	178	183	188	193	198
5′0″	92	97	102	107	112	118	123	128	133	138	143	148	153	158	163	168	174	179	184	189	194	199	204
5′1″	95	100	106	111	116	122	127	132	137	143	148	153	158	164	169	174	180	185	190	195	201	206	211
5′2″	98	104	109	115	120	126	131	136	142	147	153	158	164	169	175	180	186	191	196	202	207	213	218
5′3″	102	107	113	118	124	130	135	141	146	152	158	163	169	175	180	186	191	197	203	208	214	220	225
5′4″	105	110	116	122	128	134	140	145	151	157	163	169	174	180	186	192	197	204	209	215	221	227	232
5′5″	108	114	120	126	132	138	144	150	156	162	168	174	180	186	192	198	204	210	216	222	228	234	240
5′6″	112	118	124	130	136	142	148	155	161	167	173	179	186	192	198	204	210	216	223	229	235	241	247
5′7″	115	121	127	134	140	146	153	159	166	172	178	185	191	198	204	211	217	223	230	236	242	249	255
5′8″	118	125	131	138	144	151	158	164	171	177	184	190	197	203	210	216	223	230	236	243	249	256	262
5′9″	122	128	135	142	149	155	162	169	176	182	189	196	203	209	216	223	230	236	243	250	257	263	270
5′10″	126	132	139	146	153	160	167	174	181	188	195	202	209	216	222	229	236	243	250	257	264	271	278
5′11″	129	136	143	150	157	165	172	179	186	193	200	208	215	222	229	236	243	250	257	265	272	279	286
6′0″	132	140	147	154	162	169	177	184	191	199	206	213	221	228	235	242	250	258	265	272	279	287	294
6′1″	136	144	151	159	166	174	182	189	197	204	212	219	227	235	242	250	257	265	272	280	288	295	302
6′2″	141	148	155	163	171	179	186	194	202	210	218	225	233	241	249	256	264	272	280	287	295	303	311
6′3″	144	152	160	168	176	184	192	200	208	216	224	232	240	248	256	264	272	279	287	295	303	311	319
6′4″	148	156	164	172	180	189	197	205	213	221	230	238	246	254	263	271	279	287	295	304	312	320	328
6′5″	151	160	168	176	185	193	202	210	218	227	235	244	252	261	269	277	286	294	303	311	319	328	336
6′6″	155	164	172	181	190	198	207	216	224	233	241	250	259	267	276	284	293	302	310	319	328	336	345
	Underweight (<18.5)	Healthy Weight (18.5–24.9)						Overweight (25–29.9)					Obese (≥30)										

Find your height along the left-hand column and look across the row until you find the number that is closest to your weight. The number at the top of that column identifies your BMI. The area shaded in green represents healthy weight ranges.

Dietary Reference Intakes (DRI)

Estimated Energy Requirements (EER), Recommended Dietary Allowances (RDA), and Adequate Intakes (AI) for Water, Energy, and the Energy Nutrients

Age (yr)	Reference BMI (kg/m²)	Reference height, cm (in)	Reference weight, kg (lb)	Water[a] AI (L/day)	Energy EER[b] (cal/day)	Carbohydrate RDA (g/day)	Total fiber AI (g/day)	Total fat AI (g/day)	Linoleic acid AI (g/day)	Linolenic acid[c] AI (g/day)	Protein RDA (g/day)[d]	Protein RDA (g/kg/day)
Males												
0–0.5	—	62 (24)	6 (13)	0.7[e]	570	60	—	31	4.4	0.5	9.1	1.52
0.5–1	—	71 (28)	9 (20)	0.8[f]	743	95	—	30	4.6	0.5	13.5	1.5
1–3[g]	—	86 (34)	12 (27)	1.3	1046	130	19	—	7	0.7	13	1.1
4–8[g]	15.3	115 (45)	20 (44)	1.7	1742	130	25	—	10	0.9	19	0.95
9–13	17.2	144 (57)	36 (79)	2.4	2279	130	31	—	12	1.2	34	0.95
14–18	20.5	174 (68)	61 (134)	3.3	3152	130	38	—	16	1.6	52	0.85
19–30	22.5	177 (70)	70 (154)	3.7	3067[h]	130	38	—	17	1.6	56	0.8
31–50				3.7	3067[h]	130	38	—	17	1.6	56	0.8
>50				3.7	3067[h]	130	30	—	14	1.6	56	0.8
Females												
0–0.5	—	62 (24)	6 (13)	0.7[e]	520	60	—	31	4.4	0.5	9.1	1.52
0.5–1	—	71 (28)	9 (20)	0.8[f]	676	95	—	30	4.6	0.5	13.5	1.5
1–3[g]	—	86 (34)	12 (27)	1.3	992	130	19	—	7	0.7	13	1.1
4–8[g]	15.3	115 (45)	20 (44)	1.7	1642	130	25	—	10	0.9	19	0.95
9–13	17.4	144 (57)	37 (81)	2.1	2071	130	26	—	10	1.0	34	0.95
14–18	20.4	163 (64)	54 (119)	2.3	2368	130	26	—	11	1.1	46	0.85
19–30	21.5	163 (64)	57 (126)	2.7	2403[i]	130	25	—	12	1.1	46	0.8
31–50				2.7	2403[i]	130	25	—	12	1.1	46	0.8
>50				2.7	2403[i]	130	21	—	11	1.1	46	0.8
Pregnancy												
1st trimester				3.0	+0	175	28	—	13	1.4	+25	1.1
2nd trimester				3.0	+340	175	28	—	13	1.4	+25	1.1
3rd trimester				3.0	+452	175	28	—	13	1.4	+25	1.1
Lactation												
1st 6 months				3.8	+330	210	29	—	13	1.3	+25	1.1
2nd 6 months				3.8	+400	210	29	—	13	1.3	+25	1.1

NOTE: For all nutrients, values for infants are AI. Dashes indicate that values have not been determined.

[a]The water AI includes drinking water, water in beverages, and water in foods; in general, drinking water and other beverages contribute about 70 to 80 percent, and foods, the remainder. Conversion factors: 1 L = 33.8 fluid oz; 1 L = 1.06 qt; 1 cup = 8 fluid oz.

[b]The Estimated Energy Requirement (EER) represents the average dietary energy intake that will maintain energy balance in a healthy person of a given gender, age, weight, height, and physical activity level. The values listed are based on an "active" person at the reference height and weight and at the midpoint ages for each group until age 19. Chapter 2 (page 44), Chapter 10 (page 296), and www.ChooseMyPlate.gov provide tools to determine Estimated Energy Requirements.

[c]The linolenic acid referred to in this table and text is the omega-3 fatty acid known as alpha-linolenic acid.

[d]The values listed are based on reference body weights.

[e]Assumed to be from human milk.

[f]Assumed to be from human milk and complementary foods and beverages. This includes approximately 0.6 L (~3 cups) as total fluid including formula and drinking water.

[g]For energy, the age groups for young children are 1–2 years and 3–8 years.

[h]For males, subtract 10 calories per day for each year of age above 19.

[i]For females, subtract 7 calories per day for each year of age above 19.

Recommended Dietary Allowances (RDA) and Adequate Intakes (AI) for Vitamins

Age (yr)	Thiamin RDA (mg/day)	Riboflavin RDA (mg/day)	Niacin RDA (mg/day)[a]	Biotin AI (μg/day)	Pantothenic acid AI (mg/day)	Vitamin B_6 RDA (mg/day)	Folate RDA (μg/day)[b]	Vitamin B_{12} RDA (μg/day)	Choline AI (mg/day)	Vitamin C RDA (mg/day)	Vitamin A RDA (μg/day)[c]	Vitamin D RDA (μg/day)[d]	Vitamin E RDA (mg/day)[e]	Vitamin K AI (μg/day)
Infants														
0–0.5	0.2	0.3	2	5	1.7	0.1	65	0.4	125	40	400	10	4	2.0
0.5–1	0.3	0.4	4	6	1.8	0.3	80	0.5	150	50	500	10	5	2.5
Children														
1–3	0.5	0.5	6	8	2	0.5	150	0.9	200	15	300	15	6	30
4–8	0.6	0.6	8	12	3	0.6	200	1.2	250	25	400	15	7	55
Males														
9–13	0.9	0.9	12	20	4	1.0	300	1.8	375	45	600	15	11	60
14–18	1.2	1.3	16	25	5	1.3	400	2.4	550	75	900	15	15	75
19–30	1.2	1.3	16	30	5	1.3	400	2.4	550	90	900	15	15	120
31–50	1.2	1.3	16	30	5	1.3	400	2.4	550	90	900	15	15	120
51–70	1.2	1.3	16	30	5	1.7	400	2.4	550	90	900	15	15	120
>70	1.2	1.3	16	30	5	1.7	400	2.4	550	90	900	20	15	120
Females														
9–13	0.9	0.9	12	20	4	1.0	300	1.8	375	45	600	15	11	60
14–18	1.0	1.0	14	25	5	1.2	400	2.4	400	65	700	15	15	75
19–30	1.1	1.1	14	30	5	1.3	400	2.4	425	75	700	15	15	90
31–50	1.1	1.1	14	30	5	1.3	400	2.4	425	75	700	15	15	90
51–70	1.1	1.1	14	30	5	1.5	400	2.4	425	75	700	15	15	90
>70	1.1	1.1	14	30	5	1.5	400	2.4	425	75	700	20	15	90
Pregnancy														
≤18	1.4	1.4	18	30	6	1.9	600	2.6	450	80	750	15	15	75
19–30	1.4	1.4	18	30	6	1.9	600	2.6	450	85	770	15	15	90
31–50	1.4	1.4	18	30	6	1.9	600	2.6	450	85	770	15	15	90
Lactation														
≤18	1.4	1.6	17	35	7	2.0	500	2.8	550	115	1200	15	19	75
19–30	1.4	1.6	17	35	7	2.0	500	2.8	550	120	1300	15	19	90
31–50	1.4	1.6	17	35	7	2.0	500	2.8	550	120	1300	15	19	90

NOTE: For all nutrients, values for infants are AI.
[a]Niacin recommendations are expressed as niacin equivalents (NE), except for recommendations for infants younger than 6 months, which are expressed as preformed niacin.
[b]Folate recommendations are expressed as dietary folate equivalents (DFE).
[c]Vitamin A recommendations are expressed as retinol activity equivalents (RAE).
[d]Vitamin D recommendations are expressed as cholecalciferol and assumes minimal sun exposure.
[e]Vitamin E recommendations are expressed as α-tocopherol.

Recommended Dietary Allowances (RDA) and Adequate Intakes (AI) for Minerals

Age (yr)	Sodium AI (mg/day)	Chloride AI (mg/day)	Potassium AI (mg/day)	Calcium RDA (mg/day)	Phosphorus RDA (mg/day)	Magnesium RDA (mg/day)	Iron RDA (mg/day)	Zinc RDA (mg/day)	Iodine RDA (μg/day)	Selenium RDA (μg/day)	Copper RDA (μg/day)	Manganese AI (mg/day)	Fluoride AI (mg/day)	Chromium AI (μg/day)	Molybdenum RDA (μg/day)
Infants															
0–0.5	120	180	400	200	100	30	0.27	2	110	15	200	0.003	0.01	0.2	2
0.5–1	370	570	700	260	275	75	11	3	130	20	220	0.6	0.5	5.5	3
Children															
1–3	1000	1500	3000	700	460	80	7	3	90	20	340	1.2	0.7	11	17
4–8	1200	1900	3800	1000	500	130	10	5	90	30	440	1.5	1.0	15	22
Males															
9–13	1500	2300	4500	1300	1250	240	8	8	120	40	700	1.9	2	25	34
14–18	1500	2300	4700	1300	1250	410	11	11	150	55	890	2.2	3	35	43
19–30	1500	2300	4700	1000	700	400	8	11	150	55	900	2.3	4	35	45
31–50	1500	2300	4700	1000	700	420	8	11	150	55	900	2.3	4	35	45
51–70	1300	2000	4700	1000	700	420	8	11	150	55	900	2.3	4	30	45
>70	1200	1800	4700	1200	700	420	8	11	150	55	900	2.3	4	30	45
Females															
9–13	1500	2300	4500	1300	1250	240	8	8	120	40	700	1.6	2	21	34
14–18	1500	2300	4700	1300	1250	360	15	9	150	55	890	1.6	3	24	43
19–30	1500	2300	4700	1000	700	310	18	8	150	55	900	1.8	3	25	45
31–50	1500	2300	4700	1000	700	320	18	8	150	55	900	1.8	3	25	45
51–70	1300	2000	4700	1200	700	320	8	8	150	55	900	1.8	3	20	45
>70	1200	1800	4700	1200	700	320	8	8	150	55	900	1.8	3	20	45
Pregnancy															
≤18	1500	2300	4700	1300	1250	400	27	12	220	60	1000	2.0	3	29	50
19–30	1500	2300	4700	1000	700	350	27	11	220	60	1000	2.0	3	30	50
31–50	1500	2300	4700	1000	700	360	27	11	220	60	1000	2.0	3	30	50
Lactation															
≤18	1500	2300	5100	1300	1250	360	10	13	290	70	1300	2.6	3	44	50
19–30	1500	2300	5100	1000	700	310	9	12	290	70	1300	2.6	3	45	50
31–50	1500	2300	5100	1000	700	320	9	12	290	70	1300	2.6	3	45	50

Tolerable Upper Intake Levels (UL) for Vitamins

Age (yr)	Niacin (mg/day)[a]	Vitamin B_6 (mg/day)	Folate (µg/day)[a]	Choline (mg/day)	Vitamin C (mg/day)	Vitamin A (µg/day)[b]	Vitamin D (µg/day)	Vitamin E (mg/day)[c]
Infants								
0–0.5	—	—	—	—	—	600	25	—
0.5–1	—	—	—	—	—	600	38	—
Children								
1–3	10	30	300	1000	400	600	63	200
4–8	15	40	400	1000	650	900	75	300
Adolescents								
9–13	20	60	600	2000	1200	1700	100	600
14–18	30	80	800	3000	1800	2800	100	800
Adults								
19–70	35	100	1000	3500	2000	3000	100	1000
>70	35	100	1000	3500	2000	3000	100	1000
Pregnancy								
≤18	30	80	800	3000	1800	2800	100	800
19–50	35	100	1000	3500	2000	3000	100	1000
Lactation								
≤18	30	80	800	3000	1800	2800	100	800
19–50	35	100	1000	3500	2000	3000	100	1000

[a]The UL for niacin and folate apply to synthetic forms obtained from supplements, fortified foods, or a combination of the two.
[b]The UL for vitamin A applies to the preformed vitamin only.
[c]The UL for vitamin E applies to any form of supplemental α-tocopherol, fortified foods, or a combination of the two.

Tolerable Upper Intake Levels (UL) for Minerals

Age (yr)	Sodium (mg/day)	Chloride (mg/day)	Calcium (mg/day)	Phosphorus (mg/day)	Magnesium (mg/day)[d]	Iron (mg/day)	Zinc (mg/day)	Iodine (µg/day)	Selenium (µg/day)	Copper (µg/day)	Manganese (mg/day)	Fluoride (mg/day)	Molybdenum (µg/day)	Boron (mg/day)	Nickel (mg/day)
Infants															
0–0.5	—[e]	—[e]	1000	—	—	40	4	—	45	—	—	0.7	—	—	—
0.5–1	—[e]	—[e]	1500	—	—	40	5	—	60	—	—	0.9	—	—	—
Children															
1–3	1500	2300	2500	3000	65	40	7	200	90	1000	2	1.3	300	3	0.2
4–8	1900	2900	2500	3000	110	40	12	300	150	3000	3	2.2	600	6	0.3
Adolescents															
9–13	2200	3400	3000	4000	350	40	23	600	280	5000	6	10	1100	11	0.6
14–18	2300	3600	3000	4000	350	45	34	900	400	8000	9	10	1700	17	1.0
Adults															
19–50	2300	3600	2500	4000	350	45	40	1100	400	10,000	11	10	2000	20	1.0
51–70	2300	3600	2000	4000	350	45	40	1100	400	10,000	11	10	2000	20	1.0
>70	2300	3600	2000	3000	350	45	40	1100	400	10,000	11	10	2000	20	1.0
Pregnancy															
≤18	2300	3600	3000	3500	350	45	34	900	400	8000	9	10	1700	17	1.0
19–50	2300	3600	2500	3500	350	45	40	1100	400	10,000	11	10	2000	20	1.0
Lactation															
≤18	2300	3600	3000	4000	350	45	34	900	400	8000	9	10	1700	17	1.0
19–50	2300	3600	2500	4000	350	45	40	1100	400	10,000	11	10	2000	20	1.0

[d]The UL for magnesium applies to synthetic forms obtained from supplements or drugs only.
[e]Source of intake should be from human milk (or formula) and food only.

NOTE: A UL was not established for vitamins and minerals not listed and for those age groups listed with a dash (—) because of a lack of data, not because these nutrients are safe to consume at any level of intake. All nutrients can have adverse effects when intakes are excessive.

What's on your plate?

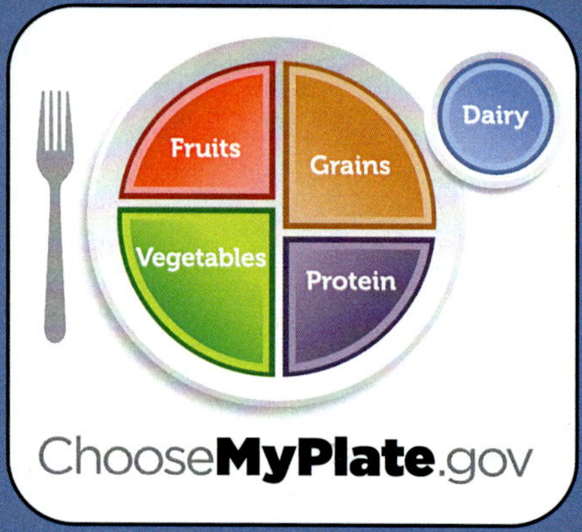

Before you eat, think about what and how much food goes on your plate or in your cup or bowl. Over the day, include foods from all food groups: vegetables, fruits, whole grains, low-fat dairy products, and lean protein foods.

- Make half your plate fruits and vegetables.
- Make at least half your grains whole.
- Switch to skim or 1% milk.
- Vary your protein food choices.

Cut back on sodium and empty calories from solid fats and added sugars.

- Look out for salt (sodium) in foods you buy. Compare sodium in foods and choose those with a lower number.
- Drink water instead of sugary drinks. Eat sugary desserts less often.
- Make foods that are high in solid fats—such as cakes, cookies, ice cream, pizza, cheese, sausages, and hot dogs—occasional choices, not everyday foods.
- Limit empty calories to less than 270 per day, based on 2,000-calorie diet.

Be physically active your way. Pick activities you like and do each for at least 10 minutes at a time. Every bit adds up, and health benefits increase as you spend more time being active.

VEGETABLES	FRUITS	GRAINS	DAIRY	PROTEIN FOODS
Eat more red, orange, and dark-green veggies like tomatoes, sweet potatoes, and broccoli in main dishes.	Use fruits as snacks, salads, and desserts. At breakfast top your cereal with bananas or strawberries: add blueberries to pancakes.	Substitute whole-grain choices for refined-grain breads, bagels, rolls, breakfast cereals, crackers, rice, and pasta.	Choose skim (fat-free) or 1% (low-fat) milk. They have the same amount of calcium and other essential nutrients as whole milk, but less fat and calories.	Eat a variety of foods from the protein food group each week, such as seafood, beans and peas, and nuts as well as lean meats, poultry, and eggs.
Add beans or peas to salads (kidney or chickpeas), soups (split peas or lentils), and side dishes (pinto or baked beans), or serve as a main dish.	Buy fruits that are dried, frozen, and canned (in water or 100% juice), as well as fresh fruits.	Check the ingredients list on product labels for the words "whole" or "whole grain" before the grain ingredient name.	Top fruit salads and baked potatoes with low-fat yogurt.	Twice a week, make seafood the protein on your plate.
Fresh, frozen, and canned vegetables all count. Choose "reduced sodium" or "no-salt-added" canned veggies.	Select 100% fruit juice when choosing juices.	Choose products that name a whole grain first on the ingredients list.	If you are lactose intolerant, try lactose-free milk or fortified soymilk (soy beverage).	Choose lean meats and ground beef that are at least 90% lean.
				Trim or drain fat from meat and remove skin from poultry to cut fat and calories.

For a 2,000-calorie daily food plan, you need the amounts below from each food group. To find amounts personalized for you, go to ChooseMyPlate.gov.

Eat 2 1/2 cups every day	**Eat 2 cups every day**	**Eat 6 ounces every day**	**Get 3 cups every day**	**Eat 5 1/2 ounces every day**
What counts as a cup? 1 cup of raw or cooked vegetables or vegetable juice; 2 cups of leafy salad greens	**What counts as a cup?** 1 cup of raw or cooked fruit or 100% fruit juice; 1/2 cup dried fruit	**What counts as an ounce?** 1 slice of bread; 1/2 cup of cooked rice, cereal, or pasta; 1 ounce of ready-to-eat cereal	**What counts as a cup?** 1 cup of milk, yogurt, or fortified soymilk; 1 1/2 ounces natural or 2 ounces processed cheese	**What counts as an ounce?** 1 ounce of lean meat, poultry, or fish; 1 egg; 1 tbsp peanut butter; 1/2 ounce nuts or seeds: 1/4 cup beans or peas